CROWLEY'S

AN INTRODUCTION TO HUMAN DISEASE

Pathology and Pathophysiology Correlations

TWELFTH EDITION

Emily G. Reisner, PhD
Durham, North Carolina

Howard M. Reisner, PhD
Professor of Pathology Emeritus
University of North Carolina
Chapel Hill, North Carolina

JONES & BARTLETT
LEARNING

World Headquarters
Jones & Bartlett Learning
25 Wall Street
Burlington, MA 01803
978-443-5000
info@jblearning.com
www.jblearning.com

Jones & Bartlett Learning books and products are available through most bookstores and online booksellers. To contact Jones & Bartlett Learning directly, call 800-832-0034, fax 978-443-8000, or visit our website, www.jblearning.com.

Substantial discounts on bulk quantities of Jones & Bartlett Learning publications are available to corporations, professional associations, and other qualified organizations. For details and specific discount information, contact the special sales department at Jones & Bartlett Learning via the above contact information or send an email to specialsales@jblearning.com.

30305-6

Production Credits
Vice President, Innovative Learning and Assessment Solutions: Ada Woo
Senior Director, Content Production and Delivery: Christine Emerton
Director, Product: Melissa Kleeman-Moy
Product Manager: Bill Lawrensen
Product Manager: Sophie Teague
Manager, Content Development: Carol Guerrero
Content Manager: Jessica Covert
Content Coordinator: Rachelle Soden
Content Management: Publishing Solutions Group
Manager, Intellectual Properties and Content Production: Kristen Rogers
Content Production Manager: Belinda Thresher
Content Production Manager, Navigate: Michael Lapera
Senior Intellectual Property Specialist (eBook): Angela Dooley
Senior Product Marketing Manager: Susanne Walker
Director, Product Fulfillment: Aaron McKinzie
Purchasing Manager: Wendy Kilborn
Composition: XBP Global
Project Management: XBP Global
Cover Design: MPS Limited
Media Developer: Faith Brosnan
Intellectual Property Specialist: Maria Leon Maimone
Cover Image (Title Page and Chapter Opener): © Kateryna Kon/Shutterstock
Printing and Binding: Lakeside Book Company

Library of Congress Cataloging-in-Publication Data
Names: Reisner, Emily G. author | Reisner, Howard M. author | Crowley, Leonard V., 1926- Introduction to human disease.
Title: Crowley's an introduction to human disease : pathology and pathophysiology correlations / Emily G. Reisner and Howard M. Reisner.
Description: Twelfth edition. | Burlington, Massachusetts : Jones & Bartlett Learning, [2027] | Previous edition was written by Leonard V. Crowley. | Includes bibliographical references and index.
Identifiers: LCCN 2025042324 | ISBN 9781284303056 paperback
Subjects: LCSH: Pathology | Diseases–Causes and theories of causation | BISAC: EDUCATION / Teaching / Subjects / Health & Sexuality
Classification: LCC RB112 .C76 2027
LC record available at https://lccn.loc.gov/2025042324

6048

Printed in the United States of America
30 29 28 27 26 10 9 8 7 6 5 4 3 2 1

This *Twelfth Edition* is dedicated to the memory of Dr. Leonard V. Crowley, the original author of this text and to those medical professionals around the world who lost their lives while treating patients with COVID-19.

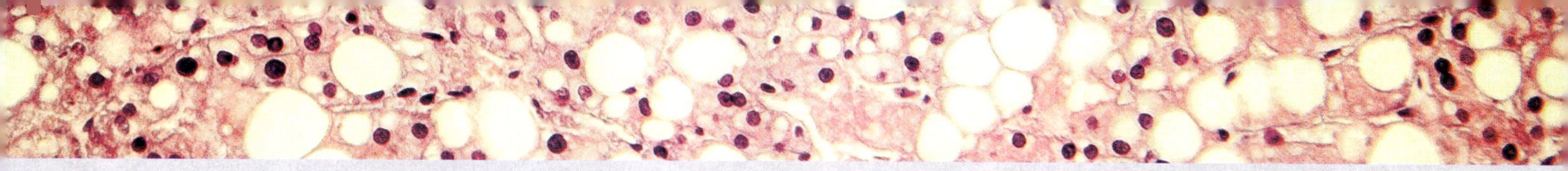

Brief Contents

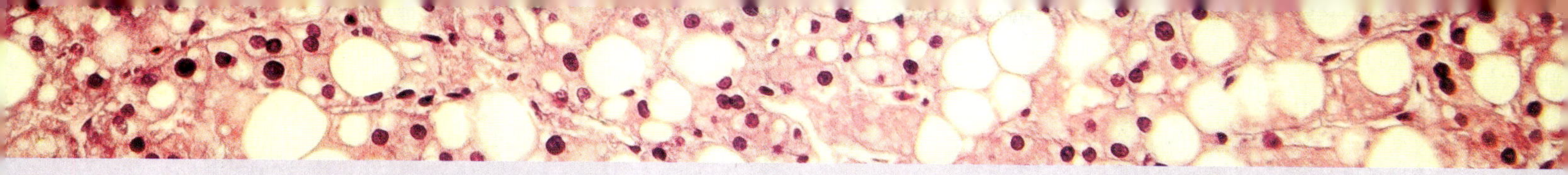

Contents

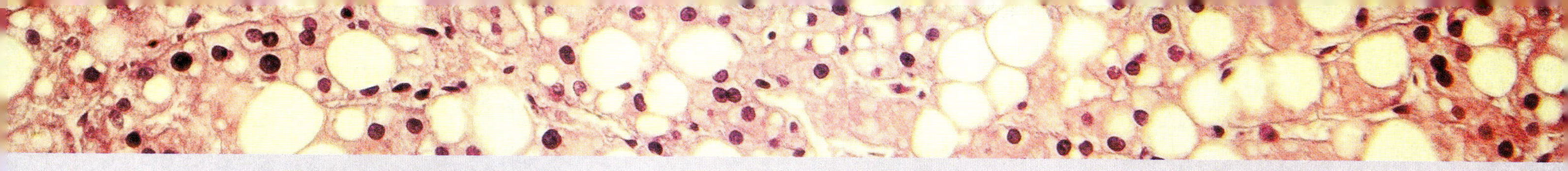

Preface

Since the COVID-19 pandemic, people realize the need for everyone to be well informed regarding the many facets of the etiology and pathogenesis of human disease. Students especially need to understand the interactions between environmental and social conditions on the body's ability to maintain health and a state of wellness. This text provides the foundational information to understand many of the most prominent human diseases. It also seeks to provide students with the skills and knowledge they will need to understand and process new information not specifically covered in this text. The textbook continues with a systemic approach. Included in this edition is a new chapter covering pregnancy and infertility. The chapter on congenital and development diseases maintains a systems approach. The genetic disease section outlines congenital and adult disorders caused by alterations within gene coding, gene expression, and chromosomal structure. The chapter on pathogenic microorganisms convers the current outbreak of measles, avian flu, and monkeypox. Additional information about cytokines and their functions is also included in the chapter on immunology.

The Audience

How did we visualize the reader of this work? We hope that any individual interested in the health sciences who wishes to understand the nature of disease would find the text informative and of interest. Specifically, this text should allow health-science students with basic knowledge of biology and mammalian physiology grasp the concepts and vocabulary to understand the consequences of when the normal processes of biology and physiology no longer function as they should.

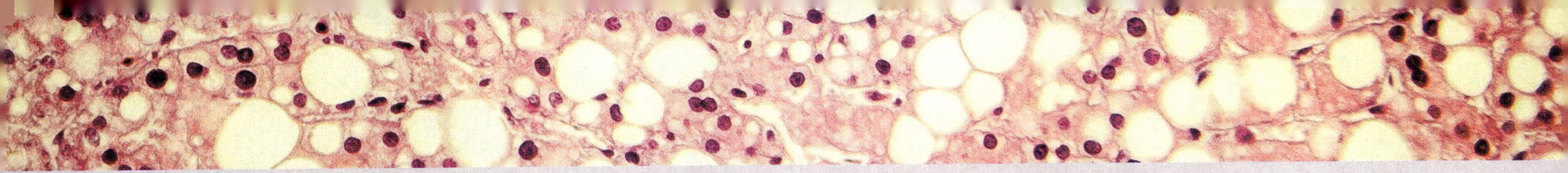

New to This Edition

The *Twelfth Edition* underwent extensive re-organization to improve the flow of information and reader experience. Some chapters from the prior edition were combined, such as the male and female reproduction chapters, and two new chapters were created: Pregnancy and Infertility and Congenital and Developmental Diseases. A selection of chapter-specific updates is listed below.

Chapter 3—Genes and Genetic Disease

- Added information on epigenetics and their impacts on gene expression
- Added information on mitochondrial diseases in humans

Chapter 5—Immunity, Hypersensitivity, Immunodeficiency, and Autoimmune Disease

- Updated information about cellular components of innate immune system
- Added information about MHC class I and class II proteins and their functions of antigen presenting
- Added information about cytokine-producing cells and types of cytokines and their related functions
- Moved HIV infection and AIDS from STD section to acquired immune deficiency in this chapter
- Added information on how to acquire adaptive immunity

Chapter 7—Pathogenic Microorganisms

- Added information on the importance of vaccines in preventing transmission of infectious diseases
- Provided information about various types of coronaviruses and the diseases they are associated with
- Added information on the current outbreaks of avian flu (H5N1) and measles
- Included information on monkeypox virus

Chapter 8—Parasitic Disease

- Included details about the life cycle of *Plasmodium malariae*
- Updated content on antimalarial drugs, highlighting the discovery and use of Artemisinin

Chapter 9—The Cardiovascular System

- Congenital cardiovascular disease has been moved to Chapter 16, Congenital and Developmental Diseases
- New figures and illustrations to promote understanding of the most commonly encountered manifestations of heart disease

Chapter 10—Diseases of Blood Circulation

- Detailed discussions concerning thrombus and embolus formation
- Additional figures and illustrations

Chapter 11—Diseases of the Lymphatic System

- All of the information regarding pathology of and white blood cells and diseases of the lymphatic system can be found in one chapter
- More information regarding the functioning and pathology of individual white blood cells included
- Additional and updated figures and illustrations

Chapter 12—Diseases of Red Blood Cells, Thrombocytes, and Hemostasis

- Discussion of diseases involving pathology of red blood cells
- More detailed information regarding blood clotting and pathology when it either clots too quickly or too slowly
- A broader discussion of disseminated clotting syndrome and its etiology

Chapter 13—The Respiratory System

- Added diagram demonstrating gases exchanges between alveolar and pulmonary capillaries
- Updated statistics of COPD disease
- Updated histologic images of diseases in respiratory system
- Added information on various types of pulmonary fibrosis and their clinical presentation

Chapter 14—The Breast

- Updated information on the genetics of breast cancer
- Undated statistical information
- Currently used clinical treatment methods

Chapter 15—Pregnancy and Infertility

- Additional information and figures concerning diseases and pathologies associated with pregnancy
- A brief discussion of maternal mortality rates in the United States
- New information regarding both female and male infertility

Chapter 16—Congenital and Developmental Diseases

- Congenital and developmental diseases for each organ system and now located in one chapter
- There is a brief discussion of the timing of the development of various organs and when they may be most vulnerable to adverse effects from environmental influences
- Discussion of the notorious teratogen thalidomide
- Discussion of several significant environmental influences on pregnancy
- Infectious disease agents which significantly impact pregnancy and the fetus are included here

Chapter 18—The Female and Male Reproductive Systems

- Extensively reorganized with the systems for both sexes covered in one place

- Updated section on sexually transmitted infections which mostly affect the reproductive system
- Discussion of infertility moved to Chapter 15 for both sexes

Chapter 20—The Pancreas and Diabetes Mellitus

- Added information on acute and chronic pancreatitis
- Updated information on diagnosis and treatment of pancreatic cancer
- Extensive discussion of cystic fibrosis including not only how it affects the pancreas but also its pathogenesis

Chapter 21—The Gastrointestinal Tract

- Updated information of HPV infection on oropharyngeal cancers and its prevention
- Provided information on irritable bowel syndrome (IBS), Crohn's disease, chronic ulcerative colitis, and gluten intolerance

Chapter 22—The Endocrine Glands

- Provided additional insights into the functions and regulation of T3 and T4 hormones
- Updated pathologic images for pituitary and thyroid gland

Chapter 23—Nervous System

- Updated epidemiology for rabies
- Moved "congenital hydrocephalus" to Chapter 16

Chapter 24—The Musculoskeletal System

- Added pathogenicity, treatment, and prevention of rickets and scurvy
- Moved "Clubfoot and hip dysplasia" to Chapter 16

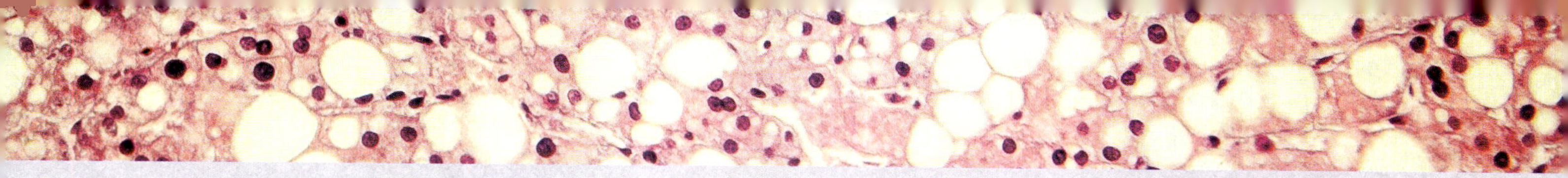

About the Authors

Howard and Emily Reisner met in graduate school and hold PhDs from Case Western Reserve University in Cleveland, Ohio. Howard is Professor Emeritus Department of Pathology at the University of North Carolina in Chapel Hill and recently retired as Professor of Pathology at the Campbell University School of Osteopathic Medicine. Emily has been a laboratory director at Duke University Medical Center and Director of Medical Writing in the pharmaceutical industry. For many years, she taught medical writing for the physician's assistant program at Duke University. Both Howard and Emily are authors or editors of numerous books on pathology and have been involved in programs for teaching pathology in the Allied Health field.

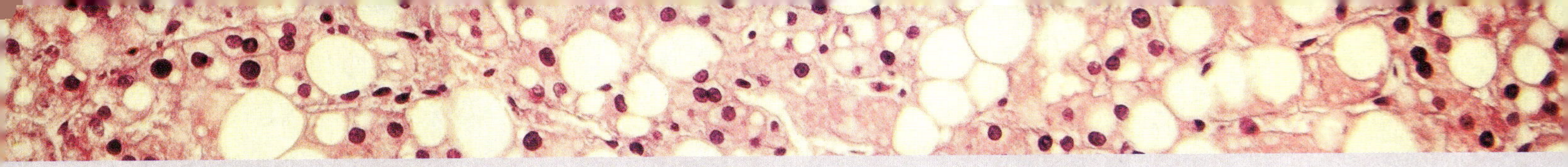

About the Contributors

Jan Reichard-Brown

Jan Reichard-Brown earned her PhD in Developmental Biology from the University of Cincinnati, Ohio. She spent 39 years on the faculty at Susquehanna University, from which she retired in December 2024 as Associate Professor Emerita of Health Care Studies and Biology. During her career, she taught courses in Human Physiology, Human Health and Disease, Human Parasites, Birth Defects, and Human Anatomy, among others. She mentored many senior research students in Biology and occasionally Neuroscience. She served as the Pre-Health Professions Advisor at Susquehanna University for 2 years. In that capacity, she published several book chapters and articles on undergraduate pre-health advising. Teaching Human Health and Disease was one of her favorite courses and she is thrilled to be able to contribute to the next edition of the textbook she used for many years.

Tong Cheng

Tong Cheng holds a PhD from University of Illinois at Chicago. She is currently a full Professor of Biology at William Rainey Harper College in Illinois. Over the years, she has taught a wide range of biology courses, including Microbiology, Fundamentals of Cellular Biology, and Human Disease. Tong also founded and advises students on the Health Career and Premed Club. Before joining Harper College, she taught at Genesee Community College and worked as a Research Assistant Professor at University of Rochester with numerous publications on Activated Protein C (APC) in treatment of ischemic stroke in humans.

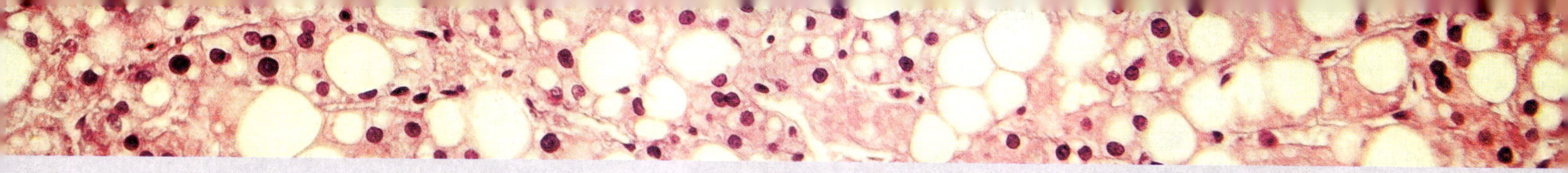

Acknowledgments

Meghan B. Schaefer MD, MS Assistant Professor, Department of Urology Medical College of Wisconsin Milwaukee, Wisconsin, reviewed and contributed to the male reproductive section of Chapter 18. Her expertise in modern male reproductive health and disease is greatly appreciated.

Tong Cheng and Jan Reichard-Brown wish to thank Jessica Covert, Jones & Bartlett Learning Content Manager, for her confidence and support as we worked on our various chapter assignments.

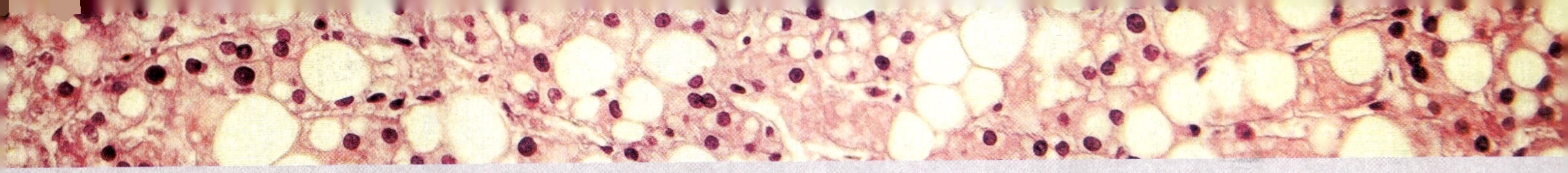

Reviewers

Dr. Brenna Bohatec, DNP, APRN, FNP-BC
DNP Director, Associate Professor and FNP Clinical Coordinator
Oral Roberts University

Laurel Glover, DHSc, MPH, RCP, RRT-NPS
Public Health Program Director
Charleston Southern University

Amanda Jones, Instructor
Doctor
Community College of Denver

Walter M. Matthews, MD, FAsMA, Col (ret) USAF, 1st Surgeon General of the United States Space Force
Clinical Professor, Pre-Medical Mentor
Baylor University Honors College

Kandice Pryor, MSN, RN
Adjunct Instructor
Paris Junior College

Peter Sayles, AAS, BA, MSc, PhD
Retired Emeritus
SUNY North Country Community College

Bill Young, NRP, EdD
Associate Professor of Paramedicine
Eastern Kentucky University

Susan Zacharia, PhD
Assistant Professor
Virginia Commonwealth University

Faith Zamamiri-Davis, PhD
Associate Professor of Biology
Union University

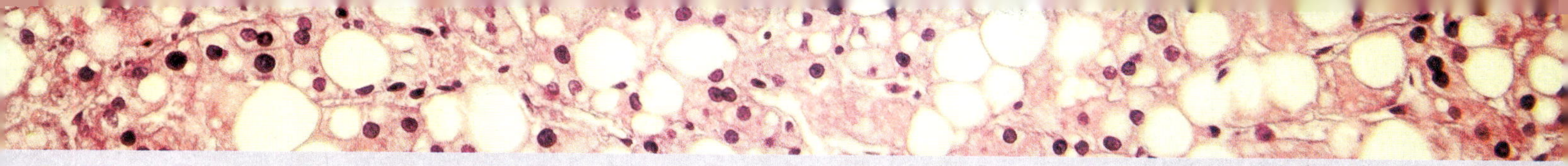

Learning and Teaching Resources

Student Resources

Each new purchase of the print textbook or Navigate course includes:

- Navigate eBook with Chapter Review Slides and Interactive Glossary
- Flashcards
- Podcasts
- Animations

Instructor Resources

Qualified instructors can receive the full suite of Instructor Resources, including the following:

- Slides in PowerPoint format
- Test Bank, including in LMS-compatible formats
- Case Studies and Answer Key
- Workbook
- Answer Key for End-of-Chapter Questions
- Image Bank

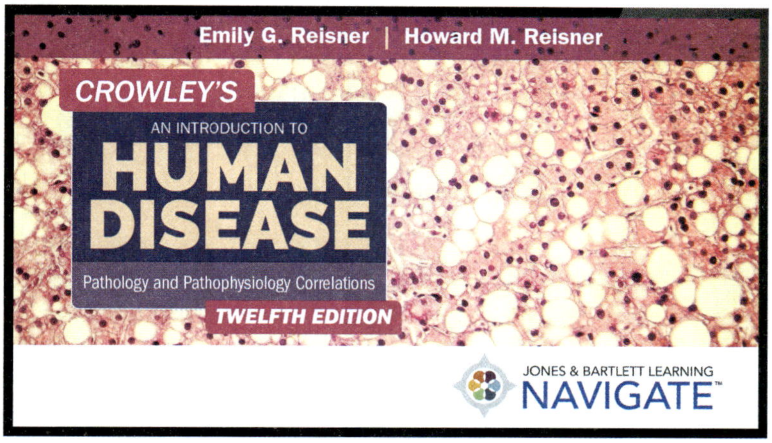

We Value Your Feedback

Do you love this text? Spot an error you'd like to report? Follow this QR code to give us your observations and suggestions for improvement.

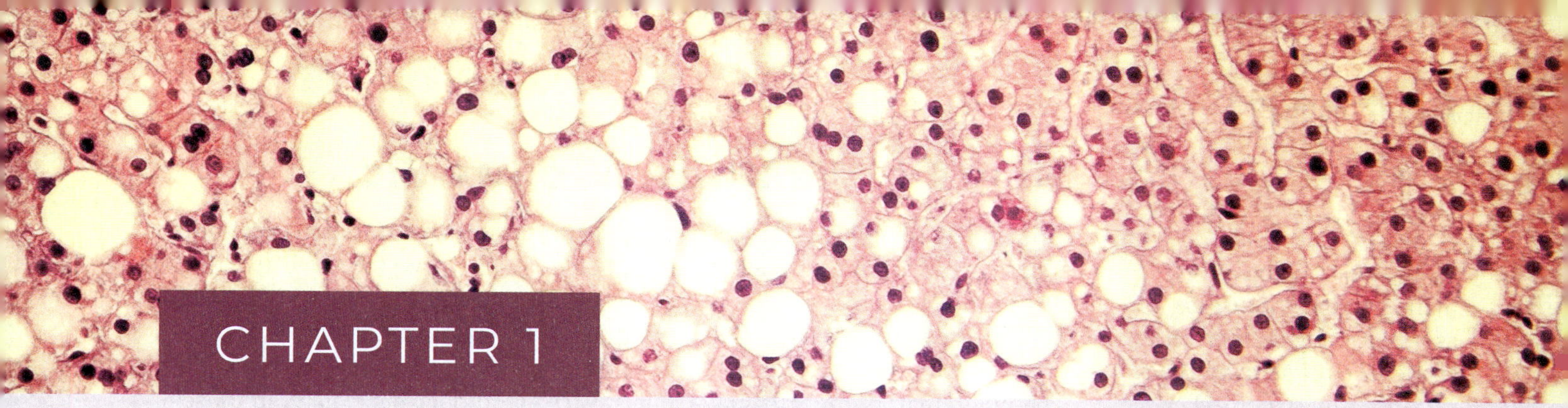

CHAPTER 1

General Concepts of Disease: Principles of Diagnosis

LEARNING OBJECTIVES

1. Define the common terms used to describe disease, including, but not limited to, lesions, symptomatic and asymptomatic disease, etiology, and pathogenesis.
2. List the major categories of human disease.
3. Outline the approach a practitioner uses to make a diagnosis and decide on a patient's treatment.
4. Describe the various types of diagnostic tests and procedures that can help the practitioner make a diagnosis.
5. Compare and contrast the imaging techniques discussed in this chapter.

What Is Disease?

Disease, in its broadest sense, includes any disturbance to normal body function, including the systems of which maintain homeostasis. However, wellness and illness constitute two extremes of a continuum. At one extreme illness can be severe, disabling, or life-threatening with concomitant effects on someone's physical and emotional well-being. At the other extreme is absolute wellness, a state of physical and mental health often sought after but rarely attained completely. Between these two extremes exists a gradient of health and disease, ranging from mild or short-term illness that limits activities to moderate good health that falls short of the ideal state. The midpoint in this continuum, in which one is neither ill nor in ideal good health, describes the state in which many people fall. Who does not suffer from an occasional cold, sprain, upset stomach, or headache? As we get older, our average position in the continuum tends to shift.

Disease Any disturbance of the structure or function of the body.

How Do We Know We Are Sick?

How do you know you are sick? This seems an obvious question, yet sometimes you do know and sometimes you don't. **Symptoms**, the subjective manifestations of disease, may be related to readily apparent **lesions** like a broken bone or a painful swelling. Often, symptoms result from the body's reaction to injury, which may stem from **trauma**, infection, or other types of pathology. The inflammatory process may manifest with symptoms, such as fever, muscle aches, and pain (see Chapter 4).

Pathologists and other healthcare providers study the **etiology** (cause) and **pathogenesis** (progression or "natural history") of disease by evaluating lesions at the level of organs, the tissues that compose the organs, the cells that form the tissues, and the molecules of which the cells are composed. The diseased tissue could be observed with the naked eye (**gross examination**) and/or with the aid of a microscope (**histologic examination**) or by the use of special methods of identifying normal or abnormal tissue components. Using biochemical or **immunological techniques**, histologic examination may be supplemented to obtain more detailed information on the tissue or cellular level. It is increasingly common to study the molecules that compose a tissue. In addition, healthcare practitioners working in the area of **laboratory medicine** study the composition of our body fluids (blood and urine, for example) to look for markers of disease.

Symptoms Subjective manifestations of disease as reported by the person (patient) experiencing them.
Lesion Any structural abnormality or pathologic change.
Trauma Injury caused by a physical extrinsic agent.
Pathologist Person who studies the structural and functional changes in the body caused by disease.
Etiology The cause of a disease.
Pathogenesis Progression of the development of a disease.
Gross examination Study of diseased organ with the naked eye.
Histologic examination Study of disease using a microscope to examine tissue.
Immunological techniques Procedures using antibody or antigen preparations, usually with chemical labels.
Laboratory medicine Analysis of clinical and biology specimens to aid in diagnosing disease.
Mnemonics Aids to memory.
Idiopathic Disease of unknown origin.
Iatrogenic Disease resulting from a medical intervention.
Clinician Health care provider having direct contact with patients.
Signs Physical manifestations of disease.

Classifications of Disease

People interested in etiology classify diseases into several large categories. Although these categories are broad, this classification helps in understanding how a disease is likely to progress and how it may affect the patient. There are several alternative systems but healthcare students (who appreciate **mnemonics**) often use the term VINDICATE'M as a scheme:

Vascular
Infectious (or **I**nflammatory)
Neoplastic
Degenerative (or **D**eficiency)
Idiopathic (or **I**atrogenic)
Congenital
Allergic (or **A**utoimmune)
Traumatic
Endocrine (or **E**nvironmental)
Metabolic

With the exceptions of **idiopathic** (of unknown origin) and **iatrogenic** (physician caused), most of these terms should be familiar and will be discussed in detail in subsequent chapters. Although the VINDICATE'M scheme is useful, many diseases fit in multiple categories or fit poorly in any.

Principles of Diagnosis

The first professional to see the patient and to diagnose the disease is the **clinician** who possesses expertise in detecting and evaluating the objective manifestations of disease (the **signs** or physical findings). However, a pathological condition may cause the affected individual no discomfort or disability (**asymptomatic** disease). Often a disease process can be asymptomatic in its early stages, implying that the patient or clinician may not notice any changes in the patient's perceived level of wellness. When disease progresses to the point where it causes observable signs (findings) prior to diagnosis, it may become more difficult, impossible, or costly to treat. Therefore, early detection of disease becomes of great importance to welfare of the public. Specialists in **public health** might design **screening** systems for early diagnosis of diseases in populations.

Determination of the nature and cause of a patient's illness by a health practitioner is called a **diagnosis**. It is based on the practitioner's evaluation of the patient's history, subjective symptoms, physical findings, signs, the results of laboratory tests, and other appropriate diagnostic procedures. Many diagnostic procedures are **noninvasive** (requiring no physical infiltration of the body, its openings, or cavities). A common example of such noninvasive diagnostic testing is the use of imaging technology (X-ray or ultrasound, for example). Sometimes diagnosis requires an **invasive** procedure. Such procedures may be relatively minor and have little discomfort associated with them. Common examples are drawing blood, obtaining a **Pap smear** (collecting a sample of cervical cells), or sampling fluid and cells from a surface-accessible lesion with a very fine needle (**fine-needle aspiration**). Somewhat more invasive are a variety of endoscopic procedures in which a tube is passed into a body opening. Laparoscopic procedures involve the introduction of devices into body cavities or obtaining samples of internal tissues. The use of sampling devices guided by imaging technology can be even more invasive but still much safer and potentially less costly than a surgical procedure.

The effort to reach a diagnosis may be minimal, requiring nothing more than evaluation of the patient's history and a physical examination, or may require multiple diagnostic procedures, including the consultation of several diagnostic specialists and more extensive testing. When clinicians reach a diagnosis, they might then offer a **prognosis**, a probability estimation of the eventual outcome of the disease. A course of therapy, often in consultation with other members of the healthcare team, may also be instituted. The basic foundation for obtaining a diagnosis starts with the patient's history and a physical examination.

Asymptomatic Without symptoms.

Public health Area of medicine concerned with the health of populations.

Screening Examining a large asymptomatic population for signs of future disease.

Diagnosis The determination of the nature and cause of a patient's illness.

Noninvasive testing Diagnostic procedure requiring no physical invasion of the body.

Invasive testing Test requiring a physical invasion of the body.

Pap smear A collection of cells from the cervix. Commonly used as a screening test for cervical cancer.

Fine-needle aspiration Sampling fluid and cells from a surface-accessible lesion.

Prognosis The probable outcome of a disease or disorder, the outlook for recovery.

The History

The clinical history is a critical initial step in the evaluation. As is the case in any interaction between individuals, this step requires the healthcare provider to establish a relationship with the patient facilitating accurate verbal transmission of information. The patient must feel enabled to present their history both fully and accurately. The clinician must be able to skillfully elicit that information and accurately interpret it without prejudgment or bias in any area. This approach is considered patient-centered. Acquiring patient-centered interviewing skills is an early and essential part of the training of a healthcare provider. A standard approach is generally used on an initial encounter to facilitate obtaining and recording an accurate, organized patient history, although it may be modified or adapted on subsequent visits. This approach consists of several parts:

1. *Chief complaint:* Why has the patient sought medical attention? Most often this is elicited in the patient's own words. Follow-up may include a brief survey of any additional issues or problems currently being experienced by the patient.

2. *History of the current illness:* The healthcare provider develops a chronological framework of the patient's illness from the first symptoms to the present. This part of the history establishes the "when, where, and how" of the chief complaint.
3. *Past medical history:* To establish the patient's general state of health, information about past illnesses, medical interventions, medications, allergies, immunizations, reproductive history, and participation in health practices should be recorded.
   a. *Family health history:* This part of the history provides background information about potential environmental or genetic influences pertinent to the patient's complaint. It may include the health status of the entire living family and historical information about deceased relatives. Family history contributes important information in diagnosing many common chronic diseases, such as diabetes and heart disease.
   b. *Psychosocial and sexual history:* The patient's education and life experiences (including personal relationships, employment, etc.), and in females the gynecological/reproductive history, may provide important information to the diagnostician. Questions are asked about potentially addictive behaviors, such as the use of alcohol, tobacco products, and recreational drugs.
4. *The review of systems:* This is often considered to be the center of the patient–physician encounter and consists of a body system–oriented, head-to-toe review of all presenting symptoms in an organized manner. The review may disclose additional symptoms not initially reported by the patient that are important to the diagnosis. A clinician's investigation of the presenting symptom of back pain, for example, may elicit the additional symptom of pain upon urination during the review, suggesting potential urinary tract disease.

The Physical Examination

The physical examination is a system-based examination of the patient in an ordered manner. The practitioner places particular emphasis on the part of the body affected by the illness, such as the ears, throat, chest, and lungs in the case of a potential respiratory infection. However, particularly in a first encounter, all body systems are examined. For example, respiratory symptoms may be associated with a range of etiologies affecting multiple body systems (e.g., allergic diseases). Any abnormalities detected on the physical examination may be correlated with the clinical history. At this point, the practitioner begins construction of a hypothesis regarding diseases or conditions that best fit with the clinical findings. Often, more than one diagnosis must be considered, and such considerations are likely to be altered by the results of laboratory and other diagnostic tests. In a **differential diagnosis**, the practitioner must consider a number of diseases that are characterized by the patient's symptoms. For example, respiratory symptoms might, based on patient history, suggest a seasonal allergy. Simple blood-based tests can aid in establishing such a diagnosis. A suggestion of renal problems in the patient could point to a serious, multisystem disease involving blood vessels (a vascular disease). Additional laboratory tests and potentially invasive procedures to sample patient tissue would be needed to support such a diagnosis.

Differential diagnosis Consideration of the different diseases possible given the patient's symptoms.

In difficult cases, the clinician may also obtain the opinion of a medical consultant (a healthcare professional with special training and experience in the type of medical problem presented by the patient). For a respiratory disease, a pathologist experienced in tissue-based diagnosis or a **radiologist** expert in the analysis of X-ray and other visualization data produced by physical methods might be consulted. The wise clinician always maintains a probabilistic approach in constructing the diagnosis. Given the patient's history, the most likely diagnosis is considered first (a respiratory infection) followed by alternatives (a seasonal allergy) and the far less likely—but potentially life-threatening—possibilities (multisystem vascular disease). In testing the diagnostic hypothesis, the clinician uses a variety of tests and procedures and considers the usefulness of possible results of the tests in the clinical reasoning process.

Radiologist Physician specializing in the use and analysis of imaging techniques and results.

Colonoscopy Procedure for examination of the colon with an endoscope.

Sensitivity Classification of diagnostic tests in regard to percentage of patients with the disease who are classified as positive by the test.

Specificity Classification of diagnostic tests in regard to the percentage of patients without the disease who are classified as negative by the test.

False negative Negative test result, which should be positive.

False positive Positive test result, which should be negative.

Diagnostic Tests and Procedures

Today a huge number of tests and procedures are available, with more than 87,000 medical and surgical diagnoses and procedures recognized in the standard coding system used in the United States (ICD-10-PCS). One major medical center lists more than 1300 laboratory tests that are available to its staff. How does the clinician choose from this massive array? Medical procedures carry a degree of risk, ranging from trivial to potentially serious. Diagnostic tests and procedures also vary in the amount of information they provide in relation to a potential diagnosis. For example, **colonoscopy** provides no information in the case of respiratory symptoms, but it may lead to a definitive diagnosis in the case of possible bleeding from the rectum. Tests and procedures differ in complexity and cost. Colonoscopy costs thousands of dollars at a major medical center, whereas determination of fecal blood (i.e., blood in stool) is trivial in cost. In a period of increased concern about the economic aspects of health care, cost must also be considered.

Choosing a Diagnostic Test

A diagnostic test can be defined in terms of a set of characteristics that help the clinician judge the usefulness of the procedure in diagnosing a specific disease. A perfect test would always be positive in a patient who has the disease in question and always negative in one who does not (see **Figure 1-1A**). Such a test does not exist. Instead, tests are classified by the terms **sensitivity** and **specificity**.

Sensitivity refers to the percentage of patients with a disease who are classified as positive by a test. Sensitivity = true positives / (true positives + false negatives). False negatives are persons who have the disease or condition that is "missed" by the test. A test with a high sensitivity will miss few people with the disease (have a low rate of **false negatives**). The other important characteristic of accurate diagnostic testing is specificity. Specificity = true negatives / (true negatives + false positives). False positives are persons without a disease who are misclassified as having the condition. Specificity refers to the percentage of patients without the disease who are correctly classified as negative by the test. Tests with a high specificity will have a low rate of **false positives** (see **Figure 1-1B**). The clinician attempts to choose a test with as high a sensitivity and specificity as possible for the diagnosis in question. Unfortunately, highly sensitive tests tend to have lower specificity (misdiagnosing people as having a disease they do not have; i.e., having a higher rate of false positives). Imagine moving the test cutoff line in Figure 1-1B. If we move the cutoff line (defining a positive test result) to the left, we decrease the number of false negatives but increase the number of false positives. The test becomes more sensitive but less

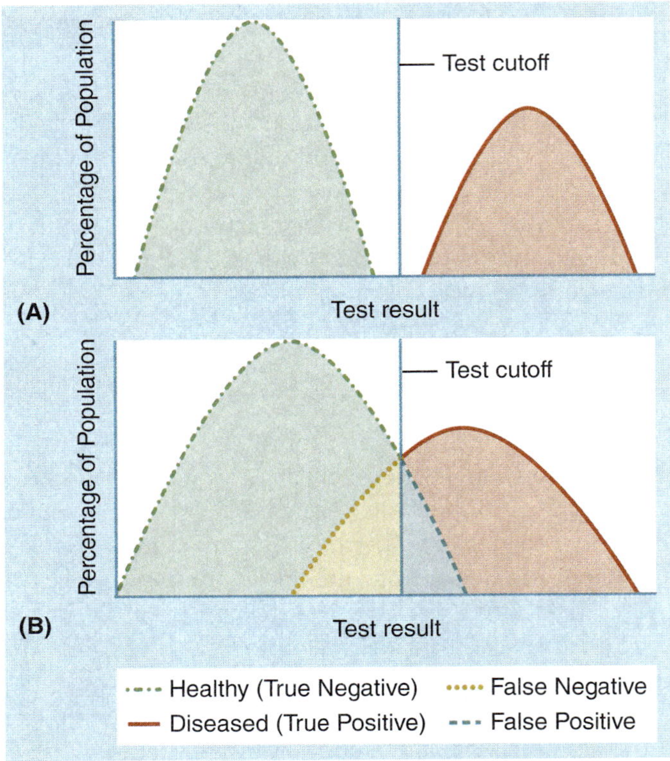

Figure 1-1 Sensitivity and specificity in a hypothetical clinical test. **(A)** A perfect test dealing with healthy and diseased populations where there is no overlap. **(B)** A "real world" example demonstrating the effect of overlapping results. The test cutoff defines the result chosen to define "positive" versus "negative" results by the clinician.

specific. If the cutoff line is moved to the right, we decrease the number of false positives but increase the number of false negatives. The test becomes more specific but less sensitive. "Missing" a disease is obviously harmful, leading to a delay in therapy and potentially a more severe illness. However, a false positive result, assuming a patient has a disease he or she does not, may also lead to anxiety, discomfort, and unneeded therapy.

Choice of test also depends on the patient population. For example, a patient in a clinic with probable disease (based on prior clinical information) is much less likely to obtain a false negative result than an individual chosen at random off the street. A healthcare provider considering an invasive, painful, or costly mode of therapy might choose to use a test with high specificity to exclude a potential false positive result and avoid putting the wrongly diagnosed patient through extensive therapy. However, choosing screening assays to be applied to a population in which the diagnostic target is a relatively uncommon, but potentially serious (possibly fatal) illness involves other considerations. The choice of a highly sensitive test (so as not to miss the uncommonly affected person), that is likely lacking specificity, could potentially increase the number of individuals incorrectly suspected of having the disease. In situations where an acceptable confirmatory test is available or if the therapy is relatively harmless, such a test might be considered for use in screening. However, if the only confirmatory test (or therapy) induces a higher level of risk, the test would be unacceptable. This is a very real problem. For example, a number of noninvasive tests have been proposed to screen for ovarian cancer, which when undiagnosed or untreated is frequently fatal. However, the currently available tests lack specificity and would expose an appreciable number of nonaffected women to invasive diagnostic procedures. Decisions regarding screening assays can often lead to controversy—even among experts. The recent discussion about the using of prostate-specific antigen (PSA) as a screening test for prostate cancer is an example of how complex such decisions are (see Chapter 18).

In summary, the clinician working with the patient makes a risk–benefit–cost determination when choosing diagnostic procedures. Which set of tests will yield the greatest information with the least risk and cost to the patient? Such determinations are part of **evidence-based medicine**, which seeks to define risk–benefit–cost ratios based on prior rigorous investigations. Going hand in hand with evidence-based medicine is **patient-centered medicine**, in which patients have a central role in decisions about their care. Patients should be fully educated about all possible risks and benefits, allowing them to make informed decisions regarding a procedure and possible alternative choices.

Evidence-based medicine The scientific method to organize and apply current data to improve healthcare decisions.

Patient-centered medicine Practice of medicine providing care that is respectful of and responsive to individual preferences, needs, and values and ensuring that people's values guide all clinical decisions.

Endoscopy An examination of the interior of the body by means of various lighted tubular instruments. Method may also be used to obtain tissue samples.

Classification of Diagnostic Tests and Procedures

Diagnostic tests and procedures can be classified into several major categories:

1. *Clinical laboratory tests,* including biochemical, immunological, and molecular-based tests (e.g., determination of gases in the blood, analysis of blood cells, and microbiological analysis)
2. *Imaging techniques,* including X-ray, ultrasound, computerized tomography (CT), magnetic resonance imaging (MRI), positron emission tomography (PET) scans, and measurement of the distribution of various radioisotopes (also called radionuclides)
3. *Cytologic and histological* studies of cells and tissues removed from the patient
4. *Endoscopy*—imaging obtained from inside the patient's body
5. *Electrical activity*—measurements of the electrical activity in portions of the body

These categories often overlap. For example, endoscopy may provide a cell or tissue sample that will be examined histologically, cultured in the clinical laboratory, or analyzed for level of specific molecules. Some endoscopic procedures require radiographic guidance. Endoscopic procedures may be used to provide imaging of internal body systems. Tests can also be classified by the medical specialty responsible for providing them. A subdivision of pathology, Clinical Laboratory Medicine, oversees a broad range of clinical laboratory tests. Anatomic pathology provides tissue- and cell-based analysis as well as autopsy service. Radiology encompasses essentially all image-based techniques and also provides a number of therapeutic procedures. **Endoscopy** covers a broad range of procedures that may be performed by specific medical specialists (e.g., gastroenterologists perform colonoscopy, cardiologists undertake a number of intravascular procedures, such as placing stents to open blocked blood vessels). Other endoscopic procedures are performed by surgical specialties. For example, cystoscopy, examination of the urinary tract, is the purview of urologists.

Clinical Laboratory Tests

Laboratory medicine provides and interprets diagnostic testing related to patient care. Clinical laboratory tests aid not only in diagnosing disease but also in searching for occult (unrecognized) disease, establishing the severity of disease, and monitoring its progression and treatment. In laboratory medicine, basic analytical science meets medical science, and it is often the place where a new aspect of biomedicine is "translated" into patient care. Hence, analytical aspects of biochemistry, immunology, microbiology, physiology, and molecular biology are used in the clinical laboratory.

The roles of the clinical laboratory and the tests it provides may not be obvious to the patient, whose experience includes having several tubes of blood drawn or providing a urine sample. However, it has been estimated that 60 to 70 percent of medical diagnoses rely on clinical tests. Almost 14 billion clinical tests are performed each year in the United States. In general, such tests are cost-efficient. A small fraction of money spent on health care in the United States covers clinical laboratory testing.

Given the large number of available tests, it is difficult to summarize the many uses of clinical tests. **Figure 1-2** provides an example of a standard set of laboratory tests along with normal ranges for the results.

Results that are "out of range" are flagged as either low or high, and it is up to the physician to determine the significance of the results. Determining the concentration of various constituents in the blood and urine is of major importance in evaluating the function of organ systems. For example, if the concentration of urea is elevated, the kidneys are not functioning properly, since urea is normally excreted by the kidneys. The concentration of hemoglobin and

Patient Name: DOE, MARY **Patient MRNO: 0000012345**

Order Number: C6140101
Collection Date: 2009-06-14 at 0400

Source:
Site:

Date Completed	Test Name	Result	Flag	Units	Range
		Individual Test(s)			
2009-06-14	SODIUM	129	L	MMOL/L	135-145
2009-06-14	POTASSIUM	4.2		MMOL/L	3.5-5.0
2009-06-14	CHLORIDE	97	L	MMOL/L	98-107
2009-06-14	CO_2	25		MMOL/L	22-30
2009-06-14	UREA NITROGEN	26	H	MG/DL	7-21
2009-06-14	CREATININE	0.82		MG/DL	0.60-1.00
2009-06-14	EST. GFR (MDRD)	>= 60		mL/min/1.73m2	>=60
2009-06-14	ANION GAP	7	L	MMOL/L	9-15
2009-06-14	BUN/CREAT RATIO	32			UNDEFINED
2009-06-14	GLUCOSE, RANDOM	108		MG/DL	65-179
2009-06-14	MAGNESIUM	1.7		MG/DL	1.6-2.2
2009-06-14	PHOSPHORUS	3.5		MG/DL	2.4-4.5
		CBC+PLATELETS			
2009-06-14	CBC+PLATELETS	:			
2009-06-14	WBC	11.7	H	×10 9th/L	4.5-11.0
2009-06-14	RBC	3.80	L	×10 12th/L	4.00-5.20
2009-06-14	HGB	11.9	L	G/DL	12.0-16.0
2009-06-14	HCT	33.1	L	%	36.0-46.0
2009-06-14	MCV	87		FL	80-100
2009-06-14	MCH	31		PG	26-34
2009-06-14	MCHC	36		G/DL	31-37
2009-06-14	RDW	13.1		%	12.0-15.0
2009-06-14	MPV	7.2		FL	7.0-10.0
2009-06-14	PLATELET COUNT	247		×10 9th/L	150-440

Figure 1-2 Example of a laboratory report.

Courtesy of Dr. Catherine Hammett-Stabler, Department of Pathology and Laboratory Medicine, University of North Carolina at Chapel Hill.

the quantity of red cells become reduced in patients with anemia. Sometimes enzyme levels in the blood are elevated; probable causes include (1) enzymes leaking from damaged cells in diseased or injured organs (liver function tests are an example), (2) increased enzyme synthesis as a result of disease, or (3) impaired excretion of enzymes due to failure of normal excretory pathways.

Clinical laboratory tests also are used to evaluate specific functions of organs. Pulmonary function tests measure the rate and efficiency with which air moves into and out of the lungs. Determinations of the concentration of oxygen and carbon dioxide in the blood can indicate pulmonary function by evaluating how efficiently the lungs oxygenate the blood and eliminate carbon dioxide. A simple device (pulse oximeter) applied to the finger can determine the amount of oxygen carried by hemoglobin in circulating blood. This is an example of a **point-of-care test**, which can be performed outside of the laboratory in the practitioner's office or at a patient's bedside. Of increasing importance are tests to detect and measure concentrations of substances that are likely to be produced by tumors growing within the body. Serial analyses of these substances can be used to monitor the response of certain tumors to treatment. Microbiologic tests detect the presence of pathologic organisms in urine, blood, bronchial secretions, and feces as well as other places. These tests also can determine the responsiveness of the organisms to antibiotics.

Point-of-care test Laboratory test that can be performed at the patient's bedside or in the physician's office.

X-ray A form of electromagnetic radiation used to generate images of the internal structures of living organisms.

Radiograph An image taken with X-rays.

Computed tomographic (CT) scan An X-ray technique producing detailed cross-sectional images of the body by means of an X-ray tube and detectors connected to a computer. Sometimes called a CAT scan.

Magnetic resonance imaging (MRI) A diagnostic procedure that yields computer-generated images based on the movement of hydrogen atoms in tissues subjected to a strong magnetic field.

Imaging Techniques

Imaging technology enables the healthcare provider to obtain a view of the body and its organ systems previously available only to the surgeon. Imaging technology permits anatomic investigation of the living patient, most often with little or no risk and minimal discomfort. The earliest, and still an important use of imaging technology, is the production of two-dimensional projected images of interior organ systems: **X-rays** or **radiographs**. However, modern computer technology now allows three-dimensional reconstruction of body systems (tomography) either using X-rays as an imaging source (**computed tomographic [CT] scans**) or using the magnetic properties of certain body constituents (most often ^{1}H in body water). To the physicist, this property is called nuclear magnetic resonance; to the physician, such studies are termed **magnetic resonance imaging (MRI)**. Of growing importance is the use of ultrasound to image accessible areas of the body. The technique depends on the differences in acoustic properties of tissue, so the movement and velocity of blood in vessels (Doppler ultrasound) is easily studied; images of the developing fetus can also safely be produced. The equipment for ultrasound analysis is relatively inexpensive and can easily be used outside of the hospital setting.

X-Ray Examination

X-ray examinations are conducted in many ways, but the basic principle is the same. X-rays (electromagnetic radiation) pass through the area of interest and are detected most commonly by a digital detecting device. The pattern of an X-ray image depends on the density of the tissue the rays pass through. Tissues of low density, such as the air-filled lungs, transmit most of the X-rays and appear black on the image. Tissues of high density, such as bone, absorb most of the rays and appear white on the image. Tissues of intermediate densities appear in varying shades of gray. The two-dimensional image produced is called a radiograph, or sometimes a "plain film" (**Figure 1-3**).

Special terminology is used for particular radiographic studies. For example, a specialized radiographic study of the breast is called a mammogram.

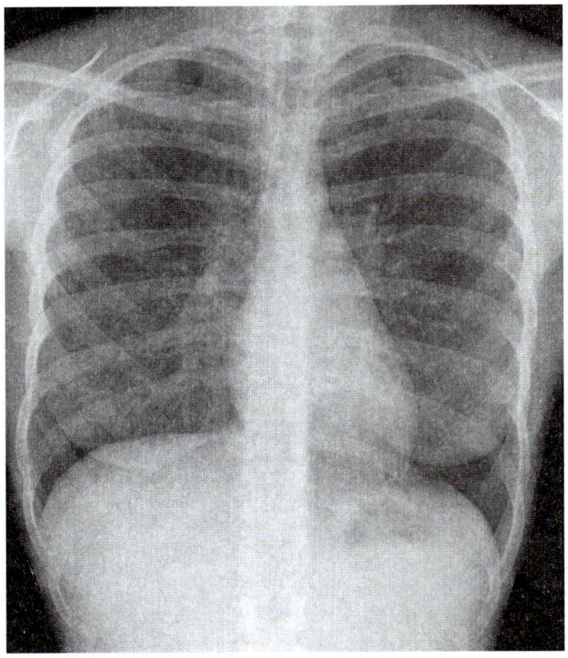

Figure 1-3 Chest X-ray (normal). Normal chest X-ray shows white bones and dark lung fields. The heart (*center of image*) and organs below the diaphragm (*bottom third of image*) are also white because of the density of the soft tissue through which the X-rays pass.

Courtesy of Dr. Donald Yandow, Department of Radiology, University of Wisconsin School of Medicine and Public Health.

The linings of some internal organ systems, such as the digestive and urinary tracts, provide little contrast. To aid in their examination, a nontoxic radiopaque substance (contrast medium) designed to coat the lining (mucosa) of the organ system may be used to outline the area of interest. For example, barium contrast media may be swallowed or given as an enema to outline portions of the gastrointestinal (GI) tract. Irregularities in the column of barium indicate alterations in the internal structure in a portion of the GI tract. After the bulk of contrast material either passes through or is expelled from the tract, the remainder coats the surface of the tract and outlines details of the internal surface, such as tumors, erosions, or ulcers (**Figure 1-4**).

Other soluble radiopaque substances can be injected into the circulation to aid in detection of irregularities or blockages in the vascular, renal, or urinary system (**Figure 1-5**). The movement of contrast agents in portions of the body also can be studied in "real time" or be recorded as a movie using a technique known as fluoroscopy.

Computed Tomographic Scans

A CT scan produces a continuous series of X-ray images of the body by rotating the X-ray tube around the patient as the patient is moved past the X-ray source. The X-ray tube rotates on a toroidal (doughnut-shaped) frame linked to an array of sensitive radiation detectors that rotate around and encircle the patient, moving through the center of the frame. As the X-ray tube and detector array move around the patient, the radiation detectors record the amount of radiation passing through the body (**Figure 1-6**).

The data from the radiation detectors are fed into a computer, which reconstructs the information into a three-dimensional image composed of a series of voxels (the three-dimensional equivalent of the two-dimensional pixels on

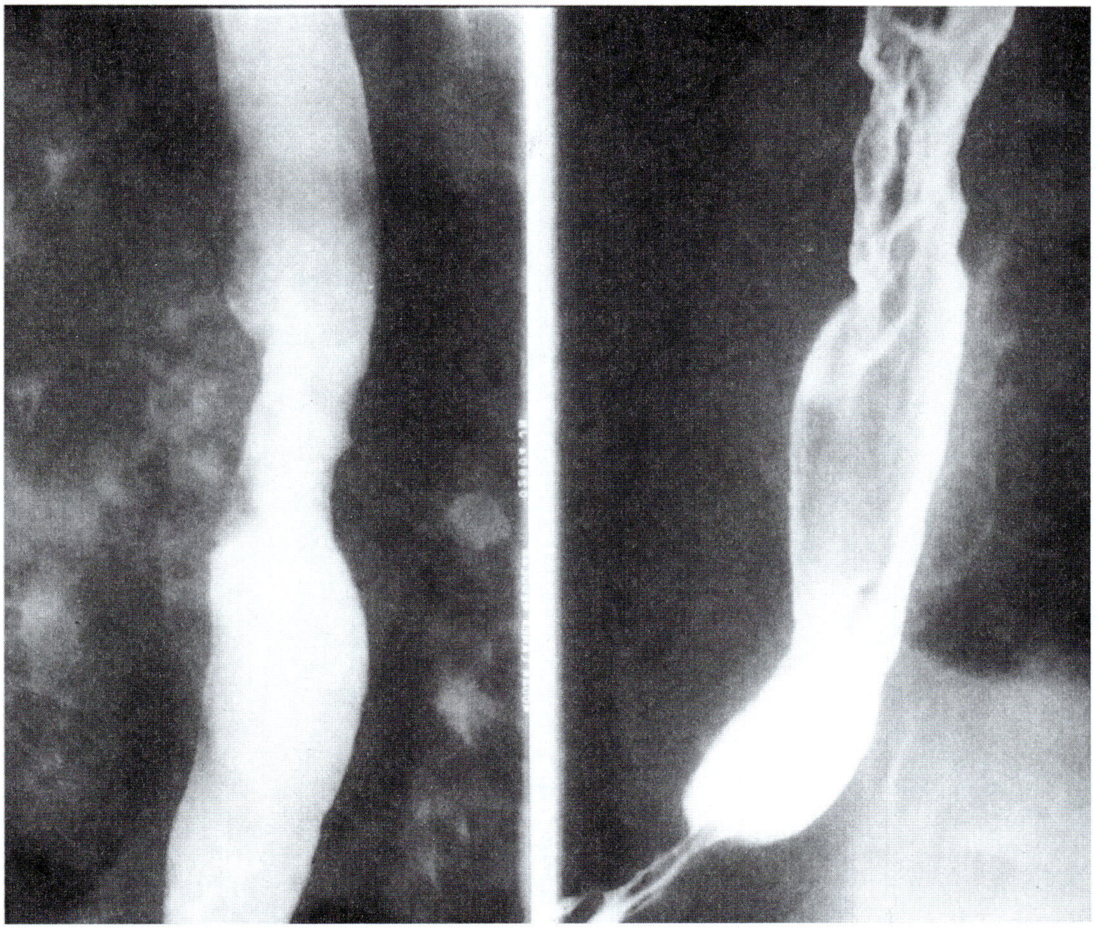

Figure 1-4 Barium contrast swallow study of the esophagus. X-ray of barium column in the esophagus showing narrowed area (*center of left image*) suggestive of an esophageal tumor (*left*). Following passage of the bulk of the barium, a coating of contrast medium outlines the mucosa, demonstrating irregularity and constriction as a result of esophageal cancer (*right*).

Image courtesy of Dr. David Warshauer, Department of Radiology, University of North Carolina at Chapel Hill.

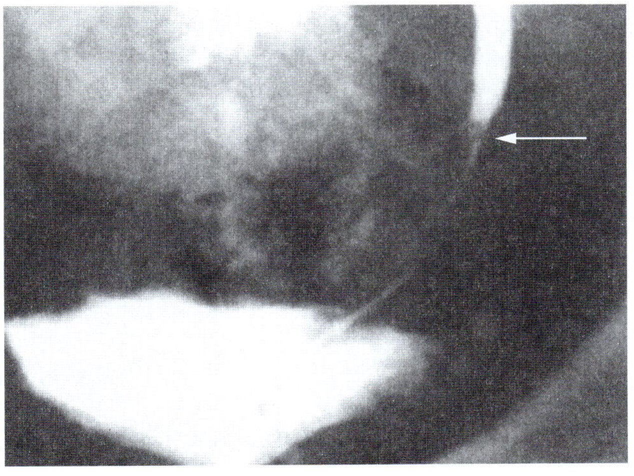

Figure 1-5 Intravenous pyelogram (IVP). Contrast media fills the bladder at the bottom of the image and the proximal (*closer to the kidney*) portion of the right ureter (*top of image*). A stone (*white arrow*) is lodged in the ureter, causing dilation of the ureter above the stone and preventing the filling of the ureter below. The dye in the bladder has come from the urine passing through the opposite ureter (*not shown*).

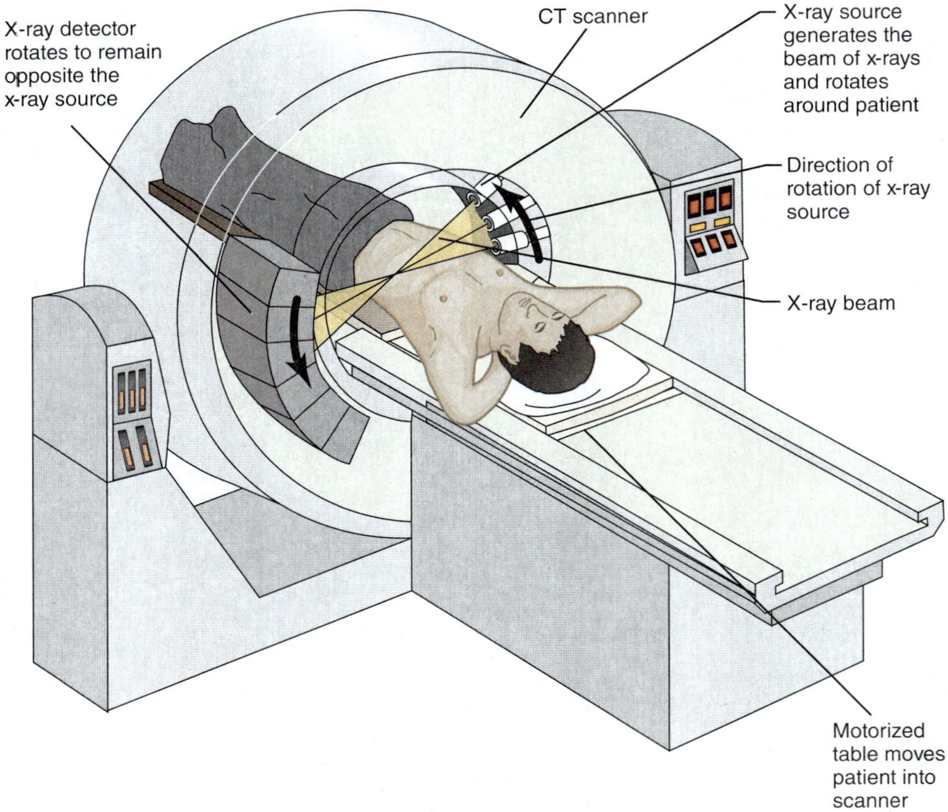

Figure 1-6 Computed tomographic (CT) scan. The patient lies on a table that is gradually advanced into the scanner. The X-ray tube mounted in the scanner rotates around the patient, and radiation detectors also rotate so that detectors remain opposite the X-ray source. Data from radiation detectors generate computer-reconstructed images of the patient's body at multiple levels.

Prone Lying on the back with feet toward the viewer.

Virtual colonoscopy A high-resolution contrast CT image of the colon. May be substituted for colonoscopy in special cases.

a computer monitor), each representing the X-ray density of a small volumetric area of the patient's body. Most often the image is displayed as a series of transverse cross-sections of the patient's anatomy (with the patient **prone**, or lying on the back with feet toward the viewer). However, the computer is just as capable of presenting information as a series of slices in any orientation. Abnormalities of internal organs that cannot be identified by means of standard X-ray examinations can often be discovered with CT scans because the geometry of an organ and the relationship of one organ to another can be seen while scanning through an entire region of the body. For example, **Figure 1-7** shows a lung tumor that might not have been obvious on a plain film.

Modern computational techniques allow entire organ systems to be reconstructed as three-dimensional images, which can be examined in great detail. In the technique of **virtual colonoscopy**, the surface mucosa of the entire colon can be reconstructed and "flown through" by the radiologist sitting at a computer who examines it for lesions, such as polyps and other mucosal growths. The technique can substitute for endoscopy in patients for whom an invasive procedure might have additional risks (**Figure 1-8**).

Magnetic Resonance Imaging

MRI scans produce computer-constructed images of various organs and tissues somewhat like CT scans. The device consists of a strong superconducting magnet capable of developing an extremely powerful magnetic field (greater than 50,000

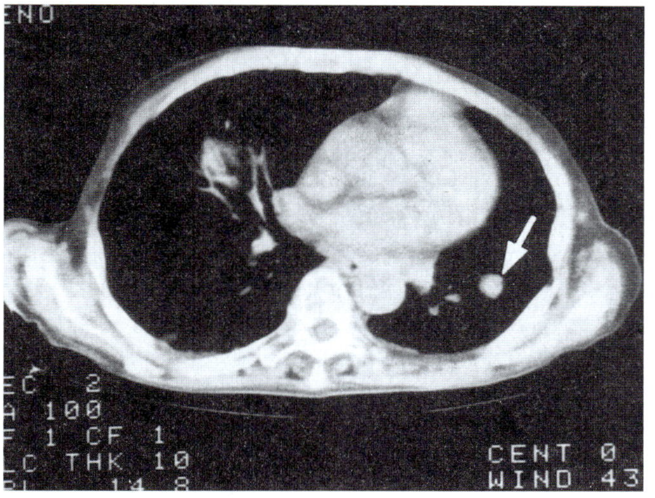

Figure 1-7 CT scan of chest. Mediastinum and heart appear white in the center of the scan, with less-dense lungs on either side. A lung tumor (*arrow*) appears as a white nodule in the lung.

Courtesy of Leonard V. Crowley, MD, Century College.

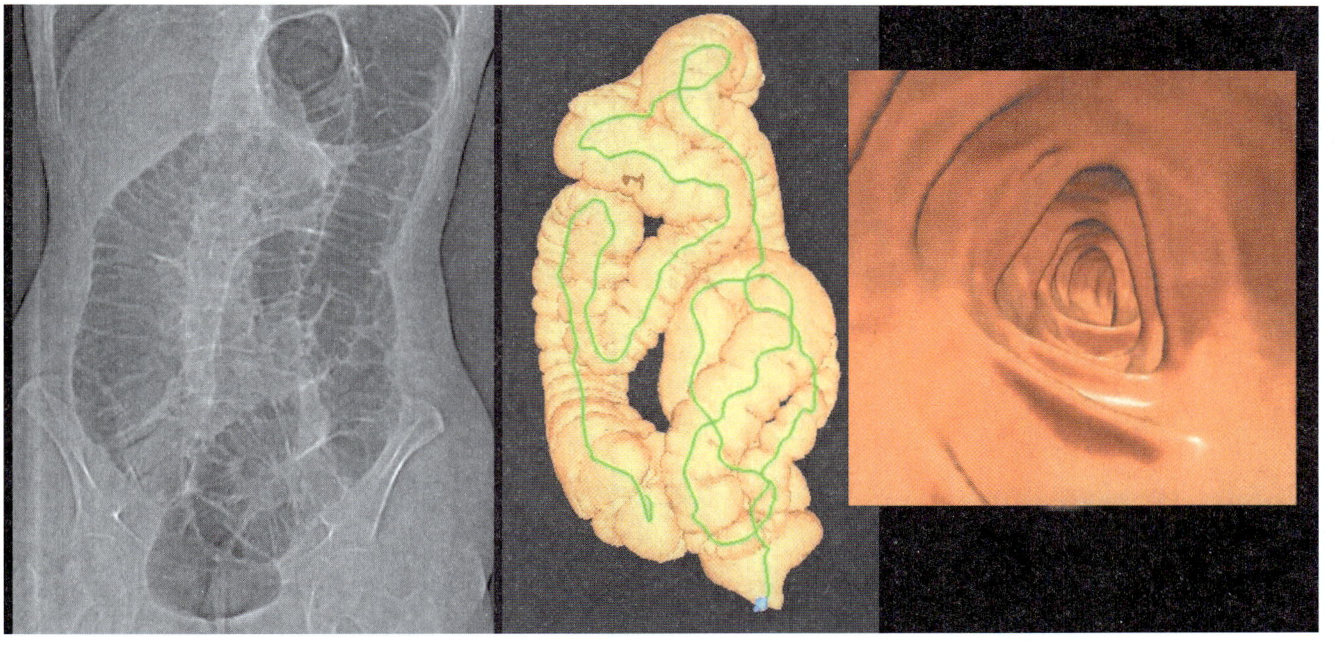

Figure 1-8 Virtual colonoscopy. A high-resolution contrast CT image of the colon is produced. The mucosa of the colon is highlighted by the contrast medium (*left*). A computer reconstruction of the entire colon in three dimensions is produced. The green line traces the center of the colon (*center*). The radiologist can "fly through" the colon and examine the mucosal surface of the interior (*right*).

Image courtesy of Dr. David Warshauer, Department of Radiology, University of North Carolina at Chapel Hill.

times that of the Earth), coils that can transmit and receive radio frequency (RF) waves, and a computer that receives impulses from the scanner and forms them into images that can be interpreted. The MRI scanner with the enclosed magnet and coils appears somewhat similar to an elongated, tubular CT scanner. The patient lies on a table that is gradually moved into the scanner, as is done in CT. The physical principles of MRI, however, are different from those of CT scanning. MRI scans most often depend on the response of hydrogen protons (positively charged particles in the nucleus around which electrons rotate) contained within the body's water molecules. Hydrogen protons behave as if they are spinning rapidly about an axis. When subjected to a strong magnetic field, the protons become aligned in the direction of the magnetic field. After a pulse of RF waves, the protons are temporarily dislodged from their orientation. As they return to their original orientation, they emit a signal (resonance) that can be measured and used to produce the computer-constructed images. Body tissues, which have a high water content, are a rich source of protons capable of excitation. The intensity of the signals produced is related to several things: the water content (and hence hydrogen ion content) of body tissues, the strength and duration of the RF pulse, plus the geometry of the applied magnetic gradient. The many combinations of RF pulse and magnetic gradients are termed MRI sequences and are chosen for particular imaging applications. For example, T2 weighted MRI is particularly useful in detecting regions in the brain and spinal cord where myelin sheaths of nerve fibers have been damaged, as in a neurologic disease called multiple sclerosis (see Chapter 23) (**Figure 1-9** and **Figure 1-10**).

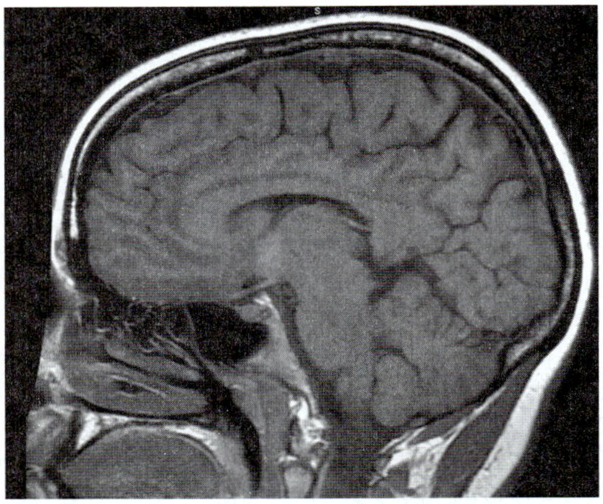

Figure 1-9 MRI normal brain sagittal view. The nose is on the left. Notice how clearly the fissures and folds over the surface of the brain can be seen, as well as the distinction between the different neural elements of which the brain is composed.

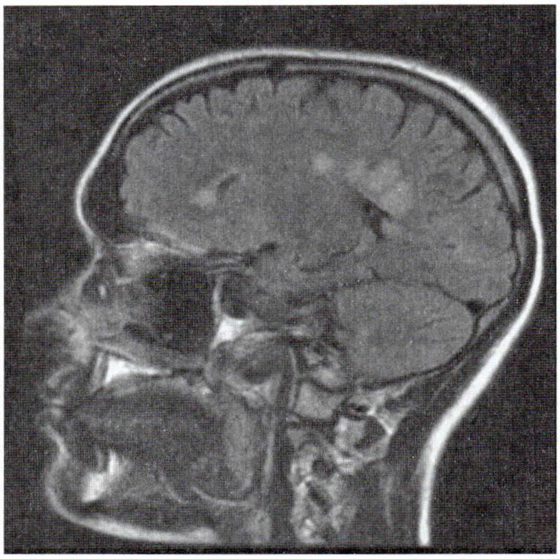

Figure 1-10 MRI of brain from a patient with multiple sclerosis in sagittal view (as in Figure 1-9). Multiple plaques (light areas) where neurons have lost their myelin coating are visible.

Because an MRI does not use ionizing radiation, the patient does not receive radiation exposure. An MRI does expose the patient to strong magnetic and RF fields. MRI appears safe provided the patient does not have implanted or embedded ferromagnetic material that might interact with the powerful magnetic field. Recent advances in the use of special contrast agents for MRI have greatly expanded the utility of the technique.

Imaging Technology to Detect Specific Molecules and Processes

There is great interest in using imaging technology to detect specific chemical constituents or metabolic activity in regions of the body. For example, Alzheimer's disease, a degenerative dementia most often associated with aging, is associated with accumulation of an abnormal protein component, beta-amyloid (Aβ), in areas of the brain. Definitive diagnosis of this disease previously required obtaining brain tissue (most often postmortem) for analysis. Modern imaging technology can now detect and localize both changes in brain metabolism and the specific abnormal protein associated with Alzheimer's disease, providing early, noninvasive diagnoses. This technology depends on detecting and localizing radiolabeled compounds injected into the patient. The location and distribution of the radiation-emitting compounds can be mapped within the body to produce a planar (two-dimensional) image using a gamma camera or to produce tomographic (three-dimensional) images using single-photon computed tomography (SPECT) or PET technology used with positron-emitting tracers.

Radioisotope Studies Using Gamma Emitters

By using specially designed radiation detectors, the uptake location and excretion of the labeled substance can be mapped. The ability of the thyroid gland to concentrate and utilize radioactive iodine is used as a measure of thyroid function and, more importantly, can be used to detect tumors within the thyroid gland. Ventilation/perfusion (V/Q) lung scans measure the distribution of an inhaled radioactive gas (xenon-133) to locate obstructions to the airways and combine it with a radiolabeled albumin injected into the circulation to measure pulmonary blood flow and to detect possible blood clots lodged within the lung (pulmonary emboli).

Phosphorus-containing isotopes are concentrated in the skeletal system. If there are deposits of tumor in bone, the isotopes are concentrated around the tumor deposits and can be easily identified (**Figure 1-11**).

Radioactive materials injected intravenously also can be used to evaluate blood flow to the heart muscle and to identify areas of damaged heart muscle. Three-dimensional tomographic techniques using SPECT or PET provide much better localization of tracers and are supplanting the use of planar gamma cameras in many radioisotope localization studies.

Positron Emission Tomography

Related to radioisotope studies using compounds labeled with gamma ray emitters is the technique of **positron emission tomography (PET)**. PET imaging uses a special class of radiolabel that emits positrons. Positrons are subatomic particles that have the same mass as electrons but carry a positive charge. They are formed when atoms, such as carbon, oxygen, or nitrogen are bombarded in a cyclotron with high-energy particles to produce a short-lived positron-emitting radio tracer. Almost all positron-emitting radio tracers are very short

Positron emission tomography (PET) scan Imaging using radioactive tracers that analyzes metabolic or biochemical functioning.

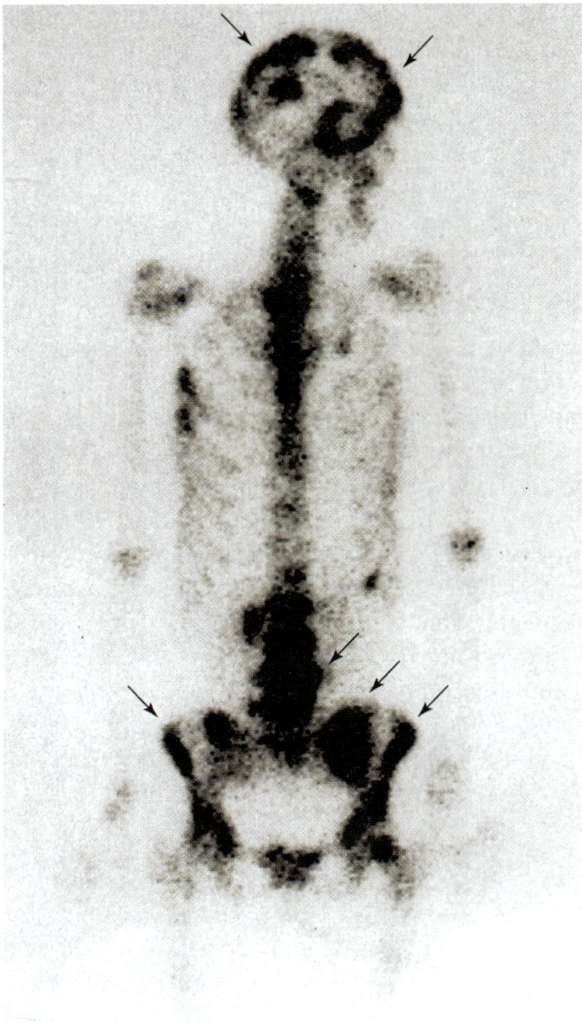

Figure 1-11 Radioisotope bone scan of head, chest, and pelvis. Dark areas (*arrows*) indicate the concentration of radioisotope around tumor deposits in bone.
Courtesy of Leonard V. Crowley, MD, Century College.

lived and produced at the imaging site using a cyclotron, thus the technology is limited to major medical centers. For example, one of the most commonly used positron-emitting radio tracers is fludeoxyglucose ^{18}F (^{18}F-FDG), which has a half-life of under 2 hours and is made by initially bombarding oxygen isotope ^{18}O-enriched water with protons to produce the positron-emitting ^{18}F, which must be incorporated into the glucose-like molecule on site. A positron escaping from the nucleus collides with a negatively charged electron in a nearby atom, simultaneously producing two gamma rays emitted 180 degrees apart. The PET scanner registers this very weak but nearly simultaneous pair of pulses while ignoring non-paired background radiation. The scanner uses this information to build a tomographic view of the distribution of the radio tracer. To further localize the source, the patient may also be CT scanned at the same time and the two images combined.

One of the most widely used applications of PET is to study the metabolic activity of areas of the body using ^{18}F-FDG, a compound that is metabolized like glucose in the patient. This provides information on the metabolic activities of the organ or tissue being studied, the site within an organ where the

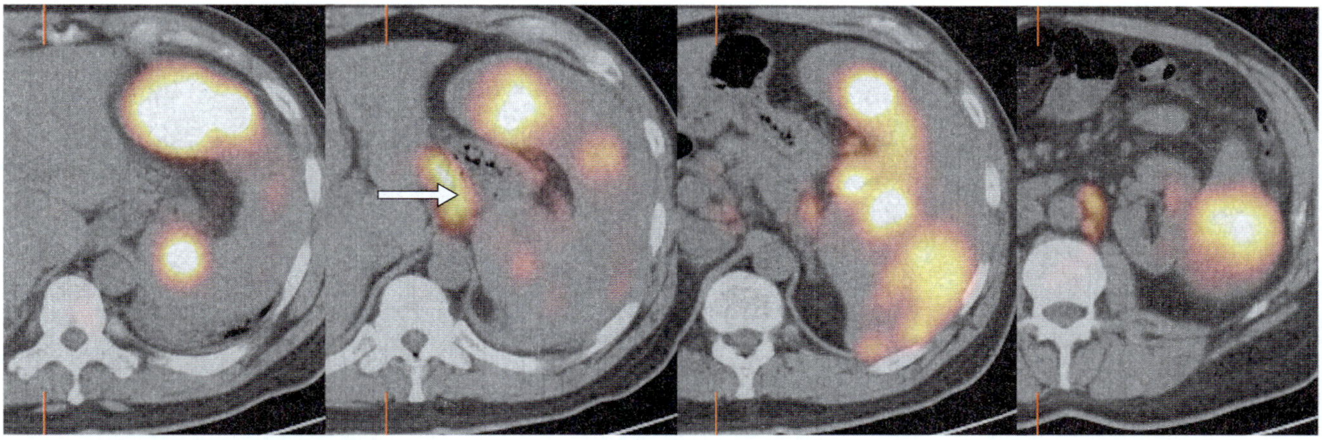

Figure 1-12 Combined PET scan and CT. Color represents PET scan results indicating distribution of ^{18}F-FDG metabolism in spleen (*large organ on right of images*) of a patient with lymphoma (cancer of lymphocytes). The PET scan has detected the spread of the cancer to adjacent lymph nodes (*arrow in second image*).

Image courtesy of Dr. David Warshauer, Department of Radiology, University of North Carolina at Chapel Hill.

compound is being metabolized, and the blood flow to the organ being studied. One can detect and measure changes in brain functions associated with various neurologic diseases, such as strokes, brain tumors, Alzheimer's disease, Parkinson's disease, and some hereditary degenerative diseases of the nervous system. This method may also be used to evaluate changes in blood flow and metabolism in the heart muscle after a heart attack. Malignant tumors often have higher metabolic rates than benign tumors. Hence, mapping the distribution and rate of ^{18}F-FDG metabolism may be used to detect and evaluate potential occult cancers, including metastases, spread throughout the body and to follow the effectiveness of therapy (**Figure 1-12**).

Even more exciting is the ability to synthesize PET radio tracers, which can bind to and localize specific abnormal molecules, such as the abnormal Aβ found in Alzheimer brains.

Ultrasound

Unlike the imaging techniques that depend on detection of electromagnetic radiation as part of the imaging process, ultrasound is a technique for mapping the reflected echoes produced by high-frequency sound waves transmitted into the body. Echoes are reflected wherever there is a change in the density of the tissue. The reflected waves are recorded on a detector, and visual images are produced, generally on a small monitor. Unlike the complex equipment needed for CT or PET scans, ultrasound devices commonly use a single handheld transducer to produce the ultrasound and record the reflected echoes. The transducers may be moved over any external area of the body (using a water-soluble gel to couple the ultrasound to the area of study) to produce a real-time image of internal organs under and within range of the acoustic beam as the transducer is moved. Although there are limits to the depth of penetration of ultrasound from the body surface, ultrasound transducers are small enough to be introduced into the rectum (to image the prostate in males), the vagina (for gynecological investigations in females), and the esophagus (to image abdominal organs, such as the pancreas). This method is widely used to study the uterus during pregnancy because it does not require the use of potentially harmful radiation and poses no risk to the fetus (**Figure 1-13**).

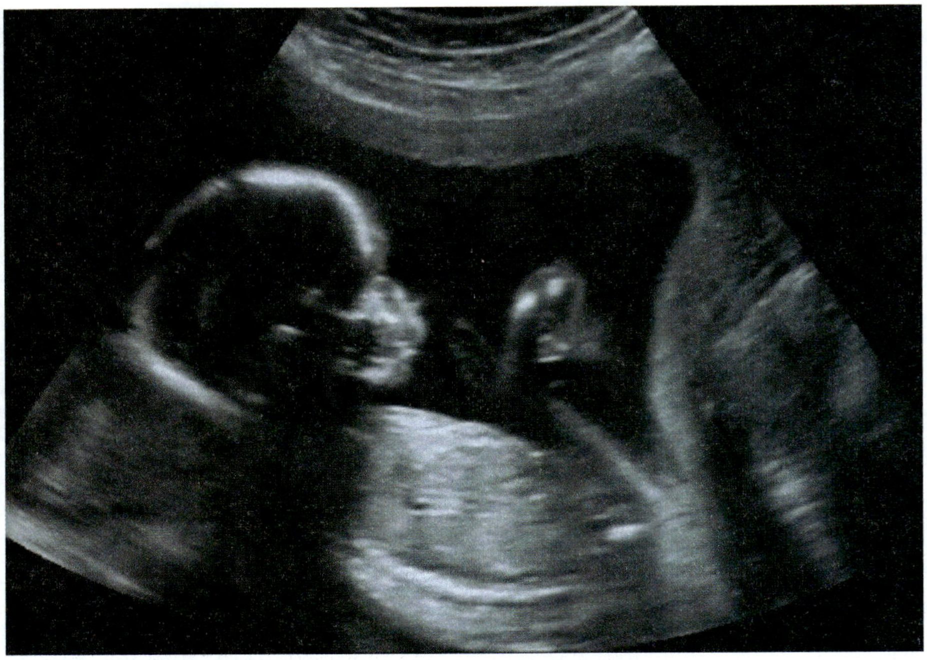

Figure 1-13 Ultrasound examination of a fetus at four months' gestation.

Echocardiogram
A record obtained from an ultrasound examination of the heart and related blood vessels; used to assist in the diagnosis of cardiovascular disease.

Ultrasound can be used to determine the position of the placenta and the fetus within the uterus. It also can identify some fetal abnormalities and detect pregnancies with more than one fetus. Ultrasound is also often used to examine the cardiovascular system. When used for this purpose, the procedure is usually called an **echocardiogram**. An echocardiogram can detect the structure and function of the heart valves as well as determine abnormal communications between adjacent cardiac chambers. Abnormal blood flow patterns characteristic of congenital or acquired valvular heart disease or other abnormalities in cardiac function can be detected in real time as the heart beats. Doppler ultrasound can determine both the direction and velocity of blood as it moves through the heart and other organs and can detect irregularities in flow. Doppler flow images are "color coded" to show flow direction in relation to the transducer (**Figure 1-14**).

Ultrasound replaced many radiology procedures because ultrasound avoids radiation, is most often not invasive (or only minimally so), and is easily performed in a doctor's office. Ultrasound devices are relatively small and inexpensive, and studies using this technology are often less expensive than those using other techniques.

Cytologic and Histologic Examinations

Cytology studies the characteristics of individual cells or small groups of cells that are either shed or sampled from body organs. Such cells may be naturally cast off into body fluids and secretions or may be removed by brushes, spatulas, or similar tools. For example, the Pap (Papanicolaou) smear mentioned previously uses a harvesting device to obtain cells dislodged from the surface of the cervix and uterine canal to screen for cancer or early precursors to this disease. Similar approaches can be used to obtain bronchial cells and cells from the bladder. Cell samples may be

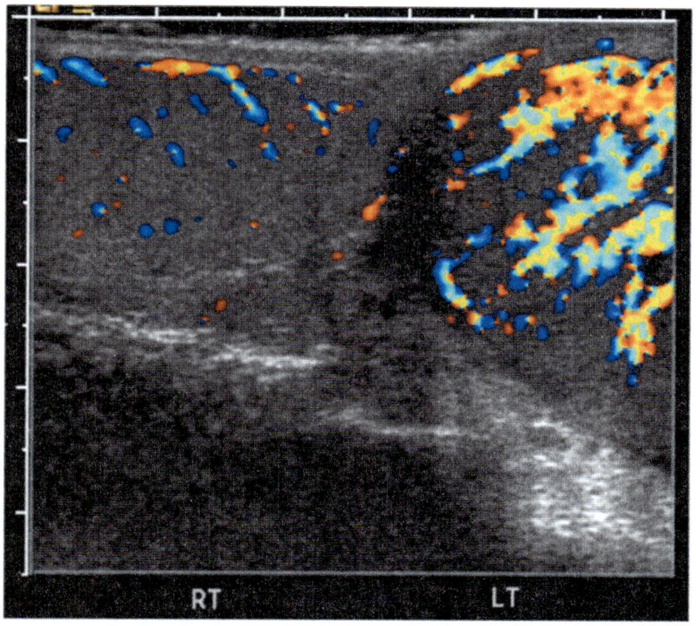

Figure 1-14 Doppler ultrasound examination of testicular mass. Left testis (LT) shows an excess of blood vessels suggestive of testicular cancer. Blue indicates blood flowing toward and red indicates flow away from the transducer placed in contact with the scrotum.

Image courtesy of Dr. David Warshauer, Department of Radiology, University of North Carolina at Chapel Hill.

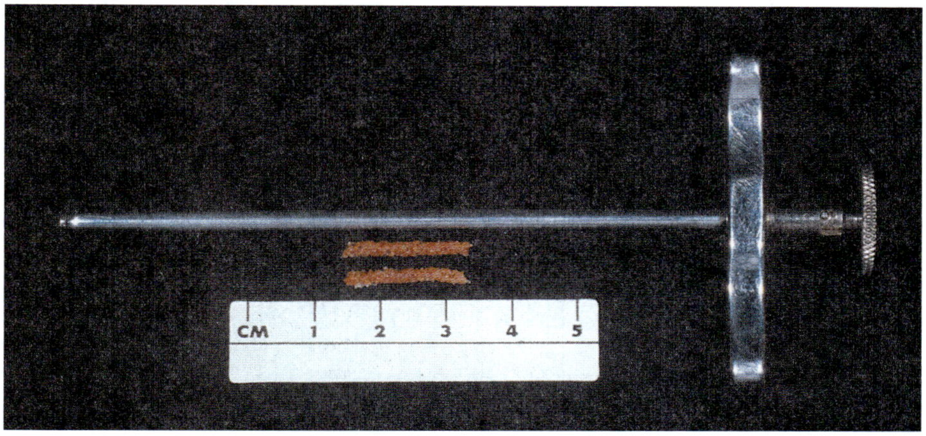

Figure 1-15 Two samples of bone marrow (*adjacent to scale*) obtained from a pelvic bone by means of a specially designed needle (*upper part of photograph*).

Courtesy of Leonard V. Crowley, MD, Century College.

obtained using very fine needles and a syringe to aspirate surface-accessible lesions. Such fine-needle aspirations (FNAs) are often painless and rapid, requiring no anesthesia. Cytological examination of blood and bone marrow (**Figure 1-15**) is critical in the diagnosis of hematologic (blood-related) diseases and is often performed to diagnose neoplastic disease in blood cell precursors found in the marrow.

Bone marrow studies are carried out by hematopathologists, who use microscopes and flow cytometers that can quickly evaluate thousands of cells for multiple parameters, such as size, internal contents, and surface characteristics as they flow past a series of detectors.

Histology examines the structure of organs and the tissues and groups of cells of which they are composed. Histopathology recognizes changes in tissues that can be indicative of disease. The tissue may be obtained as part of a surgical procedure (a surgical specimen) or the tissue may be removed from the target organ for the specific purpose of histopathological examination (a **biopsy** specimen).

Biopsy Removal of a small sample of tissue for examination and diagnosis by a pathologist.

Electrocardiogram (ECG)/electroencephalogram (EEG)/electromyogram (EMG) Tests analyzing the patterns of electrical impulses of different body parts used to evaluate function—ECG for heart, EEG for brain, and EMG for muscle. EMG only indirectly measures the nervous system.

Laparoscope A long tubular telescope-like instrument passed through the abdominal wall to examine structures within the peritoneal cavity.

Samples of tissue can be obtained from any part of the body. Gastroscopes, bronchoscopes, colonoscopes, and other instruments used for endoscopic examination, for example, are constructed so that specimens for biopsy can be obtained while the internal organs are being examined. Biopsy specimens also can be taken directly from internal organs, such as the liver or kidney by inserting a thin needle through the skin directly into the organ to produce a biopsy core. This is often done using ultrasound or other imaging techniques for guidance.

Tests of Electrical Activity

Several different tests measure the electrical impulses associated with bodily functions and activities. These include the **electrocardiogram (ECG)**, the **electroencephalogram (EEG)**, and the **electromyogram (EMG)**. The most widely used of these tests is the ECG. Electrodes attached to the arms, legs, and chest are used to measure the changes in the electrical activity of the heart during the various phases of the cardiac cycle. The ECG also identifies disturbances in the heart rate or rhythm and identifies abnormal conduction of impulses through the heart. Heart muscle injury, from a variety of causes, including a heart attack, can be recognized by means of characteristic abnormalities in the cardiogram. The EEG measures the electrical activity of the brain through attachment of small electrodes attached to different areas in the scalp. Abnormalities of cerebral structure or function may cause altered brain wave patterns. The EMG measures the electrical activity of skeletal muscle during contraction and at rest. Abnormal electrical activity is often encountered in various inflammatory or degenerative diseases involving the skeletal muscles and the nerves that control them. The test is performed by inserting a needle into the muscle that is being studied. The speed at which a nerve conducts impulses can be measured by means of electrodes taped to the surface of the skin over the nerve being tested.

Endoscopy and Laparoscopy

An endoscopy, or endoscopic examination (endo = within + skopeo = examine), is an examination of the interior of the body by means of various types of flexible tubular instruments, all of similar design, that are named according to the part of the body they are designed to examine. These instruments contain an optical system with a light source and ports through which either sampling or therapeutic devices can be guided. In addition, gas or liquid may be passed through the scope to help visualize the area studied. A **laparoscope** is used to visualize the abdominal and pelvic organs in the procedure referred to as laparoscopy. To perform a laparoscopic procedure, the peritoneal cavity is inflated first with carbon dioxide, which separates the organs so that they can be visualized more easily. Then the laparoscope is inserted through a small incision in the abdominal wall, often in or near the umbilicus. Modern laparoscopes may be used to perform surgical as well as diagnostic procedures. For example, appendectomies and gall bladder removals often are performed using laparoscopic surgical techniques (as opposed to "open" surgery).

Treatment

After diagnosis, a course of treatment is initiated. The nature and type of **specific treatment** depends upon the diagnosis as well as the cause and nature of the disease. For example, an antibiotic may be given to a patient with an infection known to be responsive to the antibiotic, or insulin may be given to a patient with a certain type of diabetes. **Symptomatic treatment** relieves the discomforts and ill effects associated with the disease but may or may not influence the course of the underlying condition. Symptomatic measures may include prescription or over-the-counter medications as well as therapeutic processes, such as icing, warming, or wrapping. Treatment regimens can overlap. Tumors may be debulked to relieve pain caused by pressure to organs, but such therapy may also prolong the life of the patient. At times, the clinician must be content with treating the debilitating manifestations of the disease, perhaps prolonging life, without being able to offer a lasting cure. Clinical medicine and patient treatment plans often involve the services and expertise of a wide range of healthcare providers. The team may contain dietitians, nurses, clinicians, physician assistants, respiratory therapists, physiotherapists, pharmacists, social workers, patient advocates, and even financial counseling.

Specific treatment Treatment of underlying cause of disease.

Symptomatic treatment Treatment to alleviate symptoms rather than underlying cause of disease.

Case 1-1

An 18-year-old college student suffers a 4-hour episode of mild abdominal pain and nausea that localizes in the **periumbilical** (near the belly button) region. She initially attributes this to "an upset stomach." As the pain continues to increase, the patient suffers severe nausea, cramping, and feels feverish. Her roommates take her to student health services. Because of the symptoms presented, the student is immediately transferred to the emergency room (ER) of a nearby hospital.

In the ER the pain continues to increase and localizes to the right lower quadrant (RLQ) of the abdominal region. On physical examination, the following is noted:

- A moderately elevated oral temperature (38.7°C).
- An elevated number of white cells in the blood (23,000 per microliter; normal is about 8,000). Most of these cells are granulocytes.
- An area of local tenderness located on a line between the umbilicus and iliac crest, closer to the **iliac crest**.
- Right-sided rectal tenderness.

Appendicitis is strongly suspected, and the patient is prepared for a CT scan of her abdomen. An axial CT scan through the upper pelvic region shows a dilated appendix containing an **appendicolith**, a calcified stone visible in the several sequential images (**Case Figure 1-1**).

The patient is prepared for laparoscopic surgery. An **edematous** (fluid-filled) red appendix is removed at surgery (**Case Figure 1-2**), which when opened contained several appendicoliths. The patient recovered uneventfully.

Periumbilical Situated in the abdominal area near belly button.

Iliac crest Area of hip bone in abdomen.

Appendicolith A calcified stone in the appendix.

Edematous Filled with fluid.

McBurney's point Localization of pain to region of abdomen specific for appendicitis.

Discussion

The combination of patient symptoms and signs provides sensitive indicators of appendicitis in young adults but lacks specificity. The elevated temperature and increased numbers of white cells (particularly granulocytes) are strong indicators of a response to tissue injury, which is most likely the result of a bacterial infection. The localization of the pain to the specific region of the abdomen (sometimes called **McBurney's point**) and the right-sided rectal tenderness suggest the infectious process may involve the appendix

(continues)

Case 1-1 *(Continued)*

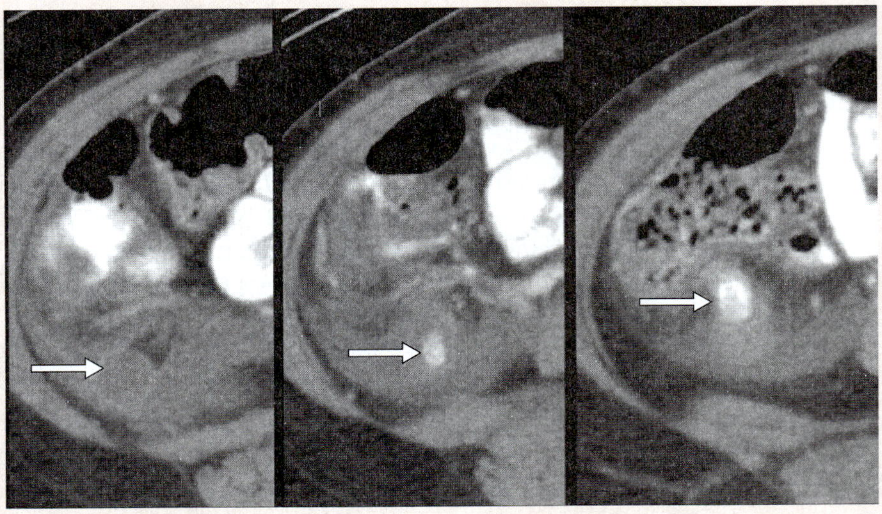

Case Figure 1-1 Sequential CT images from the upper pelvic region of a patient with appendicitis. The appendix is identified (*arrows*) and the appendicolith is visible in the last two images.

Image courtesy of Dr. David Warshauer, Department of Radiology, University of North Carolina at Chapel Hill.

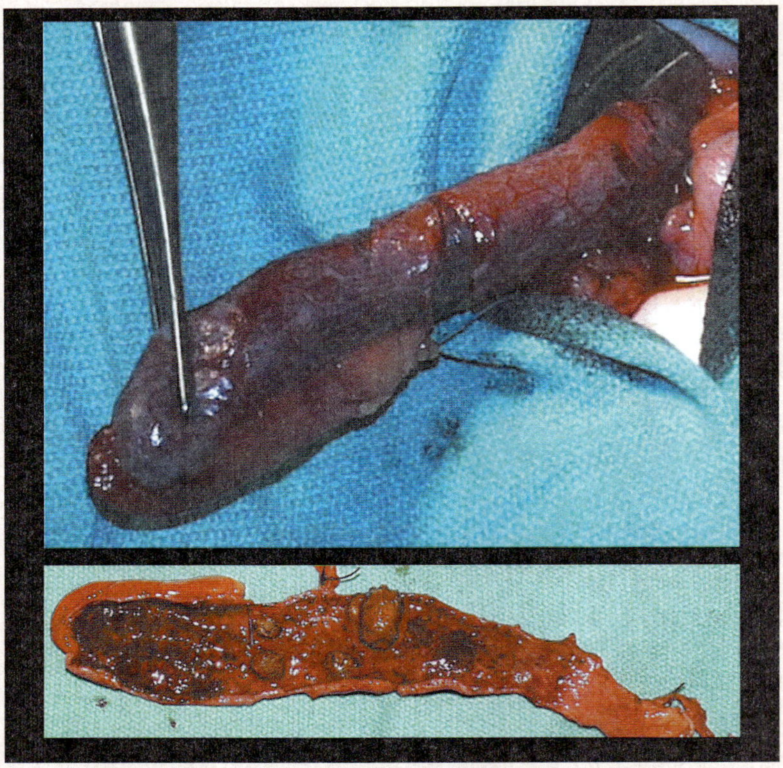

Case Figure 1-2 Inflamed appendix exposed during laparoscopic surgery (*upper image*). The removed appendix opened to reveal several appendicoliths (*lower image*).

Image courtesy of Dr. David Warshauer, Department of Radiology, University of North Carolina at Chapel Hill.

based on pelvic anatomy. However, a number of infectious diseases involving the intestine (as well as other illnesses) can present with similar signs and symptoms. The CT scan is a highly accurate test for appendicitis with a specificity approaching 95 percent. In young children, ultrasound is often used instead of CT to lower radiation exposure.

Etiology and Pathogenesis

Appendicitis is an **inflammation** of the appendix. The disease is most commonly related to blockage of the outlet of the appendix to the bowel (by stones representing calcified fecal material or sometimes by intestinal parasites). This results in bacterial overgrowth by gut microorganisms within the appendix and an inflammatory response. As you will learn in the presentation on inflammation, this response can lead to tissue injury and ultimately to rupture of the appendix (described more fully in the presentation on the gastrointestinal tract).

Inflammation An early defensive reaction by the body to tissue damage and/or infection.

Questions

1. An elevated number of white cells is a sensitive indicator of systemic inflammation present in this case. Why was a radiological study ordered prior to surgery?
2. Another patient comes to the ER complaining of pain on the center to left lower quadrant of her abdominal region. Is acute appendicitis ruled out? What are several additional potential diagnoses?
3. What are some of the potential advantages of the use of laparoscopic surgery (as opposed to "open" surgery) in this case? Consider the possibility that the diagnosis might have been uncertain.

Questions for Review

1. What are the major categories of disease?
2. What are the definitions of the following terms: etiology, symptom of disease, sign of disease, diagnosis, prognosis, and pathogenesis?
3. Describe the process of taking a patient history.
4. What principal factors does the physician evaluate in arriving at a diagnosis?
5. What is the difference between specific and symptomatic treatment?
6. What are the major categories of diagnostic tests and procedures that can help the practitioner make a diagnosis? Give some examples.
7. Compare and contrast the terms sensitivity and specificity.
8. How are cells and tissues used in diagnosis obtained?
9. What are the physical principles on which the following procedures are based: X-ray (plain film) examinations, CT scans, MRI, PET analysis, and ultrasound?

Supplementary Readings

A large number of texts are written for undergraduate pre-health professional students and may serve as useful references for this material. The texts listed here are popular and frequently updated.

A note about online material: There are many accurate, reputable online sites for information on human disease. However, it is often difficult to decide which sources are reliable. Many students turn to Wikipedia or patient-oriented sites, such as WebMD, as an initial online reference; caution is urged. Many Wikipedia articles are first rate; however, information on controversial areas must be checked against other sources and the dates of provided references carefully examined. When references from the literature (scientific papers) are cited, preference will be given to those that are freely available without subscription.

Government sources, such as the Centers for Disease Control and Prevention (www.cdc.gov), the MedlinePlus Medical Encyclopedia (www.nlm.nih.gov), and major medical centers (for example, www.mayoclinic.org /diseases/) are often a good place to start. Other specific online resources are cited as appropriate.

References

Kumar V, Abbas AK, Aster J, Deyrup AT. *Robbins & Kumar Basic Pathology*. 11th ed. Elsevier Saunders; 2023.

Rubin E, Reisner HM, eds. *Principles of Rubin's Pathology*. 7th ed. Wolters Lippincott Williams & Wilkins; 2018.

- These two books are the shorter versions of the leading pathology texts used in medical education. They serve as good general references for detailed descriptions of mechanisms of pathogenesis and disease.

Bickley L, Szilagyi PG, Hoffman RM, Soriano RP. *Bates' Guide to Physical Examination and History Taking*. 13th ed. Lippincott Williams & Wilkins; 2023.

- A classic guide to the details of physician–patient interaction.

Straus SE, Glasziou P, Richardson WS, Haynes RB. *Evidence-Based Medicine*. 5th ed. Elsevier; 2018.

- A comprehensive guide with an excellent chapter on Harm.

Bishop ML, Fody EP, Van Siclen C, et al. *Clinical Chemistry: Principles, Techniques, and Correlations*. Jones & Bartlett Learning; 2023.

- Provides an overview of the most rapidly advancing areas of laboratory medicine with clear explanations that balance analytic principles, techniques, and correlation of results with coverage of disease states.

Herring W. *Learning Radiology: Recognizing the Basics*. 5th ed. Elsevier Saunders; 2024.

- An introductory text that does a good job of providing additional background on the diseases illustrated.

Clift IC. *Clinical Immunodiagnostics: Laboratory Principles and Practices*. Jones & Bartlett Learning; 2021.

- Focuses on theoretical principles underlying different diagnostic tests performed in the clinical lab.

Moini J. *Anatomy and Physiology for Health Professionals*. 3rd ed. Jones & Bartlett Learning; 2020.

- An easy-to-read and well-illustrated text on normal human anatomy and physiology. The text is notable for its many useful tables, critical thinking questions, and correlation with pathology.

American Society for Investigative Pathology. Accessed February 26, 2025. http://www.asip.org/

- This is the major research and teaching organization (although its major focus is not clinical). It is an excellent source for those interested in educational opportunities in the area.

Testing.com. Accessed March 12, 2025. https://www.testing.com/

- Offers consumers access to laboratory testing through a network of laboratory partners and provides lab testing guides.

Geisel School of Medicine, Dartmouth Department of Medical Education. Introduction to radiology. Accessed February 26, 2020. http://www.dartmouth.edu/~anatomy/HAE/Radiology_Intro/rad_index.html

- This is an easy-to-follow, well-illustrated introduction to the area. Additional in-depth resources are available at the site.

American Cancer Society. Cancer Screening Recommendations. Accessed March 12, 2025. https://www.cancer.org/content/dam/cancer-org/online-documents/en/pdf/flyers/cancer-screenings-save-lives.pdf

- Provides recommendations for cancer screening based on age and cancer type.

Inácio V, Rodríguez-Álvarez MX, Gayoso-Diz P. Statistical evaluation of medical tests. *Annu Rev Stat Appl*. 2021;8(1):41-67.

- Provides an overview of statistical evaluation of diagnosis and prognosis using medica tests. It introduces the concept of receiver operating characteristic (ROC) curve analysis, which is critical in test optimization. The examples used are of clinical interest.

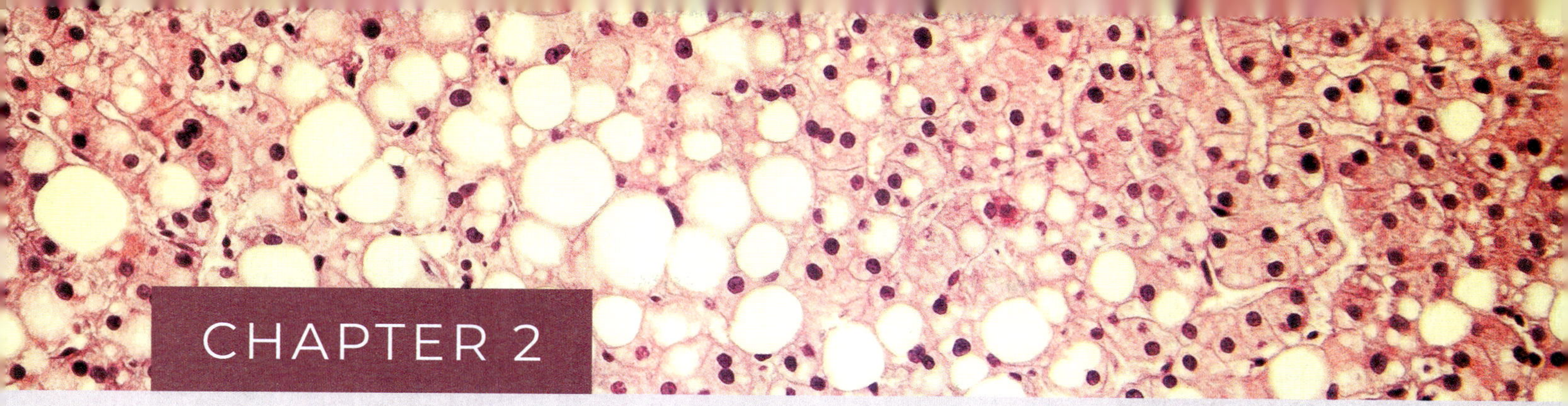

CHAPTER 2

Cells and Tissues: Their Structure and Function in Health and Disease

LEARNING OBJECTIVES

1. Make a sketch of the general structure of a typical cell.
2. Explain how cells are organized to form tissues. Diagram the fundamental structure of the four basic types of tissues: epithelium, connective, muscle, and nerve.
3. Explain how tissues are organized to form organs.
4. Write a general description of the three germ layers and their derivatives.
5. Illustrate how materials move in and out of cells.
6. List five processes by which cells adapt to changing conditions.
7. Explain the conditions under which cells might undergo the five processes by which they adapt to changing conditions.
8. Compare and contrast cell injury, cell death/necrosis, and apoptosis.
9. Explain three ways in which an aging cell becomes increasingly vulnerable to injury.

Organization of Cells

The **cell** is the basic structural and functional unit of the body. **Tissues** refer to groups of cells arranged to perform common functions. Sets of tissues, in turn, become grouped together forming **organs**, and groups of organs functioning together delineate **organ systems**. Finally, the various organ systems become integrated into a functioning organism. Communication between cells, tissues, and organs can potentially involve several processes. A cell may communicate with itself by recognizing the soluble mediator it produced (**autocrine** signaling), by direct contact between cells (**juxtacrine** signaling), by soluble mediators acting on nearby groups of cells (**paracrine** signaling), or via long-distance signaling where signal transport occurs throughout the circulation (**endocrine** signaling). Cell signal **receptors** can be found on the external or internal surface of the cell membrane or completely inside the cell, including the nuclear membrane. Interactions between cell-signaling

Cell The basic living structural and functional unit of the body.

Tissue A group of similar cells associated with each other to perform a specific function.

Organs A group of different tissues, which perform a specific function.

Organ systems A group of organs that function together as a unit, such as the various organs of the gastrointestinal tract.

Autocrine Cell signaling to itself by releasing products that act on signal receptors found associated with the cell.
Juxtacrine Cell-to-cell communication by direct contact or contact with the extracellular matrix.
Paracrine Cell-to-cell communication by soluble mediators released from a cell and acting on nearby groups of cells.
Endocrine Cell-to-cell communication by soluble mediators acting on cells that may be distant from the cell originating the signal.
Receptor Cell signal receiver.
Organelle A small structure with specific functions present inside the cell.

molecules (ligand) and receptors at any of these levels of organization contribute to maintaining homeostasis. Disruption of the communication pattern at any level of organization will cause disease.

The Cell

Although different functions of cells may be reflected in cell structure, all cells have certain features in common (**Figure 2-1**). Each cell consists of a nucleus surrounded by cytoplasm. The nucleus contains the genetic information stored in the cell, including many of the "switching mechanisms" that control the action of components of the genetic information. Gene expression directs many cellular functions that are carried out in the cytoplasm (see Chapter 3). Within the cytoplasm are numerous small structures, **organelles**, which play important roles in the functions of the cell.

The Nucleus

The nucleus contains two different types of nucleic acids combined with proteins. **Deoxyribonucleic acid (DNA)** is contained in the **chromosomes**, which are long and thin in the nondividing cell. Although the chromosomes cannot be identified as distinct structures in a nondividing cell, they form a complex structure including proteins termed **chromatin**. Unwound, the DNA in the nucleus would stretch to a length of about 2 meters, but it must be compacted to fit into the nucleus, which has a diameter of 6–10 micrometers. Most human nuclei are slightly smaller than a red blood cell. Packaging includes a **nucleosome** core consisting of nuclear proteins (**histones**) around which

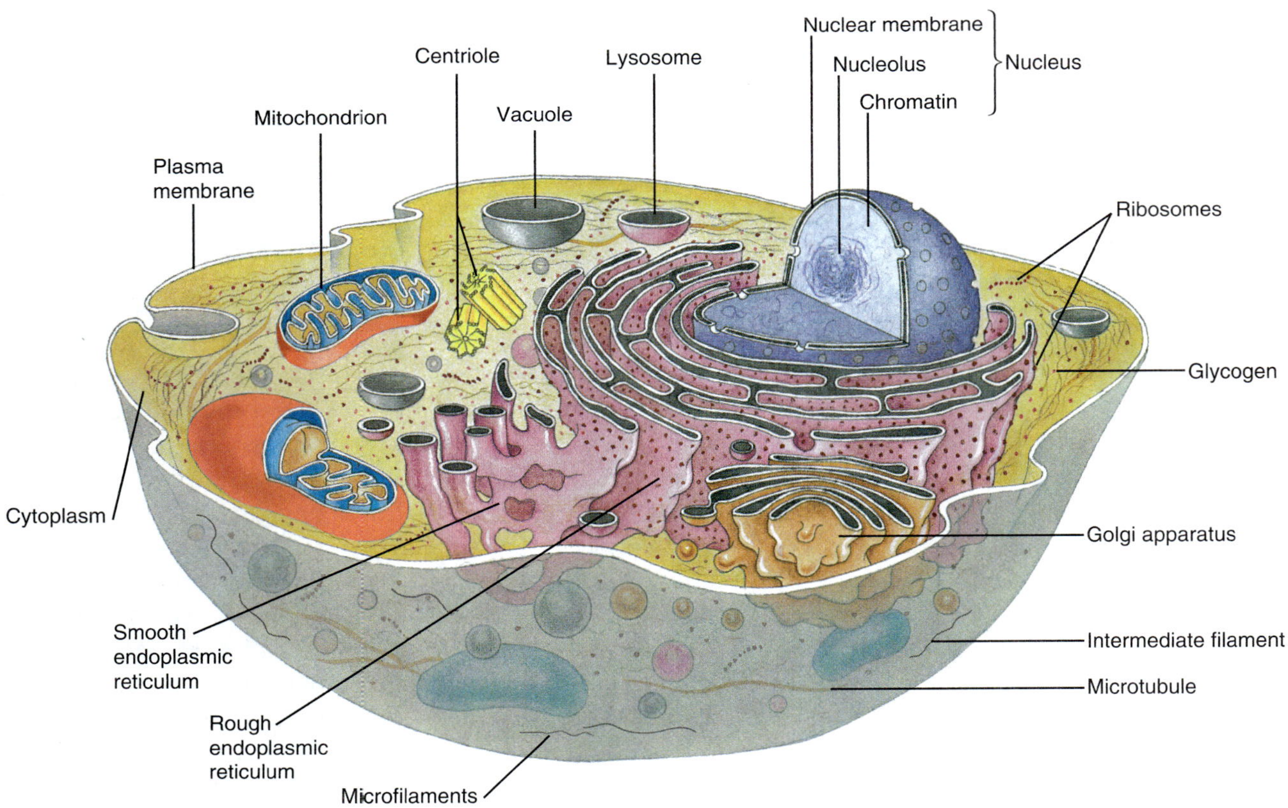

Figure 2-1 Structure of a typical eukaryotic/animal cell. Note that the cell is divided into two compartments, the nuclear and cytoplasmic. The cytoplasm contains a variety of structures, including organelles and other components.

a segment of DNA is wound. Chromatin fibers in the nucleus are formed from nucleosomes, which are connected in a continuous strand by extended stretches of DNA (often described as "beads on a string"). However, these beads on a string are further packed together and folded into loops. The geometry of DNA compaction is of great importance in determining which segments of the DNA will function (**Figure 2-2**). Further compaction of these loops forms the chromosomes, which are visible through the microscope in a dividing cell.

Deoxyribonucleic acid (DNA) The nucleic acid present in the chromosomes of the nuclei of cells that carries genetic information.

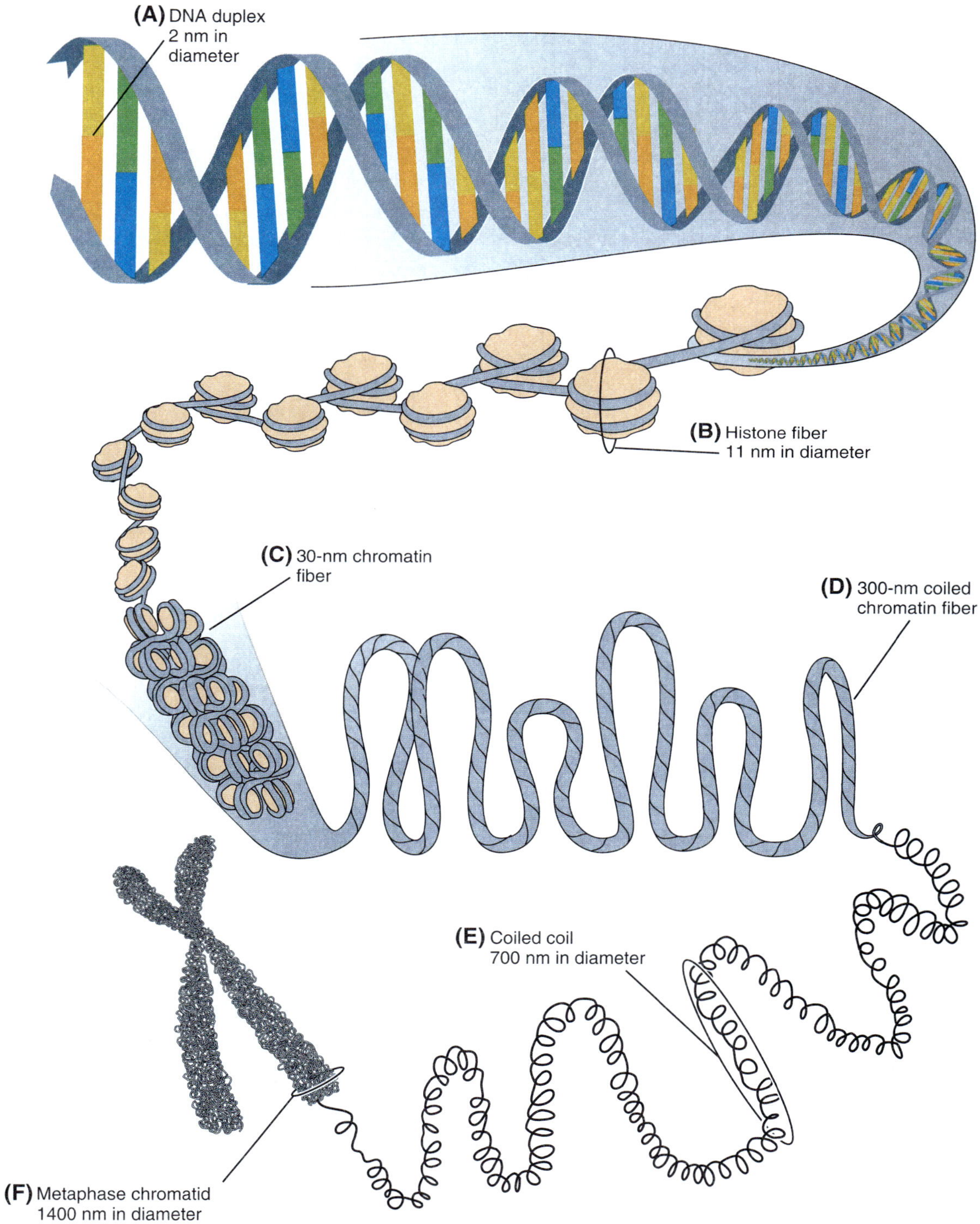

Figure 2-2 Structure of chromatin. DNA **(A)** is packaged into nucleosomes **(B)** and further folded **(C, D, E)** to form chromosomes visible in a dividing cell **(F)**.

Chromosome Cell structure organizing the molecules of DNA; individual structural units of DNA which are best seen in dividing cells.
Chromatin Tightly wound DNA in the nucleus; formed in part from nucleosomes.
Nucleosome A bead-like structure of DNA wrapped around histone and other nuclear proteins.
Histone A protein found in the nucleus, which is important in the packaging of DNA.
Ribonucleic acid (RNA) A type of nucleic acid contained in the nucleoli of cells. A component of messenger, transfer, and ribosomal RNA.
Nucleoli Structure containing RNA in the nucleus.
Mitochondria Bean-shaped structures in the cell capable of converting molecules into energy to power the cell.
Endoplasmic reticulum (ER) A mass of hollow tubular channels within the cytoplasm of the cell, frequently bordered by ribosomes. Depending on the type, ER may be associated with protein or lipid synthesis.
Golgi apparatus A group of membrane-lined sacs found in the cytoplasm of the cell near the nucleus; functions with the endoplasmic reticulum to synthesize and package secretory granules.

Ribonucleic acid (RNA) is contained in spherical intranuclear structures called **nucleoli** (singular, nucleolus). The nucleus is separated from the cytoplasm by a double-layered nuclear membrane. Small pores in the nuclear membrane permit the nucleus and cytoplasm to communicate.

The Cytoplasm

The gel-like cytoplasm contains many highly concentrated molecules, including nutrients critical for cellular function. A cell membrane envelops the cytoplasm and acts selectively to allow some materials to pass into and out of the cell while restricting the passage of others. Movement of materials across cells occurs in either a passive (requiring no energy) or active process (requiring energy) (see the section later in this chapter on movement of materials into and out of cells). The cytoplasm contains a variety of organelles, structures that have membranes, as well as particles such as ribosomes, and products that accumulate within the cell, such as glycogen and fat. The most important organelles are the **mitochondria**, **endoplasmic reticulum**, **Golgi apparatus**, **lysosomes**, **centrioles**, and the components of the **cytoskeleton**. Inappropriate or excessive accumulation of cell products or intermediate products of cellular metabolism may be an indicator of cellular dysfunction and disease. For example, excessive consumption of alcohol can lead to an abnormal intracellular accumulation of lipids, resulting in a "fatty liver," better termed alcoholic steatosis (see Case 2-1 and Chapter 19). The cytoplasm, nucleus, and organelles are surrounded by membranes composed of lipid and protein molecules, which separate these structures from one another (see Figure 2-1).

Major Cell Organelles and Their Functions

Table 2-1 lists the major cell organelles.

Mitochondria are membrane-bound, bean-shaped structures that contain enzymes capable of converting carbon-containing molecules into energy through oxidization. The mitochondria use this energy to manufacture the high-energy storage compound **adenosine triphosphate (ATP)**, the fuel that powers many chemical reactions in the cell.

The endoplasmic reticulum consists of an interconnected network of tubular channels enclosed by membranes. This network communicates with both the nuclear membrane and the cell membrane. The **rough endoplasmic reticulum (RER)** possesses numerous small nucleoprotein particles called **ribosomes** attached to the external surfaces of its membranes. The name derives from the knobby appearance that the attached ribosomes give the membranes. The RER function is to synthesize protein. Digestive enzymes and antibody proteins, for example, are produced in this way. The second type of endoplasmic reticulum lacks ribosomes and is called the **smooth endoplasmic reticulum (SER)**. Its membranes contain enzymes that synthesize lipids and some other substances.

The Golgi apparatus consists of groups of flattened membrane-like sacs located near the nucleus. These sacs are connected with the tubules of the RER. Some proteins produced by the ribosomes attached to the RER pass through the RER tubules into the Golgi apparatus. These large carbohydrate molecules are synthesized and combined with proteins, packaged into secretory granules, and eventually discharged from the cell.

Lysosomes made by the Golgi apparatus are filled with digestive enzymes that function as the "refuse removal system" of the cell. Lysosomes break

Table 2-1 Major Cell Organelles and Their Functions

Organelle	Function
Mitochondria	Generation of energy, usually in the form of adenosine triphosphate (ATP) used to power chemical reactions in the cell; also involved with detoxification and programmed cell death
Rough endoplasmic reticulum (RER)	Tubular channels that synthesize proteins when associated with ribosomes on their surface
Smooth endoplasmic reticulum (SER)	Tubular channels containing enzymes that synthesize lipids and some other compounds within the cells
Golgi apparatus	Flattened sacs located near nucleus that attach carbohydrate molecules to the proteins synthesized by RER
Lysosomes	Spherical organelles in cytoplasm containing digestive enzymes that break down worn-out cell organelles and material brought into the cell by phagocytosis. Often have a very low internal pH.
Centrioles	Short cylinders that form the mitotic spindle that separates chromosomes during cell division; also involved in the movement of cilia and flagella
Cytoskeleton	Protein tubules and filaments that form structural framework of cells and promote cell functions such as cell division, motility, and phagocytosis

down material brought into the cell by **phagocytosis**, and degrade worn-out intracellular components such as mitochondria and other organelles, consequently making the breakdown products available to be recycled or excreted from the cells. This process is called **autophagy**. When particulate material is ingested by phagocytosis, the particle becomes enclosed within a membrane-lined vacuole called a **phagocytic vacuole**. A lysosome then merges with the phagocytic vacuole and their cell membranes fuse, allowing the digestive enzymes contained in the lysosome to flow into the phagocytic vacuole and digest the engulfed material. Digestion occurs entirely within the phagocytic vacuole, which prevents digestive enzymes from leaking into the cytoplasm of the cell and causing injury to the cell (**Figure 2-3**). The same type of digestive process is involved when worn-out components are broken down within cells. In some diseases the lysosomal enzymes are unable to function properly, and incompletely digested material accumulates within lysosomes, disrupting cell functions.

Closely related to lysosomes are smaller structures called **peroxisomes**, which contain enzymes that break down potentially toxic intracellular molecules. The name of this organelle refers to hydrogen peroxide (H_2O_2), a toxic by-product of enzyme action. The hydrogen peroxide produced is used to oxidize the potentially toxic substances (such as ethanol) and is converted to water in the process. Excess hydrogen peroxide is promptly decomposed by enzymes in the peroxisome. Peroxisomes are also important in the synthesis of components of the **myelin** sheath of nerve cells.

Lysosome A cytoplasmic organelle containing digestive enzymes with an acidic pH internal environment.

Centrioles Short, cylindrical structures located adjacent to the nucleus that participate in the formation of spindle fibers during cell division.

Cytoskeleton Protein tubules and filaments that form the structural framework of cells.

Adenosine triphosphate (ATP) A high-energy phosphate-containing compound that liberates energy to power numerous cellular metabolic processes when one phosphate group is removed.

Rough endoplasmic reticulum (RER) Cell structure containing ribosomes and synthesizing protein.

Ribosome A small cytoplasmic particle that serves as the site of protein synthesis. Ribosomes are usually attached to the endoplasmic reticulum but may be free in the cytoplasm.

Smooth endoplasmic reticulum (SER) Cell structure containing enzymes and synthesizing lipids.

Phagocytosis by which the cell engulfs foreign material.

Autophagy Process by which internal cellular components are degraded and recycled by the cells.

Phagocytic vacuole Membrane-lined vacuole used to contain foreign material.

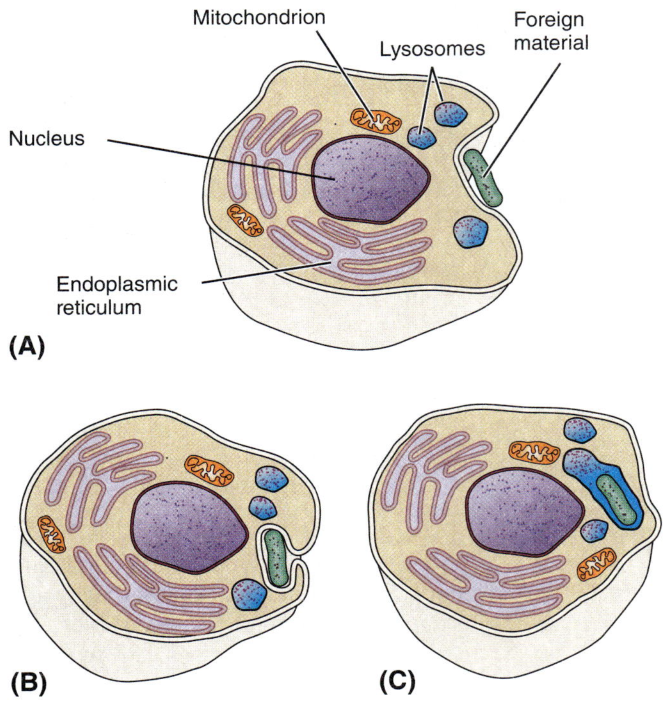

Figure 2-3 Digestion of engulfed material by lysosomes. **(A)** Extensions of cytoplasm from phagocytic cell begin to surround particulate material. **(B)** Cytoplasmic extensions engulf material and form the phagocytic vacuole containing the engulfed material. **(C)** Lysosome and phagocytic vacuole merge, and enzymes from the lysosome digest the engulfed material.

Peroxisome A cytoplasmic organelle containing various enzymes, including those that decompose potentially toxic compounds through the production of hydrogen peroxide.

Myelin Lipid based molecule secreted by some glial cells the wraps around the axon of a neuron. It provides protection and increases the rate of signal transmission.

Mitotic spindle Microtubule structure organized around the centriole during cell division.

Actin microfilament A cell framework filament made of globular proteins that polymerize, becoming filamentous actin. Actin is important in cell movement, cytoplasmic division, and muscle contraction.

Microtubule Largest type of cell framework filament.

Intermediate filaments Small, tough filaments of high tensile strength within the cell cytoplasm and nucleus.

Keratin filament Type of filament in epithelial cells.

Vimentin filament Type of filament in connective and muscle cells.

Neurofilament Type of filament in nerve cells.

Lamin filament A protein involved in nuclear structure in all cells.

Centrioles are short cylindrical structures mostly made of tubulin located adjacent to the nucleus. In cell division, they move to opposite poles of the cell and form the **mitotic spindle**. The spindle fibers attach to the chromosomes and pull them apart in the course of cell division. They also contribute to the movement of cilia and flagella.

The cytoplasm also contains three types of structural proteins that form the framework (cytoskeleton) of the cell. Actin filaments, or **actin microfilaments** (the smallest), are especially plentiful in contractile cells (such as muscle). **Microtubules** (the largest by diameter) become important during cell division and the sorting of genetic information into daughter cells. **Intermediate filaments** exhibit high tensile strength that reinforce the interior of the cell, hold the organelles in proper position within the cell, and along with the other cytoskeletal structures, contribute to the characteristic shape of each specific type of cell. Four classes of intermediate filaments exist. Three of the classes are cytoplasmic and can be identified in cells by specific histological techniques. Each of these classes is characteristic of a specific type of cell: **keratin filaments** in epithelial cells, **vimentin filaments** in connective and muscle cells, and **neurofilaments** in nerve cells. The fourth class, **lamin filaments**, is involved in nuclear structure and found in all cells.

Identification and characterization of intermediate filaments found in cells often provide both diagnostic and prognostic information. In some diseases, such as dilated cardiomyopathy, a serious disease of heart muscle (described in Chapter 9), the intermediate filaments exhibit characteristic abnormalities that help to explain the pathogenesis of the disease. Identification of the type of intermediate filaments in cells is also useful in the diagnosis of tumors (described in Chapter 6). In cases in which the originating cell of a tumor is difficult to identify, the cells are termed **anaplastic cells**. Identifying the specific type of intermediate filament in the tumor cells helps determine the type of cell from which the tumor arose. This may allow the pathologist to make a more precise diagnosis and aid the clinician in the selection of a suitable therapy.

Tissues

A tissue consists of a group of cells in close proximity performing specific functions. Tissue classification includes four major groups: epithelium, connective and supporting tissues, muscle tissue, and nerve tissue.

Epithelium

Epithelium consists of groups of cells closely joined together (**Figure 2-4**) that cover the exterior of the body and line interior body surfaces that communicate with the outside, e.g., the gastrointestinal tract, urinary tract, and vagina. Epithelium also forms glands such as the thyroid and pancreas. It also makes up the functional cells (often called **parenchymal cells** or **parenchyma**) of organs that have excretory or secretory functions, such as the liver and the kidneys. The individual cells may be flat and platelike (**squamous cells**), cube-shaped (**cuboidal cells**), or tall and narrow (**columnar cells**). Many columnar epithelial cells become specialized to absorb or secrete, and some contain fine projecting processes, **cilia**. Epithelial cells may be arranged in a single layer (simple epithelium) or may be several layers thick (stratified epithelium).

Anaplastic cell Type of tumor cell whose structure is so deranged as to make identification of origin difficult.

Parenchymal cell The functional cell of an organ or tissue.

Parenchyma The functional cells of an organ, as contrasted with the connective and supporting tissue that forms its framework.

Squamous cells Flat, platelike cells.

Cuboidal cells Cube-shaped cells.

Columnar cells Tall, narrow cells.

Cilia Specialized cytoplasmic processes on cells.

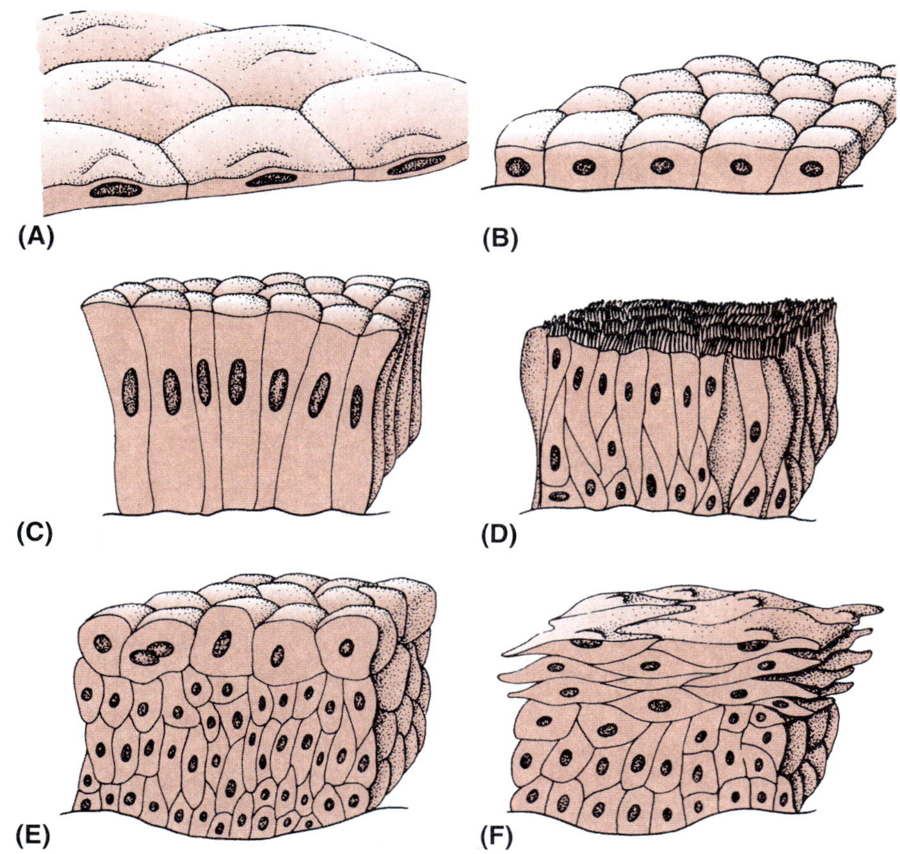

Figure 2-4 Common types of epithelia: **(A)** simple squamous, **(B)** cuboidal, **(C)** columnar, **(D)** pseudostratified columnar (ciliated), **(E)** transitional, and **(F)** stratified squamous.

Endothelium The internal lining of blood vessels and interior of the heart.

Mesothelium A layer of flat, squamous epithelial cells that covers the surfaces of the pleural, pericardial, and peritoneal cavities.

Mesoderm The middle germ layer of the embryo, which gives rise to specific organs and tissues.

Keratinization Accumulation of a fibrous protein called keratin inside cells.

Keratin An insoluble sulfur-containing protein that is the principal constituent of the hair and nails.

The interiors of the heart, blood vessels, and lymphatic vessels are lined by a layer of tissue that looks like simple squamous epithelium, **endothelium**. Endothelial tissue arises from a different embryonic germ layer than epithelial tissue, hence the different name. A similar-appearing type of epithelium lining the pleural, pericardial, and peritoneal cavities is called **mesothelium**. Although these linings are classified as types of epithelium, they arise from the middle embryonic germ layer called the **mesoderm** and are therefore much more closely related to connective tissue than to other types of epithelium. Consequently, they are considered separately and are given distinct names. Tumors arising from endothelium or mesothelium have unique patterns of behavior and are considered apart from those arising from surface, glandular, or parenchymal epithelium. This subject is considered in Chapter 6.

The Structure of Epithelium

Epithelial cells are supported by a thin basement membrane. The cells are joined to each other, and the deeper layers of epithelium are firmly anchored to molecules in the basement membrane so that the epithelial cells remain relatively fixed in position. There are no blood vessels in epithelium. Movement of materials in and out of the tissue occurs through diffusion going toward or away from the capillaries located in the underlying connective tissue. Epithelial cells may either line or cover organs or serve as secretory cells (glandular cells), depending on their primary function. Epithelium is characterized by both the shape and number of layers of cells of which it is composed.

Simple Epithelium

Simple epithelium consists of a single layer of cells. The distribution of simple squamous epithelium, composed of flat, platelike cells is limited. It forms the lining of the pulmonary air sacs, the endothelial lining of the vascular system, and the mesothelial lining of the body cavities. Simple columnar epithelium lines most of the gastrointestinal tract. Pseudostratified columnar epithelium is a type of simple columnar epithelium in which the cells are so tightly packed together that their nuclei appear to lie at different levels. This gives an appearance of stratification. Pseudostratified epithelium can often be ciliated. This type of epithelium lines most of the respiratory tract and is present in a few other areas.

Stratified Epithelium

Stratified epithelium contains multiple layers and often serves a protective function. Stratified squamous epithelium forms the external covering of the body and also lines the oral cavity, esophagus, and vagina. Stratified epithelium is named for the appearance of the most superficial cell layer. Consequently, this epithelium is designated "stratified squamous" based on the flat platelike appearance of the most superficial (exterior) layers of cells even though the deeper layers are composed of cuboidal cells (**Figure 2-5A**). The stratified squamous epithelium that forms the top layer of the skin undergoes a process called **keratinization**, in which the top layers of squamous cells accumulate a fibrous protein, **keratin**, lose their cellular structure, and eventually are shed. This fibrous protein forms a dense layer that protects the underlying cells. The deeper layers adjacent to the basement membrane consist of dividing cells that replenish the epithelial cells shed from the surface as they move upward.

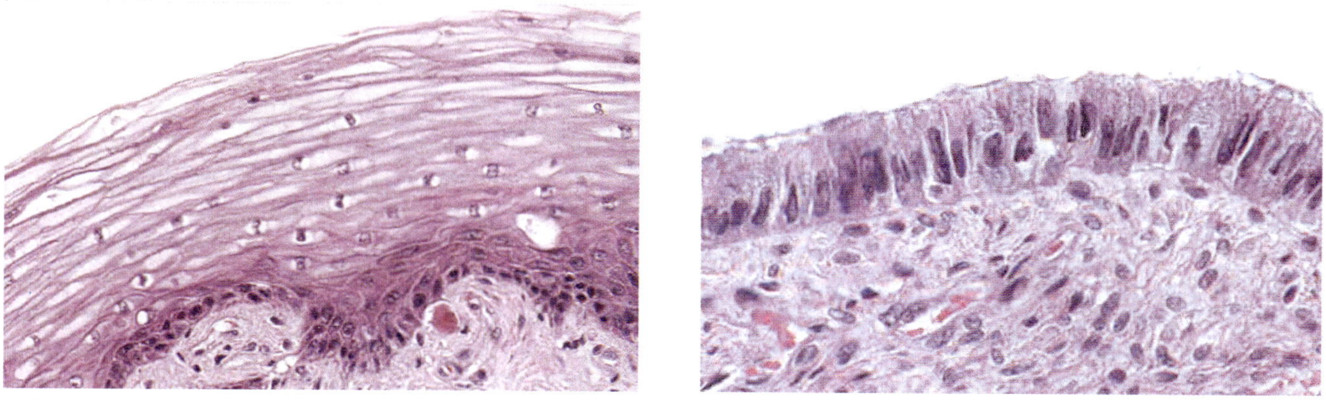

(A) (B)

Figure 2-5 Two types of epithelial cells from the cervix. **(A)** Nonkeratinized stratified squamous epithelium from the exocervix serves a protective function. **(B)** Columnar epithelium from the endocervix secretes mucus.

Courtesy of Howard M. Reisner.

Glandular epithelium is more complex. It consists of acinar cells, which serve a secretory function, and ductal cells, which transport the secreted product. Glands may be simple or compound, depending on the number of secretory units within the gland.

Transitional epithelium consists of a layer of large superficial cells covering a deeper layer of cuboidal cells. It serves as the characteristic lining of the bladder and other parts of the urinary tract. The superficial cells of transitional epithelium become flattened when the bladder is distended and resume their original shape when the bladder is empty.

Functions of Epithelium

Epithelium performs many different functions. All types of epithelium perform a protective function. Columnar epithelium, such as that lining the intestinal tract, is specialized to absorb and secrete. Other types of epithelium form glands that secrete mucus, sweat, lipid, enzymes, hormones, or other products (**Figure 2-5B**). Glands, such as the pancreas, that discharge their secretions through a duct onto an epithelial surface are designated as **exocrine glands**. **Endocrine glands**, such as the thyroid and adrenals, discharge their secretions directly into the bloodstream.

Connective and Supporting Tissues

Connective and supporting tissues consist of relatively small numbers of cells incorporated in a large amount of extracellular material generally referred to as the **extracellular matrix (ECM)**. The proportions of cells, fibers, and matrix vary greatly in different types of connective tissue. Connective tissue fibers consist of three types, each named for the predominant protein. **Collagen fibers** are long, flexible fibers. They are strong but do not stretch. **Elastic fibers** are not as strong as **collagen** but owing to the protein **elastin** in them, they stretch readily and return to their former shape when the stretching force is released. **Reticular fibers** are very similar to collagen but are quite thin and delicate and help support organs with a high density of cells. The material in which the fibers are embedded (often termed **ground substance**) contains a large amount of water bound to complex, long, and unbranched polysaccharides termed **glycosaminoglycans (GAGs)**. Some GAGs are bound to proteins to form extremely large molecules called **proteoglycans** or **mucoproteins**.

Exocrine gland A gland that discharges its secretions through a duct onto a mucosal surface.

Endocrine gland A gland that discharges its secretions directly into the bloodstream.

Extracellular matrix (ECM) Area where connective tissue cells and fibers are embedded.

Collagen fibers Fibers that are strong but do not stretch.

Elastic fibers Fibers found in the extracellular matrix.

Collagen Main constituent of fibrous proteins in the human body.

Elastin Protein made by several cell types that is capable of stretching.

Reticular fibers Very thin fibers made of collagen found in the bone marrow.

Ground substance Gel-like substance in the ECM in which fibers and cells are embedded.

Glycosaminoglycans (GAGs) Long, unbranched polysaccharides contributing to the ground substance.

Proteoglycans/mucoproteins Extremely large molecules in connective tissue.

The specific array of GAGs and connective tissue fibers defines the specific properties of the connective tissue.

Connective and supporting tissues include various types of loose and dense fibrous tissue, elastic tissue, **reticular tissue**, **adipose tissue**, **cartilage**, and bone. **Hematopoietic tissue** (blood-forming tissue) and **lymphatic tissue** (lymphoid system tissue) also are classified as types of connective tissue. Like other types of connective tissue, they originate from the mesoderm, although they are often considered separately by pathologists who specialize in their study (hematopathologists).

Fibrous connective tissue performs a variety of functions connecting and supporting many parts of the body. Loose fibrous tissue, one of the most widely distributed, forms the tissue just beneath the skin (subcutaneous tissue, dermis) and also fills in around organs. Dense fibrous tissue forms ligaments and tendons, which reinforce joints and attach muscles to bone.

Elastic tissue forms membranes that are wrapped around the walls of blood vessels and are responsible for the characteristic distensibility of large arteries. Elastic membranes also form parts of the walls of the trachea and bronchi.

Reticular tissue is a special type of connective tissue characterized by a fine meshwork of reticulin fibers that form the supporting framework of various organs, such as the liver, spleen, and lymph nodes.

Adipose tissue is a variety of loose fibrous tissue containing large numbers of fat cells. Fat is a stored form of energy and also functions as padding and insulation.

Cartilage is a type of supporting tissue in which the cells are dispersed in a dense matrix. Of the three types of cartilage, **hyaline cartilage** is the most common. It appears blue and translucent and contains only a few fine collagen fibers suspended in the abundant matrix. Hyaline cartilage covers the ends of bones where they form movable joints, form the greater part of the laryngeal and tracheal cartilages, and connect the ribs to the sternum. **Elastic cartilage** contains yellow elastic fibers in the matrix and is found in only a few locations, such as the cartilaginous portions of the ears. The elastic fibers impart a flexibility to the cartilage that is lacking in other types of cartilage. **Fibrocartilage** contains many dense collagen bundles embedded in the matrix. It is found in areas where cartilage is subjected to marked weight-bearing stresses. It forms the disks between the vertebral bodies and some of the cartilages in the knee joints; it is also present in a few other locations.

Bone is a highly specialized, rigid supporting tissue in which the matrix containing the bone-forming cells is impregnated with calcium salts (see Chapter 24 for an in-depth discussion).

Muscle Tissue

Muscle cells contain filaments of specialized intracellular contractile proteins, **actin** and **myosin**, arranged in parallel bundles. During contraction of a muscle fiber, actin filaments slide inward on the myosin filaments, somewhat like pistons, causing the fiber to shorten. There are three types of muscle fibers. **Smooth muscle** is located primarily in the walls of hollow internal organs, such as the gastrointestinal tract, biliary tract, and reproductive tract; in the walls of the blood vessels, where the muscle regulates the diameter of the vessels to control blood flow to the tissues; and in the skin, where it controls the elevation of the hairs. Smooth muscle contracts automatically and is not under conscious control. **Striated muscle** moves the skeleton (and body parts, such as eyelids and eyeballs) and is under voluntary control. **Cardiac muscle** is found only in

Reticular tissue A special type of connective tissue characterized by fine reticulin fibers.

Adipose tissue Loose, fibrous tissue containing fat cells.

Cartilage A type of flexible connecting tissue in which cells are dispersed in a dense matrix.

Hematopoietic tissue Tissue that forms the blood cells.

Lymphatic tissue Tissue that forms the lymphatic system.

Hyaline cartilage Most common type of cartilage; contains only a few fine collagen fibers.

Elastic cartilage Contains elastic fibers.

Fibrocartilage Contains many dense collagen bundles.

Actin Contractile protein, also referred to as a motor protein that enables muscle fibers to shorten and create contraction. Actin also contributes to non-muscle cell movement.

Myosin Contractile and motor protein that uses ATP to drive muscle cell contraction and relaxation cycles.

Smooth muscle Muscle that functions automatically.

Striated muscle Muscle that moves body parts under voluntary control.

Cardiac muscle Muscle found only in the heart; has features of both striated and smooth muscle.

the heart. It resembles striated muscle but has some features common to both smooth and voluntary muscle.

Nerve Tissue

Nerve tissue is composed of nerve cells, **neurons**, which transmit nerve impulses, and supporting cells termed **glial cells/neuroglia**. Neuroglial cells are more numerous than neurons. Of the three types of glial cells, astrocytes are long, star-shaped cells having numerous highly branched processes that interlace to form a meshwork. **Astrocytes** form the structural framework of the central nervous system in the way that the connective tissue fibers form the framework of internal organs. **Oligodendrocytes**, also known as **oligodendroglia** (in the central nervous system, the brand, and spinal cord) and **Schwann cells** (in the peripheral nervous system) produce the myelin covering found on the axons of myelinated neruorns. To do this, the cell wraps around the axon many times producing multiple layers of myelin. The myelin covering protects the nerve process and increases the rate of signal transduction. **Microglia** are phagocytic cells comparable to the macrophages found in other tissues.

Organs and Organ Systems

An organ is a collection of different tissues that is integrated to perform specific function(s). Generally, one tissue performs the primary function characteristic of the organ, and the other tissues perform supporting functions, such as providing the vascular and connective tissue framework for the organ. The functional cells of an organ are often called parenchymal cells, and the total mass of functional tissue is called the parenchyma. The supporting framework of the organ is the **stroma**. In the liver, for example, the parenchymal cells are formed by cords of epithelial cells that perform the many metabolic functions characteristic of the liver, such as the synthesis of protein and the excretion of bile. The cord cells are supported by a framework of connective tissue fibers. Numerous thin-walled blood vessels are interspersed between the cell cords, and the entire liver is surrounded by a capsule composed of dense fibrous tissue.

An organ system is a group of organs that performs complementary functions, such as the reproductive system, the respiratory system, and the digestive system. Finally, the various organ systems are integrated into a functioning individual.

The Germ Layers and Their Derivatives

The highly complex structure of the entire body evolves from a single cell, the fertilized ovum, also known as the zygote, by complex processes that include periods of cell multiplication, differentiation, and organization to form organs and organ systems. As the single-celled zygote undergoes repeated rounds of cell division, the cells differentiate into two groups. The peripheral group of cells is called the **trophoblast**. The trophoblast, along with maternally derived tissue, forms the placenta and other structures that will support and nourish the embryo. The inner group of cells, the **inner cell mass**, gives rise to the embryo, arranging themselves into three distinct layers called the **germ layers**. Each layer will form certain specialized tissues and organs (**Table 2-2**). The outer layer, the **ectoderm**, forms the external covering of the body and

Neuron A nerve cell, including the cell body and its processes.

Glial cells/neuroglia Supporting cells of tissue of the nervous system.

Astrocyte Participate in numerous physiological processes, such as regulation of axonal growth support, blood–brain barrier formation, and immune responses, as well as participating in higher cognitive functions, including memory.

Oligodendroglia/Oligodendrocyte/Schwann cells Types of neurogila that wrap around nerve axons within the central and peripheral nervous sytems. They provide the myelin sheath that protect the axon and speeds up nerve transmission.

Microglia Macrophage-like cells that regulate brain development, maintenance of neuronal networks, and injury repair.

Stroma The tissue that forms the framework of an organ.

Trophoblast Cell derived from the fertilized ovum that gives rise to the fetal membranes and contributes to the formation of the placenta.

Inner cell mass A group of cells derived from the fertilized ovum that are destined to form the embryo.

Germ layers The three layers of cells derived from the inner cell mass; each layer is destined to form specific organs and tissues in the embryo.

Ectoderm The outer germ layer in the embryo that gives rise to specific organs and tissues.

Table 2-2 Derivatives of the Germ Layers

Ectoderm	Mesoderm	Endoderm
Epidermis	Dermis	Lining of the digestive system
Hair, nails, sweat glands	All muscles of the body	Lining of the respiratory system
Brain and spinal cord	Cartilage	Urethra and urinary bladder
Cranial and spinal nerves	Bone	Gallbladder
Retina, lens, and cornea of eye	Blood	Liver and pancreas
Inner ear	All other connective tissue	Thyroid gland
Epithelium of nose, mouth, and anus	Blood vessels	Parathyroid gland
Enamel of teeth	Reproductive organs Kidneys	Thymus

the various organs that bring the individual into contact with the external environment: the nervous system, eyes, and ears. The inner layer, called the **endoderm**, forms the internal "lining": the epithelium of the pharynx, the respiratory tract, the gastrointestinal tract, and the organs closely associated with it (the liver, biliary tract, and pancreas), and some parts of the urogenital tract. The mesoderm layer of cells is sandwiched between the other two layers. These cells will differentiate into the various supporting tissues (connective tissues, cartilage, and bone), muscle, the circulatory system (heart, blood, and blood vessels), and major portions of the urogenital system. Each normal cell in the body is part of a community of cells and is integrated with its neighbors so that it functions along with other cells to meet the body's needs.

Endoderm The inner germ layer of the embryo that gives rise to specific organs and tissues.
Pinocytosis Process similar to phagocytosis but for the ingestion of extracellular fluid.
Diffusion The passive movement of solutes in solution from an area of higher concentration to an area of lower concentration.
Osmosis The movement of water molecules from a dilute solution to a more concentrated one.

Movement of Materials Into and Out of Cells

For any cell to function properly, oxygen and nutrients must enter the cell, and waste products must be eliminated. The proper balance of charged ions (such as Na^+, K^+, and Ca^{2+}) must be maintained between the outside and inside of the cell as well as the water balance. Materials entering and leaving the cell must cross the cell membrane, which limits the passage of some molecules and is freely permeable to others. Materials cross the cell membrane in three ways: diffusion and osmosis (the movement of water only), active transport, and non-specific methods of ingestion phagocytosis and **pinocytosis** (a process analogous to phagocytosis but in which only fluid is engulfed).

Diffusion and Osmosis

Diffusion involves the movement of dissolved particles or molecules, also known as solute, from a more concentrated environment to a more dilute one. **Osmosis** is the movement of water molecules from a dilute solution to a more concentrated solution (**Figure 2-6**). Both are passive processes that do not require the cell to expend energy. If the membrane is freely permeable to both

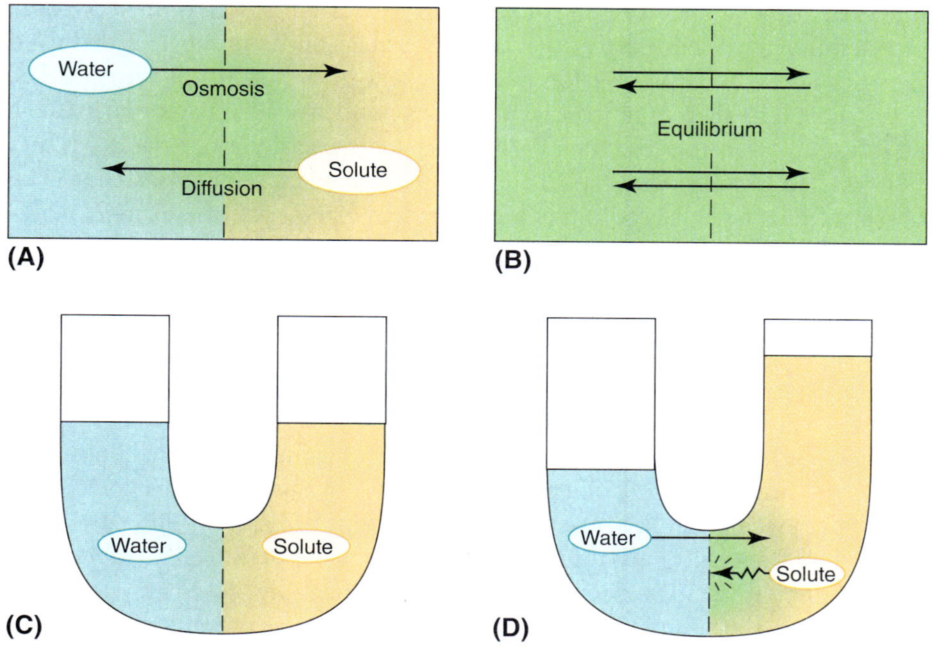

Figure 2-6 **(A)** Processes of osmosis and diffusion across a semi-permeable membrane (*dashed line*). **(B)** At equilibrium, the concentrations of water and solute molecules are equal on both sides of membrane. **(C)** The left compartment of the U tube contains water; the right compartment contains solute impermeable to the membrane. **(D)** Water molecules diffuse freely across the membrane, but solute molecules are unable to diffuse. The volume of solute is increased by diffusion of water molecules into the solute. The volume of water in the left limb of the U tube falls as water moves into the solute in the right limb of the U tube.

water and solute particles (Figures 2-6A and 2-6B), the solute particles diffuse from the higher solute concentration on the right side of the membrane into the lower solute concentration on the left side. At the same time, water molecules diffuse in the opposite direction, from the more dilute solution on the right side of the membrane into the more concentrated solution on the left side. At equilibrium, the concentrations of solute particles and water molecules are the same on both sides of the membrane if it is permeable to water and the relevant solutes. Solute and water molecules continue to move in both directions across the membrane after equilibrium is attained, but the net movement is equal in both directions, which does not change the equilibrium volume and concentration of the solutions on the two sides of the membrane.

The situation is quite different if the membrane is not permeable to the solute particles in the solution on one side of the membrane (Figures 2-6C and 2-6D). Water molecules move by osmosis from the left side of the membrane into the more concentrated solution on the right side (containing fewer water molecules). Because diffusion of solute is restricted by the membrane but movement of water molecules across the membrane is not, the volume of the solution on the right side of the membrane increases, and its solute concentration falls as the water molecules move by osmosis across the membrane.

Osmotic Pressure, Osmolarity, and Tonicity

The "water-attracting" property of a solution, which can be measured, is called its **osmotic activity/osmotic pressure**, and is related to the concentration of dissolved particles in the solution. The more concentrated the solution, the

Osmotic activity/osmotic pressure "Water attracting" property of a solution.

higher its osmotic pressure. The quantitative expression of the osmotic pressure of a solution is called osmolarity. Osmolarity reflects the number of dissolved particles in the solution, not the molecular weight or valence of the particles. For a substance such as glucose, which does not dissociate in solution, 1 mole dissolved in water to a volume of 1 liter has an osmolarity of 1 osmole per liter (abbreviated Osm/L). However, 1 mole of a substance that dissociates into two univalent ions (such as sodium chloride) has an osmolarity of 2 Osm/L. Movement of water and solute between the extracellular fluid (interstitial fluid and fluid components of blood and lymph) and the intracellular fluid (fluid within the cells) is regulated by the cell membrane, which is permeable to water and some solutes but relatively impermeable to others. The osmolarity of extracellular fluids varies from about 280 to 295 mOsm/L (1 Osm = 1000 mOsm) and the intracellular osmolarity is the same, as the two fluid compartments are in equilibrium. Most of the solutes in the extracellular fluid that contribute to its osmolarity are sodium (Na^+), chloride (Cl^-), and bicarbonate (HCO_3^-) ions. In contrast, the major intracellular ions are potassium (K^+) and phosphate (PO_4^{3-}). The sodium–potassium ion differences on the two sides of the cell membrane are controlled by the cell. A special term for osmotic pressure, **oncotic pressure**, is used when the solute is a very large molecule, such as the proteins found in the blood and other extracellular fluids. Such large proteins do not diffuse across cell membranes or exit from normal blood vessels. Blood proteins, particularly albumin, maintain the fluid content of the blood. If the level of blood protein drops, the fluid normally retained in blood vessels diffuses into tissue, resulting in **ascites**, the swelling of the abdominal area, and **edema**, swelling in other parts of the body.

The term **tonicity** is not quite the same as **osmolarity** because it is determined only by those solutes that cannot cross the membrane (most often the membrane of a cell). An **isotonic solution** is osmotically equivalent both inside and outside the cell. Clinically an isotonic solution equivalent to the tonicity of the patient's own body fluids can safely be administered intravenously to patients without causing changes in the volume of cells or fluid in the interstitium of tissue, the extracellular fluid (ECF). Generally, only isotonic solutions are used for intravenous administration. A **hypertonic solution** is more concentrated. Cells exposed to a hypertonic solution **crenate** (shrink) because water moves by osmosis from the cells into the hypertonic fluid. In contrast, a **hypotonic solution** is a diluted solution, and cells exposed to a hypotonic solution swell as water moves by osmosis from the hypotonic fluid into the cells where the osmolarity is higher. If a hypotonic solution is administered intravenously, the flow of water into cells, such as red cells, might be so great that the cell membranes become damaged, causing hemoglobin to leak from the cells, a process termed **hemolysis**.

Normally, the osmotic pressures within the cell and in the ECF are kept equal; therefore, the shape and water content of the cells do not change. This cannot be accomplished by diffusion alone. For example, in the tubules of the kidney where urine is processed, the concentration of solute (particularly sodium ions, Na^+) is much higher than that within the epithelial cells that line the tubules of the kidney. Diffusion constantly acts to increase the Na^+ concentration within the cells. This tendency is counteracted by an active transport process requiring energy (in the form of ATP) to pump the excess Na^+. If this pump fails (as happens in numerous disease states), Na^+ accumulates within the cells and water diffuses into the epithelial cells from the ECF (urine) in the tubule. If unchecked, the epithelial cells swell and ultimately die (a special type of cell death termed **oncosis**) resulting in kidney failure.

Oncotic pressure Osmotic pressure exerted by a very large molecule such as blood proteins.

Ascites A type of pneumoconiosis caused by inhalation of asbestos fibers.

Edema Accumulation of excess fluid in the interstitial tissues.

Tonicity Measure of ionic concentration determined only by solutes that cannot cross the membrane.

Osmolarity A measure of the osmotic pressure exerted by a solution.

Isotonic solution A solution having essentially the same osmolarity as body fluids so that cells neither shrink nor swell when exposed to the solution.

Hypertonic solution A solution having a greater osmolarity than body fluids, which causes cells to shrink (crenate) in such a solution because water moves by osmosis from the cells into the hypertonic solution.

Crenate Descriptive term for cell shrinkage effected by a hypertonic solution. More generally, to form a scalloped or toothed edge.

Hypotonic solution A solution having a lower osmolarity than body fluids, causing cells in the solution to swell because water moves by osmosis from the hypotonic solution into the cells.

Hemolysis Destruction of blood cells.

Oncosis Cell death due to swelling of epithelial cells caused by failure of pumping out Na^+ ions. A type of necrosis.

Active Transport

Active transport is the transfer of a substance across the cell membrane from a region of low concentration to one of higher concentration, counter to diffusion. The process requires the cell to expend energy because the substance must move against a concentration gradient. Many metabolic processes depend on active transport of ions and/or molecules. Active transport of ions is critical to many body processes, including nerve and muscle function.

Active transport Transfer of materials against a concentration gradient that is necessary to maintain proper concentration of intracellular and extracellular ions.

Atrophy Wasting of tissue due to underuse, typically due to the degeneration of cells.

Hypertrophy An enlargement or overgrowth of an organ caused by an increase in the size of its constituent cells.

Hyperplasia An increase in the number of cells.

Metaplasia Conversion of one differentiated tissue type to another.

Dysplasia Localized areas of dysregulated growth.

Physiological adaptive change Cell or organ response to changing conditions.

Adaptations of Cells to Changing Conditions

Cells respond to changing conditions in various ways, including alterations in number, size, type, and synthetic function. Common adaptive mechanisms are **atrophy**, **hypertrophy** and **hyperplasia**, **metaplasia**, **dysplasia**, and changes in enzyme synthesis.

In many instances, the adaptation enables the cells to function more efficiently. Skin cells increase in number (hyperplasia) to form a protective callus when subject to increased friction or wear. This is an example of **physiological adaptive change**. Sometimes, however, the adaptive change may be detrimental to the cell, a pathologic adaptation. The hyperplasia of skin cells in a wart is the result of inappropriate (maladaptive) hyperplasia, which is the result of a viral infection. Atrophy, hyperplasia, hypertrophy, and metaplasia may be adaptive or maladaptive. Dysplasia is always maladaptive.

Atrophy

Atrophy is a reduction in the size and number of cells (leading to changes in organ size). Atrophy occurs in response to diminished function, inadequate hormonal or neuronal stimulation, or reduced blood supply. For example, skeletal muscles are reduced in size when an extremity is immobilized in a cast for long periods or if innervation is damaged. The breasts and genital organs shrink after menopause due to inadequate estrogen stimulation. A kidney becomes smaller if its blood supply becomes insufficient. Sometimes atrophy is part of a normal physiological process; for example, the reduction in size of the uterus after childbirth and the breasts when lactation ceases.

Hypertrophy and Hyperplasia

If cells are required to do more work, they may increase either their size or their number. Hypertrophy is an increase in the size of individual cells without an actual increase in their numbers. The large muscles of a weightlifter, for example, result from hypertrophy of individual muscle fibers with little if any change in muscle cell number. The number of fibers is not increased, but the size of individual muscle cells increases. Similarly, the heart of a person with high blood pressure often enlarges as a result of hypertrophy of the individual cardiac muscle fibers. This occurs because the heart must work harder to pump blood at a higher than normal pressure (**Figure 2-7**).

Hyperplasia is an increase in the size of a tissue or organ caused by an increase in the number of cells. Hyperplasia occurs in response to increased demand. For example, the glandular tissue of the breast becomes hyperplastic

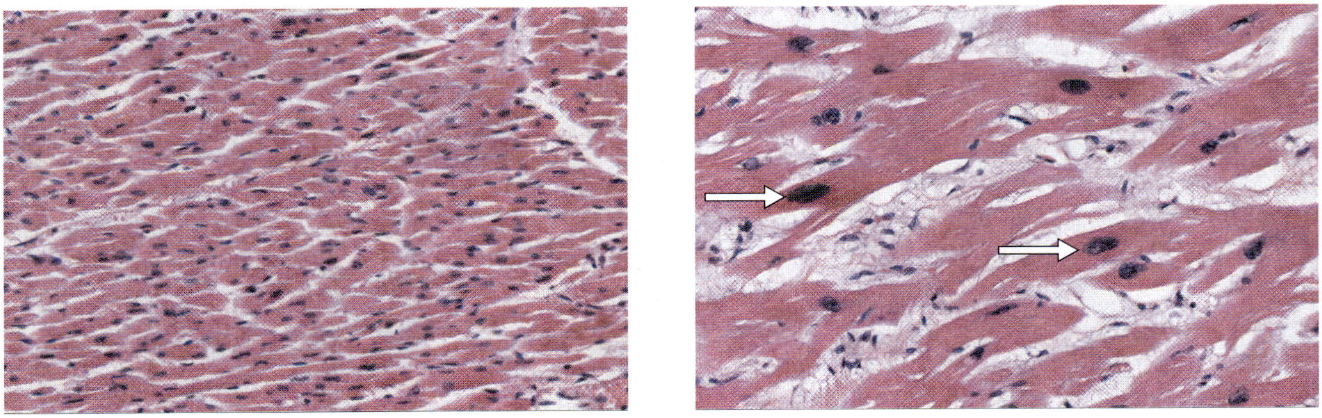

(A) (B)

Figure 2-7 **(A)** Normal cardiac muscle. **(B)** Hypertrophic cardiac muscle from an individual with high blood pressure (both images are at the same magnification). Note the greatly increased fiber size and very large nuclei (*arrows*). Although hypertrophic cardiac muscle cells do not divide, the DNA in the nuclei does, resulting in increased size.

during pregnancy in preparation for lactation. Endocrine glands such as the thyroid may enlarge in response to increased hormone demand. Hyperplasia in response to changing hormone balance may also be pathologic. An increase in the number of glandular and smooth muscle cells in the prostate results in benign prostatic hypertrophy, which often leads to difficulty in urination in elderly men.

Metaplasia

Metaplasia is a change from one type of cell to another type and may be an adaptation to adverse environmental conditions. For example, if the lining of the trachea is chronically irritated by the chemical agents in cigarette smoke, the normal ciliated columnar epithelial lining will exhibit the characteristic structure of a layer of squamous epithelium. The metaplastic epithelium is presumed to be more resistant to irritation and is better able to protect the tracheal wall. However, the metaplastic area becomes the locus at which common forms of lung cancer begin (**Figure 2-8**). The same is true of metaplasia that may occur in the esophagus (in response to acid reflux) or on the

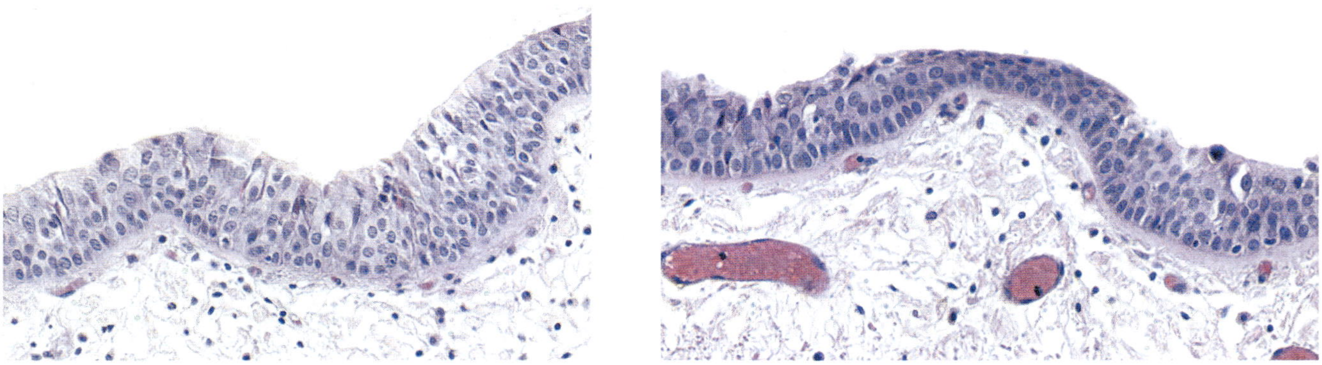

(A) (B)

Figure 2-8 **(A)** An area of normal pseudostratified ciliated columnar epithelium from the trachea of a smoker (cilia not visible at magnification). **(B)** An area demonstrating metaplasia from the same tissue sample. The tissue appears as squamous epithelium (*center*).

cervix (possibly as a protection from the acid environment of the vagina). In all cases, the metaplasia may initially be adaptive but has the potential to become the site of dysplasia.

Dysplasia

Dysplasia is a condition in which the development and maturation of cells become disturbed and abnormal. The individual cells vary in size and shape, and their relationship to one another is also abnormal. Nuclei differ from cell to cell and may show abnormal structure, termed **nuclear pleomorphism** (**Figure 2-9**). Dysplasia of epithelial cells may be associated with chronic irritation or inflammation. In some cases, dysplasia may progress to a lack of regulation of cell growth and possibly the formation of a tumor; this process is called **neoplasia**. The differentiation of dysplasia from neoplasia is often unclear. The metaplastic epithelium of the uterine cervix is a common site of dysplasia, and cervical epithelial dysplasia sometimes progresses to cervical cancer. This subject is discussed in Chapter 18.

Nuclear pleomorphism Irregular nuclear structures seen in groups of dysplastic cells.

Neoplasia A form of uncontrolled cell growth that may follow dysplasia and lead to formation of a tumor.

Changes in Enzyme Synthesis

Increased synthesis of enzymes is another adaptive change that occurs in cells. Sometimes cells' functioning involves inactivation or detoxification of drugs or chemicals using the enzymes present in the smooth endoplasmic reticulum (SER). If increased demands are placed on the cells, their response includes synthesizing more SER enzymes so that drugs or chemicals can be processed more efficiently. After the cells increase their ability to handle such chemicals or drugs, they can also rapidly eliminate other substances that are handled by the same enzyme systems. A person accustomed to heavy consumption of alcohol, for example, can metabolize the alcohol more efficiently because of this adaptive change. Such an individual may also metabolize and eliminate certain other drugs at a greatly accelerated rate. Consequently, if a clinician administers a medication that is metabolized by the same enzyme systems, the usual therapeutic doses of the medications may be less effective.

On the other hand, cells may also decrease or change the pattern of the proteins they synthesize when they encounter physiologic stress, e.g. if nutrients become scarce. This change in cellular metabolism shifts from promoting cell growth to favoring cell survival.

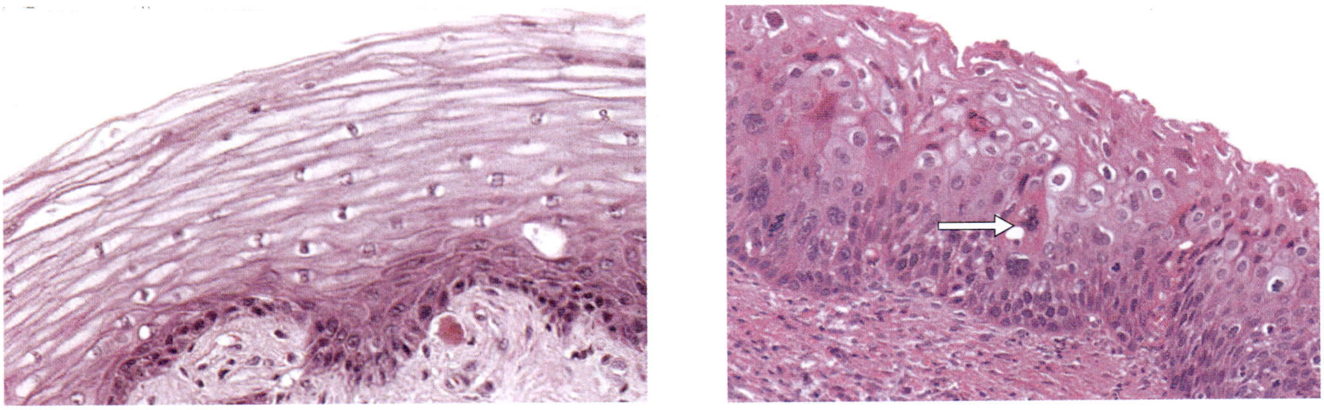

(A) **(B)**

Figure 2-9 **(A)** Comparison of normal, squamous epithelium from exocervix with **(B)** dysplastic cervical epithelium. Note the variation in nuclear size, shape, and polarity. An abnormally dividing cell is also shown.

Cell Injury, Cell Death, and Cell Necrosis

Cell Injury

Injury to a cell may be reversible when the injurious agent is removed and normal cell function is restored. For example, cell swelling and fatty change (steatosis) are common morphologic abnormalities demonstrated by injured cells. If the injury exceeds the ability of the cell to recover, the cell will die. It is not always easy to determine whether cellular injury is irreversible. The most certain sign is nuclear damage or loss, but other changes (including the nature of staining) may provide a hint.

Cell Swelling

A normally functioning cell actively transports potassium into the cell and moves sodium out. This process requires the cell to expend energy. If the cell is injured and unable to function normally, the transport mechanism begins to fail. Sodium diffuses into the cell, and water moves into the cell along with the sodium as predicted by the principles of osmosis and diffusion, causing the cell to swell. If the swelling continues, fluid-filled vacuoles may accumulate within the cell, a process sometimes called **hydropic swelling**. The process is potentially reversible if energy production recommences (**Figure 2-10**) and the cell can engage in active transport.

Hydropic swelling Cell swelling as a result of excessive water uptake by a cell. Associated with failure of active transport of ions.

Fatty Change

If the enzyme systems that metabolize or export fat are impaired, accumulation of fat droplets within the cytoplasm may occur, resulting in fatty change (steatosis). This condition is a common manifestation of liver cell injury because liver cells are actively involved in fat metabolism (see Case 2-1).

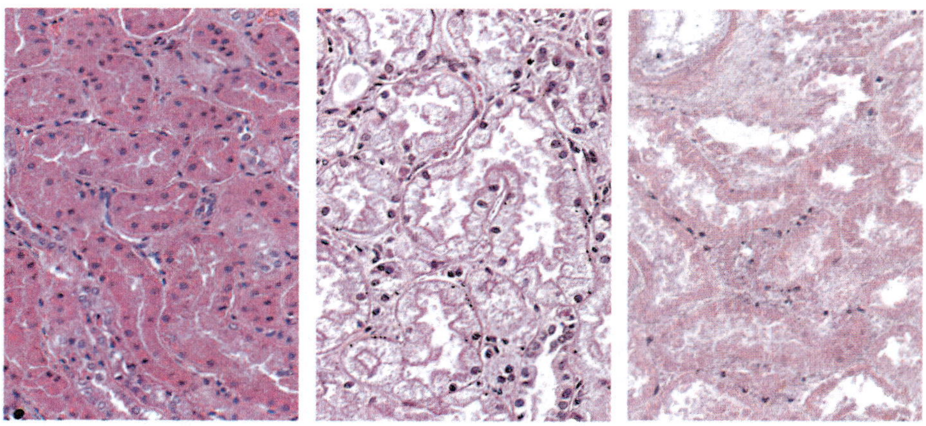

(A) (B) (C)

Figure 2-10 Comparison of **(A)** normal, **(B)** swollen (hydropic), and **(C)** necrotic renal tubular epithelial cells. The swollen cells retain normal-appearing nuclei, are intact, and remain attached to the underlying basement membrane. The necrotic cells have lost their nuclei and are no longer intact. They show blebbing (formation of small blister) of the cytoplasmic membrane and appear to be detaching from the basement membrane.

Courtesy of Department of Pathology and Laboratory Medicine, University of North Carolina at Chapel Hill.

Cell Death and Cell Necrosis

A cell dies when it has been irreparably damaged. This often occurs because of a failure in energy production by the cell. All cells ultimately depend on oxidative metabolism for energy production by the mitochondria. In the absence of an oxygen supply to the cell, such as occurs if blood circulation to the tissue is impaired (a process termed **ischemia**), the cells in the tissue will die (**infarction**). If cells in the tissue die due to other causes such as infection or toxicity, a process termed **necrosis** comes into play. For example, impairment of coronary (heart) blood circulation leads to a myocardial infarct, a "heart attack." Tissues differ in how long they can survive in the absence of an oxygen supply: the brain, minutes; connective tissue, far longer. But ultimately all cells will die without oxygen supplied by blood circulation. Lack of energy production also impairs the "ion pumps" necessary to prevent cellular swelling, resulting in a form of necrosis sometimes termed oncosis (Figure 2-10).

Ischemia Poor blood supply to cells of tissues that may lead to injury or death.

Infarction Cell and tissue death from impaired blood supply.

Necrosis Unprogrammed cell death as a result of injury and subsequent structural changes. Often results in a host response.

Apoptosis Programmed cell death that does not provoke a host protective response.

Minutes to hours after the cell dies, various structural changes begin to take place within the nucleus and cytoplasm. Mitochondria undergo a series of shape changes and may have calcium deposited within them. Lysosomal enzymes are released and begin to digest the cell, and the cell membrane may bleb or rupture. The nucleus shrinks and either dissolves or breaks into fragments. With time, visible calcium deposition may occur within the dead tissue. These structural changes are microscopically observable indicators of necrosis. All necrotic cells are dead, but a dead cell does not necessarily appear necrotic because the structural changes that characterize cell death as seen by the pathologist under the microscope take several hours to develop. With time, necrotic cells become easily recognizable on histologic examination because they appear quite different from normal cells in both their structural and their staining characteristics (**Figure 2-11**).

Programmed Cell Death: Apoptosis

Not all cell death results from cell injury. Cell death may result from a programmed, energy-requiring active process that is part of normal organism function. This form of programmed cellular self-destruction is termed **apoptosis**. Counterintuitively,

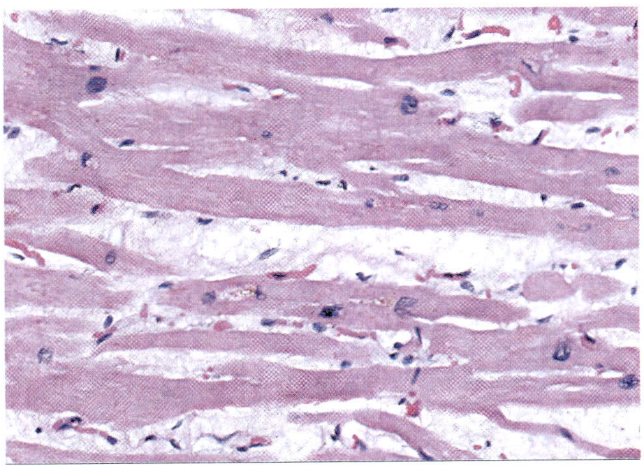

Figure 2-11 Cardiac muscle cells from a heart demonstrating chronic lack of oxygen (chronic ischemia). Many muscle fibers show either abnormal, fragmented, or absent nuclei. Compare with normal cardiac muscle cells in Figure 2-7A (same magnification).

Courtesy of Howard M. Reisner.

failure of cell death by apoptosis may result in disease because apoptosis is critical for normal development and function. During fetal development, certain body structures form and then disappear (such as webs between fingers and toes). Loss of this "unneeded tissue" is accomplished by apoptosis. The loss of uterine tissue during menstruation is accomplished by apoptosis resulting from changes in hormone balance. Death of virally infected cells may be a result of apoptosis induced in infected cells. Irremediable changes to DNA (mutations) result in the "turning on" of apoptosis within the mutated cell. If this fails, cancer may result. Certain lymphoid cells are programmed to die after a fixed number of divisions; if apoptosis fails, lymphoma (cancer of the lymphatic cells in lymph nodes) will result. Necrosis is unregulated, unwanted, and unexpected, and is recognized as injury by our host defense systems. Necrosis can lead to a variety of consequences such as, tissue damage, inflammatory response, loss of function, scarring, and systemic or chronic effects. Apoptosis does not provoke a protective host response. Apoptotic cells neatly form small membrane-bound fragments that are not recognized as injurious or foreign by our host defense systems. There are also "intermediate" forms of cell death that, although they are regulated in response to a specific event, result in a necrosis-like pattern of cell death. For example, cells may respond to some microbial pathogens by pyroptosis, a regulated form of cellular suicide that is otherwise similar to necrosis.

Aging and the Cell

All organisms grow old and eventually die. Human life expectancy has increased over the years chiefly because early deaths from infectious diseases, accidents, and other conditions have been greatly reduced; however, the human life span appears constant. Just as humans as a whole have an ultimate life span, so do our cells. Normal cells of humans (and all higher organisms) undergo a fixed number of divisions before they die (called the **Hayflick limit** in honor of the scientist who first noted it). This is related to damage that occurs at the ends of our chromosomes (telomeres) each time they divide. In the absence of an enzyme system (telomerase transcriptase complex), the damage cannot be repaired. When the Hayflick limit is reached, the DNA damage results in the cell undergoing apoptosis. Only cells that serve to continually repopulate organs (stem cells) are immune to this limit. Many cancer cells activate telomerase and hence gain the ability to divide indefinitely. Somewhat surprisingly, the Hayflick limit differs greatly between species and does not correlate well with species life span.

Hayflick limit Fixed number of cell divisions possible for a normal cell.

Progerias Diseases characterized by dramatic and premature aging.

The causes of aging are not well understood but reside within the cells themselves and are likely coded within our genetic material. A variety of mutations in single genes can result in **progerias**, diseases characterized by dramatic and premature aging in which a teenager appears to be elderly and suffers those diseases found in the aged.

The life span of an individual reflects the survival of the various populations of cells that together form the individual. Certain organ systems appear to be particularly susceptible to the effects of aging. Death and debility are often related to disease of the cardiovascular and nervous systems. Aging changes in the brain appear to be caused by the wearing out and eventual death of neurons, which are not capable of cell division. The degenerative changes in the walls of arteries, called arteriosclerosis, may result from deposition of lipids into the arterial walls, leading to a gradual failure of the endothelial cells lining the blood vessels. The common type of arthritis seen in older people involves aging-dependent change in the cartilage covering the ends of the bones. Organ systems containing constantly dividing epithelial cell populations (such as the gut) are particularly prone to cancer as one ages.

As a cell ages, many of its enzyme systems become less active, and the cell becomes less efficient in carrying out its functions. The cell becomes more susceptible to harmful chemical influences, such as **reactive oxygen species (ROS)**, which can damage and destroy the genetic material, cellular proteins, and the lipids that make up cell membranes. ROS may be environmental agents or can be products of the cell's own mitochondrial metabolism.

Reactive oxygen species (ROS) Highly reactive molecules containing oxygen that can be either environmentally- or self-produced and can damage cells.

Another example of aging related change in cells that affects the organism as a whole can be seen in our immune system. The cells of the immune system become less efficient as they age. Consequently, an aging individual becomes more susceptible to various infectious diseases, which can shorten the life span. The aging immune system also may become less able to eliminate abnormal cells that arise sporadically within the body, leading to the formation of malignant tumors that occur with increased frequency in the elderly.

In summary, cells have a finite life span. However, the less they are exposed to harmful environmental influences and the more efficient they are in repairing their own malfunctions, the greater their chances for survival to a "ripe old age."

Case 2-1

A 19-year-old female high school senior has been involved in a serious single-driver automobile accident. She is brought into a surgical trauma unit suffering from massive internal bleeding. Attempts to stabilize her prior to surgery are unsuccessful. She suffers from severe hypotension (low blood pressure) and shock and expires. Blood alcohol testing demonstrates that she was legally intoxicated. This is considered to be a likely cause of her accident. The county medical examiner requests an autopsy.

Findings Pertinent to this Case

The decedent was noted to be moderately obese. The cause of internal bleeding was discovered to be multiple sites of injury to major vessels relating to the crush injury of her thorax (chest). The autopsy was otherwise remarkable for the finding of hepatomegaly (hypertrophy of the liver). The liver weighed 2200 grams (normal about 1400 grams in a young female) and was noted to be pale and fatty appearing. Histologic investigation of the liver disclosed macrovesicular steatosis, the presence of excess lipid within hepatocytes (cells of liver parenchyma) as large vesicles. Liver cells contained large clear vesicles that displaced the position of the nucleus on routine hematoxylin-eosin (H&E)–stained material (tissue processing removes lipid). Frozen tissue sections processed to maintain lipid showed positive staining of the vesicles with a stain for lipids (**Case Figure 2-1**). No other abnormality of the liver was noted.

Discussion

Steatosis or fatty liver disease (FLD) can occur in individuals who are obese as a result of a number of metabolic diseases of the liver or with the ingestion of potentially toxic agents such as some drugs or, notably, alcohol (ethanol). FLD results when the liver's ability to export fat is lower than the intake of exogenous and/or the production of endogenous lipids. Both decreased export and increased synthesis may occur in alcoholic FLD (AFLD). AFLD is almost always found in heavy drinkers, but even modest consumption of alcohol may result in the condition. Prolonged consumption of modest amounts of alcohol (about 50 grams per day, equivalent to about

(continues)

Case 2-1 *(Continued)*

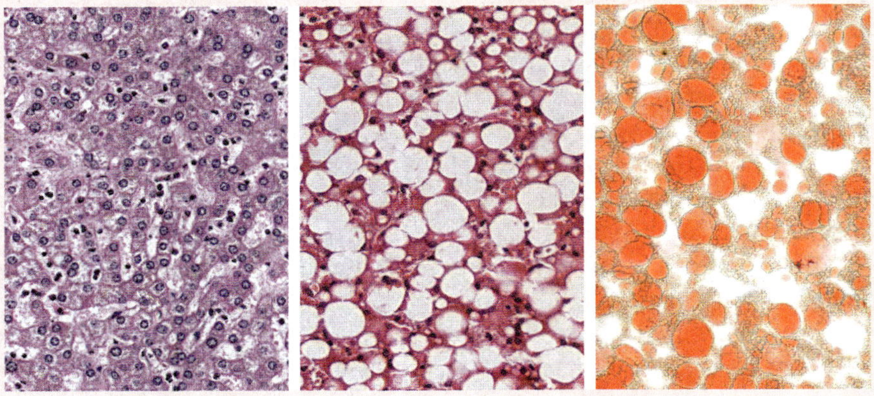

Case Figure 2-1 A section of liver from a patient with alcoholic fatty liver disease (AFLD; alcoholic steatosis). **(A)** Normal liver, routine processing (stained with hematoxylin-eosin). **(B)** Liver from a patient with AFLD. Routine processing of tissue for staining with hematoxylin-eosin removes lipids, leaving clear vesicles. **(C)** A section from the same liver processed to retain lipids (frozen section). The lipids have been stained with a special dye (oil red O).

four 12-ounce cans of beer) will result in AFLD in more than 40 percent of individuals. There is great individual variation in susceptibility to AFLD (and the more serious consequences of alcohol consumption). Females, obese people, and binge drinkers show much increased risk. Although AFLD is usually asymptomatic and is reversible with abstinence, continued alcohol consumption is likely to lead to serious and irreversible liver disease (cirrhosis; see Chapter 21).

Etiology and Pathogenesis

The etiologic agent is the toxic agent ethanol. Consumption of excess ethanol leads to derangement of liver metabolism and the deposition of lipid within the cells of the liver (alcoholic steatosis or AFLD). With continued consumption, this may progress to alcoholic hepatitis (inflammation of the liver) and alcoholic cirrhosis (scarring of the liver), resulting in hepatic failure and other systemic diseases.

Questions

1. Why are hepatocytes (liver parenchymal cells) particularly susceptible to deposition of lipid within the cells?
2. Why are frozen sections necessary to demonstrate steatosis in the liver?
3. What would have happened to the liver had the individual survived her accident and stopped drinking? What if she continued drinking?

Questions for Review

1. How does the nucleus direct the activities of the cell? What molecules are involved?
2. What are the functions of the following organelles: rough endoplasmic reticulum, ribosomes, lysosomes, and centrioles?

3. How is epithelium classified, and what are its functions? Why are mesothelium and endothelium considered separately from other types of epithelium?
4. What are the germ layers, and what are their functions?
5. What is the difference between atrophy and hypertrophy, between metaplasia and dysplasia, and between cell necrosis and apoptosis?
6. What morphologic abnormalities are manifested by an injured cell? Why do they develop?
7. What factors cause a cell to age?

References

Kumar V, Abbas AK, Aster J, Deyrup AT. Robbins & Kumar Basic Pathology. 11th ed. Philadelphia, PA: Elsevier Saunders; 2023.

Rubin E, Reisner HM, eds. Principles of Rubin's Pathology. 7th ed. Philadelphia, PA: Wolters Kluwer Lippincott Williams & Wilkins; 2019.

- These two books are the shorter versions of the leading pathology texts used in medical education. They serve as good general references for detailed descriptions of mechanisms of pathogenesis and disease.

Bickley L, Szilagyi PG, Hoffman RM, Soriano RP. Bates' Guide to Physical Examination and History Taking. 13th ed. Philadelphia, PA: Wolters Kluwer, Lippincott Williams & Wilkins; 2023.

- A classic guide to the details of physician–patient interaction.

Straus SE, Glasziou P, Richardson WS, Haynes BR. Evidence-Based Medicine. 5th ed. Edinburgh, UK: Elsevier; 2019.

- A comprehensive guide with an excellent chapter on Harm.

Bishop ML, Fodyu EP, Van Sicen C, et al. Clinical Chemistry: Principles, Techniques, and Correlations. Burlington, MA: Jones & Bartlett Learning; 2023.

- Provides an overview of the most rapidly advancing areas of laboratory medicine with clear explanations that balance analytic principles, techniques, and correlation of results with coverage of disease states.

Herring W. Learning Radiology: Recognizing the Basics. 5th ed. Philadelphia, PA: Elsevier Saunders; 2024.

- An introductory text that does a good job of providing additional background on the diseases illustrated.

Clift IC. Clinical Immunodiagnostics: Laboratory Principles and Practices. 1st ed. Burlington, MA: Jones & Bartlett Learning; 2021.

- Focuses on theoretical principles underlying different diagnostic tests performed in the clinical lab.

Moini J. Anatomy and Physiology for Health Professionals. 3rd ed. Burlington, MA: Jones & Bartlett Learning; 2020.

- An easy-to-read and well-illustrated text on normal human anatomy and physiology. The text is notable for its many useful tables, critical thinking questions, and correlation with pathology.

American Society for Investigative Pathology. Accessed February 26, 2025. http://www.asip.org/

- This is the major research and teaching organization (although its major focus is not clinical). It is an excellent source for those interested in educational opportunities in the area.

Testing.com. Accessed March 12, 2025. https://www.testing.com/

- Offers consumers access to laboratory testing through a network of laboratory partners and provides lab testing guides.

Introduction to Radiology. Geisel School of Medicine, Dartmouth Department of Anatomy. Accessed March 12, 2025. http://www.dartmouth.edu/~anatomy/HAE/Radiology_Intro/rad_index.html

- This is an easy-to-follow, well-illustrated introduction to the area. Additional in-depth resources are available at the site.

Pyeritz RE. The family history: the first genetic test and still useful after all those years? *Genet Med*. 2012;14:3-9.

Vento JM. Family history: a guide for neurologists in the age of genomic medicine. *Semin Pediatr Neurol*. 2012;19:160-166.

- Two references that go together well. The first is a history of the role of the family history in patient evaluation up to the age of molecular genetics. The second is an excellent introduction to the analysis of family history and pedigree analysis. Although the examples given involve neurological disease, it is a primer for genetic risk analysis, which has become an important component in clinical encounters.

American Cancer Society Cancer Screening Recommendations. 2023. Accessed March 12, 2025. https://www.cancer.org/content/dam/cancer-org/online-documents/en/pdf/flyers/cancer-screenings-save-lives.pdf

- Provides recommendations for cancer screening based on age and cancer type.

Vanda Inácio1 V, Rodríguez-Álvarez MX, Gayoso-Diz P. Statistical Evaluation of Medical Tests. Annual Review of Statistics and Its Application. 2021;8:41-67.

- Provides an overview of statistical evaluation of diagnosis and prognosis using medica tests. It introduces the concept of receiver operating characteristic (ROC) curve analysis, which is critical in test optimization. The examples used are of clinical interest.

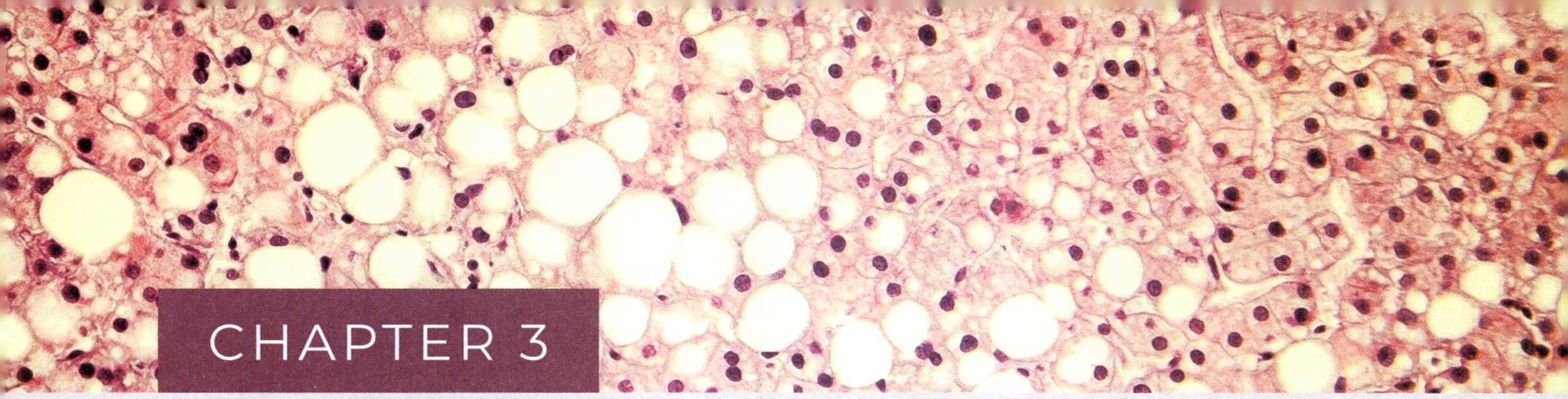

CHAPTER 3

Genes and Genetic Disease

LEARNING OBJECTIVES

1. Describe the inheritance pattern of genes and define dominant, recessive, codominant, and sex-linked inheritance.
2. Describe how chromosomes are studied. Explain how a karyotype is determined.
3. Describe some of the common genetic abnormalities and explain their methods of transmission.
4. Describe the role of chromosome deletions and translocations in inherited disease.
5. List the causes of Down syndrome and describe its clinical manifestations. Explain why it is important to identify a carrier of a 14/21 chromosome translocation.
6. List four abnormalities of sex chromosomes and describe their clinical manifestations.
7. Compare the methods of transmission and clinical manifestations of phenylketonuria and hemophilia.
8. Describe epigenetics and give examples of how epigenetics can impact gene expression.
9. Describe how recombinant DNA technology has influenced our understanding of inherited diseases.

Introduction

Transmission of genetic information was initially studied through the analysis of the inheritance of detectable traits (**phenotypic traits**) from parents through successive generations of offspring using **patterns of inheritance**. These phenotypic traits are now understood as the expression of the **genotype** of the individual; that is, the genes that are the functional manifestation of the chemical code of the **DNA** organized in **chromosomes** in the nucleus of the cell. The human **genome** contains about 20,000 genes. The information encoded by those genes in the chromosomes defines the proteins critical to the structure, metabolism, and regulation of all aspects of cellular function. This information is transmitted to each newly formed cell during cell division, either to make two identical **daughter cells** (through the process of **mitosis**) or to form sperm or ova (through the process of **meiosis**). All nongerminal cells of the body are **diploid** (have a 2N chromosome number, 46, arranged as 23 pairs in humans), with one of each pair of chromosomes derived from each parent during the fertilization of the

Phenotypic traits Characteristics apparent in the individual.

Pattern of inheritance Occurrence of detectable traits across generations in a family.

Genotype DNA/chromosome basis of inherited traits in an individual.

DNA Deoxyribonucleic acid (DNA) is the molecule carrying the coding information for genes.

Chromosome Cell structure organizing the molecules of DNA; individual structural unit of DNA, which is best seen in dividing cells.
Genome All the genes contained in a cell's chromosomes.
Daughter cell A cell resulting from the division of a single cell (called the parent cell).
Mitosis The type of cell division for somatic/body cells in which chromosomes from parent cells are duplicated and transferred to daughter cells. This type of cell division produces two daughter cells that are identical with each other and to the parent cell. The characteristic cell division found in all cells in the body except for the gametes.
Meiosis A special type of cell division resulting in gamete production (ova and sperm) in which the number of chromosomes is reduced by one-half.
Diploid Cell containing 2N (pairs) of each chromosome.
Homologous chromosomes A matched pair of chromosomes, one derived from each parent.
Reduction division Process occurring in meiosis reducing the 2N pairs of chromosomes to 1N.
Haploid Cell containing 1N of each chromosome, a gamete.
Zygote The fertilized ovum.
Autosomal chromosomes Chromosomes other than sex chromosomes. A human has 22 pairs of autosomes.

ovum by a sperm. Members of a chromosome pair are called **homologous chromosomes**. During the formation of ova (oogenesis) and sperm (spermatogenesis), a **reduction division** results in the formation of a **haploid** (has an N chromosome number, 23, with no chromosome pairs) that recombines traits from the maternal and paternal chromosome set of the individual. Fertilization restores the diploid chromosome number and produces a unique individual with a mixture of traits derived from the maternal and paternal genomes. The genome of the fertilized egg (**zygote**) also contains the blueprint for the development of the new individual, the formation of the body plan that defines us as human. In the new individual, 22 of the chromosome pairs consist of **autosomal chromosomes**, and one pair is the **sex chromosomes**, an XY pair determining a male and XX, a female. The 23 pairs of chromosomes make up the **karyotype**.

The Structure of DNA in the Chromosomes

The chromosomes are composed of DNA combined with protein. The packing of DNA into chromosomes condenses the strands of DNA as much as 10,000 times to allow the DNA to fit into the nucleus and provide structure. The chromosome strands are first wrapped around **histone** and other proteins to form a nucleosome, which appears as beads strung on the DNA strands. The **nucleosomes** become condensed into chromatin fibers and tube-like structures, which are further condensed into chromosomes (**Figure 3-1**).

The information on the DNA is referred to as the **genetic code**. The basic structural unit of DNA, called a **nucleotide**, consists of a phosphate group linked to a five-carbon sugar, deoxyribose, which in turn is joined to a nitrogen-containing compound called a base (**Figure 3-2A**). There are two different types of DNA bases: a purine base, which contains a fused double ring of carbon and nitrogen atoms, and a pyrimidine base, which contains only a single ring. There are four different bases in DNA: the purine bases are adenine and guanine, and the pyrimidine bases are thymine and cytosine. Consequently, there are four different nucleotides in DNA, each containing a different base (**Figure 3-2B**). The nucleotides are joined together in long chains, with the nitrogen bases projecting at right angles from the long axes of the chains. A DNA molecule consists of two strands of DNA held together by weak chemical attractions between the bases of the adjacent chains. The chemical structure of the bases is such that only adenine can pair with thymine and only guanine can pair with cytosine. Bases that pair in this way are called **complementary** bases, and there are 3 billion pairs of complementary bases (base pairs) in the human genome. However, less than 2 percent of the base pairs code for proteins. The base pairs that do not code for protein are important in determining when and how the protein coding genes function in the organism. The DNA chains are twisted into a double helix somewhat like a spiral staircase, with the sugar and phosphate groups forming the two railings and the complementary base pairs forming the steps (**Figure 3-2C**).

Genes and Inheritance Patterns

The alternate forms of a gene found on the maternal and paternal chromosomes pair are called **alleles**. The chromosome site of a given gene is called a **locus**. Different alleles may produce easily detectable differences in the

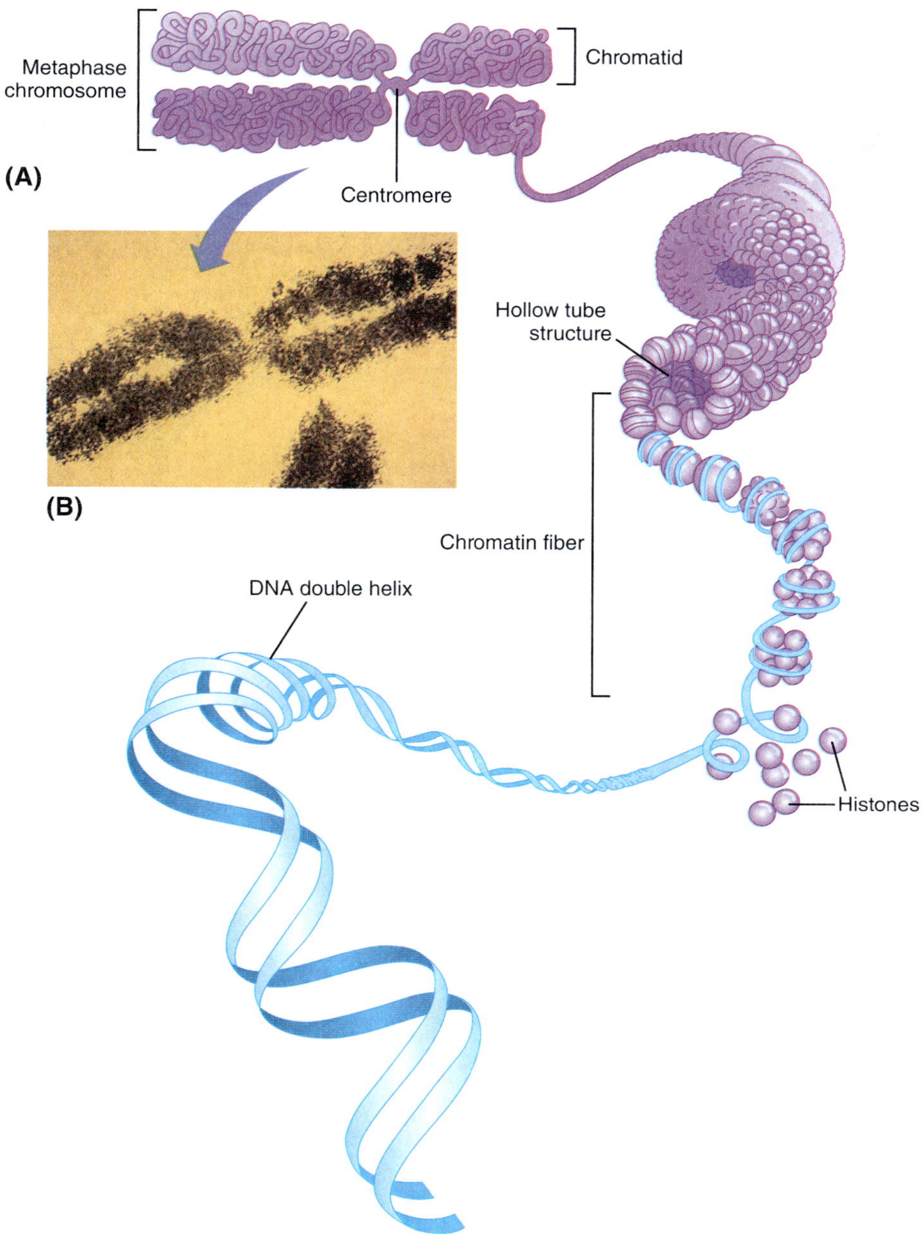

Figure 3-1 Chromosome structure. **(A)** The DNA helix wraps around the histone molecules to form a chromatin fiber. During prophase, the chromatin fibers coil tightly, forming the densely packed chromosome. **(B)** Transmission electron micrograph of a metaphase chromosome.

individual (such as eye color), more subtle differences (blood type, or the level of activity of a particular protein detectable only in the laboratory), or differences so subtle as to be undetectable in an individual. Deleterious alleles, the result of inherited alterations in the gene (**mutation**), can result in dysfunction and disease.

The common variant forms of alleles found in populations are termed **polymorphisms**. Inheritance of such polymorphisms at multiple loci is what defines us as individuals and helps define populations (which differ in the frequency of particular alleles for many genes). For example, several different alleles at a locus may be common in populations (ABO blood types are a good example). The much-misused term race represents frequency

Sex chromosomes The X and Y chromosomes that determine genetic sex. A human has one pair of sex chromosomes.

Karyotype Chromosomes from a single cell arranged in pairs in descending order according to the size of the chromosomes and the positions of the centromeres used to visualize the chromosome composition of an individual.

Histone A protein found in the nucleus, which is important in the packaging of DNA.

Nucleosome A beaded structure of DNA wrapped around histone and other nuclear proteins.

Genetic code The information carried by DNA molecules in chromosomes. The DNA basis of the phenotype/genotype.

Nucleotide Basic structural unit of DNA or RNA consisting of a phosphate group linked to a five-carbon sugar, deoxyribose or ribose.

Complementary The relationship between the base sequence of the two strands in a DNA molecule. During DNA replication, either strand can make an exact copy of the other. Complementary DNA strands bind to each other by base pairing.

Allele One of several related forms of a single gene.

Locus The location of a gene on a chromosome.

Mutation Alteration in the DNA sequence of the genome.

Polymorphism Collection of common alleles for a single gene found in populations.

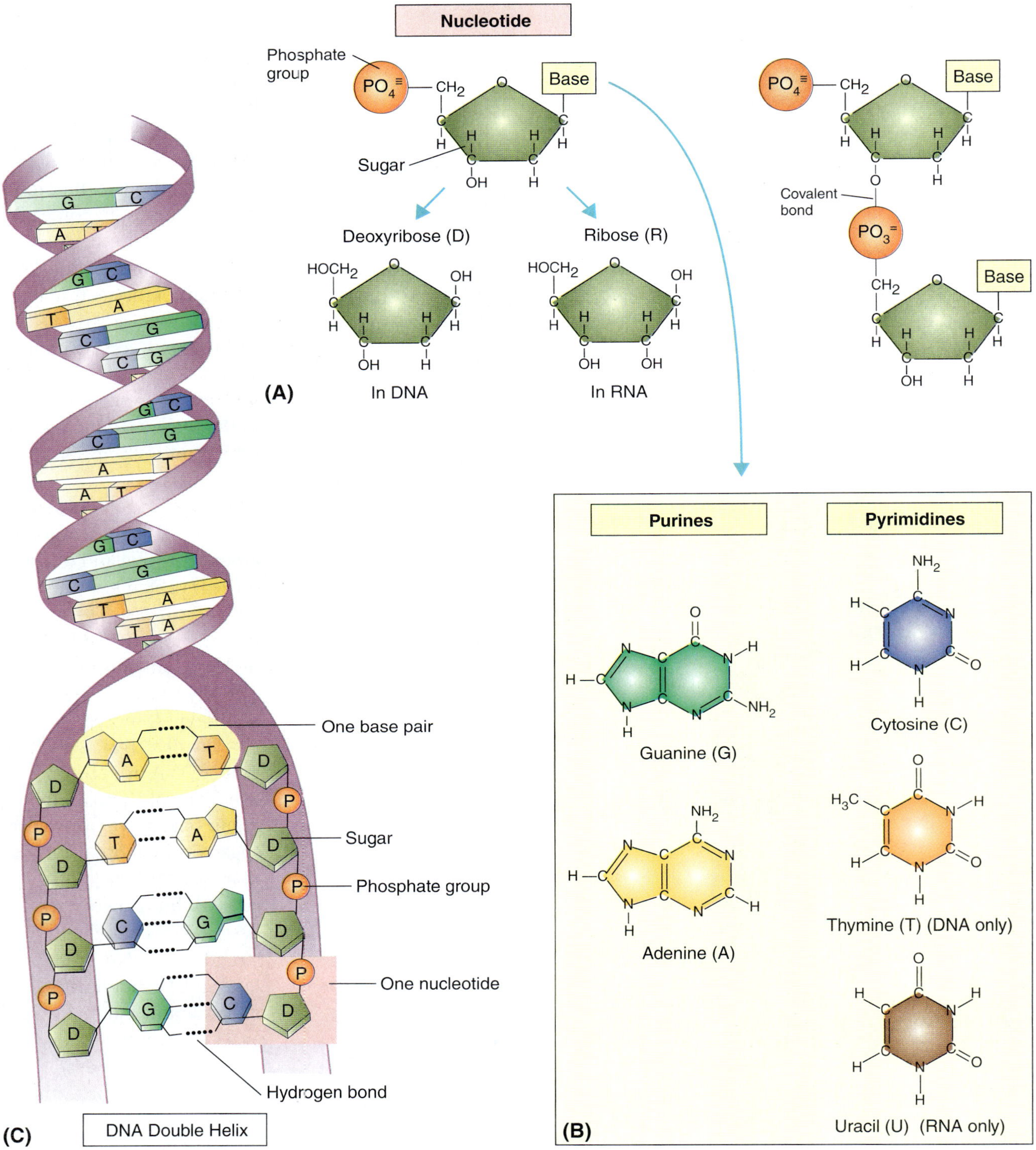

Figure 3-2 Structure of DNA molecule. **(A)** Structure of nucleotides. **(B)** Structure of purine and pyrimidine bases in DNA. Uracil (U) in RNA only. **(C)** Model of DNA double helix.

differences in many polymorphic genes that define populations historically derived from different areas. Such differences are likely to be of evolutionary significance. Populations of African origin have alleles for a number of genes that result in higher levels of skin pigment, which protect against the deleterious effects of solar ultraviolet radiation. Scandinavian populations tend to have alleles resulting in lower levels of skin pigments, perhaps to capture scanty northern solar radiation important in the biosynthesis of vitamin D.

An individual is **homozygous** for a gene if both alleles are the same and **heterozygous** if the alleles are different. Alleles of different genes differ in how they are expressed. A **recessive gene** produces a detectable **phenotype** only in the homozygous state. An example is the ABO blood group. Persons will have blood type O only if they have inherited the O allele for the ABO gene from each parent and are therefore homozygous for this allele. A **dominant gene** expresses itself in either the heterozygous or the homozygous state. The A and B alleles of the ABO blood group are dominant. Individuals inheriting either one or two A or B alleles have blood types A or B, respectively. In some cases, there are detectable differences between homozygous or heterozygous expression of a dominant allele. Such **dosage effects** can result in higher levels of expression of a gene product when two doses of a dominant allele are present. Sometimes both alleles of a pair are expressed. Such alleles are called **codominant**. If one A and one B allele is present at the ABO gene locus, the person has blood type AB, and their cells will have both the A and B alleles. Genes carried on sex chromosomes are called **sex-linked genes**; the effects they produce are called **sex-linked traits**. The small Y chromosome carries few genes other than those that direct male sex differentiation, but the much larger X chromosome carries many genes in addition to those concerned with sexual development. Most X-linked traits are recessive. The female carrier of a recessive X-linked trait is usually normal because the effect of the defective allele on one X chromosome is offset by the normal allele on the other X chromosome. The male, however, possesses only one X chromosome. Consequently, he can be neither heterozygous nor homozygous for X-linked genes and is called **hemizygous** for genes carried on the X chromosome. If the male receives an X chromosome containing a defective gene, the defective X-linked gene functions like a dominant gene when paired with the Y chromosome. Such is the case for the well-known disease hemophilia (resulting in excessive bleeding) because the genes responsible for the most common forms of this disease (hemophilia A and hemophilia B) are sex-linked. Females who inherit an allele responsible for hemophilia are most often normal because the allele is recessive. They are, however, carriers of the disease. If their offspring inherits the maternal chromosome having the defective hemophilia allele and also the Y chromosome from the male parent, the result is a male child who is hemizygous for the defective allele and has the disease hemophilia. It is of interest to note that female hemophiliacs do occur (although rarely) for reasons to be discussed. The inheritance pattern of genes can be traced through a family tree or **pedigree** (**Figure 3-3**). The pattern of appearance of a trait or disease in a pedigree offers clues to the nature of the allele studied (i.e., dominant, recessive, or sex-linked). For example, in the case of dominant inheritance, the trait (disease) is expected to appear in one of the parents of the affected child. In the recessive case, neither parent will be affected (but both will be carriers). In the case of recessive gene transmission, each parent has at least one copy of the recessive trait, which is passed to the offspring. Sex-linked (recessive) traits appear only in males. Fathers are not affected (they donate their normal Y chromosome to their male offspring), but male uncles or grandfathers are likely to show the trait.

Homozygous Having the same alleles at a given gene locus on the homologous chromosome pair.

Heterozygous Having two different alleles at a given gene locus on the homologous pair of chromosomes.

Recessive gene A gene that expresses a trait only when present in the homozygous state.

Phenotype Collection of inherited/phenotypic traits detectable in an individual.

Dominant gene A gene that expresses a trait in the heterozygous state.

Dosage effects Differing amounts of gene product in the heterozygous and homozygous states.

Codominant Products of both genes are expressed in the heterozygous state.

Sex-linked gene Gene present on the X or Y chromosome.

Sex-linked trait Product of gene present on X or Y chromosome.

Hemizygous A term applied to genes located on the X chromosome in the male.

Pedigree Formal pattern displaying the inheritance of traits or gene products through generations of a family.

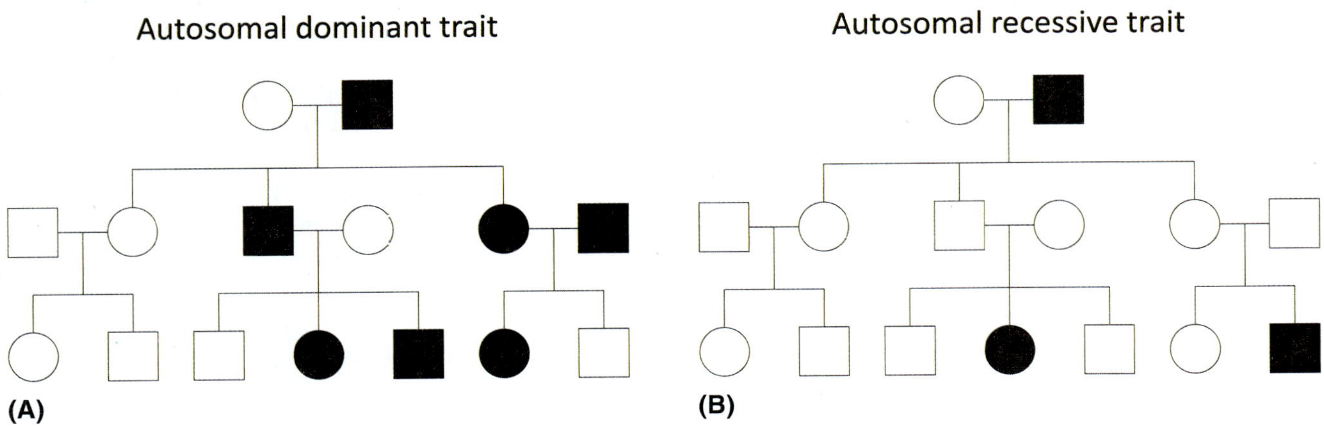

Figure 3-3 Pedigrees of dominant and recessive trait inheritance. Pedigree symbols: Male, square; Female, circle; Mating: horizontal line connecting male and female symbol. Offsprings of a mating are connected by vertical lines. Affected individuals are shown by shaded symbols. **(A)** Pedigree for a dominant trait. Note: the trait is shown in every generation. **(B)** Pedigree for a recessive trait. Note: the trait is not shown in every generation. The parents of affected individuals are most often not affected but are carriers of the trait (heterozygous).

X Chromosome Inactivation: The Lyon Hypothesis

Having the proper number of chromosomes is necessary for normal human development. Defects in the number of chromosomes, having extra or missing chromosomes (**aneuploidy**), are always associated with disease and is often fatal prior to birth. In normal individuals, all autosomal chromosomes occur in pairs. This is not the case with sex chromosomes: females who are XX appear to have twice the X chromosomal DNA of XY males. Female cells, however, function as though they contained only genetic material equivalent to that of the single X chromosome of the male. The reason for this behavior is that almost all of one of the X chromosomes is inactivated and nonfunctional. In the female, the genetic activity of both X chromosomes is essential only during the first week of embryonic development. Thereafter, one of the X chromosomes in each of the developing cells is inactivated. An exception to X inactivation occurs in a region of the X chromosome termed the **pseudoautosomal region**. Genes in this region are not inactivated but are often also found on the Y chromosome. For this reason, genes in the pseudoautosomal region have similar amounts of DNA in both males and females. With only rare exceptions, the inactivation occurs in a random manner (Figure 3-4). After the initial inactivation of an X chromosome has occurred, the same paternal- or maternal-derived X chromosome will also be inactivated in all descendants of the precursor cell. The inactivated X chromosome appears as a small, dense mass of condensed chromatin (**heterochromatin**) attached to the nuclear membrane of somatic cells.

The inactivated X chromosome can be identified in the cells of a normal female and is called a sex chromatin body or **Barr body**, after the man who first described it. Because the inactivation occurs at random, females are a **genetic mosaic** for genes that are sex-linked. If a female is heterozygous for a sex-linked gene (which has an "A" allele and a "B" allele), about half the cells in the woman would be expected to express A and half express B. Mosaicism for sex-linked coat color genes is responsible for calico cats having a splotched coat. With very rare exceptions, all calico cats are female. The situation is actually more complex and is further described in Case 3-1 and in later sections dealing with X-linked genetic diseases.

Aneuploidy Condition of having extra or missing chromosomes.

Pseudoautosomal region (of the X chromosome) The region of the X chromosome containing genes which are not inactivated

Heterochromatin Small dense mass of condensed chromatin appearing in inactivated X chromosomes.

Barr body The inactivated X chromosome attached to the nuclear membrane in the female. Sex chromatin body.

Genetic mosaic Condition of having one or more cell populations with distinct genotype and phenotype. It can affect somatic cell, germ line cell, or both.

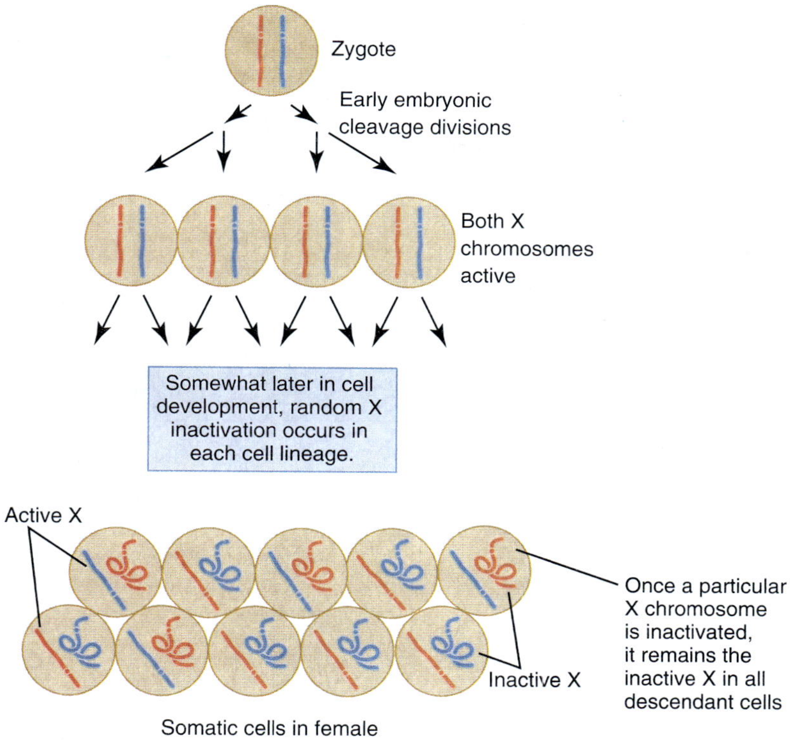

Figure 3-4 The two X chromosomes are shown in red and blue. An active X is depicted as a straight chromosome, an inactive X as a tangle. Each cell has just one active X. The particular X that remains active is a matter of chance, but it remains active in the progeny of that cell.

Chromosome Analysis

The chromosome composition (karyotype) of a human can be studied with great accuracy to determine the presence of abnormalities in chromosome number or structure. This is accomplished by using a drug to arrest dividing cells (usually from the blood) at a stage in which the chromosomes are condensed and have become separate and distinct. The complex structure of the chromosomes in such cells can be established by using special stains that allow microscopic visualization of the details of chromosome structure or by using a molecular biological technique that identifies specific regions of chromosomes using **fluorescent probes**, a technique termed "chromosome painting."

Artificially synthesized stretches of DNA that bind (hybridize) to specific chromosomes are linked to a series of fluorescent dyes in order to identify chromosomes by color. **Figure 3-5** illustrates the appearance of a cell arrested in mitosis with the chromosomes well separated. A normal dividing cell arrested in mitosis contains 46 chromosomes, each consisting of 2 **chromatids** joined at their **centromeres**. Each chromosome has its own unique structure and is classified according to size, the location of the centromere, the relative lengths of the chromatids that extend outward from the centromere (called the arms of the chromosome), and the pattern of light and dark bands along the chromosome. The separated chromosomes from a single cell are photographed and arranged in pairs in a standard pattern called a karyotype. **Figure 3-6** illustrates a karyotype produced using the technique of chromosome painting. Each pair of chromosomes is "painted" with a specific color using a fluorescent probe.

Fluorescent probes Artificial pieces of DNA labeled with a fluorescent dye.

Chromatid One of two newly duplicate chromosomes held together by the centromere.

Centromere The structure that joins each pair of chromatids formed by chromosome duplication.

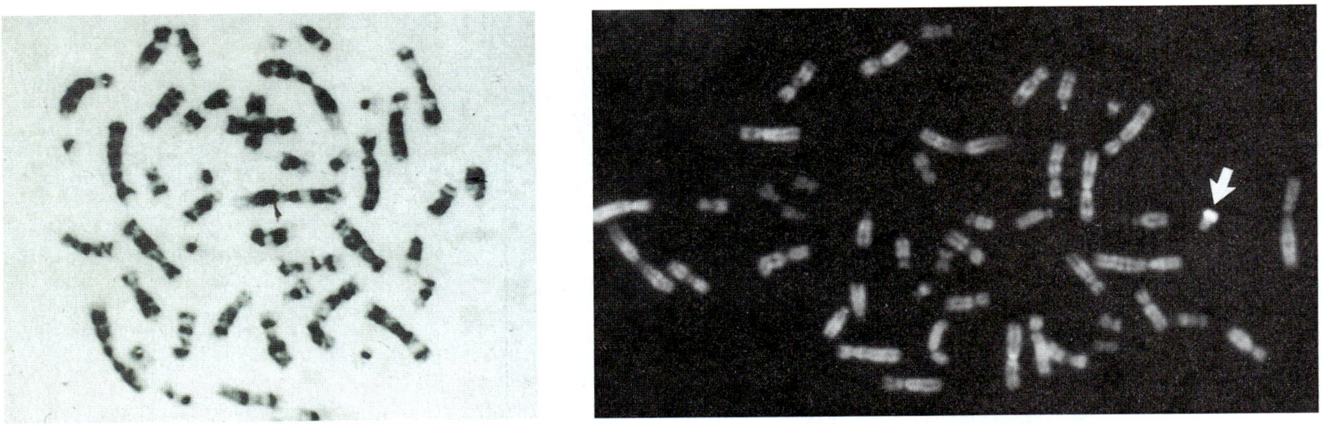

(A) (B)

Figure 3-5 The appearance of chromosomes from a single cell arrested in mitosis, illustrating the banded pattern that facilitates the identification of individual chromosomes. The two chromatids composing each chromosome lie side by side. **(A)** Giemsa stain (photograph courtesy of DR. Jorge Yunis). **(B)** Fluorescent stain showing intensely stained (*arrow*) Y chromosome (photograph courtesy of Patricia Crowley-Larsen).

Courtesy of Leonard V. Crowley, MD, Century College.

Genetic Disease

A hereditary disease or genetic disease results from a chromosome abnormality or a defective expression of a gene due to mutation within the gene or at a region important for normal gene function. Chromosomal abnormalities account for about 6 percent of genetic diseases, and all known single-gene defects (of which at least 6000 have been described) account for an additional 7.5 percent. It is likely that 20 percent to 30 percent of birth defects involve multiple genes with complex patterns of inheritance or have both a genetic and an environmental component. Relatively common defects such as congenital heart disease, cleft lip and palate, and defects in the formation of the neural tube (brain and spine)

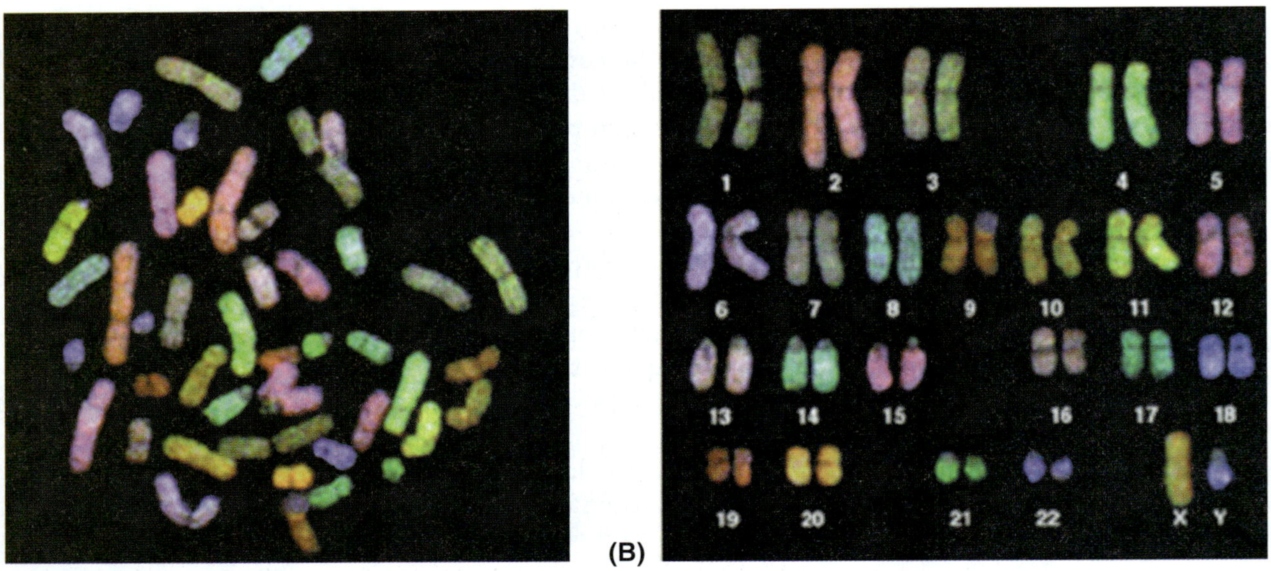

(A) (B)

Figure 3-6 Result of human chromosome painting in which each pair of chromosomes is stained a different color by hybridizing with a specific fluorescent probe. **(A)** The appearance of stained chromosomes from a single cell arrested in mitosis. Each pair can be identified by both structure and color. **(B)** A karyotype in which the chromosomes have been grouped in pairs and arranged in conventional order depending in part on size.

Courtesy of Johannes Wienberg, Ludwig-Maximilians-University, and Thomas Ried, National Institutes of Health.

fall into this category. Nongenetic, postconceptional factors such as chemical or physical agents, maternal illness and infection, and medicinal and recreational drugs (including excess alcohol consumption during pregnancy) account for an additional 5 percent to 10 percent of birth defects. About half of birth defects are of unknown cause, although undoubtedly a proportion of these are related to unrecognized defects in chromosomal structure and mutations in genes.

Chromosomal Abnormalities

Chromosomal abnormalities leading to congenital malformations may result from failure of homologous chromosomes in the germ cells to separate normally, from abnormal breaks and rearrangements of chromosomes in the germ cells as they are maturing, or at times from failure of chromosomes to separate normally in the fertilized ovum (zygote) as the cells divide by mitosis during early prenatal development.

Occasionally, homologous chromosomes in germ cells fail to separate from one another in either the first or the second meiotic division. This is called nondisjunction and leads to abnormalities in the distribution of chromosomes between germ cells (**Figure 3-7**). One of the two germ cells derived from the abnormal chromosome division has an extra chromosome, and the other cell lacks a chromosome. Nondisjunction may involve either the sex chromosomes or the autosomes. If it occurs during **gametogenesis**, one daughter cell will have 24 chromosomes and the other will have 22. If a **gamete** having an abnormal number of chromosomes fuses with a normal gamete during fertilization, the resulting zygote will either have an extra chromosome or be lacking one of the homologous pair of chromosomes, a condition termed aneuploidy. The presence of an extra chromosome in a cell is called a trisomy of the chromosome present in triplicate. Absence of a chromosome is called a monosomy of the missing chromosome. Complete monosomy for autosomal chromosomes is not viable; however, monosomy for the X chromosome

Gametogenesis The development of mature eggs and sperm from precursor cells.

Gametes Reproductive cells—egg and sperm cells—each containing 23 chromosomes, which unite during fertilization to form a zygote containing 46 chromosomes.

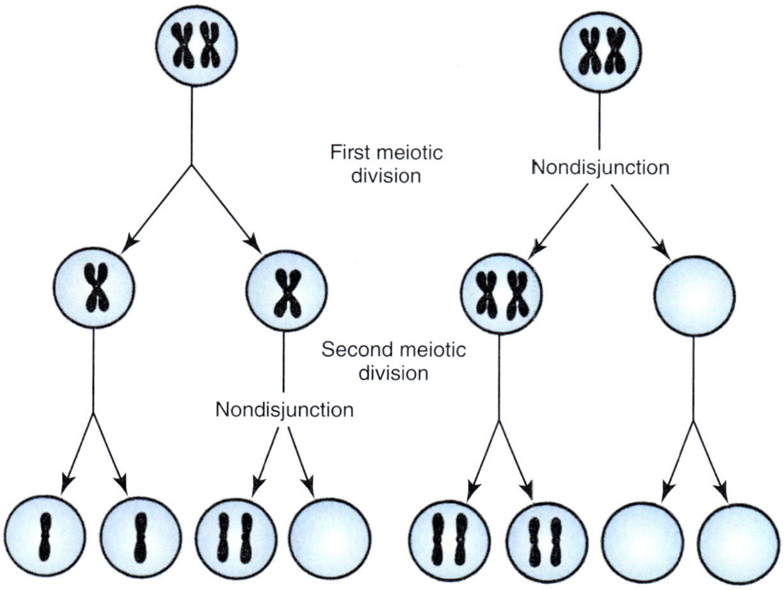

Figure 3-7 Effects of nondisjunction in meiosis, leading to formation of gametes with an extra or missing chromosome. Only the chromosome pair involved in nondisjunction is illustrated. Nondisjunction at second meiotic division (*left*). Nondisjunction at first meiotic division (*right*).

(45,X) results in an individual with Turner syndrome (although only a small percentage of 45,X conceptuses survive to term). The most common autosomal chromosomal defect resulting in a viable birth is trisomy 21, resulting in Down syndrome. Such individuals may survive into the fifth decade, albeit with significant physical and developmental defects. Fetuses with trisomy for chromosome 13 (Patau syndrome) and chromosome 18 (Edward syndrome) may survive to birth; however, unlike individuals with Down syndrome, they generally die soon after birth.

Chromosome Deletions and Translocations During Gametogenesis

Sometimes a chromosome breaks during meiosis, and the broken piece is lost from the cell. This is called chromosome deletion. In some cases, the broken piece is not lost but becomes attached to another nonhomologous chromosome with which it is carried along during meiosis. A misplaced chromosome or part of a chromosome attached to another chromosome is called a translocation. In a reciprocal translocation, pieces of chromosomes (containing different sets of genes) are reciprocally exchanged between two nonhomologous chromosomes. Such an accident may not disturb the function of the cell because there is no loss or gain of genetic material (although the expression of individual genes adjacent to break points may be affected). However, if the translocation occurs in a germ cell, an egg or sperm containing either a deficiency or an excess of chromosomal material may form during meiosis. If such a chromosomally abnormal gamete unites with a normal gamete during fertilization, the fertilized ovum (zygote) contains an abnormal amount of chromosomal material. As noted previously, most abnormal zygotes are spontaneously aborted, but some survive and give rise to abnormal fetuses. **Figure 3-8** demonstrates a case in which a chromosome 14/21 translocation may result in a case of inherited Down syndrome (**D**) or in a carrier for the disease (**C**). This is an uncommon cause of the disease (as we shall see) because most cases are not inherited.

The literature contains many descriptions of clinical abnormalities that are associated with extra chromosomes, chromosome translocation, or loss of entire chromosomes or portions of chromosomes (**Table 3-1**). Chromosomal abnormalities can be detected when abnormalities in chromosome size, configuration, or the band pattern are detected in the karyotype. Even more subtle chromosomal defects may be characterized using chromosome painting and other molecular techniques.

Chromosome Nondisjunction in the Zygote

Failures of chromosome separation are not restricted to germ cells. Sometimes the chromosomes fail to separate during mitosis in one of the cells of the zygote during prenatal development. When this occurs during mitosis, the cell lacking the chromosome is unable to survive, but the cell with the extra chromosome continues to divide along with the other chromosomally normal cells. As a result, the embryo eventually becomes composed of a population of normal cells and another population of cells having a chromosome trisomy (**Figure 3-9**). Such individuals are termed chromosomal mosaics. The relative proportions of the two cell types depend on how early in prenatal development the chromosome nondisjunction occurred and impacts on the severity of disease seen. For example, Down syndrome mosaics are often more mildly affected than those in which all cells are trisomic.

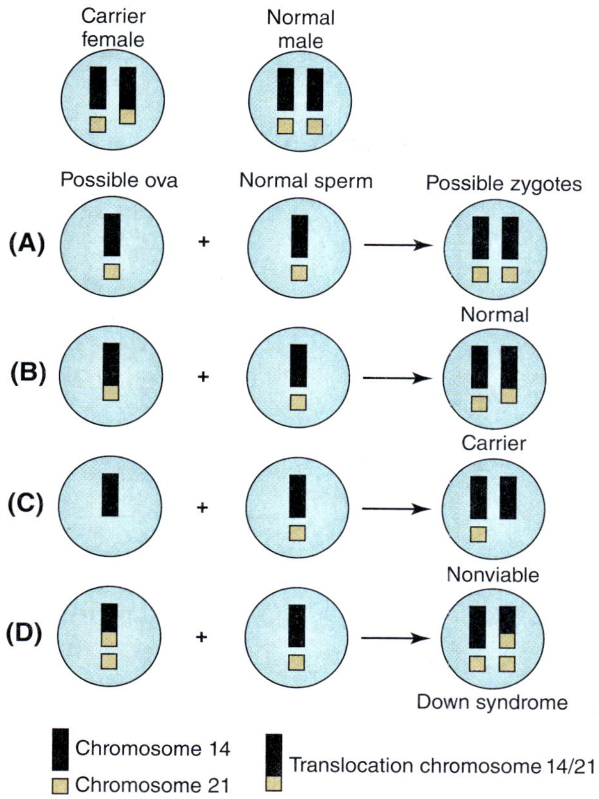

Figure 3-8 Possible ova produced by a female carrier of a 14/21 translocation chromosome and possible zygotes that could result from fertilization by normal sperm.

Table 3-1 Chromosome Abnormalities per 100,000 Recognized Human Pregnancies

Chromosome Constitution	Number Among Spontaneously Aborted Fetuses	Number Among Live Births
Normal	7,500	84,450
Trisomy	–	–
13	128	17
18	223	13
21	350	113
Other autosomes	3,176	0
Sex chromosomes	–	–
47,XYY	4	46
47,XXY	4	44
45,X	1,350	8
47,XXX	21	44
Translocations	–	–
Balanced (euploid)	14	164
Unbalanced (aneuploid)	225	52
Polyploid	–	–
Triploid	1,275	0
Tetraploid	450	0
Others (mosaics, etc.)	280	49
Total	15,000	85,000

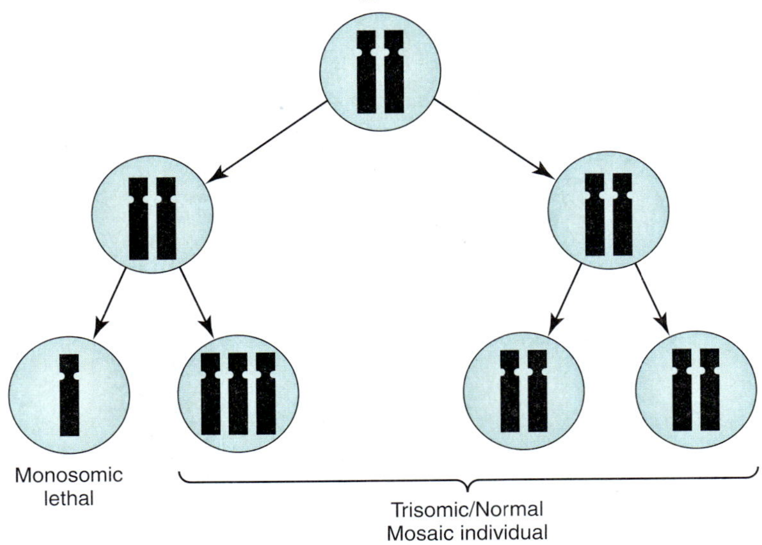

Figure 3-9 Formation of two chromosome populations (chromosome mosaic) resulting from chromosome nondisjunction during mitosis in the zygote.

Sex Chromosome Abnormalities

When detailing the number of chromosomes in a cell, it is customary to indicate first the total number of chromosomes in the cell and then indicate the sex chromosomes. For example, a normal male is designated 46,XY, and a normal female is 46,XX.

Unlike disorders of autosomal chromosome number (which most often result in fetal death or severe disease), defects in sex chromosome number are relatively mild and may be consistent with normal or near normal development into adulthood. Although most (but not all) genes on one X chromosome are inactivated in normal XX females and there are few active genes on the Y chromosome, both X- and Y-linked genes are critical for normal sexual development. If the Y chromosome is absent, the body configuration is female. Hence, it is not surprising that 45,X females (Turner syndrome) are female in body form (are phenotypically female) but do not show sexual maturation. Normal female sexual development requires two active copies of some X-linked genes (pseudoautosomal genes). The presence of one or more extra X chromosomes (Triple X syndrome) has very little effect on the female because the additional X chromosomes are inactivated. The Y chromosome directs male sexual differentiation, and its presence is almost invariably associated with a male body configuration regardless of the number of X chromosomes present. However, the presence of one or more extra X chromosomes adversely affects masculine development. Thus, 47,XXY individuals (Klinefelter syndrome) are phenotypically male but do not sexually mature and invariably have very small **gonads**. An extra Y chromosome (47,XYY, Double Y syndrome) does not cause significant changes in the appearance of the affected individual because the Y chromosome carries little genetic material other than genes concerned with male sexual differentiation. The principal characteristics of these syndromes are summarized in **Table 3-2**.

Gonad A general term referring to either the ovary or the testis.

In addition to conditions associated with abnormal numbers of sex chromosomes, fragile X syndrome, although associated with a defect in an X-linked gene, can under some circumstances be detected as an abnormal karyotype.

Table 3-2 Syndromes Resulting from an Abnormal Complement of Sex Chromosomes

	Usual Genotype	Approximate Incidence	Unusual Number of Barr Bodies	Unusual Number of Y Fluorescent Bodies	Fertility
Turner syndrome	45,X	1:2,500 females	0	0	Sterile
Triple X syndrome	47,XXX	1:850 females	2	0	Usually not impaired
Klinefelter syndrome	47,XXY	1:750 males	1	1	Usually sterile
XYY syndrome	47,XYY	1:850 males	0	2	Usually not impaired

Turner Syndrome

Turner syndrome results from either lack of or structural abnormalities in one of the X chromosomes that leads to loss of a portion of that chromosome. Sixty percent of patients have the 45,X karyotype; others have more subtle deletions in one of the X chromosomes. The reported frequency of about 1 in 2500 female births represents only the 1 percent of Turner embryos that survive to be born alive. At least 75 percent (and possibly nearly all) Turner patients are mosaic, and it has been suggested that at least some 46,XX cells must be present for viability. Severity of the syndrome is linked to the proportion of normal cells present. The most characteristic feature of Turner patients is short stature related to the absence of two copies of the X-linked SHOX gene (one of the pseudoautosomal genes that remain active on both X chromosomes of normal females). Characteristically, Turner patients, although showing normal ovarian development during fetal development, suffer what has been called "premature menopause," with loss of all **oocytes** by the age of 2. Ovaries become completely atrophic and failure of puberty and amenorrhea (lack of menses) occurs without hormonal therapy. A variety of additional developmental defects include a webbed neck, kidney malformations, and defects in the cardiovascular system. Turner syndrome patients usually have normal intelligence; only subtle defects in nonverbal learning sometimes occur.

Oocyte Germ cells in a late stage of egg development.

Triple X Syndrome

The presence of an extra X chromosome in the cells of the female is a relatively common abnormality with an incidence of about 1 in 1000 female births. There are no specific abnormalities of body form. Sexual development and fertility are usually normal. Learning disabilities and delayed motor development sometimes occur.

Klinefelter Syndrome

Having an incidence of about 1 in 750 male births, Klinefelter syndrome (usual genotype 47,XXY) is one of the most common sex chromosome abnormalities. The external genital organs are male, but the testes are atrophic and puberty is either delayed or incomplete. Defects in the structure of the penis also occur. Usually no spermatozoa are produced, and the individual is sterile. The body configuration is somewhat feminine and "long-legged," and there may be moderate breast hypertrophy. Learning disabilities and delayed language development occur, although intellectual disability is uncommon.

XYY Syndrome

The sex chromosomal abnormality known as XYY syndrome has an incidence of about 1 in 1000 male births. The individuals are usually taller than normal, but there are no specific abnormalities of body configuration or fertility. Delayed development of motor and language skills may occur along with behavioral and emotional difficulties, but intelligence is usually in the normal range. Autism disorders infrequently occur, and this may interfere with social interaction; however, individuals (contrary to early popular reports) are not aggressive.

Fragile X Syndrome

The condition called the fragile X syndrome is second only to Down syndrome as a major cause of mental retardation and is related to defects in the FMR1 (for **F**ragile X **M**ental **R**etardation-**1**), or simply fragile X, gene. The name derives from the fact that affected chromosomes show an inducible defect during karyotype studies, which cause a fragile, constricted area to form at the tip of the long arm of the X chromosome. The observed defect relates to expansion of a group of cytosine–guanine–guanine repeating sequences (CGG repeats) that occur at the beginning of the FMR1 gene (and are not translated into protein). Normal individuals have about 30 repeats, and affected individuals with full mutations have 200 to 4000 repeats. The genetics of the disease is complex and does not follow simple Mendelian rules. Carrier individuals have 60 to 200 repeats, a condition termed a premutation, and are not affected. However, premutations are unstable and tend to grow from generation to generation as they are passed from father to grandchild through a female. The tendency for a mutation to become worse with each generation is termed genetic anticipation. The disease is expressed more frequently in males with full mutations than in females (for unknown reasons). About 1 in 1600 males versus 1 in 8000 females is affected. Affected females generally have a milder form of the disease. About half of females heterozygous for a chromosome with the full mutation express the disease.

The great excess of CGG repeats causes intellectual disability because the large number of repeats blocks the function of the gene. As a result, no gene product is produced, interfering with the formation and function of synapses within the nervous system, which is the apparent cause of mental retardation. Individuals with severe forms of the disease have markedly reduced IQs, a very long face with out-turned ears, and notably very large testicles (macroorchidism). Although karyotype analysis was initially used to define the disease, modern techniques rely on molecular studies of the structure of the gene and, in particular, the number of CGG repeats.

Autosomal Abnormalities

The presence of more than two copies of an autosome (trisomy) results in severe congenital abnormalities. Absence of an autosome (monosomy) results in the loss of so many genes that development is generally not possible and the embryo is aborted. Deletion of a small part of an autosome may be compatible with development, but it usually results in multiple severe congenital abnormalities in the infant. The most common autosomal trisomy seen in newborn infants is that of the small chromosome 21, which causes Down syndrome. Less frequent trisomy of a larger chromosome, such as chromosome 13 or chromosome 18, is associated with multiple severe congenital malformations. Trisomy of other large autosomes is almost invariably lethal.

Down Syndrome

Down syndrome, the most common chromosomal abnormality, with an incidence of about 1 in 1600 births (depending in large part on the age of the mother), is characterized by mental deficiency and a characteristic facial expression caused by the upward-slanting eyes and the prominent skin folds extending from the base of the nose to the inner aspects of the eyebrows (**Figure 3-10**). Other abnormalities of body form also are seen, including a protruding tongue and abnormal palmar creases. Congenital cardiac malformations occur frequently, as do major congenital defects in other organ systems. Acute lymphoblastic leukemia is a common occurrence, and early degenerative neurological changes similar to Alzheimer's disease are seen by age 40. The reported incidence represents only the proportion of abnormal fetuses surviving to term. About 75 percent of trisomy 21 fetuses do not survive to be liveborn, and 25 percent die in the first year of life.

Down syndrome may arise from nondisjunction during gametogenesis, or translocation, or nondisjunction in zygote development. In about 95 percent of cases, Down syndrome results from nondisjunction of chromosome 21 during the first meiotic division of the oocytes in the female. Fertilization by a normal sperm produces a zygote containing 47 chromosomes, with chromosome 21 being present in triplicate. Down syndrome resulting from nondisjunction during oogenesis increases in frequency with advancing

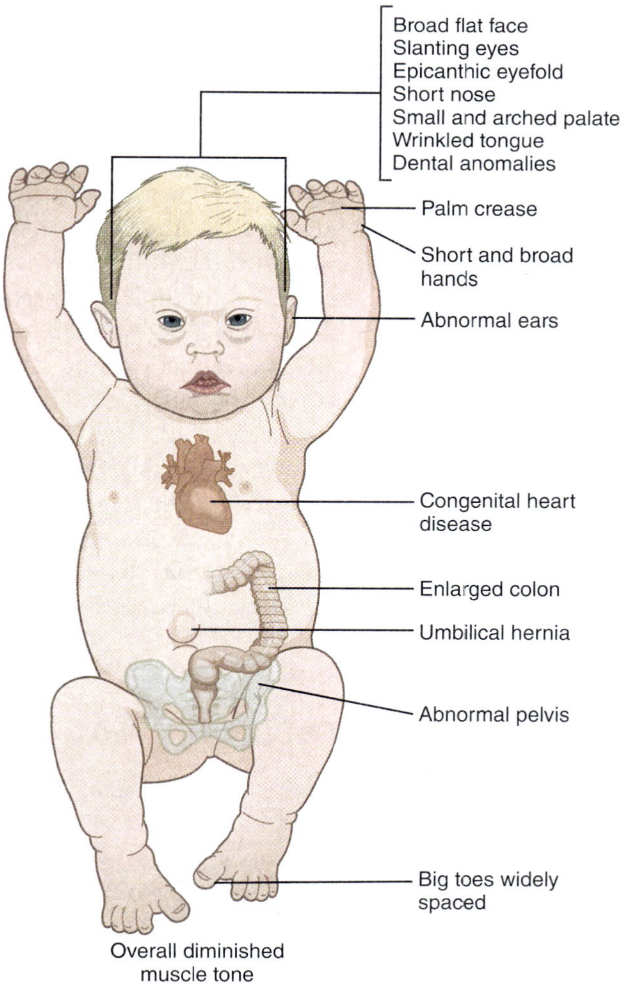

Figure 3-10 Child with Down syndrome.

maternal age. The incidence is as high as 1 in 60 in the offspring of women over 40 years of age, but even very young mothers can have Down offspring. Trisomy 21 occurs in 1 in 1000 births in women between 25 and 29 years of age.

In a small number of people with Down syndrome, the extra chromosome 21 is attached to another chromosome, usually chromosome 14. Although the total number of chromosomes is not increased in these individuals, one of the chromosomes is actually a composite chromosome resulting from the fusion of chromosome 21 with another chromosome; consequently, the affected person has extra genetic material derived from chromosome 21. The recognition of a translocation carrier is important because the carrier is capable of transmitting the abnormal chromosome to the carrier's children, resulting in translocation Down syndrome. However, the translocation chromosome is not always transmitted, as shown in Figure 3-8, which demonstrates the possible outcome of a pregnancy involving a female carrier of a 14/21 translocation chromosome.

In some individuals with Down syndrome, only some of the cells exhibit the characteristic trisomy 21 (i.e., they are mosaic for Down syndrome). Mosaic Down syndrome results from nondisjunction during mitosis of a normal cell to form a trisomy 21 cell and another cell lacking chromosome 21, which does not survive. Both the normal cells and the trisomy 21 cells continue to proliferate, and both cell populations are present in the developing embryo, as illustrated in Figure 3-9. Individuals with mosaic Down syndrome tend to suffer less disability than those in whom all of the cells contain an extra chromosome 21.

Because Down syndrome is frequent (particularly in the offspring of older mothers) and is associated with both mental and physical disabilities in the conceptus, prenatal screening for Down syndrome should be offered to all pregnant females. Such prenatal screening does not presuppose any particular choice by the parents who might choose to terminate the pregnancy or to carry the pregnancy to term. In the latter case, both the medical staff and parents are better able to cope with the difficulties associated with a Down neonate. Prenatal screening tests are complex and depend on biochemical markers in the mother's blood and imaging studies of the fetus. This combination results in an 85 percent detection rate and a 5 percent false-positive rate. Sampling the fetal material (either obtained by amniotic fluid or chorionic villus sampling) provides more definitive information using either karyotypic or molecular testing of fetal cells and has a very low risk to the fetus. Recent advances (discussed in Chapter 15) allow fetal DNA to be sampled directly from the maternal circulation, obviating the need for invasive procedures. Tests using such technology have proven extremely accurate for Down syndrome, with 99 percent detection rates and nearly undetectable false positives.

Genetically Transmitted Diseases

Genetically transmitted diseases are the result of abnormalities of individual genes on the chromosome. Most of these diseases are transmitted on autosomes. A few are carried on sex chromosomes (**Table 3-3**). The chromosomes and the karyotype appear normal; however, using modern molecular techniques, defects in chromosome or gene structure (e.g., small deletions or mutations) have been recognized in association with such diseases. Transmission of the abnormal gene is from parent to offspring, following well-established patterns of inheritance.

Table 3-3 Mode of Inheritance, Pathogenesis, and Major Manifestations of Some Common Genetic Diseases

Abnormality	Mode of Inheritance	Defect	Manifestations
Phenylketonuria	Recessive	Phenylalanine hydroxylase deficiency	Intellectual disability
Tay-Sachs disease	Recessive	Hexosaminidase A deficiency	Intellectual disability, motor weakness, blindness
Cystic fibrosis	Recessive	Dysfunction of mucous and sweat glands; thick mucus obstructs bronchioles, pancreatic ducts, and bile ducts	Chronic bronchopulmonary infections as a result of bronchial obstruction by mucus; pancreatic and liver dysfunction as a result of thick mucus obstruction of excretory ducts
Achondroplasia	Dominant	Disordered bone growth at ends of long bones (epiphyses)	Dwarfism with disproportionately short limbs
Congenital polycystic kidney disease	Dominant	Maldevelopment of nephrons and collecting tubules causes formation of multiple cysts in kidneys	Renal failure
Multiple neurofibromatosis	Dominant	Multiple tumors arise from peripheral nerves	Disfigurement and deformities caused by tumors; predisposition to malignant change in tumors
Sickle cell trait	Codominant	Red cells contain mixture of normal (A) and sickle (S) hemoglobin	None
Sickle cell anemia	Codominant	Red cells contain no normal hemoglobin	Severe anemia and obstruction of blood flow to organs by masses of sickled red cells
Hemophilia	X-linked recessive	Deficiency of protein required for normal coagulation of blood	Uncontrolled bleeding into joints and internal organs after minor injuries

Genes direct many functions within the cell. Some genes direct the synthesis of proteins. These may be proteins that form the structure of the cell (structural proteins) or enzymes that are necessary for cell function. Other genes function by regulating the activity of the genes that direct protein synthesis or are associated with the production of a variety of RNA species. Normally, genes in the germline are stable and are passed without change from parent to offspring. Occasionally, a gene undergoes a change called a gene mutation, which may occur spontaneously or as a result of exposure to chemicals or radiation. After a mutation has occurred in a germ cell, it can be transmitted from parent to offspring.

Sometimes, a gene mutation that induces only a minor change in the structure of a protein may cause a serious change in its properties. For example, sickle hemoglobin (hemoglobin S) differs from normal hemoglobin (hemoglobin A) only in a single amino acid, but it undergoes polymerization within the red blood cells when the oxygen content of the blood is reduced, leading to sickling and compromise to the circulation system.

If a mutation involves genes that control the synthesis of an enzyme, the enzyme may be defective and may lack normal functional activity. Metabolic processes regulated by the enzyme are disturbed, and the cell is unable to function normally.

The traditional diagnostic approach to genetic disease, based on the principles of classic genetics, is directed toward first identifying the abnormality in the patient; then identifying the gene product (most often a protein) that is responsible for the disease, such as an abnormal hemoglobin or an enzyme deficiency; and finally, attempting to identify the gene responsible for the abnormal gene product that caused the cell dysfunction. More recently, as a result of a better understanding of the sequence of DNA that constitutes the normal genome, there has been a shift toward molecular genetics approaches. Often the technique is to search for associations between the disease trait and other well-defined DNA markers that vary in populations (polymorphisms). Such polymorphisms occur throughout the entire human genome and serve as landmarks for such studies. For example, imagine that there is a polymorphism in a DNA sequence within or near a gene for a hemoglobin that has two detectable forms: A and B. If, within families, the presence of an unknown disease trait follows that of the marker (i.e., segregates with the marker) such that everyone in the family who has the disease also has marker A or B, it is likely that the gene for the unknown disease is located near (or perhaps contains) the marker. If we know where the marker is located in the genome (in this case hemoglobin), we then know that the gene for the new disease is near the gene for hemoglobin. The tendency for genes (or even noncoding segments of DNA) physically close in the genome to move together (i.e., to be inherited together) is termed linkage. Many complex statistical approaches are available for investigating these associations in many families and even in large groups of unrelated individuals and are called **genome-wide association studies (GWAS)**. Having identified the location of the mutation, the human genetic map is searched to determine what genes are located at that position. One can then sequence such genes from individuals with the disease to determine how they differ from the normal gene, then determine the product of the gene, and finally evaluate how the abnormal gene and its gene product disrupt the functions of the cell. This approach has led to great advances in the prenatal diagnosis of many genetic diseases, as described later in Chapter 16.

Genome-wide association studies (GWAS) Process using tests of many SNPs (single nucleotide polymorphisms) to identify genes associated with particular diseases or traits.

Autosomal Dominant Inheritance

A dominant gene expresses itself in the heterozygous state. If either parent carries an abnormal dominant gene, either the abnormal gene or the corresponding normal allele may be passed to the offspring. Consequently, there is one chance in two that the offspring will receive the abnormal gene and will be affected by the hereditary disease. A common example of a genetic disease transmitted in this manner is achondroplasia, a type of dwarfism in which the limbs are disproportionately short (discussed in Chapter 24). A second example is a type of autosomal dominant kidney disease (adult polycystic kidney disease), which is characterized by the formation of multiple cysts throughout both kidneys that progressively enlarge and eventually destroy renal function (discussed in Chapter 17). A third genetic disease of this type is multiple neurofibromatosis, a condition characterized by the formation of multiple tumors that arise from peripheral nerves (discussed in Chapter 23).

Autosomal Recessive Inheritance

A trait transmitted as an autosomal recessive is expressed only in the homozygous individual. Many diseases characterized by an enzyme deficiency within the cell are transmitted in this manner. The disease occurs only if both alleles are abnormal and no enzyme is produced. Therefore, for the offspring to be affected, both parents must carry the abnormal gene, and both must transmit the gene to the offspring. When the mutation is uncommon, it is likely that the parents are related and that the mutation is common by descent to both. Hence, inbreeding, mating with individuals who are closely related genetically, raises concerns. When both parents carry an abnormal recessive gene, there is one chance in four that the mother will give birth to an abnormal infant who is homozygous for the defective gene. If only one parent transmits the recessive gene, the infant will be a carrier of the abnormal gene but will be normal because the normal allele will direct the synthesis of enough enzymes to keep the cell functioning normally. The many recognized types of genetically determined enzyme defects are sometimes called inborn errors of metabolism. Two of the more important ones are phenylketonuria and Tay-Sachs disease.

Phenylketonuria

Phenylalanine is an essential amino acid present in dietary protein. Much of it is converted in the body to tyrosine, which the body uses to make thyroid hormone, melanin, and other important compounds. A deficiency of the enzyme phenylalanine hydroxylase, which is required for normal metabolism of the phenylalanine, causes a disease called phenylketonuria. The enzyme deficiency causes no difficulty while the infant is still within the uterus being nourished by the mother. Soon after birth, however, the infant begins to drink milk. Because milk protein contains abundant phenylalanine, which the infant is unable to metabolize, this amino acid accumulates in the infant's blood and is excreted in the urine. The affected infant is able to convert some phenylalanine into phenylpyruvic acid (and other metabolites) by means of other metabolic pathways that do not require phenylalanine hydroxylase (**Figure 3-11**). Phenylpyruvic acid accumulates in the blood and is excreted in the urine along with phenylalanine. Permanent mental deficiency results from the disturbed phenylalanine metabolism, but it can be prevented by restricting the dietary intake of phenylalanine in the developing child. Phenylketonuria can be detected in the newborn infant by means of a screening

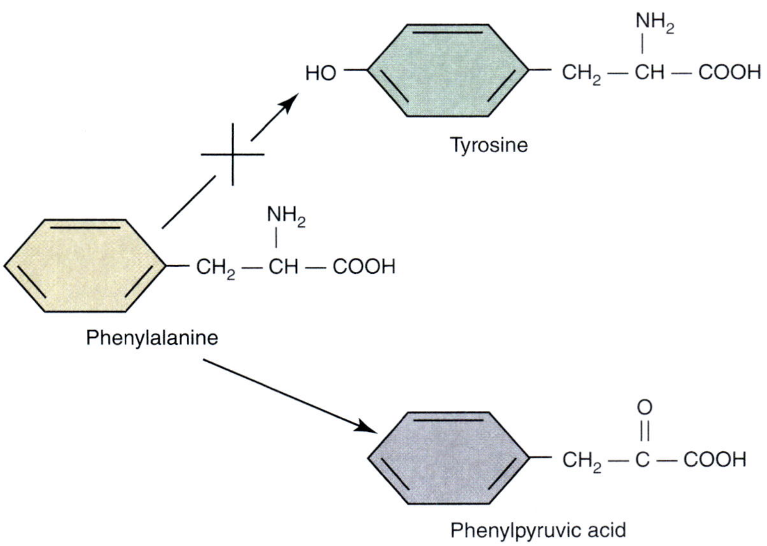

Figure 3-11 Metabolic detects in phenylketonuria. Infants with this disorder lack the enzyme phenylalanine hydroxylase, and their bodies are unable to hydroxylate phenylalanine to form tyrosine. Some phenylalanine is converted into phenylpyuvic acid (substitution of a keto group for the amino group in the molecule) by other metabolic pathways. Permanent mental deficiency results from disturbed phenylalanine metabolism and can be prevented by restricting dietary intake of phenylalanine.

laboratory test capable of detecting the elevated level of phenylalanine in the blood. Because this disease is a cause of preventable mental deficiency, a routine screening test to detect phenylketonuria (as well as many other inborn errors of metabolism) is required for all newborn infants.

Tay-Sachs Disease

Tay-Sachs disease occurs in the offspring of parents who carry the defective gene. The carrier rate is relatively high in some Jewish populations (those of Eastern European origin). In these groups, about 1 in 30 individuals carry the abnormal gene; however, other population groups also carry the gene at a high frequency (such as Cajuns and French Canadians).

The clinical manifestations result from absence of a lysosomal enzyme called hexosaminidase A. The enzyme deficiency causes a lipid called a ganglioside to accumulate within the lysosomes of nerve cells in the brain, spinal cord, autonomic nervous system, and the retina of the eye, causing cell dysfunction and, eventually, degeneration of the affected nerve cells. Clinically, the disease is characterized by progressive mental deterioration, neurologic dysfunction, and blindness. Onset of symptoms begins by about 6 months of age, and the disease is invariably fatal by the time the child is 3 or 4 years old.

Carriers of the abnormal gene can be detected by means of the low levels of hexosaminidase A in their serum and in their leukocytes. Tests for this enzyme can be used for screening. Tay-Sachs disease can be diagnosed prenatally by examining fetal cells obtained by amniocentesis.

Other Genetic Diseases

Two other relatively common and important diseases transmitted by autosomal recessive inheritance are cystic fibrosis and hemochromatosis. Cystic fibrosis is manifested by dysfunction of mucous and sweat glands related to a defective sodium ion transporter gene (cystic fibrosis transmembrane conductance regulator [CFTR]). The result of the defect is that mucous secretions in many organs of the body are abnormally viscid and tend to mechanically interfere with organ function. The most serious effect is recurrent infections of the lung that result in difficult-to-treat pneumonia and eventual loss of lung function. Plugging of the pancreas by thick secretions leads to loss of pancreatic secretions and defective digestion. Cystic fibrosis is the most common lethal autosomal recessive in White populations, with a gene frequency of about 1 in 30, but it is extremely rare in Black populations. Hemochromatosis is characterized by excessive absorption of iron that accumulates within the body and disrupts the function of the liver, heart, and other organs (discussed in Chapter 10).

Codominant Inheritance

In codominant inheritance, both alleles of a pair are fully expressed in the heterozygous state. This type of transmission is illustrated by the genes responsible for the synthesis of sickle (S) hemoglobin and other abnormal hemoglobins. These genes are abnormal alleles of the gene that directs the synthesis of normal hemoglobin. An individual heterozygous for the sickle hemoglobin gene will have approximately equal quantities of sickle hemoglobin and normal hemoglobin in the red cells. This condition is called sickle cell trait and usually causes no difficulties. Significant clinical manifestations are apparent, however, if the individual is homozygous for the sickle cell gene, resulting in no normal hemoglobin. This leads to a serious hereditary anemia called sickle cell anemia (discussed in Chapter 10).

X-Linked Inheritance

A number of hereditary diseases are transmitted on the X chromosome. The best-known examples are the two forms of the disease hemophilia (hemophilia A and B), which are caused by deficiencies of proteins necessary for normal blood coagulation (F.VIII and F.IX, respectively). Hemophilia is described in Chapter 10.

Mitochondria Inheritance and Related Diseases

Chromosomes are not the only site where genes are located in the cell. Mitochondria, the site of oxidative metabolism and ATP generation in the cell, also have small amounts of DNA containing some of the genes required for synthesis of energy-generating mitochondrial proteins. The DNA in mitochondria is circular and has several similarities to the DNA found in bacteria. These similarities have led to the suggestion that mitochondria are derived during evolution from trapped bacteria.

Although most of the genes involved in ATP synthesis are located on the chromosomes in the cell nuclei and are inherited like other genes, some of the ATP-generating components are coded as mitochondrial genes and are inherited differently from those on chromosomes. As mitochondria wear out, other mitochondria divide to replace them. Mutations occur frequently as the mitochondrial DNA duplicates (replicates). Because there are several mitochondrial DNA molecules in each mitochondrion and several hundred mitochondria in an active cell, a cell may contain a mixture of normal mitochondria and mitochondria containing mutated DNA. Mitochondrial DNA mutations do not affect cell function unless there are such a large number of mitochondrial DNA mutations that the energy-generating capability of the cells is impaired.

The human ovum contains a very large number of mitochondria, but sperm contains very few. Consequently, transmission of abnormal mitochondrial DNA is almost invariably from mother to child. A number of rare diseases result from inherited abnormalities of mitochondrial DNA, with the severity of the disease manifestations related in part to the number of mutated mitochondria. Although mitochondrial DNA is not unique to an individual, mitochondrial DNA has proven useful in identifying the relationship of an individual to a family. Because there are multiple copies of the mitochondrial genome in cells, useful samples are often obtainable from decomposed or skeletal remains.

Mitochondrial disorders often affect multiple organ systems and manifest prominent neurologic and myopathic features. Mitochondrial dysfunction can be observed in early childhood and progress throughout adulthood. Some commonly seen mitochondria-associated diseases include Leber Hereditary Optic Neuropathy (LHON), which leads to a loss of vision in both eyes; Kearns-Sayre syndrome, which is manifested as bilateral deafness, myopathy, and dementia. In Leigh Syndrome, subacute relapsing encephalopathy with infantile onset can be observed.

Epigenetics

The development of human disease cannot always be attributed to the compositions/sequences of the genes and their inheritance; other factors are also involved. **Epigenetics** is the study of identifying such factors.

Epi in Greek means "above". Epigenetics refers to the factors/mechanisms that are acting "above" the DNA by "turning on" or "turning off" genes without changing the sequence of DNA. The term was first coined by Conrad Waddington.

Epigenetics Mechanisms that control gene expression independent of the base code of DNA.

Epigenetics plays important roles in human health. In recent years, studies have shown epigenetic processes are involved in learning, stress response, and physical activities. They are also involved in disease development, including neuron degenerative disorders such as Alzheimer's and Parkinson's diseases.

How epigenetics regulates **gene expression** is not completely understood. The most studied and well accepted mechanisms include methylation of DNA, modification of histones, and interference of non-coding RNA, such as small regulatory **micro-RNA (miRNA)**. These factors, together with other unknown factors, determine genes to be in an "open" state (accessible and can be transcribed) or a "closed" state (un-accessible and cannot be transcribed).

Gene expression The production of a product by a gene.

Micro-RNA (miRNA) Small RNA molecules that regulate the activity of sets of individual genes.

Exome The totality of sequences in the genome that code for proteins.

Growth factor A soluble growth-promoting substance produced by cells that attaches to receptors on the cell membrane of other cells, which activates the receptors and initiates events leading to growth or division of the target cells.

Bioinformatics A fast-evolving field that uses tools from multiple disciplines, such as computer science, mathematics, and statistics to collect, store, analyze, and interpret data in biological systems.

Genomics Bioinformatic techniques applied to studies of human genome.

New Research on Genes

Starting with the Human Genome Project in 1990, tremendous strides have been made in our ability to determine the entire sequence of DNA in individuals. Currently, limited regions of the genome of individuals are sequenced using automated technology on a routine basis to obtain information for clinical diagnosis of disease and as an aid in selecting therapies. Major medical centers are beginning to routinely sequence multiple genes in individuals with a variety of cancers to determine genetic lesions involved in the causation and progress of the disease. It is now possible to sequence all protein coding regions of a person's genome (**exome** sequencing) and the entire genome, including all DNA base sequences for a cost of about $1,000 in a matter of days. This ability has led to the concept of personalized therapy in which specific drugs are matched to defects in genes responsible for particular diseases (so-called drugable genes). As previously noted, defects in **growth factors** and receptors may lead to unregulated cell growth and cancer. In many cases, the specific defect in the genome (mutation) responsible for unregulated growth may be determined by sequencing, allowing drugs to be tailored to inhibit the defect and slow down (although not as yet cure) the disease. Differences in how individuals respond to drugs are often related to variation in specific genes in the genome. Technology exists to detect those differences and tailor drug therapy to prevent inappropriate dosing, which can result in dangerous drug reactions.

As noted, the sequence of all expressed genes (the exome) or even the 3 billion base pairs of a single individual, can be determined. This has led to massive databases available for study and to the development of the study of **bioinformatics**. Bioinformatics as applied to studies of the human genome (**genomics** is a commonly used term for such) involves complex mathematical comparisons between data from the genome of many individuals to find base sequences that may be associated with the susceptibility to disease (or to resistance to particular diseases). Obviously, such information can be used for the prognosis, early therapy, or, potentially, the prevention of diseases in the human population. The availability of complete DNA sequences from essentially all animal species, multiple human populations, and sequence data from the preserved DNA found by paleontologists in the remains of early human (Cro-Magnon) and human-like groups (Neanderthals and Denisovans) has revolutionized our understanding of human evolution and the origin of populations.

Single Nucleotide Polymorphisms

The sequence of base pairs in the human genome is about 99.9 percent identical between humans. (In comparison, we differ from our closest primate cousin by about 4 percent.) At the gross level, human genomes appear to be nearly identical, but the remaining 0.1 percent of 3 billion base pairs (about 3 million base pairs) are different. In fact, as is familiar to all from popular media productions involving the science of forensics, no two individuals have exactly the same genome except identical twins. Determination of identity does not require complex sequencing of the genome because particular regions of DNA show great variation. Simple technology allows rapid typing of individual DNA samples (from body fluids or tissue such as hair) in a manner somewhat analogous to blood typing.

Many of the minor variations in the nucleotides contained in the individual genes of different individuals may or may not have direct significance. These variations are called **single nucleotide polymorphisms (SNPs)**, usually pronounced "snips." Some SNPs may affect how the gene functions, such as how rapidly a cell enzyme inactivates a drug or environmental toxin or repairs damage to cell DNA. Genes in individuals within specific groups having risk factors for some disease or condition can be analyzed (constructing a "gene profile") to see if there is a correlation with particular SNPs. Although some SNPs lie within genes and may directly affect how a gene functions, many SNPs occur in the 98 percent of the genome that does not contain genes expressing a protein product. Such SNPs are important because their position within the genome is known and also because they easily can be typed without the need for direct DNA sequencing. This has allowed for the ever-increasing use of genome-wide association studies (GWAS) to identify genes associated with particular diseases or traits. In such studies, the frequency of a very large number of SNPs spread across the entire genome is compared between a population with the particular condition or disease and a control population without the disease. Statistical studies are undertaken to see if the presence of particular SNPs correlates with the presence (or absence) of the disease in question. Because the position of the SNPs in the genome is known, an association suggests areas of the genome (or particular genes) that are associated with the condition. GWAS are particularly useful in studying complex chronic conditions such as heart disease and neuropsychiatric disorders that may be associated with differences in multiple genes found in different areas of the genome.

Single nucleotide polymorphisms (SNPs) Minor variations in the nucleotides contained in the individual genes of different individuals.

Recombinant DNA technology/genetic engineering/gene splicing Methods for combining a gene from one organism, such as a gene specifying insulin synthesis, with genes from another organism, such as a bacterium.

Expression vector A set of DNA sequences necessary for the expression of a foreign gene in an organism, such as a plasmid. Often engineered to promote high levels of production of the gene product.

Genes and Recombinant DNA Technology (Genetic Engineering)

Overuse of terms such as **recombinant DNA technology** (because genes from two different sources are being recombined in a single unit), **genetic engineering** (because genes are being manipulated), or **gene splicing** (because genetic material is being reassembled in a given order) has made the terms both difficult to define and of limited utility. At its heart, genetic engineering involves the techniques used to manipulate how and where individual genes and their products are expressed and to modify such genes to produce products of desired characteristics. The initial stages of the technology involved understanding how bacterial genes and their products could be manipulated. Currently gene products derived from viruses, bacteria, fungi, and higher organisms can be manipulated to be expressed in essentially any host cell desired. When the product is to be used for human therapy (such as human growth factors, or proteins involved in coagulation used to treat deficiency diseases), the source of the gene coding for the product is most often human. The source is inserted into an **expression vector**, a cassette of DNA sequences necessary for expression of the gene, which in turn is introduced into a mammalian cell grown in culture for expression. Both the gene and the expression vector are

Monoclonal antibodies Antibodies with a unique specificity for use in treating human disease, produced in tissue culture from a single clone of immune cells.

Gene therapy A process of editing a mutated gene in the cell with the objective of curing its associated diseases.

optimized to result in high levels of expression and increased stability of the desired product, which optimally will be secreted into the medium in which the mammalian cells are growing. An exception to the use of human genes is in the production of antibodies of a unique specificity (**monoclonal antibodies**) for use in treating human disease. Very often the gene may be derived from a mouse immunized to produce the desired antibody. A common example is antibodies to human inflammatory proteins used to treat diseases such as rheumatoid arthritis (which results in chronic joint inflammation). Because the use of animal proteins in a human may result in a serious immunological reaction, the mouse genes are altered to make them more "humanlike" before they are expressed, although, when available, monoclonal antibodies derived from human antibody-producing cells are preferred treatment.

It is also possible to introduce genes into living organisms or to control the expression of genes in an organism. Scientists talk about "knock-ins" and "knockouts" of genes to create experimental models of human disease by either knocking out (removing) a particular animal gene or by knocking in (adding) a defective human gene. Such models can be used to study the pathogenesis of a disease and potential therapies without endangering human patients. For example, animal models of hemophilia are widely used to study disease and potential cures. Although news accounts of animals made to "glow" by the introduction of fluorescent proteins trivialize this now widely used technique, the approach can be used to cure diseases associated with the deficiency of a protein related to a genetic mutation (so-called **gene therapy**). A prime example of this would be the introduction of the gene for a clotting factor into an individual with hemophilia. The area is complex and is only beginning to demonstrate clinical success. The obvious problems with this approach include the following:

1. One must identify and select the correct gene to insert into the cell.
2. One must choose the proper cell to receive the gene.
3. One must select an efficient means of getting the gene into the cell.
4. One must ensure that the newly inserted gene can function effectively long enough within the cell to make the therapy worthwhile and that it doesn't disrupt other important cell functions.

The gene may be expressed in a small segment of DNA that does not become a permanent part of the genome (and tends to be lost with time), or it may be integrated into the chromosome much as some viral DNAs become part of the human genome. As can be imagined, insertion of DNA into the genome at random can have serious consequences by interrupting the synthesis of other genes. In summary, although many of the pieces of this technology are present, putting the pieces together for successful human therapy is only now beginning to be achieved, most notably in the treatment of hemophilia. Proposed gene therapy in humans targets somatic cells, not the germ cells that produce eggs and sperm. Gene therapy directed at germ cells is currently not considered to be feasible, ethical, or desirable.

A recent advanced tool termed CRISPR-Cas9 has shown great promise as a "gene editing" system (and with some dismay as a possible means to "customize" the human genome so as to produce what are sometimes called "designer babies"). The system allows DNA to be cut at any desired location to insert a new DNA sequence at that site. The CRISPR part of the system contains an RNA sequence that is homologous (pairs with) the desired target DNA sequence. The Cas9 part is a bacterial nuclease (DNA-cutting enzyme) that cuts both strands of the target DNA at the desired site. The tool uses the normal DNA repair systems in cells that "fix the cut DNA," either introducing errors that result in a gene knockout or knocking in a desired DNA sequence at the target site. Although the system has been used to edit genes in a developing human fetus in a very preliminary and much criticized human experiment, animal experiments have been successful in curing a mouse model of hemophilia by inserting the correct human gene into newborn mice. The system will undoubtedly be used in the future for gene therapy.

An often ignored aspect of genetic engineering is the ability to chemically synthesize "artificial" segments of DNA or to modify segments of naturally occurring gene sequences to serve as diagnostic tools. The area is very complex but relies on the ability of DNA sequences to bind (hybridize) specifically to their complement. For example, if one wished to detect a pathogen in human samples (e.g., the TB bacteria), one would label a complementary sequence (a probe) for a common gene found in the bacterium that could detect the target organism's DNA. Thus, one can label a relatively short segment of "manufactured" DNA with an indicator (such as a fluorescent dye or enzyme) and use the probe to detect a complementary DNA sequence in a sample by its ability to bind and "light up." This technique is often used in the microbiology laboratory to diagnose the presence of an infectious agent in a human sample. Manufactured small stretches of DNA that subtend an area of the genome can be used to artificially amplify the subtended area up to millions of times, greatly increasing the sensitivity of detection. The most common amplification of technology is the **polymerase chain reaction (PCR)**. Using such technology, the HIV viral genes can be amplified to a level where even 50 copies of the viral genome can be detected in a single milliliter of patient blood.

Polymerase chain reaction (PCR) Technology used to amplify stretches of DNA.

The ability to use such technology raises difficult ethical questions, not only for the molecular biologist but for all of us who potentially might benefit. How much manipulation of human embryos is appropriate? Many would say yes to techniques aimed at curing genetic disease, but what about manipulating cosmetic factors such as attempting to increase muscle mass, height, eye color, or intelligence? Such questions most certainly will occur in the future.

Case 3-1

Hemophilia B results from a mutation of the F.IX B gene, causing a decrease in the ability of the F.IX protein to function in coagulation. At the age of 18 months, a female child (individual II.2 in the pedigree (**Case Figure 3-1**) fell while playing with her fraternal twin sister and hit her knee on a table leg. She suffered a serious bleeding event in the injured knee joint that required hospital therapy. At that time, she was found to have a F.IX level 2 percent of normal and was diagnosed as being a female with hemophilia B. She required therapy with recombinant F.IX.

The family history indicated that her father (individual I.1 in the pedigree) also has the bleeding disease hemophilia B. Because his F.IX activity is less than 1 percent of normal levels, he requires therapy with human recombinant F.IX produced using genetic engineering technology in animal cells grown in tissue culture. If not treated, he suffers from spontaneous bleeding into his joints (**hemarthrosis**), which ultimately can result in severe joint damage. He is also at risk for life-threatening hemorrhages in his brain. His wife (individual I.2) has no bleeding tendencies and has normal levels of F.IX (about 100 percent of normal). She has no family history of bleeding diseases.

Hemarthrosis Arthritic condition caused by bleeding into the joint.

The parents have two offspring (II.1 and II.3) in addition to II.2. The older sibling (II.1) is a male with normal levels of F.IX. The younger siblings are female fraternal (not identical) twins. The sister (II.3) has not suffered from

(continues)

Case 3-1 *(Continued)*

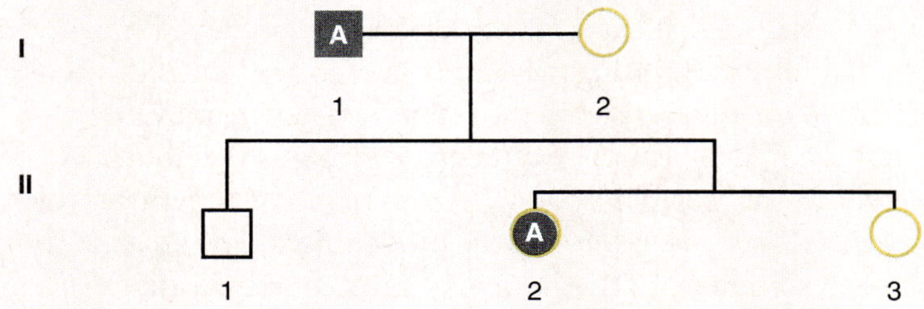

Case Figure 3-1 Case pedigree for sex-linked hemophilia B.

Courtesy of Tong Cheng.

bleeding and has a F.IX level of 60 percent, which is sufficient to provide normal coagulation. (Bleeding is usually only noted when F.IX levels are below about 20 percent of normal.) As far as could be determined, the karyotype of all members of the family (including II.2) was normal.

Discussion

The normal level of F.IX in the male sibling is expected as he would have had to inherit his father's Y chromosome (to be male) and one of the mother's two normal X chromosomes. However, because hemophilia B is a recessive sex-linked disorder, all daughters of an affected father are obligate carriers (both individuals II.2 and II.3). They must inherit their father's single X chromosome, which carries the defective gene. Even as carriers, they would be expected to be normal (in terms of hemophilia B), having inherited one of their mother's normal X chromosomes as well as their father's mutated X chromosome. However, individual II.2 is not normal.

Female hemophiliacs do occur occasionally in families in which defects of the Factor IX gene are found. There are two general reasons this might occur.

1. Suppose the mother was actually not normal but a carrier for hemophilia B. In such a case, daughter II.2 would have received her father's affected X chromosome and had a 50 percent chance of inheriting her mother's single affected X chromosome. If she had, II.2 would be homozygous for a mutation in the F.IX gene and expected to be affected. In this case, this is unlikely because the mother's family did not demonstrate a history of bleeding disease, and her normal level of F.IX strongly argues against her being an unknown carrier. However, females with homozygous hemophilia are known to occur (although very rarely).
2. A more likely reason for the low level of F.IX in II.2 is nonrandom X chromosome inactivation. As noted in this chapter, about half the cells in a female should have the paternally derived X chromosome inactivated and half the maternally derived chromosome. However, random inactivation does not always occur. A number of defects in the structure of the X chromosome (such as certain deletions and other chromosomal abnormalities) can result in the faulty chromosome being selectively inactivated. In such a case, if the structurally defective chromosome was from the mother (and hence normal in terms of the F.IX gene), the father's chromosome (carrying the hemophilia B gene) might be selectively expressed.

To determine whether nonrandom X inactivation did occur, the distribution of active maternal and paternal X chromosomes in the patient was examined using an X-linked SNP, which could differentiate the maternal and paternal X chromosomes of the patient. Ninety-seven percent of X chromosome product bearing the SNP in II.2 was from the paternal (affected) chromosome. In the unaffected twin sibling (II.3), the distribution was nearly random (about 40 percent was from the affected paternal chromosome).

Etiology and Pathogenesis

The most likely cause of female hemophilia in II.2 was extreme nonrandom X inactivation resulting in overrepresentation of the paternal X chromosome bearing a mutated Factor IX gene. However, this conclusion does not explain why this occurred in II.2 but not her sister, II.3. The great majority of female hemophiliacs result from unbalanced nonrandom X chromosome inactivation with no evidence of defects in the structure of the X chromosomes.

Questions

1. Suppose the mother in the family was a carrier of hemophilia B. How would this change the probability of disease in the offspring (and in future offspring)?
2. If the twins (II.2 and II.3) were identical, would this change your explanation for the occurrence of female hemophilia?
3. It is noted that recombinant human F.IX was used in therapy for affected individuals in the family. Why might recombinant human F.IX be preferable to F.IX isolated from pools of human blood?

Courtesy of Howard M. Reisner.

Questions for Review

1. What is meant by the following terms: homologous chromosomes, autosomes, Barr body, gene, gametogenesis, and exome?
2. What is a chromosome karyotype? How is it obtained? How is it used?
3. What pattern in a pedigree is typical of the inheritance of a recessive gene?
4. What are the consequences of chromosome nondisjunction? What is Down syndrome?
5. What are the karyotypes of an individual with Down syndrome? Klinefelter syndrome? Turner syndrome? What is fragile X syndrome?
6. What is epigenetic? Give examples of how epigenetic can impact gene expression.
7. What is a SNP? How is it used?
8. How do exomic and whole genome sequencing differ?
9. How is CRISPR-Cas9 used to edit genes?

References

The Human Genome Project. NHGRI. Accessed March 12, 2025. https://www.genome.gov/human-genome-project

- This reference provides an excellent introductory online guide to human genetics and the Human Genome Project.

Rising Tide Biology. Accessed March 12, 2025. https://www.risingtidebio.com/

Cell Gene Engineering 101. EditCo. Accessed March 12, 2025. https://www.synthego.com/resources/cell-engineering-101-ebook

- The first reference contains educational resources for those seeking more information about genetic medicine.
- The second reference is a cost-free, short e-book guide to the CRISPR-Cas9 technique that is much in the news today. It is well-illustrated and does a good job of explaining the uses and complexities of what is one of the most popular technologies currently used in gene editing.

Krebs JE, Goldstein ES, Kilpatrick ST. *Lewin's Essential GENES*. 4th ed. Jones & Bartlett Learning; 2021.

- This book provides a clear and concise overview, as well as up-to-date concepts and techniques in the area of molecular genetics. This text focuses on essential topics, background, and introductory material on the structure and function of genes and genomes and their associated cellular processes.

What are genome-wide association studies? U.S. National Library of Medicine. Accessed March 25, 2025. https://medlineplus.gov/genetics/understanding/genomicresearch/gwastudies/

Tam V, Patel N, Turcotte M, Bossé Y, Paré G, Meyre D. Benefits and limitations of genome-wide association studies. *Nat Rev Genet*. 2019;20(8):467-484.

- An introduction from the National Library of Medicine with links to other sites. The second reference is a detailed analysis of the problems associated with GWAS.

Okumura K, Fujimori Y, Takagi A, et al. Skewed X chromosome inactivation in fraternal female twins results in moderately severe and mild haemophilia B. *Haemophilia*. 2008:14(5): 1088-1093.

Snell DM, Turner JMA. Sex chromosome effects on male–female differences in mammals. *Curr Biol*. 2018;28(22):R1313-R1324.

- The first reference is the source on which the chapter case was modeled (in part) and contains additional details explaining how the pattern of X chromosome inactivation was determined in the family. The second reference provides additional information on the role of sex chromosomes in sexual dimorphism, which is far more interesting (and complex) than presented in the chapter.

Farsetti A, Illi B, Gaetano C. How epigenetics impacts on human diseases. *Eur J Intern Med*. 2023;114:15-22.

- This is a recent review about epigenetics and its role in human disease.

Wen H, Deng H, Li B, et al. Mitochondrial diseases: From molecular mechanisms to therapeutic advances. *Signal Transduct Target Ther.* 2025;10(1):9.

Aldossary AM, Tawfik, EA, Alomary MN, et al. Recent advances in mitochondrial diseases: From molecular insights to therapeutic perspectives. *Saudi Pharm J*. 2022;30(8):1065-1078.

- The first paper provides reviews of the molecular basis of mitochondrial diseases. It also lists clinical manifestations of mitochondrial diseases. The second paper discusses current therapeutic approaches, future advances, and proposed new therapeutic plans.

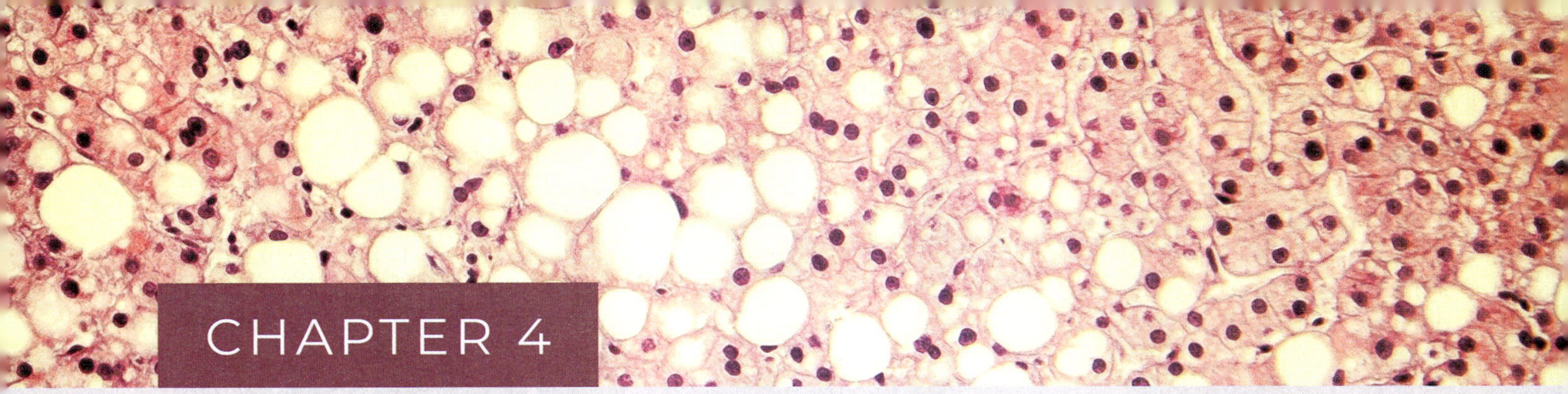

CHAPTER 4

Inflammation and Repair

LEARNING OBJECTIVES

1. Compare and contrast innate and adaptive immunity.
2. Compare and contrast acute and chronic inflammation with special attention to the timeline of the response.
3. Name the chemical mediators of inflammation. Explain how they interact to intensify the inflammatory process. Include both cell- and blood plasma–derived mediators.
4. Describe the harmful effects of inflammation. Explain why it is sometimes necessary to suppress the inflammatory process.
5. Compare inflammation and infection. Define the terms used to describe infections.

Introduction: Host Defense

The body uses two approaches to respond to cell injury: **innate immunity** and **adaptive immunity**. Both are critical, and defects in either can rapidly result in disease. Innate immunity, which an organism is born with, allows a quick response to a predetermined array of chemical signals that are associated with either invading **pathogens** (**pathogen-associated molecular patterns [PAMPs]**) or injury to cells (**damage-associated molecular patterns [DAMPs]**). The innate immune response is limited to specific PAMPs and DAMPs. DAMPs are chemicals that are released by dying or injured cells. PAMPs are a wide variety of molecules associated with pathogens. Some examples are microbial membrane components, bacterial peptides, and viral and bacterial nucleic acids. The injury-related signals are detected by specific **receptor molecules**, also called **pattern** or **pathogen recognition receptors (PRRs)**. Similar PRRs occur throughout the animal kingdom, with some related molecules that are even found in insects. There are several groups of PRRs found both on the surface and inside of human cells. A good example includes the **toll-like receptors (TLRs)**, which consist of a group of five related molecules that are integral to the cell surface and an additional group of four that are associated with intracellular components. Each TLR recognizes a specific set of PAMPs. The cytoplasmic TLRs recognize several pathogen-related components of bacteria and fungi. The intracellular TLRs recognize nucleic acids of bacteria and viruses that had reached to the cellular interior. Binding of the TLR to its specific PAMP triggers the production of a number of **cytokines**

Innate immunity Immunity present at birth and lasting a person's entire life and the first response of the body's immune system to a harmful foreign substance, non specific, no immune memory involved.

Adaptive immunity Immune response with the ability to mount an antigen specific reaction and establish immunologic memory.

Pathogens Disease-causing microorganisms.

Pathogen-Associated Molecular Patterns (PAMPs) Microbial products that stimulate innate immunity.

Damage-Associated Molecular Patterns (DAMPs) Molecules that can initiate and perpetuate immune response in the noninfectious inflammatory response.

Receptor molecules/ Pattern/Pathogen Recognition Receptors (PRRs) Receptors on cells recognizing molecular markers of disease-causing microorganism.

Toll-like receptors (TLRs) Cell surface and intracellular pathogen recognition receptors (PRRs) critical for sensing pathogens in innate immune responses.

Cytokine A general term for any protein secreted by cells that functions as an intercellular messenger and influences cells of the immune system. Cytokines are secreted by macrophages and monocytes (monokines), lymphocytes (lymphokines), and other cells.

Immune memory Enhanced and more rapid immune response upon secondary encounter with antigen in adaptive immunity.

Variable region Area on the immunoglobulin molecule specific for a particular pathogen. Amino-terminal end of the immunoglobulin chain; the part that recognizes the antigen.

Parasites Organism that lives in or on another organism, deriving nutrients at the host's expense.

Acute inflammation Earliest phase of the inflammatory response.

and interferons important in the host defense system of the cell. The second approach is termed adaptive immunity. This form of immunity can be relatively slow, but it possesses the ability to adapt itself to challenges never previously encountered by the organism. Even newly synthesized chemical toxins can be dealt with through adaptive immunity. Such new challenges trigger an immune system memory response where the adaptive response gets better with time to produce an even stronger, more specific response (**immune memory**). The PRR proteins for adaptive immunity are unique in having different **variable regions** with the potential to fit a wide variety of injurious substances. Such variable regions are found only in immunoglobulin protein molecules and on the PRRs from the T and B cells of the immune system. These adaptive immune responses are often simply termed adaptive immunity (discussed in Chapter 5). Although innate and adaptive immunity provide the "one–two punch" against tissue damage, they also often result in collateral injury to tissue or go awry and result in immune diseases.

The Inflammatory Reaction

The inflammatory reaction is part of the innate immune response to agents that cause cell injury. The agent may be physical (such as trauma, heat, or cold), chemical (such as caustic or irritating chemicals), microbiologic (such as a bacterium or virus), or **parasites**. The inflammatory reaction is characterized by predominantly local but also possible systemic effects (**Figure 4-1**).

The earliest phase of the inflammatory response, **acute inflammation**, occurs immediately after injury and lasts for 24 to 48 hours. Acute inflammation has both a vascular component (blood vessel related) and a **cellular component**, which relies on cells that circulate in the blood (**Figure 4-2**). The most important cells are **neutrophils** (polymorphonuclear leukocytes, PMNs), which are actively **phagocytic**. They engulf injurious agents (such

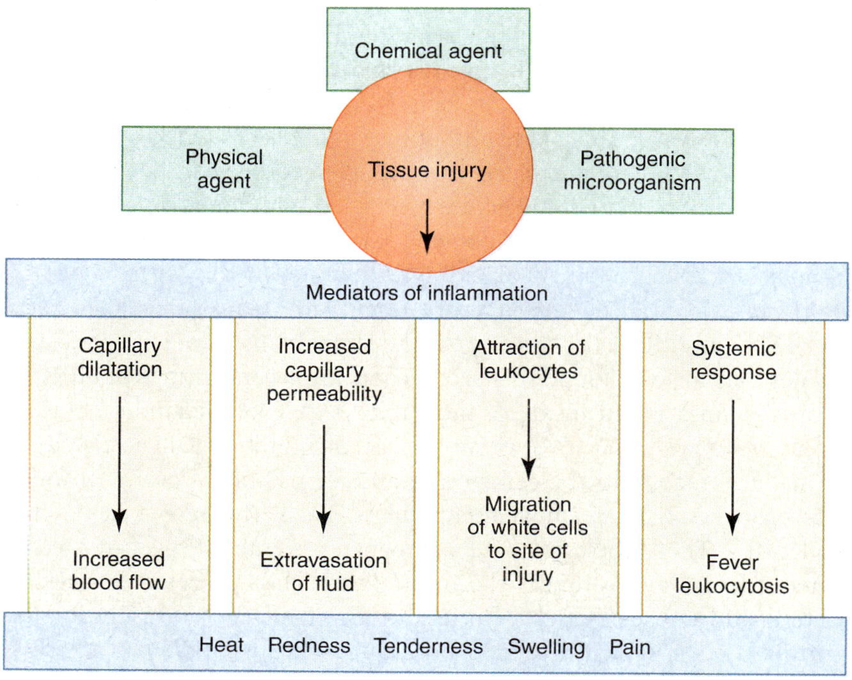

Figure 4-1 Local and systematic effects of tissue injury caused by various injurious agents.

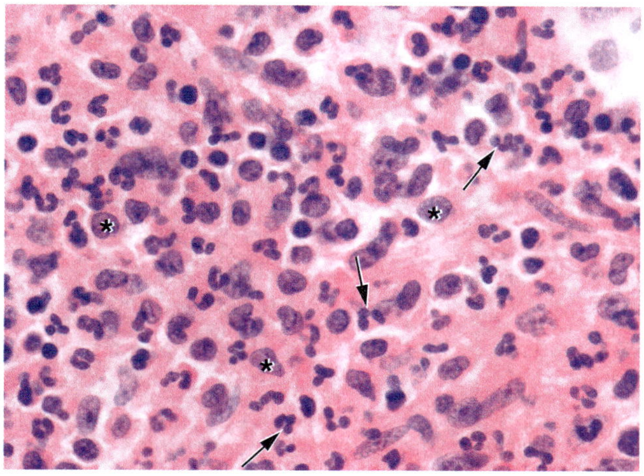

Figure 4-2 Acute inflammation is characterized by the presence of numerous neutrophils (polymorphonuclear leukocytes) (*arrows*). Several macrophages (*) are also present.

as bacteria) and attempt to destroy them. **Platelets** adhere to collagen at the site of blood vessel injury and participate in the coagulation of blood, helping to control hemorrhage related to tissue trauma. **Mast cells** found in the tissue (often in association with blood vessels) are important in the very early vascular phase of acute inflammation.

As acute inflammation runs its course, **chronic inflammation** commences and continues, to some degree, until repair is complete, sometimes for weeks or months. Chronic inflammation, unlike acute inflammation, is predominantly a cellular reaction involving **macrophage-like cells (monocytes)** from the blood and tissues that produce a variety of **chemical mediators of inflammation**. These actions clean up debris produced early in acute inflammation and also begin the healing process (**Figure 4-3**). **Lymphocytes** and related cells of the immune system contribute to adaptive immunity and also play an important role in chronic inflammation.

The earliest part of acute inflammation is the vascular phase. The characteristic effects of the vascular phase of inflammation were clearly described by

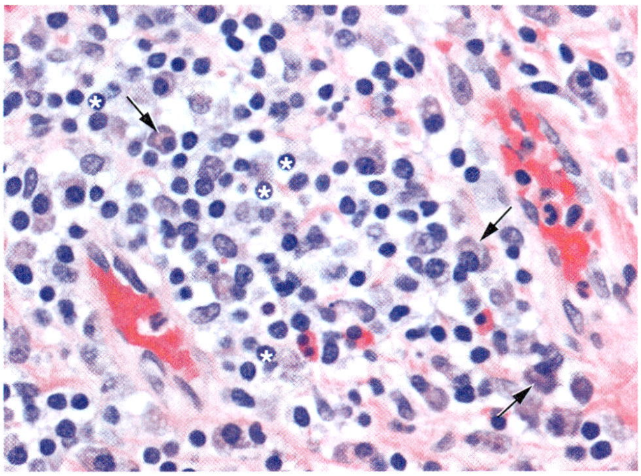

Figure 4-3 Chronic inflammation is characterized by an infiltrate composed of lymphocytes (*white**), plasma cells (*black arrows*), and macrophages. Eosinophils (demonstrating red cytoplasm) are also present, as are red cells in several capillaries.

Cellular component Circulating blood cell part of acute inflammation.

Neutrophils A type of polymorphonuclear (PMN) leukocyte that is actively phagocytic; most abundant of all leukocytes.

Phagocytic Capable of engulfing and destroying agents that are injurious to the cell.

Platelet A component of the blood; a roughly circular or oval disk formed from the plasma membrane of the megakaryocytes found in the bone marrow. Platelets are a key component in blood coagulation.

Mast cell A specialized connective tissue cell containing granules filled with histamine and other chemical mediators.

Chronic inflammation Cellular reaction leading to repair.

Macrophage-like cells (monocytes) Type of white blood cell important in the immune response.

Chemical mediators of inflammation Messenger molecule that acts on blood vessels, inflammatory cells, or other cells to contribute to an inflammatory response.

Lymphocytes A mononuclear blood cell produced in lymphoid tissue that takes part in cell-mediated and humoral immunity.

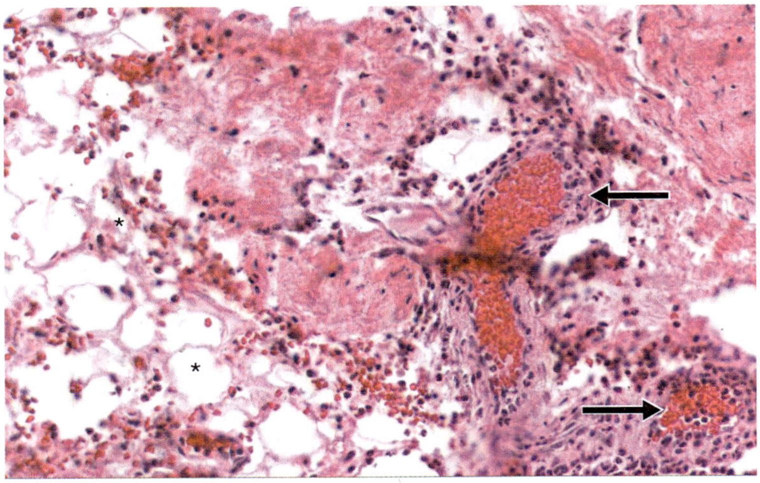

Figure 4-4 Photomicrograph of connective tissue removed during a surgical procedure illustrating neutrophils adherent to small blood vessel endothelium and migrating through the wall to the site of tissue injury. Several examples are shown at arrows. The open spaces in tissue (examples at *) represent exudation.

Courtesy of Department of Pathology and Laboratory Medicine, University of North Carolina at Chapel Hill.

the Roman writer Celsus in the first century CE (but were also described in much older Egyptian medical texts). They are termed the **cardinal signs of inflammation**: heat, swelling, redness, and pain observed at the site of injury. These signs can even be noted after a relatively minor injury such as a scratch to the skin. All of the cardinal signs result from dilatation (expansion) of blood vessels and increased vascular permeability. The increased warmth and redness of the inflamed tissues signal dilatation of capillaries and increased blood flow through the vessels (**hyperemia**). Swelling occurs because the **extravasation** (leakage) of plasma from the dilated and more permeable vessels causes the volume of fluid in the inflamed tissue to increase (**Figure 4-4**). The tenderness and pain result from irritation of sensory nerve endings at the site of the inflammatory process, with the swelling and specific chemical mediators of pain produced at the injured site contributing to the irritation.

Cardinal signs of inflammation Heat, swelling, redness, and pain observed at the site of injury.
Hyperemia Increased blood flow through vessels.
Extravasation Leakage of plasma from dilated vessels.
Emigration/diapedesis Movement of cells through walls of blood vessels.
Chemotaxis Process of active movement of inflammatory cells to the site of the injury.
Exudate The fluid, leukocytes, and debris that accumulate as a result of an inflammation.
Serous Fluid-rich exudate.
Purulent Neutrophil-rich exudate, also called pus.
Fibrinous Fibrin-rich exudate.

Local and Systemic Effects

During inflammation, a change in the permeability of venules and capillaries occurs, as well as leakage of protein-rich fluid into the tissue at sites of inflammation. PRRs on the neutrophil become activated through recognition of the PAMPs and DAMPs, inciting the inflammatory response. They are primed to adhere to the endothelium of the small blood vessels, moving between (and sometimes through) the endothelial cells lining the vessels' walls (**emigration/diapedesis**) and migrating to the area of tissue damage (Figure 4-4). In doing so, the neutrophils (and likewise the macrophage-like monocytes of chronic inflammation) react to the molecules associated with either pathogens or tissue damage and actively move toward the site of injury in a process termed **chemotaxis**. The protein-rich fluid in combination with neutrophils, either from the blood vessels or found in tissue as a result of damage to blood vessels, constitutes an **exudate**. The proportions of protein, inflammatory cells, and appearance vary in different exudates. In general, exudates can be described as **serous** exudate (fluid rich), **purulent** exudate (neutrophil rich, pus), **fibrinous** exudate (rich

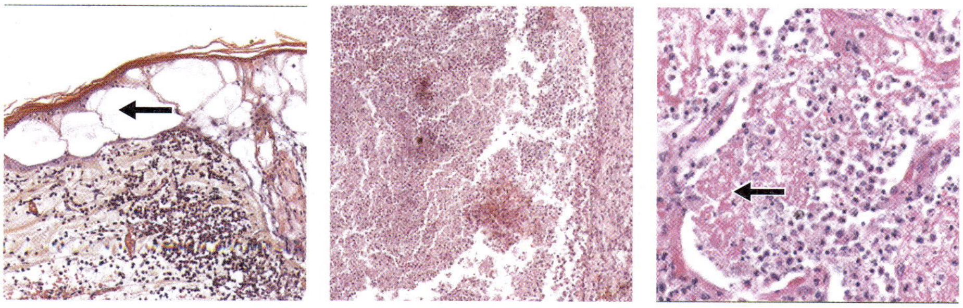

(A) (B) (C)

Figure 4-5 Examples of exudates. **(A)** Serous exudate; blister fluid in burned skin (*arrow*). **(B)** Purulent exudate; accumulation of neutrophils, many of which are necrotic in a liver abscess. **(C)** Fibrinopurulent; accumulation of neutrophils and fibrin (*arrow*) in the lung of a patient with bacterial pneumonia.

in the protein fibrin derived from **fibrinogen** in the blood), or **hemorrhagic** exudate (rich in red cells). The terms are sometimes combined, as in fibrinopurulent—rich in fibrin and cells (**Figure 4-5**).

If a fibrinous exudate involves two surfaces in close proximity, such as adjacent loops of small intestine, the surfaces may stick together. In such cases, healing may result in fibrous scar tissue, termed **adhesion**, bridging the adjacent surfaces (**Figure 4-6**).

In more severe inflammation, systemic effects become evident. The individual feels ill, and the temperature is elevated. The bone marrow accelerates production of neutrophils and monocytes, producing an elevated white blood cell count. This increased production of white blood cells can be used to monitor diseases associated with inflammation. The liver produces several proteins called **acute phase proteins** that are released into the bloodstream in response to tissue injury or inflammation. They help protect the body from the tissue injury caused by the inflammation. One of the best known of these proteins is **C-reactive protein**, which is often measured to monitor the activity of diseases characterized by tissue inflammation. Another is fibrinogen, important in blood coagulation. The proteins concerned in the coagulation of the blood

Fibrinogen An acute-phase protein important in blood coagulation.

Hemorrhagic Red cell–rich inflammatory fluid.

Adhesion Band of fibrous tissue that form subsequent to the inflammatory response, which may include scar tissue formation binding adjacent tissues together.

Acute phase proteins Proteins produced by the liver in response to inflammation.

C-reactive protein Acute phase reactant associated with inflammation.

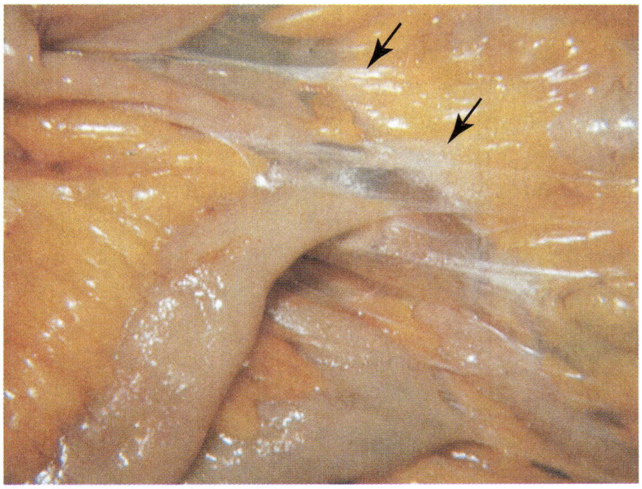

Figure 4-6 Multiple fibrous adhesions (*arrows*) between loops of small intestine resulting from previous abdominal inflammation.

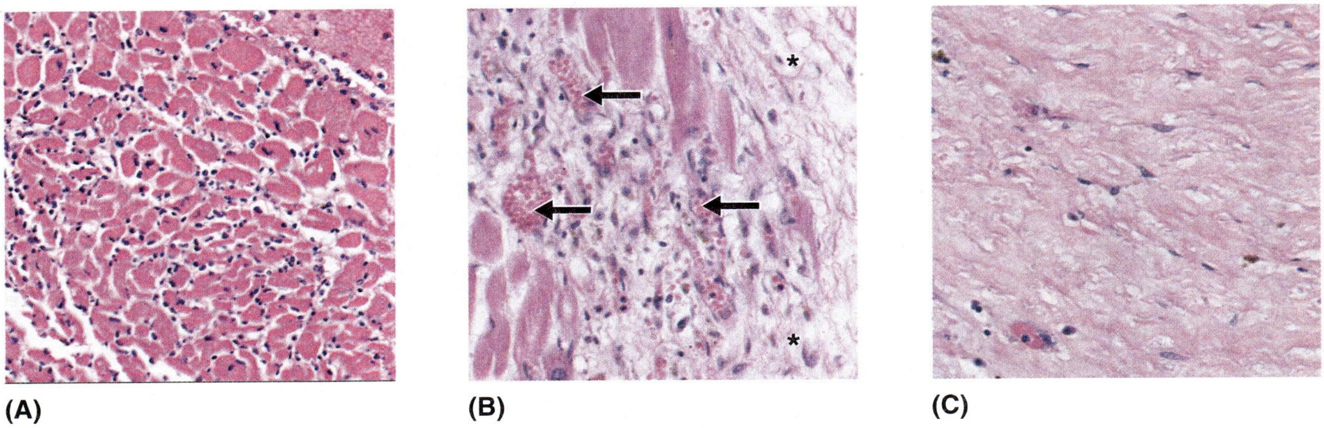

Figure 4-7 Injury and repair in a myocardial infarct (heart attack). **(A)** Acute inflammation; note presence of neutrophils in the injured tissue (24 hours post-infarction). **(B)** Healing with the formation of granulation tissue; note the formation of new blood vessels (*arrows*) and new collagen deposition (*) (10 days post-infarction). **(C)** Scar formation; note the dense fibrous (scar) tissue and lack of heart muscle cells seen in **(A)**.

Courtesy of Department of Pathology and Laboratory Medicine, University of North Carolina at Chapel Hill.

are considered in Chapter 12. Increased fibrinogen levels in the blood cause an increased sed rate, or **erythrocyte sedimentation rate (ESR)**, a measure of how quickly red cells settle out of the blood placed in a tube. The ESR detects inflammation in a patient.

The outcome of inflammation depends on the level of tissue damage resulting from the inflammation. With mild inflammation, the response soon subsides, and the tissues return to normal. This process is called **resolution**. When the inflammatory process causes more severe tissue damage, it must be repaired. During healing, damaged cells are replaced, and the framework of the injured tissue is repaired. This occurs through an ingrowth of cells producing connective tissue fibers and new blood vessels, forming **granulation tissue**. Granulation tissue signifies an intermediate step in the repair process. Scar tissue forms from the granulation tissue with the deposition of collagen in the damaged area. Sometimes, the subsequent scarring becomes so severe that function is seriously disturbed. Even though scar tissue serves as a necessary patch to heal damage to an organ, the functional cells (parenchyma) of the organ may not be replaced if they cannot divide. For example, damage to the circulation supplying the heart causes a **myocardial infarct**, also known as a **heart attack**, characterized by the death of heart muscle cells. Release of DAMPs from the dying cells results in acute and then chronic inflammation, followed by the formation of granulation tissue, which will with time become a fibrous scar. However, the heart muscle cells cannot divide to repair the damage, so the individual is left with a "patched" area of the heart, a fibrous scar made of collagen. That area of the heart cannot contract. Consequently, the heart, although repaired, can no longer function as effectively as before, and the patient may show signs of heart failure (**Figure 4-7**).

Erythrocyte sedimentation rate (ESR) A laboratory test to measure the speed red cells settle out of the blood; used to detect inflammation.

Resolution Regression of an inflammatory process without significant tissue destruction and with return of the tissues to normal.

Granulation tissue Normal part of the healing process.

Myocardial infarct/heart attack Necrosis of heart muscle as a result of interruption of its blood supply. May affect full thickness of muscle wall (transmural infarct) or only part of the wall (subendocardial infarct).

Chemical Mediators of Inflammation

The inflammatory reaction just described is a nonspecific, stereotypical response to tissue injury and functions much the same no matter the cause of the injury. The inflammatory response is not directly caused by the tissue injury but by chemical agents called mediators of inflammation. Some mediators are derived from cells, and others are formed from proteins in the blood plasma that accumulate in the injured area.

Cell-Derived Mediators

Mast cells, a major source of cell-derived mediators, are specialized cells widely distributed throughout the connective tissues of the body but often found proximate to blood vessels. Their cytoplasm is filled with preformed granules containing **histamine** and other chemicals. After tissue injury, the mast cells discharge their granules, liberating the chemicals to initiate the inflammatory process. Histamine is a potent **vasodilator** and greatly increases vascular permeability. Blood platelets also contain histamine and another mediator called **serotonin**. When platelets adhere to collagen fragments at the site of blood vessel injury, they release histamine and serotonin. Other important cell-derived mediators include **prostaglandins** and a group of similar compounds called **leukotrienes**. The cells synthesize these biologically active compounds from arachidonic acid, present in cell membranes, in response to stimuli that induce inflammation. They function as mediators that intensify the inflammatory process. Many of the cells important in the inflammatory response, including neutrophils, macrophage-like cells, and endothelial cells lining blood vessels, synthesize specific types of prostaglandins and leukotrienes. Aspirin and other **non-steroidal anti-inflammatory drugs (NSAIDs)**, such as ibuprofen and naproxen, function by inhibiting the production of prostaglandins. Cytokines, small proteins released by cells, modulate both adaptive and innate immunity reactions. They may act locally to affect nearby cells but also systemically. Cytokines may be pro-inflammatory or in some cases anti-inflammatory. **Interleukin-1 (IL-1)** and **tumor necrosis factor alpha (TNF-α)** are pro-inflammatory and act locally to help neutrophils adhere to and exit from blood vessels in injured areas. Acting systemically, they are responsible for the fever and malaise associated with inflammation and the increased synthesis of acute-phase reactants previously mentioned.

Mediators from Blood Plasma

Blood plasma contains various protein substances that circulate as inactive compounds and leak from the permeable capillaries into the area of tissue damage where they become activated by a complex process into chemical mediators. One important group of mediators formed in this way is called **bradykinins** (or simply kinins). The series of reactions that leads to the formation of bradykinins becomes triggered by one of the proteins associated with blood coagulation stimulated by tissue injury. Kinins produce vasodilation, help recruit neutrophils to injured sites, and activate pain receptors associated with inflammation.

Mediators of inflammation are also formed from another group of blood proteins called **complement**. Complement consists of at least 50 protein components, some of the best known of which are numbered as C_1 through C_9. The proteins interact in a regular sequence to yield a series of by-products, some of which function as mediators of inflammation. Complement (abbreviated as C') participates in both the nonspecific and specific responses to cell injury. It is activated when an antigen combines with an antibody in adaptive immunity (specific response) but may also be activated in other ways that do not require an antigen–antibody interaction, such as by pathogen components containing certain sugars (mannans). The various functions of the complement system are considered in connection with immunity, hypersensitivity, allergy, and autoimmune diseases.

Histamine Chemical released by mast cells.

Vasodilator A substance that dilates blood vessels.

Serotonin A vasoconstrictor mediator of inflammation released from platelets.

Prostaglandin A series of derivatives of arachidonic acid that have widespread physiologic effects.

Leukotriene A prostaglandin-like mediator of inflammation.

Non-steroidal anti-inflammatory drugs (NSAIDs) Drug such as ibuprofen and naproxen that inhibit the production of prostaglandins.

Interleukin-1 (IL-1) Pro-inflammatory cytokine, regulates immune response such as fever, leukocytes adhesion, and release of acute phase protein by the liver.

Tumor necrosis factor alpha (TNF-α) Pro-inflammatory cytokine, regulates a large group of cellular responses to injury, infection, leading to necrosis or apoptosis.

Bradykinin A chemical mediator of inflammation derived from components in the blood plasma.

Complement Group of proteins interact to produce by-products, some of which act as mediators of inflammation or cytolysis.

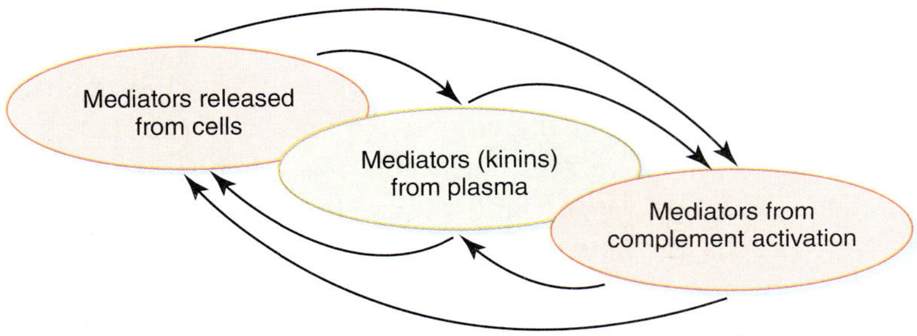

Figure 4-8 Interaction of mediators of inflammation. Activation of mediators from any source also leads to the release of mediators from other sources, which intensifies the inflammatory reaction.

Figure 4-8 illustrates how the various mediators interact. The release of mediators from any source not only initiates the inflammatory process but also induces release of more mediators from other sources, setting off a "chain reaction" that intensifies the inflammatory process.

The Role of Lysosomal Enzymes in the Inflammatory Process

The cytoplasm of phagocytic neutrophils, monocytes, and tissue macrophages attracted to the site of inflammation by chemical mediators contains organelles called **lysosomes**. Lysosomes contain potent enzymes capable of digesting the material brought into the cells by **phagocytosis**. During phagocytosis, bacteria or other foreign materials, or cellular debris, become enclosed within phagocytic vacuoles in the cell cytoplasm. The lysosomes dissolve the material by discharging their enzymes into the vacuoles, as described in the discussion on cells and tissues (**Figure 4-9**). In addition to lysosomal-mediated destruction, potent **oxidizing agents** such as hydrogen peroxide and hypochlorous acid (similar to laundry bleach) are synthesized by neutrophils and discharged into phagocytic vacuoles where they are important in destroying bacteria and fungi.

Lysosome A cytoplasmic organelle containing digestive enzymes with an acidic pH internal environment.
Phagocytosis Process by which the cell engulfs foreign material.
Oxidizing agents Chemicals that will accept electrons from other chemicals. In the inflammatory response they can be synthesized by neutrophils that help destroy bacteria and fungi.
Adrenal corticosteroid hormones/steroids Chemicals that suppress the inflammatory process.

Much of the subsequent tissue injury in an area of inflammation results from the destructive effect of the lysosomal enzymes released from leukocytes. During any inflammatory reaction, damaged neutrophils and monocytes release lysosomal enzymes. Some lysosomal enzymes and oxidizing agents also escape from intact leukocytes during phagocytosis. The tissue injury in turn generates more mediators, and this induces further inflammatory changes.

Harmful Effects of Inflammation

The tissue injury that results from inflammation is due in part to the injurious agent and in part to the inflammatory reaction itself. In most cases, the inflammatory process becomes self-limiting and subsides when the harmful agent has been eliminated. At times, however, an inflammatory process may persist and cause extensive, progressive tissue injury. If this occurs, the inflammatory process may need suppression by administering **adrenal corticosteroid hormones**, also known as **steroids**, consequently reducing the tissue damage that would result if the inflammatory process were not restrained. Milder effects are treated with NSAIDs. Suppression of the immune response is considered in Chapter 6.

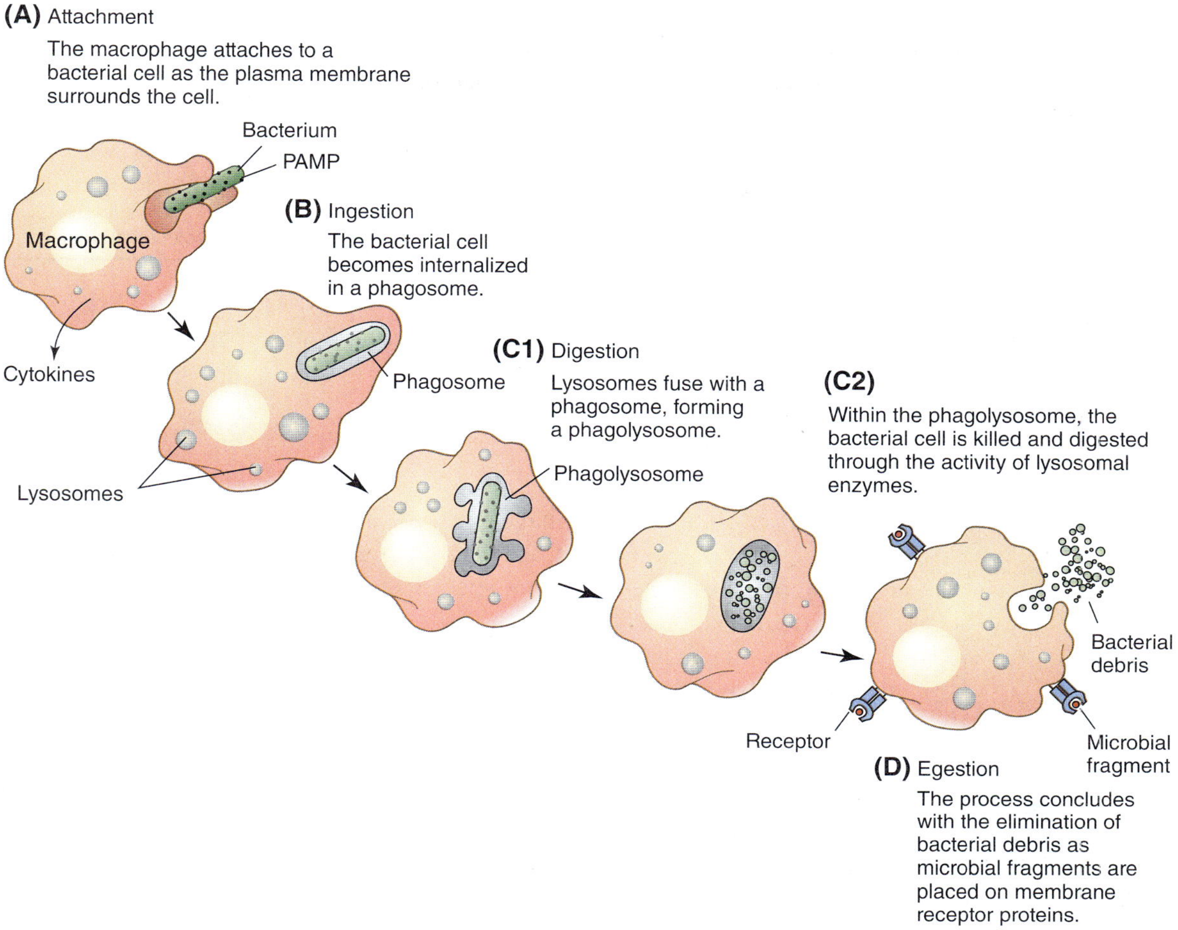

Figure 4-9 The mechanism of phagocytes: The stages of phagocytosis are shown for destruction of a bacterial pathogen.

Role of Inflammation in Infection

Factors Influencing the Outcome of an Infection

The nonspecific inflammatory process plays a role in the body's ability to fight off an **infection** caused by bacteria or other microbiologic agents. Bacteria and other microbiologic agents vary in their ability to cause disease. The term virulence refers to the speed and severity of the ensuing response with which a pathogenic organism can overcome the defenses of the body. A highly virulent organism produces progressive disease in the majority of susceptible individuals. In contrast, an organism of low virulence can only produce disease in a highly susceptible individual under certain circumstances.

The outcome of any infection depends on two factors: the **virulence** of the organism combined with the numbers (load or dosage) of the invading organisms and the resistance of the infected individual (the **host**). These may be considered balanced against one another, as indicated diagrammatically in **Figure 4-10**. When large numbers of organisms with high virulence enter into the body, especially when host resistance is lowered, the balance is quickly tipped in favor of the invader, and progressive or fatal disease develops. When the virulence or load of the organism is low or the body's resistance is high, the balance is tipped in favor of the host. The host overcomes the infection and healing occurs.

Infection Invasion by pathogens, which stimulates the hosts immune and inflammatory processes.

Virulence Assessment of the ability of a pathogen to cause disease.

Host Individual infected with a disease-producing organism.

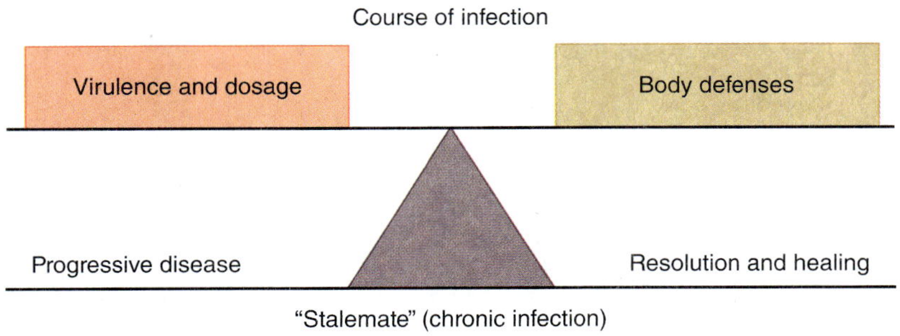

Figure 4-10 Factors influencing the outcome of an infection.

Role of Inflammatory Cells in Antimicrobial Defense

Neutrophils and macrophage-like cells (monocytes when in the blood) internalize and digest foreign material, including pathogenic microorganisms, by phagocytosis. There is some specialization as to which cell types deal with particular classes of pathogens. The acute inflammatory response characterized by the presence of neutrophils at the site of tissue injury is characteristic of bacterial disease. Viral and fungal diseases most commonly present as chronic inflammation without a preliminary acute inflammatory phase. Hence, the response to these pathogens is characterized by "mononuclear" cells, including macrophage-like cells and lymphocytes. For this reason, a healthcare provider noting a higher-than-normal level of neutrophils in the blood suspects a bacterial etiology. An increase in mononuclear cells (usually lymphocytes) suggests a viral disease. However, there are many exceptions to this rule.

Both neutrophils and macrophages are attracted to foreign material when it is coated with plasma proteins collectively called **opsonins**. Opsonins can be either derived from complement or are immunoglobulins produced as part of the adaptive host response. Microorganisms that have mechanisms to evade this process are more virulent. The role of inflammatory cells is crucial in degrading microbes but also contributes to further cell damage and inflammation resulting from release of lysosomal enzymes and oxidizing agents into tissue. The importance of these cells in antimicrobial defense is further emphasized by the frequency and severity of infections when these cells are decreased in numbers. Neutropenia can occur from cancer chemotherapy or congenital diseases or when cells are incapable of killing the phagocytosed material.

Opsonins Plasma proteins that attract neutrophils and macrophages to foreign material.

Cellulitis An acute spreading inflammation affecting the skin or deeper tissues.

Abscess A localized accumulation of pus in tissues.

Lymphangitis An inflammation of lymph vessels draining a site of infection.

Lymphadenitis An inflammation of lymph nodes draining a site of infection.

Terminology of Infection

The term *infection* denotes an inflammatory process caused by disease-producing organisms. A number of different terms are used to refer to infections in various sites. Generally, the ending *-itis* is appended to the name of the tissue or organ to indicate an infection or inflammatory process. For example, the terms appendicitis, hepatitis, colitis, and pneumonitis refer to inflammation of the appendix, liver, colon, and lung, respectively. An acute spreading infection at any site is called **cellulitis**. Usually, this term is used to refer to an acute infection of the skin and deeper tissues. The term **abscess** is used when an infection is associated with the breakdown of the tissues and the formation of a localized mass of pus. If localized infection spreads into the lymphatic channels draining the site of inflammation, the term **lymphangitis** is used. **Lymphadenitis** refers to infection in the regional lymph nodes draining the primary site of infection.

The term **septicemia** is used to refer to an overwhelming infection in which pathogenic bacteria gain access to the bloodstream.

Septicemia An infection in which large numbers of pathogenic bacteria are present in the bloodstream.

Chronic Infection

Sometimes, the organism and host are evenly matched. Neither can gain the advantage; the result is a stalemate. Clinically, this results in a chronic infection, characterized by a relatively quiet, smoldering inflammation usually associated with continued attempts at healing on the part of the host. The balance between the host and the invader is precarious. The infection may flare up at times when the pathogen obtains a temporary advantage, or it may become quiescent at other times when the defenses of the host gain the upper hand. Lymphocytes, plasma cells, and monocytes are the predominant cells in chronic inflammatory processes.

Case 4-1

Jane is an 18-year-old college freshman dressed in shorts who is playing a game of touch football on a grass field when she stumbles. She lands on a broken beer bottle and suffers a **laceration** on the **dorsal** surface of her thigh. Her friends suggest that she visit student health, but she has an examination in the afternoon. She washes the wound, places several large gauze pads on it, and wraps it to stop the bleeding. She changes the pads every day, but 5 days after the injury she notes some pus on the surface of the **eschar** (dead tissue on the surface of the wound) and an **exophytic** (mass projecting out from the surface of the wound) growing mass of tissue (**Case Figure 4-1**). Alarmed, she visits the health service. The clinician explains she has developed a minor infection in the wound. The mass is composed of granulation tissue, an excessive amount of what is a normal part of the healing process. However, because of the infection and large mass of granulation tissue, the healthcare provider **debrides** the wound. They explain that because she did not immediately seek medical attention and have the wound sutured, she is likely to be left with a large scar.

Laceration An irregular jagged wound.
Dorsal Front surface.
Eschar A layer of dead tissue that commonly forms over a wound or burn.
Exophytic Outward growing mass of tissue protruding from the wound.
Debride Remove dead, infected, and excess granulation tissue from the wound bed.

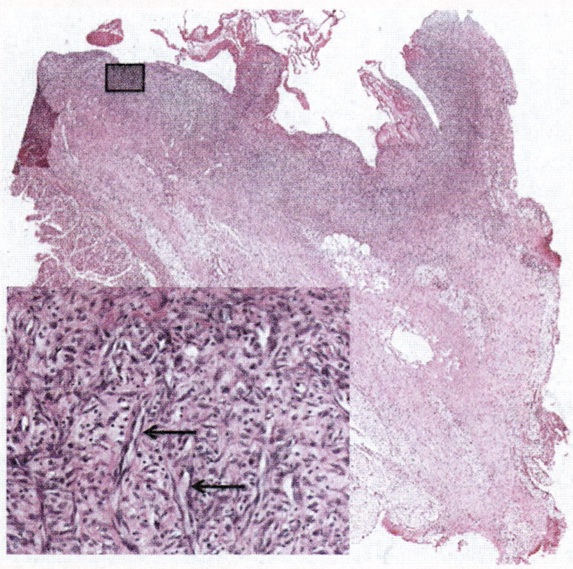

Case Figure 4-1 Debrided granulation tissue from wound. Inset (taken from boxed area) shows tissue at high power. Arrows indicate developing capillaries.

Courtesy of Department of Pathology and Laboratory Medicine, University of North Carolina at Chapel Hill.

(continues)

Fibrosis Scar formation.
Proud flesh Growth of excessive granulation tissue that can gape above the wound.
Secondary union Form of healing of a large unsutured wound.
Primary union Form of healing of a sutured wound.

Case 4-1 *(Continued)*

Discussion

During wound healing, granulation tissue is the matrix in which new blood vessels form and in which fibroblasts proliferate to produce collagen, a process termed **fibrosis** (scar formation). Case Figure 4-1 (inset) shows an area rich in the formation of small capillaries oriented upward toward the wound surface. In addition, many mononuclear inflammatory cells and the elongated nuclei of fibroblasts are present. In cases where wound healing is delayed (as it was by infection in Case 4-1), cytokine production by inflammatory cells may promote the growth of excessive granulation tissue that can gape above the wound (sometimes termed **proud flesh**). With time, the granulation tissue will be replaced by a large scar. This form of healing of a large unsutured wound is termed **secondary union**. Sutured wounds oppose the injured surfaces, leaving little space for granulation tissue to form. Such healing by **primary union** leaves a small scar (**Case Figure 4-2**). Plastic and reconstructive surgeons make a great effort to carefully suture wounds to minimize scarring and to produce esthetically satisfactory results.

Etiology and Pathogenesis

The etiology is traumatic injury (laceration) resulting in superficial bacterial infection. The pathogenesis demonstrates healing of a wound by secondary union combined with excess production of granulation tissue.

Questions

1. Suppose Jane had immediately sought medical attention. What steps might the health care provider have taken in treating the wound?
2. Granulation tissue consists of mononuclear inflammatory cells, fibroblasts, and new capillaries. What role does each play in wound healing?
3. Careful examination of Case Figure 4-1 might disclose some neutrophils in the wound bed. Why do you think this is likely?

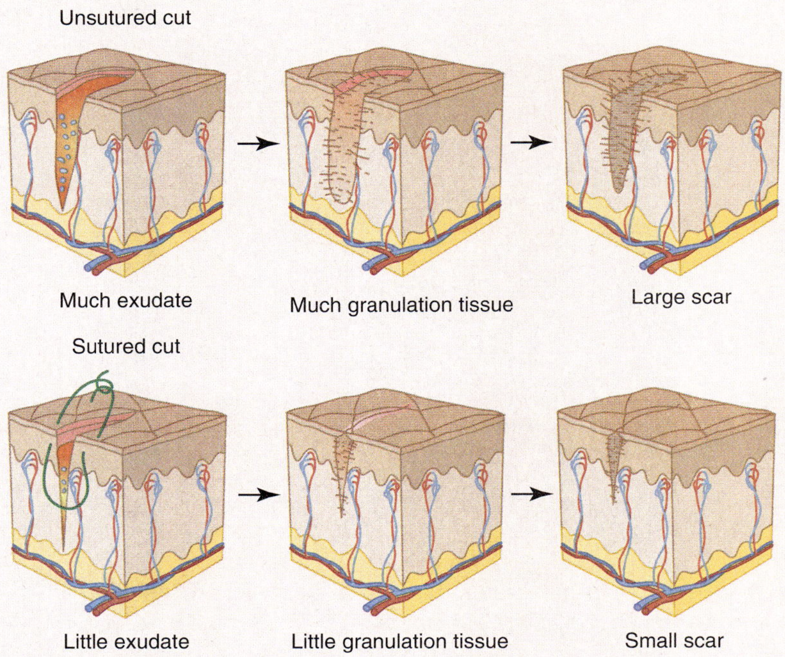

Case Figure 4-2 Repair of sutured and unsutured skin cut leading to secondary and primary union.

Questions for Review

1. What is the inflammatory reaction? What are its clinical manifestations?
2. What factors influence the outcome of an infection?
3. What are mediators of inflammation? How do they function?
4. What is meant by the following terms: chronic infection, pathogenic, complement?
5. What is the relationship between innate and adaptive immunity?

References

Murphy HS, Iskander K, Strayer DS, Remick DG, Sephel GC, Davidson JM. Inflammation and repair. In Rubin E, Reisner HM, eds. *Principles of Rubin's Pathology*. Wolters Kluwer; 2019:28-73.

- Detailed discussion of the aspects of inflammation and repair is of importance in undergraduate medical education. Hence, medical textbooks are the best source for concise and timely discussion of these complex areas. This text does a good job of presenting details in a concise manner.

IPLab. University of Alabama Pathology Education Instructional Resource. Updated January 3, 2014. Accessed March 12, 2025. http://peir.path.uab.edu/wiki/IPLab

- There are a number of web-based resources for the study of pathology. IPLab, an instructional resource for pathology education, is an excellent source for additional information and particular case studies with excellent illustrative material. "Lab 3: Inflammation and Repair" is of particular interest.

Pradeu T, Thomma BP, Girardin SE, Lemaitre B. The conceptual foundations of innate immunity: Taking stock 30 years later. *Immunity*. 2024;57(4):613-631.

- A useful historical review that defines many of the terms used in studies of innate immunity.

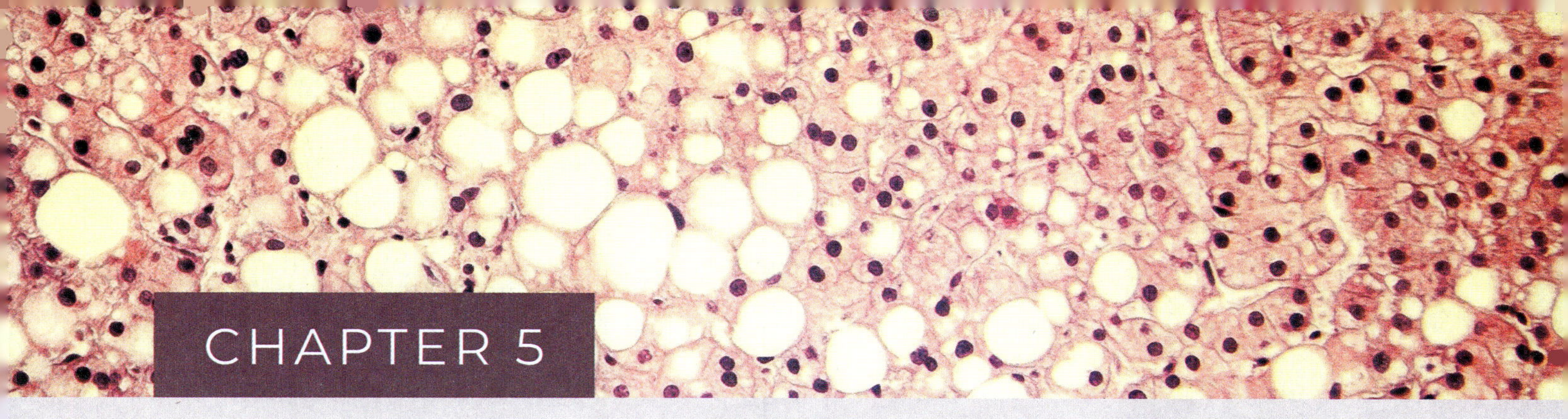

CHAPTER 5

Immunity, Hypersensitivity, Immunodeficiency, and Autoimmune Diseases

LEARNING OBJECTIVES

1. List the basic features of cell-meditated and humoral immunity. Explain the role of lymphocytes in the immune response.
2. List the five classes of antibodies and explain how they differ from one another structurally and functionally.
3. Define cytokines. Give examples of cytokines and explain their functions.
4. Study the components of complement system and its function in immune response.
5. Understand the function of NK cells.
6. Describe the four types of hypersensitivity. Describe the pathogenesis of allergic manifestations and the role of lgE in allergy. Compare the methods of treatment.
7. Explain why it is sometimes necessary to suppress the immune response and describe how this can be accomplished.
8. Describe the causes and clinical manifestation of immunodeficiency disease.
9. Compare and contrast immune tolerance and autoimmune disease, including the clinical manifestations and the methods of treatment.

Introduction: The Body's Defense Mechanisms

Innate immunity is quick to respond, but only to the predetermined array of molecular patterns associated with pathogens or those molecules characteristic of injured cells (Chapter 4). Innate immunity responds to specific challenges that frequently occurred during human evolution and is limited in its ability to respond to new challenges.

Innate immunity
Immunity present at birth and lasting a person's entire life and the first response of the body's immune system to a harmful foreign substance, non specific, no immune memory involved.

Many pathogens can quickly evolve to counter host defenses. Consider the problem posed when rapidly dividing microorganisms quickly develop

Adaptive immunity Immune response with the ability to mount an antigen specific reaction and establish immunologic memory.

Cell-mediated immunity Immunity associated with population of sensitized lymphocytes.

Humoral immunity Immunity associated with formation of antibodies produced by plasma cells.

Autoimmune disease A disease associated with formation of cell-mediated or humoral immunity against the subject's own cells or tissue components.

Interferon A broad-spectrum antiviral agent produced by various cells in the body.

antibiotic resistance. Even during the course of a single infection, organisms may evolve mechanisms that allow them to circumvent the host's innate defense mechanisms. In addition, the movement of populations and changes in the environment constantly expose us to new challenges with which innate immunity may be unable to cope.

Adaptive immunity, composed of **cell-mediated immunity** and **humoral immunity**, provides the ability to detect and adaptively respond essentially to any molecular structure foreign to us, even one never encountered. The aspects of adaptive recognition and response to foreign structures and immune memory define adaptive immunity and differentiate it from innate immunity. Innate immunity can only adapt to new challenges with evolution, whereas adaptive immunity can cope with previously unrecognized agents nearly in "real time." Unfortunately, the adaptive immune system may err, recognizing the self as foreign and resulting in **autoimmune disease**.

Innate Versus Adaptive Immunity

Innate Immunity

Innate immunity proceeds with a very rapid response, involving multiple tissues (skin and mucus membrane); classes of blood cells (**Figure 5-1**), as well as many chemical mediators, such as **interferon**, lysozyme, and more. The multiple overlapping mechanisms of the innate immune system ensure broad immune efficiency against a wide array of opportunistic pathogens. The pattern recognition receptors (PRR), such as Toll-like receptors, RIG-like receptors, and

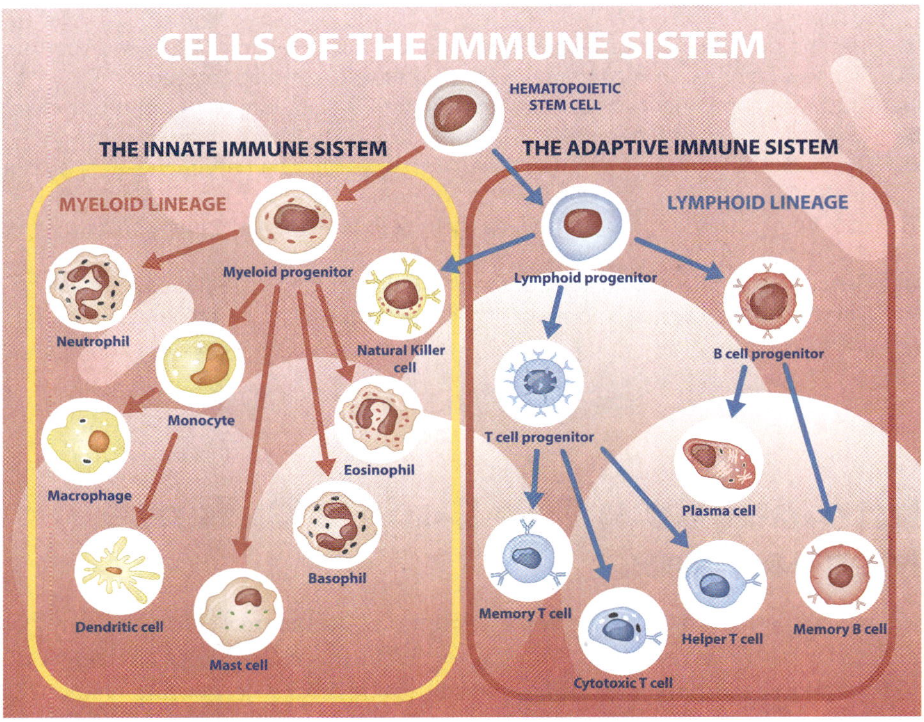

Figure 5-1 Formation of immune cells from hematopoietic stem cells in humans. Multipotent stem cells differentiate into myeloid progenitor cells or lymphoid progenitor cells. Lymphoid progenitor cells give rise to lymphatic cells, which are involved in adaptive immunity, while myeloid lineage gives rise to erythrocytes, platelets (not shown) and various white blood cells that are part of the innate immunity.

NOD-like receptors, are used by innate immunity. These receptors are found on the surface, within membrane-bound vesicles, or free in the cytoplasm of the immune cells. All of the receptors of a given type are identical and invariant, recognizing only a limited array of pathogen structures. Although the recognized pathogen structures are often essential to pathogen infectivity, they can be prone to mutation, thus allowing the pathogen to escape the innate immune system.

In summary, innate immunity is a rapidly acting first line of defense that often slows the infectious process but cannot eliminate it. Innate immunity primes the adaptive system, buying time for the adaptive system to respond as a second but highly effective line of defense.

Adaptive Immunity

Adaptive immunity can be divided into two tightly interrelated systems: humoral immunity and cell-mediated, or cellular, immunity. Lack of either system will result in susceptibility to a range of pathogens and lead to the development of life-threatening diseases. Humoral immunity absolutely requires an intact cellular immune system to function effectively.

Humoral immunity produces antibodies, soluble **immunoglobulin** proteins. Antibodies circulate in the blood and body fluids, where they bind to and eliminate foreign material. Humoral immunity provides the body's major defense against many bacteria and bacterial toxins that are predominantly extracellular. Cell-mediated immunity, on the other hand, is characterized by the formation of **T lymphocytes/T cells**. It is the main defense against invading viruses, fungi, parasites, and some bacteria, particularly those that are intracellular. Cell-mediated immunity contributes to the major mechanism by which the abnormal cells that sometimes arise spontaneously in cell division can be identified and eliminated. Consequently, it also becomes the key component during transplant rejection. A comparison of humoral and cell-mediated immunity is summarized in **Table 5-1**.

Immunoglobulin The class of proteins that includes antibodies.

T lymphocyte/T cell A type of lymphocyte associated with cell-mediated immunity.

Natural killer (NK) cells Lymphocytes capable of destroying foreign or abnormal cells, although they have not had any prior antigenic contact with the cells.

Antigen-presenting cell (APC) Cell that displays the foreign material.

Antigen Substance recognized by the immune system.

The Role of Lymphocytes in Adaptive Immunity

The key cells of the adaptive immune system are the lymphocytes, including B cells, T cells, and **natural killer (NK) cells** (Figure 5-1). B cells can recognize and bind directly to a foreign substance, broadly termed as antigen, while T cells can only recognize and bind to antigens presented by other cells, such as microphages, dendritic cells, and B cells (they are called **antigen-presenting cells, or APCs**). Both functional lymphocytes and APCs are necessary for response to an **antigen**. Antigens bind to B cell receptors (BCR, or membrane-bound immunoglobulin) to initiate humoral immunity; they can

Table 5-1 Comparison of Humoral and Cell-Mediated Immunity

Humoral	Cell-Mediated
Principal cellular agent is the B cell.	Principal cellular agent is the T cell.
B cell responds to bacteria, bacterial toxins, and some viruses.	T cell responds to cancer cells, virus-infected cells, single-cell fungi, parasites, and foreign cells in an organ transplant.
When activated, B cells form memory cells and plasma cells, which produce antibodies to these antigens.	When activated, T cells differentiate into memory cells, cytotoxic cells, suppressor cells, and helper cells; cytotoxic T cells attack the antigen directly.

T cell receptor (TCR) Antigen recognition molecule on the surface of T cells.

Immunogen Antigen that can provoke an adaptive immune response by binding to antigen receptors.

Major histocompatibility complex (MHC) A group of proteins that bind to peptide fragments derived from pathogens and display and present them to corresponding T cells. In humans, the genes coded for MHC are located on chromosome 6.

Hypersensitivity reaction A state of increased abnormal reactivity to a foreign material.

Antibody Immunoglobulin molecules produced by B cells when activated by an antigen and secreted by B cells, which mature into plasma cells.

Cytokine A general term for any protein secreted by cells that functions as an intercellular messenger and influences cells of the immune system. Cytokines are secreted by macrophages and monocytes (monokines), lymphocytes (lymphokines), and other cells.

B lymphocyte A lymphocyte associated with humoral immunity that is capable of producing antibodies, which can differentiate into antibody-secreting plasma or memory cells.

also be processed and presented to **T cell receptors (TCR)** by APCs to activate cell-mediated immunity. TCRs bind to small peptides, whereas BCRs can bind to larger proteins, carbohydrates, nucleic acids, and other substances. Some substances, such as small organic molecules, can only elicit an immune response when they are part of or chemically coupled to a larger molecule. These small molecules are termed haptens. Antigens that can provoke an immune response are termed **immunogens**.

Unlike T cell and B cells, NK cells do not have specific receptors for antigens; their functions will be discussed later in this chapter.

Cell-Mediated Immunity

T Cell Types. T cells are the major players in cell-mediated immunity. T cells are divided into classes depending on the type of **major histocompatibility complex (MHC)** they recognize. MHC can be divided into two classes. T cells that recognize class I MHC molecules become CD8+ type T cells, and those that recognize class II MHC molecules become CD4+.

The CD (cluster of differentiation) designation refers to immunologically detectable markers on the lymphocyte surface that help define the function of the cell. CD8+ cells are termed cytotoxic T cells because they function to lyse virally infected cells and possibly also tumor cells. They recognize viral peptides in combination with MHC class I molecules. Since MHC class I molecules are present in essentially all nucleated cells, any cells infected by virus can be recognized. CD4+ cells are referred to generically as T helper (Th cells). Th cells serve multiple functions and can be further divided into a number of subtypes. Th1 cells mediate inflammation via the secretion of pro-inflammatory cytokines, protect against intracellular pathogens, often by activating other cells such as macrophages, and play a role in the production of delayed **hypersensitivity reactions**. Th2 cells provide help for humoral B cell–mediated immunity and **antibody** production. A third important class of Th cells are Th17 cells, named due to their ability to secrete the potent inflammatory **cytokine** IL-17. Th17 cells are critical for defense against some infectious agents but also appear to be involved in a number of autoimmune diseases when they become dysregulated.

Antigen-Processing and Antigen-Presenting Cells. Entry of a foreign antigen into the body triggers a chain of events that involves interactions between T and **B lymphocytes** and APCs. For T cells to recognize foreign antigens, the antigen must be "processed" within the APCs, combined with MHC molecules, and presented on the APCs' surface to TCR. Macrophages, monocytes that have left the bloodstream and taken up permanent residence in the tissues, play a role in this process. However, the most important group of APCs are dendritic cells, named for their long cytoplasmic processes that resemble the dendrites of a nerve cell. These cells originated in bone marrow. Initially, dendritic cells are present in all epithelial and subepithelial sites, including the skin, Langerhans cells, respiratory system, and gastrointestinal tract, the most likely places to encounter pathogens. At epithelial sites, dendritic cells capture invading pathogens using a variety of cell surface receptors. Activation of innate immunity at such peripheral sites leads to the activation of dendritic cells. They lose their ability to adhere to epithelium and migrate into peripheral lymphoid organs that drain the epithelial sites. The activated dendritic cells process the captured antigen and move to areas in the lymph node rich in naïve T cells. Pathogens that circulate in the bloodstream are captured by APC in the spleen and are similarly presented to splenic T cells. Splenectomy (removal of the spleen) leaves people at particular risk for certain bacterial pathogens such as *Streptococcus pneumoniae*. Macrophages and B cells can also function as APC. The antigen-presenting property of B cells is of particular importance in developing humoral immunity to protein antigens (T-dependent antigen). **Figure 5-2** and **Table 5-2** present overviews of this process.

Effector Functions of T Cell Subsets. Mature T cells also function as effector cells for host defense. During the differentiation and maturation, different sets of genes become active in different T cells (e.g., the cytokine genes are activated in T helper cells, and genes for cytotoxic proteins are activated in cytotoxic T cells).

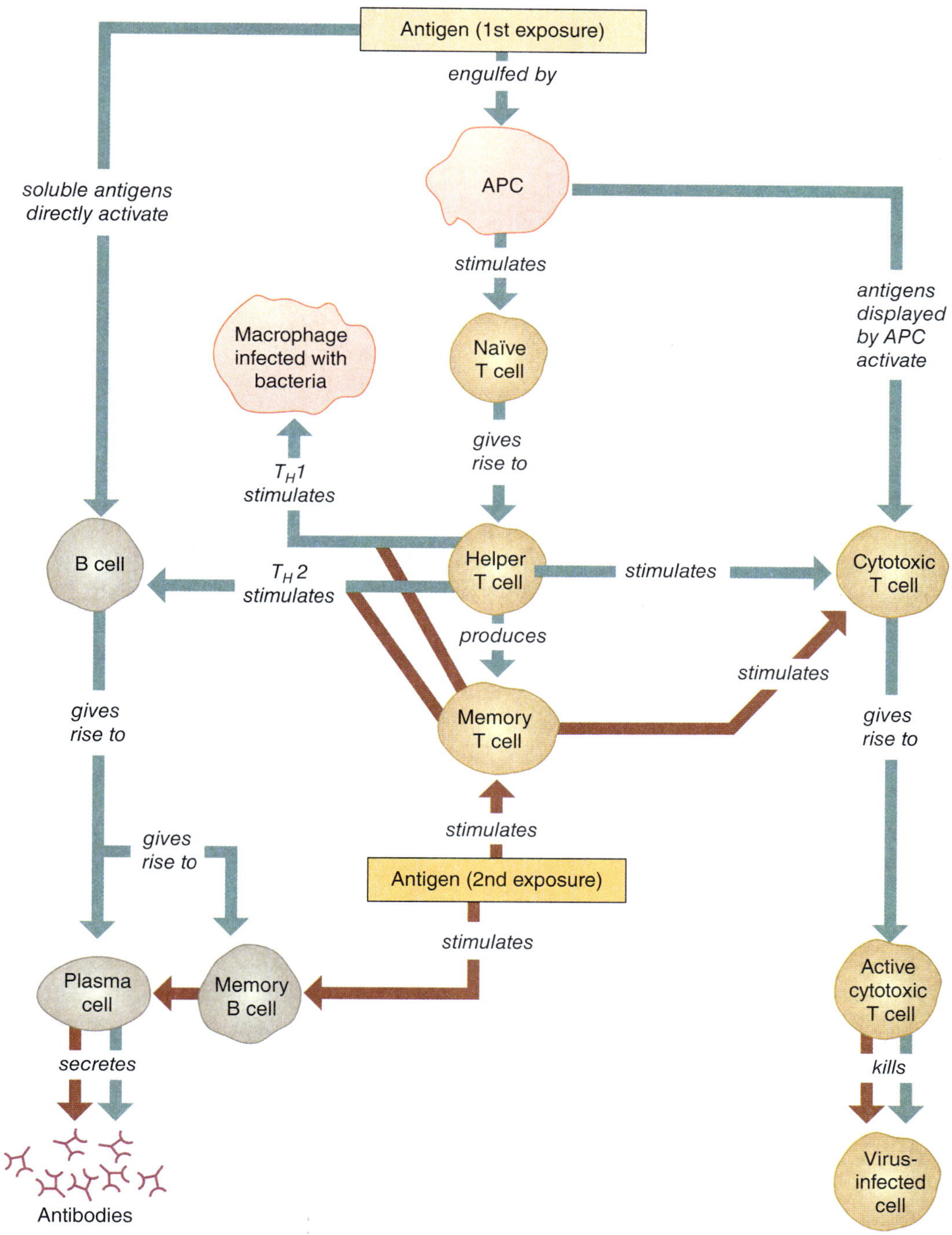

Figure 5-2 T cell and B cell activation.

Table 5-2 Classification and Functions of Immune System Cells

Cell Function	Cell Type	Action of Cell
Antigen processing	Macrophages, B lymphocytes, dendritic cells	Process antigen and present to lymphocytes
Regulate immune response	Regulator T cells (CD4+)	Cytokines regulate immune system activity
Promote cytotoxic immune response	Cytotoxic T cells (CD8+)	Produce cytokines that destroy foreign or abnormal cells displaying antigen fragments combined with MHC class I antigens
Promote delayed hypersensitivity response	Delayed hypersensitivity T cells (CD4+)	Respond to antigen-processing cells presenting foreign antigen fragments combined with MHC class II antigens; produce cytokines that activate and stimulate macrophages, cytotoxic T cells, and NK cells
Destroy virus-infected cells and cancer cells	NK cells	Cytokine-mediated cell destruction; no previous contact with antigen required
Produce antibodies	Plasma cells	Antigen processed by B lymphocytes and presented to responding T cells stimulates B lymphocytes to mature into plasma cells and make antibodies

Effector T cell Activated T cell upon exposure to foreign substance.

Delayed hypersensitivity A state of reactivity to a foreign material that takes time to develop.

For **effector T cells** (such as Th1, Th2, and cytotoxic cells) to function, they must leave the lymph node and migrate through the circulation to sites of infection or damage. For example, the surface properties of the vascular endothelial cells undergo modification during the inflammatory response to pathogens. This change in the blood vessel surface allows the adherence of effector (but not naïve) T cells at the site of inflammation, as well as their migration out of the blood vessel toward the site of inflammation. Although the migration process is not antigen specific, those effector T cells that encounter their cognate antigen tend to stick at the site of the pathogen and play a role in its destruction.

In brief, the major role of effector Th1 cells is the activation of macrophages at the site of the pathogen, which allows the macrophage to kill microbes. Activation of macrophages and the consequent release of pro-inflammatory tissue-destructive molecules at the site of reaction may result in a local, **delayed hypersensitivity** reaction.

Th2 cells secrete cytokines (Il-4 and Il-5), which promote production of a class of immunoglobulin (IgE) and activate eosinophils, both of which are important in the host defense against parasites. Th2 cells also promote a type of macrophage activation that leads to the initiation of the healing process. The particular subclass of Th cell predominant in the host defense against an organism can be critical. The most often cited example is that of leprosy, caused by the mycobacterium *M. leprae*. Certain individuals who develop leprosy cannot eliminate the bacteria. Consequently, they develop a destructive lepromatous disease associated with progressing destructive tissue lesions. These individuals are unable to mount a Th1 response (but may mount a Th2 response). Individuals who mount a Th1 response develop a generally less destructive form of the disease, called tuberculoid leprosy.

Cytotoxic T cells (CTL) attack and destroy body cells infected with viruses or intracellular bacteria. The infected cells are marked for destruction by having some of the bacterial or viral antigen debris transported to the cell surface combined with MHC class I proteins. The CTL forms a tight association with the infected cells and synthesizes the protein perforin, which dissolves the membrane of the infected cell at the point of contact, as well as the protein granzyme B, which activates apoptosis or programmed cell death leading to the death of the infected cell (**Figure 5-3**). Cancer cells displaying unique antigens that are absent from normal cells are also destroyed in a similar way. CTL also plays an important role in the rejection of transplanted organs, which contain foreign antigens. The response to foreign MHC (HLA) antigens is particularly strong because a high percentage of T cells in a nonimmune donor will recognize foreign MHC molecules.

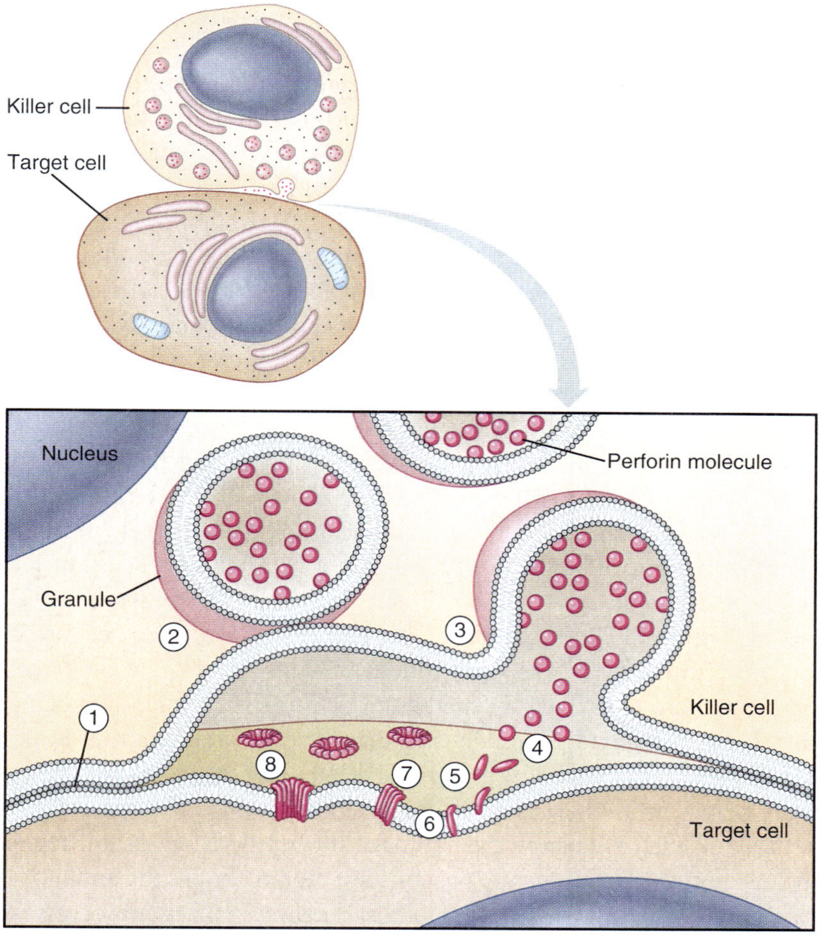

Figure 5-3 How cytotoxic T cells work. Cytotoxic T cells containing perforin-1 granules bind to their target and release perforin-1. Perforin-1 molecules form a pore in the target cell plasma membrane. Granzyme-B enters through the pore and induces the death of the target cell.

(1) Killer cell binds to target
(2) Exocytosis occurs
(3) Perforin is disgorged into space between killer cell and target
(4) Conformation of perforin molecules change in the presence of calcium
(5) Perforin molecules bind to target cell membrane
(6) Perforin molecules insert into target cell membrane
(7) Perforin monomers polymerize
(8) Perforins form pores to admit water and salts killing target cell

Reproduced from Cohn ZA and Yound JD-E. *Sci Am.* 1988;258:38-44. Illustration courtesy of Dana Burns.

Humoral Immunity

T Cell–Independent and –Dependent Humoral Responses. T cell–mediated immunity relies on close-range interactions between the immune effector T cell and the target, resulting in either the direct killing of pathogen-infected host cells or cancerous cells by cytotoxic lymphocytes or the production of a multiplicity of cytokine-like proteins by effector T helper cells. These cytokines stimulate additional cell populations (such as macrophages) to act at the site of infection. Such cytokine-mediated host defenses also amplify aspects of innate immunity, such as the inflammatory response.

Humoral immunity is different. The effector molecule of the humoral immunity, immunoglobulin (antibodies) produced by B cells, is widely disseminated through the vascular system and can be found in many parts of the human body. For this reason, humoral immunity is most effective against extracellular pathogens. B cells can respond to foreign antigens in two general ways: **T cell–independent or T cell–dependent**.

Antigens such as carbohydrates, nucleic acids, and lipids consist of chemically similar repeated components. These molecules contain multiple similar or identical **antigenic determinants (epitopes)**, each of which can react with the same antigen recognition molecule (BCR) of the naïve B cells and activate them to produce antibodies. The response by B cells to such polymeric antigens is T cell–independent. T cell–independent antigens elicit antibodies with limited properties for host defense. They are produced for a short time only and most often do not result in immune memory. These antibodies do not improve with time in their ability to bind (as do the antibodies to T cell–dependent protein antigens). T cell–independent antigens provoke a response critical in rapid host defense, but the response is limited.

Protein-based antigens are quite different. Proteins are made of chains of amino acids that differ along the length of the protein chain. Thus, they do not contain a large number of similar or identical epitopes. Rather, protein antigens contain a series of different epitopes (about 10 amino acids in length); each epitope can bind to a different B cell. These protein antigens are T cell–dependent, requiring T helper cell interaction (**T cell help**) to activate B cells and produce antibodies. T cell–dependent responses are quite different from T cell-independent ones, having several unique properties, including being very long-lived. T cell-dependent antigens result in the differentiation of B memory cells and plasma cells (antibody-producing cells) that can persist throughout the life of the host. The antibodies produced against T cell–dependent antigens can **class switch**, that is, change the nature of the antibody's constant region (Fc region). As discussed later, the type of constant region defines the antibody class, each with different effector properties in host defense. Perhaps most surprisingly, B cells can improve their affinity to a particular antigen with time, a phenomenon known as **affinity maturation**. This "fine tuning" of specificity is the result of somatic mutations of B cells at the DNA that codes for the **variable region** of the antibody that closely interacts with the antigen. A process of positive selection for strong antigen-binding B cells repeatedly occurs within an area of the **germinal center** of the lymph node, resulting in a new population of B cells producing antibodies with even higher affinity to antigen.

T cell–independent/ T cell–dependent Whether T cells are needed or not needed for a response from B cells.

Antigenic determinant/ epitope Specific molecular region from an antigen that triggers immune response.

T cell help Requirement of a T cell to stimulate a B cell to deliver humoral response.

Class switch A change in the immunoglobulin constant region using the same variable region.

Affinity maturation Band of fibrous tissue that form subsequent to the inflammatory response, which may include scar tissue formation binding adjacent tissues together.

Variable region Area on the immunoglobulin molecule specific for a particular pathogen. Amino-terminal end of the immunoglobulin chain; the part that recognizes the antigen.

Germinal center Site in lymph node where selection for strong binding B cells occurs.

Effector Molecules of Humoral Immunity: Immunoglobulins. The effector molecule of the humoral immune reaction is the immunoglobulin molecule predominantly synthesized by B plasma cells, terminally differentiated lymphocytes specialized to synthesize and secrete large amounts of protein. The term antibody should be used to refer to an Ig molecule known to react with a given antigen. Antibody and immunoglobulin tend to be used interchangeably. Although the immunoglobulin classes differ somewhat from one another in chemical composition, molecular weight, and size of their constant regions, they all have the same basic structure: two identical pairs of polypeptide (protein) chains. One pair is called **heavy chains**, each chain with a molecular weight of approximately 50 kDa. The second pair is termed **light chains**, each with a molecular weight of approximately 25 kDa. The variable regions (antigen-binding regions) are limited to the first 110 amino acids in all chains. The heavy chain variable regions are identical to each other, as are the light chain variable regions (**Figure 5-4**).

Heavy chains (H chains) Longer of two types of chains making up an immunoglobulin molecule.

Light chains (L chains) Shorter of two types of chains making up an immunoglobulin molecule.

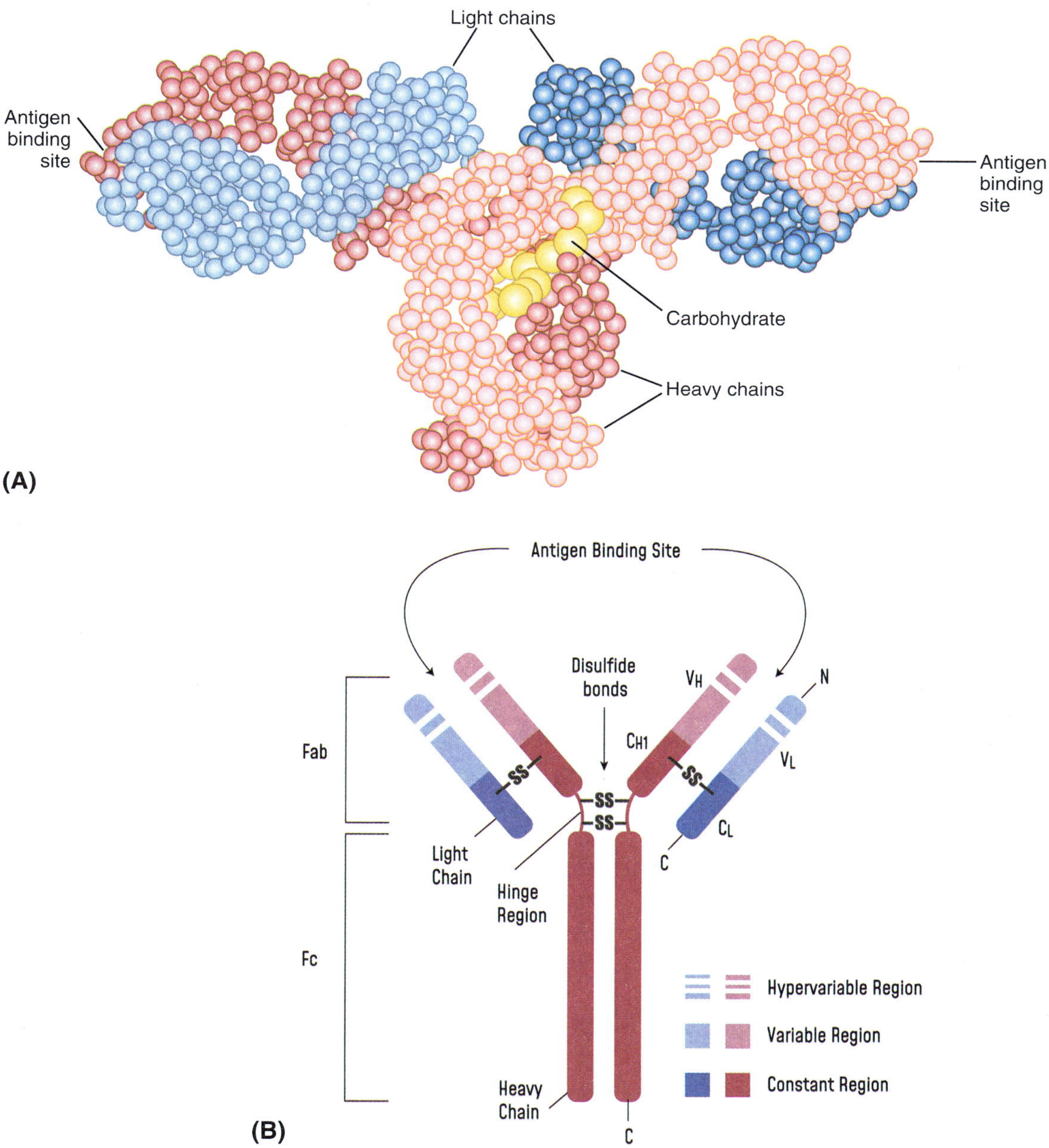

Figure 5-4 Antibody structure. **(A)** A three-dimensional model of an antibody showing the four chains. The molecule is T shaped before binding to the antigen. As it binds, it becomes Y shaped. **(B)** A diagrammatic representation of the structure of an antibody molecule that shows the four protein chains, two large (heavy chains) and two small (light chains). Note that the antigen binds to the arms of the molecule.

The class of the immunoglobulin is determined by the structure of the constant region of the heavy chain. In humans there are five classes: IgA, IgM, IgG, IgD, and IgE. In addition, the IgA and IgG classes are further divided into two and four closely related subclasses (respectively, IgA_1, IgA_2, and IgG_{1-4}). The specific effector function of the antibody is determined by the constant region of the heavy chain (i.e., the Ig class and subclass); specificity of the antibody for a given antigen, such as a pathogenic virus or bacterial toxin, is conferred by the variable region. Humoral responses, even to very simple antigens, are almost always **polyclonal antibodies**; that is, they contain antibodies produced by a large number of individual clones of B cells. The antibodies in such a response may be of several classes due to class switching. The variable regions of the antibody show great diversity and, if separated using electrophoresis, appear as a blur of overlapping proteins. In special cases antibodies may be monoclonal, the product of only a single clone of B cells. For example, if there is a cancer of the plasma cells, as in the disease multiple myeloma, such tumors derive from a single plasma cell and have a uniform variable region. On electrophoresis they form a single sharp peak (M spike). An important advance in biotechnology is the ability to produce **monoclonal antibodies** to desired antigens at will. These monoclonal antibodies have important uses in therapy and will be described later.

Polyclonal antibodies Humoral response consisting of antibodies produced by a number of clones of B cells.

Monoclonal antibodies Antibodies with a unique specificity for use in treating human disease, produced in tissue culture from a single clone of immune cells.

All Ig molecules have the same basic four-chain unit structure, but some immunoglobulins characteristically aggregate to form clusters of individual units. For example, IgM is usually a cluster of five individual units, and IgA is usually a pair of units.

An antibody molecule is not a rigid structure. The junction of its constant and variable parts, the hinge regions, is quite flexible. This feature allows the variable end of the Y-shaped molecule to adapt to the configuration of the antigen. Enzymatic treatment breaks an immunoglobulin molecule into three fragments. The variable region yields two fragments called the Fab fragments (antigen-binding fragments); each consists of a light chain and the associated part of the heavy chain. The other fragment is called the Fc fragment (constant fragment) and is in the constant region of the molecule (Figure 5-4).

IgM is present in the blood as a cluster of five individual molecules (a pentamer) joined together in a star-shaped configuration with the antigen-binding ends projecting outward and the opposite ends of the molecules directed toward the center of the cluster. It is the first antibody to be synthesized in a primary immune response because it does not require class switching. The pentamer of IgM forms a large antibody cluster that is efficient in combining with large particulate antigens such as fungi.

Monomeric IgM molecules and IgD molecules, neither of which is released from the cell, serve as the initial antigen receptors on naïve B cells. IgG, a much smaller antibody molecule, is the principal type of antibody molecule formed in response to the majority of infectious agents. IgA is produced by antibody-forming cells located in the respiratory, gastrointestinal, and genitourinary mucosa and is present in secretions from these areas. IgA apparently functions by combining with potentially harmful ingested or inhaled antigens. IgE is normally present in only small quantities in the blood of most people, but its concentration is greatly increased in allergic individuals. It binds specifically to mast cells via its Fc region, where it plays a role in defense against parasites and also in provoking certain forms of allergy. **Table 5-3** summarizes the types and functions of the various immunoglobulins.

Table 5-3 Types and Functions of Immunoglobulins

Immunoglobulin	Usual Type of Secretion	Properties and Functions
IgM	Pentamer	First Ig formed in response to foreign antigen (primary immune response). Present in bloodstream but not in tissues. Large pentamer antibody cluster very effective for combining with foreign antigen.
IgG	Monomer	Most prevalent Ig produced rapidly in large amounts (secondary immune response) to replace IgM. Found in blood and tissues. Crosses placenta protecting the fetus until infant immune system can produce antibodies.
IgA	Dimer	Present in the bloodstream, in secretions produced by mucous membranes (respiratory and GI tract), and in breastmilk providing maternal antibody protection to infant.
IgD	Monomer	Small amount in bloodstream and on surface of B lymphocytes. Undetermined functions.
IgE	Monomer	Present in the bloodstream and attaches to mast cells and basophils, which causes an allergic response when sensitizing antigen encountered. IgE evolved to protect against parasitic infections. In countries where the parasitic load is low, it is commonly associated with allergic reactions in susceptible (atopic) persons.

Immunoglobulin Effector Functions. Binding an antibody to a microbe or the toxic products of a microbe can block the ability of the microbe to infect cells or neutralize the damaging effect of the toxin. Once a pathogen is bound to the antibody via the variable region, the Fc region of the antibody serves as a signal to clear the pathogen from sites of infection; many cells that play a role in host defense have **Fc receptors** on their surface. A particular class of receptor, FcγR1 phagocytic receptor, is present on neutrophils and macrophages. Microbes coated with antibody, a process termed opsonization, are readily phagocytized by such cells via interaction with the Fc portion of the bound antibody, internalized, and destroyed. The Fc regions of IgG, in particular of IgG_1 and IgG_3, are most efficient at binding to the phagocytic receptor. Other types of Fc receptors are found on different cells important in host defense. The FcεR1 receptor found on mast cells (and the related basophils) specifically binds the Fc region of IgE molecules and plays a role in the defense against helminths (parasitic worms) as well as allergic reactions. **Figure 5-5** summarizes the several roles of antibodies in host defense.

Fc receptor Cell surface receptor for the constant region of the immunoglobulin molecule.

Acquiring Adaptive Immunity

Adaptive immunity can be established actively or passively. Active immunity is the result of exposure to antigens and developing immune responses. This process can occur naturally (e.g., you catch a flu) or artificially (e.g., you receive flu vaccine). Passive immunity is the result of obtaining protective antibody without exposure to antigen. This can also occur naturally (e.g., a woman transfers antibodies to her fetus during pregnancy) or artificially (e.g., you receive an injection of antiserum from other people or animals).

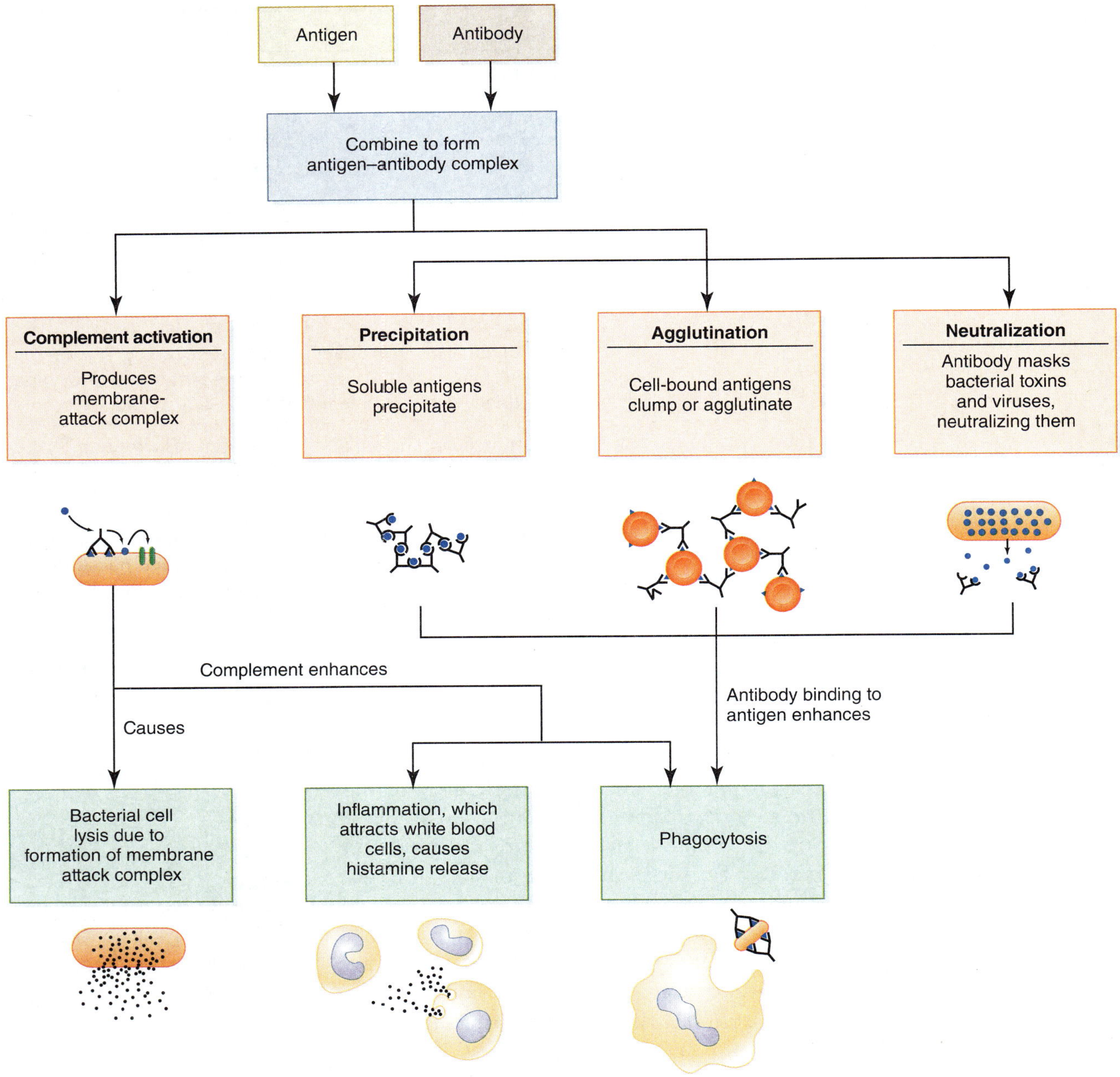

Figure 5-5 How antibodies work in host defense.

Autocrine Cell signaling to itself by releasing products that act on signal receptors found associated with the cell.

Lymphokine A soluble hormone-like substance liberated by lymphocytes.

Interleukin A type of cytokine produced by leukocytes and other body cells, involved in activation and maturation of immune cells.

Cytokines in Immune Response

Cytokines are small proteins produced by many cell populations, but they are predominantly produced by T cells and macrophages. They facilitate the interaction and communication between cells. Some cytokines act on the cells that produce them (**autocrine** signaling), others can act on the adjacent cells (paracrine signaling) or on the distant cells (endocrine). Cytokines may have specific names based on the cells that produce them, for example, monokines (produced by macrophages) and **lymphokines** (produced by lymphocytes). They may also be named based on their function, such as interferon (cytokines act by interfering with the multiplication of viruses), chemokine (cytokines with chemoattract activities), and **interleukin** (cytokines that send regulatory signals between cells of the immune system).

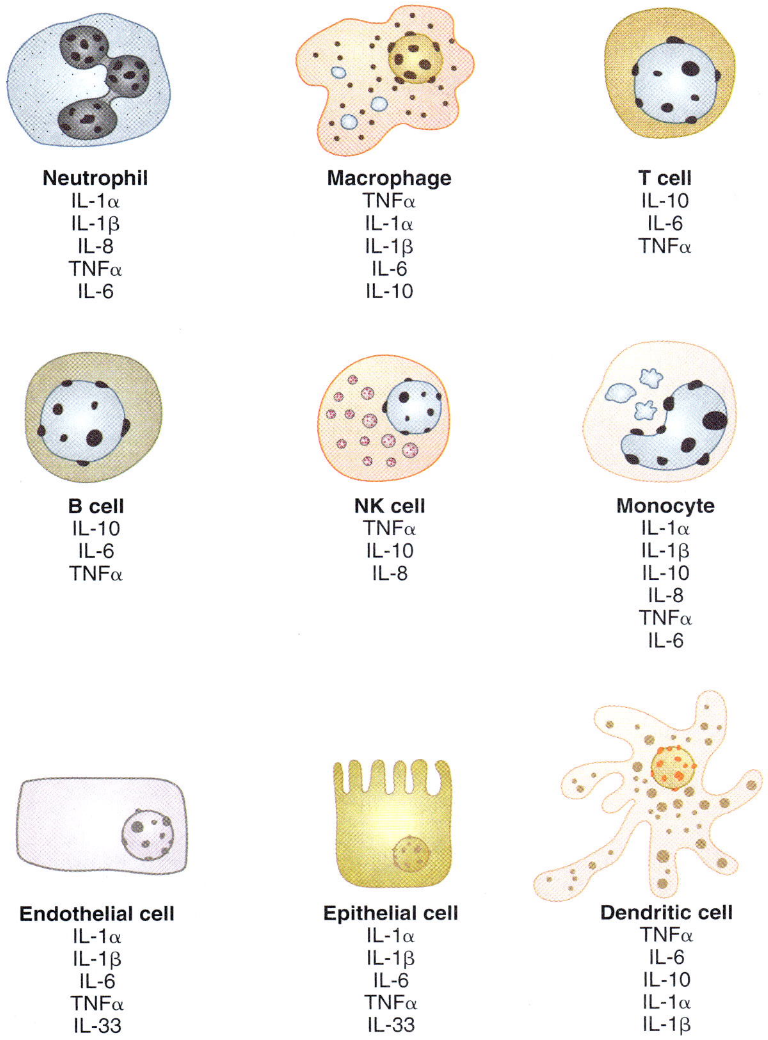

Figure 5-6 Examples of cytokines and cytokine-producing cells.

Kany, S., Vollrath, J. T., & Relja, B. (2019). Cytokines in Inflammatory Disease. International Journal of Molecular Sciences, 20(23), 6008. https://doi.org/10.3390/ijms20236008

Production of interleukin is essential for the immune cells' activation and differentiation; it regulates their proliferation, maturation, migration, and adhesion. Some interleukins also have pro-inflammatory and anti-inflammatory properties. For example, the cytokine IL-1 can promote inflammation, inducing fever. IL-2 acts as a T cell growth factor and enhances the survival of T cells. IL-4 can activate mast cells, basophile, and eosinophile, and regulate allergic responses. A list of the cytokines and cytokine-producing cells is demonstrated in **Figure 5-6**.

The Role of Complement in Immune Response

The complement system consists of a large number of interacting protein factors, which function in concert with humoral immunity to destroy or inactivate many bacterial pathogens, particularly organisms that have a capsule, such as *Streptococcus pneumoniae*, *Haemophilus influenzae*, and *Neisseria meningitidis*. Individuals lacking critical components of complement experience much higher susceptibility to these pathogens and may suffer lethal infections. Complement can be activated in several ways (see Chapter 4). The classical pathway, which is triggered by antigen–antibody interactions, is dependent on humoral immunity. Two other methods of complement activation, the alternative pathway and the lectin pathway, do not involve humoral immunity but depend on the ability of complement proteins to recognize and bind to components of the surface of microbial pathogens. When complement is activated, the complement components interact to accomplish several important host defense functions. Some components function as mediators of inflammation. Other components coat the surface of invading bacteria, which makes them easier for macrophages and neutrophils to phagocytose. Finally, the interaction of the complement components generates a group of complement molecules called an **attack complex**, which destroys the target microorganism or abnormal cell by "punching holes" in its cell membrane (**Figure 5-7**). IgM antibodies are most efficient in activating complement.

Attack complex Group of complement molecules that destroys the target microorganism or abnormal cell.

Immune complex Combination of antibody and antigen forming a lattice.

In addition to its role in host defense, complement plays an important role in clearing **immune complexes** from circulation. Immune complexes consist of antibody bound to its cognate antigen. Because there are at least two antigen binding sites on Ig molecules and most of the antigens possess multiple epitopes, antibody bound to antigen can form "lattices" of variable size. These complexes may bind to parts of the vascular system and trigger hypersensitivity reactions. Such complexes may also promote certain autoimmune diseases such as systemic lupus erythematosus (SLE). People with a genetic deficiency for certain complement components are highly susceptible to this disease.

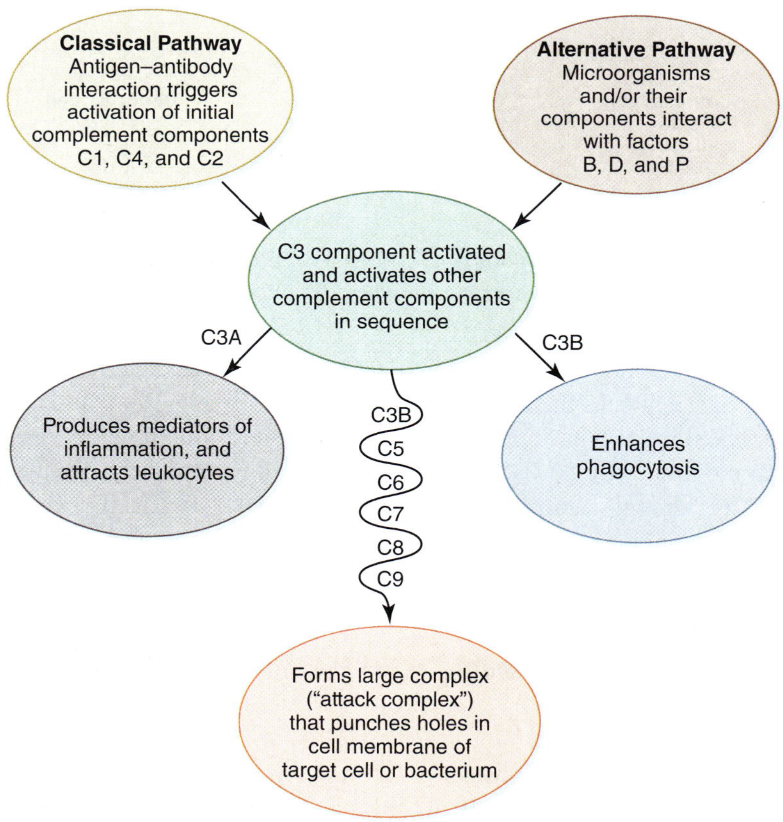

Figure 5-7 Components and pathways of complement activation that "complement" the body's immune defenses; individual components are named C1 through C9 and factors B, D, and P. Note that the lectin pathway (not shown) is similar in detail to the classical pathway, substituting a carbohydrate-binding protein (lectin) for the C1 Ig binding complex.

NK and Innate Immunity

A unique subset of lymphocytes characterized by their large size and multiple granules are natural killer (NK) cells. NK cells originate from hematopoietic stem cells in the bone marrow (**primary lymphoid organ**); they make up about 10 percent of circulating lymphocytes and those in **secondary lymphoid organs**. NK cells belong to the innate immune system, but their functions are regulated by the adaptive immune system. Although NK cells show no antigen specificity, they play an important role in detecting and killing cells that do not express class I MHC antigen, such as virally infected cells and cancer cells. NK cells also recognize the target coated with antibodies and destroy them by releasing enzymes such as perforin and granzyme A/B, a process called **antibody-dependent cellular cytotoxicity (ADCC)**.

Primary lymphoid organs Bone marrow and thymus.

Secondary lymphoid organs Lymph nodes, spleen tonsils and adenoids, and mucosal-associated lymphoid tissue.

Antibody-dependent cellular cytotoxicity (ADCC) Recognition and destruction of cells coated with antibody.

HLA system The genes of the histocompatibility complex and the antigens that they determine on the surface of cells.

HLA Types and Susceptibility to Disease

Although MHC proteins were originally considered of interest only with respect to organ transplantation, they have a much larger role in antigen presentation and are critical in the development of both cellular and humoral immunity as previously noted.

Human-version MHC molecules are known as HLA (human leukocyte antigen). The surface proteins within the **HLA system** fall into two major groups, designated MHC class I proteins and MHC class II proteins. Class I proteins are controlled by HLA-A, HLA-B, and HLA-C genes; class II proteins are controlled by HLA-D genes. More than 1200 different allelic genes can occupy the gene loci within the HLA system.

The presence of certain HLA types predisposes individuals to specific diseases. The most striking example of such an association is between HLA-B27 and a particular type of arthritis of the spine and the sacroiliac joints, ankylosing spondylitis. However, the presence of the B27 type indicates only a predisposition to the disease. It does not mean that any given individual will invariably be affected because only less than 25 percent of B27-positive people ever develop this type of arthritis. In the case of ankylosing spondylitis (and a number of related forms of arthritic disease), gastrointestinal infection with certain microbial pathogens is a likely environmental trigger for the disease in B27-positive people. Predisposition to other diseases also has been associated with this HLA type.

Similar associations exist between certain class II HLA types and specific diseases, which are considered in other chapters. The diseases include type 1 diabetes, prone to develop in children and young adults (Chapter 20), and rheumatoid arthritis (RA) (Chapter 24). These diseases tend to have an autoimmune component. The association of a particular class II HLA allele with an autoimmune disease relates to the ability of the MHC molecule specified by the gene to bind and present specific autoantigens. Certain types of RA are related to a form of post-synthetic protein modification that forms citrullinated peptides (i.e., containing the amino acid citrulline), derived from joint proteins. Such peptides bind to the particular class II MHC (HLA) alleles associated with severe rheumatoid arthritis. Smoking is also a risk factor for severe RA and results in the production of citrullinated peptides in the lung. Such peptides may be the immune trigger for RA and result in the production of humoral immunity to such modified peptides. Many (but not all) of the genes involved in propensity for a particular form of immune response, and in particular autoimmune response, are related to the HLA system.

Hypersensitivity Reactions: Immune System–Related Tissue Injury

The immune system protects us from foreign substances that could harm us, but the immune response also may damage tissues. This undesirable effect is called hypersensitivity. Hypersensitivity reactions often do not result from too much immunity but from inappropriately directed immunity or from "bystander" damage to normal tissue adjacent to the site of an immune reaction. The positive reaction to a tuberculin test (discussed later in this chapter) is a clinically mild example. A far more serious example of bystander effect is the severe liver damage in hepatitis C infection mediated by immune T cells attempting to destroy hepatocytes chronically infected with the virus.

Hypersensitivity reactions are classified based on how the immune system caused the injury using the Gell and Coombs system (named after the two immunologists who devised it) (**Table 5-4**). Four different types of hypersensitivity reactions, usually designated by Roman numerals, are recognized. The first three types are related to antibodies formed in response to antigenic material, and the fourth type is a cell-mediated hypersensitivity reaction. Although most hypersensitivity reactions involve more than one of the four defined types, and some types of hypersensitivity reactions do not fit well into any of the categories, the system is still used by clinicians to describe hypersensitivity disease.

Table 5-4 Mechanisms of Immunologic Injury

Type	Mechanism	Examples
I: Immediate hypersensitivity	IgE antibodies are fixed to mast cells and basophils. Later contact with sensitizing antigen triggers mediator release and clinical manifestations.	Localized response: Hay fever, food allergy, etc. Systemic response: bee sting or penicillin anaphylaxis, etc.
II: Cytotoxic hypersensitivity reactions	Antibody binds to cell or tissue antigen, and complement is activated, which damages the cell, causes inflammation, and promotes destruction of antibody-coated cell by phagocytosis.	Autoimmune hemolytic anemia Blood transfusion reactions Rh hemolytic disease Some types of glomerulonephritis
III: Immune complex disease	Circulating antigen–antibody complexes form, which activate complement and cause inflammatory reactions.	Some types of glomerulonephritis Lupus erythematosus Rheumatoid arthritis
IV: Delayed (cell-mediated) hypersensitivity	Sensitized (delayed hypersensitivity) T cells release lymphokines that attract macrophages and other inflammatory cells.	Tuberculosis Fungus and parasitic infections Contact dermatitis

Type I: Immediate Hypersensitivity Reactions (Allergy and Anaphylaxis)

Type I hypersensitivity reactions follow contact with foreign antigens that induce formation of specific IgE antibodies in the sensitized person. IgE has the distinctive property of attaching to the surface of mast cells (and to similar cells circulating in the blood, basophils) via the Fc region. Cross-linking of two or more IgE molecules by antigen binding to the variable region of the IgE molecule pointing away from the mast cell causes the mast cell to release preformed cytoplasmic granules filled with histamine, proteases, and cytokines, all of which serve as potent mediators of inflammation and attractants for other inflammatory cells such as eosinophils and neutrophils. Activation of mast cells by antigen binding to IgE also initiates the synthesis of other mediators in a time-dependent manner that promotes T and B cell immunity and continues to attract eosinophils to the area. Type I hypersensitivity reactions (also called immediate hypersensitivity reactions) may be localized (allergic reactions, including asthma) or may evoke a widespread systemic reaction called **anaphylaxis** (**Figure 5-8**).

Anaphylaxis A widespread systemic hypersensitivity reaction.

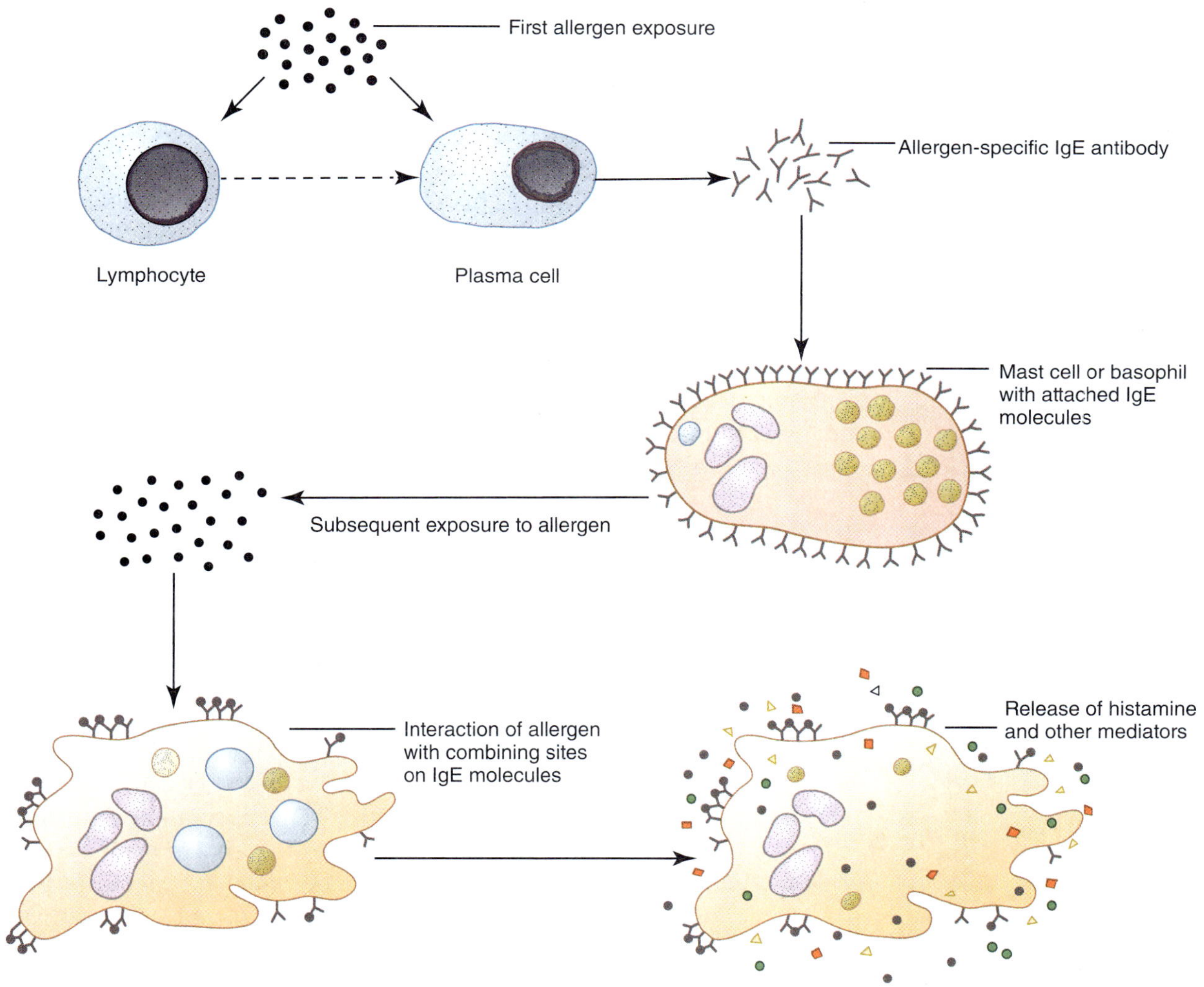

Figure 5-8 Pathogenesis of allergy. First exposure to allergen induces formation of specific IgE antibody in susceptible individual, which binds to mast cells and basophils by the nonantigen receptor end of the molecule Fc region. Subsequent exposure to the allergen leads to an dimerization of IgE antibody, liberating histamine and other mediators from mast cells and basophils. These mediators induce allergic manifestations.

Allergy

Individuals who develop localized IgE-mediated reactions are predisposed to form specific IgE antibodies, become allergic to ragweed, other plant pollens, and various antigens that do not affect others, a process termed atopic allergy. Although there is a clear genetic component to atopic allergies, the exact mechanism remains unclear, and many genes appear to play a role. The sensitizing antigen is called an allergen, and the allergic manifestations are localized to the tissues that are exposed to the allergens—for example, swollen itchy eyes, stuffy nose, and sneezing in a ragweed-sensitive person.

Because histamine is one of the mediators released from the IgE-coated cells, antihistamine drugs, blocking the effects of histamine, often relieve many of the allergic symptoms. A more specific method of treating an allergic individual consists of immunizing the person to the offending allergen by repeated subcutaneous injections of the antigen that induced the allergy, such as an extract of ragweed pollen in a ragweed-sensitive person. This method of treatment, called **desensitization**, induces the formation of IgG antibodies against the offending allergen. The IgG may act by combining with the allergen before it can affix to the cell-bound IgE, thus preventing the release of mediators, although other mechanisms such as inducing unresponsiveness (generating tolerance) in T cells may play a role.

Desensitization
Treatment for allergy that induces the formation of IgG antibodies.

Asthma

Asthma is defined by airway obstruction related to hyperresponsiveness of the smooth muscles of the bronchi. Although many pro-inflammatory triggers can result in asthma, type I (immediate) hypersensitivity involving an environmentally inhaled allergen is most often the cause. Animal dander (especially from cats), house mites, bird feathers, and seasonal allergens such as tree and grass pollens also may trigger attacks in affected individuals. Asthma can have serious consequences and can even result in death if not appropriately treated using bronchodilators, steroid drugs, and other immunosuppressive agents. Although mediators produced by activated mast cells and eosinophils (which are prevalent in the respiratory tissue of asthmatics) result in an acute attack, the initial trigger is from sensitized Th2 cells that have an IgE-type response to the inciting allergen. Individuals brought up in an environment containing numerous pathogens and allergens (such as farms) tend to be less likely to develop asthma, possibly because early exposure to environmental allergens results in a Th1 immune response, which does not stimulate IgE production and is protective. This concept has been termed the hygiene hypothesis. A little dirt in a child's environment may, in fact, be a good thing!

Anaphylaxis and Anaphylactoid Reactions

A severe generalized IgE-mediated hypersensitivity reaction, called anaphylaxis, may be life-threatening. The condition results from an initial exposure to a substance (allergen) that induces an extreme degree of sensitization in a susceptible person. Commonly implicated allergens include penicillin, bee stings, peanuts (a legume, not a true nut), tree nuts, latex products, some fruits that contain latex-like chemicals (kiwi fruit, bananas, and others), as well as various other sensitizing agents. Once sensitization has occurred, a later exposure to the sensitizing antigen triggers widespread mediator release from IgE-coated mast cells and basophils. This release may lead to a fall in blood pressure with circulatory collapse and is often accompanied by severe respiratory distress caused by mediator-induced spasm of smooth muscle in the walls of the bronchioles, restricting airflow into and out of the lungs. Prompt treatment of this immunologic catastrophe with epinephrine and other appropriate agents is essential. A similar condition, called an **anaphylactoid reaction**, resembles an anaphylactic reaction but is not caused by IgE; it is caused by direct action on mast cells or by activating complement. Aspirin, other non-steroidal anti-inflammatory drugs, some antibiotics, and radiopaque iodine containing contrast material used for X-ray examinations may trigger an anaphylactoid reaction. An unusual form of anaphylactoid reaction (scombroid poisoning) occurs when bacteria acting on improperly stored dark meat fish convert the amino acid histidine in the fish flesh to histamine and related compounds (which are not degraded by cooking). The ingested histamine can produce a severe (and occasionally fatal) reaction. The treatment for anaphylactoid reactions is the same as for an anaphylactic reaction.

Anaphylactoid reaction Immune response resembling an anaphylactic reaction but by direct action on mast cells or by activating complement.

Autoantibody An antibody formed against the host's own cells or tissue components.

Type II: Hypersensitivity Reactions

Type II hypersensitivity reactions result from the deleterious effects of antibody (most often **autoantibody**) binding to a cell or neutralizing or blocking the physiological effect of an essential protein. The injurious effects may involve complement activation, opsonization of cells and neutrophil activation, or the direct effects of antibody binding. After an IgG or IgM antibody reacts with a cell-associated antigen, complement is activated, and the products of complement activation directly or indirectly damage the target. The complement components interact to form an attack complex that directly damages the target cell membrane. Inflammatory cells such as neutrophils also are attracted and contribute to the tissue injury by releasing destructive enzymes; they may also destroy the antibody-coated target cells by phagocytosis. Examples of such type II reactions include transfusion reactions caused by administration of incompatible blood, hemolytic disease of newborn infants caused by Rh incompatibility during prenatal development, some types of chronic hemolytic anemia associated with autoantibodies directed against red blood cells in the hematopoietic and lymphatic systems, and a type of kidney disease caused by autoantibodies directed against basement membranes of glomerular capillaries in the urinary system.

In Graves' disease, autoantibodies to the TSH receptor on thyroid cells inappropriately stimulate the cells to make an excess of thyroid hormone resulting in hyperthyroidism. Autoantibodies directed to the acetylcholine receptors on motor endplates of muscle block the transmission of neuronal signals from the nerve, resulting in muscle fatigue and partial paralysis, a condition called myasthenia gravis. Patients may also develop antibodies against therapeutic proteins that inactivate them. Some individuals with severe hemophilia A totally lack the coagulation protein F.VIII. To prevent hemorrhage, these patients are treated with recombinant human F.VIII. Because the patients completely lacked the protein during development, the immune system may see the therapeutic F.VIII as foreign and produce antibodies, termed inhibitors, that render the protein useless.

Type III: Tissue Injury Caused by Immune Complexes ("Immune Complex Disease")

In type III hypersensitivity, antigen bound to antibody forms immune complexes within the circulation that can be deposited in the tissues. Because antibodies have multiple binding sites for antigen (2 on IgG, potentially 10 on IgM) and because most antigens have multiple epitopes to which antibody can bind, the interaction of antigen and antibody often forms latticelike structures, immune complexes, that differ in size and chemical properties. The ability to bind to tissue and the site of binding is determined by the properties of the immune complexes. The deposited antigen–antibody complexes activate complement, and the activated complement components, along with the inflammatory cells that they attract, damage the tissues. Often, the immunologic reaction within the tissues is quite severe and leads to thrombosis of blood vessels in the vascular system and considerable tissue necrosis in other areas.

An example of organ damage in the urinary system caused by immune complexes is a type of kidney disease called immune-complex glomerulonephritis, in which the complexes are trapped within the glomeruli as the blood flows through the kidneys. This leads to the accumulation of neutrophils within the glomerulus and destruction of the renal filtration mechanism, finally resulting in renal failure. An example of this process is acute post-infectious glomerulonephritis, which sometimes occurs following infection by β-hemolytic streptococcus infections in children. The hypersensitivity reaction usually occurs 10 days to 2 weeks after the infection starts. At this time, antibodies to the antigens derived from the bacteria are present in the circulation and bind to each other, forming complexes that deposit in glomerular capillary walls and activate complement at that site. The complement, along with neutrophils and macrophages attracted to the site, produce local inflammation and glomerular damage. The disease usually resolves spontaneously in several weeks, although in rare cases the glomerular injury may be long-lasting. Another important disease in which tissue injury is related to immune complexes is lupus erythematosus, considered in connection with autoimmune disease later in this chapter.

Type IV: Delayed (Cell-Mediated) Hypersensitivity Reactions

In type IV hypersensitivity (delayed hypersensitivity reactions), T lymphocytes rather than antibodies are responsible for the tissue injury. Unlike immediate hypersensitivity reactions, a cell-mediated inflammatory reaction requires from 24 to 48 hours to develop, the delay being the time necessary for sensitized T cells to accumulate at the site and generate an inflammatory reaction. The most common examples of delayed hypersensitivity involve the reaction of immune T helper cells recognizing a soluble antigen in tissue. This results in the recruitment of macrophages and additional lymphocytes and local damage to tissue. The reaction is usually self-limited with a peak occurring 1 or 2 days followed by subsidence. The reaction that a person previously exposed to tuberculosis experiences in response to a tuberculin test (in which a material derived from the bacteria termed tuberculin is injected into the skin) is an example of delayed hypersensitivity. Contact dermatitis (inflammation of the skin), caused by exposure to plant-derived oily resins from *Rhus* species (poison ivy, oak, and sumac), is another example with a characteristic delayed hypersensitivity reaction. On first exposure, a low–molecular weight chemical in the resin binds to a skin-derived protein on the surface of a dendritic cell present in the skin. After about a week, a population of Th1 cells is generated that will react with the plant resin when the material subsequently contacts the skin. The results are well known to those who suffer from "poison ivy" and consist of intense itching and a red blistered rash that may last for several weeks. Corticosteroids (either locally applied or taken systemically) lessen the reaction.

Suppression of the Immune Response

Cell-mediated and humoral immune responses protect against potentially harmful microorganisms and other foreign substances. However, in the case with organ transplants or misdirected immune responses creating autoimmune disease, the immune response may need to be suppressed. In such cases, a number of chemical, pharmaceutical, and biological agents can interfere with the immune response at several levels and can suppress the immune reaction.

Chemical Agents (Drugs)

Corticosteroids, derived from hormones produced by the adrenal cortex, have a broad range of anti-inflammatory effects, the most important of which is in preventing activation of neutrophils and macrophages and the production of cytokines and other chemical mediators important in inflammation. As is the case with many immunosuppressive agents, use of corticosteroids increases the risk of infection. Corticosteroids also interfere with wound healing and can lead to serious endocrine dysfunction. A number of cytotoxic drugs interfere with DNA synthesis and prevent the division of cells necessary for immune responses. Azathioprine causes a decrease in lymphocytes and NK cells by suppressing the bone marrow. There is often a fall in granulocytic cells, such as neutrophils, and platelets as well. The DNA alkylating agent cyclophosphamide has little effect on inflammation but causes dose-dependent decreases in cytotoxic and helper T cells. It is widely used to treat serious autoimmune disease and in preparing patients for hematopoietic stem cell transplants (Chapter 12). Calcineurin inhibitors, a more recently developed class of drugs, inhibit the production of the cytokine IL-2 and block the division of T helper cells. Cyclosporine and the closely related drug tacrolimus are both highly effective in prolonging graft survival and are essential for transplant procedures.

Biological Agents (Monoclonal Antibodies)

Monoclonal antibodies (mAbs) against immune cells and cytokines have been developed and used to treat inflammatory and autoimmune disease. They are also used to help prevent organ rejection. Currently, mAbs are available to inhibit activated T cells, T helper cells, B cells, and many pro-inflammatory proteins such as TNF-α. The list of mAbs is long and rapidly growing.

A major problem in the past was that many mAbs were based on murine (mouse) Ig molecules and could sometimes be recognized by humans as foreign and inactivated by our host defenses. Currently, humanized antibodies are being increasingly used. Such mAbs are 95 percent human in structure and consequently not recognized as foreign. As might be predicted, use of such potent immunosuppressive agents can be associated with susceptibility to bacterial and viral pathogens.

Pools of random human Ig given intravenously (IVIg) are often effective in treating autoimmune diseases. The exact mechanism is unknown but may involve blockading Fc receptors on cells, resulting in the more rapid destruction of endogenous antibody responsible for the disease. Eliminating a foreign antigen before the immune system can respond to the antigen is another effective way to suppress an immune response and is used routinely to prevent hemolytic disease of newborn infants caused by Rh incompatibility. Postdelivery administration of Rh immune globulin containing potent Rh antibodies to an Rh-negative mother who has given birth to an Rh-positive infant eliminates antigenic Rh-positive fetal cells that may have entered the mother's bloodstream during delivery. Because the antigenic fetal cells are rapidly removed from the mother's circulation, the mother does not form Rh antibody, preventing Rh hemolytic disease in subsequent pregnancies. This application is described in Chapter 18.

Immunodeficiency Disease

Primary immunodeficiency diseases are the result of intrinsic congenital defects that result in defects in the host immune response. Such defects may be global and result in a total lack of immune responses (severe combined immunodeficiency diseases [SCID]). The most severe form of SCID, reticular dysgenesis, is an extremely uncommon genetic disease characterized by early failure of bone marrow development, resulting in a total lack of granulocytes (such as neutrophils) and a near total lack of lymphocytes. The thymus and lymph nodes are absent or underdeveloped, and there is a lack of both innate and adaptive immunity. Severe recurrent infections in the neonatal period occur, resulting in death without hematopoietic stem cell transplantation.

Other rare genetic diseases resulting in SCID are X-linked SCID or RAG1/2. X-linked SCID, the most common, is caused by a lack of functioning receptors for a number of cytokines necessary for immune function. These receptors have a common polypeptide γ-chain that is defective in the disease. Another relatively common cause of SCID is RAG1/2. RAG enzymes are critical for the formation of both T cell receptors and Ig variable region synthesis, and affected individuals lack functioning antigen receptors. Congenital genetic defects also can result in isolated defects of either T cell or B cell development. Even in the presence of functional B cells, isolated T cell defects will result in very limited humoral immunity. SCID and isolated T cell deficiencies are generally treated by stem cell transplantation.

Primary defects in humoral immunity are somewhat more common. Common variable immunodeficiency disease is a collection of disorders that is most often associated with low IgG and IgA. The disease varies in severity and is sometimes not detected until adulthood. X-linked agammaglobulinemia (Bruton disease) is associated with a failure of B cell maturation and a lack of plasma cells. Affected individuals have little or no circulating Ig of any class. Isolated B cell defects are effectively treated by aggressive replacement of Ig, which is necessary to prevent recurrent bacterial infections. These examples represent only a selection of the most encountered of these rare but devastating conditions.

Other congenital diseases include a degree of immunodeficiency as part of a broader syndrome. DiGeorge syndrome results in an abnormal or absent thymus and defects in cellular immunity combined with cardiac and other abnormalities (such as very widely spaced eyes and defects in facial development). The disease results from a small deletion in chromosome 22. Although DiGeorge syndrome does result in immunodeficiency, it is best considered as a localized genetic developmental defect.

Acquired immune deficiency syndrome (AIDS) An infection caused by the human immunodeficiency virus. The virus attacks and destroys helper T lymphocytes, which compromises cell-mediated immunity, leading to increased susceptibility to infection and some tumors.

Secondary defects in host defense, such as **acquired immune deficiency syndrome (AIDS)**, are extensive. Malnutrition, leukemia and lymphoma therapeutic drugs, and other infectious agents all may result in some degree of immunodeficiency. Loss of proteins from the circulation, which occurs in some renal diseases (Chapter 17), or extensive burns also may result in immunodeficiency states. A common surgical intervention (splenectomy) results in greatly increased susceptibility to *Streptococcus pneumoniae* and occasionally death if the splenectomy is not considered. Immunization to pneumococcus is critical in such patients.

Human Immunodeficiency Virus Infections and AIDS

HIV Transmission

Although HIV infection often is predominantly a sexually transmitted disease, HIV may also be transmitted congenitally, parenterally, most commonly via blood-contaminated needles and improperly sterilized instruments, and, in the past, by contaminated blood products.

Infection requires the transfer of blood, seminal fluid, cervical and vaginal secretions, or breastmilk, which often contains large amounts of virus and serves as a source of infection. Urine, stool, saliva, tears, and perspiration usually contain little if any virus and are not considered a risk. Even accidental needle sticks by healthcare workers have a low probability of infection (around one percent, which can be prevented by drug prophylaxis.)

HIV-mediated disease in humans is relatively recent. Retrospective genetic studies suggest that cross-species transmission to humans occurred early in the twentieth century. The virus was probably established in the human population by the 1950s. In 1983 the scientific community identified HIV, and a blood test to detect infection became available in 1985.

HIV Life Cycle

HIV is an RNA retrovirus. It reverse-transcribes its RNA into DNA, which is then inserted into the genome of host cells as provirus. The viral RNA and an enzyme, reverse transcriptase, are enclosed within a protein coat (capsid), forming the core of the virus. The core is surrounded by an envelope, composed of a double layer of lipid molecules, acquired from the cell membrane of the infected cell as part of the budding out of the virus.

HIV targets the CD4 protein present on the cell membranes of helper T lymphocytes, as well as on monocytes, macrophages, and similar macrophage-like cells. The CD4 protein functions as a receptor and attachment point for the virus in combination with another cell surface receptor (CCR5). When the virus binds to the cell, the virus envelope fuses with the cell membrane, allowing the virus to enter the cell. Once inside the cell, the virus makes a DNA copy of its own RNA genetic material using the reverse transcriptase enzyme. The viral DNA copy is then inserted into the genetic material of the infected cell, a process assisted by another viral enzyme, HIV integrase. Integrases allow viral genes to direct the synthesis of viral-derived proteins. The final stages of virus production require a viral enzyme, HIV protease. This protease cuts and assembles the virus protein into small segments that surround the viral RNA allowing the formation of the infectious virus particles that bud from the infected cells. The newly formed virus particles attack other susceptible cells within the lymphoid tissue throughout the body. The process continues as the virus particles find more susceptible cells. Helper T lymphocytes, the primary targets for the virus, sustain damage and many are killed. Monocytes are quite resistant and survive. However, they become a reservoir where the virus continues to replicate, resulting in the release of more virus particles that infect other cells. Since monocytes circulate throughout the body, they become vehicles for transporting the virus throughout the body, including

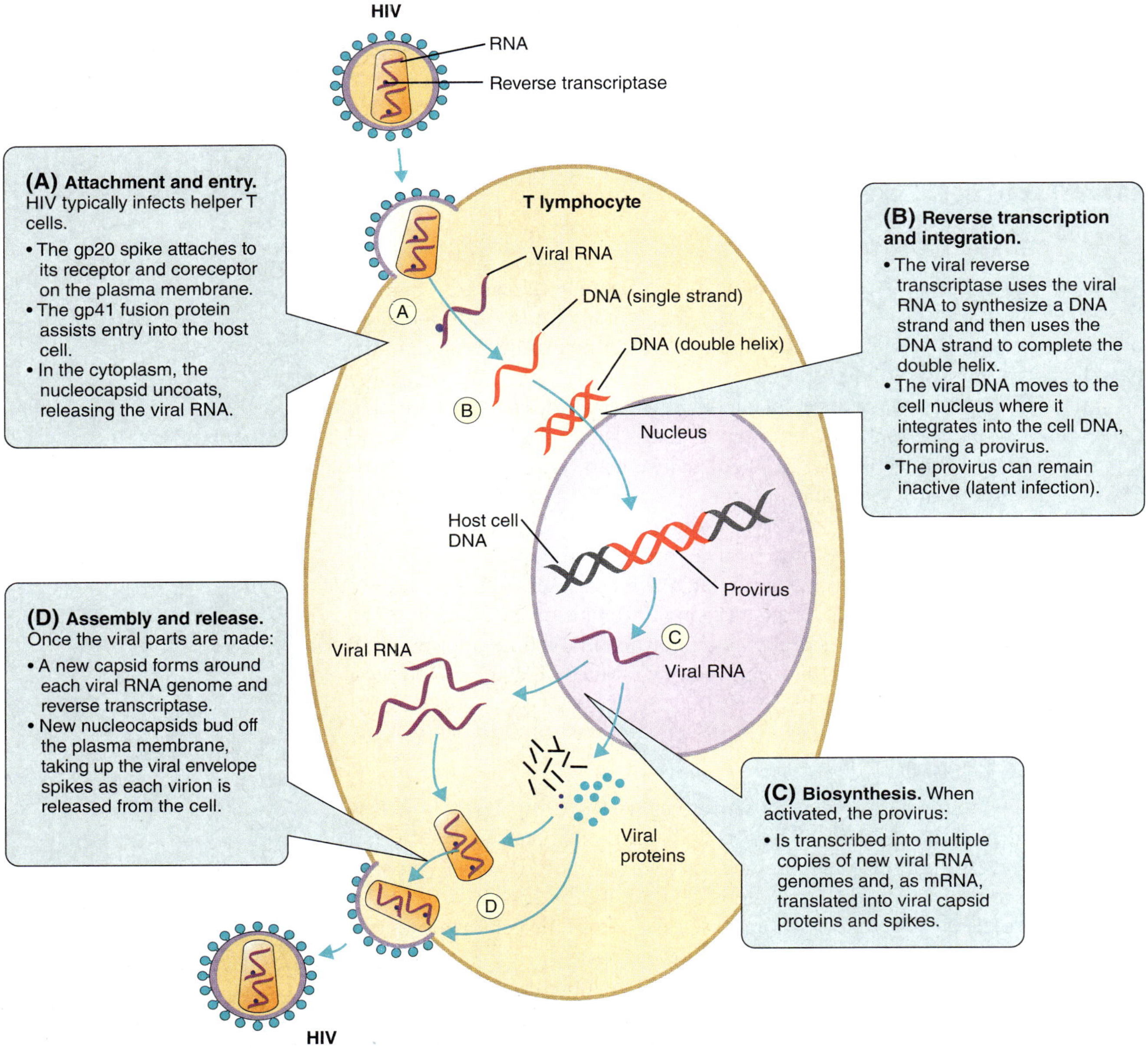

Figure 5-9 Replication cycle of the human immunodeficiency virus (HIV). Replication is dependent on the reverse transcriptase enzyme.

into the nervous system and infection of the brain (**Figure 5-9**). The viral reverse transcriptase has a very high error rate; hence HIV-1 exhibits a very high mutation rate, leading to rapid formation of viruses resistant to therapeutic drugs.

Mother-to-Infant Transmission

Maternal blood or cervical–vaginal secretions become the source of infection for newborn infants born to infected mothers. The likelihood of fetal infection depends to some extent on the maternal viral load. The level in the mother's blood and body fluids can be as high as 15–45%. Consequently, all infected pregnant people should receive highly effective antiretroviral therapy to suppress HIV multiplication. With effective antiviral therapy, the amount of virus in the maternal blood can be reduced to an extremely low level, reducing the risk of perinatal HIV transmission to less than 1%.

Manifestations of HIV Infection

During the early stages of the infection, large amounts of virus can be detected in the blood lymphocytes and body fluids. During this phase, many infected individuals develop a mild febrile illness. The body responds to the infection by forming anti-HIV antibodies and by generating cytotoxic T lymphocytes directed against the virus. Consequently, the amount of virus in the blood and body fluids declines in the acute phase of the infection. Unfortunately, the body's defenses cannot eliminate the virus. Very large numbers of virus particles are produced, continuously infecting and destroying even more CD4+ cells (helper T cells). The numbers of virus particles circulating in the bloodstream correlate with the magnitude of the infection.

The body responds to the destruction of CD4+ cells by increasing production of CD4+ cells. Cytotoxic (CD8) T cells directed against HIV proliferate and dampen viral multiplication and helper T cell destruction. Eventually, the rate at which CD4+ cells can be replaced cannot keep up with rate of destruction, and subsequently, the functions of the immune system begin to decline (**Figure 5-10**).

Unfortunately, the anti-HIV antibodies cannot completely eradicate the virus or reduce the level of infectivity. A confirmed positive test for anti-HIV antibodies indicates infection with HIV and the potential for transmission to others. Their immune system is at risk.

There are many different strains of HIV. Some can be quite aggressive, with rapid progression of the disease and the development of AIDS. In contrast, a few strains appear to be relatively benign; the individuals infected with these HIV strains for many years do not show evidence of immune system damage.

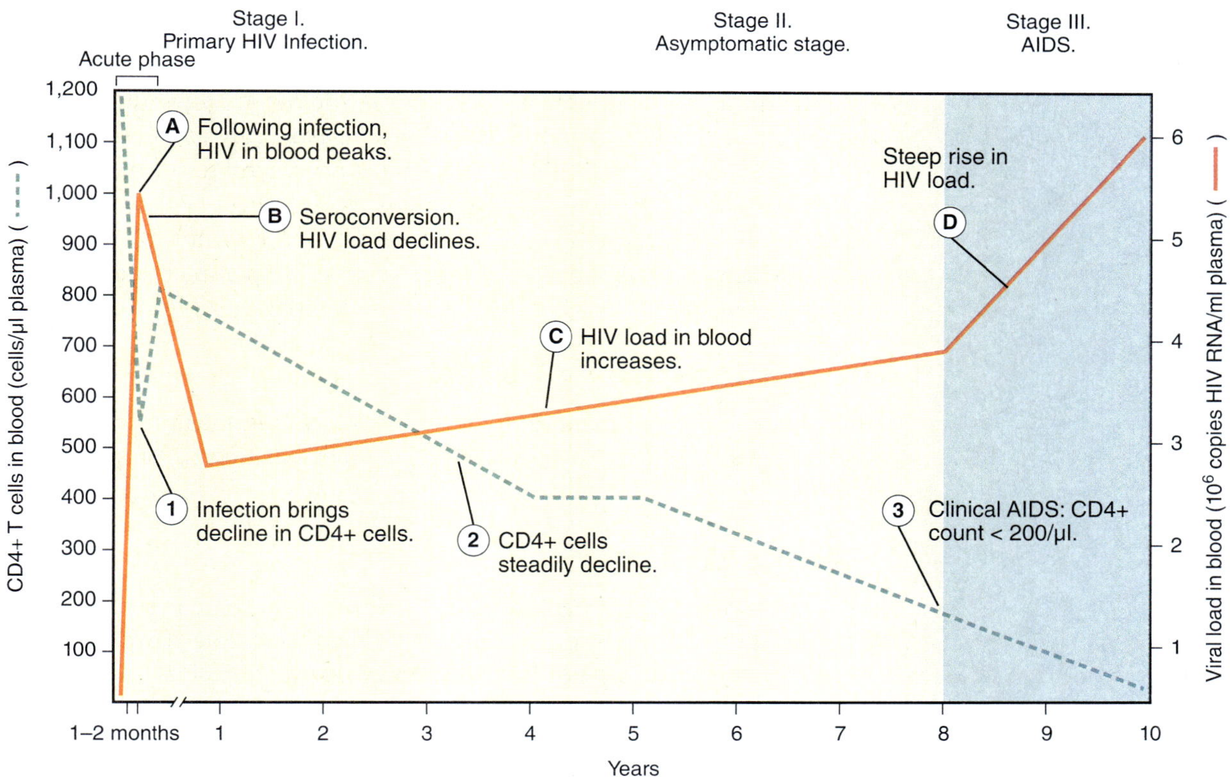

Figure 5-10 HIV infection and AIDS. Once infected with HIV, the immune response brings about an abrupt drop in circulating HIV virus particles, which will rise as the immune system fails (A–D). Without antiretroviral therapy, the T cell count slowly drops (1–3) and clinical AIDS occurs.

Table 5-5 Sequence of Events in HIV Infections and Their Significance

Event	Significance
HIV invades CD4+ cells and becomes part of cell DNA	Individual is infected for life
Virus proliferates in infected cells and sheds virus particles	Virus presents in blood and body fluids
Body forms anti-HIV antibody	Antibody is a marker of infection but is not protective
Progressive destruction of helper T cells	Compromised cell-mediated immunity
Immune defenses collapse	Opportunistic infections Neoplasms

Table 5-5 summarizes the sequence of events in HIV infection and their significance.

Measurement of Viral RNA and CD4 Lymphocytes as an Index of Disease Progression

Although HIV replicates in lymphocytes in the lymph nodes, the amount of viral RNA in the blood reflects the extent of viral replication throughout the body. An acute infection presents with over a million virus particles per milliliter of blood plasma. Successful treatment reveals extremely low levels of HIV particles in the patient. Currently, measuring the level of viral RNA using quantitative PCR-based techniques indicates disease progression and reflects the efficacy of therapy.

The number of helper T lymphocytes in the blood allows an estimation of the extent of damage to the immune system. Normally, there are from about 800 to 1200 helper T (CD4+) lymphocytes per microliter of blood, with this number declining progressively as the disease advances. Below 500 cells per microliter of blood, the patient becomes at risk of opportunistic infections, and when the helper T lymphocyte count falls below 200 per microliter, the infected person experiences a very high risk of major complications from the disease.

Complications of AIDS

Impaired cell-mediated immunity leads to two very serious problems: a greatly increased susceptibility to infection and a predisposition to various malignant tumors.

Infections

Many of the viruses, fungi, parasites, and other pathogens that attack AIDS patients do not usually cause disease in healthy people. (Infections of this type are often called **opportunistic infections**.) Formerly, one of the most common AIDS-related opportunistic infections was pneumocystis pneumonia, caused by the fungal parasite *Pneumocystis jirovecii*. Another relatively common and serious systemic infection is caused by a normally nonpathogenic acid-fast bacterium called *Mycobacterium avium* complex. Other serious infections are the parasitic infections (of) *toxoplasmosis* and *cryptosporidiosis*, described in Chapter 8.

Opportunistic infection Infection in an immunocompromised person caused by an organism that is normally nonpathogenic or of limited pathogenicity.

Table 5-6 Common Infections in HIV Patients

Viruses	Herpes, cytomegalovirus, Epstein-Barr virus (infectious mononucleosis)
Fungi	Histoplasmosis, coccidioidomycosis, aspergillosis, *Candida* infections, *Pneumocystis jiroveci* pneumonia
Protozoa	Amoebiasis, cryptosporidiosis, toxoplasmosis
Mycobacteria	Tuberculosis, *Mycobacterium avium-intracellulare* infections

AIDS patients, as immunocompromised patients, are at risk for acquiring widespread, rapidly progressive tuberculosis or histoplasmosis infections. Many of the symptoms exhibited by patients with AIDS, such as fever, cough, shortness of breath, weight loss, and enlarged lymph nodes, result from severe opportunistic infections. **Table 5-6** lists some of the more common, severe, and often life-threatening infections in AIDS patients.

Malignant Tumors

The malignant tumors common in AIDS patients also are related to failure of the immune system. The most common malignant tumor in AIDS patients, which is rare in other people, is Kaposi sarcoma, caused by a herpes virus designated human herpesvirus 8. This tumor, which is composed of immature connective tissue cells (fibroblasts) and blood capillaries intermixed with inflammatory and phagocytic cells, forms hemorrhagic nodules in the skin, mouth, lymph nodes, and internal organs (**Figure 5-11**). Malignant tumors of B lymphocytes also are common, as are cancers of the mouth, rectum, and uterine cervix.

Treatment of HIV Infection

Infections and tumors in AIDS patients can be treated, but treatment of the underlying viral infection has been hampered by lack of a drug(s) that can eliminate the virus. The viral life cycle offers a number of potential drug targets.

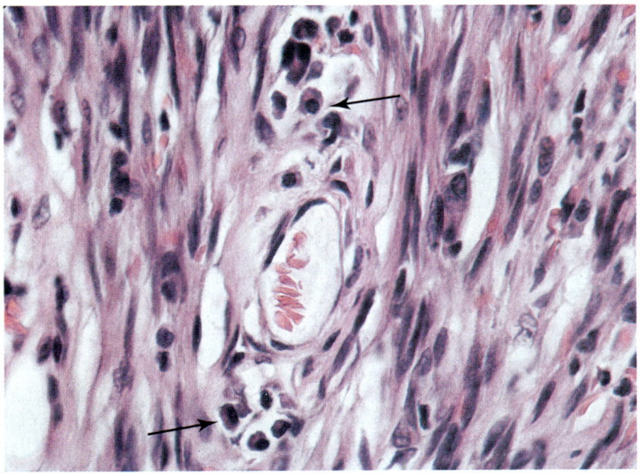

Figure 5-11 Kaposi sarcoma, illustrating proliferating spindle-shaped connective tissue cells (fibroblasts) surrounding a small blood vessel in the center of the field. Plasma cells (**arrows**) are intermixed with connective tissue cells (original magnification ×400).

Courtesy of Leonard V. Crowley, MD, Century College.

Currently HAART (highly active antiretroviral therapy) uses a combination of drugs directed against several different viral targets. HAART has greatly improved the outcome of an HIV infection, which now can often be controlled for many years by appropriate treatment. Analysis of the infective strain can be used to target virus-specific mutations. When medical care is limited, the best combination of drugs based on efficacy, cost, and availability is chosen.

Unfortunately, although the proliferation of the virus and associated damage to the immune system can often be suppressed, antiviral drugs available now cannot completely eliminate the virus, which persists indefinitely in the tissues of the infected host. Current drug therapy has changed HIV infection from a relatively rapidly progressing fatal disease to a slowly progressive chronic disease that can be controlled but cannot be cured.

How to Treat

Intensive treatment of HIV (HAART) should be started as soon as infection is diagnosed to arrest disease progression. HAART has nearly eliminated mother-to-child transmission and has much reduced the risk of transmission of HIV to an uninfected partner.

Drug resistance often occurs, especially if the treatment regimen doesn't include multiple drugs acting on different stages of the infection process. Current guidelines suggest starting antiretroviral therapy regardless of CD4 T lymphocyte count. Delay in therapy is associated with treatment failure. The anti-HIV drugs are classified into groups based on the phase of the viral life cycle inhibited by the drugs:

- Non-nucleoside reverse transcriptase inhibitors bind to reverse transcriptase, blocking DNA polymerase that converts RNA to DNA.
- Nucleoside reverse transcriptase inhibitors are nucleoside analogs that resemble the normal nucleosides a virus uses to construct DNA. Synthesis is disrupted when the analog substitutes for the required nucleoside.
- Protease inhibitors block the enzyme that cuts the viral protein into segments and assembles them around the viral RNA to form the infectious virus particle.
- HIV fusion/entry inhibitors block the binding entry and fusion of HIV with the target cell.
- HIV integrase inhibitors block the enzyme responsible for inserting the HIV viral DNA into the cell DNA.
- Entry inhibitors (CCR5 co-receptor antagonists) are drugs that prevent the CCR5 receptor on CD4 T cells from interacting with an HIV protein,
- CD4 post-attachment inhibitors bind to the CD4 receptor and prevent the virus from attaching to CCR5.

Tolerance and Its Failure: Autoimmune Disease

Mechanisms of Tolerance Generation

The process of self-recognition, immunological tolerance, is central to the properly directed function of host defense. Failure results in self-reactivity and autoimmune disease. Self-recognition lymphocytes (both T cells and B cells) are eliminated or become **anergy** by mechanisms of central and peripheral tolerance. **Central tolerance** of T cells occurs in the thymus. Like all cells in the body, thymic cells have MHC molecules as a surface component; they

Anergy Continued non-responsiveness of immune cells to a host or foreign antigen.

Central tolerance Part of the development of cellular and humoral immunity; cells reacting against self-antigen are removed during development; takes place in primary lymphoid organs.

also express a multitude of other small peptides found throughout the body. In the cortex of the thymus, immature T cells capable of binding to these small peptides presented by MHC molecules (pMHC, peptide major histocompatibility complex) are an example of **positive selection** (for the presence of CD molecules/markers) and move to further development. If binding does not occur, the lymphocyte self-destructs. The next step, **negative selection** (which occurs in the medulla of the thymus), is to eliminate lymphocytes with TCRs that have strong binding to self-pMHC. Central tolerance of B cells occurs in the bone marrow. Immature B lymphocytes with high affinity to self-antigen will be deleted, inactivated or undergo BCR editing. Some self-recognition lymphocytes might escape the central tolerance; they will be deleted or inactivated through the **peripheral tolerance** process. For this to function properly, self-antigen must be expressed in those locations during immune development. This is not universally the case. Self-antigens from poorly vascularized tissue or structural proteins such as collagen or cartilage may not generate **self-tolerance**, and a low level of autoreactivity to these proteins (not associated with disease) is sometimes detected. Antibodies directed toward the proteolytic products of Ig breakdown are universally present in normal individuals and may play a physiological role in removing these products from the circulation. A more striking example is that of sperm antigens, which are not present in fetal development and, consequently, not presented to developing T cells in the thymus. Traumatic or surgical damage to the testes or spermatic ducts in an adult can expose sperm-related antigens to the immune system and result in immune reactivity toward the host sperm. Sperm autoantibodies occasionally result in male sterility after such interventions.

Positive/negative selection Selection of lymphocytes with receptors recognizing self MHC molecules (positive selection)/deletion of lymphocytes that strongly bind to self-antigen (negative selection).

Peripheral tolerance A process to further eliminate self-reactive T cells and B cells that escaped from central tolerance; takes place in secondary lymphoid organs.

Self-tolerance Selection process to remove ability to recognize self.

Autoimmunity Immunological activity against self-antigen markers.

Regulatory T cells Type of T cells that modulate the extent of immune response and prevent autoimmune activity.

The development of autoimmune disease in three percent of the population suggests that an ongoing process must occur and that failure results in self-recognition. Certain groups of individuals are more prone to developing **autoimmunity**. Women are up to eight times more susceptible to certain autoimmune conditions than men, which may be related to endocrine hormone production. (There are some exceptions to this. The previously mentioned HLA-B27–related disease ankylosing spondylitis presents far more commonly in men.) There is a clear genetic component to the development of autoimmune disease, and these diseases run in families. In some cases, the genes of the MHC (HLA) system are implicated, but in many cases the nature of the genetic factors responsible is unclear.

At some level, autoimmune disease is likely to be related to a failure in ongoing peripheral T and B cell tolerance, which appears to be a continuing active process during life. Anergy is the continued non-responsiveness of T cells to a host or foreign antigen that occurs when the antigen is presented to the T cell without necessary costimulatory signals, B7 cell receptors, from an antigen-presenting cell. APCs express B7 in limited locations, primarily lymph nodes, but not in tissue. A T cell encountering a self-antigen in tissue (outside the lymph node) will become anergic and be unable to respond to the self-antigen. During thymic development, a population of long-lived **regulatory T cells** develop that are specific for self-antigens. These cells block activation of autoreactive T cells, perhaps by producing inhibitory cytokines or possibly by capturing IL-2 necessary for T cell activation. An uncommon genetic disease that ablates the development of this regulatory cell population results in IPEX, which is an autoimmune disease directed toward multiple endocrine glands. Exposure of T cells to self-antigen may trigger apoptotic cell death, although the mechanism remains unclear. Although different in detail, the mechanisms for peripheral B cell tolerance have a similar function.

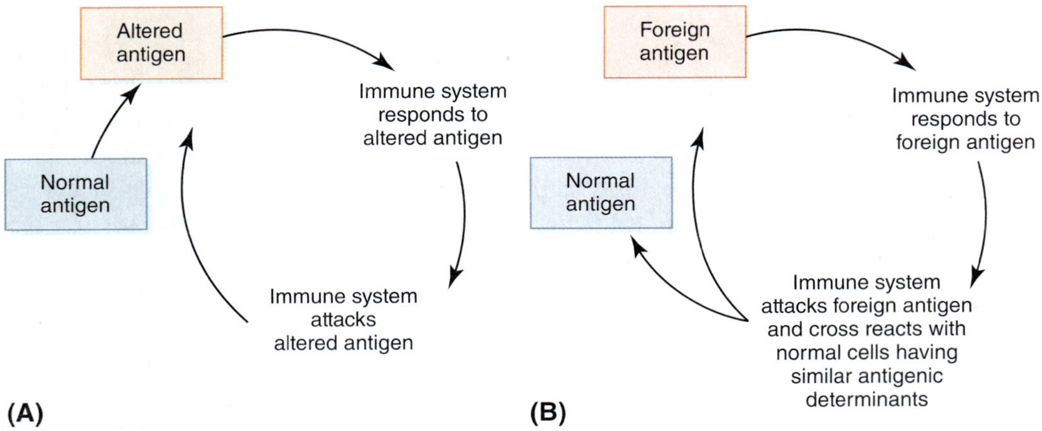

Figure 5-12 Two mechanisms postulated to induce autoimmunity. **(A)** Normal self-antigens altered, generating an immune response. **(B)** Immune response directed against foreign antigen cross reacts with similar antigenic determinants in normal self-antigens.

Failure of Tolerance: Autoimmune Disease

The reasons an individual forms an autoantibody to their own cells or tissue components are not well understood. Unfortunately, after an individual develops an autoimmune disease, it usually "doesn't go away." Although the affected person experiences periods when the disease is in remission or the manifestations are controlled by treatment, the disease persists and often progresses. Several mechanisms have been postulated to explain the pathogenesis of autoimmune diseases. As previously noted, many autoimmune diseases have a genetic component, which is often complex. Localized infections may provoke an autoimmune disease by allowing inflammatory antigen-presenting cells to present necessary costimulatory signals normally not present at the tissue site. Experimentally it is possible to induce self-reactive antibodies in animals by presenting either a self-antigen or a closely related antigen along with potent inflammatory chemicals. Molecular mimicry can occur when a foreign antigen is sufficiently similar to a self-antigen (cross reactive to a self-antigen) that autoimmunity can occur. The group A streptococcal M protein is likely to result in the autoimmune reaction responsible for rheumatic fever. Cross-reactive viral proteins may play a role in type 1 diabetes, which is clearly an autoimmune disease (Chapter 20). Certain drugs may induce autoimmune destruction of cells by altering their surface properties to promote immune recognition (**Figure 5-12**).

Table 5-7 summarizes the features of some of the more important diseases in which autoantibody formation appears to play a role. A presentation of lupus erythematosus follows; the other diseases are considered in greater detail in discussions of the appropriate organ systems.

Table 5-7 Etiology and Clinical Manifestations of Common Autoimmune Diseases

	Probable Pathogenesis	Major Clinical Manifestations
Rheumatic fever	Antistreptococcal antibodies cross-react with antigens in heart muscle, heart valves, and other tissues.	Inflammation of heart and joints

	Probable Pathogenesis	Major Clinical Manifestations
Glomerulonephritis	Some cases caused by antibodies formed against glomerular basement membrane; other cases caused by antigen–antibody complexes trapped in glomeruli.	Inflammation of renal glomeruli
Rheumatoid arthritis	Immunity to environmentally altered (citrullinated) proteins in joints and possibly lung.	Systemic disease with inflammation and degeneration of joints
Autoimmune blood diseases	Autoantibodies formed against platelets, white cells, or red cells; in some cases, an antibody apparently is formed against altered cell antigens, and the antibody reacts with both altered and normal cells.	Anemia, leukopenia, or thrombocytopenia, depending on nature of antibody
Lupus erythematosus, scleroderma, and related collagen diseases	Various autoantibodies, often to DNA or other nuclear components, cause widespread injury to tissues and organs.	Systemic disease with manifestations in several organs
Thyroiditis (Hashimoto thyroiditis)	Antithyroid antibody causes injury and inflammatory cell infiltration of thyroid gland.	Hypothyroidism
Diffuse toxic goiter (Graves' disease)	Autoantibody mimicking thyroid-stimulating hormone (TSH) causes increased output of thyroid hormone.	Hyperthyroidism
Diabetes (type 1)	Autoantibodies and activated T lymphocytes destroy pancreatic islet beta cells.	Diabetes mellitus caused by insulin deficiency
Pernicious anemia	Autoantibodies destroy gastric mucosa cells.	Macrocytic anemia and nervous system damage resulting from inadequate absorption of vitamin B_{12}
Vasculitis (various types of blood vessel inflammation)	Autoantibody-mediated damage to small, medium, and large blood vessels.	Blood vessel damage interferes with blood vessel function and blood supply to tissues
Various skin conditions and diseases causing loss of skin pigment or skin blisters	Some autoantibodies damage pigment-producing cells in skin; others attack intercellular connections among skin cells.	Pigment cell loss causes areas of skin depigmentation (vitiligo); blisters result from loss of skin intercellular connections
Myasthenia gravis	Autoantibodies destroy acetylcholine receptors at muscle–nerve junctions.	Muscle weakness resulting from inadequate transmission of impulses from nerves to muscles

Lupus Erythematosus

Lupus erythematosus, one of the most common and serious autoimmune diseases, is seen most frequently in young women and is characterized by widespread damage to the vasculature in the skin, articular tissues, heart, serous membranes (pleura and pericardium), and kidneys. The skin rash often has a characteristic appearance and is called a malar rash because it affects both cheeks (mala = cheek) joined by an extension across the bridge of the nose. The rash is also sometimes called a butterfly rash from its fancied resemblance to a butterfly with spread wings (**Figure 5-13**). The hemolytic anemia, leukopenia, and thrombocytopenia that are frequent hematologic manifestations of lupus are caused by autoantibodies. Patients may die of renal failure resulting from the severe renal glomerular injury.

Patients with lupus develop a variety of autoantibodies directed against nuclear components of the cell, including double-stranded DNA and a variety of nucleoproteins and phospholipids. Circulating antigen–autoantibody complexes (immune complexes) containing these nuclear antigens form and are deposited in kidney glomeruli and blood vessels in many locations. The malar rash is related to immune complex deposition in the skin (**Figure 5-14**).

Complement is activated, which generates an inflammatory reaction where the immune complexes are deposited. Renal disease (lupus glomerulonephritis) is one of the most serious consequences of the disease (and can result in rapid renal failure), but neurological and vascular disease, inflammation of the linings of organs, and arthritis all occur, likely as a result of the systemic deposition of immune complexes. These complexes interact with complement in promoting tissue damage. Decreases in the levels of complement components in the circulation of an SLE patient herald disease exacerbation. Diagnosis of the disease depends on the detection of the types of autoantibodies most characteristically associated with SLE, such as autoantibodies to double-stranded DNA and other nuclear components.

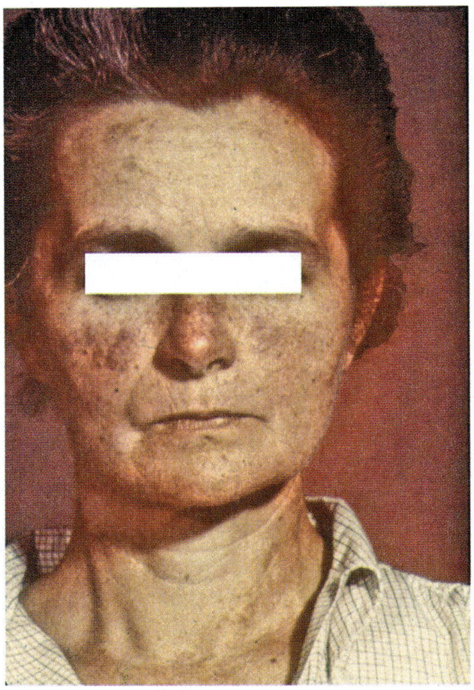

Figure 5-13 Characteristic butterfly rash in woman with lupus erythematosus.

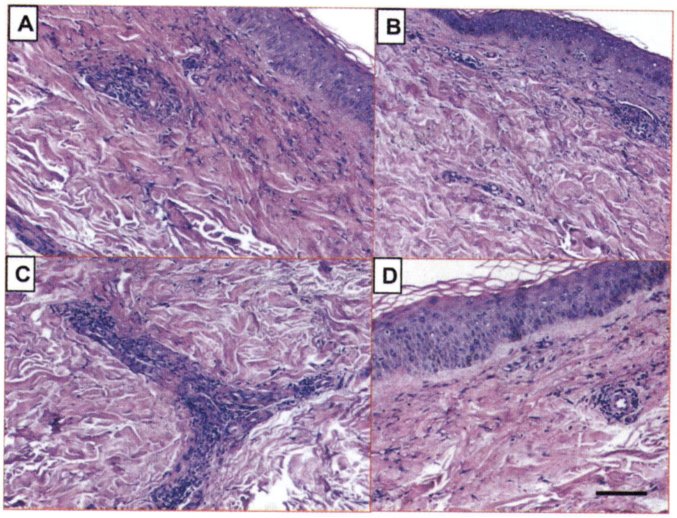

Figure 5-14 Vasculitis (vascular inflammation) of skin biopsy from SLE patients. Inflammation is demonstrated as nuclear dust and subepithelial myxoid degeneration in perivascular derma. **(A, B)** Original magnification: 40×, scale bar: 50 μm, **(C, D)** original magnification: 100×, scale bar: 25 μm.

Leone, P., Prete, M., Malerba, E., Bray, A., Susca, N., Ingravallo, G., & Racanelli, V. (2021). Lupus Vasculitis: An Overview. Biomedicines, 9(11), 1626. https://doi.org/10.3390/biomedicines9111626

The pathogenesis of lupus is not well understood but appears to be related to a failure in cellular mechanisms that clear immune complexes (hence the strong association of SLE with genetic defects in early complement components important in binding to immune complexes). These complement components are likely to also play a role in clearing cellular debris and degraded DNA. Solar damage to the skin can provoke dermal disease in a patient with SLE, probably because of UV's ability to cause photodamage to cells (and specifically DNA). Variations in genes important in innate and adaptive immunity increase the risk of SLE, but no one gene has a strong effect. A combination of multiple genetic factors and intrinsic factors (including the presence of estrogen in females) plays a role in the pathogenesis of the disease. Many other diseases are also autoimmune in etiology (see Table 5-7).

Case 5-1

George was sort of a hard luck guy. Now 18 years old, he had a history of repeated sinus infections, and his pediatrician previously had concerns about potential chronic bronchial infections caused by common bacteria. (The medical records mentioned *Haemophilus influenzae* and *Strep pneumoniae*.) His mother told him that when he was very young (about 2 years old), he had a series of "crouplike" episodes (inflammation of the larynx and trachea with "noisy" breathing) that seemed resistant to antibiotics. These were diagnosed as viral and became less frequent as George got older. Because George had repeated cases of bacterial respiratory infections through puberty, his pediatrician considered the possibility of immunodeficiency and evaluated him further at age 13. He had a mildly elevated neutrophil count along with a normal lymphocyte count with a normal ratio of B and T cells. His total immunoglobulin level was slightly low (on the lower borderline of normal). At that time, levels of individual immunoglobulin classes (IgG, IgA, and IgM) were not done. George mentioned that he was extremely sensitive to poison ivy, and, based on that, the pediatrician assumed that delayed

(continues)

Case 5-1 *(Continued)*

hypersensitivity reactions (dependent on T cell and macrophage function) were normal. The pediatrician considered the possibility that George had a mild deficiency in B cell function (humoral immunity). She prescribed a course of broad-spectrum antibiotics, gave George an intramuscular injection of "gamma globulins" (a crude preparation of Ig prepared from pooled plasma), and asked George to return in 2 months for further evaluation and possible gamma globulin therapy. George felt much better over the next month with no further sinus or respiratory problems. He did not care for the gamma globulin injection and did not return for further evaluation. George did relatively well over the next 4 years. He had far fewer sinopulmonary infections but did develop an allergy to a variety of pollens that progressed to mild asthma, which was treated with occasional use of bronchodilators. At age 17 George began to have mild gastrointestinal problems with bloating, cramping, and diarrhea. His girlfriend Shelly had given up gluten-containing products and suggested George try it. George was a skeptic, but to his surprise a gluten-free diet helped. It was clear that eating grain products made his gastrointestinal problem worse. George's pediatrician was doubtful but agreed to order testing when George showed her a food diary that linked his symptoms to gluten consumption. She ordered a TTG-IgA test (which is both highly specific and sensitive for the presence of celiac disease), and it was negative. The pediatrician diagnosed a mild food intolerance (but not celiac disease). George continued his low-gluten diet, which made his gastrointestinal condition better (and pleased his girlfriend Shelly).

Now George's luck has become worse. While riding on his motorcycle, he hit a wet patch on the road, skidded, and slid into a tree. His blood pressure was low when the emergency responders arrived, and George was rushed to the local hospital. His blood pressure remained low, and he was evaluated for internal bleeding as a result of splenic rupture. His surgeon ordered that blood be available for transfusion should it be needed. There was considerable bleeding during surgery, and a transfusion was required post-surgery. Immediately on starting the transfusion, the nurse noted wheezing, hypotension, flushing, and signs of shock. An anaphylactic transfusion reaction was diagnosed, the transfusion was immediately stopped, and intravenous epinephrine and hydrocortisone were administered. George responded satisfactorily and recovered from surgery without further problems.

Discussion

Transfusion reactions can occur from a wide variety of causes (both immune- and nonimmune-mediated); however, such reactions are uncommon, occurring in about 0.24 percent of all transfusions in the United States. Anaphylactic transfusions are rare, with a reported incidence of 0.005 percent of all units transfused. Death from anaphylaxis related to transfusion is possible but has only been recorded once in the literature (as of 2015, the latest date available). Nevertheless, such reactions are of great concern to transfusion services and are investigated with care. Significant effort is expended to prevent this. So, what was George's problem?

Samples of George's blood plasma were obtained after the reaction and tested for levels of immunoglobulin. He had normal levels of IgG (and associated IgG subclasses), somewhat high IgM, but less than 0.07 g/l IgA (nondetectable at the limit of test sensitivity). Normal levels in an adult have a lower limit of about 0.7 g/l IgA. Based on this, George was diagnosed as having selective IgA deficiency (SIgAD), by far the most common primary immunodeficiency disease. Individuals with SIgAD have no detectable IgA in their blood and secretions. Considering that IgA is the Ig isotype produced in the greatest amount (and second only to IgG in plasma level) and that it is believed to have a critical role in mucosal immunity to bacteria, it is surprising that 90 percent of individuals with SIgAD are asymptomatic. This figure may underestimate the morbidity associated with SIgAD because several careful recent studies in Scandinavia indicate a relatively higher mortality in SIgAD individuals as younger patients (within the first 10 to 15 years of diagnosis).

Individuals with SIgAD have a tenfold or greater prevalence of diseases with an autoimmune component, such as celiac disease or type I diabetes, and also have a greater prevalence for several others, including SLE and rheumatoid arthritis. There is also a less certain indication that allergic disease and possibly certain cancers occur at a somewhat elevated rate. The mechanism for such a propensity for immune disease in SIgAD remains unknown.

Although SIgAD is often familial, the mechanism of inheritance remains uncertain. It is likely in some cases to be linked to the HLA locus, and a number of other genes have been implicated, but this remains controversial. The B cell defect seems to reside in a stem cell population: (inadvertent) transplantation of hematopoietic stem cells from an SIgAD donor into a previously normal donor resulted in an IgA defect in the recipient, whereas transplantation of normal stem cells into an SIgAD recipient cured the disease.

George had no IgA (presumably this was a congenital condition), so he has no self-tolerance to IgA. SIgAD patients are considered to be at risk of anaphylaxis following exposure to IgA-containing materials. George's early exposure to pooled Ig (gamma globulin) probably resulted in the formation of IgE antibodies to human IgA present in the blood transfusion. The demonstration of such antibodies in SIgAD patients following anaphylaxis is often unsuccessful, possibly due to a technical issue, as IgE antibodies can be difficult to detect. (In any case, George was not tested post-transfusion.) Although there is controversy over how likely anaphylaxis is in SIgAD patients following transfusion it certainly does occur; hence, transfusion services make a great effort to prevent the exposure of such patients to IgA. For example, red cells to be transfused into SIgAD patients are repeatedly washed to remove plasma IgA. Some blood transfusion services prepare low IgA preparations for use in therapy.

George demonstrates the characteristic set of diseases expected in an SIgAD patient. In particular, celiac disease would not be unlikely. Why was George's test for the disease negative? The best test for celiac disease depends on finding IgA autoantibodies to a protein termed TTG. Because George has no IgA, his test was negative. Other tests that detect IgG autoantibodies might have been positive (but these tests are considered less reliable than those detecting IgA antibodies). George now wears a med-alert bracelet to warn of his sensitivity to plasma therapy and remains on a gluten-free diet.

Etiology and Pathogenesis

Primary immunodeficiency, isolated IgA deficiency, and consequent impaired immunity to sinorespiratory infections. Increased susceptibility to autoimmune disease with celiac disease probable.

Questions

1. Suppose SIgAD had been diagnosed at age 13. What difference (if any) would this have made in George's medical history?
2. How would George's medical condition have differed if he had X-linked (Bruton) agammaglobulinemia?
3. It is expected that an initial (primary) immunization is necessary prior to the occurrence of anaphylaxis. In many cases of transfusion-related anaphylaxis, no primary exposure to an antigen can be demonstrated. What are some potential explanations for this finding?
4. George objected (with good reason) to intramuscular gamma globulin injections, which can be quite painful. What alternative form of medication is currently in common use to treat humoral immunodeficiency?
5. Why might autoimmune diseases such as celiac disease be more common in individuals with SIgAD?

Questions for Review

1. What is meant by the following terms: adaptive immunity, cell-mediated immunity, humoral immunity, and hypersensitivity?
2. What is the role of the lymphocyte in adaptive immunity? What is the role of the macrophage?
3. How is the body's immune reaction manipulated to allow transplantation?
4. What is meant by the following terms: B lymphocyte, T lymphocyte, and lymphokine?
5. What are immunoglobulins? What is their basic structure? How do they function?
6. What is meant by the following terms: anaphylaxis, allergy, and immune deficiency?
7. How can tolerance be induced?
8. What is an autoantibody? What are some of the postulated mechanisms that result in autoantibody formation? What is the effect of autoantibody directed against the patient's own blood cells?
9. What are antigen–antibody complexes? How do they cause tissue injury?
10. How can the immune response be suppressed? Why is this sometimes necessary?

References

Loeffler AG, Hart MN. *Introduction to Human Disease*. 7th ed. Jones & Bartlett Learning; 2018.
Abbas AK, Lichtman AH, Pillai S. *Basic Immunology*. 7th ed. Elsevier Saunders; 2023.
Rich RR. *Clinical Immunology: Principles and Practice*. 6th ed. Elsevier; 2022.

- The area of immunology is so complex that specialized texts are a sensible place to start a search for additional information on the subjects covered in this chapter. For the first reference, Chapter 27 in Loeffler is a useful introduction to the basics of immunology and immune disease, which is an excellent starting place. The second reference is a short version of a much-used immunology text with excellent diagrams that will walk you through some of the complexities not dealt with in this chapter. The third covers rapidly expanding research and clinical advances.

Introduction to Immunology. The Allen Institute. https://alleninstitute.org/resource/introduction-to-immunology/

- This educational guide provides a series of well selected links to basic areas of immunology that are available on the web. A student and instructor guide are included.

Yazdani R, Azizi G, Abolhassani H, Aghamohammadi A. Selective IgA deficiency: Epidemiology, pathogenesis, clinical phenotype, diagnosis, prognosis and management. *Scand J Immunol*. 2017;85(1):3-12.

Koenen MH, van Montfrans JM, Sanders EAM, Bogaert D, Verhagen LM. Immunoglobulin A deficiency in children, an undervalued clinical issue. *Clin Immunol*. 2019;209:108293. Accessed March 14, 2020. doi:10.1016/j.clim.2019.108293

Immune Deficiency Foundation. Accessed March 14, 2020. https://primaryimmune.org/

- Three sources for Case 5-1. The third resource is a great go-to source for information on all forms of immunodeficiency, including selective IgA deficiency.

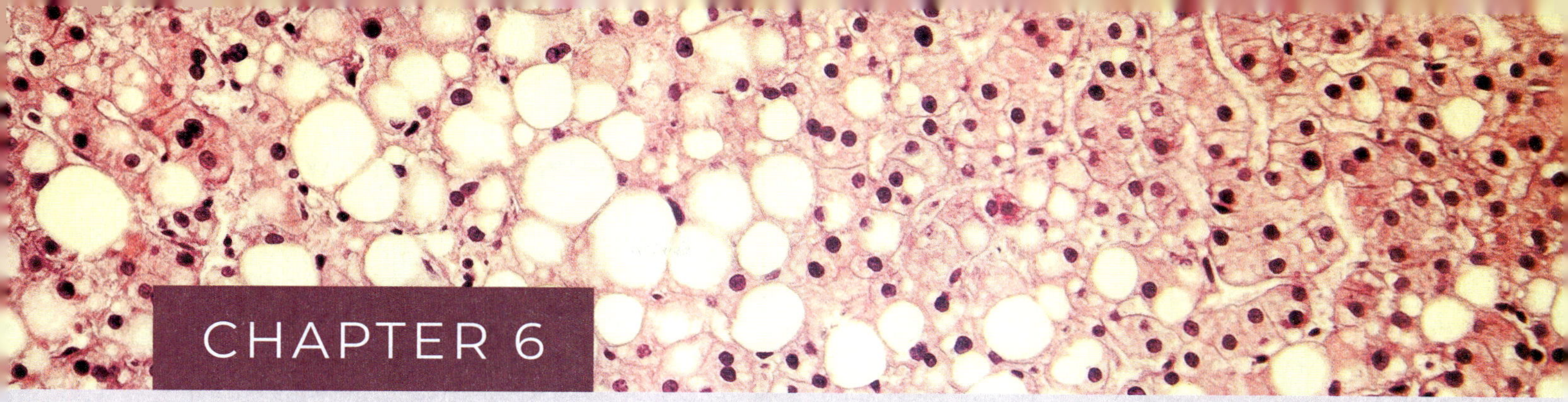

CHAPTER 6

Neoplastic Disease

LEARNING OBJECTIVES

1. Compare the general characteristics of benign and malignant tumors. Explain how tumors are named.
2. Describe the stepwise process for the development of malignancy.
3. Differentiate between infiltrating and in situ carcinoma.
4. Understand the role of activated oncogenes and disturbance in suppressor gene function on the pathogenesis of tumors.
5. Understand how susceptibility to cancer can be inherited.
6. Explain the mechanisms of the body's immunologic defenses against tumors.
7. Summarize the principal modulators of tumor treatment, including physiology, advantages, disadvantages, and common side effects of each technique.
8. Compare the incidence and survival rates for various types of malignant tumors. Explain the mechanisms of late recurrence. Describe the role of adjuvant therapy in preventing late recurrence.

Introduction

All cells in the body are subject to control mechanisms that regulate their growth rate. Some cell populations continually divide. These **labile cell populations**, such as those found in the gut, undergo constant renewal. Other populations remain stable and show little cell division, but with the potential for rapid renewal from a specialized cell population when needed. Hepatocytes in the liver serve as a good example. Yet other cell populations are **permanent** and have no (or perhaps extremely limited) ability to divide or be renewed, as is the case with cardiac myocytes. In all cases, the process of cell division, maturation, and, in many cases, cell death is under physiological control. In contrast, a neoplasm (neo = new + plasm = growth) results from the growth of cells without the control mechanisms that normally regulate cell growth and differentiation. Neoplasms often do not resemble the tissue from which they are derived. Neoplasms represent **clonal** cell growth. They derive from a single cell and perpetuate the genetic alteration that leads to the loss of growth control. The alteration, usually somatic, occurs in a nongerminal cell of the body, and is not inherited. However, sometimes the genetic changes associated with the development of cancer can be inherited mutations.

Labile cell populations Cells that divide continually.

Permanent Type of population of cells that have no ability to divide.

Clonal Derived from a single cell.

Tumor A benign or malignant overgrowth of tissues that serves no normal function, which is no longer under homeostatic control.

Dysplasia Localized areas of dysregulated growth.

Benign Quality of neoplasms that do not invade surrounding tissue or spread to sites distant from their origin.

Malignant Quality of neoplasms that spread to sites distant from their origin.

Metastasize The spread of cancer cells from the primary site of origin to a distant site within the body.

Solid Tumor Type that is embedded in host tissue.

Invasive Tumor Type that infiltrates host tissue.

Leukemia A neoplastic proliferation of leukocytes.

Lymphoma A neoplasm of lymphoid cells limited to lymph nodes and sometimes spleen.

Well-circumscribed Tumor with a clear border.

Grade Term in cancer diagnosis describing how closely the neoplasm resembles host tissue.

Classification and Nomenclature

The terms neoplasm and **tumor** are often used interchangeably but should not be. The root for the word tumor derives from the Latin word for swelling. Although it is true that in common usage tumors are most often neoplasms, many (perhaps most) neoplasms do not start as tumors but as localized areas of **dysplasia**. Such lesions often found in flat areas of epithelium may or may not protrude above the normal tissue but do differ in visual or histologic appearance from the surrounding tissue. A good example is melanoma, a neoplasm of epithelial pigment cells. Melanomas start out as flat, pigmented lesions and certainly would not initially be termed tumors. With time, many neoplasms grow and displace normal cells and then warrant being described as tumors. Neoplasms may be categorized as either benign or malignant (**Table 6-1**). **Benign** neoplasms do not spread to sites distant from their origin. However, a benign neoplasm can certainly cause local injury and in some cases become lethal. A neoplasm of the meninges of the brain may be classified as benign in the sense that it will remain localized to that tissue layer within the brain. However, if it cannot be completely removed, it may grow large enough to become lethal by occupying space within the skull. **Malignant** tumors can **metastasize**. Usually the cells migrate through the lymph system or bloodstream to other sites where they can divide and continue to grow. The term *cancer* is used to refer to malignant neoplasms. The distinction between benign and malignant neoplasms can become confusing and, at times, pivot on the specifics of a given case. Depending on their location, tumors can be **solid** and, while embedded in the host tissue, remain a discrete entity. **Invasive** tumors grow within the host tissue. Blood cell or blood cell precursor neoplasms will be found in the circulation (**leukemia**) or in the lymph nodes or spleen (**lymphoma**).

Comparison of Benign and Malignant Tumors

Generally, a benign tumor grows slowly and remains localized. Although it pushes surrounding normal tissue aside, it does not infiltrate surrounding tissues, being **well-circumscribed**. It does not spread via blood or lymphatic channels to distant sites. A benign tumor often can be completely removed surgically without difficulty, depending upon the location (**Figure 6-1**, **Figure 6-2**, and **Figure 6-3**). Histologically, the cells in a benign tumor typically appear mature and closely resemble the normal cells from which the tumor was derived. The **grade** of the tumor refers to how closely the neoplasm resembles the cell of origin as determined by the pathologist examining the tumor tissue. Benign tumors are generally low grade because they most often closely resemble the cell of origin.

Table 6-1 Comparison of Typical Benign and Malignant Tumors

	Benign Tumor	Malignant Tumor
Growth rate	Slow	Rapid
Character of growth	Expansion	Infiltration
Tumor spread	Remains localized	Metastasis by bloodstream and lymphatics
Cell differentiation	Well differentiated	Poorly differentiated

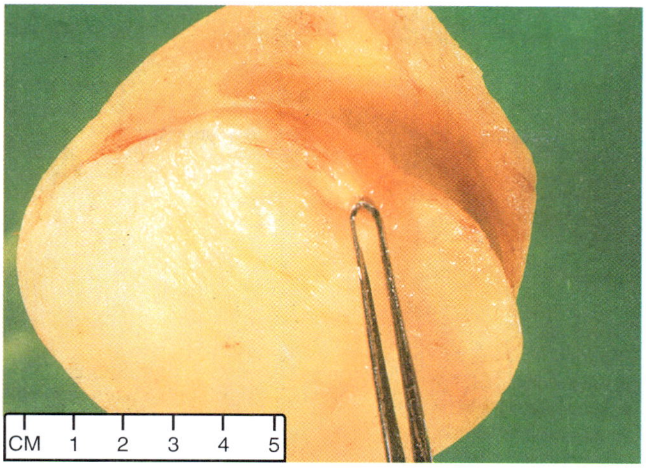

Figure 6-1 Well-circumscribed benign tumor. The capsule of the tumor is held by a clamp. Surrounding normal tissues have retracted, indicating an absence of infiltration.

Courtesy of Leonard V. Crowley, MD, Century College.

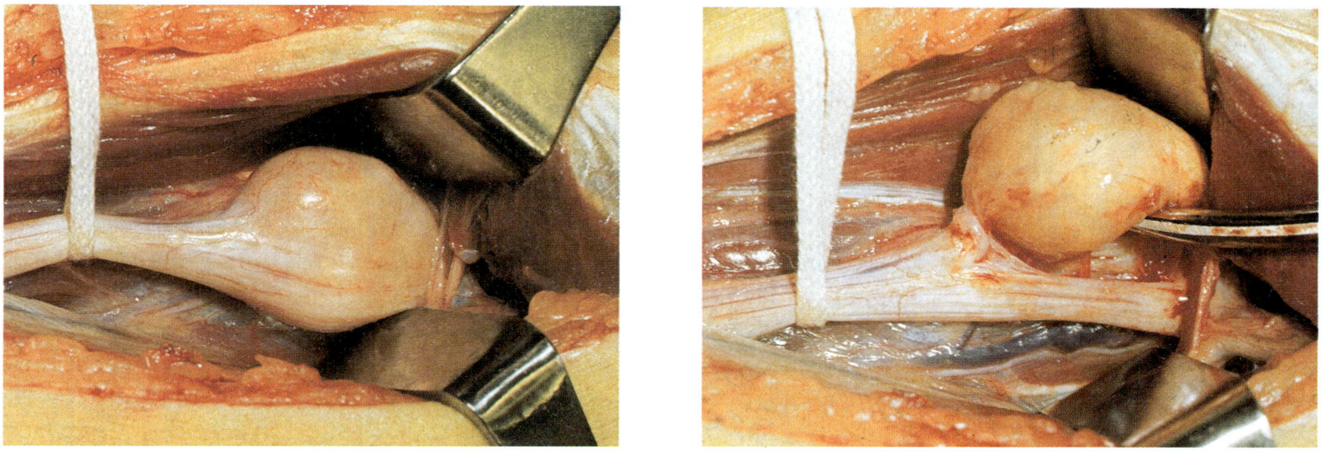

(A) (B)

Figure 6-2 **(A)** Benign tumor (neuroma) arising from the sciatic nerve. **(B)** Tumor dissected from surrounding nerve. The cleavage plane is easily established, indicating that the tumor is sharply circumscribed and does not infiltrate the adjacent nerve.

Courtesy of Leonard V. Crowley, MD, Century College.

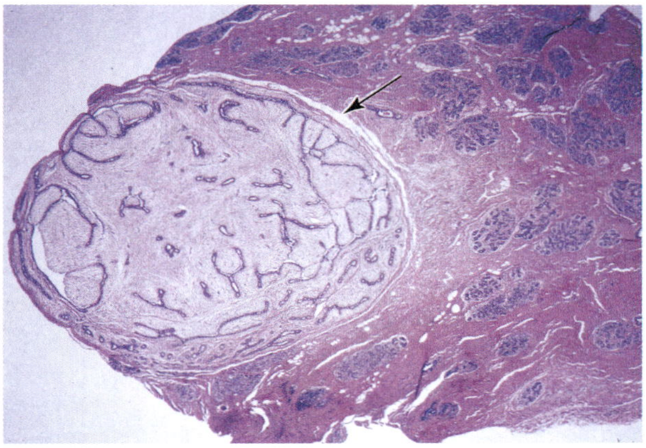

Figure 6-3 Low magnification photograph of benign breast tumor (fibroadenoma). Note the sharp demarcation between the tumor and surrounding breast tissue (*arrow*).

Courtesy of Leonard V. Crowley, MD, Century College.

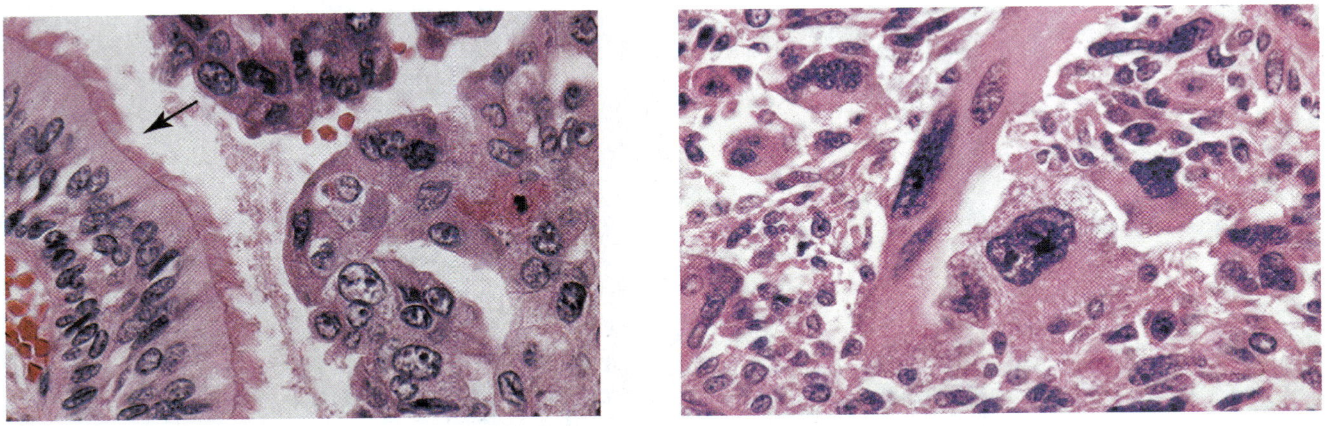

(A) (B)

Figure 6-4 Cellular abnormalities in malignant tumors. **(A)** Biopsy of bronchus from a patient with lung carcinoma, comparing normal respiratory epithelium (*arrow*) with clusters of neoplastic cells from a lung carcinoma. Cancer cells grow in a haphazard pattern and exhibit great variation in size and structure. **(B)** Malignant tumor of smooth muscle (leiomyosarcoma), illustrating large, bizarre, elongated tumor cells showing little resemblance to normal smooth muscle cells from which the tumor arose.

Courtesy of Leonard V. Crowley, MD, Century College.

In contrast, a malignant neoplasm contains less well-differentiated cells, is often characterized as a higher grade (**Figure 6-4**), grows more rapidly, and infiltrates the surrounding tissues (**Figure 6-5**). Frequently, the infiltrating strands of a tumor find their way into the vascular and lymphatic channels. Tumor cells from the **primary site** may establish **secondary sites** of metastatic tumor growth not connected with the original tumor (**Figure 6-6** and **Figure 6-7**). If a malignant tumor is not eradicated promptly, it may eventually become widely disseminated throughout the body. For example, a primary tumor of the colon may metastasize via the blood to the liver. Multiple secondary metastatic tumors grow in the liver, occupy space, and injure hepatocytes, ultimately resulting in liver failure and death. Unfortunately, this may occur even if the primary colonic tumor had been removed. The staging of a malignant tumor defines how far the tumor has progressed; is it invading locally or

Primary site Tissue of origin for neoplasm.

Secondary site Site of tumor following metastatic growth.

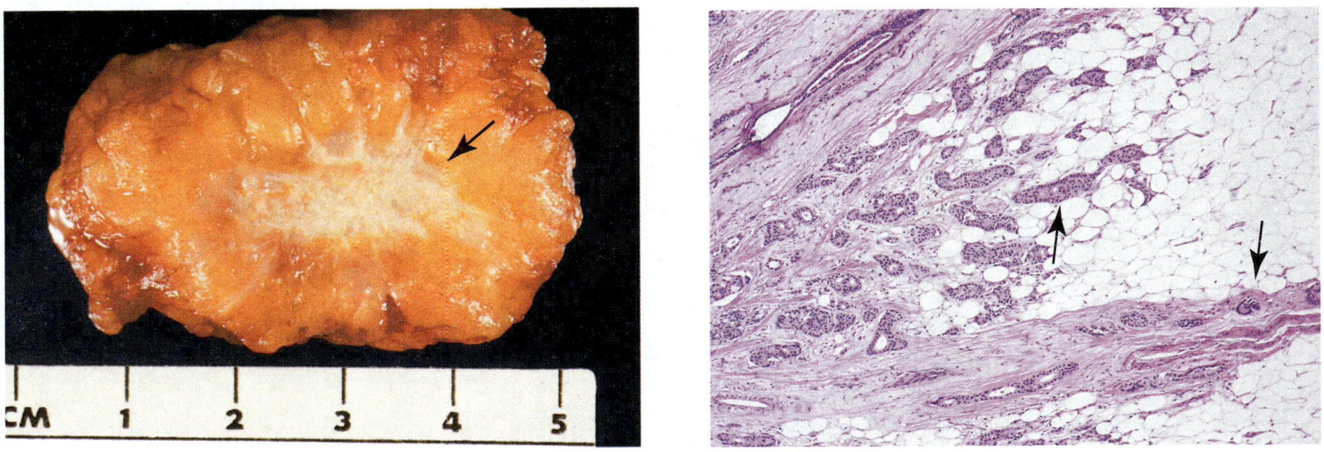

(A) (B)

Figure 6-5 Breast carcinoma. **(A)** Breast biopsy illustrating breast carcinoma (*arrow*) infiltrating adjacent fatty tissue of the breast. There is no distinct demarcation between tumor and normal tissue. **(B)** Low-magnification photograph illustrating the margin of infiltrating breast carcinoma. Small clusters of tumor cells (*arrows*) infiltrate adipose tissues of breast (original magnification ×20).

Courtesy of Leonard V. Crowley, MD, Century College.

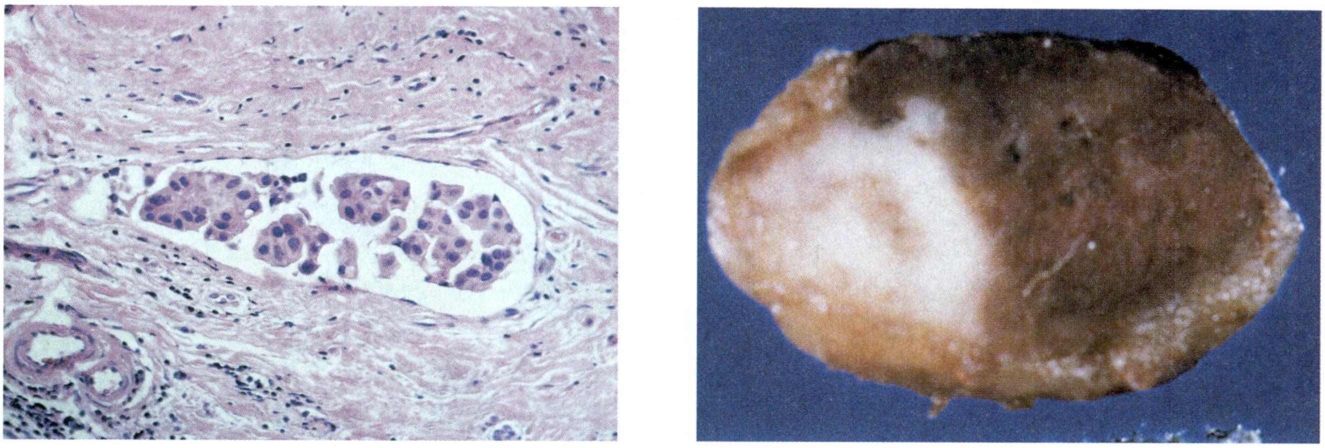

(A) (B)

Figure 6-6 Lymphatic spread of carcinoma. **(A)** Cluster of tumor cells in lymphatic vessel (original magnification ×400). **(B)** Deposit of metastatic carcinoma (white mass within node) that has spread via lymphatic channels into a small regional lymph node.

Courtesy of Leonard V. Crowley, MD, Century College.

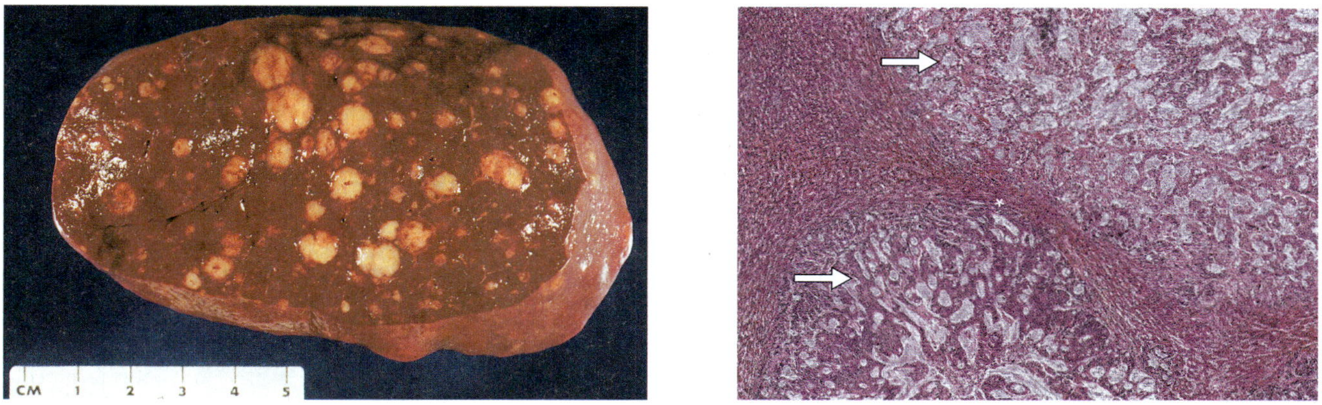

(A) (B)

Figure 6-7 **(A)** Multiple nodules of metastatic carcinoma in spleen. **(B)** Multiple nodules of metastatic adenccarcinoma in the liver (*arrows*). Liver cells show damage from expanding nodules (pressure atrophy) (*).

(A) Courtesy of Leonard V. Crowley, MD, Century College; **(B)** Courtesy of Department of Pathology and Laboratory Medicine, University of North Carolina at Chapel Hill.

are there distant metastases? Stage is often determined by the surgeon during tumor resection and the pathologist examining the tissue.

The primary factor used to classify any tumor involves the cell or tissue of origin. Consequently, understanding primary tissue types, including their structures and functions, provides a basis for understanding tumor nomenclature. Although not completely uniform, with historical names or jargon being included, certain generalizations are possible.

Benign Tumors

A tumor that projects from an epithelial surface is usually termed a **polyp/papilloma** (**Figure 6-8**). Papillomas are wart-like benign growths often resulting from human papillomavirus (HPV) infection. The term polyp usually refers to epithelial lesions that project from the surface of an organ into the lumen, such as colonic and uterine polyps. Benign neoplasms are named by adding the suffix *-oma* to the prefix that designates the cell of origin, as shown in **Table 6-2**. For example, a benign tumor arising from glandular epithelium is termed an

Polyp/papilloma Wart-like benign tumor often associated with viral infection.

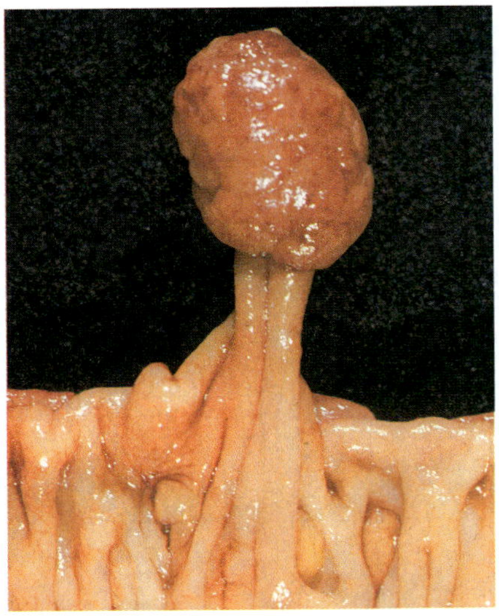

Figure 6-8 Benign polyp of colon.

Courtesy of Leonard V. Crowley, MD, Century College.

adenoma. A benign tumor of blood vessels is an angioma, one arising from cartilage is designated a chondroma, and one from bone is an osteoma.

Malignant Tumors

Sarcoma A malignant tumor arising from connective and supporting tissues.

Carcinoma A malignant tumor derived from epithelial cells.

There are many types of malignant tumors (cancers), but most can be classified based on their tissue of origin into three groups: (1) carcinoma (from epithelium), (2) **sarcoma** (from connective tissue), or (3) leukemia/lymphoma (from blood cells or their precursors).

A **carcinoma** is any malignant tumor arising from surface, glandular, or parenchymal (organ) epithelium. (The term is not applied, however, to malignant tumors of endothelium or mesothelium, which behave more like malignant connective tissue tumors.) A carcinoma is classified further by designating the type of epithelium from which it arose and whether it is of glandular or epithelial origin. For example, a malignant tumor arising from the urothelium of the urinary bladder is termed a urothelial carcinoma of the bladder. A carcinoma arising from

Table 6-2 Common Prefixes Used to Name Tumors

Prefix	Meaning
Adeno-	Gland
Angio-	Vessels (type not specified)
Chondro-	Cartilage
Fibro-	Fibrous tissue
Hemangio-	Blood vessels
Lymphangio-	Lymph vessels
Lipo-	Fat
Myo-	Muscle
Neuro-	Nerve
Osteo-	Bone

the glandular epithelium of the pancreas is termed an adenocarcinoma of the pancreas (aden = gland), and a tumor arising from the squamous epithelium of the esophagus is termed a squamous cell carcinoma of the esophagus.

Sarcoma is a general term referring to a malignant tumor arising from connective tissue. The exact type of sarcoma is specified by prefixing the term designating the cell of origin. For example, a malignant tumor of cartilage is designated as a chondrosarcoma. Fibrosarcoma, liposarcoma, myosarcoma, osteosarcoma, and angiosarcoma indicate, respectively, malignant tumors of fibroblasts, fat cells, muscle cells, bone-forming cells, and blood vessels.

The term leukemia is applied to any neoplasm of blood-forming tissues found in the bone marrow or circulating in the blood. Neoplasms arising from the precursors of white blood cells usually do not form solid tumors. Instead, the abnormal cells proliferate within the bone marrow, where they overgrow and crowd out the normal blood-forming cells. The neoplastic cells also "spill over" into the bloodstream, where large numbers of abnormal cells can circulate in the peripheral blood. In some cases, these neoplastic cells may populate lymph nodes and spleen rather than circulate. Then the term lymphoma is used (For more detailed information, see Chapter 11).

There are some inconsistencies and exceptions to the general principles of nomenclature. As mentioned previously, melanomas are malignant tumors derived from melanocytes. Benign neoplasms of these cells are termed benign nevi (singular, nevus). Seminomas are malignant testicular tumors. A **teratoma** is a germ cell–derived tumor of multiple tissue types and may be either benign or malignant. Pediatric malignant neoplasms are sometimes denoted with the suffix "blastoma," some examples being retinoblastoma and nephroblastoma (commonly termed Wilms tumor). These cancers are derived from primitive (immature) retinal and renal cells, respectively. It can be helpful to know the embryonic germ layer from which a tissue derives since neoplasms from the same germ layer can display similar properties. **Table 6-3** summarizes the general principles used to name malignant tumors.

Teratoma A tumor of mixed cell components.

Table 6-3 Names of Malignant Neoplasms

Cell or Tissue of Origin	Name
Epithelium	
Site not specified	Carcinoma
Squamous epithelium	Squamous cell carcinoma
Basal cells of epithelium	Basal cell carcinoma (unique to skin)
Colonic mucosa	Adenocarcinoma of colon
Breast glands	Adenocarcinoma of breast
Bronchial epithelium of lung	Bronchogenic carcinoma
Prostatic glands	Adenocarcinoma of prostate
Bladder mucosa	Urothelial carcinoma
Endometrium	Adenocarcinoma of endometrium
Cervix	Squamous cell carcinoma of cervix
Stomach mucosa	Adenocarcinoma of stomach
Pancreatic ducts	Adenocarcinoma of pancreas

(continues)

Table 6-3 Names of Malignant Neoplasms *(continued)*

Cell or Tissue of Origin	Name
Connective Tissue and Muscle	
Site not specified	Sarcoma
Lymphoid tissue	Lymphoma
Bone marrow	Leukemia
Plasma cells in bone marrow	Multiple myeloma
Cartilage	Chondrosarcoma
Bone	Osteosarcoma
Fibrous tissue	Fibrosarcoma
Smooth muscle	Leiomyosarcoma
Other	
Site not specified	Malignant neoplasm
Glial cells	Glioma
Melanocytes	Malignant melanoma
Germ cells	Teratoma

Development of Malignant Neoplasms

Studies of the development of epithelial neoplasia of the cervix, colon, lung, and breast indicate the development of cancer is a stepwise process—an ongoing series of genetic changes. However, leukemia and lymphoma development appears to be different. This concept is important from a clinical point of view because the progress of neoplasia from an initial event to the development of a cancer that can widely metastasize may take years. This slow progression gives the **oncologist** a window of time to diagnose and treat the disease in some situations.

Oncologist Physician specializing in treatment of cancer.

Metaplasia Conversion of one differentiated tissue type to another.

Cervical intraepithelial neoplasia (CIN) Precancerous condition characterized by cervical dysplasia in mucosa of cervix.

Precancerous Describing an area of dysplasia in early stages of cancer development.

Many neoplasms arising from surface epithelium remain localized within the epithelium for many years before evidence of spreading into the deeper tissues or to distant sites occurs. This has been well documented for squamous cell carcinoma of the cervix (**Figure 6-9** and **Figure 6-10**). Most often cervical cancer begins in an area of the cervix (the transition zone) where the columnar, mucin-producing epithelial cells of the cervical canal leading to the uterus meet the squamous epithelial cells that line the face of the cervix. During sexual maturation, the transition zone moves further onto the face of the cervix, exposing the secretory cells to the acidic environment of the vagina. Perhaps as a response to injury, the columnar secretory cells undergo **metaplasia** and become squamous cells. This area of metaplasia is susceptible to the initiation of the processes of neoplasia. It begins with the development of cervical dysplasia, a combination of abnormal cytological appearance and abnormal tissue architecture in the mucosa that defines early **cervical intraepithelial neoplasia (CIN)**. In a strict sense, the area of dysplasia is **precancerous** until the neoplastic cells traverse the basement membrane into the body of the cervix. The pathologist defines increasing degrees of dysplasia (CIN I to CIN III) by whether the neoplasia subtends more of the thickness of the epithelial layer.

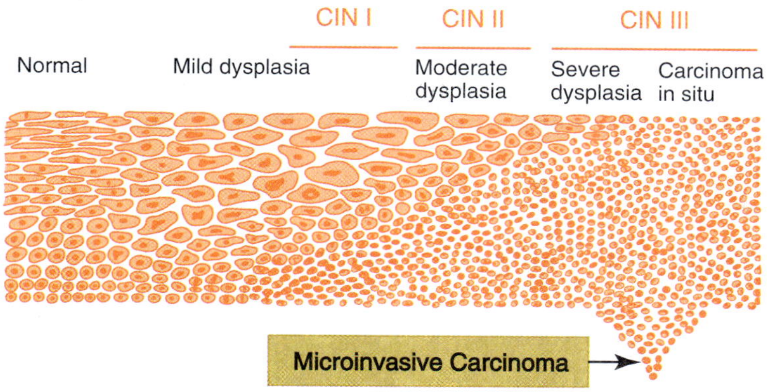

Figure 6-9 Cervical intraepithelial neoplasia (CIN). Drawing illustrates progressive changes in cervical epithelium with time, leading to carcinoma *in situ*.

Courtesy of Department of Pathology and Laboratory Medicine, University of North Carolina at Chapel Hill.

When dysplastic cells occupy the full thickness of the epithelium, the lesion is termed CIN III or **carcinoma *in situ***. An abnormal Pap test indicates the detection of dysplastic epithelial cells scraped from the surface mucosa of the cervix. However, once the neoplastic cells traverse the basement membrane, metastasis to distant sites becomes possible and the disease is no longer CIN but cervical cancer. Although most clearly demonstrated in the cervix, the gradual progression of metaplasia to dysplasia to carcinoma *in situ*, followed by invasion and metastasis, can also describe cancer pathogenesis in the breast, bronchus and lung, urinary tract, and skin. The slow progression of histological changes is accompanied by the neoplastic cells gaining additional mutations, contributing to an increasing degree of malignancy. A similar progression can be described in the colon cancer as well.

Carcinoma *in situ* Neoplasm occupying full thickness of the epithelium.

Actinic keratosis A precancerous scaly proliferation of squamous epithelial cells in sun-damaged skin.

Leukoplakia A white patch of hyperplastic and usually atypical squamous epithelium on the oral mucosa or genital tract mucosa.

Although a pathologist determines the level or degree of dysplasia based on changes seen at the cell or tissue level, certain precancerous neoplasms can be visually recognized. Recognizing them becomes important since the lesions could eventually develop into cancer. Prolonged exposure to sunlight, for example, not only causes premature aging of the skin but also causes small, crusted, scaly patches to develop on sun-exposed skin, a condition termed **actinic keratosis** ("actinic" refers to sun rays). Untreated, many keratoses eventually develop into skin cancers. Precancerous, thick, white patches descriptively termed **leukoplakia** (leuko = white + plakia = patch) can develop in the mucous membranes of the mouth as a result of exposure to tobacco tars from pipe or cigar smoking or from use of smokeless tobacco (snuff and chewing tobacco). They potentially may give rise to squamous cell

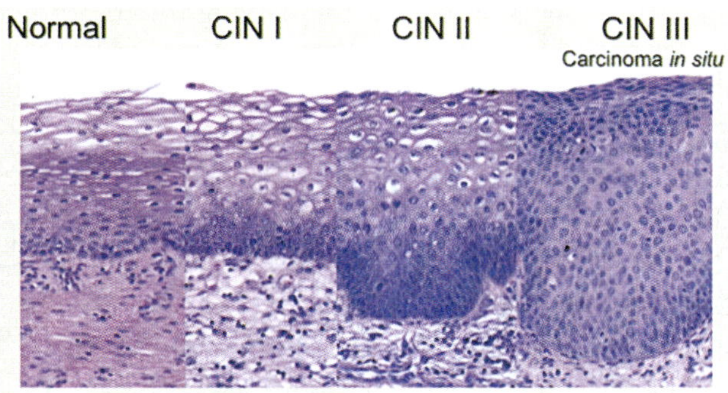

Figure 6-10 Cervical intraepithelial neoplasia (CIN). Cervical biopsies from four patients illustrating progressive stages of CIN.

Courtesy of Department of Pathology and Laboratory Medicine, University of North Carolina at Chapel Hill.

cancers of the oral cavity (see Chapter 23). Somewhat similar precancerous changes may take place in the epithelium of the vulva and may develop into vulvar cancer (Chapter 18). These neoplastic precancerous conditions should always be treated appropriately to prevent malignant change, which occurs in many, but not all, cases.

Growth of Neoplasms

Stem cells A self-renewing pool of cells that normally give rise to mature differentiated progeny.
Apoptosis Programmed cell death that does not provoke a host protective response.
Angiogenesis The formation of new blood vessels.

The great majority of neoplasms derive from a single cell with clonal expansion that perpetuates the genetic change responsible for the uncontrolled growth. Some neoplasias appear to be initiated in a population of cells that serves as a continuing source of differentiated cells to replace cells in that tissue, which become damaged or die, often referred to as **stem cells**. Stem cells may undergo a mutational event, giving rise to cancer stem cells (CSC). The CSCs can produce malignant progeny, which continue the propagation of the malignancy or contribute to the reappearance of the malignancy, as in a relapse. These CSC populations exhibit a low rate of cell division, rendering them resistant to many anticancer drugs, which demonstrate the best efficacy with rapidly dividing cells. Hence, eradication of the entire population becomes difficult.

Although a neoplasm starts from a single cell, the population of cells within the tumor can vary widely, termed tumor heterogeneity. As the tumor grows, additional mutations occur. The cells with mutations that enable rapid growth, extended survival, poor immune cell recognition, or resistance to therapeutic drugs will predominate. The acquisition of mutations that prevent DNA repair or interfere with **apoptosis**, contributes to the cells' increasing level of mutations and increased malignancy.

Although there are many exceptions, malignant lesions generally grow more rapidly than benign lesions. However, the apparent sudden expansion of tumors results from exponential growth. It may take 30 cell-doubling times for a tumor to be just detectable (about 1 gram or 2^{30} or 10^9 cells); only 10 more cell-doubling times would result in 10^{12} cells, having a weight of 1 kg, and perhaps only a month more to grow to a lethal cell number and mass. However, rapidly dividing and growing tumor cells will be subject to physiological constraints, such as outgrowing their blood supply.

Necrosis in Tumors

Tumors derive their blood supply from the tissues they invade but may outgrow that blood supply. Malignant tumors frequently induce **angiogenesis**. When the blood supply is no longer sufficient, the parts of the tumor with the poorest blood supply undergo necrosis (**Figure 6-11**). If the tumor grows within an organ, such as the lung or kidney surrounded by normal tissue, the blood supply will be richest at the junction of the tumor and adjacent normal tissue, and poorest in the center of the tumor, which often degenerates. In contrast, if the malignant tumor is growing outward from an epithelial surface, such as the colon, the best blood supply is at the base of the tumor. The poorest blood supply is at the surface, which frequently becomes necrotic and sloughs, leaving a shallow crater covered with degenerated tissue and inflammatory exudate (**Figure 6-12**). Exposed small blood vessels in the ulcerated base of the tumor may bleed, eventually leading to anemia from chronic blood loss. This is the basis for the use of stool blood tests to detect colon cancer. More recent tests, however, look for altered DNA. Sometimes the ulcerated tumor may be the source of a severe hemorrhage.

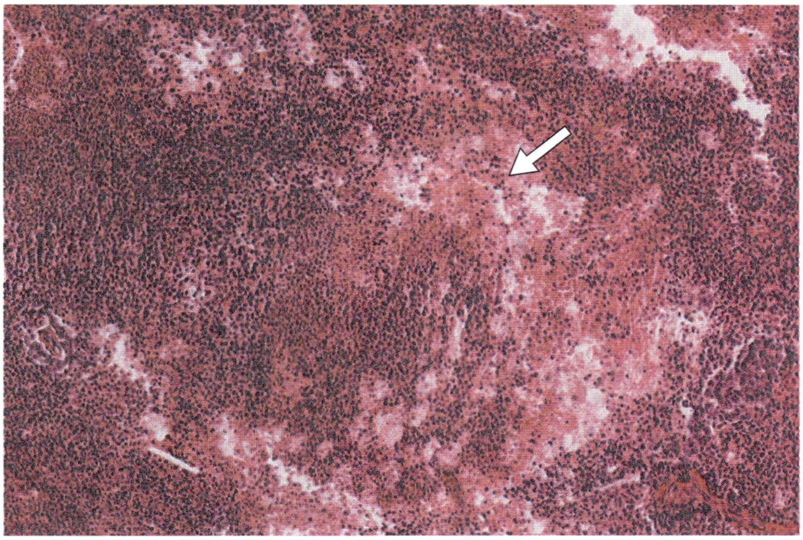

Figure 6-11 Central area of necrosis in a rapidly growing small cell carcinoma of the lung. (*arrow*).

Genetic Change in Neoplastic Disease

In the body, billions of cells are dividing all the time. They are also continually subjected to injurious agents; radiation, chemical carcinogens, viruses, and even some of the products of cellular metabolism can alter the structure of genes. Although the genome contains robust error correction systems, these systems are not failsafe, and uncorrected mutations can accumulate in the DNA. The increase in the rate of many types of cancer with increasing age probably reflects both the accumulation of errors and a gradual failure of the error correction systems. Although mutations can be in the germline cell resulting in inherited dispositions to cancer, the somatic mutations occurring in dividing cell populations are far more common.

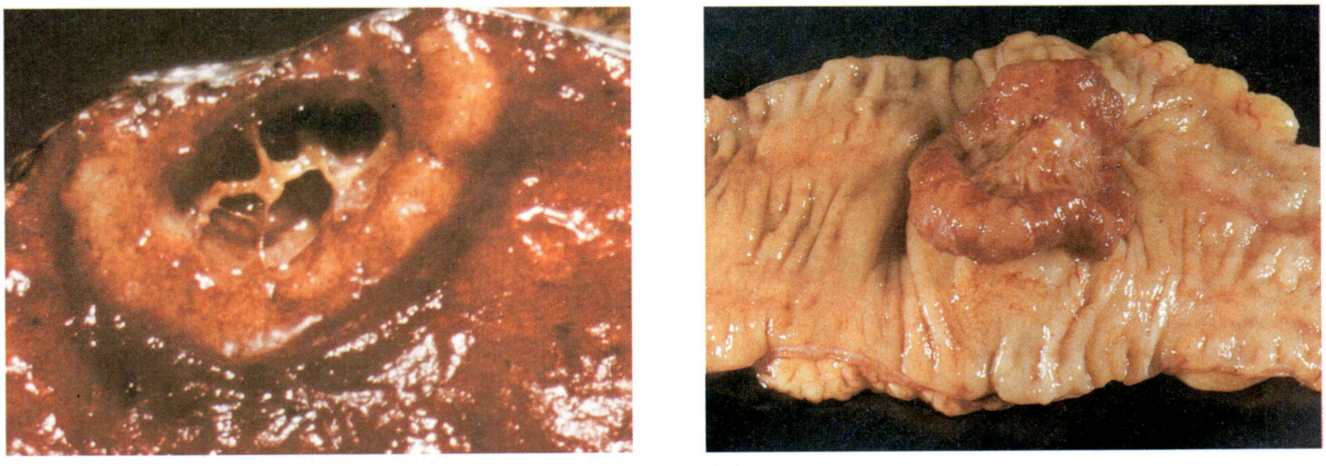

(A)

(B)

Figure 6-12 **(A)** Carcinoma of lung with central necrosis. **(B)** Carcinoma of colon exhibiting superficial ulceration.

Table 6-4 Gene Mutations that Disrupt Cell Function

Gene	Normal Function	Malfunction
Proto-oncogenes	Promote normal cell growth	Point mutation, amplification, or translocation forms an oncogene, resulting in unrestrained cell growth.
Tumor suppressor genes	Inhibit cell proliferation	Both alleles inactivated in same cell promotes cell proliferation.
DNA repair genes	Correct errors in DNA duplication	Gene inactivation increases mutation rate.

Mutations that can lead to cancer occur in genes with functions such as controlling cell growth, programmed cell death, or DNA repair. The cells may be able to undergo unlimited divisions without undergoing cellular senescence (as discussed in Chapter 2). They may gain the ability to stimulate prolonged angiogenesis, preventing outgrowing the blood supply. Mutations in genes required for triggering apoptosis, or continuing its suppression, can allow cells to continue to grow and divide indefinitely, when usually DNA damage would activate apoptotic pathways resulting in cell death. Mutations in genes required for DNA repair and genome stability allow the neoplastic cell to accumulate additional mutations that further promote malignancy. In addition, secondary mutations may result in cells able to invade tissues and metastasize to other locations. Alteration of cell surface properties, changing the cell's ability to adhere to neighboring cells, and new or increased secretion of enzymes capable of breaking down normal cell and tissue barriers could also potentially contribute to increased malignant activity.

Genes in which derangements are associated with **carcinogenesis** are classified into three large groups: **proto-oncogenes**, **tumor suppressor genes**, and **DNA repair genes** (**Table 6-4**).

Carcinogenesis Development of cancer.

Proto-oncogenes A gene promoting cell growth, differentiation, or mitotic activity associated with neoplasia.

Tumor suppressor gene Gene that normally functions to suppress abnormal cell growth.

DNA repair gene Gene that normally functions to repair DNA.

Oncogene An abnormally functioning gene that causes unrestrained cell growth leading to formation of a tumor. Results from mutation or translocation of a proto-oncogene.

Gene amplification Generation of multiple copies of a gene, increasing gene activity.

Proto-oncogenes

Human chromosomes contain a number of normal "growth genes" (proto-oncogenes) that promote aspects of cell growth, differentiation, or mitotic activity. They are closely related to genes carried by viruses that cause tumors in experimental animals and are named after those viruses they resemble. A proto-oncogene regulates some normal growth function in a cell; however, a proto-oncogene can be converted into an **oncogene** (onkos = tumor), an abnormally functioning gene that stimulates excessive cell growth leading to unrestrained cell proliferation. An oncogene is a gene that is important in causing cancer.

Conversion of a proto-oncogene into an active oncogene may occur with a single point mutation, or chromosomal changes may generate multiple copies of the same gene, termed **gene amplification**, which increases the activity of the gene. Translocation of a proto-oncogene to another chromosomal location may form a new oncogene because of the ways in which the regulatory components may now be interacting in the new location. Alternatively, the translocation may bring the proto-oncogene to a new location adjacent to another gene that stimulates its functions. Mutations that create oncogene mutations are dominantly gain-of-function mutations, since the oncogenes' altered function interferes with normal control of cell growth and replication.

A straightforward example is the oncogene c-Sis (named for the simian sarcoma virus). In normal cells, the proto-oncogene for c-Sis codes for a growth factor (beta PDGF, platelet-derived growth factor), which is under physiological control. It is synthesized only when needed to support the generation of new blood vessels during tissue repair. The oncogene c-Sis becomes mutated so that beta PDGF is produced constantly. This mutation results in clonal cell growth, with each "daughter" cell also constantly producing excess growth factor. This type of **autocrine** loop is found in many cancers, particularly glioblastomas, and is responsible in part for uncontrolled growth and tumor formation.

The best-known chromosomal abnormality resulting in gene activation, the Philadelphia chromosome (named after the city where it was discovered), can be demonstrated in the white blood cells of patients with chronic granulocytic leukemia. The abnormality stems from a reciprocal translocation of end pieces between chromosomes 9 and 22. In this translocation, a proto-oncogene (abl) on chromosome 9 is moved to a position on chromosome 22. There it becomes fused with another gene (bcr) to form a composite gene (bcr/abl). The composite gene directs the uncontrolled synthesis of extremely active **tyrosine kinase**, producing multiple effects involving cell growth and cell division. The excessive unregulated activity of this enzyme stimulates the unrestrained proliferation of white blood cells, a typical characteristic of chronic granulocytic leukemia (**Figure 6-13**). The same type of translocation also occurs in some patients with acute lymphocytic leukemia, but the composite gene bcr/abl is slightly different, leading to a different and more aggressive type of disease.

Autocrine Cell signaling to itself by releasing products that act on signal receptors found associated with the cell.

Tyrosine kinases A family of enzyme that produces multiple effects concerned with cell growth and cell division by phosphorylation of selected tyrosine residues in a protein.

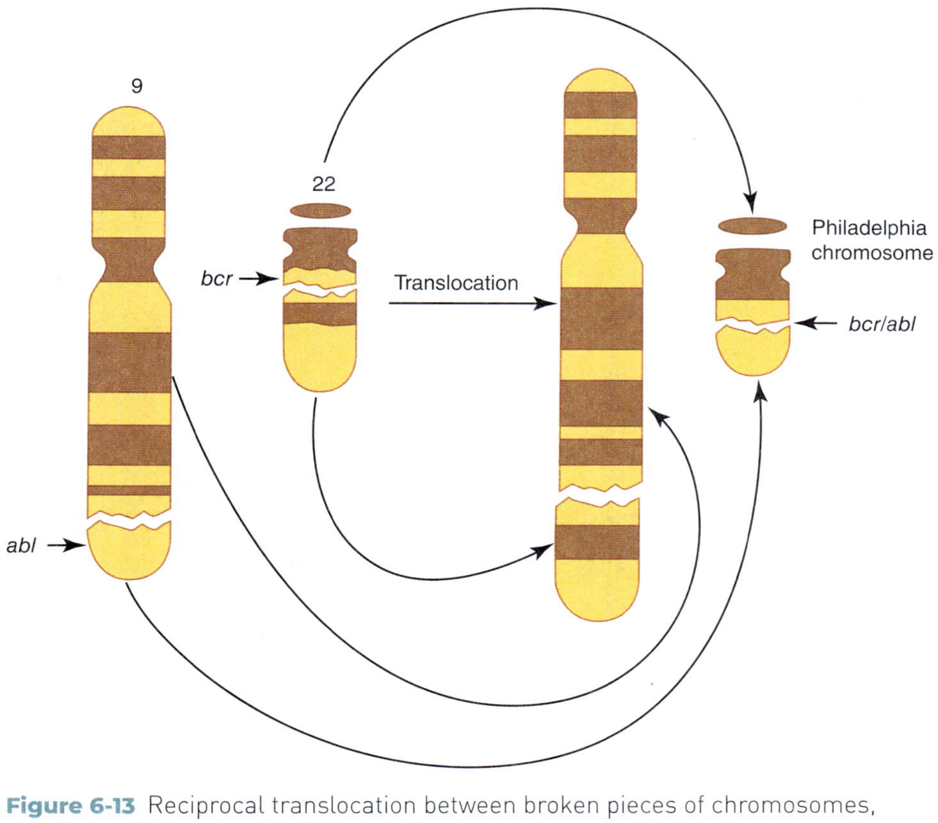

Figure 6-13 Reciprocal translocation between broken pieces of chromosomes, e,g., 9 and 22, forming the Philadelphia chromosome containing the composite gene that disrupts normal cell functions.

Tumor Suppressor Genes

Tumor suppressor genes are groups of different genes that suppress cell proliferation. Loss of suppressor gene function by mutation or other event disrupts cell functions and can lead to unrestrained cell growth. Tumor suppressor genes often function by preventing cells from undergoing unlimited DNA replication and thereby completing mitosis in an uncontrolled manner. In the absence of a functioning tumor suppressor gene, the cell may repeatedly divide without restraint and form a malignant tumor. Tumor suppressor genes exist as paired alleles at corresponding gene loci on homologous chromosomes; consequently, both alleles must cease functioning before the cell malfunctions. However, a heterozygote for a mutation at this locus possesses a greatly increased risk of developing cancer because a somatic mutation in a single cell could inactivate the one functioning copy of the tumor suppressor gene leading to potential tumor formation. Tumor suppressor genes may also inhibit "pro-growth" metabolic pathways, be part of DNA repair mechanisms, or help maintain stability of the genome. Loss of function of specific tumor suppressor genes has been correlated with specific tumors, and the suppressor genes are often named from the tumors with which they have been associated.

The classic example is retinoblastoma, an uncommon childhood tumor illustrated in **Figure 6-14**. Retinoblastoma is a malignant tumor of primitive retinal cells occurring in infants and children caused by loss of function of a tumor suppressor gene termed RB. Normal RB genes exist as alleles, one on each of the homologous pair of chromosome 13. Both RB genes must be nonfunctional in a retinal cell before a tumor arises. About 40 percent of retinoblastomas are hereditary; the rest occur sporadically. The hereditary form of retinoblastoma occurs if a child inherits a defective, nonfunctional RB allele from a parent. Consequently, the child possesses a single functioning RB allele in each of the somatic cells, including those in the retina. The single functioning RB allele maintains control of cell functions. However, if by chance a mutation occurs in this functional RB allele within a retinal cell, loss of all RB gene function in the affected cell occurs. The affected cell proliferates, forming a clone of unregulated cells, eventually becoming a malignant retinal tumor. Hereditary retinoblastomas may occur in both eyes

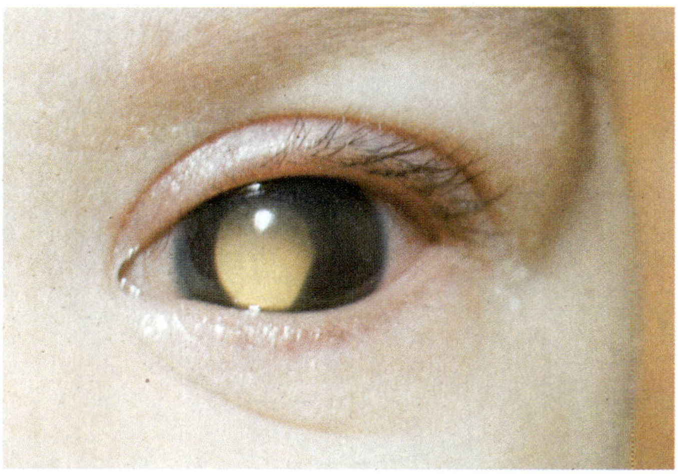

Figure 6-14 Retinoblastoma of an eye that appears as a pale mass of tissue seen through the dilated pupil.

Courtesy of Leonard V. Crowley, MD, Century College.

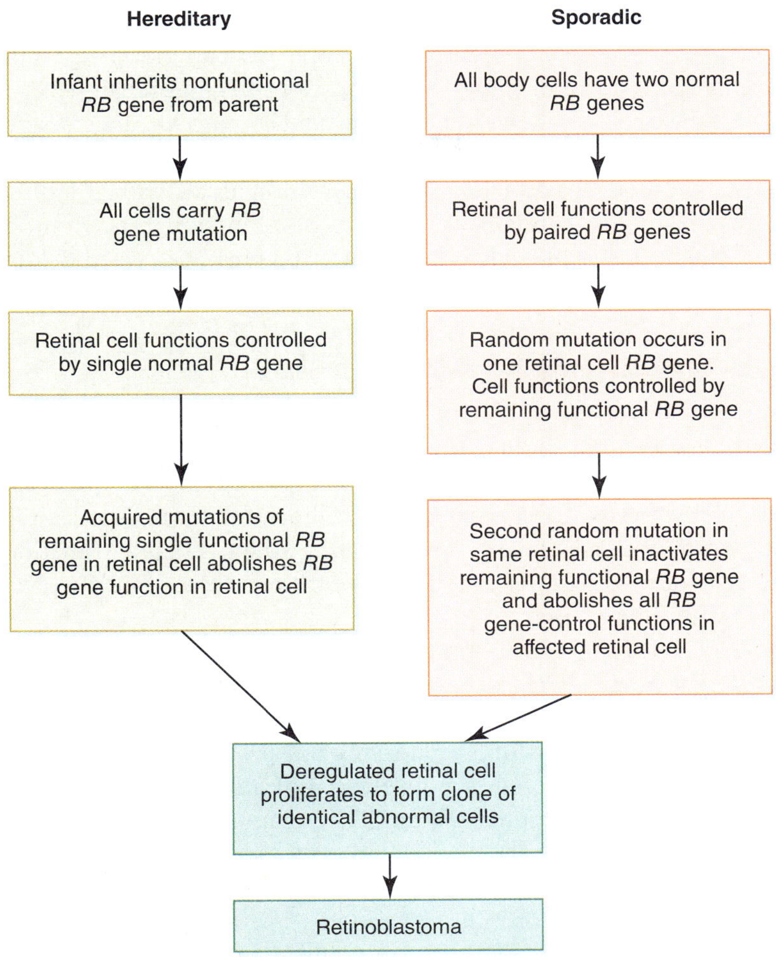

Figure 6-15 Pathogenesis of retinoblastoma.

because retinal cells in both eyes are equally vulnerable to similar random RB gene mutations. In the sporadic form of retinoblastoma, both RB alleles in the same retinal cell must undergo mutation to deregulate cell function and give rise to a retinoblastoma; consequently, tumors in both eyes are unlikely. **Figure 6-15** summarizes the pathogenesis of this tumor. The hereditary form of retinoblastoma is transmitted as a Mendelian dominant trait because the transmission of a single defective RB allele from parent to child places the child at very high risk of developing this tumor, even though the second RB allele must become nonfunctional in a retinal cell before the neoplasm arises.

DNA Repair Genes

DNA repair genes are part of the cell's "quality control" and repair system. These genes regulate the processes that monitor and repair any errors in DNA duplication that may occur during cell division. These repair genes also repair DNA damaged by radiation, chemicals, environmental agents, or by-products of cellular metabolism. Understandably, repairing gene misfunction increases the likelihood of DNA mutations being maintained and passed on to daughter cells arising from any affected cell. A high rate of uncorrected mutations within individual cells predisposes the individual to tumors because some of the mutations may affect cell functions resulting in unrestrained cell growth.

Again, both alleles must become nonfunctional before the repair functions regulated by the genes are compromised. People with an inherited mutation of a DNA repair gene are at increased risk. Mutations in DNA repair genes may be related to increased risk for developing particular types of cancer. Xeroderma pigmentosum results from an inability of skin cells to repair a particular class of mutations caused by ultraviolet radiation. Individuals with the disease are extremely sensitive to sunlight and readily develop skin cancer. Individuals inheriting mutations in BRCA1 or BRCA2 are at a greatly elevated risk for early onset breast and ovarian cancer.

Genes Regulating Apoptosis

Another group of genes plays a more limited but nevertheless important role in regulating cell functions influencing the survival time of cells. Normal cells live for a variable period of time, depending on the cell type. The predetermined death of a cell, referred to as programmed cell death, or apoptosis, is regulated by genes within the cell. If the genes regulating apoptosis fail to function properly, the cells don't die as they should and continue to accumulate, eventually resulting in forming a tumor.

The gene BCL2 on chromosome 18 produces a regulator of apoptosis. If BCL2 undergoes a translocation next to the gene for the immunoglobulin heavy chain, it becomes dysregulated and is synthesized in excess. The excess of BCL2 inhibits apoptosis in a class of lymphocytes and promotes an accumulation of inappropriately long-lived cells within the lymph node. This results in a lymphoid tumor (follicular lymphoma) caused by a failure of cell death rather than by excess proliferation of cells.

The most commonly mutated gene in human cancers, TP53, is a tumor suppressor that is critical for inducing apoptosis in cells with irreparable DNA damage. Referred to as "the guardian of the genome," TP53 provides the final protection against neoplasia by inducing apoptosis in cells that cannot be repaired. Mutations in TP53 occur in about half of all cancers. Individuals who are heterozygous for a single mutation in TP53 have Li-Fraumeni syndrome and a 25-fold increased risk of developing cancer, in a manner analogous to that seen with mutations in RB. Because loss of TP53 function allows rapid additional accumulation of mutations in neoplastic cells, it is often associated with the occurrence of **high-grade disseminated cancer**, cancer cells that are poorly differentiated (aggressive) and extensively spread throughout the body. Because many anticancer drugs work by inducing apoptosis in cancer cells, tumors with inactivation of p53 function may become resistant to the drug's anticancer activity.

High-grade disseminated cancer Cancer cells that are poorly differentiated (aggressive) and extensively spread throughout the body.

Multistep Progression of Genetic Changes Leading to Cancer

In most cases, cancers do not result from mutation of a single gene. Rather, they result as a consequence of multiple genetic "insults" to the genome characterized by activation of oncogenes along with loss of function of one or more tumor suppressor genes. The transition, for example, from a benign polyp of the colon to an invasive colon cancer requires activation of an oncogene (ras) and inactivation of three distinct tumor suppressor genes (APC, DCC, and TP53) (**Figure 6-16**).

Once a cell becomes deregulated and forms a tumor, additional random genetic changes may take place in the tumor cells, which now possess a very unstable genome. Individual genes may undergo additional mutations, or they

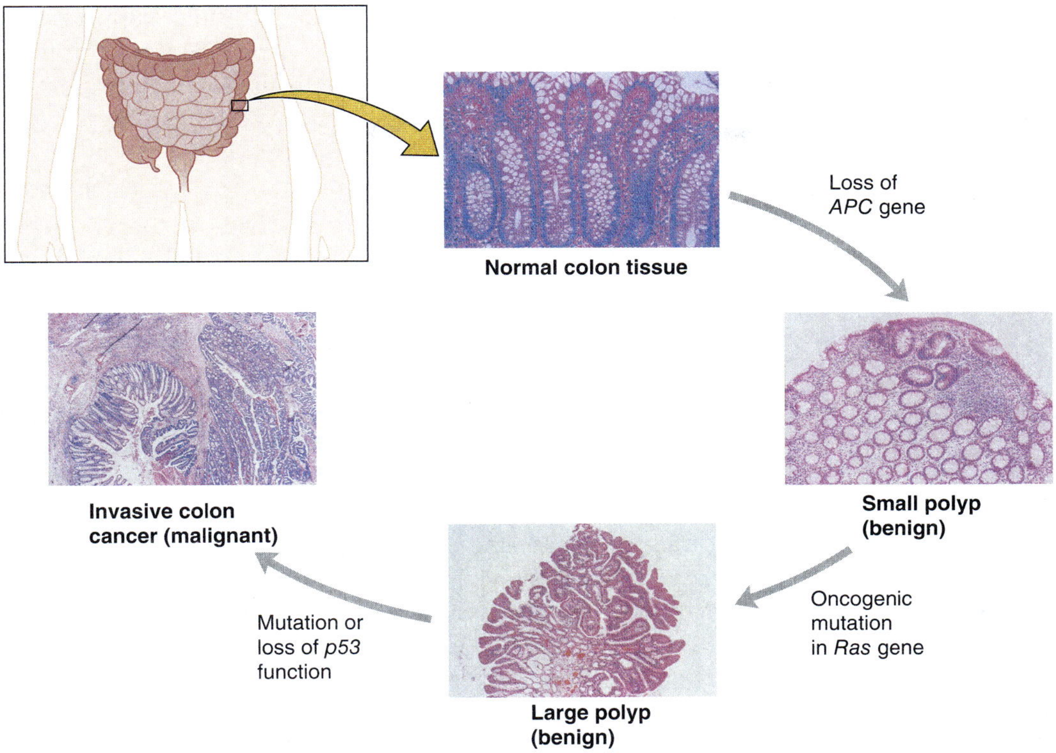

Figure 6-16 Somatic mutations and cell morphography in the progression of colon cancer. (Loss of *DCC* is not shown.)
Photographs courtesy of Dr. Kathleen R. Cho, University of Michigan Medical School.

may replicate, creating many copies in the genome by gene amplification. Chromosomes can fragment, with pieces of chromosomes being lost from the cells or translocated to other chromosomes. Some of these mutations in the unstable tumor cell genome may produce new mutant cells that exhibit more aggressive growth than the original tumor cells. The new mutant may eventually outgrow the other cells in the tumor. Clinically, this event can be manifested in more rapid growth and aggressive behavior of the tumor; often the tumor may become less responsive to the anticancer drugs that formerly could control it. Leukemias present an exception to the pattern of stepwise accumulation of mutations associated with malignancy because a single chromosomal translocation and associated oncogene activation can result in the production of aggressive disease.

Viruses

Many types of tumors in animals are caused by viruses and can be readily transmitted to animals of the same or a different species. In some instances, a single type of virus is capable of causing many different types of tumors in various species of animals. Some of the cancers in humans also appear to be caused by viruses. Unusual types of leukemia and lymphoma are caused by a virus termed the human T cell leukemia–lymphoma virus (HTLV-1), which is related to the virus that causes the acquired immune deficiency syndrome (AIDS). The HTLV-1 genome contains a gene termed tax that has an oncogene-like action in T lymphocytes. Some strains of the human papillomavirus (HPV) that cause genital condylomas (Chapter 18) are responsible for cervical carcinoma and for some squamous cell carcinomas of the mouth, throat, and larynx (oropharyngeal carcinomas). Oncogenic strains of HPV integrate into the host cell genome and secrete proteins that inactivate the tumor suppressor genes RB and TP53. Chronic viral hepatitis (Chapter 21) predisposes to primary carcinoma of the liver. Kaposi's sarcoma, which occurs predominantly in immunodeficient patients, is caused by a herpes virus, designated human herpesvirus 8 (HHV-8). Some types of nasopharyngeal carcinoma and some types of lymphoma appear to be related to infection with Epstein-Barr virus, the same herpes virus that causes infectious mononucleosis. The mechanism by which herpes viruses result in cancer is complex and not entirely clear, but viral genes may function both to activate oncogenes and to inactivate tumor suppressors. In addition, host immunosuppression acts as a cofactor for the development of cancer.

Chemical Carcinogens

Many chemical agents found in the environment are capable of causing cancer through a two-step process. Initiation occurs when a highly reactive chemical targeting DNA produces a nonlethal mutation in the genome that cannot be repaired. In many cases, the mutation occurs at random in the DNA and will result in cancer only, if by chance, the mutation occurs within a critical gene. However, some chemical agents exhibit a degree of specificity in their action. For example, the carcinogen aflatoxin B_1 is produced by a mold that infects improperly stored grains and nuts. The toxin is either directly ingested by humans or enters the food chain and inadvertently contaminates foodstuffs. In the southern United States, contaminated feed for cows results in aflatoxin levels in milk; the toxin may also contaminate peanut products. Aflatoxin tends to mutate a particular codon in the gene for TP53 that ultimately may result in hepatocellular carcinoma (liver cancer). This cancer is far more frequent in areas where ingestion of contaminated products is common. Contact with an initiating carcinogen alone is not sufficient to cause cancer; a promoter that stimulates the growth of those contacted cells must also be present. Promoters may be exogenous agents that do not, in themselves, cause cancer but do encourage cell division, including substances such as certain drugs and hormone preparations. Endogenous promoters include persistent inflammation and excess production of estrogen-like hormones.

Failure of Immunologic Defenses

A neoplasm may produce proteins and cell surface components (glycolipids and glycoproteins) that are either not present or altered from those found in the healthy cell. These new or altered products may be produced by mutated genes directly involved in carcinogenesis or may be overly or abnormally expressed by cellular genes induced by neoplasia. For example, some tumors produce **oncofetal antigens**, proteins normally synthesized at high levels only during fetal development, that reappear in high amounts in some cancers. Such cell products can sometimes be recognized as abnormal by the immune system and activate various cell-mediated mechanisms for their removal, but this is not always the case.

Oncofetal antigens Proteins normally synthesized only during fetal development and associated with neoplasia.

The role played by the immune system in surveillance and destruction of neoplastic cells is still unclear. Immunocompetent people do get cancer, so the system is not absolute. In part the failure of the immune system may be related to immune checkpoint genes, which usually serve to control the immune response and prevent autoimmune reactions (Chapter 5), but they can also prevent targeting of cancer cells. Severely immunocompromised individuals are at much increased risk for some, but not all, cancers. The majority of the high-risk cancers are mature B cell neoplasms (lymphomas), often associated with an Epstein-Barr virus infection.

Cancer cells may mutate and no longer express antigens necessary for immune killing and may lose expression of HLA molecules necessary for recognition by immune cells. The cells may secrete immunosuppressive agents or turn on cellular pathways that inhibit immune activation. Cancer cells may exploit immune checkpoints, as noted previously, to prevent immune destruction. A major goal in developing new cancer therapies is to learn how to better use the immune system to destroy cancer cells and to circumvent the mechanisms expressed by the cancer cell that result in poorly functioning immune-mediated killing.

Heredity and Tumors

Although well-defined hereditary (germline) mutations are responsible for a small proportion of all cancers, individuals bearing these mutations are at greatly increased risk. A person whose parent or sibling has been afflicted with a breast, colon, or lung carcinoma has about three times greater risk of developing a similar tumor than do other people. The predisposition is apparently the result of a multifactorial inheritance pattern. The individual at risk has inherited sets of genes that influence some hormonal- or enzyme-regulated biochemical process within the body that slightly increases the susceptibility to a specific cancer. The increased risk may be caused by genetic differences in various biochemical or physiologic activities that influence cell functions. Such differences may include circulating hormone levels that could influence cell growth rates, variations in the rate at which the cell can metabolize and inactivate cancer-causing chemicals, variations in the ability to repair DNA that has been damaged by injurious agents, or variations in the efficiency of the immune system in eliminating abnormal cells as they arise.

The best known of these hereditary-based neoplasms involve autosomal dominant mutations of tumor suppressor genes. Hereditary gene mutations are responsible for a small percentage of breast carcinomas, with the affected individuals also at increased risk of ovarian carcinoma as well. Two different genes are involved. Some hereditary breast and ovarian carcinomas can be traced to an inherited mutation of a tumor suppressor gene designated BRCA1 (breast carcinoma 1), which has been localized to chromosome 17. Other cases are related to a mutation of a second tumor suppressor gene designated BRCA2 (breast carcinoma 2), which is located on chromosome 13. The pathogenesis of hereditary breast and ovarian carcinoma related to either a BRCA1 or BRCA2 mutation is comparable to that of hereditary retinoblastoma caused by an inherited mutant RB gene (see Figure 6-15). BRCA mutations are considered to be inherited as dominant traits because the inheritance of a single BRCA mutant gene from either parent is responsible for the increased susceptibility to both breast and ovarian carcinomas. Most (but not all) cases of breast cancer in BRCA1- or BRCA2-positive females are related to loss of heterozygosity as described previously. Men carrying BRCA mutations are also at increased risk of breast, prostate, and other cancers.

A condition termed multiple polyposis of the colon, also a dominant trait, is characterized by the formation of multiple polyps throughout the colon, and usually one or more of them eventually becomes malignant. Another condition transmitted as an autosomal dominant trait is multiple neurofibromatosis (Chapter 23). Many of the nerves throughout the body give rise to benign tumors termed neurofibromas, and often one of these tumors eventually undergoes malignant change. Another hereditary tumor syndrome, also an autosomal dominant transmission, is multiple endocrine adenomatosis, which is characterized by the formation of adenomas arising in several different endocrine glands, as the name indicates.

There are many other examples of tumors related to hereditary gene mutations, but it is important to remember that they make up only a small fraction of the benign and malignant tumors afflicting humans.

Diagnosis of Tumors

Early Recognition of Neoplasms

The American Cancer Society publicizes a number of signs and symptoms that should arouse suspicion of cancer (**Table 6-5**). In general, any abnormality of form or function may be an early symptom of a neoplasm and should be investigated by a healthcare provider. For example, a lump in the breast, an ulcer on the lip, or a change in the character of a wart or mole may be considered an abnormality of form. Vaginal bleeding in a postmenopausal woman or a change in bowel habits manifested by constipation or diarrhea is an abnormality of function. Early diagnosis of specific cancers is furthered by routine screening tests such as mammograms and routine fecal stool blood tests and colonoscopy in selected groups at increased risk, most often persons above a particular age.

A complete medical history and physical examination by the clinician are the next steps in evaluating suspected abnormalities. The physical examination and laboratory work may include special studies specific to the presenting sign(s).

If a tumor is discovered, exact diagnosis requires biopsy or excision of the suspected tumor. Histologic examination of the tissue by the pathologist provides an exact diagnosis and serves as a guide to further treatment. If the tumor is benign, simple excision is curative. If the tumor is malignant, a more extensive operation or additional types of treatment may be required.

Cytologic Diagnosis of Neoplasms

Tumors shed abnormal cells from their surfaces, and these cells can be detected in the body fluids and secretions. Often the abnormal cells can be recognized when the neoplasm is only microscopic in size and is still confined to the surface epithelium. These observations have been applied to the cytologic diagnosis of tumors of the cervix. The method is named after the physician who played a large part in developing and applying cytologic

Table 6-5 American Cancer Society Warning Signals

Change in bowel or bladder habits
A sore that does not heal
Unusual bleeding or discharge
A thickening or lump in the breast or elsewhere
Indigestion or difficulty in swallowing
An obvious change in wart or mole
A nagging cough or hoarseness

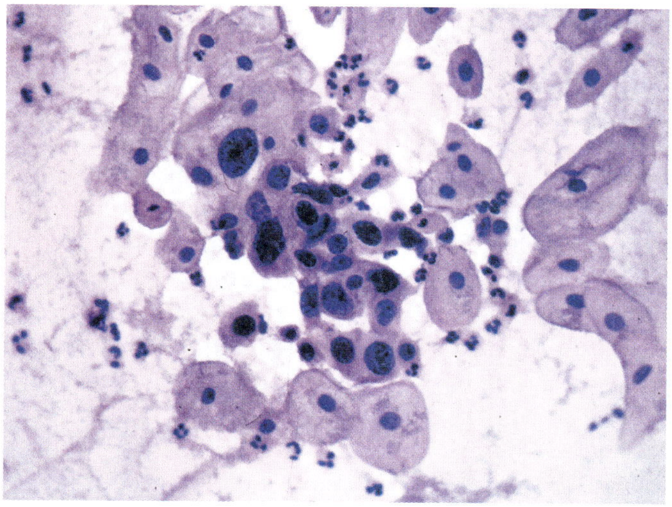

Figure 6-17 Photomicrograph of Pap smear, illustrating a cluster of abnormal cells from in situ carcinoma of the cervix. Cells appear much different from adjacent normal squamous epithelial cells.

Courtesy of Leonard V. Crowley, MD, Century College.

methods, Dr. George Papanicolaou. The microscopic slides of the material prepared for cytologic examination are termed a Papanicolaou smear, or simply **Pap smear** (**Figure 6-17**).

Pap smear A collection of cells from the cervix. Commonly used as a screening test for cervical cancer.

Cytologic methods can also be applied to the diagnosis of neoplasms in other locations by examining sputum, urine, breast secretions, and fluids obtained from the pleural or peritoneal cavities.

Fine Needle Aspiration

Cells for cytologic and histopathologic study can also be examined by aspirating material from organs or tissues by means of a fine needle attached to a syringe and preparing slides from the aspirated material (fine needle aspiration [FNA]). This technique can be used to evaluate nodules in the thyroid or breast. Often the nature of the nodule can be determined by the appearance of the aspirated cells, avoiding the need for a biopsy. However, many fine needle aspirations require a follow-up biopsy to better determine whether a neoplasm is benign or shows signs of malignancy. Suspected tumors in the lung, liver, pancreas, kidney, and other internal organs can be examined by fine needle aspiration. When attempting aspiration from internal organs, the precise location of the suspected tumor must be determined by imaging procedures. The needle is then inserted into the suspected tumor under X-ray or ultrasound guidance. In general, the diagnostic accuracy of fine needle aspiration is not as good as a biopsy but may be adequate for diagnosis, avoiding a more extensive biopsy procedure. Because FNAs are less traumatic to the patient, safer, and often provide results rapidly and at less expense, these procedures are widely used in the initial diagnosis of suspicious lesions.

Circulating Tumor Cells

There is increasing interest in detecting, isolating, and characterizing tumor cells found circulating in the blood (circulating tumor cells [CTC]). The technique depends on the availability of devices that can specifically capture and concentrate the relatively rare tumor cells in the blood. Such cells can then be characterized using a variety of molecular techniques to help provide prognostic and diagnostic information about the cancer. Although the technique is, at present, still in development, it shows great promise for noninvasive detection and characterization of a wide variety of tumors.

Frozen-Section Diagnosis of Neoplasms

Many times, it is important that a surgeon learn immediately whether a tumor discovered in the course of an operation is benign or malignant because the extent of surgery performed may depend on the nature of the neoplasm. The surgeon must also find out during the operation whether a tumor has been excised completely and whether it has spread to lymph nodes or distant sites. A pathologist can provide the surgeon with a rapid **intraoperative** histologic diagnosis and other information by means of a special technique termed a **frozen section**. In this method, a portion of the tumor or other tissue to be examined histologically is frozen solid at a subzero temperature. A thin section of the frozen tissue is cut by means of a special instrument termed a cryotome, and slides are prepared and stained. The slides can then be examined by the pathologist, and a rapid histologic diagnosis can be made. The entire procedure takes only a few minutes as compared to routine histologic diagnosis, which can take several days.

Intraoperative During surgery.

Frozen section A method of rapid diagnosis of tumors used by the pathologist; tissue is frozen solid, cut into thin sections, stained, and examined microscopically.

Tumor-associated antigen An antigen associated with growing tumor cells that serves as an indicator of tumor growth in the body.

Carcinoembryonic antigen (CEA) A tumor-associated antigen that resembles the antigen secreted by the cells of the fetal gastrointestinal tract.

Alpha fetoprotein (AFP) Protein produced by fetal liver early in gestation. Sometimes produced by tumor cells. Level is elevated in amnionic fluid when fetus has a neural tube defect resulting in abnormally high levels in the maternal serum.

Human chorionic gonadotropin (hCG) A hormone made by the placenta in pregnancy with actions similar to pituitary gonadotropins. Same hormone is made by neoplastic cells in some types of malignant testicular tumors.

Tumor-Associated Antigen Tests

As discussed earlier in this chapter, some cancers secrete substances termed **tumor-associated antigens**. These are either absent from normal mature tissues or present only in trace amounts. Many tumor-associated antigens are glycoproteins that are secreted on the external surface of the cancer cells. Some of the glycoproteins gain access to the circulation, where they can be detected by means of specialized laboratory tests performed on the blood of patients with cancer.

A well-known tumor-associated oncofetal antigen is **carcinoembryonic antigen (CEA)**, so named because it resembles a glycoprotein antigen secreted by the cells lining the fetal intestinal tract. CEA is produced by most but not all malignant tumors of the gastrointestinal tract and pancreas and by many cancers of the breast and lung as well as other cancers. Moreover, elevation of CEA levels is not specific for any one type of cancer. CEA is usually not elevated in the blood of people with small, early cancers, and it also occurs at low levels in diseases other than cancer. For these reasons, it is not a useful screening test. However, CEA levels are related to tumor size and may be very high in people with large tumors or tumors that have metastasized. The level of CEA falls after the tumor has been removed and often rises again if the tumor recurs or metastasizes (**Figure 6-18**). If CEA falls after removal of the tumor and later becomes elevated, this usually means the tumor has recurred and additional treatment is needed.

Other products secreted by tumor cells that can be used to monitor tumor growth (Chapter 18) include **alpha fetoprotein (AFP)**, a protein produced by fetal tissues but not normally produced by adult cells, and **human chorionic gonadotropin (hCG)**, the hormone normally produced by the placenta in pregnancy, which are often elevated in patients with testicular carcinoma and in females with certain gynecologic tumors. Alpha fetoprotein is frequently elevated in patients with primary carcinoma of the liver. Prostatic-specific antigen (PSA), produced by prostatic epithelial cells, often is elevated in the bloodstream of men with prostatic carcinoma. The PSA test is used to detect early prostate

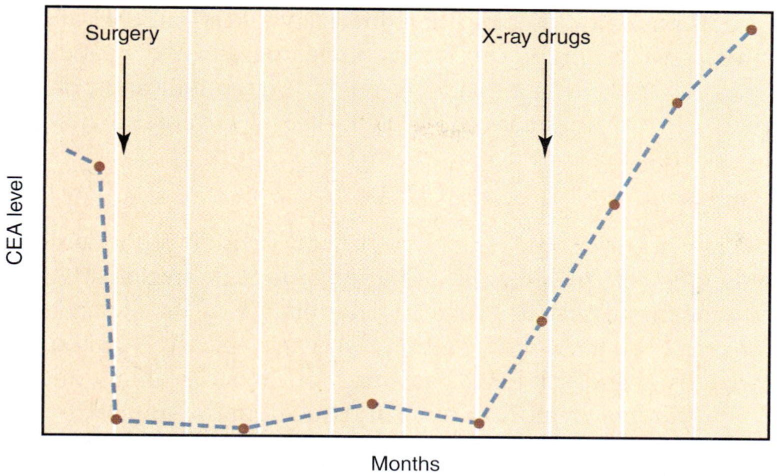

Figure 6-18 The use of CEA to monitor the response to therapy. An elevated CEA level falls after resection of colon cancer and then rises when tumor recurs, indicating the need for additional treatment.

carcinoma before symptoms develop and to monitor the response to treatment. Many other tumor-associated substances have been described, which are used to monitor patients with various types of lung, breast, and ovarian carcinoma.

Treatment of Tumors

Benign tumors may be completely cured by surgical excision, although some have a tendency to reoccur if great care is not taken to remove all traces. Malignant tumors are much more difficult to treat. Four major forms of treatment directed against malignant tumors are surgery, radiotherapy, hormone treatment, and chemotherapy/**immunotherapy**.

Immunotherapy Treatment given to retard growth of a disseminated malignant tumor by stimulating the body's own immune defenses.

The method of treatment depends on the type of tumor and its extent, and often several methods are combined. In many cases, treatment eradicates the cancer, and the patient is cured. In less favorable cases, a cure is no longer possible, but the growth of the cancer is arrested, and life is prolonged. Before a course of treatment is selected, further information obtained by grading and staging the tumor is needed.

Grading and Staging Malignant Tumors

After a biopsy has established the diagnosis of a malignant tumor, selection of the appropriate treatment is based on the characteristics of the tumor cells and the extent of the tumor. Grading the tumor predicts the behavior of the tumor. Grading evaluates the differentiation of the tumor cells, their growth rate based on the number of mitoses, and any characteristics of the tumor cells that would influence the type of treatment selected. Such characteristics may include the response of the tumor cells to estrogen in the case of a breast carcinoma. Staging of the tumor determines whether the tumor is still localized or has spread to regional lymph nodes or distant sites, providing important additional information to guide selection of the best treatment. The characteristics of a tumor identified by staging usually are expressed in a classification termed the TNM system. The T refers to the size of the primary tumor, with T0 indicating an *in situ* lesion, and T1 through T4 indicating increasing size. N refers to the spread of tumor to regional lymph nodes, with N0 indicating no spread, and N1 through N3 indicating progressively greater lymph node spread. M refers to distant metastasis, with M0 indicating no distant spread, and M1 and M2 indicating progressively more extensive distant metastases. Grading and staging are useful not only for selecting treatment but also as an indication of prognosis. In addition, they are important in evaluating the effectiveness of new therapies.

Surgery

Many malignant tumors are treated by surgical excision of the tumor and the surrounding tissues, possibly including removal of the regional lymph nodes that drain the tumor site. The surgeon determines how much surrounding tissue must be excised to ensure removal of all cancer cells. The pathologist, using frozen sections, will check for the adequacy of surgical margins, and, if necessary, the surgeon may remove additional tissue from the surgical area. Surgical excision is successful if the tumor has not already spread to distant sites. Unfortunately, many cancers have already metastasized prior to detection and may no longer be curable by surgery alone. Other methods of treatment must be used frequently in combination with surgery.

Radiotherapy

Malignant lymphomas and some other tumors are quite radiosensitive and can be destroyed by radiotherapy alone or in combination with surgical excision. In some cases, antibodies can be used to deliver radiotherapy to the tumor cells. For example, radiation may be administered preoperatively to reduce the size of a tumor, thereby facilitating its surgical resection. In other instances, radiotherapy is given after a malignant tumor has been resected to destroy any cancer cells that may remain. Radiotherapy is also used to control the growth of widespread tumors and to treat deposits of metastatic tumors that cause pain and disability. The treatment relieves symptoms and makes the patient more comfortable, even though the cancer is not curable. Radiotherapy may be delivered from an external source (X-rays being a common example) or by implanting radioactive "seeds" or pellets at the site of the tumor, a technique used in treating prostate cancer.

Hormone Therapy

Some malignant tumors require hormones for their growth and are termed hormone responsive; these tumors regress temporarily if deprived of the required hormone. For example, many prostate tumors require testosterone and are inhibited by removal of the testes (eliminating the source of testosterone) or by administration of drugs that suppresses testosterone secretion. Many breast carcinomas in postmenopausal women are estrogen responsive and can be controlled by drugs that block estrogen so that the tumor cells are no longer stimulated by estrogen.

Adrenal cortical hormones (corticosteroids) also inhibit the growth of many malignant tumors. Corticosteroids inhibit protein synthesis, thereby suppressing the growth and division of the tumor cells. Tumors of the lymphatic tissues are especially susceptible to the effects of corticosteroids.

Anticancer Drugs

Chemotherapy of cancer is an extraordinarily complex and rapidly changing area. At a basic level, the chemotherapeutic agent most useful in cancer therapy interferes with some metabolic pathway in a cancer cell without causing unacceptable damage in normal cells. Broadly speaking, such drugs are selectively **cytotoxic** (causing cell death) to cancer cells as opposed to other cells in the body. An **antimetabolite** is a drug that interferes with some well-defined metabolic target within the cell, and the cause of its cytotoxicity is usually well known. Surprisingly, the reason a particular antimetabolite is specific for cancer cells is often unclear because the target metabolic pathway is present in both normal and cancer cells. The goal of designing chemotherapeutics is to produce agents that have near absolute specificity for a mutated protein involved in cancer production. If a drug specific for the mutated product responsible for malignant transformation of a cell can be found, that drug would be specific for treating the cancer, with no side effects (or much reduced side effects) on normal cells. Such agents are now available for some cancers and are used in the clinic.

Cytotoxic Causing cell death.

Antimetabolite A substance that competes with or replaces another substance (metabolite) required for cell metabolism.

Alkylating agent An anticancer drug that disrupts cell function by binding DNA chains together so they cannot separate.

The various drugs differ in their mechanisms of action. Some inhibit the synthesis of either DNA or RNA. Others alter the structure of DNA or disturb its function. Still others inhibit protein synthesis or prevent the mitotic spindle from forming so the cell cannot divide. Frequently, several different anticancer drugs are administered simultaneously, each drug blocking a different phase in the cell's metabolic processes. Another group of anticancer drugs acts by suppressing the proliferation of the blood vessels that nourish the tumor, thereby inhibiting tumor growth by interfering with its blood supply.

Most anticancer drugs work best against fast-growing tumors that contain large numbers of actively growing and dividing cells. They are usually less effective against slowly growing tumors because only relatively small numbers of the tumor cells are in the stages of cell growth or division susceptible to the injurious effects of the drugs. However, even within a rapidly growing tumor, many cells have a very low rate of division. Although rate of cell division may play a role in the selectivity of anticancer drugs, this cannot be the only answer.

One important group of anticancer drugs is **alkylating agents**. These drugs interact with both strands of the paired DNA chains in the nucleus and bind them together so they cannot separate. This reaction is termed cross linking of the DNA chains. It disrupts the function of DNA because the chains must separate for duplication of the DNA chains and for synthesis of RNA. In contrast to most anticancer drugs, these agents are effective against nondividing ("resting") cells as well as actively growing cells. Similarly, some drugs chemically alter one of the DNA bases (often guanine) within the DNA strands. These changes are not removed by the DNA repair process and can lead to apoptotic cell death. For this reason, inactivation of the tumor suppressor TP53 interfering with the death of mutated cells can lead to resistance to such agents.

Although they have some degree of selectivity for cancer cells, most anticancer drugs are quite toxic to normal cells as well. Therefore, they must be administered very carefully to ensure maximum damage to tumor cells without irreparable injury to normal cells. Lymphoid tissue is quite susceptible to the destructive effects of these potent drugs; consequently, one unavoidable side effect of anticancer drugs is impairment of cell-mediated and humoral immunity (see Chapter 5).

Recently, several less toxic and more cell-specific anticancer drugs have been developed that block the action of specific cell components that stimulate the tumor cells. Some of those drugs suppress tumor growth by blocking growth factor receptors on the surface of the tumor cells so that growth factors produced by normal cells cannot attach to the receptors and stimulate the tumor cells. For example, antibodies directed against HER2, which are overexpressed on the surface of some breast cancer cells, is an effective therapy for HER2-positive breast cancer. Other drugs inhibit the functions of important intracellular proteins, such as the tyrosine kinases that act as oncoproteins (active oncogene products) in some cancers.

No matter how effective the drug, cancer cells ultimately develop resistance to chemotherapeutic drugs, relating to the large number of cancer cells and their propensity to mutate. If, by chance, a single cell in a tumor mutates and develops resistance to a drug, the cell and all its progeny will be at a growth advantage and ultimately lead to resistance. One way around this is to use multidrug therapies. It is unlikely that a single cancer cell will simultaneously become resistant to several agents. Another is to design additional drugs capable of acting against the mutant cells.

Early detection of localized cancers certainly can result in cures, but this is unlikely in most cases of widespread cancer. Although life span can be prolonged, ultimately the cancer becomes resistant and leads to death.

Adjuvant Chemotherapy

Sometimes surgical resection of a cancer appears to be successful, but metastases appear several years later and eventually prove fatal. The operation failed to eradicate the tumor because small, unrecognized metastases had already spread throughout the body. Even though the main tumor had been removed, the minute metastases continue to grow until eventually they form many large, bulky deposits of metastatic tumor that kill the patient.

To forestall the development of late metastases, a current trend is to administer a course of anticancer drugs either immediately before or after surgical resection of some tumors. This is termed adjuvant chemotherapy (adjuvare = to assist). The drugs destroy any small, undetected foci of metastatic tumor before they become large enough to produce clinical manifestations. In many cases, **adjuvant chemotherapy** combined with surgery appears to achieve better results than surgery alone (Chapter 14). Anticancer drugs are quite toxic, and the potential benefits of adjuvant chemotherapy must be weighed against the harmful effects of the drugs on normal tissues.

Adjuvant chemotherapy Anticancer chemotherapy administered before or after surgical resection of a tumor in an attempt to destroy any small, undetected foci of metastatic tumor before they become clinically detectable.

Immunotherapy

The immune system evolved a number of ways to deal with abnormal cells that can proliferate and form tumors and to deal with established tumors. Cytotoxic T cells recognize antigens on tumor cells that are displayed along with the cells' own MHC class I proteins and can damage the tumor cells by secreting destructive lymphokines. Natural killer lymphocytes can attack and destroy tumor cells without prior antigenic stimulation. Some killer lymphocytes specialize in attacking antibody-coated tumor cells. Activated macrophages can destroy tumor cells by phagocytosis and by secreting tumor necrosis factor along with other cytokines that stimulate lymphocytes to attack tumor cells. Antibodies formed against tumor cell antigens can attach to tumor cells and activate complement; products of complement activation attract lymphocytes and macrophages and form destructive attack complexes that damage the cell membranes of the tumor cells.

Despite this array of immunologic defenses, many tumors circumvent or overwhelm the body's immune defenses, which then become ineffective and no longer retard the growth of the tumor. Treatment of tumors by stimulating the body's immune defenses is termed immunotherapy. Nonspecific immunotherapy is directed toward bolstering the patient's own immune defenses to help the patient deal more effectively with the tumor. Specific immunotherapy directs the immune system against the specific antigens present in the patient's own tumor.

Nonspecific Immunotherapy

Recent approaches for immunotherapy administer various cytokines that either stimulate cells of the immune system or act directly against the tumor cells. The two cytokines used with greatest success against tumors are **interferon alpha** and **interleukin-2 (IL-2)**.

Interferon alpha A broad-spectrum antiviral agent produced by various cells in the body.

Interleukin-2 (IL-2) A lymphokine that stimulates growth of lymphocytes.

In general, interferon consists of a group of carbohydrate-containing, "broad-spectrum" antiviral protein substances produced by cells in response to viral infection. It can regulate the functions of the immune system and inhibit the growth of rapidly dividing cells. Interferon proved useful in treating some types of leukemia, multiple myeloma, malignant melanoma, and kidney cancer. Interferon is much less toxic than many anticancer drugs, and treatment by subcutaneous injection several times per week is usually well tolerated, although flulike symptoms and disorders in the production of red blood cells and platelets are common.

Interleukin-2, a lymphokine produced by T cells, stimulates natural killer cells and cytotoxic T cells that can destroy tumor cells, but it has no direct effects against the tumor cells. Interleukin-2 administered in multiple courses has produced beneficial effects in the treatment of metastatic melanoma and renal cell carcinoma. High doses of interleukin-2 produce a variety of serious toxic effects that limit its use.

Specific Immunotherapy

Specific immunotherapy targets the patient's own tumor cells for attack. Four different approaches appear promising: (1) administration of cytotoxic T lymphocytes directed against the tumor, which are termed tumor-infiltrating lymphocytes; (2) administration of tumor vaccines; (3) administration of antitumor antibodies; and (4) "blockading" (inhibiting) immune checkpoints, which inhibit the role of the immune system in destroying tumor cells.

Adoptive T cell transfer therapy uses cytotoxic T cells isolated from within a patient's tumor. The cells are grown in the laboratory using a variety of cytokines, including interleukin-2. The expanded cytotoxic T cells are then reinfused into the patient. The cells may also be genetically modified before reinfusion to allow them to specifically attach to a cell surface component of the tumor. Although initially used to treat malignant melanoma, the technique shows promise for use in treating a number of tumors.

Immunotherapy, like chemotherapy, is more successful when the therapeutic agent can be directed specifically against the cancer cells. Chimeric antigen receptor T cell therapy (CAR T) harvests the patient's own T cells to use in developing a "living drug." This specifically expanded population of CAR T cells kills the antigen-containing cancer cells to which the CAR T cells bind. It takes approximately three to five weeks from the initial T cell harvest to infusion of the CAR T cells into the patient. The chimeric antigen receptor (CAR) contains two domains. The external portion found on the surface of the T cell contains sections and fragments of antibodies which recognize cell surface proteins on the targeted cell. The interior part of the CAR can signal the T cell and stimulate it to multiply. The CAR T cells, after being infused, will continue to multiply within the patient's system when they encounter the targeted antigen. The procedure shows real promise with blood-borne cancers like leukemias and lymphomas. The technology for developing CAR T cells against solid tumors has been moving much more slowly due to the variability of solid tumor markers from patient to patient and the fact that some solid tumor cells produce local immune suppressive environments, which hamper the work of the CAR T cells.

Tumor vaccines prepared from the patient's own tumor also have been used to immunize the patient against the tumor in an effort to reduce the likelihood that the tumor will recur or metastasize after it has been resected. Tumor cells are obtained from the resected tumor, grown in the laboratory, and then killed so they cannot proliferate in the patient but can still generate an immune response. They are then used to prepare a vaccine that will stimulate an immune response to the resected tumor. Tumor vaccines have been used as an additional treatment after resection of a malignant melanoma or a colon carcinoma when the patient is considered at high risk of recurrence.

For tumor antibody therapy, antibodies are prepared against tumor cell antigens, and then linked to an antitumor drug or toxin that can kill tumor cells. The antibodies with attached drug or toxin are then infused back into the patient to seek out and destroy the tumor cells without damaging normal cells.

Immune checkpoint blockades prevent tumors from shutting down the immune response by inappropriately activating physiological pathways that regulate and control the immune response. Blockading immunosuppressive receptors with monoclonal antibodies "reactivates" the patient's immune system and has had impressive success in treating tumors with vaccines directed against specific tumor antigens.

Although the results of immunotherapy have been mixed to date, the combination of immune checkpoint blockade with additional modes of therapy is promising. There have been some notable successes, such as in the use of interferon therapy for one type of leukemia termed hairy cell leukemia, or in cases involving specific types of widespread tumors when no other methods of treatment are available to control the tumor. No single method works against all types of tumors. Unfortunately, most patients treated with immunotherapy have advanced diseases, and often the body's immune defenses are incapable of dealing with such large amounts of tumor even when stimulated by immunotherapy.

Case 6-1

John is a 70-year-old who has not been seen by his primary care physician for several years. He has noticed increasing fatigue and weight loss of about 10 pounds in the last 2 months. He is concerned that he may have seen signs of rectal bleeding in the past year (but attributed them to hemorrhoids). The physician orders a stool blood test, which is positive and detects iron deficiency anemia. John also has a moderate elevation in blood CEA levels. The physician notes that John has not had any of the recommended screening procedures for the detection of colorectal cancer such as colonoscopy or flexible sigmoidoscopy and is concerned about the possibility of such. John is unaware of any history of colorectal cancer in his large number of relatives. The patient is scheduled for a colonoscopy, to which he objects, but the physician notes that other diagnostic procedures such as a double contrast barium enema or CT-based colonography also require preliminary bowel preparation and are likely to require subsequent colonoscopy either for definitive diagnosis or therapy. John undergoes a successful colonoscopy during which several small polyps are found in the descending colon and removed. However, the endoscopist is unable to fully examine the colon because the lumen of the colon is stenosed (constricted) in the ascending portion, preventing further passage of the scope. The stenosed area appears to be associated with a large tumor that cannot be removed using the endoscope. The endoscopist tattoos the area with ink to note the area of concern and refers the patient for surgery. The surgeon notes a suspicious lesion of the right (ascending) colon and performs a right

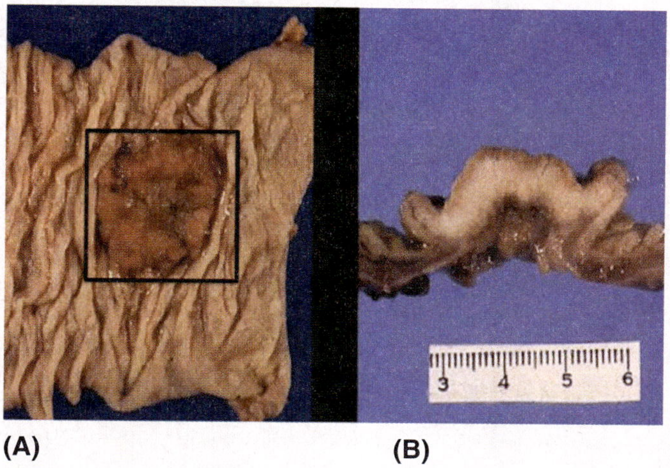

Case Figure 6-1 **(A)** Opened loop of the colon removed at colectomy showing lesion (*boxed*). **(B)** Cross section of lesion seen on edge. White-tan tumor infiltrates into the bowel wall.

Courtesy of Department of Pathology and Laboratory Medicine, University of North Carolina at Chapel Hill.

hemicolectomy, removing the lesion and the right colon, reattaching the small intestine to the transverse colon to preserve bowel function. During surgery, the surgeon also removes adjacent lymph nodes for analysis. The surgical specimen and nodes are sent to pathology for evaluation (**Case Figure 6-1**). Microscopic analysis indicates the lesion to be an adenocarcinoma that has infiltrated through almost the entire colon (**Case Figure 6-2**). No tumor is detected in lymph nodes. John is given a course of adjuvant chemotherapy with a cytotoxic agent. The patient remains healthy. His CEA level fell to normal and has shown no elevation in the 5 years since surgery.

Discussion

John is lucky. The only potential cure for colon cancer is surgical removal of the lesion. TNM analysis of his lesion would be T3; cancer has grown through the muscular layers but has not penetrated beyond the outer layer, or serosa,

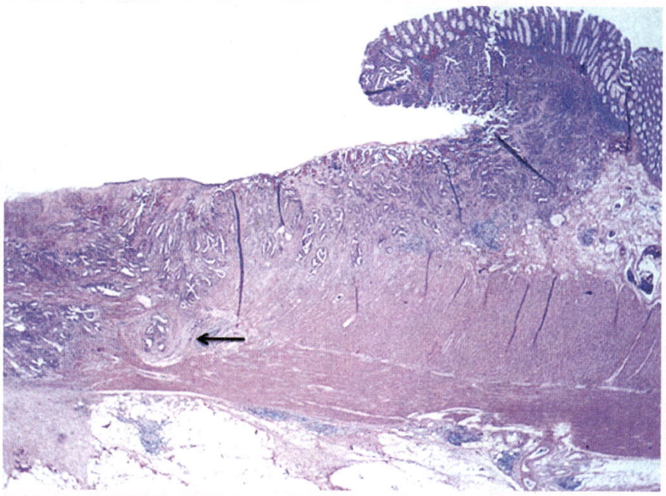

Case Figure 6-2 Microscopic examination of lesion in Case Figure 6-1 showing adenocarcinoma infiltrating into the muscular wall (muscularis) (*arrow*).

Courtesy of Department of Pathology and Laboratory Medicine, University of North Carolina at Chapel Hill.

(*continues*)

Case 6-1 *(Continued)*

of the colon. N0 (no cancer in adjacent nodes), and M0 (no distant spread). T3N0 disease has almost an 80 percent 5-year relapse-free survival rate. Adjuvant chemotherapy is not always used with John's stage of disease but is likely to improve relapse-free survival. However, there is a moral to this case. It is extremely likely that John would never have had colon cancer had he followed routine cancer screening guidelines. Colon cancer peaks in both sexes at about age 65. Hence, screening for polyps in the colon and rectum should start at age 45 (in the absence of other risk factors such as a strong family history or a defined hereditary disease). Because most colon cancer starts as a detectable precancerous lesion, removal of these lesions (colon and rectal adenomatous polyps) via endoscopy prevents colon cancer from occurring. Even removal of lesions showing marked dysplasia or localized cancer is likely to be curative.

Because colon cancer progresses slowly, screening tests need not be undertaken frequently if no suspicious lesions are found. Colonoscopy at 10-year intervals allows examination of the entire colon and cecum and is considered to be the most sensitive screening test. It also allows for therapeutic removal of lesions. Alternatively, flexible proctosigmoidoscopy every 5 years is recommended. This procedure (unlike colonoscopy) generally does not require anesthesia and is often done by a trained physician rather than a gastroenterologist. It is less costly than colonoscopy and requires less patient preparation (generally two disposable enemas as opposed to the thorough bowel cleaning needed for colonoscopy). However, proctosigmoidoscopy (as the name implies) can examine only the descending colon. Detection of multiple polyps in this region suggests the presence of additional undetected polyps in the transverse or ascending colon, necessitating colonoscopy. Several other techniques are available for use in special cases (CT-based colonography, double contrast barium enema, and, recently, examination of the colon by orally ingested camera-containing capsules). None of these techniques allow for removal of lesions, and suspicious findings require follow-up colonoscopy. Annual fecal blood testing and tests that detect DNA mutations in the stool that derive from colonic cells may also be of value.

Etiology and Pathogenesis

Colonic adenocarcinoma T3N0 treated by surgery and adjuvant chemotherapy with no signs of recurrence 5 years post-operation.

Questions

1. There is dispute over the cost-effectiveness of colonoscopy versus proctosigmoidoscopy. What factors should be taken into account in establishing the procedure that should be recommended?
2. Stool-based DNA testing has been licensed for use in the detection of colon cancer. What potential advantages and disadvantages does such a test have?
3. There is some controversy about the use of adjuvant chemotherapy in this patient's disease. What factors might argue for and against its use?

Questions for Review

1. What are the major differences between a benign and a malignant tumor?
2. How are tumors named? What are the common prefixes used in naming tumors?
3. What are proto-oncogenes, tumor suppressor genes, DNA repair genes, and genes regulating apoptosis? What is their role in the development of neoplasms?
4. What is the role of viruses in causing cancer?

5. How does the body defend itself against abnormal cells that arise spontaneously in the course of cell division? What is the consequence of failure of these defense mechanisms?
6. What is a lymphoma? What is the difference between a nevus and a melanoma? What is a teratoma?
7. What is the significance of a Pap smear containing atypical cells?
8. What is a frozen section? How is it used in the diagnosis of tumors?

References

Strayer DS, Saffitz JE, Rubin E. *Rubin's Pathology*. 8th ed. Wolters Kluwer; 2019.

Weinberg RA. *The Biology of Cancer*. 3rd ed. W. W. Norton & Company; 2023.

- The area of neoplastic disease is so broad and intensely studied that the interested individual would be wise to read an overview prior to undertaking detailed reading. The first resource presents an up-to-date pathologist's view of cancer in its Chapter 5, Neoplasia. The second reference provides a detailed text on all aspects of neoplastic disease; strong on experimental concepts.

National Institutes of Health, National Cancer Institute. CAR T Cells: Engineering Patients' Immune Cells to Treat Their Cancers. Updated February 26, 2025. Accessed May 2, 2025. https://www.cancer.gov/about-cancer/treatment/research/car-t-cells

- This resource from the National Cancer Institute describes a form of immunotherapy that has generated a lot of excitement: CAR T-cell therapies.

American Cancer Society. ACS Research Highlights on Top Cancers. Accessed May 2, 2025. https://www.cancer.org/research/acs-research-highlights.html

- This website highlights recent discoveries from American Cancer Society researchers.

Centers for Disease Control and Prevention. Cancer Research. https://www.cdc.gov/cancer/research/index.html

CDC's Division of Cancer Prevention and Control's latest cancer research is highlighted.

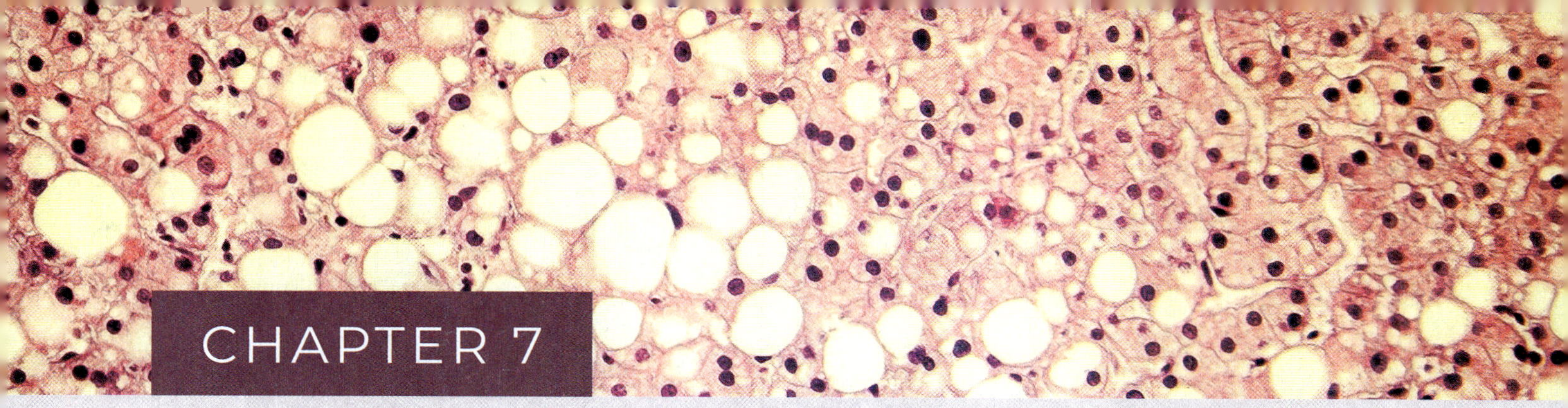

CHAPTER 7

Pathogenic Microorganisms

LEARNING OBJECTIVES

1. Explain how bacteria are classified. List and describe the major groups of pathogenic bacteria.
2. Describe the mechanism by which antibiotics inhibit the growth and metabolism of bacteria.
3. Explain the adverse effects of antibiotics.
4. Explain the mode of action of virus infections and describe how the body's response to viral infection leads to recovery.
5. List the common infections caused by chlamydiae, mycoplasmas, and rickettsiae.
6. Discuss the spectrum of infections caused by fungi. Explain the factors that predispose people to systemic infections. Describe the methods used to treat fungus infections.
7. Give examples of how the development of a vaccine contributes to the disease control.

Introduction

Of the wide spectrum of microorganisms found in nature, only a relatively small proportion cause disease in humans. These pathogenic microorganisms are classified into several large groups: bacteria, viruses, chlamydiae, rickettsiae/ehrlichiae, mycoplasmas, and fungi. In addition, humans serve as host to a number of animal parasites capable of causing illness or disability. A small number of microbiologic agents are extremely **virulent**. Such virulence is often associated with specific genes; **virulence** factors may be part of the bacterial chromosome or be inherited as a plasmid, most often a small circular DNA element in the bacterial cytoplasm that can replicate and be transmitted independently of the bacterial chromosome. Others are of very low virulence and are capable of causing disease only when the body's normal defenses have been weakened by a debilitating illness.

Virulence/virulent Ability to cause disease.
Virulence Assessment of the ability of a pathogen to cause disease.
Coccus Spherical bacteria.

Classification of Bacteria

Historically, bacteria have been classified on the basis of four major characteristics: shape, Gram stain reaction, antigenic structure, and biochemical and cultural characteristics. A bacterium may be spherical (**coccus**) or

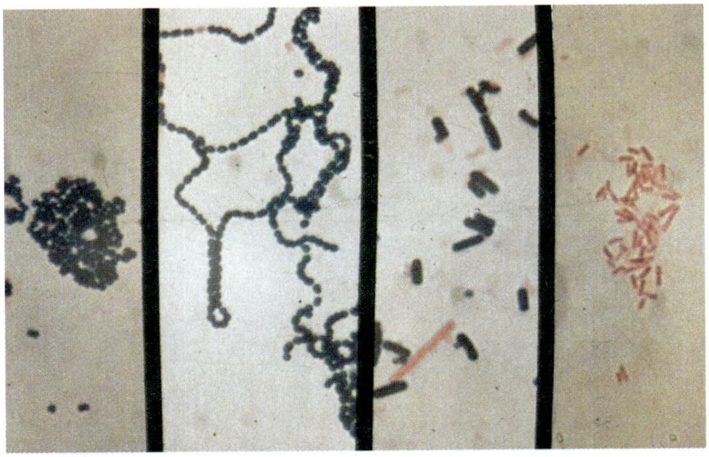

Figure 7-1 Appearance of bacteria as seen in Gram stains. From left to right; Gram-positive cocci in clusters (staphylococci), Gram-positive cocci in chains (streptococci), Gram-positive bacilli, Gram-negative bacilli (original magnification ×1000).

Bacillus Rod-shaped bacteria.

Gram stain Staining process used to differentiate the cell wall structure of bacterial cells.

Flagellum/flagella A whiplike process that propels an organism or sperm.

Media Solid, liquid, or gel-sol substances created to support the growth of organisms *in vitro*.

Aerobic organisms Microbes that grow best in the presence of oxygen.

Anaerobic organisms Microbes that grow best in the absence of oxygen.

Spores A unit of asexual reproduction found in life cycles of many plants, algae, fungi and protozoa that can remain viable even under extreme conditions.

rod-shaped (**bacillus**) or have a spiral or corkscrew shape. Cocci may grow in clusters (staphylococci), in pairs (diplococci), or in chains (streptococci). Gram staining is a standard procedure to classify and identify unknown bacterial cells. After Gram stain, Gram-negative cells will appear as pink under the microscope (**Figure 7-1**). The **Gram stain** reaction is based on differences in the structure of the bacterial cell wall between the two classes of bacteria, which reflect certain significant biochemical properties of the bacteria, such as susceptibility to host defense mechanisms and particular antibiotics (**Figure 7-2**).

Each type of bacterium contains a large number of antigens associated with the cell body, the capsule of the bacterium, and the **flagella** (in the case of motile organisms). The antigenic structure can be determined by special methods, defining a system of antigens unique for each group of bacteria. Some bacteria are quite fastidious and can be grown only on enriched **media** under carefully controlled conditions of temperature and acidity (pH). Other bacteria are hardy and capable of growing on relatively simple culture media under a wide variety of conditions. Many bacteria grow best in the presence of oxygen (**aerobic organisms**). Some bacteria are able to grow only in the absence of oxygen or under extremely low oxygen tension. These are called **anaerobic organisms** (without oxygen). Others grow equally well under either aerobic or anaerobic conditions.

Many bacteria have special structural characteristics. Some bacteria have flagella: hairlike processes covering their surface. Flagella can give a bacterium motility. Some bacteria form **spores**, which may be spherical or ellipsoidal in shape. Endospores develop inside the mother cell. Exospores develop outside the parent cell. Endospores are produced by bacterial genera such as *Bacillus* and *Clostridium*. Exspores are formed by *Actinomyces, Streptomyces and Actinobacterial*, for example.

Most bacteria have distinct biochemical characteristics. Some types of bacteria are capable of fermenting carbohydrates and can promote many different biochemical reactions under suitable cultural conditions. Each type of bacterium has its own "biochemical profile," which aids in its identification. This biochemical profile can be determined by growing the bacteria on differently modified media.

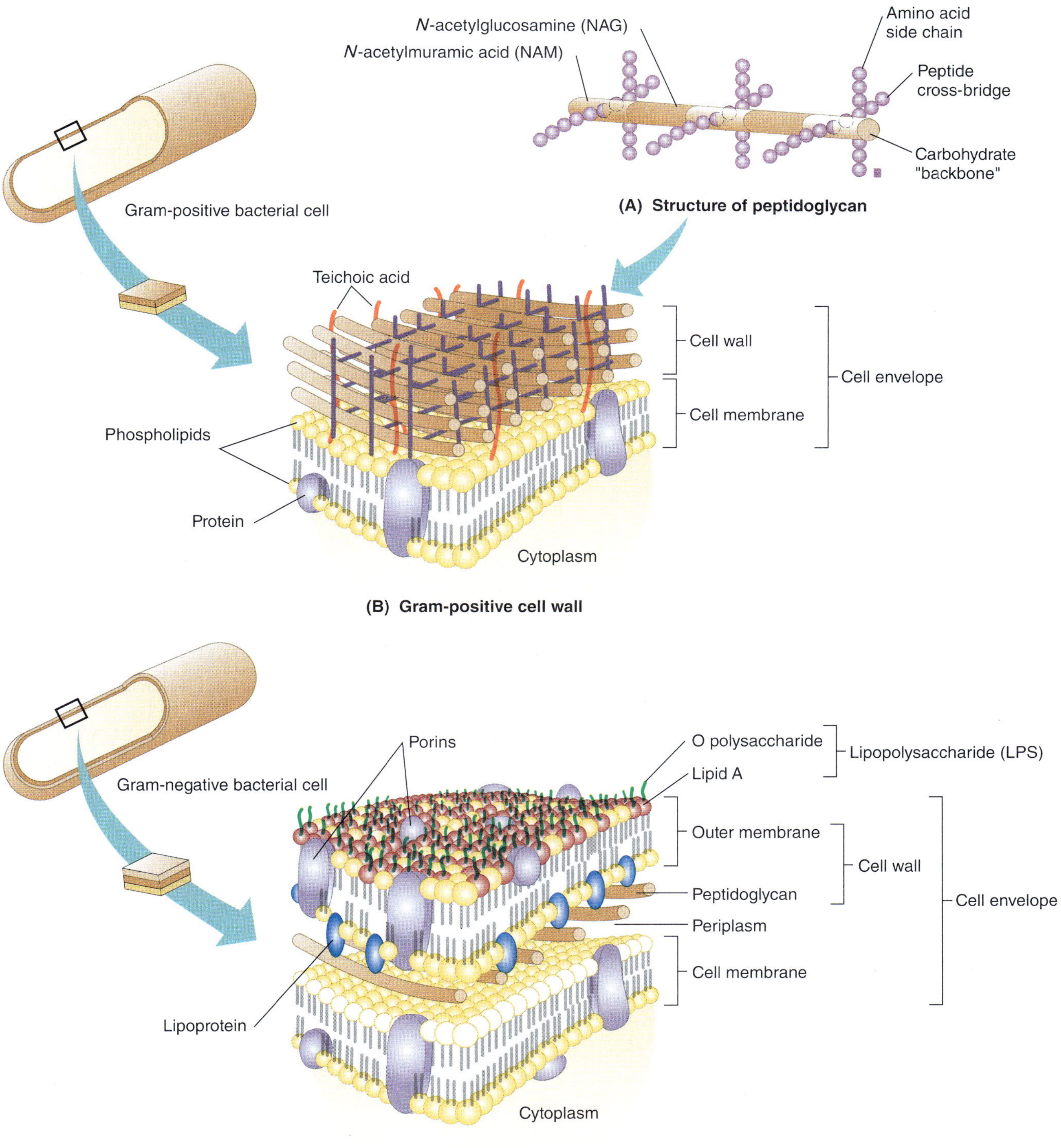

(C) Gram-negative cell wall

Figure 7-2 A comparison of cell walls of Gram-positive and Gram-negative bacterial cells. **(A)** The structure of peptidoglycan of the cell wall is shown as units of NAG and NAM joined laterally and vertically by amino acids. **(B)** The cell wall of a Gram-positive bacteria is composed of multiple peptidoglycan layers combined with teichoic acid (a bacterial polysaccharide). **(C)** In the Gram-negative cell wall, the peptidoglycan layer is much thinner and lacks teichoic acid. In addition, the cell wall has an outer membrane. Gram-negative bacteria are also unique in having lipid A (a lipopolysaccharide important in bacterial virulence) and unique proteins called **porins** in the outer membrane that contribute to the resistance of this class of bacteria to certain antimicrobial agents.

Porins Unique proteins on G-bacteria's outer membrane that contribute to resistance to antimicrobial agents.

Since the introduction of molecular technology for the study of microbiology, the taxonomy of bacteria is now based on genomic sequence, predominantly that of the 16S ribosomal RNA gene, a gene found in all prokaryotes. The use of this technology has resulted in an extensive array of data defining bacterial species as well as "superspecies and subspecies." The current hierarchy of bacterial species is complex. (Information is available online at lpsn.dsmz.de/.)

Major Classes of Pathogenic Bacteria

This section summarizes important bacteria that infect humans along with the principal diseases they cause. These major groups of pathogenic bacteria and their Gram stain reactions are shown in **Table 7-1**. The diseases caused by these organisms are described in the following section and summarized in **Table 7-2**.

Staphylococci

Blood agar plates Bacteria media incorporating red blood cells.

Hemolysis Destruction of blood cells.

Staphylococci, normal inhabitants of the skin and nasal cavity, are generally not pathogenic. Some staphylococci are pathogens and may be extremely virulent. Pathogens usually can be distinguished from nonpathogenic staphylococci by the appearance of their colonies on media containing blood (**blood agar plates**). Pathogenic staphylococci produce zones of complete **hemolysis** around the growing colonies (**Figure 7-3**) in contrast to nonpathogenic staphylococci, which do not hemolyze red blood cells.

Table 7-1 Important Pathogenic Bacteria

	Gram-Stain Reaction	
Type	**Gram-Positive**	**Gram-Negative**
Cocci Spherical single or chained	Staphylococci Streptococci Pneumococci	Gonococci Meningococci
Bacilli Rod-shaped, single, or chained	*Corynebacteria* *Listeria* *Bacilli* *Clostridia*	*Haemophilus* *Gardnerella* *Francisella* *Yersinia* *Brucella* *Legionella* *Salmonella* *Shigella* *Campylobacter* Cholera bacillus Colon bacillus (*Escherichia coli*) and related organisms
Spiral organisms Helical shapes		*Treponema pallidum* *Borrelia burgdorferi*
Acid-fast organisms Special staining response	Tubercle bacillus Leprosy bacillus	

Table 7-2 Summary of Major Bacterial Pathogens and the Diseases They Cause

Pathogen	Disease
Gram-positive Cocci	
Staphylococcus aureus	Various localized and systemic infections.
Beta hemolytic streptococcus, Group A	Pharyngitis, systemic infections, skin and muscle necrosis. Hypersensitivity response to organism causes rheumatic fever, nephritis.
Beta hemolytic streptococcus, Group B	Urinary tract and wound infections, and systemic infection. Newborn infection acquired from vaginal organisms in mother.
Streptococci, other groups	Wound and urinary tract infections.
Streptococcus pneumoniae (Pneumococcus)	Middle ear and sinus infections. Systemic infection. Lobar pneumonia. Meningitis.
Gram-negative Cocci	
Neisseria gonorrhoeae (Gonococcus)	Genital tract infections (see Chapter 18 Sexually Transmitted Infections). Bacteremia causing endocarditis, osteomyelitis, and septic arthritis.
Neisseria meningiditis (Meningococcus)	Meningococcal meningitis.
Aerobic Gram-Positive Rods	
Corynebacterium diphtheriae	Diphtheria. Clinical manifestations caused by toxin production.
Listeria monocytogenes	Systemic infection. Pregnant women may infect fetus. Persons with impaired immune system are very susceptible.
Aerobic Spore-Forming Rods	
Bacillus anthracis	Primarily a disease of animals. People infected from contact with wool or animal products. Localized and systemic infection. Potential germ warfare agent.
Anaerobic Spore-Forming Rods	
Clostridium perfringens	Gas gangrene. Muscle necrosis and hemolytic anemia caused by toxin. Gas formation in infected tissues.
Clostridium tetani	Tetanus (lockjaw) caused by toxin-induced spasm of voluntary muscles.
Clostridium botulinum	Botulism. Neuroparalytic toxin produced in improperly processed or canned foods.
Clostridium difficile	Antibiotic-associated colitis. Loss of normal intestinal flora caused by antibiotics allows overgrowth of Clostridia. Toxin produced by Clostridia damages bowel mucosa.
Gram-Negative Rods	
Haemophilus influenzae	Pulmonary infections. Meningitis in susceptible children.
Yersinia pestis	Plague. Disease of wild rodents transmitted to humans by fleas. Causes systemic infection. Can spread person to person if infection spreads to lungs (pneumonic plague).
Brucella species	Brucellosis. Febrile illness from contact with infected animals or consumption of raw milk from infected animals.
Francisella species	Tularemia. Febrile illness acquired from flesh of infected animals, usually wild rabbits, or transmitted to humans by bite of infected ticks or deer flies.
Legionella pneumophila	Legionnaires' disease. Organisms live in water and cause pulmonary infection in persons who inhale aerosolized droplets from showers, air conditioners, or other water sources. No person-to-person spread.

(continues)

Table 7-2 Summary of Major Bacterial Pathogens and the Diseases They Cause *(continued)*

Pathogen	Disease
Salmonella species	Gastroenteritis and systemic infections. Infection acquired from contaminated food or water sources.
Shigella species	Dysentery with frequent watery stools. Spread by person-to-person contact or by contaminated food and water.
Campylobacter species	Gastroenteritis. May cause systemic infection. Infects many animals. Humans are infected from contaminated water, raw shellfish harvested from contaminated water, undercooked meat or poultry, or contact with infected animals.
Escherichia coli	Gastroenteritis, urinary tract, and systemic infections. Some strains (0157:H7) produce toxins that cause hemolytic anemia and kidney damage.
Spirochete	
Treponema pallidum	Syphilis. Considered in the discussion on communicable diseases. See also Chapter 18, Sexually Transmitted Infections.
Borrelia burgdorferi	Lyme disease, transmitted from rodents to humans by ticks. Causes febrile illness and arthritis with lesion at site of tick bite.
Acid-Fast Bacteria	
Mycobacterium tuberculosis	Pulmonary tuberculosis. Considered in the discussion on the respiratory system.
Mycobacterium avium complex	A normally nonpathogenic organism that may cause an opportunistic infection in AIDS patients.

Pathogenic staphylococci (and in particular *Staphylococcus aureus*) are a very common cause of boils, other skin infections, and postoperative wound infections. Occasionally, staphylococci cause serious pulmonary infections, infections of the bones and joints or heart valves, and other types of systemic infections. Staphylococci infections can be difficult to manage in hospitals where patients have undergone recent surgical operations or have various chronic diseases associated with impairment of the body's normal defenses

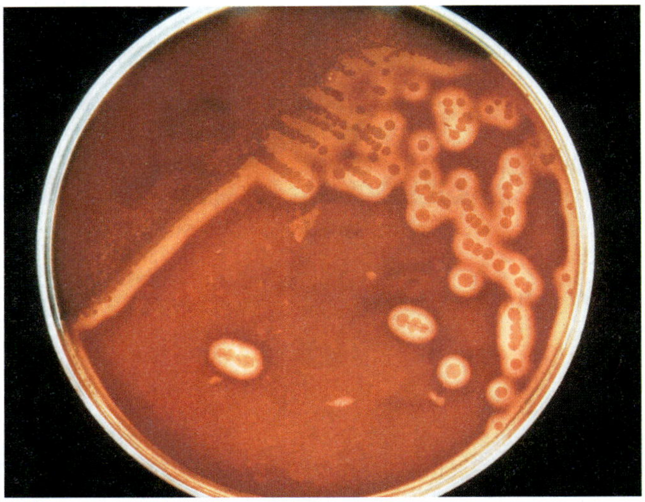

Figure 7-3 Bacteriologic culture plate (blood agar) containing colonies of hemolytic staphylococci. Enzymes produced by the bacteria break down (hemolyze) the blood cells in the culture medium, which causes the clear zones surrounding the colonies.

Courtesy of Leonard V. Crowley, MD, Century College.

against bacterial infection. Some strains of staphylococci are highly resistant to antibiotics, and infections caused by antibiotic-resistant staphylococci are extremely difficult to treat. Toxins produced by *S. aureus* are the cause of toxic shock syndrome (discussed in Chapter 18) and some cases of food poisoning.

Streptococci

Streptococci are classified on the basis of their serologic group designated by a capital letter and on the type of hemolysis the organism produces when grown on a solid medium containing blood. Generally, both the letter group and the type of hemolysis are specified when describing a streptococcus.

The serologic classification, called the Lancefield system, divides the streptococci into 20 major groups based on differences in the carbohydrate antigens present in their cell walls. These groups are designated A through H and K through V, with most of the streptococci of medical importance in groups A, B, and D. The classification based on hemolysis describes the organisms as producing either alpha hemolysis (partial hemolysis associated with a green pigment production), beta hemolysis (complete hemolysis), or no hemolysis on blood agar plates. Usually both the Lancefield group and the type of hemolysis are specified when describing streptococci.

Alpha hemolytic streptococci (or simply alpha streptococci) produce green discoloration of the blood immediately around the colony and are often called *Streptococcus viridans* because of this growth characteristic (*viridans* = green). These organisms are normal inhabitants of the mouth and throat and usually are not pathogenic, although *Strep mutans* is a common cause of dental caries (tooth decay). Some alpha hemolytic streptococci cannot be classified in the Lancefield system because they lack the carbohydrate antigen possessed by other streptococci.

Beta hemolytic streptococci (or simply beta streptococci) produce a narrow zone of complete hemolysis around the growing colony. One of the most important beta streptococci is in Lancefield group A and is called a group A beta streptococcus (sometimes called *S. pyogenes*). Many group A beta streptococci are extremely pathogenic, causing streptococcal sore throat, scarlet fever, serious skin infections, and infections of the uterus after childbirth. Some produce a toxin that causes a toxic shock syndrome similar to that caused by toxin-producing staphylococci. One particularly virulent toxin-producing group A beta streptococcal strain causes a rapidly progressive, destructive infection of the subcutaneous tissues and the fibrous tissue (fascia) covering the adjacent muscles. This condition, called **necrotizing fasciitis**, may be complicated by necrosis (**gangrene**) of the overlying skin and by necrosis of the muscles in the infected area (streptococcal myositis).

In addition to causing infections in various tissues, some strains of group A beta streptococci are capable of inducing a state of hypersensitivity in susceptible individuals, leading to development of **rheumatic fever** or a type of kidney disease called **glomerulonephritis**. These diseases are considered in greater detail in the sections on the circulatory system (Chapter 10) and kidneys (Chapter 17). Fortunately, group A beta streptococci still remain quite sensitive to penicillin and other antibiotics.

Beta streptococci in other Lancefield groups are also of medical importance. Group B beta streptococci *S. agalactiae* may cause urinary tract and wound infections, but they are of greatest importance as a cause of serious infections in newborn infants. They often inhabit (colonize) the rectum and vagina of pregnant women, and the infant may become infected during labor and delivery.

Necrotizing fasciitis Destruction of subcutaneous tissues in beta streptococcal infection.

Gangrene Tissue death caused by bacterial infection or lack of blood circulation.

Rheumatic fever A disease caused by hypersensitivity to antigens of the Group A beta-hemolytic streptococcus, characterized by fever, joint pains, and inflammation of heart valves and muscle.

Glomerulonephritis An inflammation of the glomeruli caused by either antigen–antibody complexes trapped in the glomeruli or by antiglomerular basement membrane antibodies.

Because of the potential hazard of a life-threatening infection in an infant born to a mother colonized by group B beta streptococci, routine rectal and vaginal cultures to detect the organism are recommended for all pregnant women late in pregnancy. Those women who are colonized are treated with intravenous antibiotics during labor to reduce the risk of a serious group B beta streptococcal infection in the infant.

Group D streptococci and streptococci of other Lancefield groups may also cause various types of infections, but it is the group A beta streptococcus that is responsible for almost all of the late immunologic complications: rheumatic fever and glomerulonephritis.

Closely related to group D streptococci but classified separately are organisms that inhabit the intestinal tract called enterococci (*enteron* = bowel). These organisms are often very resistant to multiple antibiotics. Consequently, a wound or urinary tract infection caused by an enterococcus may be very difficult to treat.

Pneumococci

Pneumococci (*Streptococcus pneumoniae*) are Gram-positive cocci and are classified with the streptococci. They grow in pairs and short chains and have certain biochemical characteristics setting them apart from other streptococci. Pneumococci are a common cause of bacterial pneumonia, middle ear infections, and sinusitis and are one of the most common human pathogens.

Gram-Negative Cocci

Most Gram-negative cocci are nonpathogenic members of the genus *Neisseria* and are normal inhabitants of the upper respiratory passages. This group has two pathogenic members. The meningococcus (*Neisseria meningitidis*) causes a type of meningitis (inflammation of the membranes surrounding the brain and spinal cord) that frequently occurs in epidemics. The gonococcus (*Neisseria gonorrhoeae*) causes gonorrhea. This disease is transmitted by sexual contact and is discussed in greater detail in Chapter 18.

Gram-Positive Bacilli

There are several important groups of Gram-positive rod-shaped bacteria that can be subdivided on the basis of their oxygen requirements and on their ability to form spores. Two important groups of *non-spore-forming* aerobic bacteria are *Corynebacteria* and *Listeria*. The two important groups of *spore-forming* organisms are *Bacilli*, which are aerobic microorganisms, and *Clostridia*, which are anaerobic organisms.

Aerobic Non-Spore-Forming Gram-Positive Organisms. *Corynebacteria* are a large group of microorganisms. Most are nonpathogenic inhabitants of the skin and other squamous epithelium-lined body surfaces (mucous membranes). However, one member of this group (*Corynebacterium diphtheriae*) causes diphtheria. The organism causes an acute ulcerative inflammation of the throat and produces a potent toxin that can injure heart muscle and nerve tissue.

One important member of the *Listeria* group of microorganisms, called *Listeria monocytogenes*, can cause a very serious infection. The organism is widely distributed in nature: in the soil, on plants, and in the intestinal tract of people and animals. The organism may contaminate dairy products, raw vegetables, and other food products such as soft cheeses, hot dogs, and delicatessen foods. People become infected by eating *Listeria*-contaminated foods, and those at greatest risk for serious infections are infants and older people, pregnant women, and people whose immune system is impaired. *Listeria* infection is a very serious systemic illness that may be complicated by the spread of the organism to the brain and meninges, causing meningitis or a brain abscess. In pregnant women, the organism may also spread through the placenta to infect the unborn infant, leading to intrauterine fetal death or life-threatening infection of the infant.

Aerobic Spore-Forming Gram-Positive Organisms. Spore-forming aerobic bacteria include the genera *Bacillus*. Only one member of this group is highly pathogenic. This organism is *Bacillus anthracis*, which causes anthrax.

Anthrax is primarily a disease of animals that is rare in the United States but is a more common animal infection in some other countries. Anthrax spores are highly resistant, can survive for many years in the soil, and can contaminate the hair, wool, or other tissues of animals from countries where anthrax is prevalent. If anthrax spores enter the body of a susceptible animal or person, the spores can germinate to form very large numbers of rapidly growing bacteria, which causes the disease anthrax.

Inhalation of anthrax spores from spore-contaminated wool, yarn, or other animal products causes a severe life-threatening pulmonary and systemic infection with extremely high mortality. The spores germinate within the pulmonary alveoli, actively proliferate, and produce lethal toxins that cause extensive tissue destruction. Other spores are ingested by macrophages and transported to regional lymph nodes, where they continue to germinate and produce toxins. A vaccine to immunize against anthrax has been available for many years, and it is recommended for people at high risk of exposure to anthrax, such as veterinarians and employees of textile mills that process imported wool or similar animal products.

Concerns about the use of anthrax spores as a bioterrorism germ warfare agent became a reality in 2001 when a letter containing anthrax spores was mailed to a U.S. senator, processed at a postal facility in Washington, DC, and opened in a senate office building. The spores contaminated the postal facility and senate office building, causing acute inhalation of anthrax in five postal workers who worked in the facility where the letter was processed. Also exposed were a number of people who worked in the office building. Currently anthrax is a very rare disease, with one case or less reported per year. Two unusual cases have been reported in association with imported goat skins used to make drums.

People who may have been exposed to anthrax spores require a prolonged course of antibiotics to prevent development of pulmonary anthrax. Antibiotics effective against the germinated form of the anthrax bacillus are not effective against the spore form of the organism, and many spores do not germinate as soon as they are inhaled. Some are ingested by macrophages and transported to the regional lymph nodes, where they may continue to germinate for as long as 2 months after the initial exposure. The long course of antibiotics is required to destroy the antibiotic-sensitive vegetative bacteria as they germinate at various times from antibiotic-resistant spores.

Anaerobic Spore-Forming Gram-Positive Organisms. Anaerobic spore-forming bacilli belong to the genus *Clostridia*. These are normal inhabitants of the intestinal tract of animals and humans and are also found in the

Botulism Food poisoning caused by ingestion of a neurotoxin produced by an anaerobic spore-forming bacillus, *Clostridium botulinum*, growing in improperly canned or preserved food.

soil. Members of this group produce potent toxins and cause several diseases. Species of *Clostridia* cause gas gangrene, tetanus (lockjaw), and **botulism**, and others cause an intestinal infection.

Gas gangrene, caused by *Clostridium perfringens* and related organisms, develops in dirty, spore-contaminated wounds. These anaerobic organisms germinate and proliferate in dead or devitalized tissues, especially in wounds where considerable necrosis of tissue has taken place. The *Clostridia* produce large amounts of gas by fermenting the necrotic tissues, and they also release powerful toxins that destroy tissues and cause widespread systemic effects.

Another clostridial species, *Clostridium tetani*, produces a potent toxin that causes spasm of voluntary muscles. The common term lockjaw comes from the marked rigidity of the jaw muscles that is a common feature of the disease. Tetanus may be fatal because of respiratory failure resulting from spasm of the muscles concerned with respiration.

Clostridium botulinum produces a potent neuroparalytic toxin. Botulism can generally be traced to eating improperly processed or canned foods in which the organism has grown and produced toxin. Botulism is a poisoning caused by the ingestion of toxin in food rather than a bacterial infection. Although botulism was more common when home canning was prevalent, outbreaks of botulism have also been traced to contamination of home-cured ham, some meats, and even raw carrot juice left unrefrigerated for several days. Infantile botulism can occur when infants consume contaminated honey or corn syrup resulting in the toxin being absorbed from bacteria proliferating in the intestine. For this reason, even commercially produced honey should not be fed to infants.

Clostridium difficile is the organism responsible for the intestinal infection called antibiotic-associated colitis that sometimes follows use of broad-spectrum antibiotics and is considered in Chapter 21.

Gram-Negative Bacteria

There are many Gram-negative organisms of clinical importance. Several different species or genera cause important diseases in humans. These are named *Haemophilus*, *Francisella*, *Yersinia*, *Brucella*, and *Legionella*. Members of the genus *Haemophilus* are normal inhabitants of the respiratory tract. One member of this group, *Haemophilus influenzae*, sometimes causes meningitis in infants and young children. Occasionally, it produces respiratory infections in patients with chronic lung disease. Another closely related organism was previously classified as *Haemophilus* but has been renamed *Gardnerella*. In conjunction with other bacteria, this organism causes a common vaginal infection called nonspecific vaginitis (discussed in Chapter 18). One member of the genus *Yersinia* is responsible for bubonic plague. A member of the genus *Francisella* produces a somewhat similar illness called tularemia. Members of the genus *Brucella* cause disease in cattle, goats, and hogs that can be transmitted to people from contact with meat or other tissues from infected animals or from drinking unpasteurized milk from infected cows or goats. In humans, the disease is a febrile illness without any specific features and responds to appropriate antibiotics. *Legionella* causes a serious respiratory illness called Legionnaires disease.

Other Gram-negative organisms of medical importance include a number of closely related organisms that live in the gastrointestinal tract of people and animals. Other members of this group are free-living organisms, widely distributed in nature. Important pathogenic members of the group include the genera *Salmonella*, *Shigella*, *Campylobacter*, and the cholera bacillus (*Vibrio cholerae*).

These organisms cause various types of febrile illness and gastroenteritis. The organisms are excreted from the gastrointestinal tract in the feces of infected patients and are then transmitted by contaminated food or water.

An organism closely related to *Campylobacter* but now designated *Helicobacter* is of medical importance because it appears to cause chronic inflammation of the stomach lining (chronic gastritis) and stomach ulcers. This organism is considered in connection with the gastrointestinal tract (discussed in Chapter 21).

Other members of this large group are of only limited pathogenicity but sometimes produce disease when they are outside of their normal habitat in the gastrointestinal tract. These organisms may cause wound infections, urinary tract infections, and pulmonary infections in susceptible individuals. The best-known enteric bacterium is the colon bacillus (*Escherichia coli*), which is the predominant organism found within the intestinal tract of humans and animals. Some strains of the colon bacillus can produce various toxins that can cause intestinal symptoms ranging from a cholera-like diarrhea to a dysentery-like acute inflammation of the intestinal tract. One well-known pathogenic strain is designated *E. coli 0157:H7*, the numbers referring to the antigens contained in the bacterial cell wall and its flagella. This organism's toxin causes an acute inflammation of the colon characterized by bloody diarrhea and abdominal pain. Sometimes there is also an associated destruction of the patient's red blood cells, with marked anemia and impaired renal function with renal failure, called the hemolytic uremic syndrome. This pathogenic organism is present in the intestinal tract of infected cattle, and people usually become infected by consuming contaminated, incompletely cooked beef or by drinking raw milk. Recent outbreaks were caused by consumption of improperly cooked hamburgers prepared from beef contaminated with the organism and by consumption of leafy vegetables contaminated in the field. In 2011 almost 4000 Europeans were infected by a closely related E. coli organism, resulting in more than 50 deaths. The organism *E. coli 0104:H4* contaminated fenugreek seed–derived beansprouts.

Spirochete Organisms

The spirochete bacteria can cause a wide variety of illnesses. The best-known member of this group is *Treponema pallidum*, which causes syphilis—one of the sexually transmitted infections (STI). These diseases are considered in Chapter 18. Another organism in this group is *Borrelia burgdorferi*, which causes **Lyme disease**. Named after a town in Connecticut where the disease was first recognized, it is now widespread in North America, Europe, and Australia. Transmission to humans is by the bite of an infected tick (*Ixodes dammini* and other *Ixodes* species). Most infections occur in the summer, when exposure to ticks is frequent. Untreated Lyme disease typically progresses through three stages. In the first stage, a roughly circular, localized skin rash appears at the site of the tick bite and is frequently associated with flulike symptoms of fever, chills, and headaches, along with muscular and joint aches and pain. The rash and other manifestations eventually subside, but weeks or months later many patients develop various neurologic, cardiac, and joint manifestations, which characterize the second stage of the disease. The third stage, which eventually develops in some untreated patients, is characterized by chronic arthritis and various neurologic problems. Diagnosis is usually made by means of various serologic tests, and the disease is commonly treated with a tetracycline antibiotic.

Lyme disease A tick-borne systemic infection caused by a spirochete, *Borrelia burgdorferi*, characterized by neurologic, joint, and cardiac manifestations.

Acid-Fast Bacteria

Acid-fast bacteria have a waxy capsule that is stained with difficulty by means of certain red dyes (carbol fuchsin). After the organism has been stained, the stain-impregnated capsule resists decolorization with various acid solvents. This property, attributable to the capsule, is the reason for the term *acid-fast*, used to refer to this type of organism. Acid-fast bacteria cause a special type of chronic inflammatory reaction, called a chronic granulomatous inflammation, rather than the polymorphonuclear inflammatory reaction usually seen with bacterial infections.

The best-known acid-fast bacterium is the tubercle bacillus (*Mycobacterium tuberculosis*) responsible for tuberculosis. Mycobacteria other than the tubercle bacillus may at times cause a tuberculosis-like disease affecting lungs, lymph nodes, or skin, and some may cause severe systemic infections in immunocompromised individuals. (Disseminated infection caused by *Mycobacterium* avium complex in people with the acquired immune deficiency syndrome is described in Chapter 18.) Another acid-fast bacterium (*Mycobacterium leprae*) causes leprosy.

Obligate Intracellular Bacteria

Obligate intracellular bacteria, such as *Chlamydia* spp., *Rickettsia* spp., and *Ehrlichia* spp., can only replicate exclusively inside host cells. The chlamydiae are very small, Gram-negative, nonmotile bacteria once thought to be large viruses. They are deficient in certain enzymes and can live only as parasites inside of the cells of the individual that they infect. They are taken into the cells of the host by phagocytosis, where they divide to form large intracytoplasmic clusters of organisms called **inclusion bodies**. These resemble inclusion bodies formed in some viral diseases. Their growth can be inhibited by various antibiotics that inhibit protein synthesis.

Inclusion bodies Spherical structures in the nucleus or cytoplasm of virus-infected cells or intracytoplasmic clusters of organisms such as Chlamydiae within a cell.

Chlamydiae cause several different types of diseases. The most common chlamydial disease affects the genital tract and is transmitted by sexual contact. In the male, it causes an inflammation of the urethra called nongonococcal urethritis. In the female, it causes an inflammation of the uterine cervix that may spread to the fallopian tubes and ovaries as well. If a pregnant person has a chlamydial infection of the cervix, infected secretions may get into her infant's eyes during childbirth and cause an inflammation called inclusion conjunctivitis. The name is based on the fact that characteristic inclusions can be demonstrated in the infected cells of the infant's conjunctiva. Other chlamydiae cause pulmonary infections. One species causes a disease of birds called psitticosis that is transmissible to humans and is manifested clinically as a type of pneumonia. Another species of chlamydiae causes an uncommon sexually transmissible infection called lymphogranuloma venereum. This disease is characterized by marked enlargement and inflammation of the lymph nodes in the groin and around the rectum (see Chapter 18).

Rickettsiae are very small intracellular bacteria that can only multiply within the cells of an infected person. Many small animals and dogs are infected. The rickettsiae are transmitted to humans by insect bites (often from ticks), and they multiply in the endothelial cells of small blood vessels, which become swollen and necrotic, leading to thrombosis, rupture, and necrosis. Clinically, a rickettsial infection usually causes a febrile illness, often associated with a skin rash. Typhus and Rocky Mountain spotted fever are the most common rickettsial diseases. These organisms are sensitive to some antibiotics. Similar organisms transmitted by ticks infect white blood cells rather than endothelial cells and are called Ehrlichiae (named after an early immunologist, Paul Ehrlich). There are several species. Some infect neutrophils and others infect monocytes. The infected white cells contain small, compact clusters of organisms called morulae (singular, morula), which can be identified in blood smears. Ehrlichiosis is a febrile illness similar to infections caused by rickettsiae and may be associated with a skin rash. Ehrlichiosis can be treated successfully with antibiotic therapy.

Wall-less Bacteria

Mycoplasmas are very small bacteria that are very fragile because they lack a cell wall. One member of this group, *Mycoplasma pneumoniae,* causes a type of pneumonia called primary atypical pneumonia (or sometimes "walking pneumonia"). Mycoplasmas respond to several antibiotics such as tetracycline.

Antibiotic Treatment of Bacterial Infections

The discovery of antibiotic compounds and their widespread use to treat various types of infections has been one of the great advances in medicine. Antibiotics are substances that destroy bacteria or inhibit their growth. They are useful clinically because of their ability to injure bacterial cells without producing significant injury to the patient.

The bacterial cell is a complex structure containing genetic material, a protein-synthesizing mechanism, numerous enzyme systems concerned with intracellular metabolic functions, a semipermeable cell membrane, and a rigid cell wall. The bacterial genetic material is arranged as a circular DNA molecule that is attached to the cell membrane. Some bacteria also contain smaller circular DNA molecules, called plasmids, that contain genes coding for various properties useful to bacteria but often harmful to the people infected by the bacteria. Such properties include resistance to antibiotics, toxin production, and formation of soluble factors that inhibit growth of normal bacterial flora, so the plasmid-bearing bacterium has a growth advantage over the bacterial flora with which it must compete. Antimicrobial substances act by interfering with the structure or function of the bacterial cell in one or more ways (**Figure 7-4**).

Inhibition of Cell-Wall Synthesis

The bacterial cell has a high internal osmotic pressure, and the rigid outer cell wall maintains the shape of the bacterium. In some respects, the function of the cell wall can be compared with a corset or belly band supporting the enclosed cell. Penicillin and several other antibiotics act by inhibiting the synthesis of the bacterial cell wall so that the cell body is exposed. Because of the high osmotic pressure inside the bacterium, the relatively unsupported cell swells and eventually ruptures.

Inhibition of Cell-Membrane Function

The cell membrane is a semipermeable membrane surrounding the bacterial protoplasm. It controls the internal composition of the cell by regulating the diffusion of materials into and out of the cell. Some antibiotics act by inhibiting various functions of the cell membrane. Loss of the selective permeability of the cell membrane leads to cell injury and death.

Inhibition of Metabolic Functions

Some antibiotics interfere with nucleic acid or protein synthesis by bacteria so that the organisms are unable to carry out essential metabolic functions.

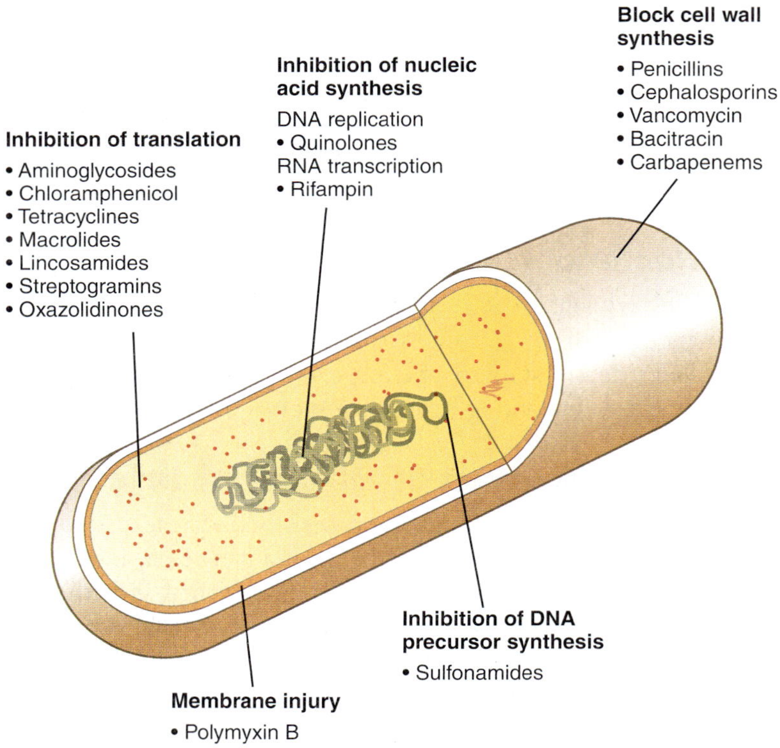

Figure 7-4 The targets for antibacterial agents. There are five major targets for antibacterial agents: the cell wall, cell membrane, ribosomes (protein synthesis), nucleic acid synthesis (RNA and DNA synthesis), and metabolic reactions vital to the bacteria.

Inhibition of Nucleic Acid and Protein Synthesis

A large number of antibiotic agents inhibit bacterial protein synthesis by binding to either the 30s or 50s subunits of the bacterial ribosome and interfering with their activity. One of the most commonly used classes of antibiotics (the fluoroquinolones) blocks DNA synthesis in both Gram-positive and Gram-negative organisms.

Antibiotic Sensitivity Tests

In selecting antibiotics to treat a bacterial infection, the practitioner is aided by laboratory tests called antibiotic sensitivity tests. These tests measure, under standardized conditions, the ability of the antibiotic to inhibit the growth of the organism isolated from the patient. One method, called a tube dilution sensitivity test, consists of preparing various dilutions of antibiotics in test tubes and inoculating the tubes with the organism to be tested. The tubes are then incubated for a period of time to permit growth of the organism. Finally, determination of the highest dilution of antibiotic that inhibits the growth of the organism indicates the sensitivity of the organism to the drug.

Another method of sensitivity testing consists of inoculating the organism on a bacteriologic plate containing a culture medium. Several filter paper disks are then placed on the plate, each containing a standardized concentration of a different antibiotic. Next, the plate is incubated to allow the organism to grow. During incubation, the antibiotics in the disks diffuse into the surrounding culture. If the antibiotic is capable of inhibiting the organism, the organism is unable to grow in the area around the disk, and a circular clear zone free of bacterial growth appears (**Figure 7-5**). The organism is said to be sensitive to the antibiotic. On the other hand, if the growth of the organism is not influenced by

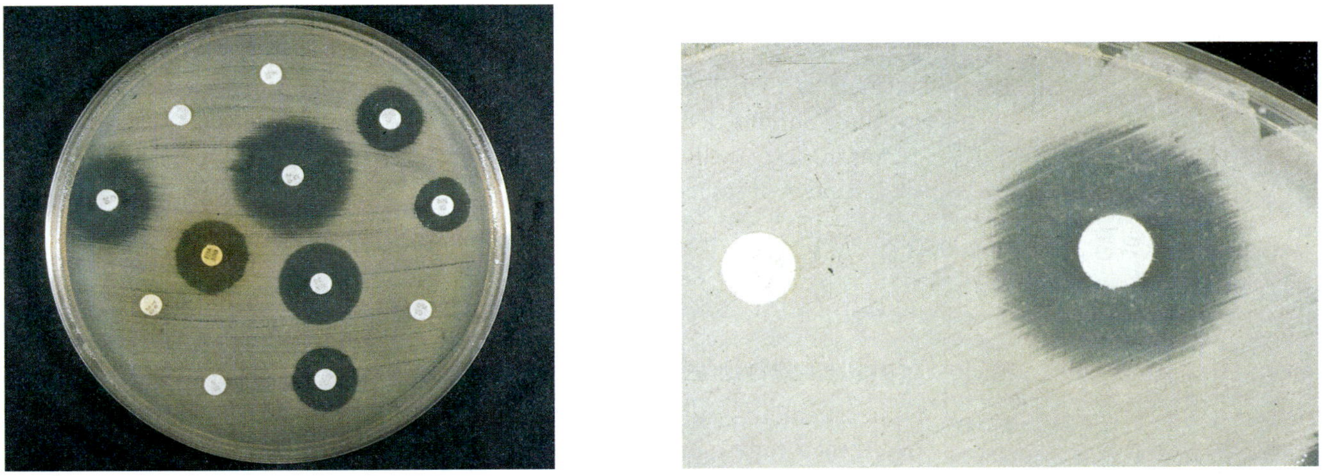

(A)

(B)

Figure 7-5 **(A)** Sensitivity test, illustrating antibiotic-impregnated filter paper disks on the surface of a culture plate. The clear zone around the disk indicates that the antibiotic in the disk has inhibited bacterial growth. **(B)** Closer view of two disks on a plate. The antibiotic contained in the disk (*left*) fails to inhibit growth of the organism, which is *resistant* to the antibiotic. The clear zone around the antibiotic (*right*) indicates that the antibiotic in the disk inhibits the growth of the organism, which is *sensitive* to the antibiotic.

Courtesy of Leonard V. Crowley, MD, Century College.

the antibiotic, growth will not be inhibited around the disk, and the organism is said to be resistant to the antibiotic. The diameter of the zones of inhibition around the disks further indicates the sensitivity of the organism. The tube dilution and disk diffusion sensitivity test methods yield comparable results. The two methods are standardized so that the diameter of the zone of inhibition obtained by the disk diffusion method correlates with the antibiotic concentration required to inhibit the organism, as measured by the tube dilution method.

A bacteriology laboratory report that the organism is sensitive to a given antibiotic means that the organism probably can be inhibited by giving the patient the usual therapeutic dose of that drug. A report that the organism is resistant to an antibiotic indicates that a therapeutic dose of antibiotic is unlikely to inhibit the growth of the organism.

It should be emphasized, however, that the sensitivity of an organism to an antibiotic is only one factor influencing a patient's response to an infection. Other factors include the patient's own resistance and the antibiotic's ability to diffuse in sufficient quantities into the site of the infection.

Traditional methods, such as tube dilution and disk diffusion tests assess antimicrobial sensitivity/resistance phenotypically. In contrast, molecular-based technique took a different approach. Methods such as Polymerase Chain Reaction (PCR), DNA microarray, and Whole Genome Sequence (WGS) enable scientists to detect genetic determinants responsible for antimicrobial across various bacterial species. These approaches are usually faster with high throughput and can be used as alternatives to or in combinations with conventional antimicrobial susceptibility tests.

Adverse Effects of Antibiotics

Toxicity

Antibiotics are useful because they are much more toxic to bacteria than they are to the patient. Antibiotics vary in their effects on people, but all are toxic to some degree. Some injure the kidneys; others injure nerve tissue or the blood-forming tissues. Penicillin and other antibiotics that act by interfering with bacterial cell-wall synthesis are relatively nontoxic, probably because the body cells have no structure comparable to the bacterial cell wall. Some antibiotics that interfere with bacterial metabolic functions can sometimes produce similar derangements in the patient's own metabolic functions. For example, tetracycline is a relatively nontoxic antibiotic, excreted chiefly by the kidneys. If renal function is impaired, very high blood levels of antibiotic may develop after administration of the usual therapeutic doses of the drug; this may cause severe and often fatal impairment of the patient's own cellular metabolic functions.

Hypersensitivity

Some antibiotics induce a marked hypersensitivity that can lead to a fatal reaction if the drug is later administered to a sensitized patient. Penicillin is capable of inducing extremely severe anaphylactic reactions, although the antibiotic itself has a very low toxicity.

Alteration of Normal Bacterial Flora

The normal bacterial flora in the oral cavity, the colon, and other locations may be altered by antibiotics. If the normal bacteria are destroyed, there may be overgrowth of resistant bacteria and fungi previously controlled by the normal flora. These resistant organisms may cause infections in susceptible patients.

Development of Resistant Strains of Bacteria

Some bacteria that are initially sensitive to antibiotics eventually become resistant. There are two ways in which an organism becomes resistant. It may undergo a spontaneous mutation that conveys resistance, or it may acquire a plasmid that contains resistance genes from another bacterium.

Spontaneous mutations do not occur frequently in cell division, but many bacteria divide so rapidly that spontaneous mutations can present a problem if the rapidly dividing bacteria are not quickly eliminated by the antibiotic. After a mutation that conveys antibiotic resistance occurs, the mutant organism has an advantage over its antibiotic-sensitive counterpart because it can flourish in the presence of the antibiotic while the antibiotic-sensitive organisms are eliminated.

Plasmid-acquired resistance can be a major problem because the transferred plasmid may convey resistance to multiple antibiotics, and plasmid transfers can take place between bacteria of different types. In this process, a bacterium (the donor) with antibiotic-resistant genes carried on one of its plasmids extends a thin cytoplasmic tube to contact another bacterium (the recipient), "reels in" the bacterium that it has contacted, and passes a copy of its plasmid to the recipient bacterium. Now both bacteria possess antibiotic-resistance plasmids, which they in turn can pass to other bacteria.

There are a number of mechanisms by which resistant bacteria can circumvent an antibiotic's effect. Such mechanisms include (1) developing enzymes to destroy the antibiotic, (2) either changing their cell-wall structure so that the antibiotic is unable to get into the cell or developing mechanisms to expel the antibiotic as soon as it enters the cell and before it can disturb bacterial functions, or (3) changing their intracellular "metabolic machinery" so that the antibiotic is no longer able to disturb bacterial functions.

A few examples serve to illustrate the ingenious adaptations of bacteria that thwart our efforts to eliminate them. A bacterium that is penicillin sensitive may develop an enzyme, penicillinase, that inactivates the antibiotic and allows the bacterium to survive in the presence of the drug. An antibiotic that acts against an enzyme required for a bacterial function, such as constructing a cell wall, may be rendered ineffective if the bacterium slightly alters the structure of its enzyme so that the antibiotic can no longer bind to the enzyme and inactivate it. An antibiotic that attaches to bacterial ribosomes, preventing protein synthesis, may be rendered ineffective if the bacterium slightly changes the structure of the ribosome so that the antibiotic can no longer act against it.

Widespread use of an antibiotic predisposes to the development of resistant strains. This may complicate the treatment of patients who become infected with antibiotic-resistant organisms. Staphylococci, in particular, have raised this problem because many strains isolated from hospital patients have been found to be highly resistant to a large number of antibiotics. Treatment of gonorrhea also has been complicated by the development of a high degree of penicillin resistance in many strains of gonococci; consequently, prolonged courses of therapy and much larger doses of antibiotics are required to eradicate the infections. Even the pneumococcus is no longer uniformly sensitive to penicillin, as it was in the past. Some strains are resistant to penicillin and other drugs normally used against them. Resistant strains of tubercle bacilli also have developed, hindering treatment of tuberculosis with antituberculosis drugs. On the other hand, some bacteria still remain quite sensitive to antibiotics. For example, group A beta streptococci remain sensitive to penicillin, despite widespread use of penicillin to treat streptococcal infections. *Treponema pallidum*, the organism responsible for syphilis, also has remained quite sensitive to penicillin, even though the drug has been used to treat syphilis for many years.

There is current concern over the use of antibiotic additives in livestock production. The use of antibiotics in raising meat animals increases weight at slaughter and prevents disease in herds. However, such antibiotics lead to the generation of bacteria with antibiotic resistance that may either directly infect humans or serve as a source of resistance-bearing plasmids, which may be transferred to human pathogens.

Viruses

Viruses are the smallest infectious agents. A typical virus consists of a molecule of nucleic acid (either DNA or RNA), its genome, enclosed within a protein shell called a **capsid**. The capsid is made of subunits called **capsomeres**, which are arranged in a precise geometric fashion around the genome. Many viruses are also covered by an outer lipid envelope acquired from the cytoplasm of the host cell when the virus buds from the cell that it has infected. Projections from the surface of the virus allow the virus to attach to the cell that it will infect. Viruses vary greatly in size. The smallest are only slightly larger than protein molecules, whereas the largest viruses approach the size of a bacterium.

Capsid The protein covering the central nucleic acid core of a virus.

Capsomere One of the subunits that make up the protein shell (capsid) of a virus.

The nucleic acid of the virus genome may be arranged in either a single or a double strand, and the complexity of the viral genome varies. Some viruses have as many as 400 genes within their nucleic acid structure, whereas others have as few as 8. Viruses have few metabolic enzymes and therefore must rely on the cells of the infected person to carry out their activities. When a virus invades the cell, the viral genome directs the metabolic processes of the cell to synthesize more virus particles. In many respects, the virus may be likened to a criminal who takes over a business, forcing it to function for the criminal's benefit rather than for the benefit of the owner. Viral infection of a cell may be

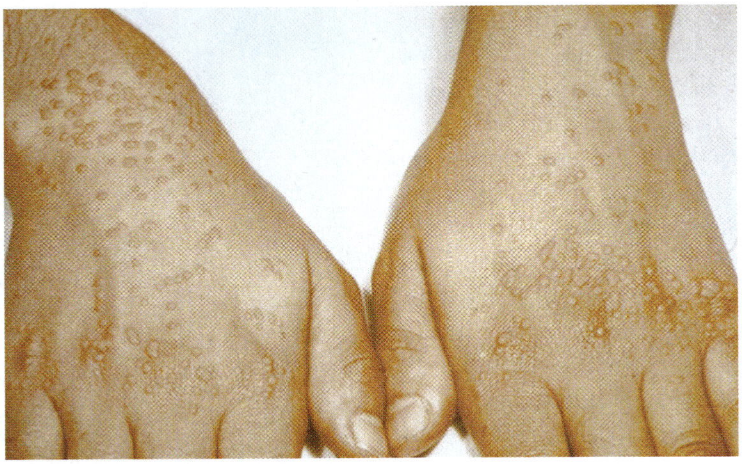

(A)

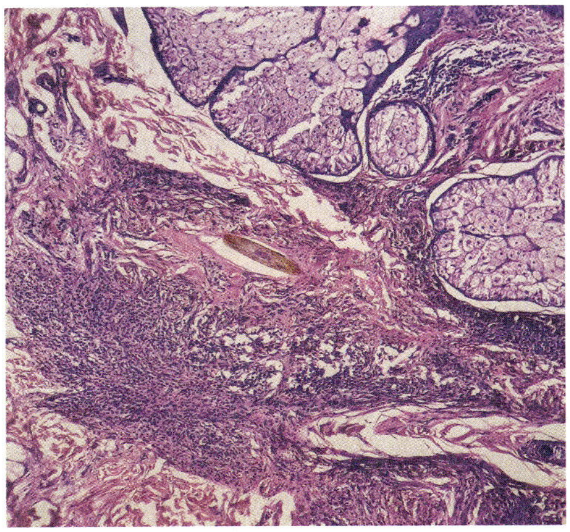

(B)

Figure 7-6 **(A)** Multiple dermal warts on the skin of hands. **(B)** Photomicrograph of a dermal wart demonstrates hyperplasia of the epidermis and dilated capillaries. Multiple clefts that give warts their characteristic appearance are also shown.

(A) Courtesy of Leonard V. Crowley, MD, Century College; (B) © Babul Hosen/Shutterstock

Papilloma Otherwise known as a wart, a neoplasm produced after human papilloma virus infection.

latent and produce no symptoms at the time of infection, only to reactivate and cause disease in the future. Viruses may cause either acute cell necrosis or a slow progressive injury. In addition, a viral infection may cause cell hyperplasia and may ultimately lead to a malignant neoplastic disease. For example, warts (**papillomas**) are a benign neoplasm commonly found on the hands and feet that are caused by strains of the human papillomavirus (**Figure 7-6**). Other strains of the papillomavirus are associated with venereal warts and cervical and penile cancer.

Classification of Viruses

An older classification of viruses was based on the major clinical features of the viral infection, and viruses were classified on the basis of the portion of the body or organ system in which the viral infection produced the most prominent clinical manifestations. A more modern classification categorizes viruses on the basis of their nucleic acid structure, size, structural configuration, and biologic characteristics. In this classification, several large groups of viruses are recognized, and a large number of viruses are identified in each group. **Table 7-3** presents a simplified classification of viruses and the diseases they cause.

Hemorrhagic Fevers

Hemorrhagic fevers include Ebola and Marburg fevers, the former now a major public health problem in West Africa. Ebola is caused by infection with one of the four infectious strains of Ebola virus. In earlier outbreaks, approximately 80 percent of infected people died. Uninfected people can be exposed to the virus by direct contact with the blood or secretions of symptomatic infected people or through contact with contaminated objects. The Ebola virus damages endothelial cells, causing massive internal bleeding and hemorrhage. The infected individual often suffers from severe fluid loss or bleeds to death before an immune response can be mounted. Although still uncertain, bats appear to be the animal host of the virus, particularly the Marburg virus. Infected primates

Table 7-3 Common Viruses Infecting Humans

	Virus	Disease
DNA viruses	Adenoviruses	Respiratory infections
	Hepatitis B virus	Hepatitis B
	Herpes viruses	
	Herpes simplex type 1	Cold sores
	Herpes simplex type 2	Genital herpes
	Epstein-Barr virus	Infectious mononucleosis
	Varicella-zoster virus	Chickenpox, herpes zoster (shingles)
	Cytomegalovirus	Mononucleosis-like illness, hepatitis
	Herpesvirus 8	Kaposi's sarcoma
	Papilloma virus	Warts, condylomas (benign tumors)
RNA viruses	Arboviruses	Encephalitis
	Noroviruses	Gastroenteritis
	Coronavirus	Respiratory infections
		Severe acute respiratory syndrome (SARS)
	Hantavirus (bunyavirus)	Acute respiratory illness
	Hepatitis viruses	
	Hepatitis A virus (picornavirus)	Hepatitis
	Hepatitis C virus (flavivirus)	Hepatitis
	Hepatitis D virus (coated with HbsAg)	Hepatitis
	Hepatitis E virus (calicivirus)	Hepatitis
	Myxoviruses	
	Influenza viruses	Influenza
	Parainfluenza viruses	Respiratory infections, croup
	Respiratory syncytial viruses	Respiratory infections
	Measles virus	Measles
	Mumps virus	Mumps
	Picornaviruses	
	Coxsackie viruses	Pharyngitis, myocarditis, pericarditis
	Echoviruses	Respiratory infections, gastroenteritis
	Hepatitis A virus	Hepatitis A
	Polioviruses	Poliomyelitis
	Rhinoviruses	Respiratory infections
	Rabies virus (rhabdovirus)	Rabies
	Retroviruses	
	HIV	AIDS
	HTLV 1	Adult T-cell leukemia
	Rubella virus (togavirus)	German measles

used as a food source may also contribute to epidemics. Poor and overcrowded neighborhoods in urban centers have led to outbreaks of epidemic proportion and the collapse of public health and medical facilities in the worst affected countries. Marburg fever was first identified in green monkeys imported into Germany from Africa. Recent outbreaks have been traced to exposure to fruit bats. Symptoms are similar to those for Ebola.

Coronavirus

Coronaviruses (CoVs) are single-stranded RNA viruses. The host cells for CoVs varied from humans to other animals and avian species. Most human CoVs, such as HCoV-229E, HCoV-OC43, HCoV-NL63, and HCoV-HKU1, were known to cause mild respiratory tract infection with signs and symptoms like the "common cold." Some other strains, however, including severe acute respiratory syndrome coronavirus (SARS-CoV), Middle East respiratory syndrome coronavirus (MERS-CoV), and SARS-CoV-2 (etiology for COVID-19), can cause severe life-threatening respiratory infection and lung damages.

COVID-19 started to plague the world in 2019. Signs and symptoms of COVID-19 varied from asymptomatic, pneumonia-like, acute respiratory distress symptoms, to death. According to WHO (World Health Organization), by the end of 2023, more than 700 million people had been infected, and more than 6 million people had died from the infection.

Different approaches have been used to treat and prevent COVID-19. In 2021, the FDA approved an antiviral drug, Paxlovid, developed by Pfizer, to treat patients with mild to moderate signs and symptoms. Messenger RNA (mRNA)-based vaccines against SARS-CoV-2 were also quickly developed and approved by the FDA for emergency use during the COVID-19 pandemic.

Avian Flu Virus H5N1

Influenza A virus is an enveloped RNA virus with many subtypes delineated by their H and N antigens. Many of the subtypes have caused several documented pandemics in human history. This includes the 1918 pandemic (also known as Spanish flu, caused by H1N1 subtype); the 1957 pandemic (also known as Asian flu, caused by H2N2 subtype); the 1968 pandemic (also known as Hong Kong flu, caused by H3N2 subtype); and the 2009 pandemic (also known as swine flu, caused by H1N1 subtype).

Since 2021, a highly pathogenic subtype, H5N1, a cause of avian flu, started to draw public attention. H5N1 was a significant problem for poultry farmers historically; it was not recognized as a human pathogen until 1997, when the first cases of H5N1 infection in humans were confirmed in Hong Kong. The outbreak primarily occurred in the poultry market, and it resulted in 18 human infections, with six deaths. The outbreak was ultimately contained by culling.

Starting from 2020, H5N1 has begun spreading worldwide and infecting new mammal species, posing great threats to wildlife, agriculture production, and human health. In March 2024, an H5N1 outbreak in the United States dairy cattle was reported in Texas and was quickly spread to other states, probably caused by interstate transport of infected animals. From April to May 2024, more than thirty percent of pasteurized milk samples from 12 states were tested positive for H5N1. The same virus was also found in other species, including cats, racoons, and humans. As of March 16th, 2025, CDC has reported 70 confirmed human cases and one death since the outbreak. The situation is highly concerning. As the influenza virus is notorious for its swift mutation through antigenic drift or antigenic shift, if the virus continues to circulate, reassortment between a human seasonal flu virus and H5N1 might occur, resulting in a virus that is both pathogenic and transmissible between humans. This might lead to future pandemics.

Important practices should be adopted to reduce the overall risk of developing a new pandemic. Vaccinating agriculturally important animal species against H5N1 could be an effective strategy to reduce viral circulation and the risk of zoonotic transmission. Dairy farm workers, healthcare professionals, and other at-risk individuals should use personal protective equipment and receive the seasonal flu vaccine. These precautions will help prevent co-infection and decrease the likelihood of viral genome reassortment.

Mpox Virus

The Mpox virus belongs to the genus *Orthopoxvirus*, the family *Poxviridae*. Other viruses in this group include variola (smallpox) and cowpox. MPXV has a broad host range, including various animals and humans, a fact that might contribute to its prolonged zoonotic circulation in the world. MPXV was first isolated from infected cynomolgus monkeys in 1959. Human infection by MPXV was first recognized in 1970.

MPXV infection can be transmitted through oropharyngeal, nasopharyngeal, intradermal routes, and sexual contact. The incubation period lasts from 1 to 3 weeks. MPXV infection has two phases. In the invasion period, patients experienced sore throat, shortness of breath, fever and enlarged lymphadenopathy (a hallmark for Mpox infection). In the eruption period, skin lesions progressed from macular phase to popular, vesicular, and pustular phase. Mpox infection is usually self-limiting; severe complications such as encephalopathy and retropharyngeal abscess can occur.

Mpox has remained endemic in Central and Western Africa since 1970. However, starting from 2022, the virus has re-emerged and spread to non-endemic regions. According to WHO, between January 2022 to August 2025, the virus spread to over 120 countries, causing more than 100,000 confirmed infections with 220 deaths among the confirmed cases. In the United States, CDC reported 33,791 confirmed infections and 139 death cases since January 2024. The fast pace of the outbreak brought a new public concern about the rise of another viral pandemic and public health threat.

The outbreak may be due to several factors. The discontinuation of smallpox vaccination may play a role. It has been reported that the smallpox vaccination provides approximately 85% protection against Mpox infection. Other factors may include, but are not limited to, growing consumption of animals' meat (which may serve as a potential MPXV reservoir), increased population density, and frequent traveling.

To contain the current Mpox outbreak, essential measures, such as active surveillance, thorough contact tracing, increasing public awareness and understanding of the illness, along with early detection and prompt interruption of the transmission chain are necessary.

Measles Virus

The measles virus is a member of the genus *Morbillivirus*. It is highly contagious with R0 from 12 to 18. It is transmitted through droplet and aerosol. Measles viruses can lead to serious infections and complications, including pneumonia, encephalitis, and, in rare cases, subacute sclerosing panencephalitis (SSPE)—a condition characterized by gradual, progressive brain degeneration that can be fatal.

Before the MMR (measles, mumps, rubella) vaccine became available in 1964, there were between 3 to 4 million people infected with measles annually in the United States. In 2000, the United States declared elimination of measles, defined as absence of continuous disease transmission for more than 12 months. In 2017, the United Kingdom also declared measles elimination; however, such status was revoked in 2018 due to the large number of confirmed cases.

In 2024, European regions reported 127,350 measles cases, the highest number in more than 25 years. Meanwhile, in the United States, CDC reported a total of 1046 confirmed and 3 death cases in 2025 (as of May 22nd). All cases were identified from within close-knit communities with low measles vaccination coverage.

The resurgence of measles has become a significant public health concern. Several factors may contribute to these outbreaks, including a decline in vaccination rates during or after the COVID-19 pandemic, general vaccine hesitancy, unsupported lingering concerns about a possible link between the MMR vaccine and autism, and a diminished awareness of the seriousness of the disease.

To prevent the resurgence and spread of measles, it is essential to raise public awareness about the dangers of measles infection and to implement and promote vaccination programs worldwide.

Mode of Action

A distinction is sometimes made between a viral infection and a viral disease. A condition in which a virus infects a cell without causing any evidence of cell injury is considered a latent viral infection. Many viruses are capable of coexisting with normal cells in lymphoid tissue and the gastrointestinal tract, and probably in other sites, without causing cellular injury. Such viruses are able to live for long periods within the cells of the infected host while they continually discharge virus particles. Other viruses are more virulent and regularly produce cell injury, manifested by necrosis and degeneration of the infected cell. This is called a cytopathogenic effect. Some viruses induce cell hyperplasia and proliferation rather than cell necrosis (Figure 7-6B). Many viruses induce various combinations of cell damage and cell hyperplasia.

Under certain circumstances, a latent asymptomatic viral infection may become activated, leading to actual disease. The herpes virus, which infects both the oral cavity and the genital tract, may persist in the tissues of the host for many years. The virus periodically becomes activated and causes crops of painful vesicles that may recur during an intercurrent febrile illness when the patient's immunologic defenses have been disrupted by a neoplasm or by various other diseases, or sometimes for no apparent reason (**Figure 7-7**).

Another member of the herpes group of viruses is the varicella-zoster virus, named from its two different manifestations. The initial contact with the virus causes chickenpox (varicella), which is an extremely contagious disease characterized by an itchy skin rash that usually soon subsides, almost always without any serious complications. A person who has had chickenpox develops an immunity and cannot contract chickenpox again. However, the virus is not eradicated by the immune system and remains dormant within sensory nerve ganglia. Sometimes the virus becomes active again within a sensory ganglion many years later and then travels in the nerve associated with the ganglion to the skin, where it causes a characteristic bandlike vesicular skin rash in the segment of skin supplied by the sensory nerve. The recurrent infection is **herpes zoster**, which is often called **shingles**, from a Latin word, cingulum, which means a belt or belly band. The term refers to the belt-like band of skin vesicles along the course of a spinal nerve that partially girdles the trunk, as illustrated in **Figure 7-8**.

Herpes zoster A virus that causes chicken pox.
Shingles Another name for herpes zoster flare in adults who were infected with chicken pox as children.

Herpes zoster is a late complication of the varicella-zoster virus (VZV) infection and is often complicated by chronic pain in the distribution of the previously affected nerve, which is called post-herpes-zoster neuralgia. Chickenpox had been a very common disease before the introduction of an attenuated virus

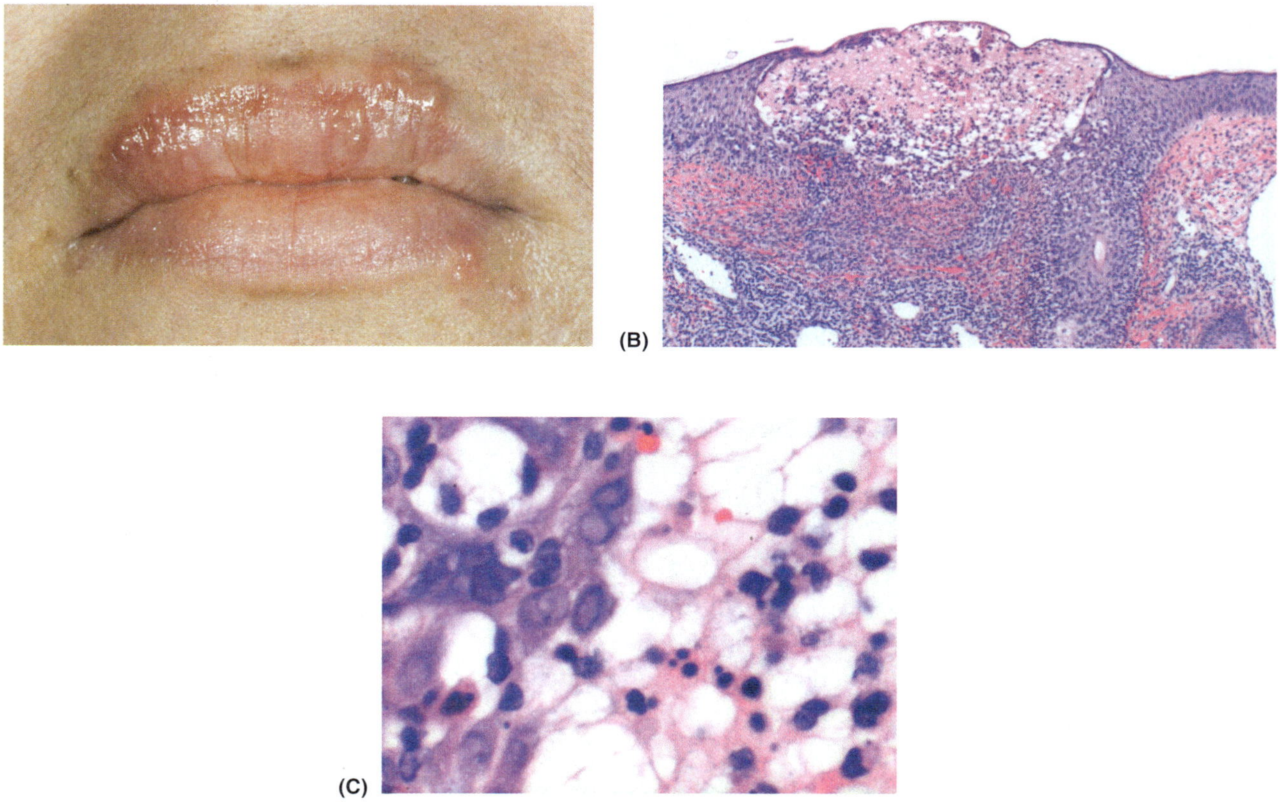

(A) (B) (C)

Figure 7-7 Herpes virus infection. **(A)** Recurrent oral herpes is most often caused by herpes virus type 1. **(B)** Section of small herpes blister showed acantholysis with solidary keratinocytes within the blister cavity. **(C)** Viral inclusions presented as small pink deposits with a clear halo seen within the nucleus.

(A) Courtesy of Leonard V. Crowley, MD, Century College; **(B-C)** Reproduced with permission from ©DermNet dermnetnz.org 2024.

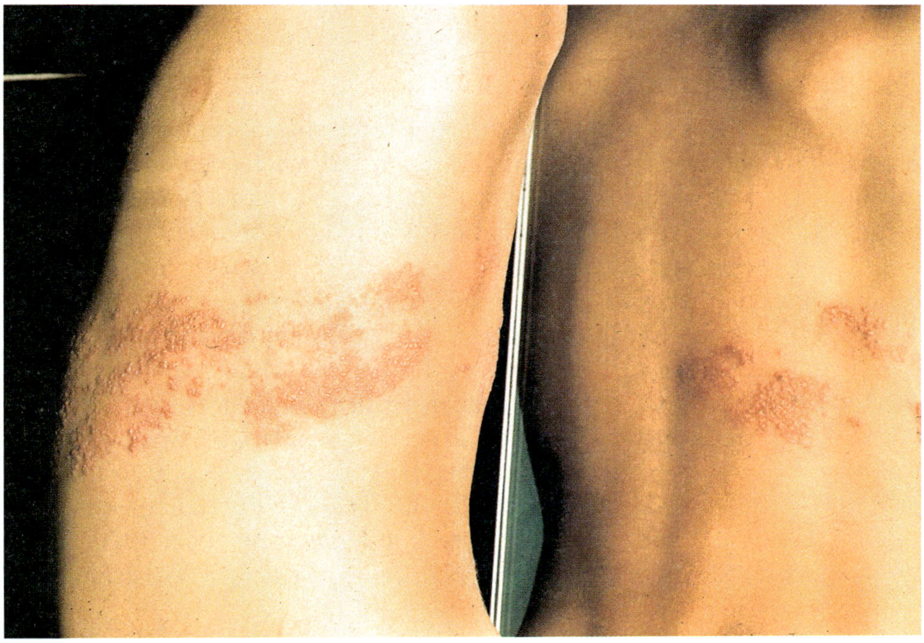

Figure 7-8 One type of herpes virus infection (called shingles or herpes zoster) characterized by clusters of vesicles that occur in a segment of skin (dermatome) supplied by a sensory nerve. The subject was photographed beside a mirror to illustrate the bandlike distribution of the rash in the segment of skin supplied by a spinal nerve.

Courtesy of Leonard V. Crowley, MD, Century College.

varicella-zoster vaccine in 1996. More than 95 percent of people living in the United States had developed chickenpox by the time they were 20 years old, and they were at risk for later reactivation of the virus followed by development of herpes zoster. However, they had also developed a cell-mediated immune response resulting from chickenpox, which tended to suppress reactivation of the latent virus. The cell-mediated immunity of previously infected adults declines as they age, which increases the risk that the latent virus might become activated to cause herpes zoster and its associated complications. A high dose form of the attenuated virus varicella-zoster vaccine helps to prevent herpes zoster and is recommended for older adults to help boost their immunity against VZV. The vaccine is over 60 percent effective, but it is not effective once herpes zoster has developed. To treat patients with herpes zoster, a number of medications similar to acyclovir (used to treat oral and genital herpes) are helpful to shorten the duration and severity of herpes zoster and may also reduce the pain often associated with the skin rash.

Inclusion Bodies in Viral Disease

Tissues infected with virus frequently contain spherical, densely staining structures called inclusion bodies (Figure 7-7C) that are also illustrated in the presentation of congenital and genetic diseases. They are present within the nucleus or the cytoplasm, or in both locations. Inclusion bodies consist of masses of virus or products of virus multiplication. The presence of inclusion bodies may be of considerable diagnostic aid in recognizing viral infection and determining the type of viral disease present.

Bodily Defenses Against Viral Infections

The body responds to a viral infection by forming a protein substance called **interferon** and by activating **humoral immunity** and **cell-mediated defense mechanisms**.

Interferon A broad-spectrum antiviral agent produced by various cells in the body.

Humoral immunity Immunity associated with the formation of antibodies produced by plasma cells.

Cell-mediated defense mechanism The defense against foreign antigens provided by a population of T lymphocytes that can attach and destroy the foreign antigens.

Formation of Interferon

Interferon is a general term for a group of carbohydrate-containing proteins produced by cells in response to viral infection and was named from its ability to "interfere" with viral multiplication. Interferon functions as a nonspecific, broad-spectrum antiviral agent. It induces the production of antiviral protein in uninfected cells and thus stops the spreading of viral infection. This is in contrast with the behavior of a specific antiviral antibody, which reacts only to the virus that induced its formation. Many cells are capable of producing interferon, but monocytes and lymphocytes are the primary sources. Several different interferons are produced, each designated by a Greek letter. Interferons provide a rapid "first-line" defense against a viral infection. By slowing viral replication during the early phase of the infection, time is gained to mobilize humoral and cell-mediated responses directed against the invading virus.

In addition to their antiviral activity, interferons have other actions concerned with regulation of the immune system and cell growth. These functions are considered in Chapter 5.

Humoral and Cell-Mediated Immunity in Viral Infections

The body also forms specific antiviral antibodies capable of inactivating viruses and destroying virus particles in the presence of complement. Antiviral antibodies cannot combine with the virus, however, unless the virus particles are discharged into the extracellular fluid where they are exposed to the action of the antibody. Consequently, antiviral antibodies are relatively inefficient in combating viruses that spread directly from cell to cell because the virus particles remain within the infected cells and are protected from the antibody. For example, people who have recurrent fever blisters caused by the herpes virus possess antibodies to the virus, but the antibody is often unable to eradicate the intracellular virus particles.

In addition to producing specific antiviral antibodies, the immune defenses of the host are directed against the virus-infected cells. This occurs because viruses that invade cells often induce the formation of new antigens on the surface of the infected cells. These antigens are recognized as foreign by the host's immune defenses and induce both humoral and cell-mediated immune reactions directed against the virus-infected cells. Antibodies are formed that affix to the infected cells and destroy them in the presence of complement. Sensitized lymphocytes release lymphokines, which damage the cells, and they also produce interferon, which inhibits the multiplication of viruses. Chemical mediators that induce an acute inflammatory reaction also are liberated (see discussion on inflammation and repair). In many viral infections, much of the tissue injury is caused not by proliferation of the virus within the cells of the host but by the inflammation and tissue destruction caused by the body's attempts to rid itself of the virus-infected cells.

Treatment with Antiviral Agents

Because viruses are simple structures lacking a cell wall, a cell membrane, and the complex "metabolic machinery" of bacteria, they are not susceptible to the disruptive actions of antibiotics. Some chemotherapeutic agents that are active against viruses have been developed, however. Some antiviral agents active against DNA viruses either block synthesis of DNA or induce the formation of an abnormal, nonfunctional DNA, thereby preventing virus multiplication. Another agent active against RNA viruses causes the formation of an abnormal messenger RNA that disrupts viral multiplication. Unfortunately, many compounds that block viral multiplication by such mechanisms also have a similar adverse effect on the host cells and may be as toxic to the host as to the virus. For this reason, antiviral agents have had limited application in the treatment of most viral diseases. They are, however, the mainstay in the treatment of HIV. Because the reverse transcriptase enzyme is found only in virally infected cells, many anti-HIV drugs use the reverse transcriptase as a target (see Chapter 5). The drug acyclovir is effective against some infections caused by the herpes group of viruses. The drug is activated within the virus-infected cells by a viral enzyme to yield the active antiviral compound that selectively inhibits synthesis of viral DNA within the cells in which the virus is replicating.

Fungi

Fungi are eukaryotic heterotrophs (cannot make their own food), including yeasts, rusts, smuts, mildews, molds, and mushrooms. Molds can form large colonies composed of multiple branching filamentous structures called **hyphae** (singular, hypha). The matted mass of hyphae, which is called a **mycelium**, is responsible for the characteristic appearance of the colony (**Figure 7-9**). Some pathogenic fungi exhibit two different growth phases, forming typical mycelial colonies on laboratory culture media but forming small yeastlike structures in the tissues of the infected individual.

Hyphae Filamentous branching structures formed by fungi.

Mycelium Matted mass of hyphae forming a fluffy colony characteristic of fungi.

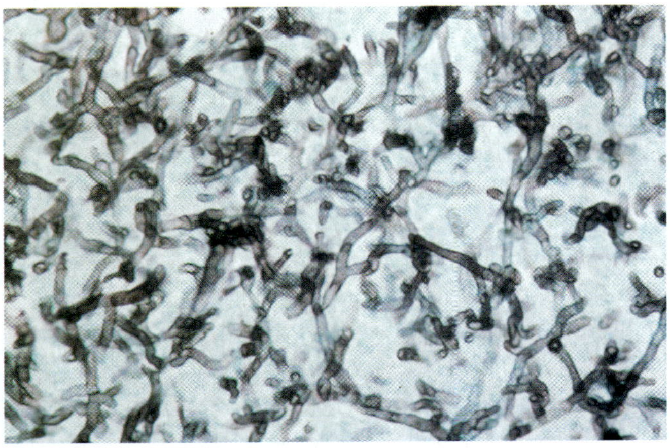

(A)

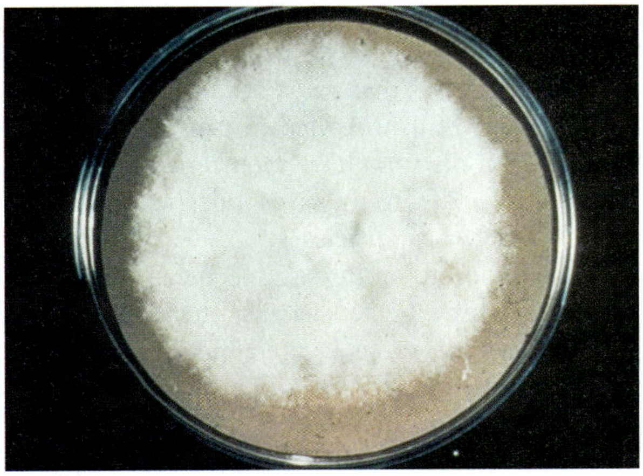

(B)

Figure 7-9 **(A)** A low magnification photomicrograph illustrating a cluster of fungal hyphae. **(B)** Appearance of fungus colony growing on a laboratory culture medium.

Courtesy of Leonard V. Crowley, MD, Century College.

Some fungi live on the skin and only occasionally cause minor discomfort. Others are found in small numbers in the oral cavity, gastrointestinal tract, and vagina, where they live in harmony with the normal bacterial flora. Most fungi have a limited ability to cause disease. Under special circumstances, however, fungi may produce serious localized or systemic infections in susceptible individuals. Two major factors predispose to systemic fungal infections: disturbance in the normal bacterial flora and impaired immunologic defenses.

After intensive therapy with broad-spectrum antibiotics, the normal bacterial flora of the oral cavity, colon, vagina, and other areas may be altered or completely eradicated, disturbing the normal balance between the bacterial flora and fungi. Normally, the predominance of the bacterial flora holds the fungi in check. When the bacteria are eliminated, the fungi may proliferate and cause disease.

Patients with various types of chronic debilitating diseases may be susceptible to fungal infections. Infections of this type are also encountered in patients whose immunologic defense mechanisms have been depressed by various drugs and chemicals or by radiation therapy. Patients with certain types of cancer, particularly those treated with cytotoxic drugs, may also develop systemic fungal infections.

Superficial Fungal Infections

Dermatophyte A fungus that causes a superficial infection of the skin.

Thrush Superficial infection of mouth caused by *Candida albicans*.

The common superficial fungal infections of the skin are caused by a group of fungi called **dermatophytes**. They cause itchy, scaling skin lesions on the scalp and on other parts of the body. Some have been given such descriptive, popular names as "athlete's foot" and "jock itch." A common superficial fungal infection of the mucous membranes is caused by a yeastlike fungus called *Candida albicans*. This organism is a common cause of superficial infections of the tongue, mouth, and esophagus (termed **thrush**) in the newborn and in immunosuppressed individuals (**Figure 7-10**). Vulvovaginal infections, producing symptoms of itching and vaginal discharge, are common in pregnant women and those taking broad-spectrum antibiotics. A number of antifungal drugs are available that can be applied locally to treat infections caused by dermatophytes and *Candida*.

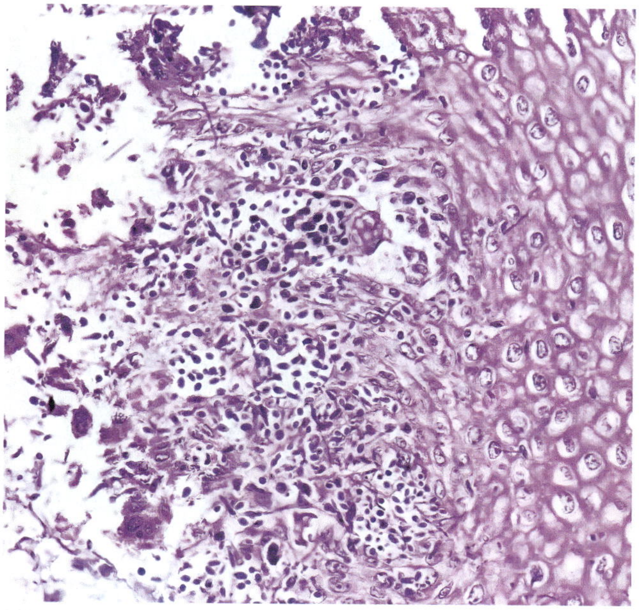

(A)

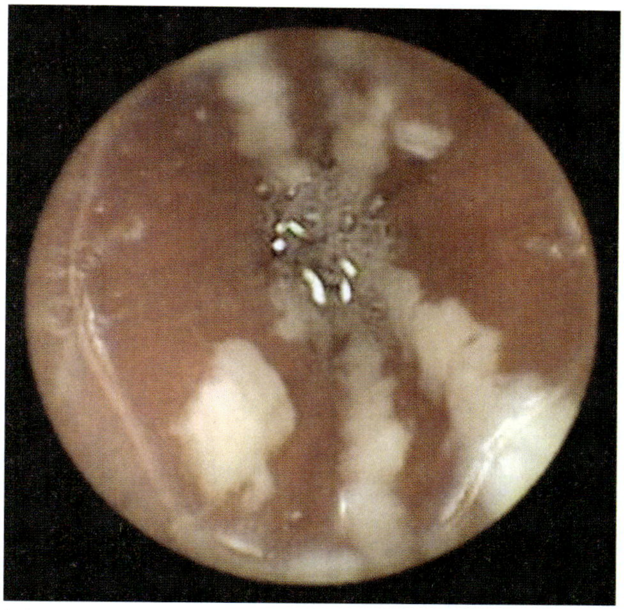

(B)

Figure 7-10 Esophageal candidiasis in an immunocompromised patient. **(A)** Histopathologic studies identify esophageal mucosas containing *Candida* spore and pseudohyphae. (Grocott's methenamine silver stain, ×400). **(B)** Endoscopic appearance of multiple whitish plaques.

Highly Pathogenic Fungi

Although most fungi are at best only potential pathogens of low virulence, several are highly infectious and frequently produce disease in humans. They can be identified by biopsy or by culture of infected tissues.

Various species of the fungus *Aspergillus* (most often *Aspergillus fumigatus*), a common fungus found in decaying plant material in the soil, can cause both pulmonary disease from inhaled spores and serious, potentially fatal systemic disease in immunocompromised individuals. In the lung, the fungus is responsible for allergic bronchopulmonary aspergillosis, a condition that complicates (and may contribute to) allergic asthma. Individuals with pulmonary cavities (as may occur in those who have had tuberculosis) may develop aspergillomas, fungal balls that reside in such spaces but generally do not invade lung tissue. Invasive aspergillosis most often occurs in severely immunocompromised patients with very low numbers of circulating neutrophils (**Figure 7-11**).

The fungus *Histoplasma capsulatum*, which is found in many parts of the United States, causes the disease **histoplasmosis**. This organism is found in the soil. People become infected by inhaling dust containing spores of the fungus. In most cases, the fungus produces an acute, self-limited respiratory infection. Less commonly, the organism causes a more chronic pulmonary infection similar to tuberculosis. In some cases, a progressive, disseminated, sometimes fatal disease develops. Another fungus, *Coccidioides immitis*, which is found in parts of California and elsewhere in the southwestern part of the United States, causes the disease coccidioidomycosis. As in the case of histoplasmosis, humans become infected by inhaling dust that contains fungus spores. The symptoms are similar to those of histoplasmosis. Coccidioidomycosis is usually manifested as an acute pulmonary infection, but sometimes the fungus causes chronic or severe progressive systemic disease.

Histoplasmosis An infection caused by the fungus *Histoplasma capsulatum*.

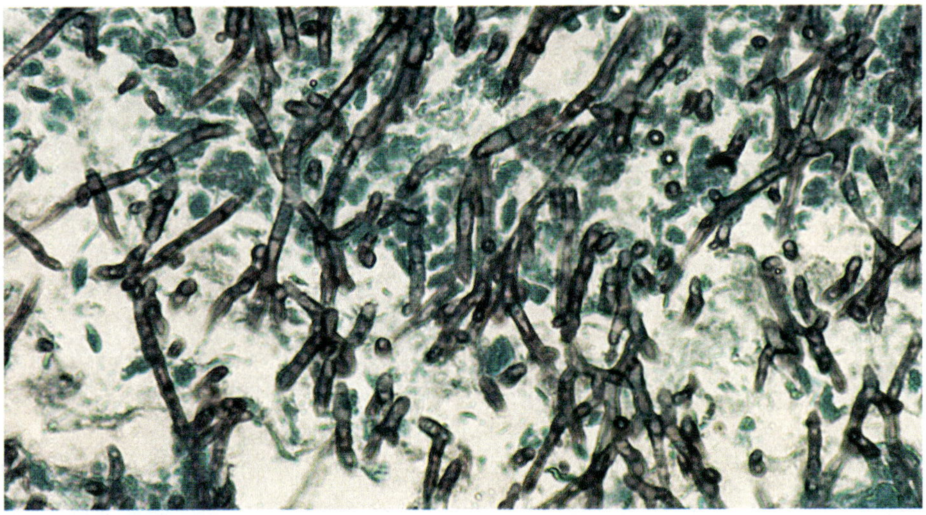

Figure 7-11 Histology from patient with pulmonary *Aspergillus* infection. The acutely branching dark blue elongated hyphae of *Aspergillus* are visible. *Aspergillus* organisms have a tendency to invade blood vessels.

Blastomycosis A systemic fungus infection caused by the fungus *Blastomyces dermatiditis*.

Coccidioidomycosis A disease caused by the pathogenic fungus *Coccidioides immitis*.

Other Fungi of Medical Importance

Two other pathogenic fungi of medical importance are *Blastomyces dermatitidis*, which causes the disease **blastomycosis**, and *Cryptococcus neoformans*, which causes cryptococcosis. Infections caused by these organisms are less common than either histoplasmosis or **coccidioidomycosis**. Both organisms are found in the soil, and infection is caused by inhalation of dust containing the organisms.

Clinically, blastomycosis is similar to histoplasmosis and coccidioidomycosis. Most infections are acute and self-limited. Occasionally, the fungus causes a more chronic pulmonary infection or a widespread systemic disease.

Cryptococcus neoformans is a yeastlike organism that has a large mucoid capsule. The organism initially causes a pulmonary infection but then may be transported in the bloodstream to the meninges of the brain, where it causes chronic meningitis. The organisms can be identified in smears and cultures of spinal fluid.

Treatment of Systemic Fungal Infections

Acute pulmonary infections caused by fungi frequently subside spontaneously and do not require treatment. Chronic or progressive systemic fungal infections are treated with various systemic antifungal antibiotics; local superficial infections are treated topically.

Vaccine and Human Infectious Diseases

The development and administration of vaccines has offered great benefit to human health. Mainly, vaccination is known to limit the transmission of diseases within a population (herd immunity), reduce the morbidity and mortality of infectious diseases and more. In 1980, the World Health Assembly declared the eradication of smallpox, which could not have occurred without the intervention of the smallpox vaccine. Similarly, the development of polio vaccines, IPV (inactivated polio vaccine) and OPV (oral polio vaccine, attenuated), made it possible to eradicate serotype 2 and 3 polio virus infections globally. Currently, endemic incidences of serotype 1 occur only in Afghanistan and Pakistan. In 2006, the FDA approved the use of Gardasil (Merck & Co) to prevent the infection and transmission of Human Papilloma Virus (HPV). The administration of Gardasil bivalent (2vHPV), quadrivalent (4vHPV), and nonavalent vaccines (9vHPV) offered a promising outcome for the reduction of cervical cancer development in females and other cancers in both males and females.

Case 7-1

A 6-year-old male child attending a small private preschool is noted to have a high fever (103°F). He has malaise (is tired) and has lost his appetite (anorexia). His mother notes that his eyes appear red (conjunctivitis), and he has a cough and runny nose (coryza). When the child complains of pain on eating, spots are noted on the mucosa of his mouth opposite his molars (Koplik spots). Soon after, an itching rash appears initially behind his ears that within a day spreads to cover much of his body. The child complains of itching. The rash is "dusky" red and maculopapular (has large red areas not raised above the skin that have small raised bumps also termed "morbilliform," which look similar to measles) (**Case Figure 7-1A**). The child's pediatrician diagnoses measles (rubeola). The child appears to recover over the next 5 days. However, on day 6 he develops a croup-like cough and earache that by day 7 progresses to respiratory distress diagnosed as measles pneumonia (**Case Figure 7-1B**). Aggressive respiratory support is provided, but the child dies. The clinical history notes that 10 days before the onset of illness the family was visited by a 10-year-old cousin from Central Africa. On questioning, the relatives' parents state that their child had also suffered from a "measles-like" illness but had recovered.

Discussion

Measles is an extremely contagious viral disease spread by droplets. The virus initially infects tracheal and bronchial epithelia but spreads via lymphatics systemically. The **viremia** produces a notable general immunosuppression that can outlast the acute disease for weeks. The immunosuppression may lead to progressive fatal disease in patients who have preexisting compromise of their immune system. Although measles is considered a benign disease by many, this is not the case. In developing countries, particularly in areas with childhood malnourishment, measles is a major cause of childhood death. Most of these deaths have occurred in Africa and Southeast Asia in areas with poor vaccination programs. It is also a major cause of blindness. In this case, the medical history indicated the child was under therapy for childhood allergic asthma using inhaled corticosteroids, and the child's parents had refused measles vaccination. The asthma therapy may have produced sufficient immunosuppression to account for the progressive viral pneumonia. Other complications of measles are not uncommon and occur in about 30 percent of cases. These complications include ear infection and subsequent hearing loss, diarrhea, and, as noted, pneumonia, which can occur in 5 percent to 10 percent of cases. Viral encephalitis is an uncommon complication, and, more rarely, a fatal neurodegenerative disease (subacute sclerosing panencephalitis [SSPE]) may occur 5 to 10 years following measles infection.

Viremia Presence of large numbers of viral particles in the bloodstream.

Vaccination against measles early in childhood is an extremely effective method of disease prevention. However, the unfounded rumors and inaccurate information that have linked measles vaccination to childhood autism and other diseases have led to a decline in vaccination rates and a resurgence of measles in the United States. Since 2013 there has been a marked increase

(continues)

Case 7-1 (Continued)

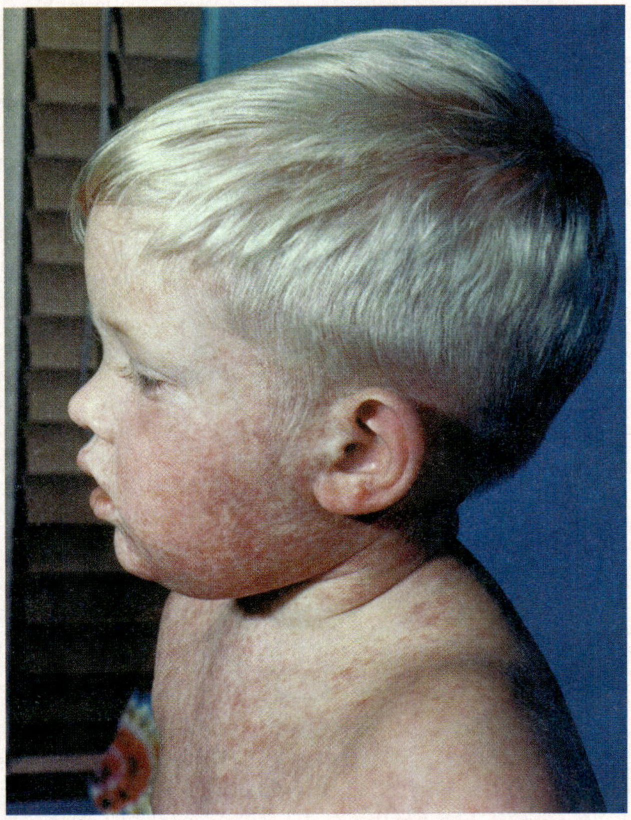

(A)

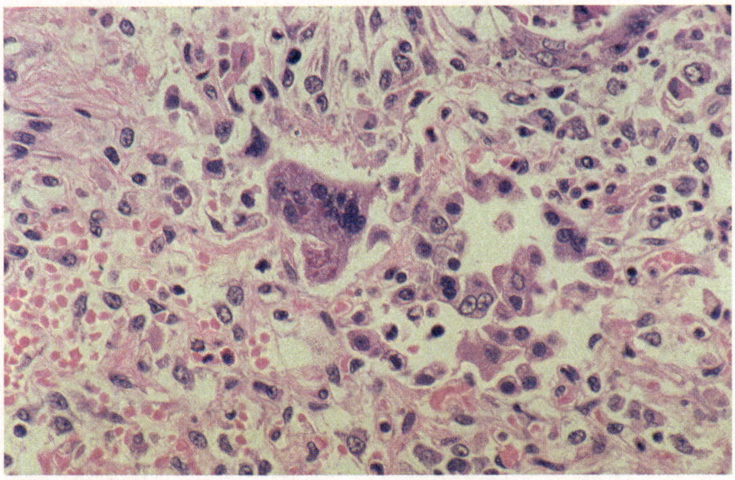

(B)

Case Figure 7-1 **(A)** Maculopapular (morbilliform) rash of measles. **(B)** Histopathology of measles pneumonia, large number of mononuclear cells and giant cell with intracytoplasmic inclusions.

(A) Courtesy of CDC; (B) Courtesy of CDC/ Dr. Edwin P. Ewing, Jr.

in reported cases of measles, resulting in localized outbreaks in more than 20 states. In the first 8 months of 2014, 600 cases of measles were reported, compared to fewer than 100 in 2012. During the measles outbreak in 2025, by September 24, the CDC reported 1514 confirmed cases with three deaths, and a 12% hospitalization rate. Ninety-two percent involved unvaccinated or unknown vaccination individuals. It is important to realize that in the case of effective vaccination programs, the small number of unvaccinated individuals are protected by herd or community immunity. Nevertheless, the unvaccinated remain at high risk of disease by imported infections.

Etiology and Pathogenesis

The etiologic agent is the RNA measles virus, a paramyxovirus closely related to that causing canine distemper. The virus causes systemic infection and immunosuppression, leading to a significant incidence of secondary infections and complications.

Questions

1. A mother asks you why it is necessary to immunize her child against measles, as it is a very mild disease. How would you answer her?
2. Over 95 percent of cases of measles in the United States result from disease imported from outside the country. Why is this?
3. The term *herd* or *community immunity* is used in the case discussion. What does the term mean?

Questions for Review

1. By what standards are bacteria classified? Name the classifications.
2. What important diseases are caused by the following bacteria: staphylococci, beta streptococci, pneumococci, gonococci, and acid-fast bacteria?
3. What is meant by the following terms: *granulomatous inflammation*, *Gram-positive organism*, and *Legionella*?
4. How do antibiotics inhibit the growth of bacteria? How does penicillin kill bacteria?
5. How do bacteria become resistant to an antibiotic?
6. What are some of the potential harmful effects of antibiotics?
7. What is meant by the following terms: *sensitivity test*, *resistant organism*, and *cell membrane*?
8. How does a viral infection affect a susceptible cell?
9. What is a latent (asymptomatic) viral infection? Give an example.
10. What is meant by the following terms: *inclusion body*, *chlamydiae*, and *mycoplasma*?
11. What factors render a patient susceptible to an infection by a fungus of low pathogenicity?
12. What are the names of the two highly pathogenic fungi? What type of disease do they produce?
13. A young woman receives a course of antibiotics and soon afterward develops a vaginal infection caused by a fungus. Why?

References

Shors T. *Understanding Viruses*. 2nd ed. Jones & Bartlett Learning; 2011.

- This book contains additional information on all aspects of virology, including HIV and Ebola.

Pommerville JC. *Fundamentals of Microbiology*. 10th ed. Jones & Bartlett Learning; 2013.

- This book contains additional information on all aspects of microbiology; in particular, Ebola, which is also covered in Chapter 16.

Alby K, Gilligan PH. Identification of pathogens by classical clinical tests. In: Rosenberg E, DeLong EF, Lory S, Stackebrandt E, Thompson F, eds. *The Prokaryotes*. 4th ed. Vol. 5: *Human Microbiology*. Springer-Verlag Berlin Heidelberg; 2013.

- Detailed information on identification of organisms using microscopic examination and culture methods is included in this article on pages 1-45.

Omer SB, Salmon DA, Orenstein WA, Dehart MP, Halsey N. Vaccine refusal, mandatory immunization, and the risks of vaccine-preventable diseases. *N Eng J Med.* 2009;360(19): 1981-1988.

- The success of an immunization program depends on high rates of acceptance and coverage. Rates of refusal of immunization are increasing, and clustering of refusals leads to outbreaks of vaccine-preventable diseases. Children with exemptions from school immunization requirements, which is a measure of vaccine refusal, are at increased risk for measles and pertussis. In turn, they can infect others who are too young to be vaccinated, cannot be vaccinated for medical reasons, or were vaccinated but did not achieve a sufficient immunologic response. Clinicians can play a crucial role in promoting vaccination by respectfully listening to parents' concerns and discussing the risks and benefits of immunization.

Chen SP. Measles. Medscape. Updated June 3, 2015. http://emedicine.medscape.com/article/966220-overview

- The details used to construct the case and additional detailed information on the disease can be found here.

Centers for Disease Control. Ebola Disease Basics. Published April 23, 2024. http://www.cdc.gov/vhf/ebola/index.html

- The ongoing Ebola outbreak in Central West Africa has led to a large number of publications detailing the epidemiology and clinical details of the disease as well as the molecular biology of the virus. An excellent starting place for detailed information can be found here.

Gajic I, Kabic J, Kekic D, et al. Antimicrobial Susceptibility Testing: A Comprehensive Review of Currently Used Methods. *Antibiotics (Basel).* 2022;11(4):427. Published 2022 Mar 23. doi:10.3390/antibiotics11040427

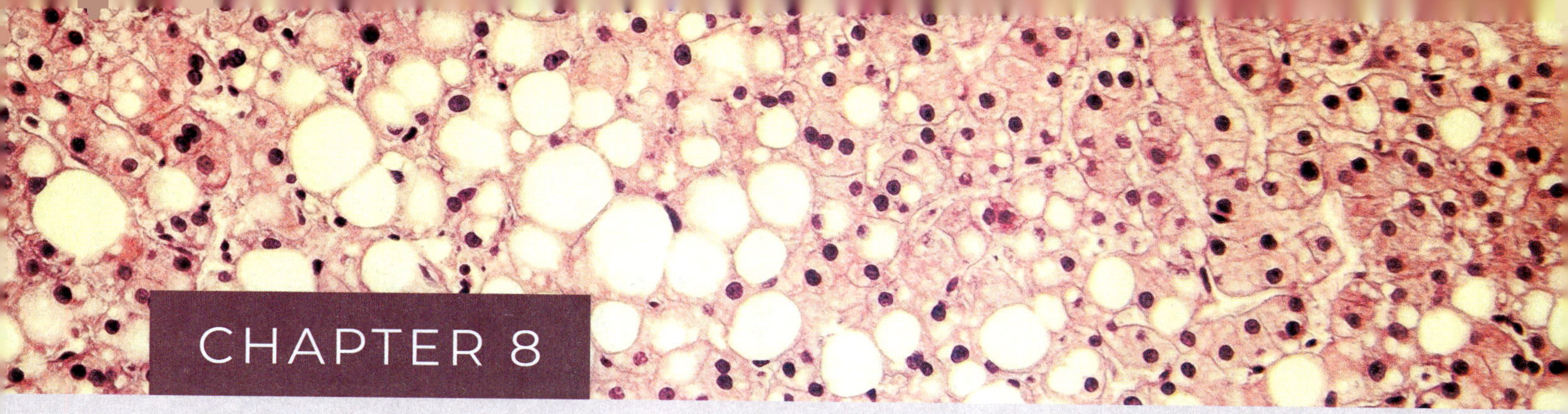

CHAPTER 8

Parasitic Disease

LEARNING OBJECTIVES

1. List the common types of parasites and their associated human infections.
2. Compare and contrast parasitic disease in humans and animals.
3. Study the life cycle of malaria and understand why it is hard to eradicate malaria infection.
4. Explain how these infections are acquired.

The Parasite and Its Host

Parasitism involves a close relationship between organisms, where the parasite, from one species, is completely dependent upon an organism of another species, the **host**. Many animal parasites display complex life cycles. An immature form of a parasite may spend part of its cycle within the body of one animal (the **intermediate host**), while the mature parasite eventually takes up residence within the body of another animal, the final host (the definitive host). Because many animal parasites live in the intestinal tract and discharge eggs into the feces, transmission is favored by conditions of poor sanitation as well as poor food and water quality. Insect **vectors** may transmit a parasite from the intermediate or **definitive host** to humans. In some situations, humans may serve as an **opportunistic host** (accidental host).

Parasites are classified into three large groups: **protozoan parasites**, which are simple, one-celled organisms; **metazoan parasites**, which are more complex, multicellular structures; and ectoparasites, which are often small insects living on the external surface of the host. Parasitic diseases, particularly those involving helminths (worms), may be accompanied by eosinophilia (excess amount of eosinophils produced). These white blood cells may play a role in the host defense against such parasitic agents.

The Centers for Disease Control and Prevention (CDC) notes that parasitic diseases can infect anyone. There is no doubt that parasitic diseases are a major health burden in some nations, malaria being a prime example. A parasitic disease affecting a significant number of individuals may be considered a severe disease. In some cases that disease can be easily prevented and treated. In this chapter, five neglected parasitic infections (NPIs) listed by

Host Individual infected with a disease-producing organism.

Intermediate host Organism that harbors an immature stage of a parasite.

Vectors Transmission agents of a parasite; may be insects or other animals.

Definitive host Organism in which a parasite reaches final maturity.

Opportunistic host Accidental host of parasite, often humans.

Protozoan parasite Simple one-celled animal parasite, such as the plasmodium causing malaria.

Metazoan parasite Complex multicelled animal parasite, such as worms and flukes.

the CDC and other parasitic diseases of importance will be discussed. Those five NPIs include: Chagas disease, neurocysticercosis, toxocariasis, toxoplasmosis, and trichomoniasis.

Infections Caused by Protozoa and Related Organisms

Some of the more important protozoal infections in humans include malaria, caused by various species of *Plasmodium*; amoebic dysentery, caused by a pathogenic amoeba, *Entamoeba histolytica*; Chagas disease (American trypanosomiasis caused by *Trypanosoma cruzi*), a systemic disease causing serious damage to the heart; leishmaniasis, caused by various species of the protozoan *Leishmania*, resulting in ulcerating skin lesions and a multisystem visceral disease termed kala azar; trichomonad infections of the genital tract, caused by the parasite *Trichomonas vaginalis*; giardiasis, caused by *Giardia lamblia*, which infects the small intestine; toxoplasmosis, caused by ***Toxoplasma gondii***, which may infect the fetus and cause congenital malformations; and cryptosporidiosis, caused by the parasite, *Cryptosporidium parvum*, which parasitizes the intestinal tract and can cause severe diarrhea (**Table 8-1**).

Toxoplasma gondii A small intracellular parasite of birds, animals, and humans. Causes the disease toxoplasmosis.

Table 8-1 Some of the More Common Protozoal Diseases in Humans

Disease	Some Representative Etiological Agents	Geographical Localization	Clinical Features
Malaria	*Plasmodium falciparum, P. vivax, P. ovale*	Over 100 countries in the tropic and subtropics	Fever, shivering, cough, respiratory distress, pain in the joints, headache, watery diarrhea, vomiting, convulsions, severe anemia
African trypanosomiasis	*Trypanosoma brucei*	36 countries in sub-Sahara Africa	Initial haemolytic phase (fever, joint pains followed by neurological disorder, somnolence
Chagas disease	*Trypanosoma cruzi*	From northern Mexico to South Argentina	Acute phase (fever and splenomegaly) Chronic phase (irreversible damage to heart, esophagus, and colon)
Leishmaniasis	*Leishmania donovani, L. major, L. mexicana, L. braziliensis*	Over 88 countries in tropic and subtropics	Skin ulcers, mucocutaneous complications, and viscera. diseases (hepatosplenomegaly)
Toxoplasmosis	*Toxoplasma gondii*	Worldwide	Blindness and mental retardation can result in congenitally infected children. Immunosuppressed patients can present more severe symptoms: splenomegaly, polymyositis, dermatomyositis, chorioretinitis, myocarditis, pneumonitis, hepatitis, encephalitis, and multisystem organ failure.
Trichomoniasis	*Trichomonas vaginalis*	Worldwide	Vaginal discharge, odor, and edema or erythema.
Intestinal protozoan infection	*Giardia lamblia, Entamoeba histolytica, Cryptosporidium parvum, Cyclospora cayetanensis*	Worldwide	Hematuria, anemia, and impaired growth. Renal, hepatic, and spleen failure

Monzote L, Siddiq A. Drug development to protozoan diseases. *Open Med Chem J.* 2011;5:1–3. doi:10.2174/1874104501105010001. Epub 2011 Mar 9. PMID: 21629506; PMCID: PMC3103878.

This list is not exhaustive. Other protozoal diseases may have serious consequences in animal husbandry and occasionally infect humans who serve as an opportunistic host when exposed to infected animals and insect vectors. An example is babesiosis, which is most often asymptomatic or produces only mild disease in humans. The organism can cause a malaria-like disease, destroying erythrocytes in asplenic or immunocompromised people. The primary host of the protozoan parasite (*Babesia* species) is rodents, most often deer mice in the United States. Deer ticks serve as a vector, and increased deer populations result in increased risk, although the disease is seen in limited regions, including Cape Cod and the coastal area and islands of New England and Long Island.

Malaria

Malaria is caused by several species of the protozoan parasite *Plasmodium*. There are five species of human malaria parasite: *P. falciparum*, *P. malariae*, *P. vivax*, *P. ovale*, and *P. knowlesi*. They all cause debilitating diseases, but only one, *P. falciparum,* is deadly. The parasite is transmitted to humans by the bite of the *Anopheles* mosquito, which breeds in free standing water. The name malaria dates to the time when, in Italy, the disease was thought to be caused by breathing night air near lowland marshes and swampy areas (malo = bad + aria = air).

The life cycle of *Plasmodium* is quite complex (**Figure 8-1**). The female mosquito takes a blood meal from an infected person and ingests the malaria parasite. The sexual stage of the parasite (gametocytes) reproduces within the insect host, producing the infectious stage of the parasite (sporozoites). Following delivery by a mosquito bite, the sporozoites begin their development within the liver and after several weeks invade the red blood cells of the host. Inside the RBCs they multiply, feeding on the hemoglobin, which becomes degraded to a product called malaria pigment. The infected RBCs rupture and release masses of new parasites along with cell debris and malaria pigment into the circulation. This event triggers the inflammatory response resulting in an elevated temperature and a shaking chill, "chills and fever." The newly liberated parasites attack other red cells, continuing the cycle of invasion–multiplication–red cell destruction. The time required for each species of parasite to complete its cycle is constant, so the episodes of chills and fever tend to occur at regular intervals every 48 or 72 hours, depending on the species of malaria. In addition to suffering repeated, periodic chills and fever, infected individuals frequently become anemic because of the excessive red blood cell destruction. Often their spleens and livers enlarge when phagocytic cells in the spleen proliferate and become filled with debris and malarial pigment. In one type of malaria, clumps of infected red blood cells may plug small blood vessels in the brain (cerebral malaria), heart, or other vital organs. This serious complication impedes blood flow to the affected organs and may be fatal. Diagnosis of malaria is established by demonstrating the parasite inside the RBCs of the infected individual. The slides need to be properly prepared and stained to visualize the protozoan invader (**Figure 8-2**).

Malaria is a major health problem in many parts of the world, including parts of Africa, Asia, Central America, and South America. According to the World Health Organization (WHO), globally in 2022, there were an estimated 249 million malaria cases and 608,000 malaria deaths in 85 countries. The WHO-designated African Region carries a disproportionately high share of the global malaria burden. In 2022, the Region was home to 94% of malaria cases (233 million) and 95% (580,000) of malaria deaths. Children under 5 accounted for about 80% of all malaria deaths in the Region. Few infectious

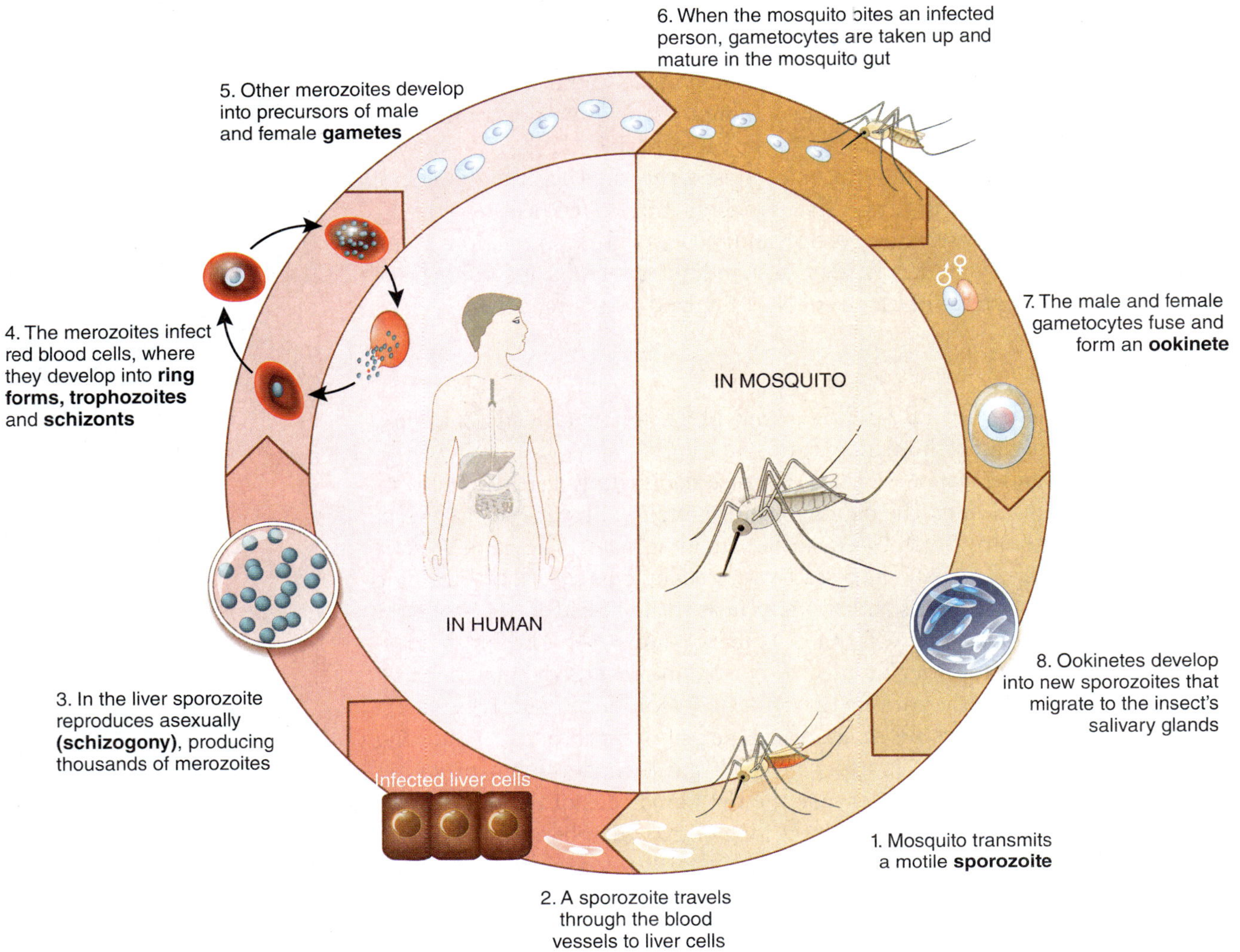

Figure 8-1 Life cycle of malaria parasite.

diseases have had such a profound effect on the social and economic development of countries. Various antimalarial drugs have been developed to treat the disease (**Figure 8-3**). According to the WHO Model List of Essential Medicines, 14 medicines are currently used for curative treatment of malaria, among which artemisinin-based combinations are the most effective. Artemisinin was first isolated from the plant *Artemisia annua* in 1971 by Tu Youyou, who was awarded the Nobel Prize in Physiology or Medicine in 2015 for "her discovery concerning a novel therapy against malaria." Artemisinin has been very effective in treating many drug-resistant forms of *P. falciparum*.

Malaria is no longer a major public health problem in the United States, Canada, and Europe. Most of the 2000 cases of malaria diagnosed in the United States were contracted by people who have traveled to or have emigrated from areas where malaria occurs frequently. Medications are available to prevent infection when traveling in an endemic area and to treat an established infection. Unfortunately, drug resistance makes effective treatment more difficult.

It is also worth noting that the global temperature has increased significantly over the past 100 years. This change, together with increased global travel, will increase the transmission of mosquito-borne diseases, including malaria. Surveillance and preparedness for malaria control need to be reintroduced and emphasized, not compromised.

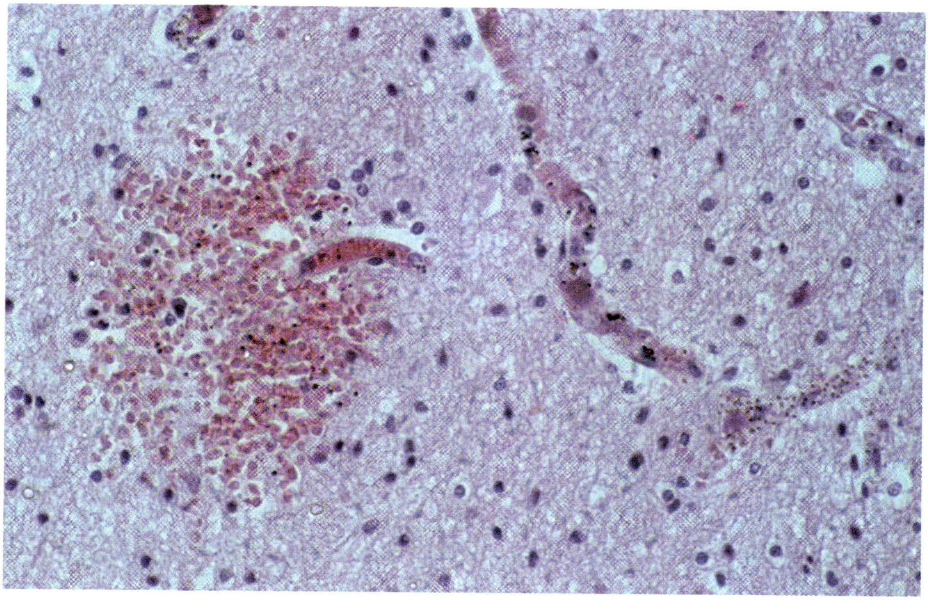

Figure 8-2 Cerebral malaria: histopathology This image is a medium-power view of a section of white matter of the brain from a patient with cerebral malaria. It shows capillaries engorged with parasitized red blood cells. On the left, one vessel has ruptured and produced a surrounding hemorrhage. H&E stain.

Courtesy of Wellcome Collection.

Amoebiasis

Amoebiasis is an infection of the intestinal tract by a pathogenic amoeba, *Entamoeba histolytica*. The life cycle of the parasite includes an active, motile, vegetative phase (called a **trophozoite**) and a relatively resistant cystic phase.

Trophozoite Active, motile vegetative phase of a parasite.

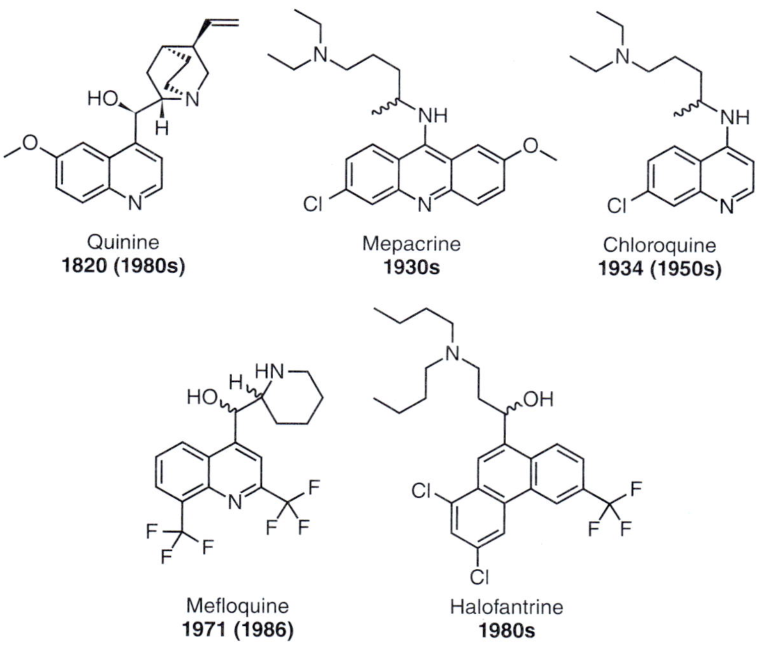

Figure 8-3 Well-known antimalarial medicines were discovered between 1820 and the 1980s. Some are still used today, while some have been rendered ineffective due to the development of resistant strains or the emergence of undesirable side effects. Dates of first reported resistance are shown in brackets.

Tse EG, Korsik M, Todd MH. The past, present and future of anti-malarial medicines. *Malar J.* 2019;18:93. https://doi.org/10.1186/s12936-019-2724-z

Humans become infected by ingesting cysts of the parasite in contaminated food and water. The motile phase of the parasite develops from the cyst and invades the mucosa of the colon, producing mucosal ulcers and causing symptoms of inflammation of the colon. Occasionally, the amoebas are carried to the liver in the portal circulation and may cause amoebic hepatitis or amoebic liver abscess (**Figure 8-4**).

Amoebic Meningoencephalitis

Meningoencephalitis
A serious disease of the brain and its linings, which can be caused by amoebic infections from freshwater sources.

Although very uncommon, the free-living ameba *Naegleria fowleri* produces a devastating infection of the brain and its linings, known as primary amoebic **meningoencephalitis** (PAM), when it enters the nasal cavity and migrates up the olfactory nerve to the brain. PAM is a rare disease that is almost always fatal. In the United States, there have been 157 PAM infections from 1962 through 2022 with only four survivors. These infections have primarily occurred in southern-tier states, with almost half of the infections occurring in Texas and Florida. The organism requires warm fresh water to propagate, and the majority of the cases were associated with aquatic sports in which water can be forcibly introduced into the nose, such as diving and white-water rafting.

Chagas Disease (American Trypanosomiasis)

Chagas disease is caused by the protozoan *Trypanosoma cruzi*, which produces an endemic infection in both wild and domestic animals. The disease is transmitted to humans by a vector (triatomine insects, "kissing bugs"). The parasite and insect vector are present in animal populations in the Southwest of the United States, but the disease is most common in South and Central America, where infection is associated with living conditions that allow insects entry into dwellings. The overwhelming majority of people with Chagas disease in the United States were infected in Mexico, where the prevalence of the disease is

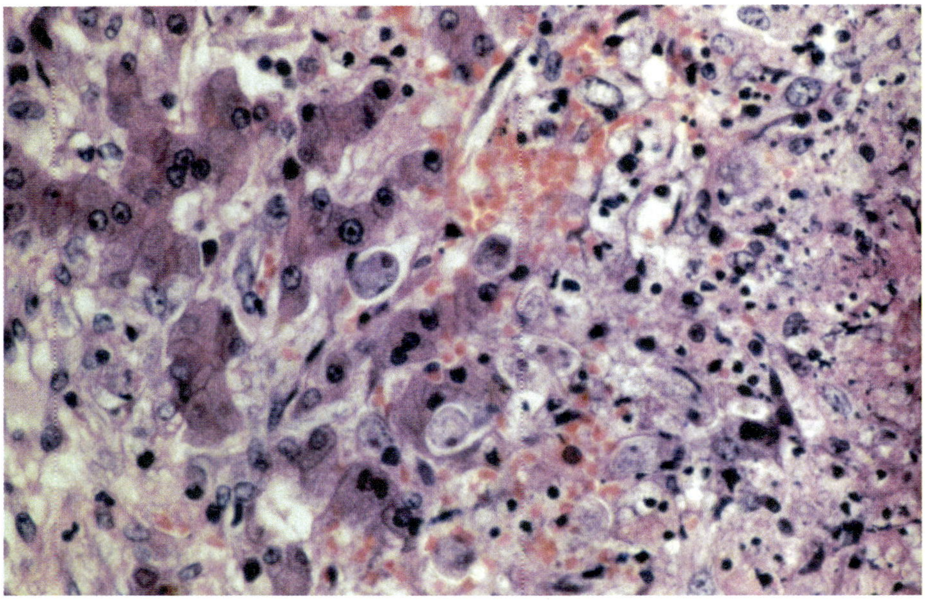

Figure 8-4 Microscopy features of amoebic liver abscess with trophozoites (H & E. 100×). Granular and eosinophilic necrosis with nuclear debris is also evident.

Courtesy of SB Lucas/Wellcome Collection.

about one percent. Overall, the CDC estimates about 300,000 individuals in the United States suffer from chronic Chagas disease, most of whom were infected in Latin America. The organisms spread systemically after entry and parasitize muscle, most frequently the heart, resulting in severe acute myocarditis and necrosis of affected tissue. The disease may cause a chronic infected state with progressive heart failure and disease of the gastrointestinal tract. Chagas disease may also be transferred by blood products. Active insect eradication programs and screening of blood products have reduced disease frequency in many South American countries. Effective antiparasitic drug therapy is also available.

Leishmaniasis

Leishmaniasis occurs as a variety of syndromes in different geographic areas depending on the particular infecting species. The disease is endemic in a variety of animal populations and is transmitted to humans by the bite of phlebotomus sandflies. The disease is found in a cutaneous form, which produces ulcerating skin lesions (oriental or tropical sores) that often heal spontaneously. The disease can be found in the Middle East, Asia, tropical and North Africa, and Central and South America. Rare cases occurred in Texas and Oklahoma, but 75 percent of those diagnosed among civilians in the United States were acquired at tourist destinations such as Costa Rica. The mucocutaneous form of the disease, found predominantly in Central and South America, produces progressive and disfiguring ulcers where the mucous membrane and skin meet, e.g., in the nasal septum and mouth, and requires antiprotozoan therapy. Visceral leishmaniasis, kala azar, is a systemic form of the disease with massive enlargement of the spleen and liver. The name comes from the Hindi for "black fever" because of a characteristic darkening of the skin in severely affected individuals. This form of the disease occurs predominantly in the Indian subcontinent and Brazil. Without treatment, kala azar leads to severe wasting and death. Although uncommon in the United States, there are an estimated 1 million cases of cutaneous and 0.3 million cases of visceral disease per year worldwide.

Trichomonal Genital Tract Infections

The trichomonads are small motile parasites. One species, *Trichomonas vaginalis*, sometimes causes an acute inflammation of the vagina and urethra (**Figure 8-5**). Refer to Chapter 18 for more information.

Giardiasis

Giardiasis is caused by the protozoan *Giardia duodenalis*, also known as *G lamblia* and *G intestinalis*. Infected animals excrete cysts into freshwater, which remain infective and viable for weeks to months. Human infection occurs through ingesting cysts via contaminated water or direct person-to-person contact, with transmission heavily influenced by inadequate hygiene and sanitation practices. Daycares have emerged as epicenters of infection due to insufficient handwashing protocols, especially during diaper handling and changing. Within the intestinal system, cysts undergo excystation, giving rise to trophozoites. Several epidemics caused by contaminated water supplies have occurred, most frequently in the western mountain regions of the United States. Giardiasis is a nationally notifiable disease, meaning healthcare providers must report cases to their departments of public health.

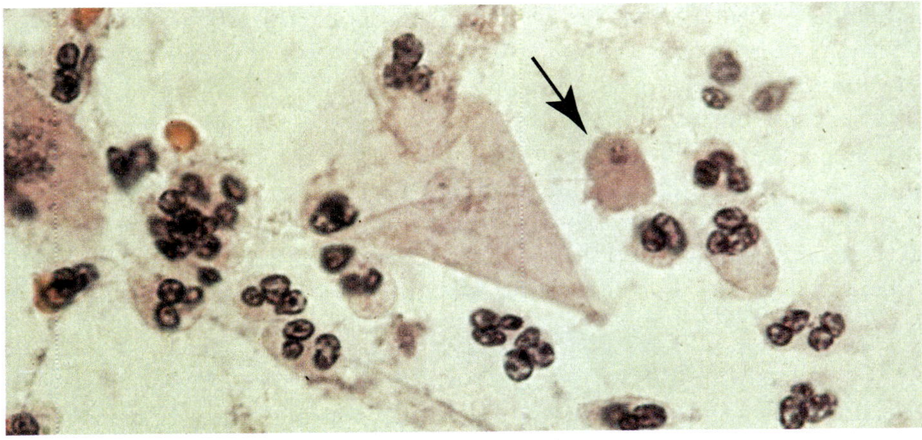

Figure 8-5 Vaginal secretions from women with trichomonad infection, illustrating parasite (*arrow*) and many neutrophils.

Courtesy of Leonard V. Crowley, MD, Century College.

Toxoplasmosis

Oocyst Infectious form of a parasite that contains the zygote.

Toxoplasma gondii is a small intracellular parasite that infects a large number of birds and animals as well as humans. Many cats are infected with the parasite and excrete an infectious form of the organism in their stools. The parasite is frequently present in the flesh of cattle and many other animals. People acquire toxoplasma infections by ingesting raw or partially cooked meat that is infected with the parasite or by contact with the feces of infected cats, which may contain an infectious form of the parasite called an **oocyst**. Usually, the infection does not cause symptoms in healthy adults. About 50 percent of the adult population has had a previous inapparent infection and is immune. The importance of toxoplasmosis is related to its effect on the fetus (Chapter 16). If a susceptible (nonimmune) woman acquires a toxoplasma infection during pregnancy, the parasite may be transmitted to the fetus. Infection of the fetus causes severe injury to fetal tissues and often leads to congenital malformations (Chapter 16).

Toxoplasmosis, like other parasitic diseases, is of increased risk to immunocompromised individuals. In these people, toxoplasmosis most commonly manifests as a disease of the brain, toxoplasmosis encephalitis (**Figure 8-6**). The disease may result either from a first exposure to the parasite or from reactivation of an infection acquired many years previously.

Cryptosporidiosis

Cryptosporidium parvum, Cryptosporidium hominis, and several other species found commonly in animals are protozoal parasites related to toxoplasma and are an important cause of severe diarrhea in both immunocompetent and immunocompromised people. Cryptosporidiosis became well-known when nearly half a million people in Milwaukee, Wisconsin, developed the disease in 1993. Many large outbreaks have occurred subsequently in the United States and in England and other European countries. The organism infects cattle, other farm animals, and people, who excrete large numbers of the infectious forms of the parasites called oocysts in their feces. Fecal material from farm animals can contaminate surface water flowing into rivers and lakes, and oocysts have been identified in 65 percent to 85 percent of surface water samples tested throughout the United States. The infectious oocyst has a thick wall and is quite small, only about half the size of a red blood cell. It is highly resistant to chlorination

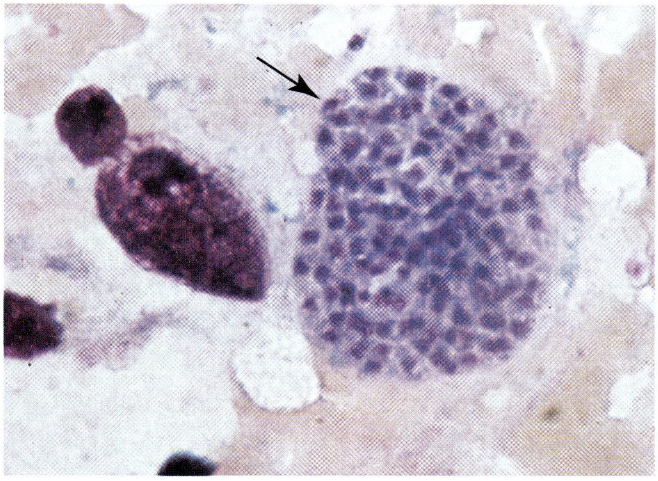

Figure 8-6 Cerebral toxoplasmosis demonstrated by brain biopsy. The cyst (*arrow*) is composed of a large cluster of organisms.

Courtesy of Leonard V. Crowley, MD, Century College.

and must be removed from municipal water supplies by filtration. People can become infected by ingesting oocysts in unfiltered municipal water supplies, from oocyst-contaminated recreational water (the most common source of outbreaks), or by person-to-person fecal–oral transmission in the same way that other intestinal infections are transmitted. The infection is easily transmitted from person to person in households and in child daycare facilities.

When oocysts are ingested, the cyst wall disintegrates in the intestinal tract, releasing the infectious parasite, which multiplies and infects the intestinal epithelial cells. Only a few oocysts are enough to cause an infection, and people with diarrhea excrete large numbers of oocysts in their stool. People with normal immune defenses experience an acute self-limited diarrhea, but people with AIDS and other immunocompromised people develop a severe chronic life-threatening diarrheal disease. Antiparasitic therapy is of limited utility but appears to shorten the duration of the disease.

Metazoal Infections

The three large groups of metazoal helminthic parasites are roundworms (nematodes), tapeworms (cestodes), and flukes or flatworms (trematodes). Some of the more common diseases caused by helminths are summarized in **Table 8-2**.

Roundworms

A number of nematodes are intestinal parasites in humans. For the most part, parasitemia does not lead to clinical symptoms until the parasite load becomes very large. Intestinal nematodes are of greatest concern in tropical areas and regions of poor sanitation where shed eggs are passed in the feces from person to person, most often infecting children. The overall health burden of such infestation is high; it results in growth retardation and malnutrition with associated developmental problems. Fortunately, drug therapy is safe, effective, and inexpensive. However, hundreds of millions of people remain infected, particularly in developing countries, along with millions of individuals in the United States, particularly in the Southeast. The most important roundworms that parasitize the human intestine are the roundworm *Ascaris*, the **pinworm**

Pinworm A small parasitic worm infecting humans. Lives in the lower bowel and causes perianal pruritus.

Table 8-2 Some Common Diseases Caused by Helminths

Organism	Disease	Route of Infection	Infected Organ(s)	Disease Manifestations
Schistosoma sp.	Schistosomiasis (Bilharzia)	Infected water, across the skin	▪ Skin ▪ Liver ▪ Bladder ▪ Intestine ▪ Kidney ▪ CNS	▪ Chronic disease ▪ Anemia, malnutrition ▪ Destruction of liver, portal hypertension ▪ Cystitis and ureteritis, progressing to bladder cancer
Enterobius vermicularis	Pinworm	Fecal–oral	▪ Intestine	▪ Anal itching
Trichinella spiralis	Trichinosis	Undercooked meat (pork)	▪ Muscle ▪ Heart	▪ Muscle pain
Taenia solium	Cysticercosis	Undercooked meat (pork)	▪ Brain	▪ Encysted larvae in brain cause seizures, headaches
Echinococcus granulosus	Echinococcosis	Food contaminated by dog feces	▪ Liver	▪ Hydatid cysts
Ascaris lumbricoides	Ascariasis	Fecal–oral	▪ Lung ▪ Intestine	▪ Pneumonitis ▪ Intestinal obstruction
Trichuris trichiura (whipworm)	Trichuriasis	Fecal–oral	▪ Intestine	▪ Abdominal pain ▪ Anemia ▪ Appendicitis ▪ Rectal prolapse
Wuchereria bancrofti (and others)	Filariasis	Mosquito bites	▪ Lymphatic system	▪ Lymphatic obstruction, lymphedema, elephantiasis

Enterobius, the whipworm *Trichuris*, the threadworm *Strongyloides*, and a variety of hookworms. The tissue nematode *Trichinella spiralis*, although uncommon in the United States, is also discussed.

Ascaris

Ascaris lumbricoides is the most commonly encountered parasitic worm, infecting an estimated one billion people worldwide. The roundworm is about the size of a large earthworm, lives in the intestinal tract, and discharges eggs in the feces. Direct person-to-person transmission of *Ascaris* eggs does not occur because the eggs expelled in feces are immature, and a maturation period of about a week is required before the eggs become infectious. Maturation of the immature eggs usually occurs in the soil when fecal material is defecated on the ground or when fecal material is used to fertilize soil. The mature eggs can survive in the soil for up to 2 years. Contact with egg-contaminated soil may transfer the eggs to hands, then to food or beverages, and finally into the intestinal tract.

When mature *Ascaris* eggs are ingested, the larval worms are released from the eggs within the intestinal tract, and burrow through the intestine, where they enter the circulatory system of the liver and then the lungs, potentially producing pneumonia-like symptoms. They are expectorated (coughed up) and eventually are swallowed, finding their way again into the small intestine, where they grow to maturity. At times, mature worms may enter and block the bile or pancreatic ducts or plug the appendix. Rarely, a large mass of worms

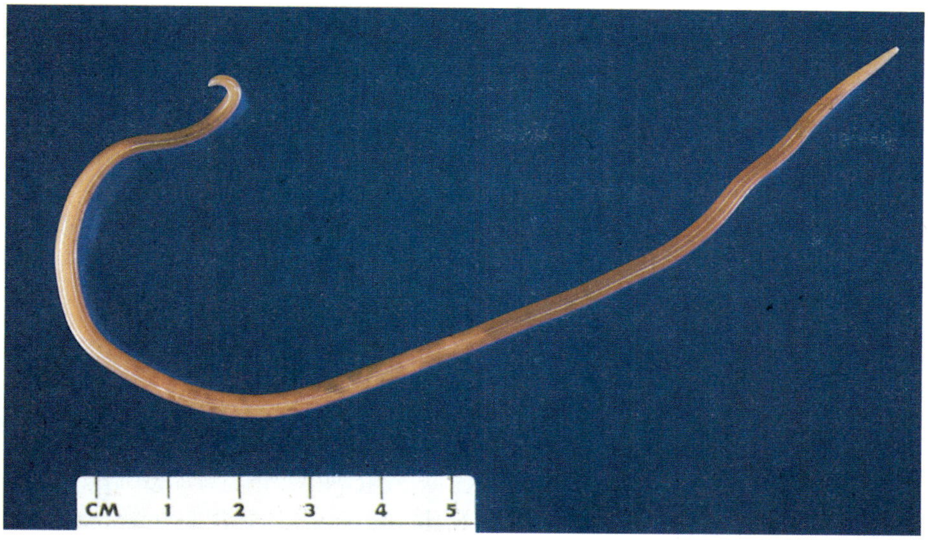

Figure 8-7 Large *Ascaris* that migrated into the back of the patient's throat and was coughed up.

Courtesy of Leonard V. Crowley, MD, Century College.

may completely block the lumen of the small intestine. Mature worms may also be expectorated (**Figure 8-7**). The mature worm has a limited life span, so persistent infections are the result of re-exposure. An *Ascaris* infection is identified by detecting worm eggs in the fecal material of an infected person or by identifying an adult worm.

Dogs and cats may be infected with a similar type of roundworm that occasionally causes disease in humans. Infection by the animal worm is most common in children who are in close contact with an infected animal. The children transfer the eggs to their mouths by contaminated hands, toys, or other objects.

Whipworms (Trichuriasis)

Trichuriasis, caused by parasitization with *Trichuris trichiura*, is extremely prevalent in warm, moist regions, and nearly a billion people may be infected worldwide. The disease is common in the Southeast of the United States, infecting several million. As has been seen with other nematodes, whipworm is transferred from fecally contaminated soil by ingestion of eggs. The eggs hatch in the intestine, and adult forms reside in the cecum and ascending colon. The worms burrow into the colonic mucosa, and if infection is heavy, they may cause colitis (although light infections are asymptomatic). Eggs shed by the female worm pass into the feces.

Pinworms

The small roundworm *Enterobius vermicularis*, called simply the pinworm because of its small size, generally measures less than one cm in length. Pinworm infections are very common, second only to *Ascaris* infections in frequency, and often infect children, who may harbor a large number of worms in their intestinal tract. Often the infection spreads from the child to the rest of the family members. The infection is acquired from ingesting worm eggs that are transferred to the hands from contaminated bedclothes or other objects. The worms hatch in the duodenum and then travel to the ileocecal region, where they take up residence. Female egg-laden worms migrate out of the colon through the anus, often at night while the child is asleep, and deposit their eggs on the perianal skin. The main symptoms of pinworm infection are intense anal and perianal itching caused by irritation resulting from the migration of the worm. Increased incidences of appendicitis have been observed as the result of infection. Intravaginal infections can occur in females. Pinworm eggs are usually not found in fecal material. The diagnosis of a pinworm infection is made by identifying the eggs deposited by migrating worms on the perianal skin.

Hookworms

Hookworm disease is caused by *Necator americanus* (American hookworm) and several species of *Ancyclostoma*. Infection was once common in the American Southeast but is now nearly eradicated. Parasitic infection is extremely common in many subtropical and tropical areas. It has been estimated that 30 percent of the population of sub-Saharan Africa is infected. Unlike many other parasitic nematodes, hookworm infection occurs by direct contact with larvae in soil contaminated with human feces. Initially the larvae are inactive, but over time they mature into a stage that can rapidly penetrate undamaged skin, usually the hands and feet, where they often provoke extreme itching (ground itch). The larvae migrate through the bloodstream into the lungs where they enter the alveoli, move up the respiratory tract, and are swallowed, eventually arriving in the small intestine. During their journey they may cause pulmonary symptoms, sore throat, and cough. The worms mature and develop a specialized attachment organ (the **buccal plate**) and use this to attach themselves to the mucosa of the small intestine. They cause local bleeding by damaging vessels and secreting digestive enzymes and an anti-coagulant substance. Sexually mature worms produce eggs that pass into the stool. Intestinal blood loss is the major clinical effect, which may lead to iron deficiency anemia, malnutrition, and potentially low levels of blood proteins because of worm ingestion in severe cases.

Buccal plate Specialized attachment organ of hookworms. Also refers to a thin layer of bone in the mouth which supports teeth and facial structure.

Strongyloidiasis

Strongyloidiasis (threadworm) infection by the nematode *Strongyloides stercoralis* has similarities to hookworm in mode of infection via intact skin. Most cases are asymptomatic; however, immunosuppressed individuals may suffer from hyperinfection syndrome, where dissemination of parasites can occur and result in a critical illness requiring immediate therapy.

Trichinella

Another small roundworm, *Trichinella spiralis*, causes a severe parasitic infection called trichinellosis (formerly trichinosis). The organism parasitizes not only humans but also a wide variety of animals. Larval forms of the *Trichinella* are encapsulated as small cystic structures within the muscles of the infected human or animal host. People formerly became infected by eating improperly cooked meat (usually pork) containing *Trichinella* larvae. The disease is very uncommon in the United States today and is usually related to ingestion of undercooked wild game (bear meat being a common source). After the infected meat has been ingested, the larvae are released from their cysts and develop into mature parasitic worms in the small intestine. The worms then burrow into the intestinal mucosa and produce larvae, which gain access to the circulation and are carried throughout the body. They are filtered out in various tissues, where they incite an intense inflammatory reaction. The parasites that lodge in the muscles of the infected individual become encapsulated, forming small

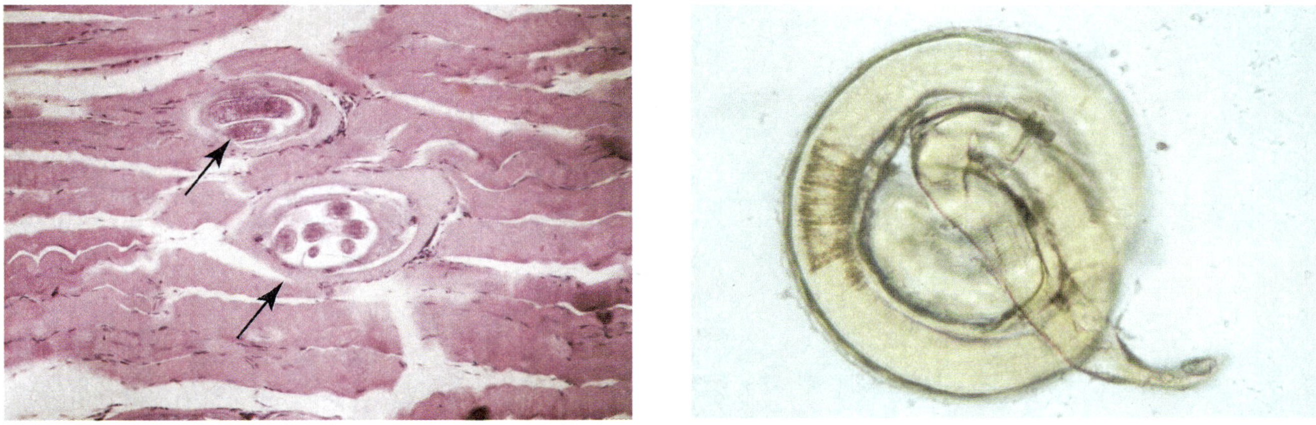

(A) (B)

Figure 8-8 Trichinellosis. **(A)** Biopsy of skeletal muscle showing encysted larvae surrounded by fibrous capsules. Each cyst measures about 1 mm in diameter (original magnification × 100). **(B)** Higher magnification view of unstained coiled larva with the capsule removed (original magnification × 400).

Courtesy of Leonard V. Crowley, MD, Century College.

cysts within the muscle (**Figure 8-8**). These cysts represent the infectious form of the parasite. The phase of larval migration is associated with severe systemic symptoms, and there may also be symptoms referable to disturbed function of organs that have been heavily infiltrated by the parasites. The disease is usually self-limited and ranges from mild to severe depending on parasite load. Initial symptoms (within days of ingestion) relate to gastrointestinal distress. With time, muscle pain and, less commonly, heart problems may occur.

Tapeworms

Tapeworms, long, ribbonlike worms that sometimes grow to a length of several feet, can inhabit the intestinal tract. In general, tapeworms cause no great inconvenience to the individual carrying them except for depriving the host of the food that nourishes the worm. Three species of tapeworms are recognized: the pork tapeworm, the beef tapeworm, and the fish tapeworm. Humans become infected by eating the flesh of an infected animal that contains the larval form of the parasite. Accidental ingestion of pork tapeworm (*Taenia solium*) ova can result in several forms of infection. Taeniasis denotes an intestinal tapeworm infection. Cysticercosis involves an immature form, the cysticercoid, which creates lesions in muscle. Neurocysticercosis is a parasitic disease of the nervous system that often leads to the development of acquired epilepsy. Infection can result from a human carrier or from contaminated food products. Treatment of the disease is complex and depends on the stage of the infecting organism; it may require surgical removal of cysts from brain spaces and symptomatic therapy to reduce neurological consequences.

Flukes

Flukes are thick, fleshy, short worms provided with suckers for attachment to the host. They have a complex life cycle involving one or more intermediate hosts. Flukes are classified according to the area of the body in which the adult fluke matures and the eggs are deposited. Some species of flukes live in the intestinal tract, others live in the liver, and one species lives in the lung. Some flukes live in the portal venous system and its tributaries or in the veins draining the bladder, where the eggs cause severe inflammation and damage to

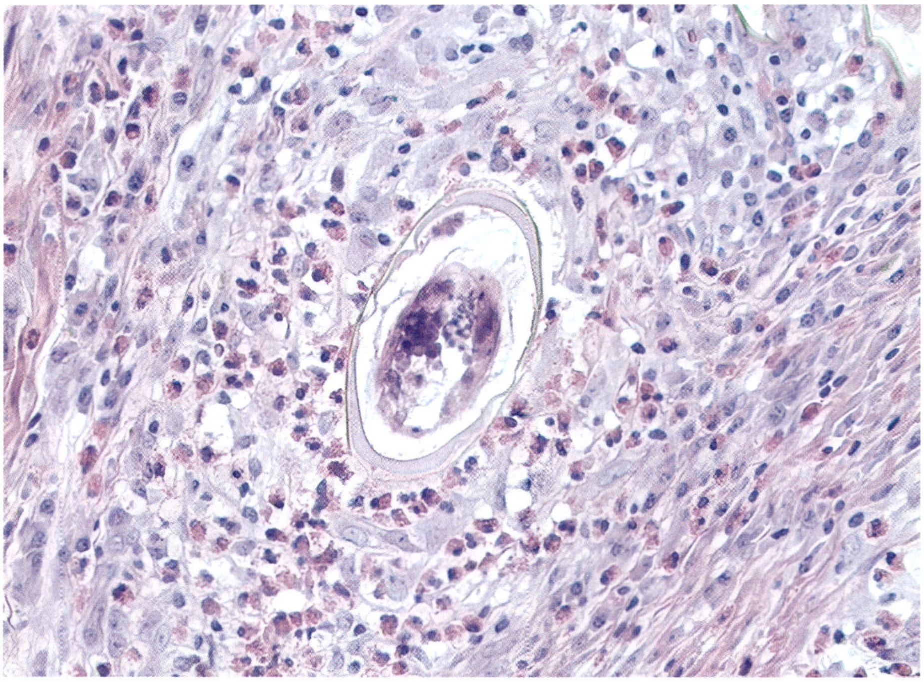

Figure 8-9 An active hepatic Schistosoma granuloma around a central ovum, with a refractile eggshell, surrounded by a giant cell (multinucleated macrophage) and inflammatory cellular infiltrate formed of eosinophils, lymphocytes, and few histiocytes (H&E stain, ×400)

Reproduced with permission from Jamal M, Rayes O, Samuel L, Tibbetts R, Pimentel JD. The Brief Case: Benign Rectal Polyp with Schistosoma mansoni. *J Clin Microbiol.* 2017;55(4):992-995. doi.org/10.1128/jcm.01402-16

the bladder and ureters, which is a major risk factor for development of bladder cancer (**Figure 8-9**). Fluke infections are an important cause of illness and disability in some Asiatic countries, but human fluke infections are not seen in the United States or Canada. Infection with flukes belonging to the genus *Schistosoma* is often referred to as schistosomiasis.

Although human fluke infections do not occur in North America, some animal schistosomes can infect humans, becoming more a nuisance than a cause of serious illness. Birds and mammals, infected with their own specific species of schistosomes, excrete them in their droppings into lakes and other bodies of water, where they develop into the infectious form of the parasite. People who swim in bird or animal schistosome–contaminated lakes may be "attacked" by the parasites, which can penetrate the skin of the swimmers. The parasites cause discrete areas of acute pruritic inflammation at the site where they entered the skin. They cannot cause a systemic infection, however, because humans are not the normal host for the parasite, and the parasites are destroyed in the skin by the body's immune defenses. The condition is called schistosome dermatitis but is more commonly referred to as "swimmers itch." Many lakes in North America and some saltwater beaches are contaminated by bird or animal schistosomes.

Arthropod Invertebrate animal with jointed limbs and segmented body, such as insect and spider. Important arthropods that parasitize humans include the crab louse and the organism causing scabies.

Arthropods

Two common parasitic skin infestations caused by **arthropods**—scabies and lice—are transmitted by close physical contact and often are spread by sexual contact. Both infestations respond promptly to treatment with antiparasitic medications applied to the skin.

Scabies

Scabies is caused by a small parasite called *Sarcoptes scabiei*, which burrows in the superficial layers of the skin, where it lays eggs that hatch in a few days. The infestation causes intense itching. The tracks made by the parasites as they burrow in the skin appear as fine, wavy, dark lines measuring from one mm to one cm in length. Common sites of involvement are the base of the fingers, the wrists, the armpits, the skin around the nipples, and the skin around the belt line.

Crab Louse Infestation

The most common and best-known infectious louse is the **crab louse**, *Phthirus pubis*, which lives in the anal and genital hairs. The organism also causes intense itching. The louse lays eggs that become attached to the hair shafts. Diagnosis is established by identifying either the parasite or the eggs.

Crab louse A parasite of the pubic area; causes intense itching.

Case 9-1

The patient is an 18-year-old female who initially noted a swollen, warm area on her left cheek accompanied by a low-grade fever, headache, muscle aches, and other nonspecific symptoms. Two days later she was alarmed when her right eye became pruritic, swollen, and painful. The condition progressed, and the patient consulted with an ophthalmologist who believed the condition to be either an allergic reaction or a bacterial infection of the conjunctiva and eyelid. Antibiotics were prescribed. The patient did not respond to the therapy and 3 days later sought attention at a local emergency room for increasing fever and headaches, lack of energy, and shortness of breath with no additional symptoms. In the ER the attending physician inquired about recent travel. The patient noted that she had returned about 2 weeks before from an eco-tour to Costa Rica. She had slept in a modern facility under insect netting in Puerto Viejo Limon but had gone on a several-day raft trip up the Pacure River. During this trip she slept on an open platform covered with an insecticide-treated net. She noted that the net appeared old and had several torn areas. She did not apply insect repellent (as she had been instructed) because what was available was "not organic." She was referred to the infectious disease department for additional workup. Initial blood cultures and eye swabs showed only normal skin bacteria. Liver function tests noted a borderline abnormality. However, both electrocardiogram and transthoracic ultrasound disclosed a number of abnormalities suggestive of mild myocarditis. Analysis of her peripheral blood smear showed *Trypanosoma cruzi* organisms. The results were confirmed by the Centers for Disease Control and Prevention using PCR analysis. The patient was treated for 4 months with antiparasitic agents. The patient became negative by PCR analysis following 3 months of therapy.

Discussion

The case demonstrates a typical presentation of acute Chagas disease in a returning traveler from Central America. Chagas disease (American trypanosomiasis) is caused by parasitization by the protozoa *T. cruzi*. It is a zoonotic infection with a multiplicity of both wild and domesticated mammalian hosts. The disease vector is triatomine insects (kissing bugs), which transmit the disease between animal hosts and humans. Triatomines are nocturnal obligate blood-feeding insects that defecate after feeding. Infection occurs when infected feces are deposited on mucosal surfaces or at the site of the bite. Triatomine insects tend to infest thatch roofs, adobe and brick homes, and substandard dwellings. Oral transmission of fecally contaminated food,

(continues)

Case 8-1 *(Continued)*

congenital infections, and transmission via infected blood products (now much reduced by blood screening) can also occur. In this case, the initial swelling was likely the site of an insect bite (a chagoma), which may show local parasite infection or may be the result of an immune reaction to the bite. Such swellings are of minor medical concern. Unilateral eye swelling is a typical sign/symptom of disease and infection of the conjunctiva by the organism. Of more concern is systemic infection by the organism, which can produce acute myocarditis and infection of the brain and its coverings. Treatment is critical as the disease may become chronic and lead to severe cardiac and gastrointestinal disease that is difficult or impossible to treat.

Chagas disease is prevalent in South and Central America, where it may produce more disability than malaria. Aggressive insect eradication programs for dwellings and donor blood screening programs have reduced disease frequency; however, deforestation has led to increased movement of insects to more heavily inhabited areas. Only a handful of autochthonous (indigenous) cases of insect-vectored Chagas disease have been reported in the United States. This is quite surprising, as both the insect vector and infected sylvatic (not domesticated, "wild") mammalian animal hosts, which are the disease reservoirs, are common in the southern United States. In the Southeast raccoons, opossums, and armadillos serve as infected hosts; in the Southwest, woodrats and many other small mammals are infected. In addition, infected domestic dogs have been found in the South. Sylvatic animal dens are often colonized by the vector triatomine insects. Hence, the lack of "native" U.S. disease is likely related to the quality of housing and rarity of vector insect infestation. It is of interest that several of the "native U.S. cases" demonstrated triatomine insects in the dwelling.

Etiology and Pathogenesis

Travel-related infection by *Trypanosoma cruzi*, producing acute Chagas disease, is characterized by cutaneous and ocular symptoms and mild myocarditis.

Questions

1. An essential part of taking a patient's history is to question recent travel outside of the United States. Why is this information of particular relevance in cases of suspected parasitic disease?
2. Parasitic infestation is often considered to be insignificant in the United States. Cite examples of protozoal parasitic disease that have caused significant public health problems in the United States.
3. Several roundworm (nematode) parasites still frequently occur in the United States, particularly in children. What simple precautions can be taken to prevent infestation?

Questions for Review

1. What are some of the more important protozoal infections?
2. How is malaria transmitted?
3. What is trichinellosis? How is it transmitted?
4. What are the more important worm infestations? What are their manifestations?
5. What parasitic diseases are acquired from unclean water sources? From chlorinated water sources?
6. How do people become infected with pinworms? How do they acquire an *Ascaris* infection?
7. What is the source of most parasitic disease in the United States?

References

Parasites. Centers for Disease Control and Prevention. http://www.cdc.gov/parasites/

- A large number of texts discuss the study of parasitic disease (parasitology) in great detail. However, the CDC is an authoritative source that is readily available, up to the minute, and should always be consulted first.

Yellow Book and Travelers' Health. Centers for Disease Control and Prevention. www.cdc.gov/travel/

- This site has definitive information on travel-related health and provides links to the definitive "Yellow Book" with information on disease risks country by country.

Bern C, Kjos S, Yabsley MJ, Montgomery SP. *Trypanosoma cruzi* and Chagas' disease in the United States. *Clin Microbiol Rev.* 2011;24(4):655-681.

Carter YL, Juliano JJ, Montgomery SP, Qvarnstorm Y. Case report: Acute Chagas disease in a returning traveler. *Am J Trop Med Hyg.* 2012;87(6):1038-1040.

Edwards MS, Stimpert KK, Bialek SR, Montgomery SP. Evaluation and management of congenital Chagas disease in the United States. *J Pediatric Infect Dis Soc.* 2019;8(5):461-469. doi:10.1093/jpids/piz018

- Three useful references to *Trypanosoma cruzi* and Chagas disease with particular reference to the United States. (Note: The case is in part based on the second reference.)

Dorny P, Praet N, Deckers N, Gabriel S. Emerging food-borne parasites. *Vet Parasitol.* 2009;163(3):196-206.

Dunn N, Juergens AL. Giardiasis. StatPearls - NCBI Bookshelf. Published February 12, 2024. https://www.ncbi.nlm.nih.gov/books/NBK513239

Ito A, Budke, CM. Culinary delights and travel? A review of zoonotic cestodiases and metacestodiases. *Travel Med Infect Dis.* 2014;12(6):582-591.

Shamsi S, Sheorey H. Seafood-borne parasitic diseases in Australia: Are they rare or underdiagnosed? *Intern Med J.* 2018;48(5):591-596.

- Three references for those interested in exotic foods, fish, and the parasites therein. The last is of particular interest to sushi lovers (even outside of Australia).

Alonso PL, Brown G, Arevalo-Herrera M, et al. A research agenda to underpin malaria eradication. *PLoS Med.* 2011;8(1):e1000406.

- An excellent series of articles on the current status of attempts to eradicate malaria. The supplement referenced contains a number of short review articles. Malaria is an increasing worldwide problem and is becoming harder to control because the organisms are becoming resistant to antimalarial drugs. About 1000 new cases are reported annually in the United States, usually acquired outside the country by travelers, military personnel, and immigrants from malaria-endemic countries, but a small number of cases are acquired in the United States.

Oo WH, Gold L, Moore K, Agius PA, Fowkes FJI. The impact of community-delivered models of malaria control and elimination: A systematic review. *Malar J.* 2019;18(1):269.

- Public health interventions at the community level are critical in malaria control. Which models of community-based interventions work best? Of particular relevance to those interested in international public health.

Fernando SD. Climate Change and Malaria—A Complex Relationship. United Nations. https://www.un.org/en/chronicle/article/climate-change-and-malaria-complex-relationship

- This article discusses how climate change will impact malaria control.

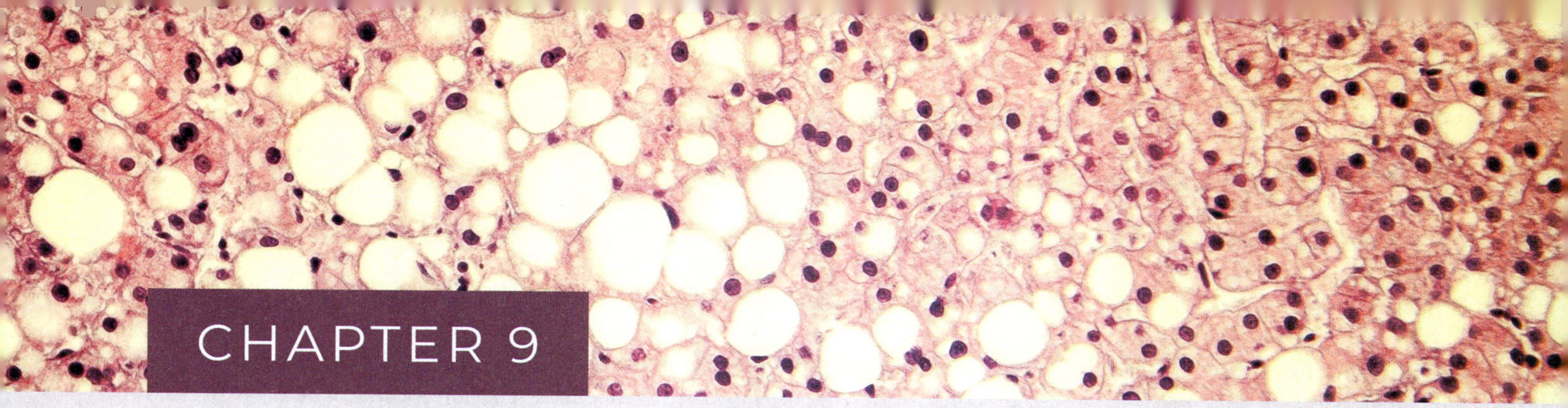

CHAPTER 9

The Cardiovascular System

LEARNING OBJECTIVES

1. Explain the basic anatomy and physiology of the heart and relate information to the common types of heart disease.
2. Explain how the heartbeat is generated and sustained.
3. Describe the pathogenesis of primary myocardial disease.
4. Describe the development and treatment of cardiac arrythmias.
5. Describe the pathogenesis of myocardial ischemia. Describe the clinical manifestations of coronary heart disease. Explain the methods of treatment and their rationales.
6. List the major complications of myocardial infarction and describe their clinical manifestations.
7. Explain the general principles applied to the diagnosis and treatment of coronary heart disease and myocardial infarction.
8. Compare and contrast myocardial ischemia and myocardial infarction.

Cardiac Structure and Function

The heart is a muscular pump that propels blood through the lungs and to the peripheral tissues via the vasculature. Heart disease results from a disturbance in the function of the cardiac pump due to an intrinsic defect of pump function, a defect of the vasculature, or a combination of both. A working knowledge of the normal structure and function of the heart is essential to gaining understanding of the various manifestations of heart disease. The heart is a cone-shaped muscular pump weighing about 350 g. It's enclosed within a fibrous sac termed the **pericardium** located in the **mediastinum**, the middle compartment of the thorax. The pericardium is lined by a layer of mesothelial cells that is continuous with a similar layer of mesothelial cells covering the external surface of the heart. The heart is composed of three layers: the **epicardium**, a layer of mesothelial cells overlying a small amount of loose fibrous and adipose tissue on the external surface of the heart; the **myocardium**, a thick layer of cardiac muscle forming the bulk of the heart; and the **endocardium**, a thin layer of endothelial cells lining the chambers and covering the surfaces of the heart valves. The heart consists of four chambers

Pericardium Fibrous sac enclosing the heart.

Mediastinum Middle compartment of the thorax.

Epicardium/myocardium/endocardium Three layers of the heart moving from the external surface to the internal.

Atrium/atria Upper chambers of the heart.
Ventricle One of two lower chambers of the heart.
Fibrous framework Layer of dense fibrous tissue located between the atria and the ventricles.

divided by septae (singular septa or septum). The two upper chambers, the right and left **atria** (singular, **atrium**) are separated by the interatrial septum. The right atrium receives venous blood returning to the heart; the left atrium receives oxygenated arterial blood returning from the pulmonary circulation. The two lower chambers become separated by the interventricular septum into the right and left **ventricles**. The right ventricle pumps venous (deoxygenated) blood through the pulmonary artery to the lungs. The oxygenated blood returns to the left atrium and then passes to the left ventricle, which pumps oxygen-rich blood throughout the body. The blood circulated throughout the body collects into veins and eventually returns to the right atrium. The right and left cardiac chambers work together, but normally no direct communication exists between the chambers on the right and left sides of the heart. It can be clinically convenient to consider each half as an independent structure. The "right heart" pumps deoxygenated venous blood into the pulmonary artery, which then courses through the lungs (the pulmonary circulation), and the "left heart" receives oxygenated blood from the pulmonary vein and pumps blood through the aorta for distribution to the various organs and tissues in the body (the systemic circulation) (**Figure 9-1**).

The atrial and ventricular musculature encircles the heart and attaches to a layer of dense fibrous tissue termed the **fibrous framework**. The framework is located between the atria and ventricles extending into the upper part of the interventricular septum surrounding the openings of the cardiac valves. The fibrous framework separates the atrial muscle fibers from those in the ven-

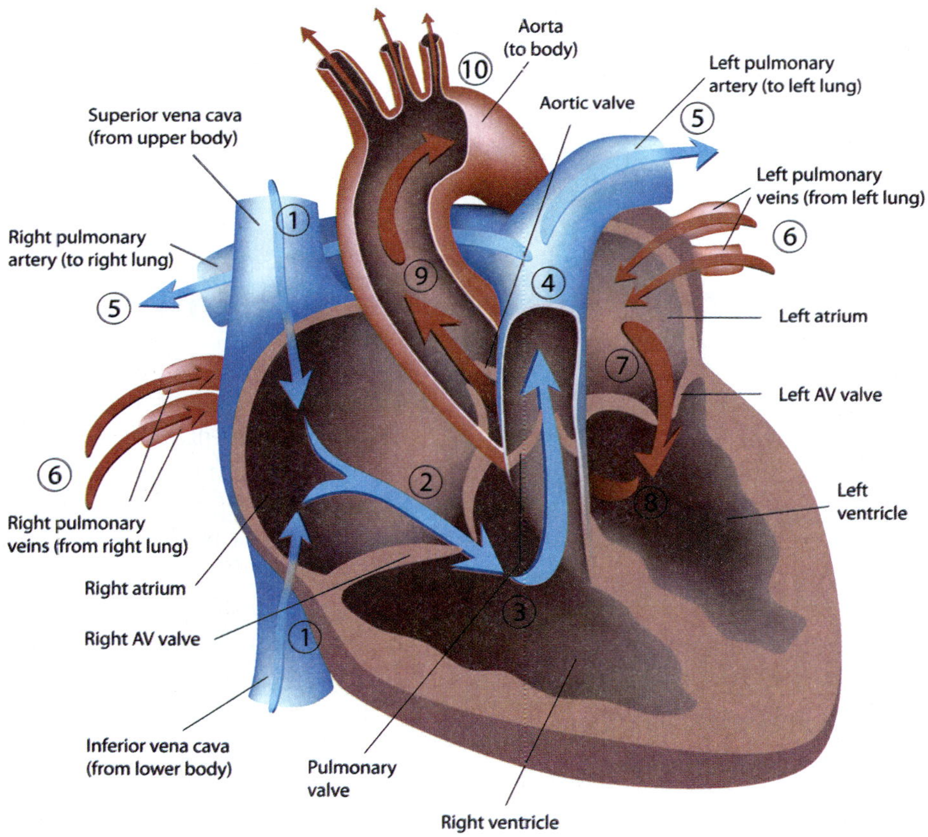

Figure 9-1 Blood flow in the heart is normally unidirectional, with the tricuspid valve on the right and the bicuspid valve on the left preventing backflow from the ventricles into the atria.

tricles, allowing the atrial and ventricular muscles to function independently. Contraction of cardiac muscle reduces the size of the chambers, compressing the blood inside and squeezing it out of the chambers. The fibrous framework provides a firm support to which the heart valves can attach and contains a small opening for the passage of the atrioventricular bundle (bundle of His), which carries electrical impulses to the ventricles.

Cardiac Valves

The controlled flow of blood into and out of the cardiac chambers is regulated by a system of four valves permitting blood flow in only one direction. The flaplike **atrioventricular (AV) valves** permit blood flow from the atria into the ventricles. The **tricuspid valve** moderates the right atrium and ventricle; the **mitral valve** (so named because of its resemblance to a bishop's mitre) separates the left atrium and ventricle. The free margins of the valves are connected to the papillary muscles of the ventricular walls by narrow, stringlike bands of fibrous tissue termed the **chordae tendineae** (in layman's terms, the heartstrings) (**Figure 9-2A**). These bands prevent the valves from prolapsing (falling back) into the atria during **ventricular systole** (the period of ventricular contraction). The **semilunar valves** surrounding the orifices of the aorta (the **aortic valve**) and pulmonary artery (the **pulmonary valve**) are positioned so that the free margins of the valves face upward. This structural arrangement creates cuplike pockets between the free margins of the valves and the roots of the blood vessels to which the valves are attached (**Figure 9-2B**).

When the heart relaxes in **diastole** (the relaxed phase of the cardiac cycle, when the chambers fill with blood), the chordae produce tension on the valves and pull the atrioventricular valves apart. When the ventricles contract in systole, the chordae are no longer under tension, and the force of the blood flow pushes the valves together so that no blood flows "backward" from the ventricles into the atria. During ventricular contraction, the semilunar valves are forced apart by the increased intraventricular pressure of blood, allowing blood to leave the ventricles. When ventricular contraction ceases, the weight of the volume of ejected blood forces the valves back into position, closing the valves,

Atrioventricular (AV) valves The flaplike heart valves located between the atrium and the ventricle.

Tricuspid valve AV valve separating the right atrium and ventricle.

Mitral valve AV valve, also called the bicuspid valve, separating the left atrium and ventricle.

Chordae tendineae Bands of fibrous tissue connecting the margins of the valves to papillary muscles.

Ventricular systole Period of ventricular contraction.

Semilunar valve The cup-shaped valve located between the ventricles and the aorta or pulmonary artery.

Aortic valve Semilunar valve surrounding the orifices of the aorta.

Pulmonary valve Semilunar valve surrounding the orifices of the pulmonary artery.

Diastole Ventricular relaxation.

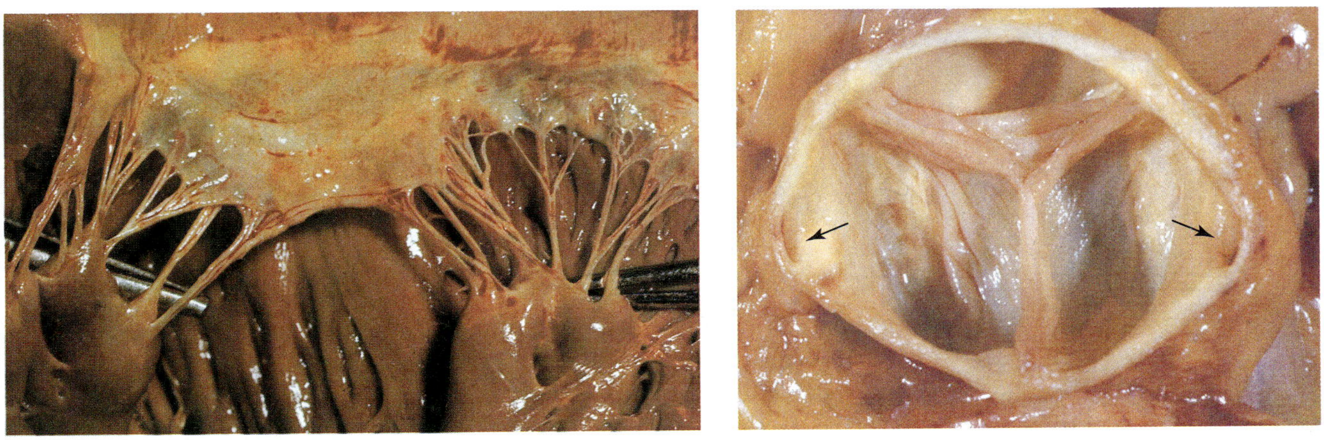

(A) (B)

Figure 9-2 **(A)** Normal mitral valve, illustrating thin chordate extending from valve leaflets to papillary muscles. **(B)** Aortic valve viewed from above, illustrating a cup-shaped configuration of valve leaflets. Note the openings of coronary arteries (*arrows*) arising from the base of the aorta adjacent to the aortic valve leaflets.

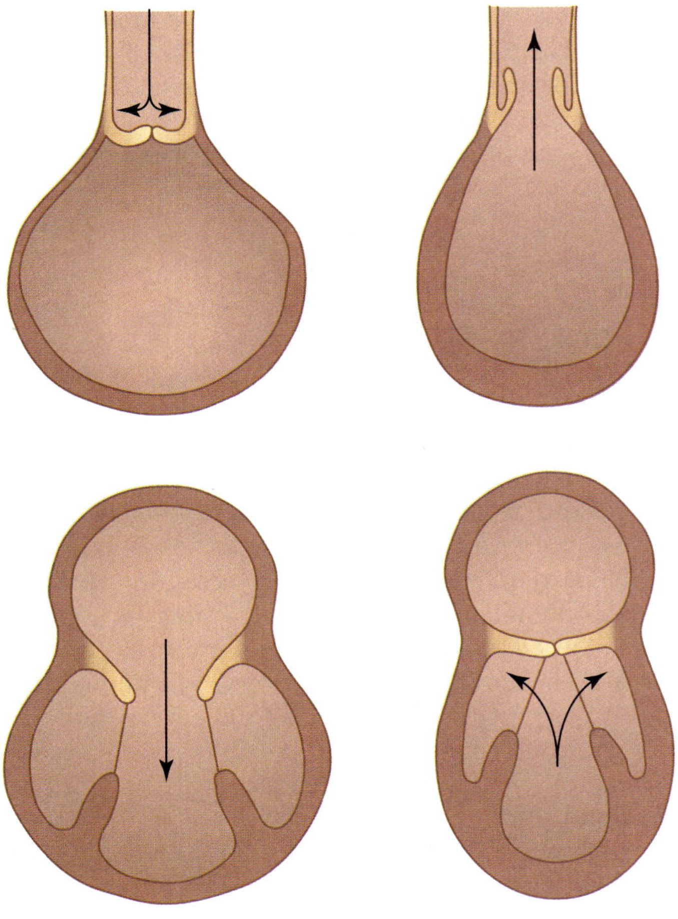

Figure 9-3 Reciprocal action of atrioventricular and semilunar valves, resulting in unidirectional blood flow.

thereby preventing reflux of blood into the ventricles during diastole. The atrioventricular and semilunar valves function reciprocally, meaning, ideally, when one set of valves is open, the other set is closed. Ventricular contraction relaxes tension on the chordae, causing the atrioventricular valves to close while the increased intraventricular pressure of blood in the ventricles forces the semilunar valves to open. Closure of the semilunar valves during diastole (heart muscle relaxed and chambers are filling with blood) is associated with opening of the atrioventricular valves. **Figure 9-3** illustrates the reciprocal action of the two sets of valves, which is responsible for the unidirectional flow required for normal cardiac function.

Blood Supply to the Heart

The heart is supplied by the coronary arteries that arise from the aortic sinuses at the root of the aorta (**Figure 9-4**), meaning that the heart muscle itself receives blood almost as soon as it is pumped out of the left ventricle. The left coronary artery is a short vessel that divides into two major branches. The left anterior descending artery supplies the front of the heart and the anterior part of the interventricular septum. The circumflex artery swings to the left (circum = around + flex = bend) to supply the left side of the heart. The right coronary artery swings to the right, supplying the right side of the heart, and then descends to supply the back of the heart and the

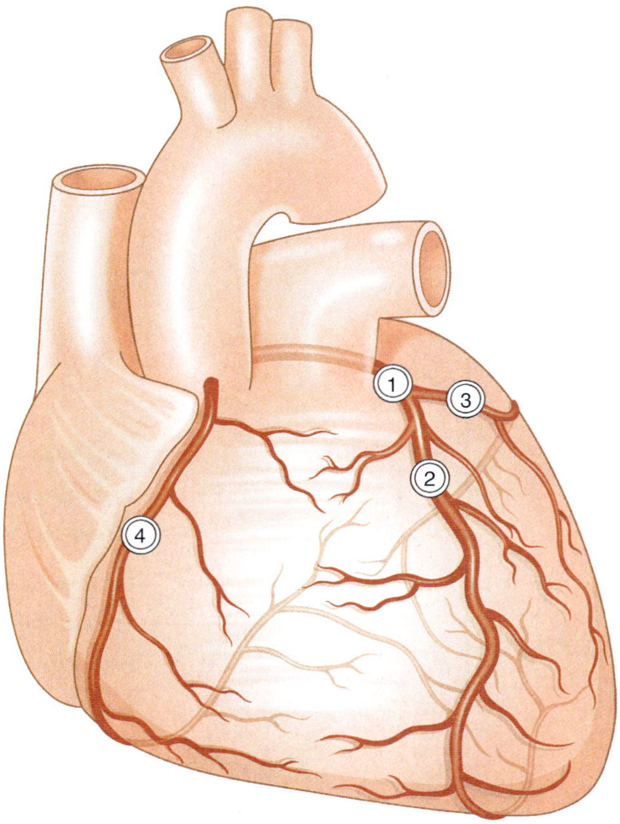

Figure 9-4 The vessels that supply blood to the cardiac muscle: (1) left main trunk, which splits into three supporting arteries; (2) left anterior descending artery; (3) left circumflex artery; and (4) right coronary artery.

posterior part of the interventricular septum. Each coronary artery divides into many branches that supply the heart muscle. The terminal branches of the coronary arteries frequently connect within anatomical arrangements termed anastomoses (singular, **anastomosis**). These anastomoses become important when obstruction of one of the arteries or its branch could impede the blood flow to the tissues normally served by that artery. When an anastomosis is present, blood flow to the area served by the vessel does not necessarily become completely interrupted. The **collateral circulation** reduces the risk of injury and damage.

If blood flow is not sufficient to support the metabolic function of heart cells, ischemia occurs as a consequence of diminished delivery of oxygen to the cells resulting from reduced blood flow. If this continues, a segment of cardiac myocytes will eventually die and undergo necrosis (an infarct). The infarcted area may heal, but adult cardiac cells do not divide. Consequently, non-contractile scar tissue will replace the cardiac myocytes in the areas of damage.

Conduction System of the Heart

The impulses that stimulate the heart to beat are initiated and propagated by groups of specialized muscle cells collectively referred to as the conduction system of the heart (**Figure 9-5**). Impulses generated in the sinoatrial (SA) node, located in the right atrium near the opening of the superior vena cava, result from **spontaneous depolarization**. This automatic change in cell membrane potential occurs without stimulation from other cells and proceeds

Anastomosis A communication between two blood vessels or other tubular structures. Also refers to a surgical connection of two hollow tubular structures, such as the divided ends of the intestine or a blood vessel (surgical anastomosis).

Collateral circulation An accessory circulation capable of delivering blood to a tissue when the primary circulation is blocked, as by a thrombus or embolus.

Spontaneous depolarization The automatic change in cell membrane potential that occurs without stimulation from other cells.

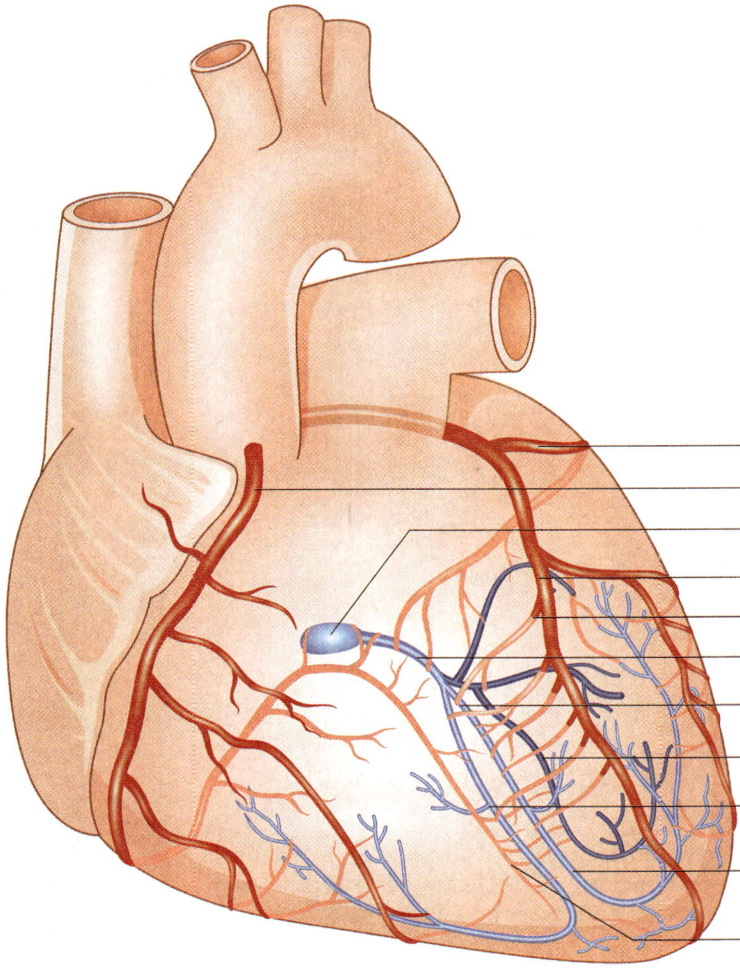

Figure 9-5 Cardiac conduction system and its blood supply The cardiac impulse originates in the SA node and proceeds to the ventricles via internodal tracts of conduction fibers.

in a rhythmic pattern. The conduction system passes the impulses throughout the heart. Small bundles of fibers termed internodal tracts connect the SA node to the atrioventricular (AV) node, located posteriorly in the lower part of the atrial septum. The atrioventricular bundle (bundle of His) continues from the AV node, transmitting the impulse to the ventricles passing through a small opening in the fibrous framework mentioned previously. After entering the interventricular septum, the AV bundle divides into right and left bundle branches, which descend in the septum and extend into the ventricles, where they terminate as Purkinje fibers that activate the heart muscle. The depolarization rate is also influenced by the autonomic nervous system. Sympathetic nervous system impulses increase the rate, and parasympathetic impulses slow it. The normal rhythm established by the cardiac conduction system is often termed a normal sinus rhythm to emphasize that the normal cardiac rhythm is controlled by the sinoatrial node (which is often termed simply the sinus node).

Although any part of the conduction system can depolarize spontaneously and generate an impulse, the SA node normally functions as the cardiac pacemaker because it depolarizes about 60 to 70 times per minute, which in turn stimulates depolarization of the other parts of the conduction system, which depolarize at a slower rate. However, if impulse transmission from the SA node is interrupted by damage to the conduction system, the AV node, which discharges at about 50 times per minute, can take over, and if this system fails, then the bundle or bundle branches can initiate impulses but at a still slower rate of about 30 to 40 times per minute.

The Cardiac Cycle

The sequence of events that occurs during a single contraction and relaxation of the cardiac chambers is referred to as the cardiac cycle. During diastole, both the atria and ventricles are relaxed, the chambers are dilated, and the pressure of the blood within the chambers is very low. Normally at rest, each ventricle in diastole contains about 120 mL of blood, and much of the blood that fills the ventricles flows passively into the ventricles through the open atrioventricular valves. Later in diastole, initial atrial contraction (the beginning of atrial systole) expels an additional 30 mL of blood into the ventricles. For a heart at rest with a normal heart rate, the additional blood pumped into the ventricles by atrial contractions is not essential for reasonably normal cardiac function. The extra volume makes a greater contribution to ventricular filling when the heart beats rapidly.

The ventricles contract following completion of atrial systole, the left ventricle ejecting blood into the aorta at high pressure and the right into the pulmonary artery at much lower pressure. Both ventricles contract at the same time with the heart muscle undergoing a wringing motion. Each ventricle ejects the same volume of blood. The stroke volume (SV) is the amount of blood ejected from the ventricle with each heartbeat. Normal stroke volume averages 60–80 mL, which is only a portion of the 120 mL of blood that filled the chamber. Consequently, the percentage of the ventricular volume ejected during systole is termed the **ejection fraction**, a measurement that is often used when evaluating heart function. The total blood volume pumped over time will be influenced by the heart rate (HR) measured in beats per minute.

Ejection fraction Percentage of the ventricular volume ejected during systole.

Cardiac output (CO) is the output of blood from a single ventricle in one minute and can be calculated by the formula CO = HR × SV. The CO for most cardiac-healthy adults is close to 5 L/min; 5 L is equivalent to the blood volume of an average adult. During vigorous activity, the normal heart of a healthy young person can double the stroke volume and greatly increase the heart rate, increasing cardiac output from four to seven times the resting cardiac output.

Blood Pressure

The flow of blood in the arteries is a result of the force of ventricular contraction. The pressure within the arteries varies rhythmically with the beating of the heart. The highest pressure is reached during ventricular contraction as blood is ejected into the aorta and its branches (systolic pressure). The pressure is lowest when the ventricles are relaxed and filling (diastolic pressure); the recoil of the stretched arteries provides the force to propel the blood between contractions. The peripheral arterioles regulate the rate of blood flow into the capillaries by adjusting the radius of the arteriole. If the smooth muscle in the arteriole contracts, the radius becomes smaller. If the muscle is not contracted, the radius becomes larger. The muscles in arteries and veins do offer some resistance, so the blood pressure during cardiac diastole does not fall to zero but declines slowly as blood leaves the large arteries and enters the arterioles and then the capillaries (**Figure 9-6**).

The elasticity of the large arteries also influences the systolic pressure. Some of the pressure rise caused by the blood ejected from the ventricle is absorbed by the stretch of the arteries, so the systolic pressure does not rise as high as it would if the arteries were more rigid and unable to stretch normally. In

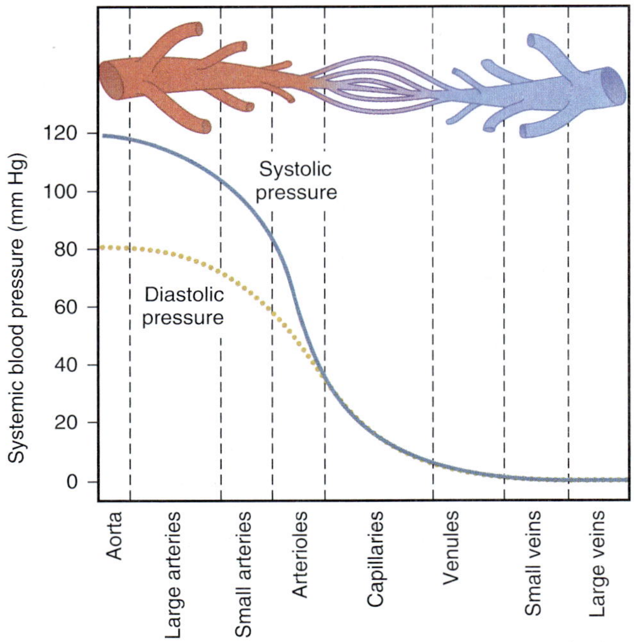

Figure 9-6 Changes in blood pressure as distance from the left ventricle increases.
Data from Shier, D.N., Butler, J.L., and Lewis, R. *Hole's Essentials of Human Anatomy & Physiology*, Tenth Ecition. McGraw Hill Higher Education, 2009.

summary, blood pressure depends on cardiac output and the resistance of the peripheral vascular system. The systolic blood pressure is a measure of the force of ventricular contraction as blood is ejected into the large arteries and the resistance of the arterial system (sometimes termed the tone of the system). The diastolic pressure is a measure of the pressure in the arteries between heart beats, which is governed in part by the peripheral resistance caused by the small arterioles throughout the body. The mean (average) pressure of blood in the large arteries is approximately midway between systolic and diastolic pressure. Both cardiac output and vascular resistance are regulated by multiple physiologic systems to accommodate the body's needs, as discussed in Chapter 12.

Tools to Examine Cardiovascular Function

The Electrocardiogram

Electrocardiogram (ECG) A technique for measuring the serial changes in the electrical activity of the heart during the various phases of the cardiac cycle. (Often termed ECG or EKG.)

The **electrocardiogram (ECG)** is a measure of the electrical activity of the heart as measured on the surface of the body by means of electrodes attached to the legs, arms, and chest. Voltage differences are recorded as a series of upward (positive) and downward (negative) deflections that form a characteristic pattern of deflections named in order: P, Q, R, S, and T. The P wave reflects the initial wave of depolarization associated with atrial systole. The Q, R, and S waves, collectively termed the QRS complex, reflect the depolarization of the ventricles, which is followed by ventricular systole. The T wave represents repolarization of the ventricles during diastole. The time interval from the beginning of the P wave to the beginning of the QRS complex, which is termed the PR interval, reflects the time required for the depolarization wave to pass through the AV bundle from the atria to the ventricles (**Figure 9-7**).

In most modern clinical settings, the ECG tracing will be displayed on a fluorescent screen. When the recordings need to be saved as a hard copy or

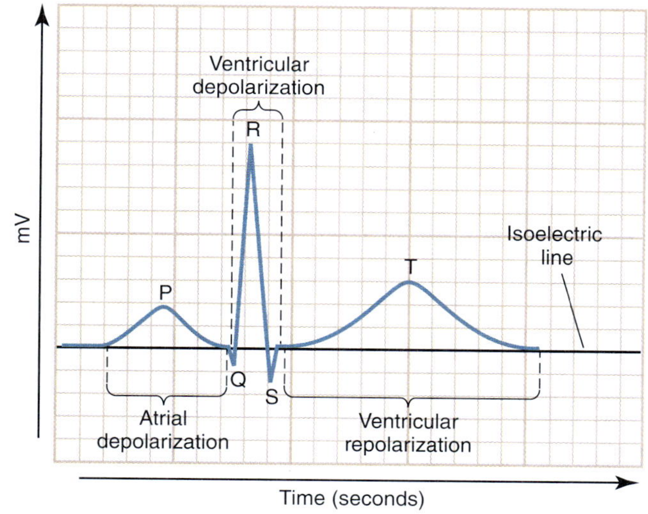

Figure 9-7 Characteristic features of a normal electrocardiogram.

transported non-electronically, a printout can be generated on a long strip of graph paper with regularly marked intervals. The printout can undergo closer examination to analyze heart rhythm. Some electronic systems will display the results in traditional graph paper style format with some of the vital measurements calculated on the paper.

The ECG is a valuable diagnostic aid that can identify characteristic disturbances in the heart rate or rhythm and abnormalities in the conduction of impulses through the heart. The ECG can also identify heart muscle injury, as occurs following a heart attack, and can contribute to determining the extent of the damage to the heart muscle (**Figure 9-8**).

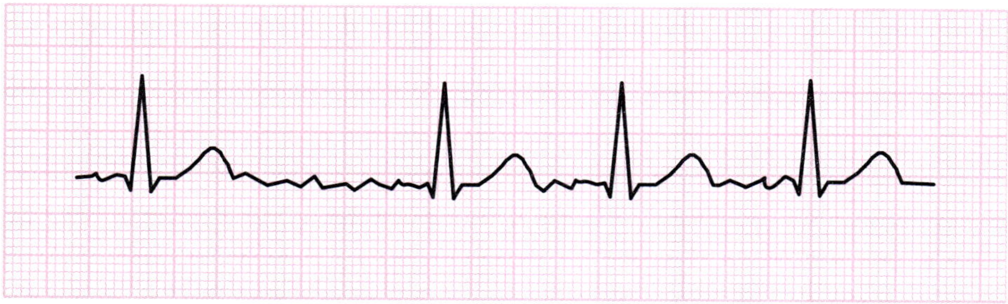

(A)

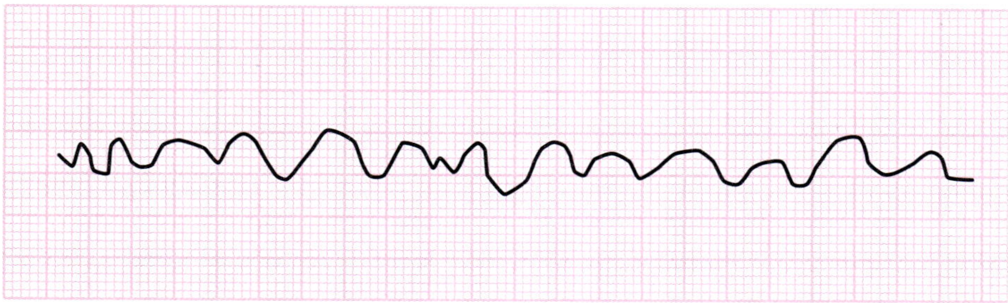

(B)

Figure 9-8 **(A)** Atrial fibrillation illustrating absence of distinct P waves together with irregular ventricular rate, usually 140 to 160 beats per minute. **(B)** Ventricular fibrillation illustrating extremely abnormal chaotic cardiac rhythm without any evidence of synchronized electrical impulses.

Garcia TB, Holtz NE. *Introduction to 12-Lead ECG*. Boston, MA: Jones and Bartlett Publishers; 2003

Echocardiography

Echocardiogram A record obtained from an ultrasound examination of the heart and related blood vessels; used to assist in the diagnosis of cardiovascular disease.

Arrhythmia An irregularity of the heartbeat.

Ultrasound examinations, described in Chapter 1, have many applications in medicine. An ultrasound examination of the cardiovascular system is usually termed an **echocardiogram**. Echocardiography can visualize and evaluate many different alterations in cardiac function. It can detect heart valve abnormalities resulting in heart murmurs. Blood clots, which may have formed inside the heart as the result of an **arrhythmia**, trauma, or heart attack, can be identified and managed before they leave the heart and create pathology elsewhere. An echocardiogram can document fluid buildup in the pericardium, tumors, and problems with the aorta, and provide real-time visualization of the heart's responses to certain treatments as well. The most common type is transthoracic echocardiography. A transducer is placed on the chest, which sends ultrasound waves through the chest wall to the heart. As the ultrasound waves bounce off of the structures in the heart, they are converted by a computer within the echo machine to images. A stress echocardiogram will use either pharmaceuticals or exercise to make the heart beat faster and work harder. A transesophageal echocardiogram gets a closer look at the heart because the transducer is actually passed down the esophagus, so it is in very close proximity to the heart.

Cardiovascular Disease: An Introduction

Cardiovascular disease refers to any disease or pathology that affects the heart or the blood vessels. Heart disease refers to diseases affecting the blood supply to the heart, also referred to as coronary heart disease (**Figure 9-9**). According to the CDC, approximately one in five deaths in the United States is associated with heart disease. When thinking about the etiology of cardiovascular disease and the subsequent pathology, it is important to remember that the heart functions as a biological version of some forms of mechanical pumps that may be encountered in everyday life. A pump needs a regulatory system. For cardiac function, that includes the coronary conduction system combined with the electrical overrides provided by the autonomic nervous system. Any pump needs a mechanism to create enough force to push the material being pumped through the system. In the heart, that would be the cardiac muscle and the processes that provide energy and support to the cardiac muscle. To work at maximum efficiency, a pump needs a steady reliable supply of the material that it's designed to pump. The heart pumps blood; consequently, adequate venous blood returning to the heart is important for maintaining healthy heart function. When considering the pathologies discussed as follows, it may be useful to stop and think about which part(s) of the pump mechanism seem to be malfunctioning.

According to the Center for Disease Control and Prevention (CDC), heart disease is the number one cause of death for both men and women in the United States. The World Health Organization (WHO) lists cardiac disease and pulmonary disease as the top two causes of non-violent deaths worldwide. Understanding and controlling cardiovascular disease will lead to better national and international health outcomes.

Cardiovascular disease can result from congenital (and sometimes inherited) defects in the structure of the heart or in the contractile apparatus of cardiac myocytes (Chapter 16). Infectious agents may damage heart valves and cardiac myocytes. Atherosclerotic disease of the coronary arteries will lead to compromised blood supply to the heart, termed coronary ischemia. If severe, ischemia will result in cardiac necrosis. The formation of necrotic tissue defines

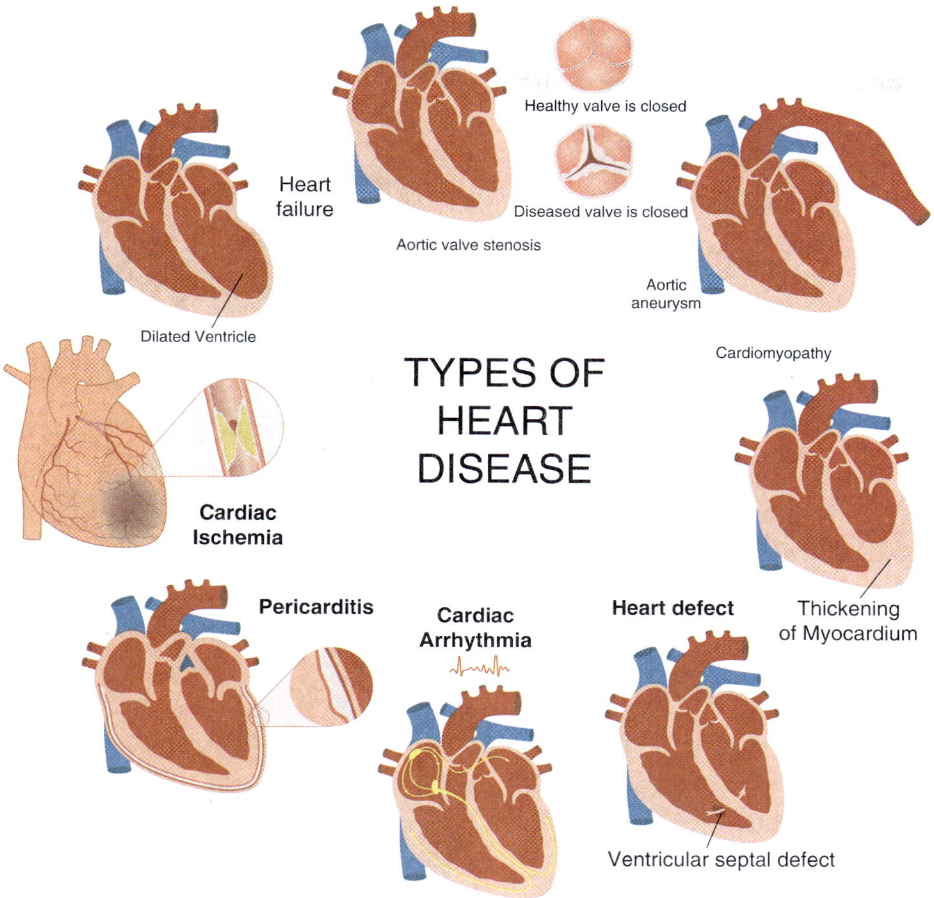

Figure 9-9 Heart disease constitutes a collection of symptoms and pathologies that contribute to the etiology of those symptoms. Many of the pathologies noted in this figure will be covered in more detail.

a myocardial infarct (heart attack) with sequelae that may result in sudden cardiac death or some degree of chronic heart disease and heart failure. Systemic hypertension (excessive systemic blood pressure) will cause the heart to compensate by undergoing left ventricular hypertrophy. Ultimately, the heart may not be able to compensate for the extra workload and can eventually result in heart failure. Some forms of cardiac pathophysiology will be discussed in more detail as follows.

Myocarditis

Myocarditis describes an active inflammation in the heart muscle associated with injury, which may lead to necrosis of individual muscle fibers. In the United States, most cases are caused by viruses: coxsackievirus, parvovirus B19, and human herpesvirus 6 (**Figure 9-10**). Rarely, myocarditis may be caused by parasites, such as *Trichinella* or *Trypapnosoma cruzi,* the pathogen of Chagas disease (see Chapter 8). The parasites lodge in the myocardium and cause inflammation. Occasionally, other pathogens, such as the fungus causing histoplasmosis, invade the cardiovascular and pulmonary systems. Histoplasma infections arise more frequently in immunocompromised patients. Some cases of myocarditis result from a hypersensitivity reaction, such as myocarditis associated with acute **rheumatic fever** (discussed later in this chapter) and some drug reactions.

Rheumatic fever A disease caused by hypersensitivity to antigens of the Group A beta-hemolytic streptococcus, characterized by fever, joint pains, and inflammation of heart valves and muscle.

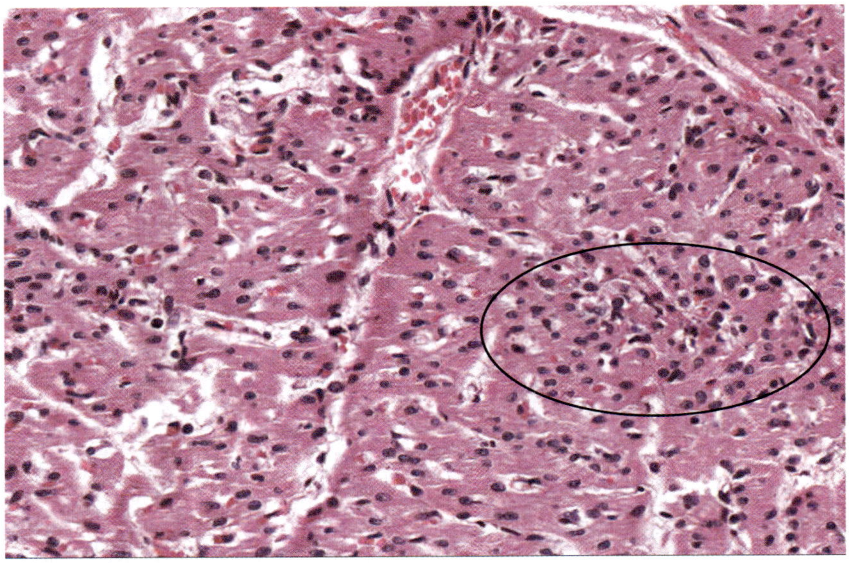

Figure 9-10 Photomicrograph of acute viral myocarditis in a child. There is infiltration of the heart by mononuclear inflammatory cells in response to the viral infection. The highlighted area shows a locus of inflammatory cells and destruction of cardiac myocytes.

Courtesy of Department of Pathology and Laboratory Medicine, University of North Carolina at Chapel Hill.

The onset of myocarditis is usually abrupt and may lead to acute heart failure. Fortunately, in most cases, the inflammation subsides completely and the patient recovers without any permanent heart damage. There is no specific treatment other than treating the underlying condition that caused the myocarditis and decreasing cardiac work by bed rest and limited activity until the inflammation subsides.

Cardiomyopathy

The general term *cardiomyopathy* encompasses several different conditions of which dilated cardiomyopathy (DCM) and hypertrophic cardiomyopathy (HCM) are most important (**Figure 9-11**). One-third of DCM cases are hereditary and most are transmitted as dominant traits. More than 50 genes are associated with the disease. DCM can also be associated with alcohol and cocaine abuse and some anti-cancer agents. Dilated cardiomyopathy is characterized by enlargement of the heart and dilatation of its chambers. The pumping action of the ventricles is greatly impaired, which leads to chronic heart failure. For most cases of DCM, the disease is considered to be idiopathic, with the acknowledgment that a genetic component does probably play a role.

Approximately only one in five people with hypertrophic cardiomyopathy (HCM) get diagnosed. The main reason is that they appear to be asymptomatic, though their heart muscle has thickened. In these cases, the thickening hasn't affected blood flow, and symptoms don't show up if oxygen-rich blood is reaching all parts of the body. Sometimes thickening of the heart muscle is detected when people have imaging tests for other health-related issues. About 80 percent of the time, HCM is caused by mutations in heart-associated genes, with eight genes being more predominant and displaying an autosomal dominant inheritance pattern. The responsible gene mutations can be identified by genetic tests. Hypertrophic cardiomyopathy is characterized by disarray of the cardiac muscle fibers, causing them to intersect at odd angles with no apparent organized pattern, which can result in marked hypertrophy

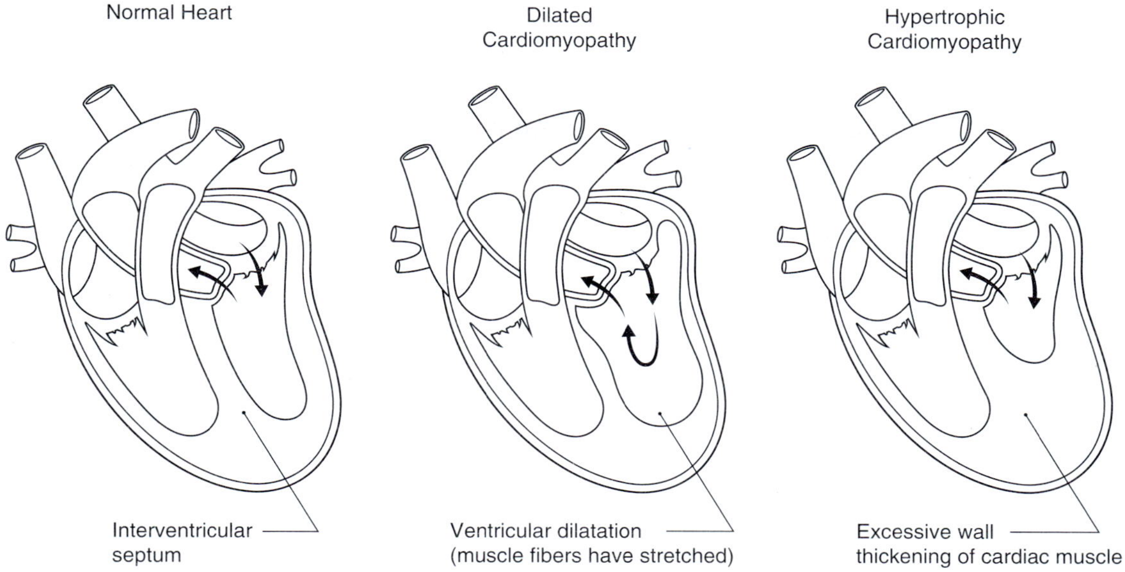

Figure 9-11 With dilated cardiomyopathy, the muscle fibers become stretched and the ventricle walls become thin and the heart chambers enlarged, making heart contractions less efficient. Patients with hypertrophic cardiomyopathy have increased thickness in cardiac muscle fibers and scar tissue resulting in reduced capacity inside the heart chambers.

of heart muscle to such an extent that the thick-walled chambers become greatly reduced in size and do not dilate readily in diastole. Frequently, the muscle of the septum is hypertrophied to a greater extent than the rest of the myocardium and hinders outflow of the blood from the ventricle into the aorta. At times, the thick septum may actually impinge on the anterior mitral valve leaflet, intermittently completely blocking the outflow of blood from the left ventricle (HCM with outflow tract obstruction) (**Figure 9-12**).

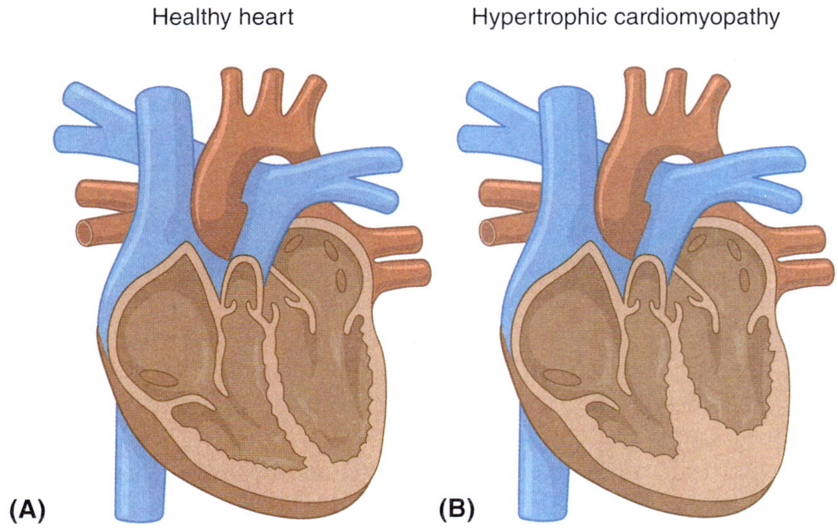

Figure 9-12 A comparison of normal cardiac function with malfunction characteristic of hypertrophic cardiomyopathy. **(A)** Normal heart, illustrating unobstructed flow of blood from left ventricle into aorta during ventricular systole. **(B)** Hypertrophic cardiomyopathy, illustrating obstruction to outflow of blood from left ventricle by hypertrophied septum, which impinges on anterior leaflet of mitral valve.

Patients with HCM that show outflow tract obstruction frequently exhibit manifestations related to inadequate cardiac output, such as episodes of excessive fatigue and lightheadedness related to exertion. The characteristic myocardial hypertrophy with greatly thickened septa can be identified by echocardiography (see Figure 9-12). Treatment consists of administering drugs that slow the heart, allowing more time for ventricular filling, and that reduce the force of ventricular contraction, which tends to reduce the degree of obstruction caused by the hypertrophied septum. Commonly used drugs are those that block the sympathetic nerve impulses that normally increase heart rate and the force of contraction (beta blockers) and those that decrease myocardial contractility by impeding the flow of calcium into myocardial cells (termed calcium channel blocking agents). People who do not respond to medical treatment may require surgical resection of part of the thickened septum.

Valvular Heart Disease

Conditions that cause valve malfunction contribute to valvular heart disease. These may include various degenerative conditions of the aortic valve and an abnormality of the mitral valve that causes it to prolapse into the atrium during ventricular systole.

Rheumatic Fever and Rheumatic Heart Disease

Rheumatic valvular heart disease has markedly declined, along with the incidence of rheumatic fever. Rheumatic fever is a complication of infection by the group A beta hemolytic streptococcus, the bacteria responsible for streptococcal sore throat and scarlet fever. Clinically, the affected individual has an acute arthritis affecting multiple joints (which is why the disease is called "rheumatic" fever) and evidence of inflammation of the heart.

Rheumatic fever is not a bacterial infection but the result of a hypersensitivity reaction induced by various antigens present on the streptococcus. This reaction develops several weeks after the initial streptococcal infection. Some individuals form antibodies against antigens present on the streptococcus, which cross-react with similar antigens in the individual's own tissues, a process known as molecular mimicry. The antigen–antibody reaction occurring on the tissues of the body injures the tissue. The inflammatory response resulting from this injury causes the fever and other associated symptoms. Fortunately, rheumatic fever develops in only a small proportion of people with group A beta-hemolytic streptococcal infections.

Patients with acute rheumatic fever rarely die as a result of severe inflammation of the heart and consequent acute heart failure; generally the fever and signs of inflammation eventually subside, although healing is often associated with some degree of scarring. In the joints and in many other tissues, scarring causes no difficulties, but scarring of heart valves may produce deformities that impair their function.

Rheumatic heart disease is caused by scarring of the heart valves subsequent to the healing of a rheumatic inflammation. This complication is relatively common and primarily affects the valves of the left side of the heart, the mitral and aortic valves (**Figure 9-13**). If the valve does not close properly, blood refluxes back through it (**regurgitation**). Frequently, the damaged valve also does not open properly, and the valve orifice is narrowed. This is called valvular **stenosis**. Valve lesions impair cardiac function. When valvular stenosis is

Regurgitation Backward flow of blood in the heart because of a valve does not close properly.
Stenosis Abnormal narrowing of a passageway.

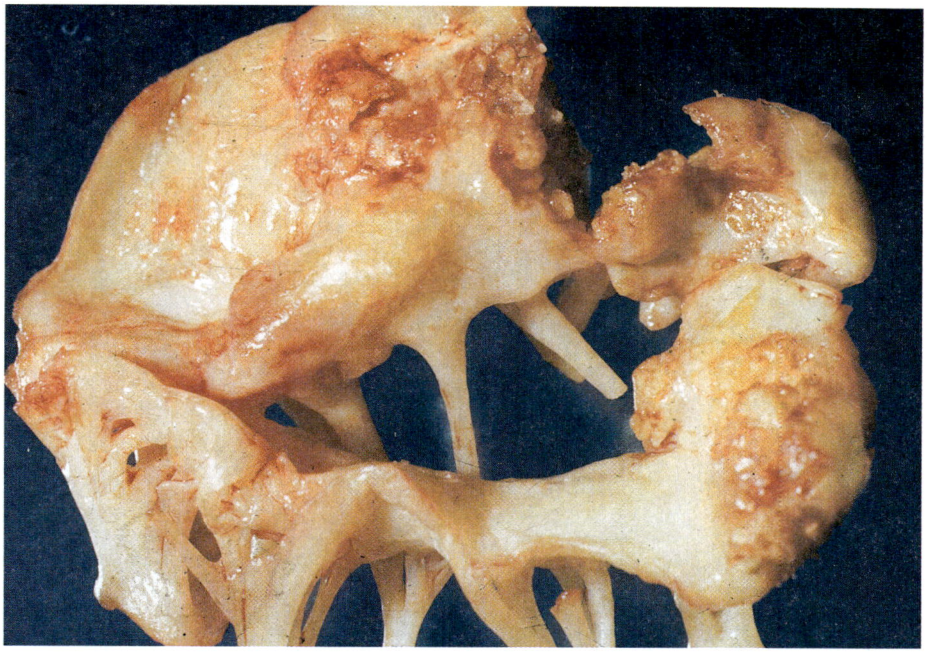

Figure 9-13 A poorly functioning scarred and calcified mitral valve resulting from valve damage caused by prior rheumatic fever. The valve was excised and replaced by an artificial heart valve.

Courtesy of Leonard V. Crowley, MD, Century College.

present, the heart must exert more effort than normal to force blood through the narrowed orifice. In regurgitation, a portion of the ventricular output is not expelled normally and leaks through the incompetent valve. This is a serious disadvantage because the heart must repump the volume of regurgitated blood to deliver the same amount of blood to the peripheral tissues.

When a person is seriously disabled by a rheumatic valvular deformity, it is possible to excise the abnormal, scarred heart valve surgically and replace it with an artificial valve (discussed later in this chapter).

Nonrheumatic Aortic Stenosis

Nonrheumatic aortic stenosis can be caused by aortic stenosis secondary to an abnormal aortic valve or by the aging of the valve. In about two percent of people, the aortic valve has two rather than the usual three cusps. This abnormality is called a congenital bicuspid aortic valve. The valve functions satisfactorily for a time but is subjected to unusual stress during opening and closing because of its bicuspid configuration. As a result, the valve gradually becomes thickened and may eventually become calcified after many years, leading to marked rigidity of the valve, often when a person reaches middle age (**Figure 9-14**). This condition is called aortic stenosis secondary to bicuspid aortic valve.

Fibrosis and calcification of the valve leaflets of a normal three-cusp aortic valve may also occur. Often the inflammatory response triggers the development of scar tissue. In some people the valve may become so rigid that it is unable to open properly. A valve with significant calcification leading to stiffening and malfunction can be described as calcific aortic stenosis (**Figure 9-15**).

Mild degrees of aortic stenosis may not greatly compromise cardiac function, but severe aortic stenosis places a great strain on the left ventricle, which must expel blood through the significantly narrowed and rigid valve orifice. This condition can lead to marked left ventricular hypertrophy and eventual

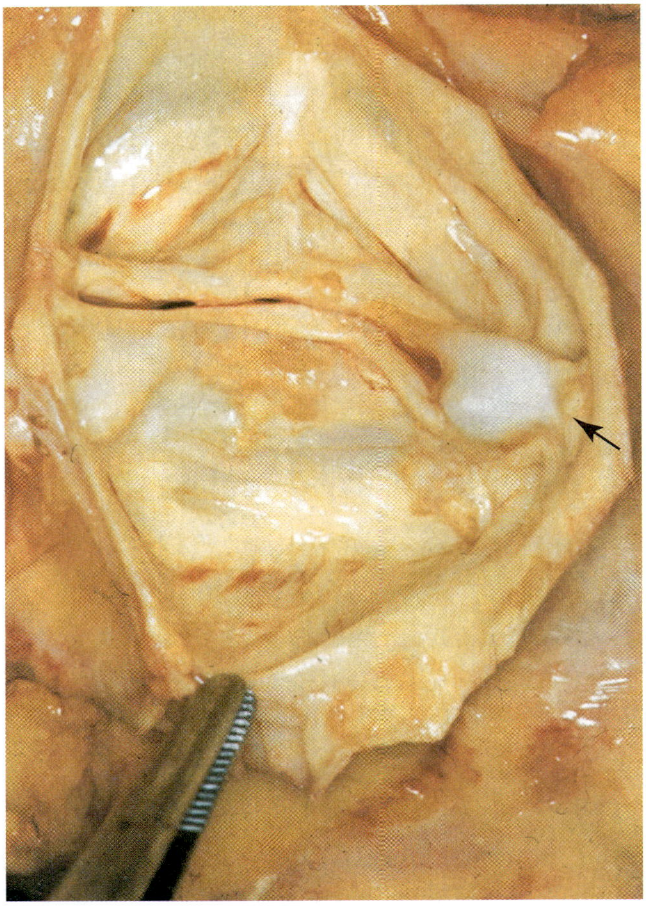

Figure 9-14 A congenital bicuspid aortic valve viewed from above. Beginning scarring is seen at the right margin of the valve (*arrow*).

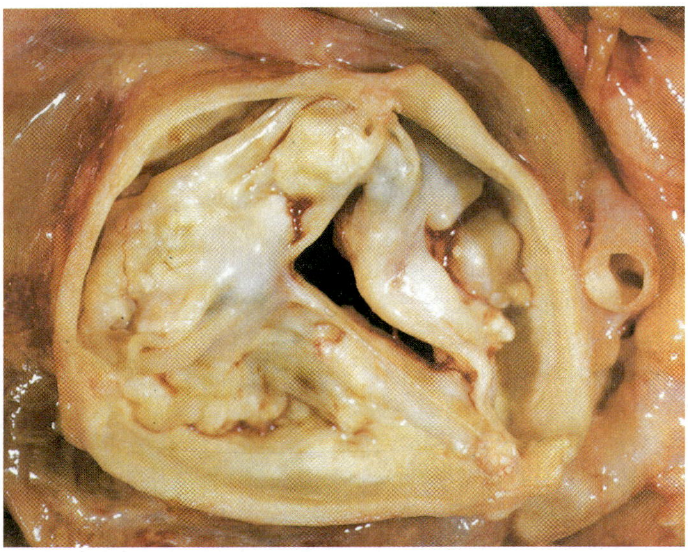

(A)

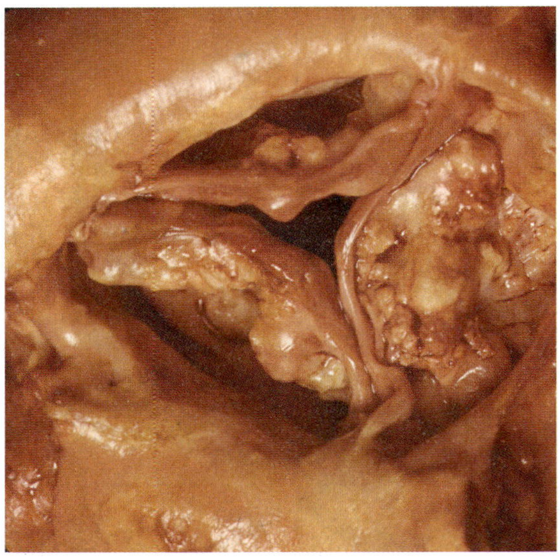

(B)

Figure 9-15 An aortic valve viewed from above, illustrating marked thickening and nodularity of valve leaflets. **(A)** Partial fusion of valve cusps (*left*). A normal coronary artery is seen in a cross section at right of aortic valve. **(B)** Severe calcific aortic stenosis. Extensive calcium deposits within cusps severely limit valve mobility.

heart failure. Treatment of severe aortic stenosis consists of surgically replacing the stenotic valve with an artificial heart valve.

Aortic stenosis usually is considered to be caused by degenerative changes in valve leaflet connective tissue, which are similar to those seen in atherosclerotic disease (discussed in Chapter 10). As a population ages, aortic stenosis is becoming one of the most common types of valvular heart disease.

Mitral Valve Prolapse

Although mitral valve prolapse is a common condition, only a very small percentage of people experience any problems related to the prolapse. In this condition, one or both mitral leaflets are enlarged and prolapse into the left atrium during ventricular systole. Sometimes, the prolapsing free margins of the valve leaflets do not fit together tightly, allowing some blood to leak across the closed mitral valve into the atrium, termed mitral regurgitation. The amount of blood that leaks into the left atrium through the prolapsing valve depends on how tightly the free margins of the prolapsing valve leaflets come together during ventricular systole (**Figure 9-16**).

In some cases, the prolapse appears to be caused by degenerative changes in the connective tissue of the valve leaflets, which permits the affected valve leaflets to gradually stretch as a result of the degeneration of the valve connective tissue. Eventually, one or both leaflets may become enlarged. When this occurs, the stretched prolapsing mitral valve, held at its margin by the chordae, resembles an open parachute (**Figure 9-17**); a significant amount of blood may reflux into the left atrium. The prolapsing valve may also produce excessive strain on the chordae and papillary muscles, which may provoke bouts of ventricular arrhythmia. Sometimes the excessive stress causes one of the chordae to rupture. Mitral regurgitation may be related to any defect in the structure of the valve (e.g., caused by rheumatic disease or by certain tumors or drugs that increase the circulating level of serotonin) and, if severe, can be associated with acute and chronic disease. Surgical valvular repair or replacement may become necessary.

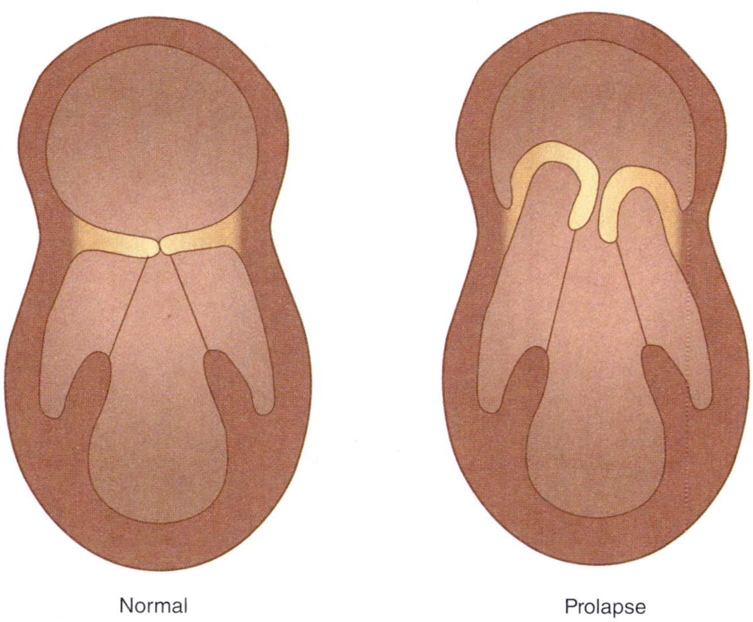

Figure 9-16 Normal mitral valve leaflets (*left*) compared with prolapsing mitral leaflets associated with mild mitral insufficiency (*right*).

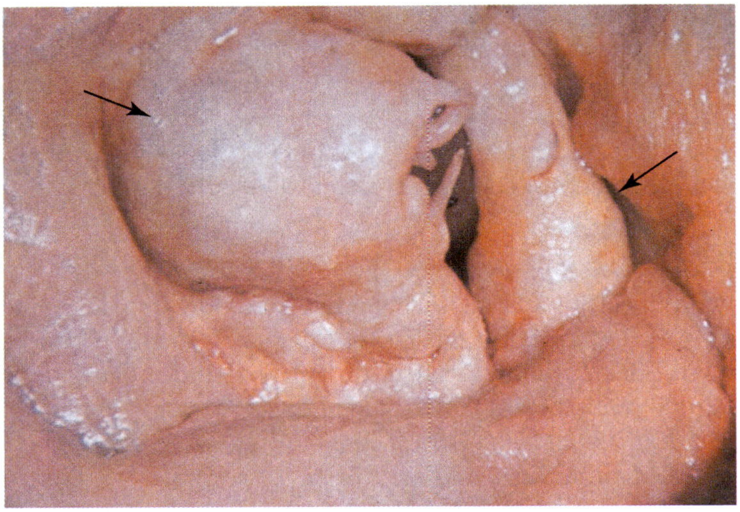

Figure 9-17 The interior of the left atrium viewed from above, illustrating prolapsing mitral valve leaflets ballooning into the left atrium (*arrows*). Prolapse was complicated by a rupture of mitral valve chorda tendinea.

Prosthetic (Artificial) Heart Valves

A heart valve that has been so badly damaged by disease that it no longer can function adequately can be replaced by an artificial valve, termed prosthetic heart valve (prosthesis = replacement).

Infective Endocarditis

Infective endocarditis is an infection of a heart valve, usually caused by bacteria but occasionally by other pathogens (**Figure 9-18**). Infective endocarditis may arise from several types of pathogens. Most significant is the infection of the

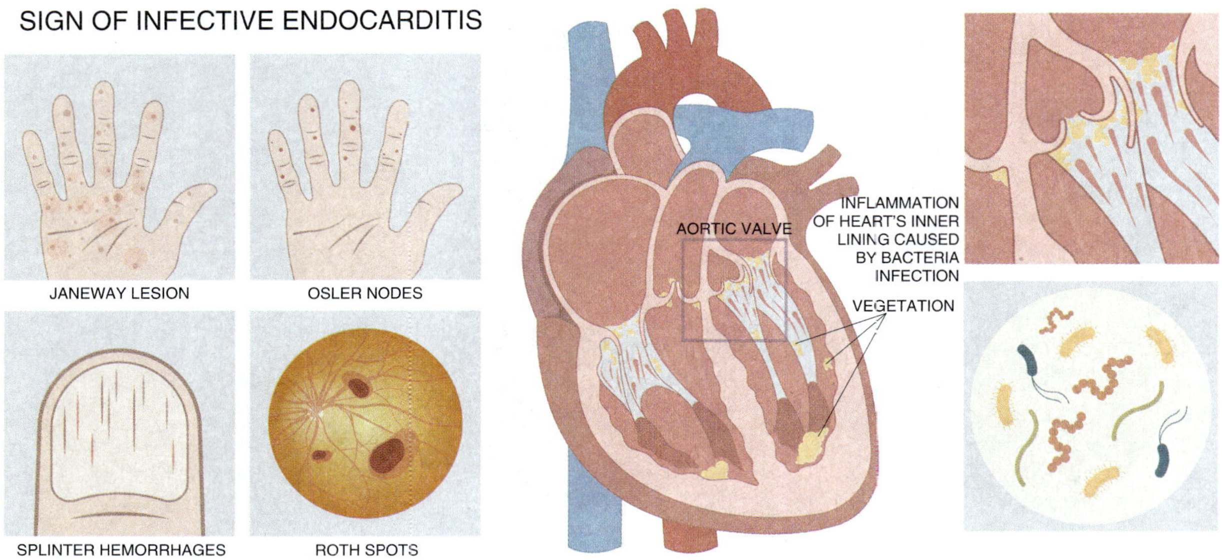

Figure 9-18 Infective endocarditis: Signs, symptoms, and manifestations.

endocardial layer of the heart. Other signs and symptoms may be present as well. In most cases, the infection is in the mitral and aortic valves on the left side of the heart. It is customary to classify infective endocarditis as either subacute or acute infective endocarditis. The subacute form is caused by organisms of low virulence, meaning the organism doesn't pose an alarming infectious threat by itself. However, many pathogens with low virulence may not strongly stimulate the immune system, meaning they contribute to a chronic low-level infection. Any type of valvular heart disease may contribute to infective endocarditis. Acute infective endocarditis, caused by highly virulent organisms that infect previously normal heart valves, presents the symptoms of a severe systemic infection.

Subacute Infective Endocarditis

An abnormal or damaged valve is susceptible to infection because small deposits of aggregated platelets and fibrin may accumulate on the roughened surface of the valve, serving as a site for implantation of bacteria. In people with healthy heart valves, transient bacteremia causes no problems because the organisms are normally destroyed by the body's defenses. However, an individual with a damaged valve runs the risk that bacteria may become implanted on the valve and cause an inflammation (**Figure 9-19**). Frequently, thrombi (blood clots) form at the site of the valve infection, and bits of thrombus may be dislodged and carried as emboli to other parts of the body, producing infarcts in various organs.

Acute Infective Endocarditis

Acute infective endocarditis results when highly pathogenic organisms spread into the bloodstream from an infection elsewhere in the body and infect a previously normal heart valve. Virulent staphylococci are a common cause of acute endocarditis and may cause considerable destruction of the affected valve (**Figure 9-20**).

A group at particularly high risk are intravenous drug abusers; in this group, the infection is usually in the tricuspid valve rather than the valves on the left side of the heart. Infection results from the use of unsterile materials

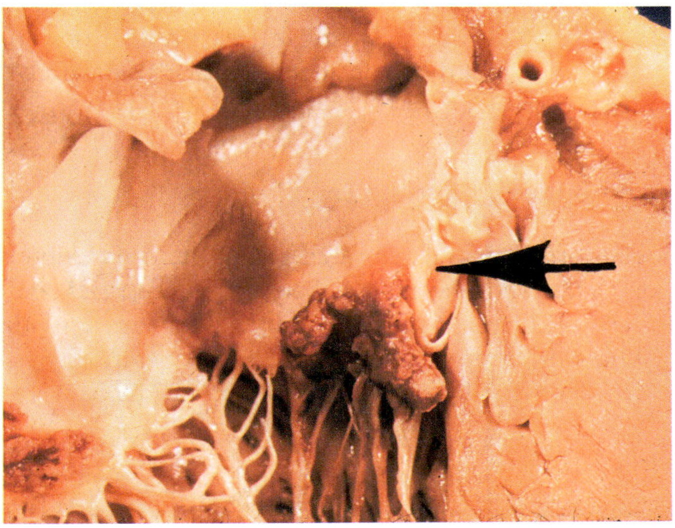

Figure 9-19 Bacterial endocarditis illustrating vegetations on mitral valve leaflet (*arrow*). Normal coronary artery is seen in cross section (*upper right*).

Courtesy of Leonard V. Crowley, MD, Century College.

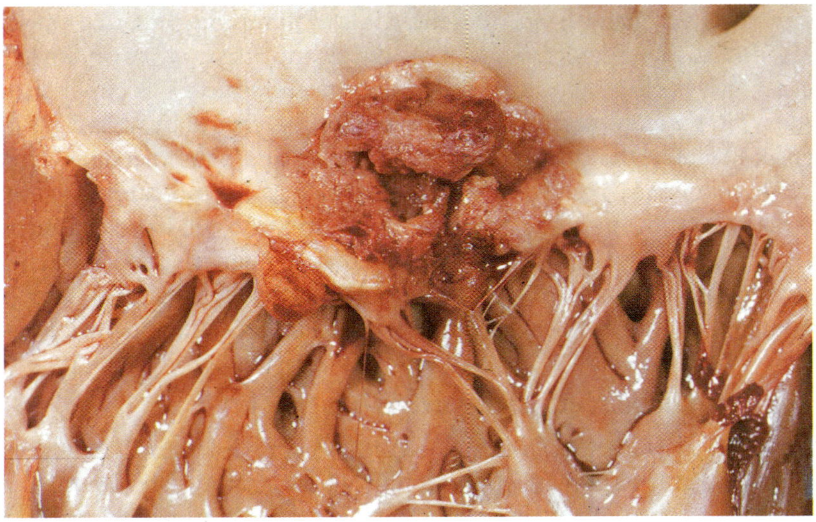

Figure 9-20 Severe bacterial endocarditis caused by staphylococcal infection of a normal mitral valve; infection has caused extensive destruction and perforation of the valve leaflet.

Courtesy of Leonard V. Crowley, MD, Century College.

to dissolve and inject the drug and from the normal skin flora, which may be introduced during the needle stick.

Antibiotic Prophylaxis to Prevent Endocarditis

Infective (bacterial) endocarditis is relatively uncommon, but it is a very serious disease. Individuals with damaged heart valves or other cardiac abnormalities are at increased risk. Some surgical procedures and many dental procedures, such as cleaning and removal of dental plaque, tooth extractions, and root canal treatment, may cause a shower of bacteria to be discharged into the bloodstream, becoming a potential risk to patients with damaged or abnormal heart valves. The American Heart Association provides guidelines regarding who should receive antibiotic prophylaxis, the types of surgical procedures requiring antibiotic prophylaxis, the recommended antibiotics to use, and the recommended dosage and duration of antibiotic treatment. Recent studies published by the American Heart Association indicate that antibiotic prophylaxis should be considered for at-risk patients undergoing non-dental invasive procedures.

Cardiac Arrhythmias

The orderly depolarization and repolarization of the conduction system that directs the contraction and relaxation of the atria and ventricles does not always function perfectly, leading to disturbances in the heart rate or rhythm, called a cardiac arrhythmia. Such problems include atrial or ventricular fibrillation or heart block. See Figure 9-7 for explanation of a normal ECG.

Atrial Fibrillation

One of the more common abnormal cardiac rhythms is called atrial fibrillation (AF), in which the atria contract in an irregular pattern at a very rapid rate. Fibrillation refers to the uncoordinated contraction of muscle fibers. The condition often occurs more frequently as people age. It is found in higher instances in people with cardiovascular disease or chronic pulmonary disease. AF can also be associated with hyperthyroidism, Type II diabetes, smoking, and a few other conditions. AF may include a genetic component as the tendency toward developing AF seems to run in families. Occasionally, AF occurs in apparently normal healthy individuals for no apparent reason.

AF starts as an abnormal focus of electrical activity in the atrium, which abruptly evolves into multiple areas of depolarization throughout the atria that stimulate atrial muscle fibers to contract in a continuously haphazard, disorganized manner at a very rapid rate that can reach up to 400 impulses per minute. The intense disorderly stimulation of multiple groups of atrial muscle fibers causes the atrial muscle to quiver ineffectively instead of contracting normally. This allows blood to "pool" in the atria, which may result in thrombus formation. The abnormal electrical impulses are also relayed to the AV node. The AV node cannot respond to such a large number of stimuli. Only a relatively small number of impulses are able to travel through the AV node and AV bundle (bundle of His) to reach the ventricles. Consequently, the ventricles beat irregularly, often at rates much higher than the patients average heart rate (Figure 9-8A). At such a fast ventricular contraction rate, the duration of diastole is very short. The duration of diastole also varies from beat to beat because the rate at which impulses can be delivered to the ventricles from the quivering atria is not uniform. As a result, the time available for ventricular filling in diastole also varies from beat to beat, which causes the volume of blood filling the ventricles and ejected during each ventricular contraction (stroke volume) to vary. Some of the ventricular contractions occur before the ventricles are adequately filled with blood, and the volume of blood ejected may be insufficient, resulting in **hypotension** (abnormally low blood pressure) and **pulmonary congestion** (pooling of blood in the lungs). The diagnosis of atrial fibrillation is made by examination of the ECG, which reveals a lack of P waves (an indication that the atria are not contracting normally) along with some variability in the QRS complexes related to the variable ventricular stroke volumes (Figure 9-8A).

Hypotension Abnormally low blood pressure.

Pulmonary congestion Pooling of blood in the lungs.

Treatment of Atrial Fibrillation

The first treatment step is to administer drugs that help regulate AV node function. This can be accomplished by giving medications that impede transmission of impulses through the AV node and bundle so fewer impulses reach the ventricles. The drugs include beta blockers, calcium channel antagonists, and sometimes digitalis [digoxin], which decrease heart contractility.

When the heart rate has been slowed, the next step is to restore a normal heart rhythm by terminating the fibrillation. This can be accomplished either by an electrical cardioversion, which involves the application of an electrical shock by paddles applied to the patient's chest to terminate the arrhythmia, or by pharmacologic therapy, which uses drugs that terminate the arrhythmia by interfering with some phase in the abnormal impulse formation to "break up" the arrhythmia. Endoscopic techniques that ablate areas of the heart around the AV node may also be attempted if these therapies fail. Once the normal rhythm is restored, the patient may need to continue taking some medication to maintain the normal rhythm.

Ventricular Fibrillation

In contrast to atrial fibrillation, ventricular fibrillation is incompatible with life because the ventricles are unable to contract normally and the circulation ceases (Figure 9-8B). Ventricular fibrillation sometimes occurs following a heart attack.

If recognized promptly, it is often possible to stop the fibrillation by delivering an electric shock to the heart by means of electrodes applied to the chest. The procedure usually causes the ventricles to resume normal contractions.

Heart Block

Heart block is a delay or complete interruption of impulse transmission from the atria to the ventricles. Usually, the condition results from arteriosclerosis of the coronary arteries, in which parts of the conduction system fail to receive an adequate blood supply. In the mildest form, heart block is manifested only as a delay in the conduction of impulses from the atria to the ventricles. In a more marked degree of block (incomplete heart block), not all the SA node impulses are conducted through the damaged AV bundle. Every second, third, or fourth impulse may fail to reach the ventricle. In the most severe form (complete heart block), conduction of impulses through the AV bundle is completely interrupted. Impulses originating in the SA node cause the atria to contract normally, but the impulses are not transmitted normally to the ventricles. When this occurs, the conduction system distal to the block "takes over" as the source of impulses to activate the ventricles, but the impulses are generated at a much slower rate of 30 to 40 per minute. The extremely low ventricular rate may not provide sufficient blood flow to the brain, resulting in periodic episodes of dizziness or loss of consciousness. Complete heart block is treated by implanting an artificial pacemaker that consists of a small electrode inserted into the heart through a vein and positioned in the ventricle. The electrode is connected to a small device containing a battery that is implanted beneath the skin of the chest. The device can be programmed to generate impulses that stimulate ventricular contractions at a predetermined rate. Many different types of pacemakers are available, each having specific applications.

Myocardial Ischemia and Its Complications: A "Heart Attack"

Several mechanisms may trigger a heart attack in a patient with coronary artery disease. Sudden blockage of a coronary artery may occur by thrombus formation on the surface of an atheromatous plaque (atheroma), a process termed **coronary thrombosis** (**Figure 9-21**). This is most often related to some change in atheroma, such as hemorrhage into the plaque (further narrowing the vessel's lumen), plaque rupture, or sudden damage to the plaque surface exposing the contents of the plaque to the blood (**Figure 9-22A**). Platelets accumulate at the site of the altered atheroma, followed by activation of the blood coagulation mechanism and formation of a thrombus at the site of plaque rupture (**Figure 9-22B**). Vigorous activities, such as running, snow shoveling, or sports activities that abruptly increase cardiac output, thereby raising myocardial oxygen consumption, can precipitate a myocardial infarct because atherosclerotic coronary arteries with their reduced blood flow are incapable of delivering an adequate blood supply to the heart muscle. Severe **myocardial ischemia** (inadequate blood flow reaching the heart muscle) then develops. Severe and prolonged myocardial ischemia may precipitate an acute episode called a "heart attack" (see **Figure 9-23** and **Figure 9-24**). This event may be manifested as damage and necrosis of heart muscle, a myocardial infarction. Cessation of normal cardiac contractions, called a **cardiac arrest**, frequently follows.

Coronary thrombosis Thrombus formation on the surface of a plaque blocking the coronary artery.

Myocardial ischemia Inadequate blood flow through the coronary arteries to the heart muscle.

Cardiac arrest Complete cessation of cardiac activity.

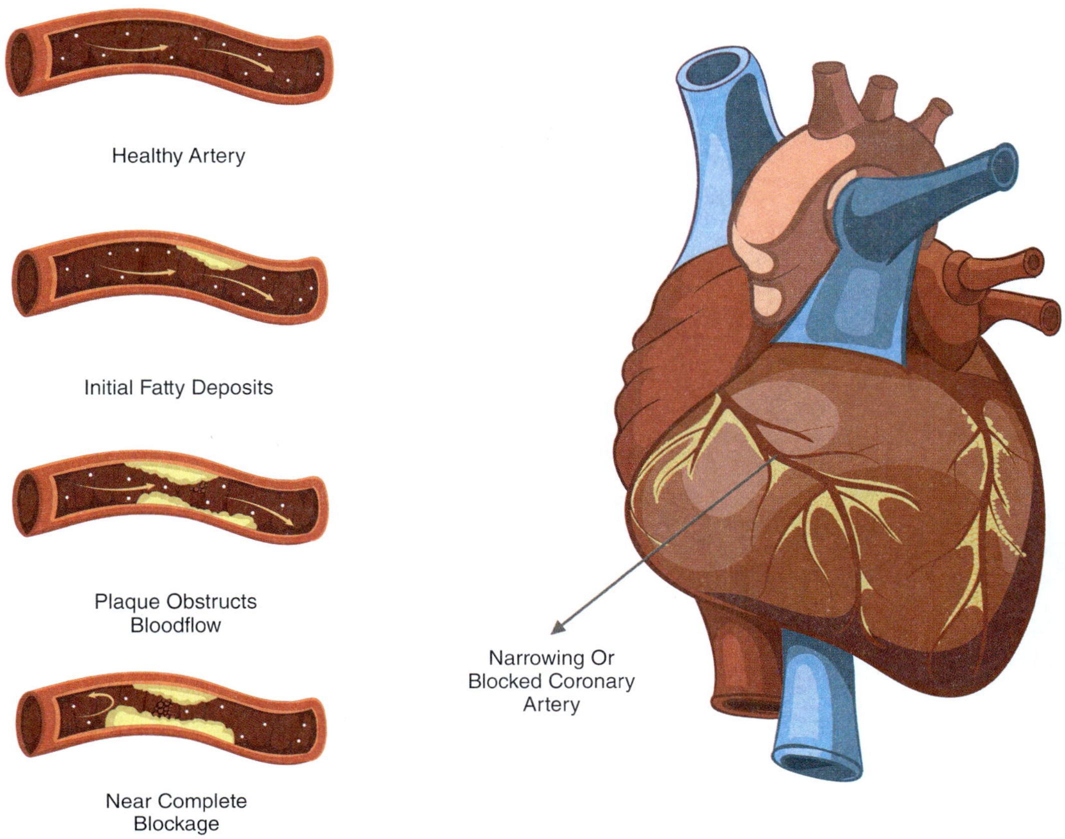

Figure 9-21 Coronary artery disease. The heart pumps continually and therefore it is imperative that it has an adequate and well-functioning blood supply. Coronary artery disease puts the health of the heart tissue at great risk.

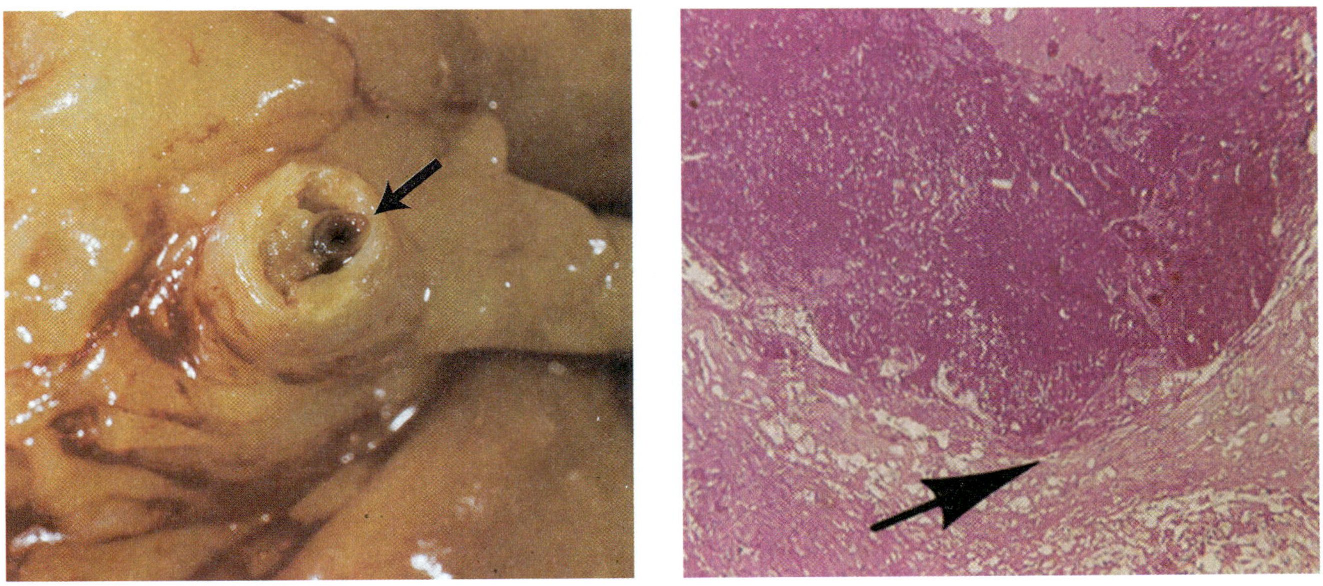

(A) **(B)**

Figure 9-22 **(A)** Marked atherosclerosis of the coronary artery with a thrombus blocking the artery (*arrow*). **(B)** Photomicrograph illustrating thrombosis of the coronary artery at the site of a ruptured unstable atheromatous plaque. Note the absence of fibrous tissue (*arrow*) covering the inner surface of the plaque.

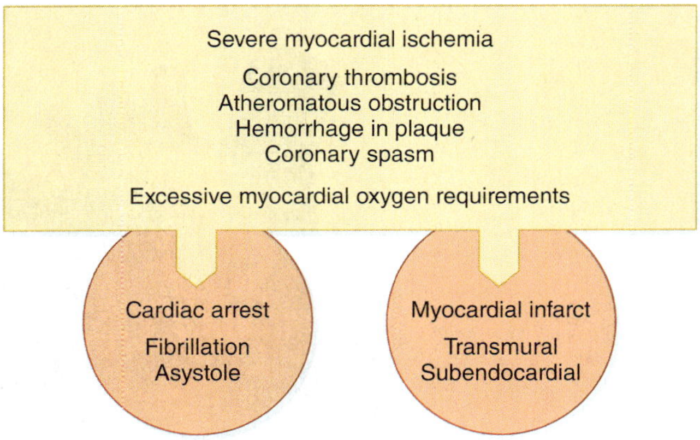

Figure 9-23 Causes and effects of severe myocardial ischemia, as described in the text.

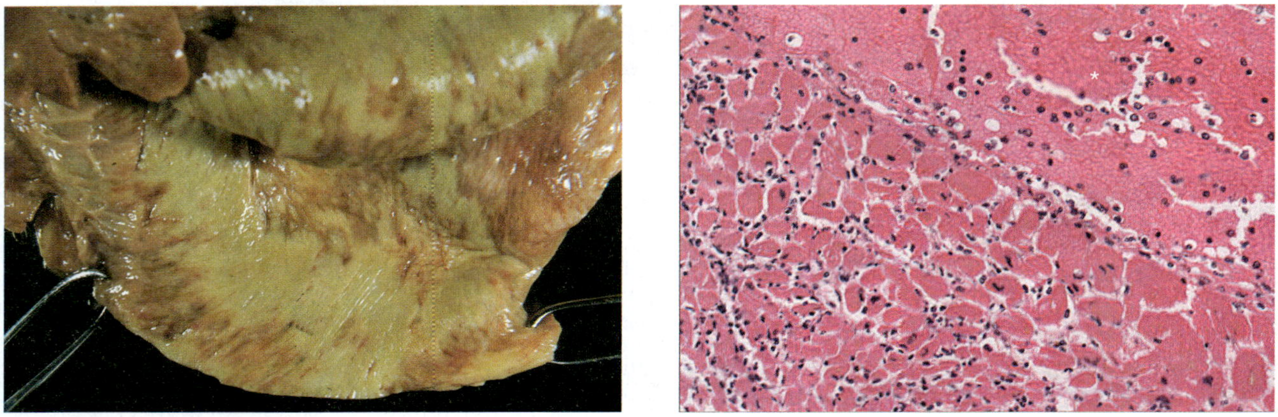

(A) **(B)**

Figure 9-24 **(A)** Longitudinal section through infracted heart muscle, illustrating the pale zone of necrotic muscle that has been infiltrated by inflammatory cells. **(B)** Photomicrograph of a 36-hour-old myocardial infarct demonstrating necrotic myocytes and infiltrating inflammatory cells. Upper right of the image (*star*) is an area of hemorrhage into the heart tissue.

(A) Courtesy of Leonard V. Crowley, MD, Century College; **(B)** Courtesy of Department of Pathology and Laboratory Medicine, University of North Carolina at Chapel Hill.

Cardiac Arrest

Myocardial ischemia may lead to disturbances of cardiac rhythm called cardiac arrhythmias (see previous section). Damage to the conduction pathways of the heart, accumulation of toxic metabolites, and stimulation by the autonomic system all can play a role. Sudden cardiac arrest (SCA) occurs when there is an immediate loss of heart activity. The etiology may be an arrhythmia, severe myocardial ischemia, trauma, or a combination of events. The patient may be experiencing symptoms prior to the cardiac arrest, or the arrest may lead to collapse. Supportive measures, such as CPR (cardiopulmonary resuscitation), need to be undertaken until the heart can be restored to a normal rhythm. The application of an electric shock may stimulate the heart's electrical system to return to a normal rhythm. In cases of ventricular fibrillation, which occurs without warning, the timeframe for restoring normal rhythm can be minutes. Unfortunately, in many cases, the patient dies before medical attention can be obtained. Even in the absence of total arrest, the ischemic heart will demonstrate impaired ventricular contraction because of the loss of functioning cardiac myocytes and lack of synchronous contraction, which should be visible on an ECG. Damaged portions of the ventricle may be **akinetic** (lacking contraction) or **hypokinetic** (showing reduced contraction).

Akinetic/hypokinetic
Lacking or showing reduced contraction.

Acute Coronary Syndrome

The manifestations of a myocardial infarct result from partial to complete obstruction of a coronary artery, making the prognosis related to the amount of muscle damage. The level of muscle damage can be minimized by prompt treatment to restore blood flow to the damaged heart muscle. Compromised coronary function due to coronary thrombosis results in a pattern of injury of increasing severity. Stable angina is considered a chronic condition characterized by predictable chest pain or discomfort during physical exertion or stress. The pain is usually resolved with rest or nitroglycerin. It can often be managed by lifestyle changes and medication. **Acute coronary syndrome (ACS)** is a broad term which refers to several diseases where blood to the heart decreases. It can be classified based on therapeutic criteria, anatomic classification, or electrical activity based upon ECG patterns. ACS includes unstable angina, myocardial infarction, and cardiac death.

Partial chronic blockage of the coronary vasculature results in **stable angina**. This leads to temporary chest pain during stress and exertion that is relieved by rest or vasodilating drugs (such as nitroglycerin) and is not considered part of ACS as it is chronic in nature. The onset of the acute coronary syndrome occurs with a sudden increase in angina of prolonged duration that is resistant to therapy. This delineates **unstable angina** and is associated with an acute worsening in the nature of coronary thrombosis. The anginal chest pain is a direct result of hypoperfusion of the heart muscle analogous to the cramping muscle pain people experience from over exertion of skeletal muscles. The patient requires treatment with anti-angina drugs but also anticoagulant and antiplatelet drugs (blood thinners) to prevent aggregation of platelets that may initiate a coronary thrombosis. Without treatment, unstable angina is likely to progress to non-ST-elevation myocardial infarction (NSTEMI), which is related to the nature of ECG changes observed. ST refers to two of the peaks on an ECG. A myocardial infarction (MI) results from necrosis of heart muscle subsequent to ischemia. Non-ST-elevation MI can be seen as a "mild MI," but one in which death of cardiac myocytes can be detected through laboratory analysis. The ECG may show minor abnormalities but does not reveal the ST-segment elevation of a large infarct.

ST elevation MI (STEMI) results from more severe cardiac necrosis related to total obstruction of the coronary artery and is often associated with shock and collapse. The extensive myocardial injury causes a characteristic elevation of the ST segment in the ECG and is also associated with marked elevation of cardiac muscle enzymes in the blood. An ST elevation myocardial infarction is a medical emergency and should be treated by an angioplasty or thrombolytic drugs to unblock the artery as soon as possible. The faster the blood flow can be restored through the blocked artery, the less severe the heart muscle damage and the better the prognosis. Acute coronary syndromes are diagnosed on a continuum related to the severity of cardiac ischemia and degree of myocyte necrosis (**Table 9-1**).

An infarct may involve the full thickness of the muscular wall or only part of the wall. A full-thickness infarct extending from endocardium to epicardium is called a transmural infarct (trans = across + muris = wall) and is usually the result of thrombosis of a major coronary artery. If only part of the wall undergoes necrosis, the term subendocardial infarct is used.

The healthcare team can assess the amount of heart muscle damage by correlating the changes in the ECG (**Figure 9-25**) with cardiac enzyme test results and the patient's clinical condition. This information helps guide proper treatment and provides insight into the patient's prognosis.

Acute coronary syndrome (ACS) A broad classification of diseases arising from inadequate flow of blood to the heart, falling into one of three separate groups (unstable angina, myocardial infarction, and cardiac death). Subcategories of ACS are differentiated based upon ECG and other laboratory testing.

Stable angina Temporary chest pain during stress or exertion caused by partial chronic blockage of the coronary vasculature, usually relieved by rest or nitroglycerin.

Unstable angina Angina of prolonged duration resistant to therapy.

Table 9-1 Acute Coronary Syndrome (ACS) Classification of Coronary Heart Disease

Condition	ECG	Enzymes	Evaluation and Treatment
Unstable angina	ST depression during angina returns to normal when angina subsides	Not elevated	Treat angina. May progress to minor myocardial damage. Consider adding antiplatelet and anticoagulant drugs. Minimize cardiovascular risk factors.
Non ST-segment elevation myocardial infarction	ST-segment depression	Troponin elevated Creatine kinase not elevated if the test is performed	Minor myocardial damage caused by atheromatous debris from ruptured coronary plaque blocking distal branches of artery, or artery partially blocked by thrombus. Treat with anticoagulant and antiplatelet drugs to keep the artery open. Consider angioplasty (percutaneous coronary intervention) if anticoagulant-antiplatelet treatment is not successful.
ST-segment elevation myocardial infarction	ST-segment elevation	Troponin elevated Creatine kinase is also elevated if the test is performed	Artery completely blocked. Identify the site of the block by arteriogram and the open blocked coronary artery, preferably by angioplasty (percutaneous coronary intervention), as quickly as possible to salvage as much cardiac muscle as possible. If facilities are not available for angioplasty, attempt to dissolve the clot with thrombolytic drugs.

Diagnosis of Myocardial Infarction

Diagnosis of myocardial infarction encompasses evaluation and interpretation of the medical history, physical examination, and laboratory data. The clinical history may at times be inconclusive because severe angina can present similarly to the pain of a myocardial infarction. Conversely, many patients who develop subendocardial myocardial infarcts may report minimal symptoms. A physical examination will usually not be abnormal unless the patient exhibits evidence of shock, heart failure, or a heart murmur as a result of papillary muscle dysfunction. Consequently, the healthcare provider must rely on specialized diagnostic studies to properly diagnose infarction of the heart muscle. The most helpful diagnostic aids are the electrocardiogram (discussed previously) and determination of blood levels of various enzymes that leak from the damaged heart muscle.

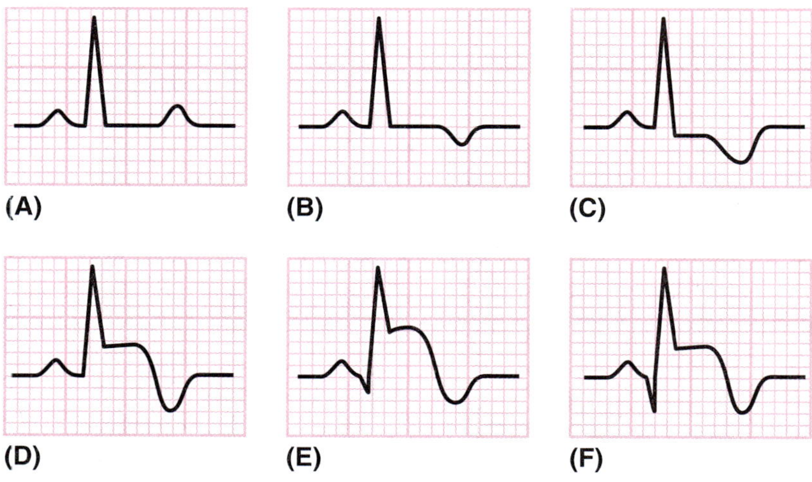

Figure 9-25 ECG ischemia and infarction patterns. **(A)** Normal ECG for comparison. **(B)** Mild ischemia demonstrated by inverted T wave. **(C)** Moderate ischemia demonstrated by slight ST-segment depression and inverted T wave. **(D)** and **(E)** ST-segment elevation myocardial infarction. **(F)** ST-segment myocardial infarction with a prominent Q wave indicating more severe myocardial damage.

Slightly modified from Garcia TB, Holtz NE. Introduction to 12-Lead ECG. Boston, MA: Jones and Bartlett Publishers; 2003.

Blood Tests to Identify Cardiac Muscle Necrosis

Heart muscle is rich in proteins and enzymes that regulate the metabolic activities of cardiac muscle cells. When heart muscle is damaged, some of these components leak from the injured cells into the bloodstream, where they can be detected by laboratory tests. A combination of cardiac proteins can be detected and used to evaluate heart muscle damage. Cardiac enzymes (including troponin and creatine kinase), C-reactive protein (CRP), fibrinogen, homocysteine, lipoproteins, triglycerides, brain natriuretic peptide (BNP), and prothrombin all contribute to understanding the extent of the MI and creating a timeline for the event. Important proteins used as diagnostic tests of muscle necrosis are called cardiac troponin T (cTnT) and troponin I (cTnI). These are not detectable in the blood of people without heart damage. Elevated troponin blood levels appear within 3 hours after muscle necrosis, with the highest levels attained within 24 hours. The elevations may persist for as long as 10 to 14 days. In general, the larger the infarct, the higher the troponin elevation and the longer it takes for the levels to return to normal. The pattern of rapid troponin rise and subsequent fall over the succeeding days is characteristic of myocardial necrosis. Troponin tests are so sensitive that even very small areas of muscle necrosis are sufficient to produce a positive test. Consequently, the troponin tests have become the preferred blood tests for evaluating patients with a suspected myocardial infarct because the tests can detect a very small area of heart muscle damage as well as a large myocardial infarct, and elevated levels can be detected within hours of the suspected MI.

Another diagnostic test for heart muscle damage is measurement of the creatine phosphokinase (CK) enzyme present in heart muscle, termed CK-MB. The test is less sensitive than troponin tests but usually becomes positive when a large amount of heart muscle has been damaged. Muscle and other tissues have low levels of CK-MB, and hence the test is not as specific nor as sensitive as the use of troponins.

Treatment of Acute Coronary Syndrome (Unstable Angina and Myocardial Infarcts)

Initial treatment may use drugs that decrease the heart's demand for oxygen. These include the previously mentioned nitroglycerin as well as beta-blocking agents (to reduce sympathetic nervous system stimulation) and calcium channel antagonists, which decrease heart rate and contractility.

A new family of antiplatelet agents that block ADP-dependent platelet aggregation (P2Y12 inhibitors), including drugs such as ticagrelor and prasugrel, contributes greatly to managing acute coronary syndrome and post-MI therapy. Such agents are often used in combination with aspirin (although some current studies question the utility and safety of aspirin in combined therapy).

This conservative drug-based therapy may be sufficient for dealing with unstable angina or NSTEMI. However, STEMI or progressing NSTEMI requires therapy to reestablish blood flow to the myocardium and limit cardiac damage. Two different methods can be used to reestablish blood flow through a thrombosed coronary artery; each has advantages and limitations. One method is fibrinolytic (clot dissolving) treatment, which attempts to dissolve the clot, and the second is a procedure called percutaneous coronary intervention (often abbreviated PCI). This angioplasty procedure opens the artery and places a short expandable metal mesh stent at the site of the **occlusion** to hold the artery

Occlusion Blockage or closing of an open blood vessel or hollow organ.

open. The angioplasty procedure is more effective than thrombolytic therapy but requires a medical center staffed by personnel experienced with PCI procedures.

Fibrinolytic Treatment

Fibrinolytic therapy offers the advantage of ready availability. Various fibrinolytic drugs are available for intravenous administration. Their mechanism of action is based on recombinant human tissue plasminogen activator. The drugs act by binding to the fibrin within the clot and converting plasminogen into plasmin. Plasmin degrades the fibrin, which allows the clot to dissolve (see Chapter 14).

Fibrinolytic therapy can be performed quickly in a hospital or emergency room setting, while the angioplasty procedure requires skilled personnel. Additionally, extra time would be needed to transfer the patient to a coronary care facility, which would delay opening the artery and could lead to further myocardial necrosis. Rapid use of this therapy is critical for success. The benefit of thrombolytic therapy decreases progressively as the time interval between coronary thrombosis and clot lysis lengthens. After about 6 hours, administration of a thrombolytic drug is of little benefit because by this time the heart muscle has progressed from ischemia to complete infarction, and it can no longer be salvaged by restoring blood flow through the occluded vessel. The disadvantages are that up to 30 percent of patients are not suitable for fibrinolytic therapy because bleeding may be a serious side effect of therapy. Postsurgical or other patients for which bleeding might be expected to have serious consequences are not candidates for fibrinolytic therapy. The procedure is less effective than percutaneous coronary intervention.

Percutaneous Coronary Intervention

European and U.S. guidelines currently recommend primary percutaneous coronary intervention (pPCI) as the preferred reperfusion method when it is performed in a timely fashion by an experienced team. Compared to fibrinolytic therapy, survival improves and the rate of recurrent MI and intracranial hemorrhage (ICH) is lower. However, there is a steep incremental increase in mortality when pPCI cannot be delivered promptly, particularly with delays in first medical contact to PCI longer than 60 minutes. The procedure is quite similar to the angioplasty procedure used to dilate stenotic coronary arteries (see Chapter 10). Generally, blood flow through the artery can be restored in about 90 percent of patients, which compares favorably with dissolving the clot using thrombolytic drugs. This results in a 70 percent to 80 percent success rate. Unfortunately, although good flow is restored through the blocked artery, the PCI procedure may dislodge small bits of thrombus and atherosclerotic plaque debris from the arterial wall when the artery is opened, which is carried downstream to block small arterioles and capillaries. Coronary care units in many hospitals can evaluate a suspected myocardial infarction patient and proceed with a PCI if necessary in as little as 1 hour. Ultimate success of the PCI procedure depends on the time between when the artery endured obstruction and when the patient reached the coronary care unit. Many patients delay seeking treatment for several hours after the onset of symptoms, which reduces the chance of a successful outcome in patients with an ST elevation myocardial infarction. In cases where PCI therapy is not available, fibrinolytic therapy followed by transfer to a center where PCI is available is optimal.

Subsequent Treatment and Prognosis of Myocardial Infarction

It can be expected worldwide that 17.9 million people will die annually due to cardiovascular diseases (CVDs), with those under 70 constituting one-third of those deaths. Of the survivors, approximately two-thirds will not make a full recovery and return to the life they had lived previously. This equals 330 million years of life lost due to the premature death and 35.6 million years of life with disabilities. The expected survival rate for women is less than for men. These diseases impose a high cost on countries' healthcare systems. The survival rate of patients experiencing myocardial infarct depends on many factors. The most important relates to the size of the infarct, which correlates with how rapidly the blood flow to the damaged muscle can be restored; the patient's age; the development of complications; and the presence of other diseases that would adversely affect the patient's survival.

Long-term survival rates are highly dependent on variables such as patient age. Overall, 5-year survival rates are about 80 percent. Major causes of death after myocardial infarction are fatal arrhythmia, heart failure, and cardiac rupture. Coronary care units staffed by specially trained personnel reduce the mortality from cardiac arrhythmias, which often occur in the first several days after myocardial infarction. However, these facilities and access to high-level care do not affect the rates of death from heart failure or cardiac rupture.

Survival data usually do not include patients with small infarcts that may not be detected clinically. Many small myocardial infarcts cause relatively mild symptoms and heal without complications. The patients may ascribe their chest discomfort associated with the infarction to indigestion or other causes and never seek medical attention. Some studies indicate that as many as 25 percent of all patients with myocardial infarcts have very few symptoms and do not consult a healthcare provider.

After as much myocardium as possible has been salvaged by restoring flow through the occluded artery, further treatment of myocardial infarction consists of initial bed rest, gradually progressing to limited activity, and then to full activity. Sometimes, the injured heart is quite irritable and prone to abnormal rhythms. Therefore, healthcare providers may prescribe drugs to decrease the irritability of the heart muscle. Reversal of heart block may require insertion of a cardiac pacemaker. Myocardial infarction may lead to development of intracardiac thrombi if the endocardium is injured, with reduced activity also contributing to the potential for thrombi in leg veins. As noted previously, the use of antiplatelet agents decreases the likelihood of thromboses and emboli. If the patient shows evidence of heart failure, drugs may be administered to sustain the failing heart.

Patients recovering from a myocardial infarct are at increased risk of sudden death from a fatal arrhythmia or a subsequent second infarct, and the risk is greatest within the first 6 months after the infarct. Many postinfarct patients receive treatment for at least 2 years with beta blockers, which interact with sympathetic nervous system receptors and consequently reduce myocardial irritability. If recommended by a healthcare professional, ingesting a small amount of aspirin (details in a subsequent section) daily can help prevent a first MI or stroke in adults less than 60. Aspirin use can generate some serious side effects including GI bleeding. An aspirin regimen should only be initiated after consultation with trained healthcare professionals. As mentioned earlier, antiplatelet agents make it less likely that platelets will adhere to roughened atheromatous plaques and initiate thrombosis in the coronary artery. Insertion of a cardioverter-defibrillator in postinfarct patients considered at high risk of a cardiac arrest or fatal arrhythmia may also be recommended. The device continually monitors the patient's heart rhythm. In cases of ventricular fibrillation and ventricular tachycardia, the device automatically administers an electric shock to terminate the arrhythmia. The defibrillator does not control atrial fibrillation.

Location of Myocardial Infarcts

Myocardial infarcts most commonly involve the muscle of the left ventricle and septum. Only rarely are the walls of the atria or right ventricle involved. This is because the left ventricle is much more vulnerable to interruption of its blood supply than are other parts of the heart. The left ventricular wall is much thicker than the walls of the other chambers and pumps blood at high pressure into the systemic circulation. Consequently, it requires a very rich blood supply. In contrast, the other chambers have much thinner walls, pump blood under much lower pressures, need a less abundant blood supply, and can usually "get by" by means of collateral blood flow if a major coronary artery is blocked.

The size and location of myocardial infarcts depend on both the location of the obstructions in the coronary arteries and the amount of collateral blood flow. Generally, an obstruction of the left anterior descending artery leads to an infarct of the anterior wall and often of the adjacent anterior part of the interventricular septum as well. If the circumflex artery is blocked, it is usually the lateral wall that is damaged. Occlusion of the right coronary artery generally causes an infarction of the back wall of the left ventricle and adjacent posterior part of the interventricular septum. A block of the main left coronary artery, which fortunately is quite uncommon, causes an extensive infarction of both the anterior and the lateral walls of the left ventricle and is frequently fatal.

Major Complications of Myocardial Infarcts

Patients who sustain a myocardial infarct can be subject to an array of complications. These include the previously discussed arrhythmias, cardiac rupture, intracardiac thrombus formation, and chronic heart failure. The latter is often called congestive failure because of the association with pulmonary congestion, which arises due to related increased intrapulmonary pressure caused by left ventricular failure. Complications are not inevitable, and prompt restoration of blood flow through the blocked artery can reduce the damage sustained by the heart muscle and improve the patient's prognosis. On the other hand, the ventricle may be so badly damaged that it is unable to maintain normal cardiac function, and the heart fails. Heart failure may develop abruptly (acute heart failure) or more slowly (chronic heart failure), as described in a subsequent section, and may be difficult to treat.

Intracardial Thrombi

If the infarct involves the endocardium, thrombi may form on the interior of the ventricular wall and cover the damaged endocardial surface, particularly in areas that are akinetic. These are called mural thrombi. Bits of the thrombus may break loose and be carried as emboli into the systemic circulation, causing infarctions in the brain, kidneys, spleen, or other organs. Some treatment protocols attempt to forestall this complication by administering anticoagulants when a patient has sustained a severe infarction.

Cardiac Rupture

If a patient sustains a transmural infarct, a perforation may occur through the necrotic muscle (**Figure 9-26**). This permits blood to leak through the rupture into the pericardial sac, and as the blood accumulates, it compresses the heart so the ventricles cannot fill in diastole, a condition called **cardiac tamponade**. Eventually, the circulation ceases because the heart is no longer able to pump blood.

Cardiac tamponade Fluid accumulation in the pericardial sac, which compresses the heart and impairs heart function.

Risk Factors for Coronary Artery Disease

Coronary artery disease is the overriding risk factor for the acute coronary syndrome and concomitant occurrence of myocardial infarction. The risk of coronary artery disease (and specifically atherosclerosis, the formation of atheromatous plaques within the coronary vessels) is strongly related to blood lipid (cholesterol) levels, hypertension, diabetes, and smoking. Such risk factors are discussed in relation to atherosclerosis (see Chapter 10).

Taking Aspirin to Reduce the Risk of Cardiovascular Disease

Aspirin regimens can reduce the risk of heart attacks and strokes. Aspirin works by interfering with platelet function by permanently inactivating a platelet enzyme (acetylation) needed to produce a chemical compound called thromboxane A_2 that is released by platelets when they adhere to a roughened surface. Thromboxane A_2 causes platelets to clump together and start the clotting process (discussed in Chapter 14). Blocking platelet function by taking aspirin reduces the likelihood that platelets will adhere to the roughened surface of an atherosclerotic plaque in a coronary or cerebral artery and cause a blood clot to plug the artery. As little as 30 mg per day (less than one-half a baby aspirin)

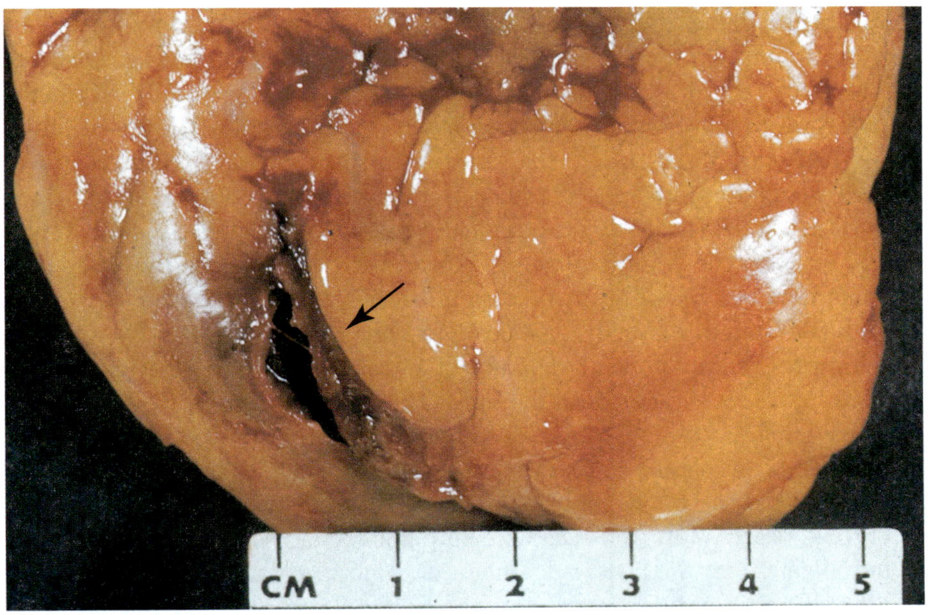

Figure 9-26 Rupture of heart (*arrow*) through large transmural myocardial infarct.

Courtesy of Leonard V. Crowley, MD, Century College.

inhibits thromboxane A_2 production, which persists for the entire 10-day life span of the platelets. Because about 10 percent of the circulating platelets are replaced every 24 hours, after about 10 days functionally normal platelets are probably no longer present in the circulation.

Although taking aspirin to inactivate platelet function reduces the risk of cardiovascular disease as well as strokes caused by blood clots in cerebral blood vessels, aspirin significantly increases the risk of major bleeding events. For example, one study found that 4 of 1200 persons taking aspirin for 5 years for primary prevention of cardiovascular disease would suffer four fewer MIs and three fewer strokes but three additional intracranial bleeds and eight additional major bleeding events. However, it should also be noted that aspirin use is reported to reduce overall risk of mortality from all causes, including cancer. Although there is little dispute about the value of antiplatelet drugs (and possibly aspirin) in cases of acute coronary syndrome or post-MI, the prophylactic use of aspirin to reduce the risk of cardiovascular disease needs evaluation on a risk–benefit basis. The possibility that aspirin may be of prophylactic value in certain selected populations having specific risk factors for cardiovascular disease remains.

Recreational Drug Use and Cardiovascular Disease

Many drugs which fall into the "recreational drug" category influence myocardial function and their use can lead to CVD. Drugs that stimulate the sympathetic nervous system can lead to complications involving increased heart rates and subsequent arrhythmias. When the parasympathetic nervous system becomes triggered, the heart rate can slow down, leading to bradycardia and inadequate blood flow to other parts of the body.

Heart Failure

Heart failure exists whenever the heart is no longer able to pump adequate amounts of blood to the tissues (**Figure 9-27**). It may result from any type of heart disease. Rapid failing of the heart, when a large portion of muscle undergoes infarction, is called acute heart failure. In most cases, however, cardiac failure develops slowly and insidiously, creating chronic heart failure. When the heart begins to fail, the pumping capability of both ventricles slowly declines, but initially not necessarily to the same extent. A disproportionate decline of left ventricular output causes the lungs to become engorged with blood, which is called left heart failure. Right heart failure is when the right ventricle cannot "keep up" with the volume of venous blood being returned to the heart. The increased venous pressure in the distended veins causes the body tissues to accumulate fluid that usually is detected most easily in the feet and legs. When one compresses the swollen (edematous) skin with a fingertip, the indentation persists for a few minutes until the fluid refills the depression, which is called pitting edema. Because the most prominent feature in chronic heart failure is congestion of the tissues and at times the lungs as a result of engorgement by blood, the clinician often uses the term congestive heart failure when referring to chronic heart failure and its attendant clinical manifestations. Although the term indicates that the heart is failing, it does not necessarily indicate a severe life-threatening condition. Chronic heart failure is a slowly progressing condition, so many patients respond well to effective treatment and can live comfortably in reasonably good health for many years.

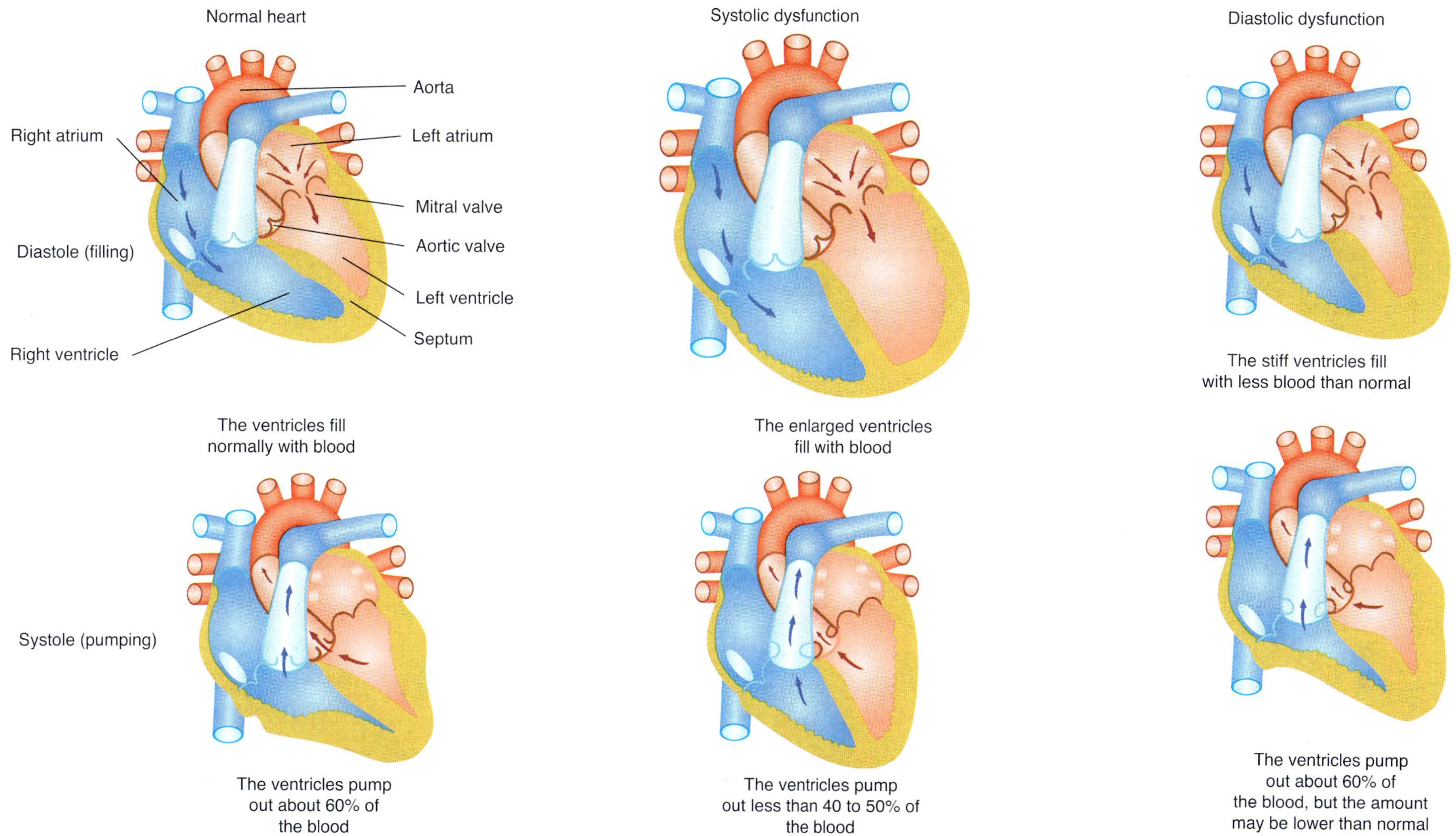

Figure 9-27 Heart failure is often categorized as diastolic or systolic heart failure. Both categories address the pumping activity of the heart.

Pathophysiology and Treatment

Heart failure is often categorized as being associated with either left or right ventricular failure (although left-sided failure will ultimately also affect the right side of the heart). The most common symptom of left ventricular failure is exertional dyspnea (shortness of breath on exertion). It may result from "back-up" of venous blood in the lungs (exacerbated when the patient is in a prone position, such as during sleep) and hence poor oxygenation, or from insufficient cardiac output to muscles involved in respiration. Reduced cardiac output may also result in fatigue, altered mental status, and decreased kidney function. Right-sided failure results in increased systemic venous pressure with abdominal discomfort. The high venous pressure and high capillary pressure cause excessive transudation of fluid from the capillaries, leading to edema of the tissues. In backward failure, the inadequate output of blood is considered to cause "backup" of blood within the veins draining back to the heart, leading to increased venous pressure, congestion of the viscera (leading to abdominal pain), and edema. **Figure 9-28** illustrates the interrelation of the various factors concerned in the development of cardiac failure. Treatment consists of diuretic drugs, which promote excretion of excess salt and water by the kidneys, thereby lowering blood volume. In addition, digitalis preparations are sometimes administered. They act to increase the efficiency of ventricular contractions. Other medications called ACE inhibitors are also frequently used. These drugs block an enzyme called angiotensin-converting enzyme (ACE), which is part of a renal regulatory mechanism called the renin–angiotensin–aldosterone system (see Chapter 19) that promotes retention of salt and water by the kidneys and raises blood pressure. Both of these effects are undesirable in heart failure patients, and blocking this mechanism by an ACE inhibitor has been shown to improve survival of patients with congestive heart failure. The

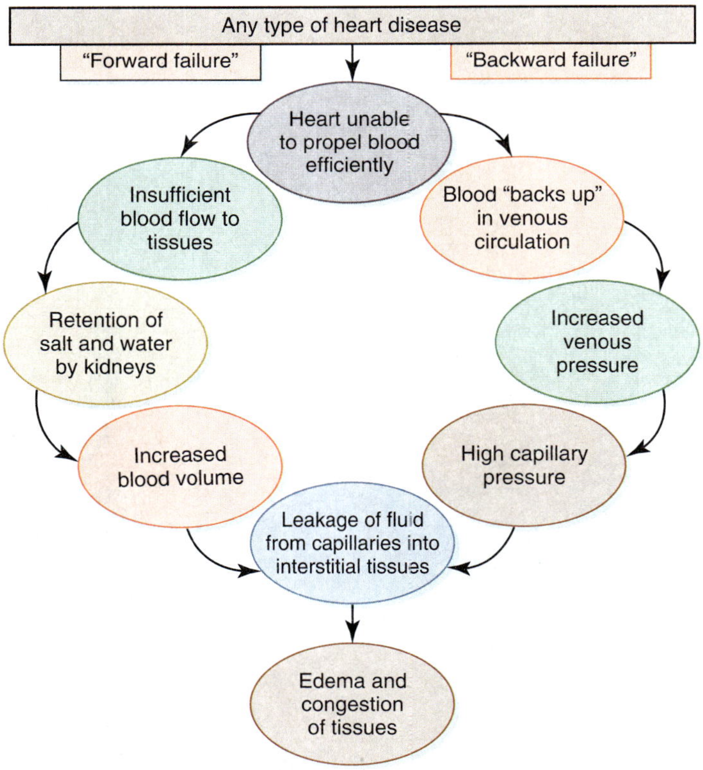

Figure 9-28 Mechanisms in the pathogenesis of congestive heart failure.

use of left ventricular assist devices, implanted mechanical devices that assist a chronically failed heart, may be lifesaving in selected cases, such as a person waiting for a heart transplant or someone who is terminally ill and is not a candidate for transplantation.

Acute Pulmonary Edema

Acute pulmonary edema is a manifestation of acute heart failure and a very serious life-threatening condition that requires immediate treatment. The output of blood from the ventricles becomes altered. If the output of blood from the left ventricle is temporarily reduced more than the output from the right ventricle, the right heart will pump blood into the lungs faster than the left heart can deliver the blood to the peripheral tissues. This rapidly engorges the lungs with blood, raises the pulmonary capillary pressure, and produces transudation of fluid into the pulmonary alveoli. The patient becomes extremely short of breath as the fluid accumulates within the alveoli, and oxygenation of the blood circulating through the lungs cannot happen efficiently. The edema fluid becomes mixed with inspired air, forming a frothy mixture that "overflows" into the bronchi and trachea, filling the patient's upper respiratory passages. Treatment consists of supplementary oxygen, intravenous diuretics, and other medications to improve cardiac function by reducing the circulating blood volume and morphine to relieve anxiety. Measures directed toward correcting the underlying condition that precipitated the acute heart failure need to be undertaken as well.

Types of Heart Failure

The efficiency of ventricular function in heart failure patients determines whether the heart failure results primarily from inadequate ejection of blood from the ventricles during systole or from inadequate filling of the ventricles in diastole (heart failure with preserved ejection fraction, **diastolic heart failure**). Most patients with heart failure demonstrate **systolic heart failure**; the failing ventricles are distended with blood but are unable to expel a normal volume of blood during systole. Consequently, the left ventricular ejection fraction is significantly reduced and may fall as low as 20 percent.

In contrast, the main problem in some heart failure patients is not with the impaired ejection of blood in systole but with inadequate filling of the ventricles during diastole. In this condition (diastolic heart failure), the volume of blood contained in the ventricles during diastole is lower than it should be, and the pressure of the blood within the chambers is elevated. This condition may occur in individuals with marked hypertension in whom the thick hypertrophied left ventricular wall cannot relax enough in diastole to allow the left ventricular chamber to expand normally. Consequently, less blood can flow into the ventricle. Some other less common conditions in which the ventricles are unable to relax normally in diastole may also reduce ventricular filling and raise intraventricular pressure. In all of these conditions, the left ventricle is underfilled in diastole (low-end diastolic volume), and the stroke volume is also low because there is a smaller volume of blood available in the chamber to be ejected. However, the ejection fraction is normal because both end diastolic volume and stroke volume are reduced proportionately. Nevertheless, the cardiac output is inadequate to supply the body's needs. The clinical manifestations and methods of treatment of both systolic and diastolic heart failure are similar, although diuretics are the preferred treatment for patients with diastolic heart failure.

Diastolic heart failure Heart failure caused by inadequate filling of the ventricles during diastole, in contrast to systolic heart failure in which ejection of blood from the ventricles during systole is inadequate.

Systolic heart failure Heart failure caused by inadequate ejection of blood from the ventricles during systole, in contrast to diastolic heart failure, in which filling of the ventricles in diastole is inadequate.

Natriuretic Peptides in Heart Failure

In heart failure patients, the unfavorable physiologic effects of the renin–angiotensin–aldosterone system resulting from reduced renal perfusion are counteracted to some extent by peptide hormones called natriuretic peptides that are released from cardiac muscle fibers when the fibers are stretched. As the name indicates (natrium = sodium + uresis = urination), the peptides promote urinary loss of salt and water and also reduce blood volume and pressure, opposing those caused by activation of the renin–angiotensin–aldosterone system. The peptides are called atrial natriuretic peptides (ANP), released from the atria, and B-type natriuretic peptides (BNP), released from the ventricles. Because ventricular pressures are higher than atrial pressures, the ventricular muscle cells are subjected to greater stretching forces. Consequently, BNP is of greater physiologic significance than ANP.

A blood test to measure the level of BNP in a seriously ill patient who is very short of breath may help determine whether the patient's marked dyspnea (shortness of breath) is caused by heart failure or by some other condition, such as lung disease. In heart failure, BNP is very high because the ventricular muscle fibers of the failing heart are overstretched. If BNP is not significantly elevated, the diagnosis of heart failure is unlikely, and other conditions must be considered to explain the patient's symptoms. BNP has been prepared for clinical use by recombinant technology and is sometimes used to treat patients with acute heart failure who are very short of breath. The intravenously administered BNP preparation promotes fluid loss and improves the patient's dyspnea.

Case 9-1

John Strelow is a 15-year-old male child with no prior history of serious illness. He is a freshman at Brementown High School (ninth grade) and is interested in participating in the school's highly competitive athletics program. He wishes to join the school's freshmen football team. As a requirement for participation, he goes for a preparticipation health screening at his local pediatrician. The physician does a cardiac examination looking for heart murmurs and checks John's blood pressure in a sitting position, all of which are normal. He asks John if he has ever experienced chest pain, shortness of breath, or palpitations. John answers in the negative. Finally, the pediatrician asks John about heart disease or unexplained early death in his family. John replies that his father died in a farm accident, having been crushed in a combine at age 40, and that he has no other known paternal relatives. John's mother has been diagnosed with mild hypertension and elevated blood lipids but is otherwise healthy. John has a younger sister (age 12) who has only minor medical problems. The pediatrician approves John's participation but warns him about adequate fluid intake and the danger of excessive exercise during periods of high heat and humidity.

John begins a preparticipation workout session at the school on a hot, humid September day and tells the coach he feels a bit dizzy and that his vision temporarily "grayed out." The coach instructs him to rest in the shade for a few minutes. Feeling better, John continues his workout, telling the coach he feels fine. On returning home, John mentions the episode to his mother, who is concerned. John has not told the coach (or his mother) that he felt short of breath for the entire workout. John participates in several additional training sessions and has several more episodes of shortness of breath, coming close to fainting twice. He hides this from the trainer and coach, wanting to participate in the first freshmen team game against Muenster High. During the game, John collapses suddenly. Paramedical aid is on hand, but John cannot be resuscitated. He is pronounced dead on arrival at Saint Ann Regional Hospital.

His autopsy, requested by the county medical examiner, shows cardiac abnormalities. There is asymmetric thickening of the left ventricle with excess septal wall hypertrophy. The ventricular chamber is small, and there is a suggestion that vascular outflow from the left ventricle might have been impeded. A tissue sample from the left ventricle is examined and disorganization of the cardiac myocytes is noted. The medical examiner records the case as sudden cardiac death related to presumptive hypertrophic cardiomyopathy, resulting in cardiac arrhythmia.

Discussion

Sudden cardiac death (SCD) in preadolescent and adolescent children is a tragic event and comes to general attention when those deaths are involved in school athletic programs. Because of understandable publicity, these deaths appear common when, in fact, they are unusual. The U.S. Registry of Sudden Death in Athletes has collected data for over 30 years. There are about 75 cardiovascular deaths per year in young athletes, compared to about 115 deaths among young athletes from all causes. The overall incidence of cardiac death in young athletes is estimated to be between 0.5 and 0.7 deaths per 100,000 person-years. Deaths from motor vehicle accidents are 2500 times more common in the same age group. It should be noted that estimates of SCD in school athletes have been criticized because they are difficult to interpret based on the large number of variables in these studies. Some believe the true figures to be twice as high (1 death per 100,000) or perhaps even higher. However, for U.S. high school students, the incidence of sudden cardiac death among athletes as compared to nonathletes was over 3.5 times higher. Clearly, participatory high school athletics does present an elevated risk for SCD, but the overall risk is very small when compared to the more common causes of death among the young (notably trauma by accident, homicide, or suicide).

What is responsible for the increased risk of SCD in young athletes? In the previously noted registry, hypertrophic cardiomyopathy (HCM), defined as increased asymmetric left ventricular wall thickness in the absence of other causes, was the most common cause of SCD in athletes, being responsible for 35 percent of deaths. Other studies report the incidence of proven and possible HCM in cases of SCD ranging from 11 percent (in NCAA athletes) to 7 percent (in the U.S. military) to 37 percent (in athletes in the United Kingdom). Myocarditis, often cited as a cause of SCD in young athletes, was less common (6 percent of deaths in the U.S. Registry).

The variation in frequency of HCM in SCD is likely related to differences in diagnostic criteria and, more important, to the fact that at least 60 percent of HCM cases are genetic in origin, with mutations in three genes being responsible for over 80 percent of cases. The disease is most often dominant, and familial clusters of affected individuals may have a strong effect on observed frequencies. The disease is common, with a prevalence of 1 in 500 and although many cases are asymptomatic, 10 percent of patients ultimately develop heart failure. Stress accentuates symptoms in HCM patients, and in some cases the risk for SCD may be as high as 4 percent to 5 percent per year. Although certain high-risk HCM mutations have been defined, the correlation between mutations and the presence and severity of cardiac disease is poor. Hence, there is considerable controversy about the utility of genetic analysis (although it may be useful in some families).

Considering the relatively high frequency of HCM in at least some populations and the publicity and trauma attendant with SCD in a young athlete, proposals have been made to increase screening criteria. Currently, a 14-element preparticipation screen is suggested by the American Heart Association for competitive athletics (**Case Table 9-1**). Some, but not all, of these elements were utilized in this case. Major problems are standardization between screenings and qualifications for the person doing the screening. Even with effective screening, not all cases of HCM will be detected. Also, youth might be expected

(continues)

Case 9-1 *(Continued)*

Case Table 9-1 American Heart Association Recommendations for Preparticipation Cardiovascular Screening for Competitive Athletes

Athlete's physical exam should include checking for evidence of the following:

- Heart murmur
- Marfan syndrome
- Abnormalities in blood pressure while sitting
- Pulse in the femoral artery

Examine the athlete's medical history for the following (The list is not all-inclusive.)

- Chest pain
- Shortness of breath when exercising
- Unattributed exhaustion
- Unexplained fainting
- Evidence of high blood pressure or prior heart murmur

Take a look at the Athlete's Family History for Evidence of the following:

- Sudden death due to heart disease
- Congenital heart defects and disease

to be less than forthcoming in reporting symptoms. Screening using 12-lead ECG, which is effective in detecting ventricular hypertrophy, has been suggested as a mandatory component to screening. However, the test is costly and controversial in terms of specificity and sensitivity, and is technically challenging. Mandatory screening with 12-lead ECG is not recommended for young athletes and nonathletes by the American Heart Association or the American College of Cardiology because there is no evidence of benefit. Serious ethical concerns exist regarding the provision of specialized screening solely to athletes when, in aggregate, there are far more cases of HCM in the nonathlete population.

When HCM is suspected, highly effective, specialized, noninvasive diagnostic procedures are available (two-dimensional echocardiography and cardiac MRI investigations). Today these procedures are far too costly and too technically demanding for use in screening normal populations. Finally, a diagnosis of HCM need not prevent a person from engaging in a program of physical activity of a stress level appropriate to the specifics of their particular case.

Etiology and Pathogenesis

Sudden cardiac death likely from cardiac arrhythmia as a result of hypertrophic cardiomyopathy.

Questions

1. The case notes that there are far more cases in aggregate of HCM in nonathletes than in athletes. Why is this? Given that fact, would you support mandatory screening for high school athletes?
2. There are racial and sex-based differences in SCD frequency in athletes (not discussed in this case). What could be some of the factors responsible for these differences?
3. Based on the content in this chapter, suggest a plausible pathophysiological explanation for SCD in HCM.
4. Based on the case description, how thorough was the preparticipation screening given to John?
5. Under what circumstances might genetic screening for mutations be useful in evaluating the risk of HCM?

Questions for Review

1. How do the heart valves function to provide unidirectional blood flow? What factors determine the level of the systolic and diastolic blood pressure?
2. What are the major causes of heart disease? What is the difference between rheumatic fever and rheumatic heart disease?
3. What is infective endocarditis? How does it arise? How is it prevented?
4. What is coronary heart disease? What are its manifestations? What is the difference between angina pectoris and myocardial infarction?
5. What is the effect of high blood pressure on the heart and the blood vessels?
6. What are the major complications of a large myocardial infarction?

References

Lilly LS. *Pathophysiology of Heart Disease: An Introduction to Cardiovascular Medicine*. 8th ed. Wolters Kluwer; 2025.

- This book provides an in-depth overview of the topics covered in this chapter. The interested reader is urged to consult this resource for additional information on the cardiovascular system and, in particular, current clinical and therapeutic approaches to heart disease. The area of heart disease is so broad (and so detailed) that no set of readings can fully do it justice. This text presents a readable and somewhat technical overview aimed at medical and advanced undergraduate students. It is an excellent single source for additional background for this chapter. It is particularly strong on therapy.

American Heart Association. Accessed May 2, 2025. http://www.heart.org/

AHA Research. American Heart Association. Accessed May 2, 2025. https://professional.heart.org/professional/ResearchPrograms/UCM_316889_Research.jsp

- The American Heart Association website is an essential resource for any area of cardiovascular disease. The first entry is for the homepage, and the second entry provides a portal for scientific information. AHA statements and guidelines (which can be accessed on the site) are authoritative and carefully reviewed by all healthcare professionals. In-depth overviews of the topics covered in the chapter can be found at these websites. The interested reader is urged to consult them for additional information on the cardiovascular system and, in particular, current clinical and therapeutic approaches to heart disease.

American College of Cardiology. Accessed May 2, 2025. https://www.acc.org

American College of Cardiology. New USPSTF Recommendation on Aspirin in CVD: No For Primary Prevention, Yes For Secondary Prevention. Published April 27, 2022. Accessed May 2, 2025. https://www.acc.org/Latest-in-Cardiology/Articles/2022/04/27/20/41/New-USPSTF-Recommendation-on-Aspirin-in-CVD

- The American College of Cardiology website has a wealth of material, and much of it is updated immediately. It also acts as a gateway to scientific publications of extremely high quality, and many are publicly available. The second selection describes current thinking about the use of aspirin to prevent cardiovascular disease. The interested reader should also examine the next set of references for a somewhat different view.

Maron BJ, Winkel BG, Tfelt-Hansen J. Perspectives on cardiovascular screening. *JAMA*. 2015;313(1):31-32.

Maron BJ, Friedman RA, Kligfield P, et al. Assessment of the 12-lead ECG as a screening test for detection of cardiovascular disease in healthy general populations of young people (12-25 Years of Age): A scientific statement from the American Heart Association and the American College of Cardiology. *Circulation*. 2014;130(15):1303-1334.

Maron BJ, Friedman RA, Caplan A. Ethics of preparticipation cardiovascular screening for athletes. *Nat Rev Cardiol*. 2015;12(6):375-378.

Harmon KG, Drezner JA, Wilson MG, Sharma S. Incidence of sudden cardiac death in athletes: A state-of-the art review. *Heart*. 2014;100(16):1227-1234.

Wolf CM. Hypertrophic cardiomyopathy: Genetics and clinical perspectives. *Cardiovasc Diagn Ther*. 2019;9(Suppl 2):S388-S415.

- This set of five readings presents an overview of current thought on aspects of sudden coronary death in young athletes and the utility of additional preparticipation tests. The articles should be read with care by anyone is involved in participatory athletics in an academic setting. These readings (and several others) were used in Case 9-1 preparation. The fifth selection is an updated review of hypertrophic cardiomyopathy.

National Institute of Health National Heart, Lung, and Blood Institute. Heart Tests. Accessed May 2, 2025. https://www.nhlbi.nih.gov/health/heart-tests

Centers for Disease Control and Prevention. National Center for Health Statistics. Deaths and Mortality. Accessed May 2, 2025. https://www.cdc.gov/nchs/fastats/deaths.htm

- The first resource provides information about heart tests used to diagnose cardiovascular disease. The second resource provides up-to-date statistics on mortality, detailing heart disease as the leading cause of death in the United States.

Konno T, Chang S, Seidman JG, Seidman CE. Genetics of hypertrophic cardiomyopathy. *Curr Opin Cardiol*. 2010;25(3):205-209. https://pmc.ncbi.nlm.nih.gov/articles/PMC2932754/

Baddour LM, Janszky I, Thornhill M, et al. Nondental invasive procedures and risk of infective endocarditis: Time for a revisit: A science advisory from the American Heart Association. *Circulation*. 2023;148(19):1529-1541. https://www.ahajournals.org/doi/epdf/10.1161/CIR.0000000000001180

Bayat S, Hashemi Nazari SS, Mehrabi Y, Sistanizad M. Long-term Survival Rate Following Myocardial Infarction and the Effect of Discharge Medications on the Survival Rate. *J Res Health Sci*. 2022;22(4):e00567. doi:10.34172/jrhs.2022.102. PMID: 37571938; PMCID: PMC10422162.

Ghuran A, van Der Wieken LR, Nolan J. Cardiovascular complications of recreational drugs. *BMJ*. 2001;323(7311):464-466. doi:10.1136/bmj.323.7311.464. PMID: 11532824; PMCID: PMC1121066.

- These four readings provide current insight into genetics, treatments, survival rate, and complications related to cardiovascular disease.

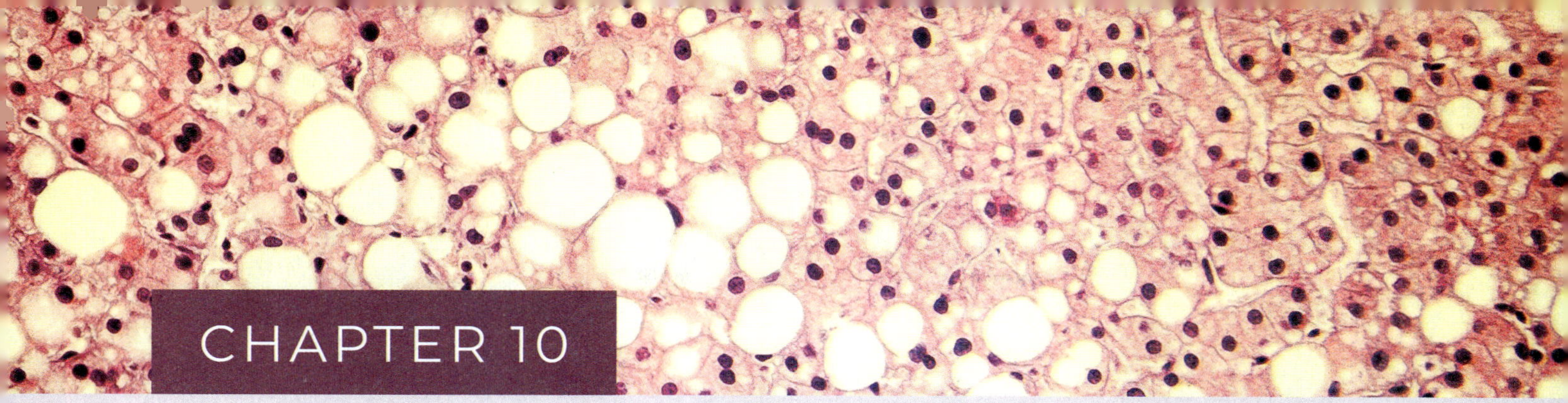

CHAPTER 10

Diseases of Blood Circulation

LEARNING OBJECTIVES

1. Describe the types of blood vessels and their pattern of blood flow.
2. List the factors regulating the circulation of fluid between capillaries and interstitial tissue.
3. Describe the causes and types of circulatory disturbances.
4. Describe the causes and effects of venous thrombosis.
5. Explain the pathogenesis of pulmonary embolism. Describe the clinical manifestations and compare the techniques of diagnosis.
6. List factors that predispose people to thrombus formation in leg veins. Describe the major complications of venous thrombi.
7. Explain the major clinical disturbances leading to edema.
8. Describe the factors leading to shock.
9. Describe the causes and effects of arterial thrombosis
10. Describe the pathogenesis of the hypercoagulable state sometimes seen in patients with carcinoma.
11. Describe the natural history of atherosclerosis.
12. Explain the current concepts regarding risk factors for coronary heart disease.
13. Describe the adverse effects of hypertension on the cardiovascular system and the kidneys.
14. Differentiate between the pathogenesis and clinical manifestations of arteriosclerotic and dissecting aneurysms of the aorta. Explain the principles of treatment.

Blood Vessels

The heart pumps blood into a system of vasculature in which the vessels exhibit differences in structure and function. It is convenient to consider the system which distributes blood away from the heart in four categories: the elastic arteries, the muscular arteries, the arterioles, and the capillaries. Blood returning to the heart travels through venules and veins.

The large elastic arteries distend as the heart ejects blood during systole. During diastole the recoil of the arteries applies pressure to blood and contributes to maintaining flow between contractions and reducing pulsations. The muscular arteries distribute blood from the large elastic arteries into individual organs. These smaller vessels with muscular walls regulate flow and reduce

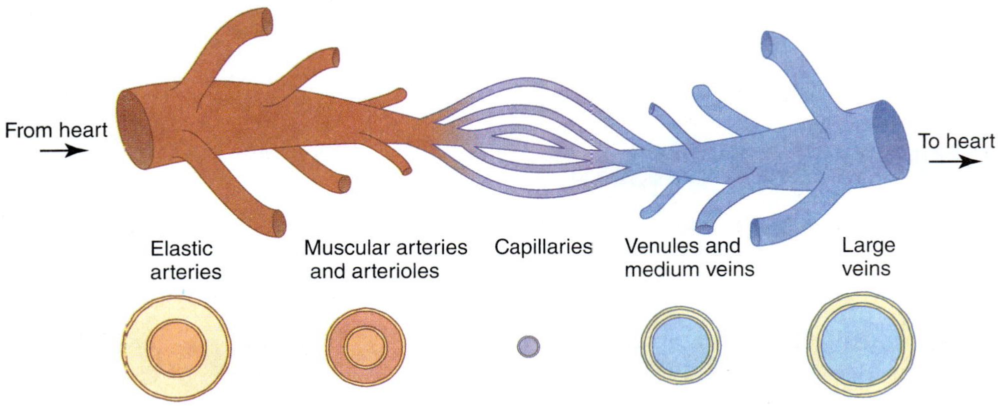

Figure 10-1 The composition and diameter of blood vessel walls vary with the type of blood vessel.

blood pressure from the large arteries into the capillaries. They also contribute to maintaining systemic blood pressure by controlling resistance to flow, mainly by changing vessel diameter. The arterioles are the smallest component of the arterial system and lack an elastic layer. Smooth muscle cells in their walls regulate blood flow into capillaries. Contraction narrows the size of the lumen, increasing resistance with the potential to increase blood pressure. Relaxation increases the size of the vessel, lowering resistance and decreasing blood pressure. The capillaries deliver nutrients and fluids to the tissues and remove waste products. These functions may be accomplished by several different processes. In some tissues, the endothelial cells of the capillaries are leaky, and materials move in between the cells. Capillaries in some organs have fenestrations, or pores, allowing for maximal exchange of nutrients and waste.

The venous return system often functions against gravity. Consequently, some veins contain a series of one-way valves that prevent backflow of blood away from the heart. Veins return blood to the heart under low pressure and often are found near the corresponding artery (**Figure 10-1**). Veins serve as reservoirs for blood and help regulate systemic blood pressure even in the case of a loss of large volume as a result of hemorrhage. The total fluid capacity of the vascular system exceeds the actual total blood volume. Regulation of blood flow to the tissues and blood return from the tissues is one factor determining the volume of blood capable of being pumped with each heartbeat.

A separate system of channels carrying fluid retrieved from the tissues, called lymph, constitutes part of the lymphatic system. The functions of the lymphatic system and its interactions with the circulatory system contribute to circulatory disturbances. These topics are included later in this chapter.

Factors Regulating Fluid Flow Between Capillaries and Interstitial Tissue

The flow of fluid through the interstitial space between arteries and veins depends on capillary hydrostatic pressure, capillary permeability, osmotic pressure of blood proteins, and the presence of open lymphatic channels. The capillary hydrostatic pressure provides the physical force that drives fluid from the blood through the capillary endothelium and into the tissues. The selectively permeable capillary endothelium regulates what may pass out of the capillary and into the surrounding tissues. Large molecules such as proteins require a specific biological mechanism that enables them to cross the endothelium. Osmotic pressure relies on selective permeability in membranes. Two of the

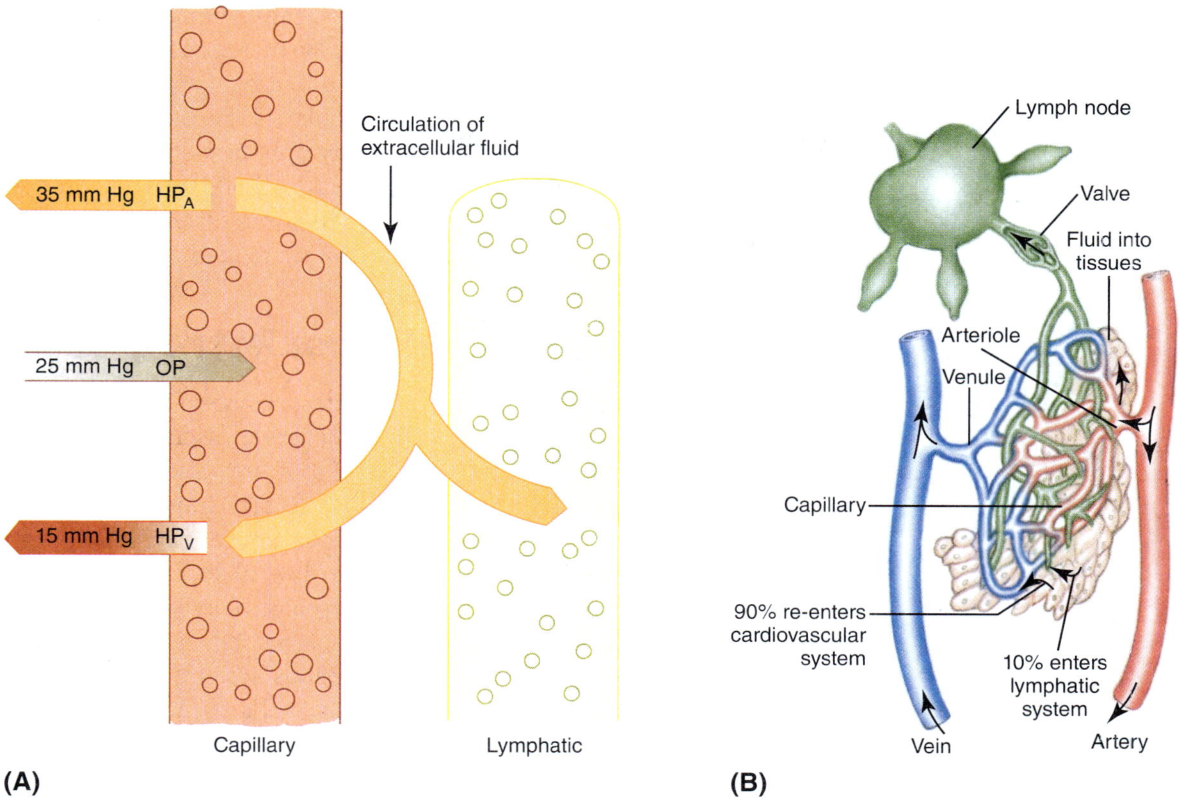

Figure 10-2 **(A)** Factors regulating the flow of fluid through the interstitial tissues. HP_A, hydrostatic pressure at the arterial end of the capillary. HP_V is hydrostatic pressure at the venous end of the capillary. OP, osmotic pressure. Pressures are indicated in millimeters of mercury (mm Hg). Fluid is forced from the arterial end of the capillary because the hydrostatic pressure exceeds the osmotic pressure. At the venous end of the capillary, the hydrostatic pressure is lower than the osmotic pressure. **(B)** Excess tissue fluid is also picked up by lymphatics that drain into larger vessels. Lymph nodes are interspersed along the vessels and act to filter the lymph.

major ions of the extracellular fluid, Na^+ and Cl^-, move rapidly between plasma and interstitial fluid spaces; consequently, they make ineffective osmotic agents. Proteins, by contrast, are mostly restricted to the plasma compartment. Consequently, their usually higher concentration in the plasma compared to the interstitial spaces would create an osmotic gradient where water from the interstitial space (where protein concentration is low) moves to the plasma compartment (where protein concentration is higher (colloid osmotic pressure)). The osmotic pressure of the plasma depends primarily on the concentration of the plasma proteins (termed the **plasma oncotic pressure**). Because generally capillaries are impermeable to protein, the colloid osmotic pressure results in water leaving the interstitial fluid through osmosis. However, changes in capillary permeability (i.e. during the inflammatory response) may allow proteins to leak into tissue, reducing the plasma oncotic pressure. Lymphatic channels collect some of the fluid (water, dissolved solutes, and larger molecules) that has leaked out of the capillaries. Eventually that fluid would return to the circulation. **Figure 10-2** illustrates the mechanism by which fluid flow is regulated through interstitial tissues.

Plasma oncotic pressure The likelihood of osmotic movement of water from the surrounding tissues into the plasma is mostly driven by the concentration of the plasma proteins in blood.

Flow of Fluid Into and Out of Capillaries

The pressure of the blood at the arterial end of the capillary is higher than the colloid osmotic pressure, causing water and dissolved solutes to be filtered through the endothelium of the capillaries into the interstitial space.

The capillary endothelium acts as a semipermeable membrane and limits the rate at which fluid is filtered from the blood. At the venous end of the capillary, the hydrostatic pressure is lower than the colloid osmotic (oncotic) pressure, and fluid tends to diffuse back into the capillaries. Excess fluid found in the interstitial tissues and spaces also enters the lymphatic system. Ultimately, fluid containing dissolved nutrients is carried from the blood into the interstitial tissues to nourish the cells, and waste products are returned to the circulation either directly or through lymphatics for processing and eventual excretion.

Vascular Disturbances: Introduction

Often pathology associated with the cardiovascular system discusses issues with the heart and the vasculature together. This chapter discusses diseases associated with the blood vessels, while Chapter 9 discusses diseases associated with the heart. Often disturbances of one will also affect the functioning of the other.

The etiology of disturbances to the vascular system encompasses a variety of contributing factors. Disturbances to the flow of blood result from either complete or partial blockage of vessels. Normally, blood does not clot within the vascular system. Under unusual circumstances, however, **thrombosis**, or intravascular clotting, may occur. In the venous system, this is the result of slowing or stasis of blood flow, damage to the walls of the blood vessel, or an increase in the coagulability of the blood. These three factors leading to venous thrombosis is sometimes referred to as Virchow's Triad. Intravascular thrombi can also form within arteries and occasionally within the heart itself. Most commonly, arterial thrombi arise in relation to **atherosclerosis**, the formation of lipid-rich plaques in large and medium arteries. Any clot within the vascular system may become detached and carried throughout the circulation. Such a clot, termed an embolus (embolus = plug or stopper), may come to rest when the caliber of the blood vessel is smaller than the diameter of the clot. Embolization refers to the formation of circulating clots. Depending on the anatomic origin of the blood clot, the embolus may be carried into either the pulmonary circulation or, less commonly, the systemic arterial circulation. Tissue downstream from where the clot lodged suffers ischemia, a loss of tissue oxygen, and may become damaged or undergo necrosis if the collateral blood supply is inadequate. The area of tissue breakdown is termed an **infarct**; the process of the tissue becoming damaged is labeled infarction.

Blood vessels may also undergo excessive damage to their walls. An aneurysm, or outpouching, can rupture and result in hemorrhage. **Varicosities** present as excessive tortuosity and dilation of blood vessels, commonly veins. Changes in the permeability properties of vessels can lead to leakage of fluid from the blood vessel into the tissue, resulting in **edema** or swelling.

Shock occurs when low systemic blood pressure from any cause progresses to circulatory failure and collapse. Conversely, **hypertension** (excessively high systemic blood pressure), if prolonged, will result in damage to the heart and blood vessels in many organ systems.

Thrombosis The formation of blood clots (thrombi plural, thrombus singular) within the vascular system.

Atherosclerosis Formation of lipid-rich plaques in large and medium arteries, which result in stiffening of the vessel in the area of the plaque.

Infarct Necrosis of tissue caused by interruption of its blood supply.

Varicosities Outpouching and excessive tortuosity and dilation of blood vessels, often found in veins.

Edema Accumulation of excess fluid in the interstitial tissues.

Shock A general term for any condition leading to receiving an inadequate amount of oxygen, most often caused by acute blood loss or severe infection (sepsis).

Hypertension Excessively high systemic blood pressure.

Venous Thrombosis and Pulmonary Embolism

The formation of blood clots within leg veins results primarily from slowed blood flow, or stasis. Contributing factors can include periods of prolonged bed rest or remaining in a fixed or cramped position for a long period of time. Such a situation can occur with prolonged airplane travel or riding in a car for long uninterrupted periods of time. Under these circumstances, the "milking action" of the leg musculature, which normally promotes venous return, decreases, leading to stasis of the blood. Varicose veins or any condition preventing normal emptying of veins predisposes an individual to thrombosis through venous stasis.

Postoperative thrombosis in leg veins is a common problem. The surgical patient is susceptible to venous thrombosis due to the combined effects of inactivity and increased blood coagulability resulting from the additional release of coagulation factors as a result of surgery or other trauma. In general, blood coagulation factors usually increase as a result of tissue injury or necrosis from any cause.

A venous thrombus may partially block venous return in the leg, causing the leg to swell, and the site may become painful. However, the major complication of venous thrombosis relates to detachment of the clot from the wall of the vein. If the thrombus is not firmly attached to the vein wall, it may break loose, forming an embolus that can be carried rapidly up the inferior vena cava into the right side of the heart. Right ventricle ejection of the thrombus into the pulmonary artery can occur, where it may become lodged in either the main pulmonary artery or one of its branches. The clinical manifestations of a pulmonary **embolism** depend on the size of the embolus and where it lodges in the pulmonary circulation. Complications can range from mild pulmonary damage and pain to occlusion of the main pulmonary artery leading to sudden death.

Embolism A condition in which a blockage composed of a detached clot, mass of bacteria, or other foreign material (embolus) occludes a blood vessel.

Post-surgical care often includes the use of pressure-driven cuffs placed around the legs, which pulsate and promote blood flow to reduce stasis and inhibit thrombus formation. Venous thrombosis is treated by elevation of the leg, heat, and most importantly, by anticoagulant drugs. The anticoagulation stops the progression of the intravascular clotting process while the body's normal protective mechanisms remove the clot. The clot is dissolved by activation of the fibrinolytic mechanism associated with the blood clotting process (Chapter 9) and by ingrowth of connective tissue from the vein wall (see Chapter 12). Damage to the vein wall and its valves after an episode of venous thrombosis may disturb venous return and predispose the individual to later development of varicose veins.

Large Pulmonary Emboli

According to the CDC, up to 900,000 people per year experience venous thromboembolism. A large pulmonary embolus (PE) ranks as the third most common cause of cardiovascular death, resulting in 60,000–100,000 deaths in the United States per year. About 25% of the time the first symptom of untreated PE is sudden death. PE that completely blocks the main pulmonary artery or its two major branches will obstruct the flow of blood through the lungs (**Figure 10-3**). The right side of the heart becomes overdistended with blood because blood cannot be expelled into the lungs. The pulmonary artery proximal to the obstructing embolus also becomes overdistended with the rising pressure in the pulmonary artery. Since less blood flows through the lungs into the left side of the heart, the left ventricle is unable to pump an adequate volume of blood to maintain adequate oxygenation of the brain and other vital organs. Consequently, the systemic blood pressure falls, and the patient may go into shock and die. Blood still flows into the lungs from the bronchial arteries, which arise from the descending aorta and interconnect with the pulmonary arteries by means of collateral channels. This flow may lessen the degree of infarction, but also allows blood to flow into the damaged tissue, leading to pulmonary hemorrhage in the damaged area (**Figure 10-4**).

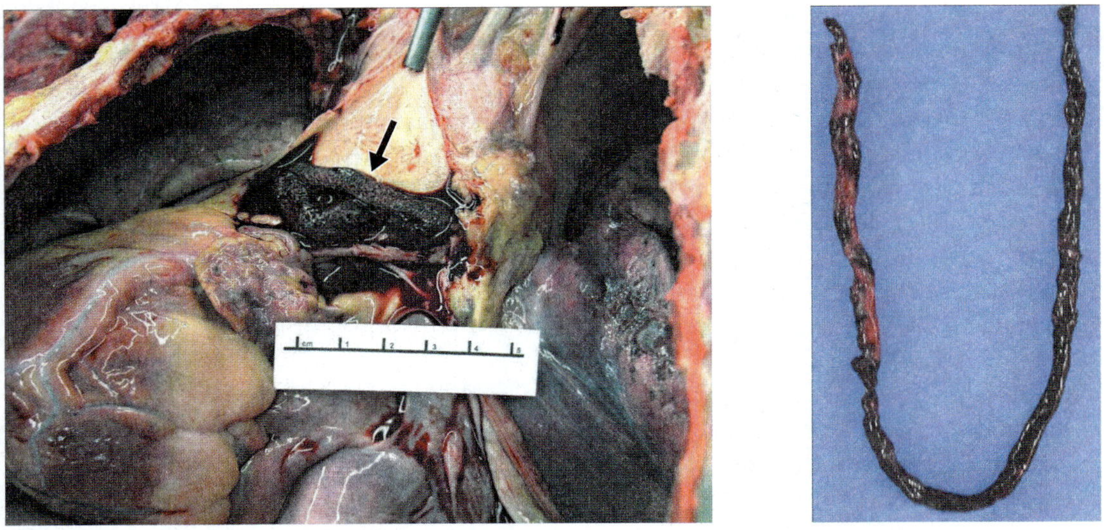

(A) (B)

Figure 10-3 Massive pulmonary embolism. **(A)** Main pulmonary artery occluded by an embolus (*arrow*). The embolus resulted in sudden death of the patient. **(B)** Extracted embolus from the case is illustrated in the figure.

Courtesy of Vincent Moylin Department of Pathology and Laboratory Medicine, University of North Carolina at Chapel Hill.

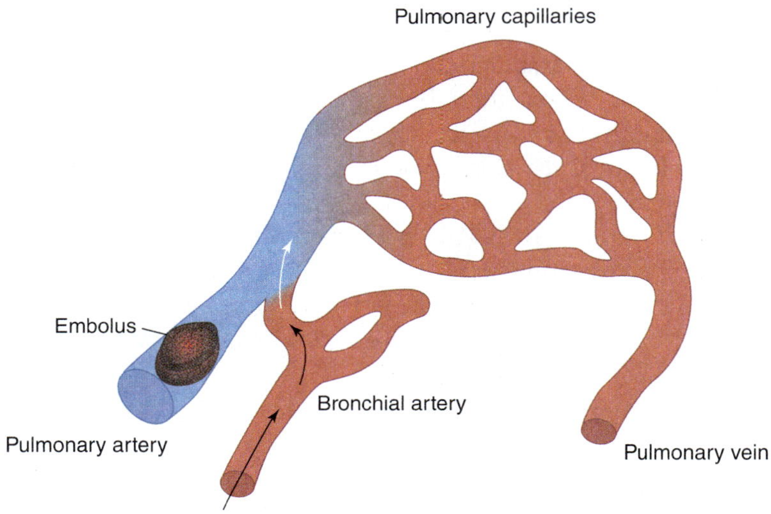

Figure 10-4 Anastomoses between bronchial and pulmonary arteries. The presence of an alternative pathway for blood flow often prevents infarction of the lung when the pulmonary artery is blocked by an embolus.

Clinically, the patient becomes very short of breath and suffers chest pain, and the skin and mucous membranes assume a bluish coloration (cyanosis) because of inadequate blood oxygenation. If the massive embolism is not immediately fatal, some blood may flow around the embolus and circulate through the lungs. Overdistension due to the restricted blood flow can cause the caliber of the pulmonary artery to increase, with the increased arterial pressure forcing blood around the site of obstruction. In favorable circumstances, the embolus eventually dissolves via the body's normal clot-dissolving mechanisms, restoring blood flow through the pulmonary artery. In unfavorable outcomes, thrombus material builds up on the surface of the obstructing embolus, enlarging it. The sluggishly flowing blood in the branches of the pulmonary artery distal to the obstructing embolus may also become thrombosed, further impairing pulmonary blood flow and may ultimately lead to death several days after the initial embolization.

Small Pulmonary Emboli

Small emboli may pass through the main pulmonary arteries and become impacted in the peripheral branches, often in the arteries supplying the lower lobes of the lungs. Smaller emboli impede the flow of blood through the lungs and raise pulmonary artery pressure. Frequently, the segment of lung supplied by the branch of the obstructed pulmonary artery undergoes necrosis, resulting in a pulmonary infarct. The alveolar septa break down, and blood flows from the ruptured capillaries into the pulmonary alveoli, causing distension by the excess blood. The typical infarct is a wedge-shaped hemorrhagic area extending to the pleural surface (**Figure 10-5**). Infarction does not always follow a pulmonary embolism because anastomoses between the bronchial artery and pulmonary artery distal to the obstruction can provide an alternative pathway for blood flow. If the pulmonary venous pressure is elevated, as occurs in heart failure or when the lungs are poorly expanded, an adequate collateral circulation often does not develop and the lung becomes infarcted.

The clinical manifestations of smaller pulmonary emboli are quite variable and frequently minimal if the lung does not become infarcted. Common symptoms of pulmonary infarction are difficulty breathing (dyspnea), pleuritic chest pain, cough, and expectoration of bloody sputum. Chest pain occurs because the pleura overlying the infarct become inflamed and rub against the overlying parietal pleura as the lung expands and contracts during respiration. The cough results from irritation of the bronchi in the injured area. The bloody sputum appears because blood escapes from the infarcted segment of the lung into the bronchi and is subsequently expectorated (coughed up).

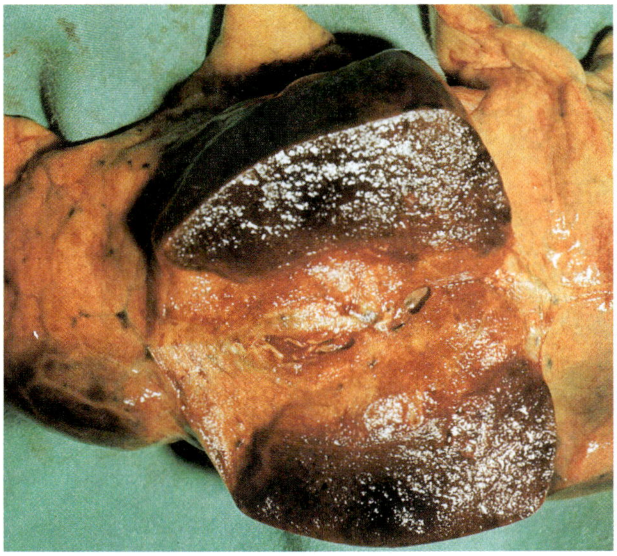

(A)

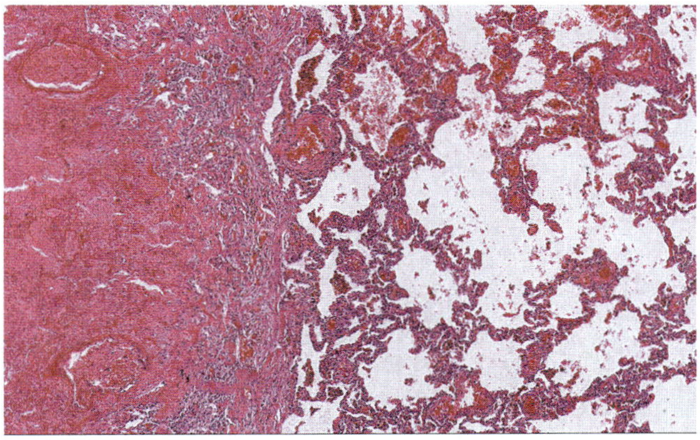

(B)

Figure 10-5 **(A)** Cut surface of a pulmonary infarct, illustrating the hemorrhage in the infarcted lung segment and the sharp demarcation between infarct and adjacent normal lung tissue. **(B)** Photomicrograph of a several days' old pulmonary infarct. Infarcted hemorrhagic area (*left third*) is shown as well as the adjacent lung tissue (*right*), which is spared.

(A) Courtesy of Leonard V. Crowley, MD, Century College; **(B)** Courtesy of Department of Pathology and Laboratory Medicine, University of North Carolina at Chapel Hill.

Diagnosis of Pulmonary Embolism

Unexplained dyspnea, cough, dizziness, heart palpations, pleuritic chest pain, or syncope may be manifestations of a pulmonary embolism. These symptoms should alert the healthcare provider to undertake further diagnostic studies, particularly with evidence of venous thrombosis in the leg (a deep-vein thrombosis, or DVT). A blood test is a critical aid to help confirm the healthcare provider's clinical impression of a possible pulmonary embolism. The test (termed the D-dimer test) measures a by-product formed when fibrin within a blood clot is being broken down (fibrinolysis) by the body's normal clot-dissolving process, activated in response to an intravascular thrombus or embolus. The D-dimer test is over 80% sensitive in the detection of pulmonary emboli; hence, if the D-dimer concentration is not elevated, the possibility of a pulmonary embolism is much less likely. Although an elevated D-dimer concentration supports the healthcare provider's clinical evaluation, it is not sufficient for diagnosis, as the test has a high level of false positive results and further studies are required.

Tools for Diagnosis

The definitive diagnostic method to identify a pulmonary embolism is **computerized tomography pulmonary angiography (CTPA)**. This is a specialized type of CT test in which a dye is injected into the vascular system to allow visualization of the blood vessels entering the lung. The test has a greater than 90 percent sensitivity and specificity for detecting pulmonary emboli.

Computerized tomography pulmonary angiography (CTPA) This is a specialized type of CT test in which a dye is injected into the vascular system to allow visualization of the blood vessels in the lung.

An intravenous catheter is inserted into a vein in the arm, and radiopaque material is injected through the catheter. The flow of the material through the pulmonary arteries is visualized by means of a specialized computed tomography technique that allows three-dimensional reconstruction of the pulmonary vasculature. If the pulmonary artery or one of its branches is completely obstructed by an embolus, no contrast material flows into the blocked vessel (**Figure 10-6**).

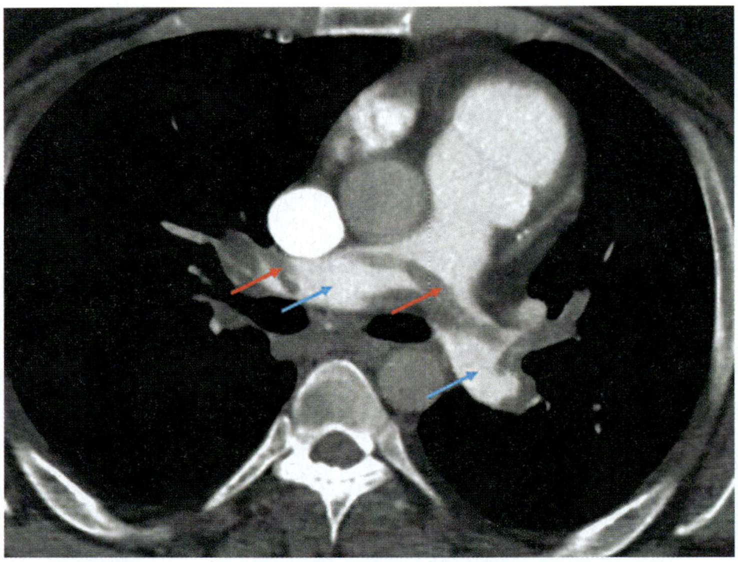

Figure 10-6 A CTPA study to identify a pulmonary embolism illustrated by a view of the right and left pulmonary arteries after radiopaque contrast material has been injected into the vascular system. Flow of contrast material is almost completely blocked (*red arrows*) in both the right and left pulmonary arteries by a large pulmonary embolus (*blue arrows*). The lungs are the large dark areas on the right and left of the images and are not seen.

Courtesy of Leon Bacchus, Chief of Cardiothoracic Imaging at the University of North Carolina at Chapel Hill.

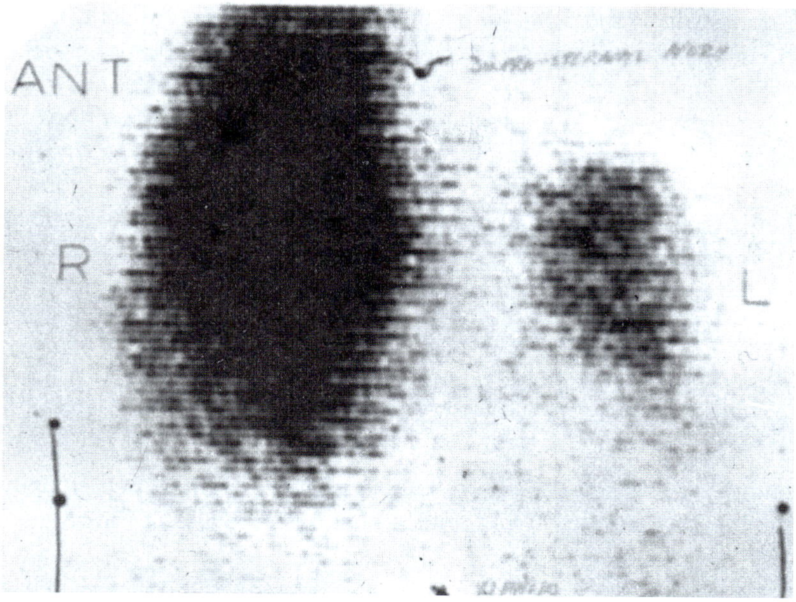

Figure 10-7 Lung scan illustrating impaired blood flow to the left lung (*right*), representing decreased radioactivity. Radioactivity of the opposite lung is normal (uniform dark appearance), indicating normal pulmonary blood flow. This represents the perfusion phase of a V/Q scan.

Courtesy of Leonard V. Crowley, MD, Century College.

If the embolus does not completely obstruct the artery, some contrast medium flows around the embolus. This appears as a filling defect in the column of contrast material within the partially occluded vessel. If the embolus caused pulmonary infarction, a routine chest X-ray may demonstrate the infarct, appearing as a wedge-shaped area of increased density in the lung. Routine chest X-rays are not useful for the detection of pulmonary emboli, as they demonstrate very poor sensitivity (10–20 percent).

A **ventilation/perfusion scan (V/Q scan)** may be used with patients where CTPA cannot be performed (often because of allergy to the dye or kidney problems) or is inconclusive. The test has two parts. First, a radioactive gas or aerosol preparation is inhaled (the ventilation phase). The distribution of the tracer is detected using a gamma ray camera to determine the area of the lung that is ventilated. In the subsequent perfusion phase, a solution of specially prepared albumin labeled with a radioisotope is injected into a peripheral vein. The injected material flows through the lung and is filtered out in the pulmonary capillaries. The radioactivity in the lungs, related to pulmonary blood flow, is likewise recorded. An area of the lung that shows a ventilation–perfusion mismatch (i.e., an area of the lung ventilated but not perfused by blood) is highly indicative of a pulmonary embolism. The V/Q study does not demonstrate the embolus; it only indicates part of the lung can be ventilated but has a reduced blood supply, which is highly indicative of a PE (**Figure 10-7**). Consequently, the lung scan will be abnormal even when the lung is not infarcted.

Ventilation/perfusion scan (V/Q scan) Procedure used to detect a pulmonary embolus.

Treatment of Pulmonary Embolism

Treatment of patients with pulmonary embolism includes general supportive care, including oxygen administration and administration of anticoagulants. The purpose of anticoagulant therapy is twofold: to prevent recurrent pulmonary emboli by preventing the formation of more thrombi in leg and pelvic veins and to prevent thrombus formation in branches of the distal pulmonary artery to the embolism. If the patient sustained a massive embolus and blood flow through a main pulmonary artery is blocked, rapid dissolution of the embolus by administering thrombolytic drugs may be undertaken. These are frequently the same drugs given to a heart attack patient to dissolve a thrombus blocking a coronary artery (see Chapter 9).

If the patient continues to have pulmonary emboli despite adequate anticoagulant therapy, a filter may be placed in the inferior vena cava percutaneously (through a skin incision). Such filters trap emboli and prevent them from reaching the lung. The filter may be removed at a later date if necessary.

Embolism as a Result of Foreign Material

Most emboli are caused by blood clots, but other materials occasionally gain access to the circulation. Fat, air, and foreign particles within the vascular system sometimes cause serious difficulties.

Fat Embolism

After a severe bone fracture, fatty bone marrow and surrounding adipose tissue may be disrupted. The emulsified fat globules can be sucked into the veins and carried into the lungs, leading to widespread obstruction of the pulmonary capillaries. Some of the fat may be carried through the pulmonary capillaries and reach the systemic circulation, eventually blocking small blood vessels in the brain and other organs (**Figure 10-8**).

Amniotic Fluid Embolism

This condition is an uncommon but devastating complication of pregnancy. It usually occurs during labor when the pressure of uterine contractions forces a large volume of amniotic fluid released through a tear in fetal membranes into a torn uterine vein. The amniotic fluid, containing desquamated fetal epithelial cells, hair, fatty material (vernix), debris from the fetal respiratory and gastrointestinal tracts, and thromboplastic (blood clot–promoting) material, can be carried through the maternal venous circulation to the lungs. In the lungs, the pulmonary capillaries become obstructed with contents of the amniotic fluid.

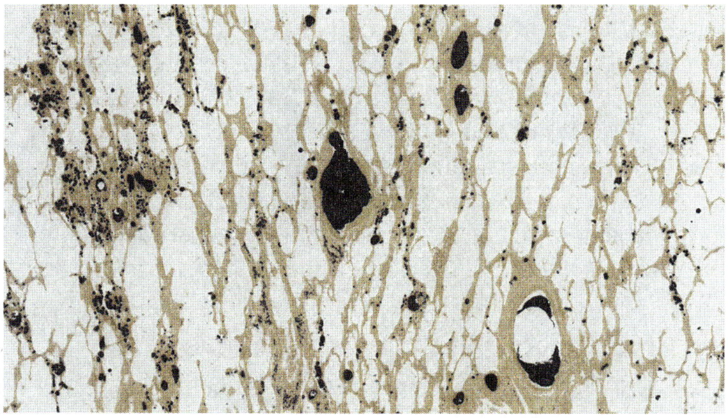

Figure 10-8 Multiple fat emboli in cerebral vessels of a patient who suffered severe lower limb trauma. Intravascular fat emboli are stained black using a fat-specific stain.

Courtesy of Department of Pathology and Laboratory Medicine, University of North Carolina at Chapel Hill.

Manifestations are severe dyspnea, shock, and often an acute disseminated intravascular coagulation syndrome (see Chapter 12) induced by the thromboplastic material in the amniotic fluid.

Air Embolism

Sometimes a large amount of air is introduced into the venous circulation after a chest wound with injury to the lung. Air can also be accidentally injected during venipuncture procedures. Consequently, care must be taken when administering IV therapy and intravenous therapies. The air is carried to the heart and accumulates in the right heart chambers, preventing filling of the heart by returning venous blood. As a result, the heart is unable to pump blood, and the individual dies rapidly of circulatory failure. In cases where a smaller air bubble has been introduced into the venous circulatory system, the bubble can become lodged in a blood vessel, blocking it in the same way a thrombus might. The amount of air resulting in a fatal outcome is generally over 100 ml, but this depends on the location of the embolism, the cerebral circulation being very sensitive.

Embolism of Particulate Foreign Material

Various types of particulate material may be injected into veins through "recreational" drug use. Crushed pharmaceutical tablets incompletely dissolved in solution might be injected intravenously. Street drugs can be cut with insoluble materials that remain as solids in the solution. Sharing needles can also lead to dirt and tissue debris accumulating within the needle, where it can be inadvertently injected as well. The material is usually trapped within the small pulmonary blood vessels, producing symptoms of severe respiratory distress caused by obstruction of the pulmonary capillaries by the foreign material, or may, with time, result in pulmonary fibrosis (lung scarring).

Varicose Veins

Dilated, tortuous veins are termed "varices" or "varicose veins." (Varix is a Latin word meaning dilated vessel; the plural term is varices.) Varicosities occur most often in leg veins but may occur in other veins as well. Venous thromboses can form in abnormally dilated vessels due to the slowing of blood flow through the area. Inflammation of a vein is termed **phlebitis** (phleb = vein + itis = inflammation). If there is an associated thrombosis of the affected vein, the term thrombophlebitis is used (**Figure 10-9**).

Phlebitis Inflammation of a vein.

Veins, both deep veins and superficial veins, return blood from the lower limbs, with the deep veins carrying most of the venous return. These veins accompany the major arteries and drain into the iliac veins, which in turn empty into the inferior vena cava. The superficial veins form a network of intercommunicating channels that travel beneath the skin in the subcutaneous tissue and eventually drain into the deep veins and constitute the saphenous system. Both the superficial and deep veins contain cup-shaped valves that are interposed along the course of the veins. The arrangement of the valves ensures one-way blood flow. Blood can flow toward the heart in the veins but cannot flow in the reverse direction. The superficial and deep venous systems are also interconnected with short communicating branches containing valves arranged so that blood normally flows only from superficial to deep veins and not in the reverse direction.

Blood is propelled upward within the deep veins by contraction of the leg and thigh muscles, which intermittently compress the veins and force the blood within the veins against gravity, while the valves prevent retrograde flow.

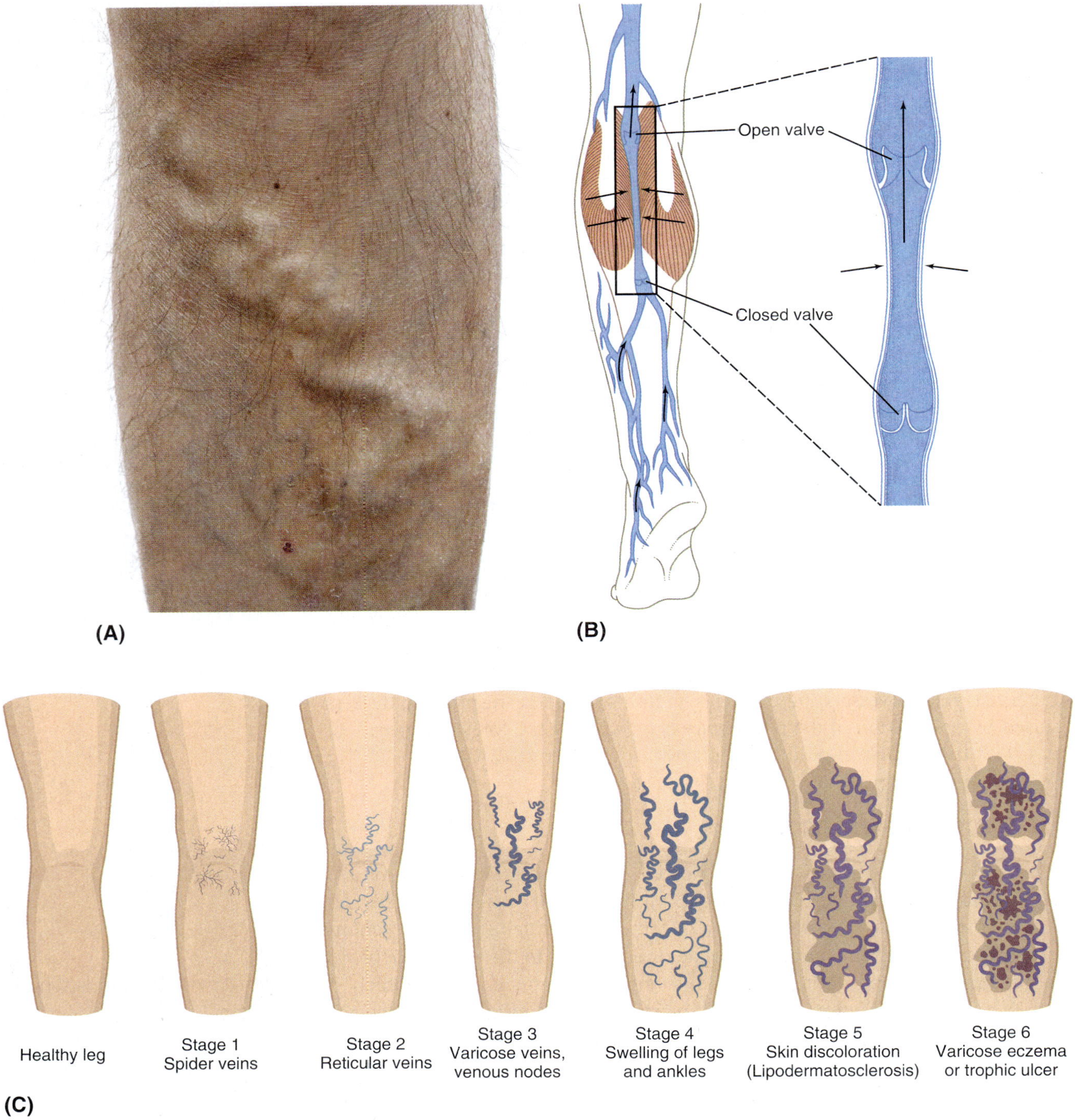

Figure 10-9 **(A)** Varicose veins result from a restriction of venous blood flow to the heart. **(B)** Valves in veins. The slight hydrostatic pressure in the veins and the contraction of skeletal muscles propel the blood along the veins back toward the heart. The oneway valves stop the blood from flowing backward. **(C)** Stages of varicose veins: the progression of the development of varicose veins.

(A) © Audie/Shutterstock; (C) © Olga Bolbot/Shutterstock

In contrast, the superficial veins are relatively unsupported, and venous return is much less efficient (Figure 10-9B).

Varicose veins result if the saphenous veins become dilated and their valves become incompetent. As a result, the blood tends to stagnate in the veins instead of flowing back to the heart, causing the veins to become elongated and tortuous.

The condition is common, affecting 15 percent of people, and tends to run in families, suggesting that the basic cause is an inherited weakness of the vein wall or its valves, which predisposes them to the varicosities. Varicose veins increase with age and are more common in women, particularly those who have been pregnant. Continued upright posture, including standing for long amounts of time, and obesity are also risk factors.

Varicose veins of the saphenous system also may develop if the deeper veins become blocked or if their valves become damaged by previous thrombophlebitis. As a result of damage to the deep veins, more of the venous return is shifted to the unsupported superficial veins, which are unable to accommodate the increased flow and become varicose.

Complications of Varicose Veins

Complications result from stasis of blood in the veins, leading to poor nutrition of the tissues caused by chronic venous engorgement. The skin of the distal leg and ankle becomes thin and atrophic and quite susceptible to infection. Skin ulcers may develop and heal poorly. The dilated veins are easily injured and may rupture, leading to extravasation of blood and chronic discoloration of the skin. Stasis of blood in the veins also predisposes individuals to repeated bouts of thrombophlebitis.

Treatment of Varicose Veins

Varicosities of the saphenous veins are treated by elastic stockings to support the veins and elevation of the legs whenever possible to promote more efficient venous return. Sometimes surgical removal of the varicose veins may be required. This is usually performed in conjunction with ligation of the communicating veins that interconnect the superficial and deep venous systems.

Varicose Veins in Other Locations

Dilated veins around the rectum are termed **hemorrhoids** and are described in the discussion on disorders of the gastrointestinal tract. Varicose veins of the esophagus often occur in patients with cirrhosis of the liver. Esophageal varices may rupture and cause profuse life-threatening hemorrhage. Their pathogenesis and treatment are considered in the discussion on the liver and the biliary system. Varicose veins of the spermatic cord appear as a mass of vessels in the scrotum above the testicle. The condition is termed a varicocele (varix = vein + cele = swelling). The varicosities usually do not cause symptoms but at times may cause mild scrotal discomfort. Rarely they may impair fertility in some men. Usually no treatment is required (discussed in Chapter 18).

Hemorrhoids Dilated veins around the anus and the rectum.

Thrombosis at Nonvenous Sites

Arterial Thrombosis

Blood flow in arteries is rapid and intravascular pressure is high, so stasis of blood is not a factor in arterial thrombosis. The main cause of arterial thrombosis is injury to the wall of the vessel, usually secondary to atherosclerosis. The effects of arterial thrombus formation depend on the location and size of the artery that has become obstructed. Blockage of a coronary artery frequently causes infarction of the heart muscle and consequent "heart attack" (see Chapter 9). Peripheral arterial disease resulting in thrombi in the vessels supplying the leg (aortoiliac disease of the iliac arteries) may result in claudication, pain, or weakness in the legs on walking. If a major artery supplying the leg is completely occluded, the extremity undergoes

Gangrene Tissue death caused by bacterial infection or lack of blood circulation.

necrosis, often referred to as **gangrene**. This type of gangrene differs from "gas gangrene" caused by a bacterium species, *Clostridium*. Occlusion of an artery to the brain leads to infarction of a portion of the brain, commonly termed a "stroke."

Intracardiac Thrombosis

Occasionally, blood clots may form within the heart itself. With abnormal heart function, thrombi may form within the atrial appendages. Heart failure and arrhythmias such as atrial fibrillations can lead to abnormal atrial contractions predisposing the patient to intracardiac thrombi. Thrombi can form on the surface of heart valves damaged as a result of disease. Occasionally, thrombi may form on the internal lining of the ventricle adjacent to an area where the heart muscle is infarcted. Such thrombi, which adhere to the endocardium (inner layer of heart), are termed mural thrombi (mural is Latin for "wall") (**Figure 10-10**). Intracardiac thrombi can be dislodged and carried into the systemic circulation, leading to infarctions in other tissues, such as the spleen, kidneys, brain, or other organs. The symptoms produced depend on the size and location of the infarction.

Thrombosis in Patients with Cancer

Many patients with advanced cancer are predisposed to both venous and arterial thromboses. This tendency results from the release of thromboplastic (prothrombotic) materials into the circulation from the tumor. The same basic mechanism induces hemorrhage in patients with a disseminated intravascular coagulation syndrome (discussed in Chapter 12).

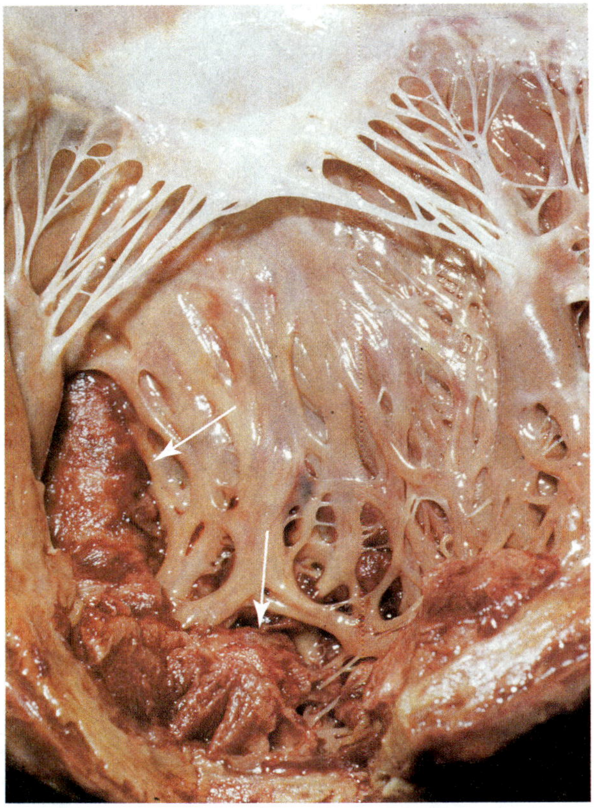

Figure 10-10 Interior of heart chamber (left ventricle), illustrating a mural thrombus adherent to the wall (endocardium) adjacent to the myocardial infarct (*arrows*). A normal heart valve (the mitral valve) and its components are seen at the top of the photo.

Edema

The term *edema* refers to the accumulation of fluid in the interstitial tissues (**Figure 10-11**). Edema is most conspicuous in the skin and subcutaneous tissues of the dependent (lower) parts of the body and is usually noted first in the legs and ankles. When the edematous tissue is compressed by indenting the tissue with the fingertips, the fluid is pushed aside, leaving a pit or indentation that gradually refills with fluid. This characteristic is responsible for the common term *pitting edema*. Fluid may also accumulate in the pleural cavity (**hydrothorax**) or in the peritoneal cavity (**ascites**).

Edema may result from any condition in which the circulation of extracellular fluid between the capillaries and the interstitial tissues becomes disturbed.

Hydrothorax Accumulation of fluid in the pleural cavity.
Ascites A type of pneumoconiosis caused by inhalation of asbestos fibers.

Pathogenesis and Classification of Edema

Increased Capillary Permeability

Normally, the endothelium of the capillaries limits the amount of fluid filtered from the blood. If the capillaries are excessively permeable, filtration of fluid into the interstitial space is greater than normal. Increased capillary permeability is responsible for the swelling of the tissues associated with acute inflammation, such as a boil or a severe sunburn. Some systemic diseases also cause a generalized increase in capillary permeability, which leads to widespread edema of the subcutaneous tissues (**Figure 10-12**).

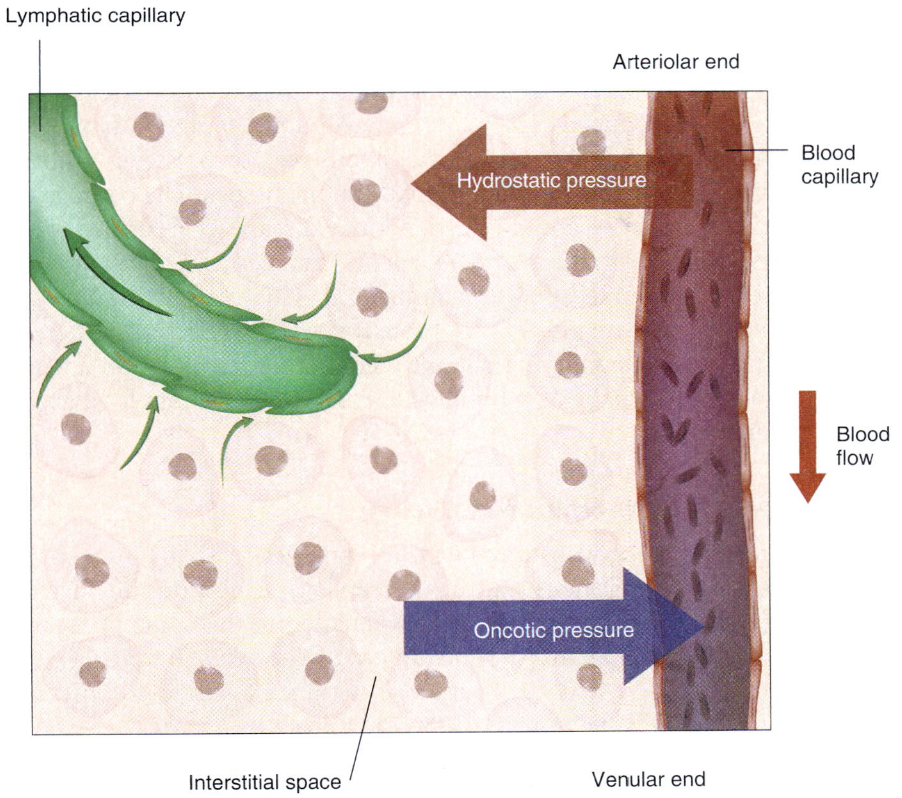

Figure 10-11 Fluid homeostasis in the body involves the cardiovascular system and the lymph system. Changes in protein, ion, and other solute concentrations in the blood and interstitial fluid drive osmosis between those compartments.

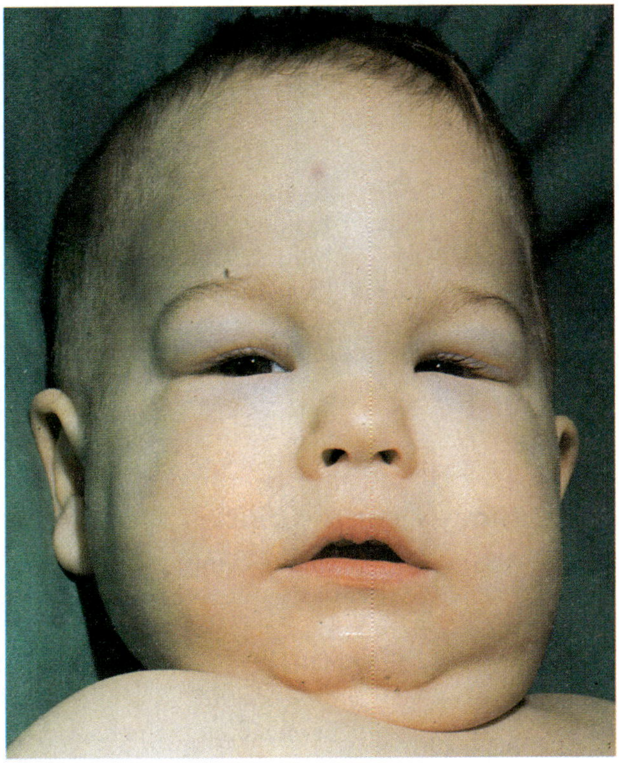

Figure 10-12 Edema as a result of increased capillary permeability. Note the swelling of the eyelids and face.

Courtesy of Leonard V. Crowley, MD, Century College.

Low Plasma Proteins

If the concentration of plasma proteins is decreased, the colloid osmotic (oncotic) pressure is reduced correspondingly. Albumin, a protein synthesized in the liver, is the major contributor to the blood's oncotic pressure. When the oncotic pressure of blood is low, fluid remains in the tissues. The pathogenesis of low blood protein levels could include kidney disease when urine contains plasma proteins that normally are not excreted. In some cases, the synthesis of plasma proteins is inhibited due to malnutrition, starvation, or liver disease. Hypoproteinemia, resulting from poor protein intake, may be encountered in patients with chronic debilitating disease who are unable to eat an adequate amount of food and in patients with intestinal diseases in whom food absorption is impaired.

Superior vena cava syndrome This syndrome occurs with blockage or compression of the superior vena cava, the vessel that carries blood from the head, neck, upper chest, and arms. This results in fluid accumulation in those areas.

Inferior vena cava syndrome This syndrome occurs with blockage or compression of the inferior vena cava and results in edema of the lower extremities.

Increased Hydrostatic Pressure

Increased pressure in the veins draining the capillaries leads to a higher-than-normal pressure at the venous end of the capillaries, resulting in increased fluid filtration from the capillaries and accumulation in the tissue. A localized increase in venous pressure may be encountered if the veins draining a part of the body become compressed (for example, by a tumor), twisted, or obstructed by a blood clot that fills the lumen. **Superior vena cava syndrome** occurs with blockage or compression of that vessel, leading to fluid accumulation in the areas it drains: the head and neck, upper chest, and arms. Likewise, **inferior vena cava syndrome** leads to edema of the lower extremities. More commonly, increased venous pressure is a manifestation of heart failure, and the pressure is elevated in all the systemic veins (**Figure 10-13**).

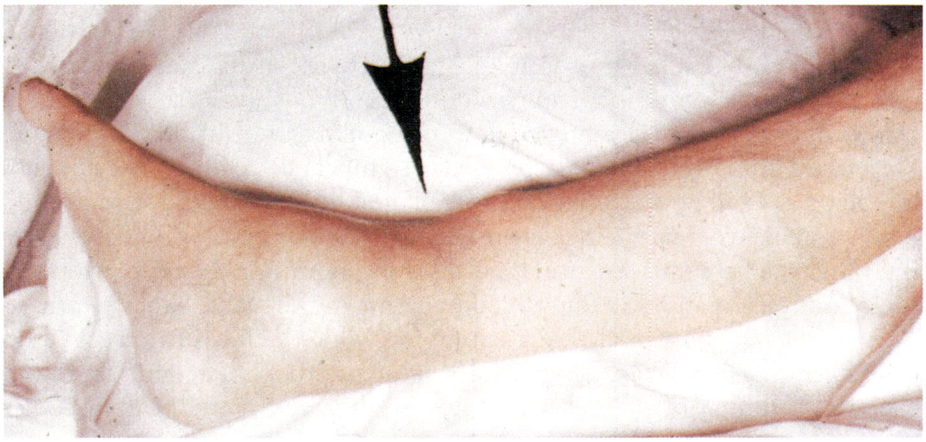

(A)

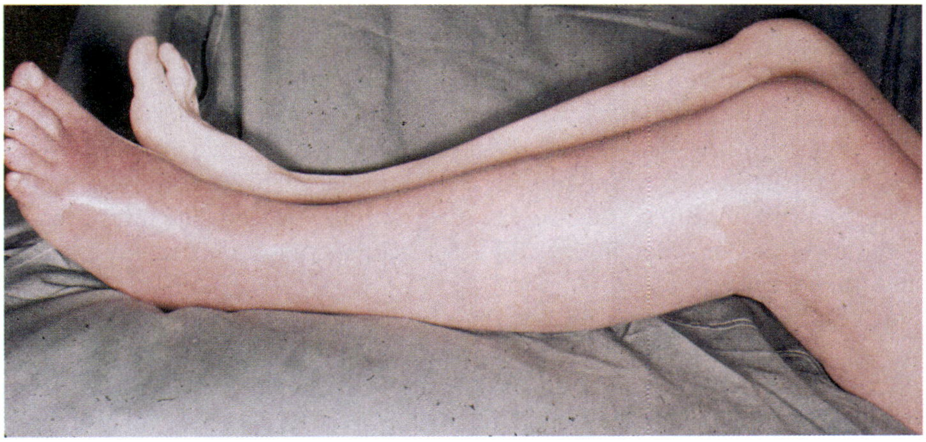

(B)

Figure 10-13 **(A)** Marked pitting edema of leg (*arrow*) as a result of chronic heart failure. **(B)** Localized edema of left leg caused by venous obstruction. Right leg appears normal.

Courtesy of Leonard V. Crowley, MD, Century College.

Lymphatic Obstruction

Sometimes, lymphatic channels draining a part of the body become obstructed. The obstruction blocks a pathway by which fluid is returned from the interstitial space into the circulation and leads to edema in the region that is normally drained by the obstructed lymphatic vessels.

Shock

Shock is a general term describing any condition in which the blood pressure is too low to provide adequate blood flow to the body cells and organs. It is a serious, potentially life-threatening condition. Shock occurs because the total capacity of the circulatory system is larger than the actual blood volume. Blood pressure falls if the volume of blood filling the circulatory system falls or if marked dilation of blood vessels expands the capacity of the vascular system to such an extent that the existing blood volume is insufficient to fill the vessels adequately and venous return to the heart becomes inadequate.

Classification

Shock can be classified into four categories based on its cause: hypovolemic, cardiogenic, septic, or anaphylactic shock. Hypovolemic shock is caused by low blood volume, leading to a corresponding drop in blood pressure. Most cases result from a large hemorrhage significantly reducing the circulating blood volume, but any excessive depletion of body fluids, such as fluid losses from an extensive burn, severe diarrhea and/or vomiting, and excessive fluid loss due to increased urination resulting from, for example, excessive use of diuretics, can also reduce blood volume. Cardiogenic shock is caused by inadequate or impaired cardiac pumping, which reduces cardiac output. Cardiogenic shock often accompanies a myocardial infarction. However, effective pumping of the heart can also be impaired if the heart becomes compressed by accumulation of blood or fluid within the pericardial sac, a condition termed "cardiac tamponade." When the pericardial sac accumulates blood or other fluid, the filling of the heart during diastole becomes impeded, causing acute heart failure. Septic shock results from the release of inflammatory mediators in response to infection. The infection often results from gram-negative organisms that release endotoxins, potent inflammatory mediators. These mediators can increase capillary permeability, resulting in the decrease of plasma oncotic pressure as substances leak from the capillary into the surrounding tissues. The drop in plasma oncotic pressure then leads to a shift in fluids from the vasculature to the tissues. The infection can promote endothelial cell injury and accompanying vasodilation as a result of endothelial cell stimulation.

Anaphylaxis results from a reaction to a foreign substance to which a person has an allergy (for example, peanuts, tree nuts, and bee stings are often implicated). Anaphylactic shock (described in Chapter 5) results from excessive vasodilation caused by the widespread release of inflammatory mediators from mast cells and basophils. Circulatory collapse often follows anaphylactic shock.

Prognosis and Treatment

The outcome of shock depends on its cause and how quickly it is recognized and treated. Treatment consists of administering drugs that raise blood pressure (vasopressive agents), restoring blood volume by intravenous fluids or blood transfusion, and treating the underlying condition that led to the shock response. The prognosis depends upon the overall health of the patient and other comorbidities, but the condition has a high mortality of over 30% even with prompt treatment.

Atherosclerosis

The Response to Injury Hypothesis

Atherosclerosis is a chronic and progressive, degenerative disease of large-to medium-sized arteries. Examples include the thoracic and abdominal aortae, the femoral and popliteal arteries, the internal carotids, various cerebral arteries, and the coronary arteries. The disease is believed to be triggered by endothelial injury, which leads to a gradual accumulation of cells, connective tissue, and lipids. The lipids consist of mostly free cholesterol and cholesterol esterified to long-chain fatty acids. These accumulations occur within the intima (innermost layer) of the vessel wall (**Figure 10-14**).

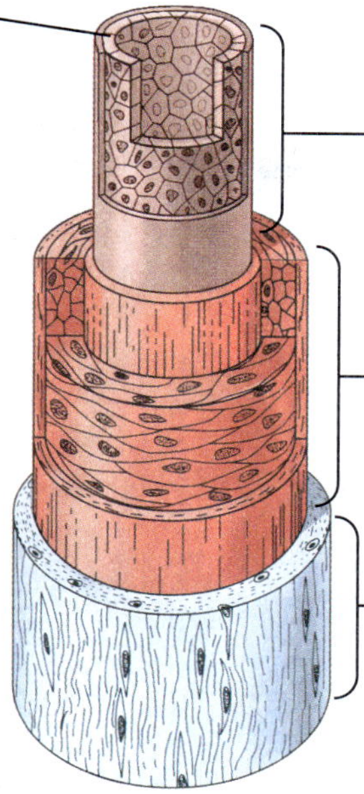

Figure 10-14 General structure of the blood vessel. The artery shown here consists of three major layers: tunica intima, tunica media, and tunica adventitia.

The normal artery consists of several layers: the tunica intima closest to the lumen, the tunica media, and the tunica adventitia, the outermost layer. The nonthrombogenic single layer of endothelial cells (the endothelium) lining the lumen constitutes the innermost layer of the artery (tunica intima), which is predominantly collagenous in nature and contains few fibroblasts or smooth muscle cells. The tunica media (middle layer) contains multiple concentric layers of smooth muscle cells that are rich in elastin in an elastic artery. The outer surface of the artery is the tunica adventitia, composed of connective tissue. During the process of atherosclerosis, inflammatory and immune cells accumulate in the tunica intima, as do smooth muscle cells, which migrate from the tunica media in response to cytokines liberated by inflammatory responses and immune cells. Damage to the endothelial cells occurs in part due to friction, lipid products, inflammatory mediators, and possibly pathogens and their products. The endothelial permeability barrier changes, allowing lipids to penetrate into the tunica intima from the blood. In addition (and critical to the process), damaged endothelial cells express cell surface molecules that facilitate adherence of blood monocytes/macrophages to the damaged endothelium. These cells adhere and then migrate into the arterial wall. The macrophages carry lipids (as a component of **low-density lipoprotein (LDL)**) from the blood into the intima, where they accumulate as lipid-rich **foamy macrophages**. The macrophages also release cytokines and growth factors, which stimulate smooth muscle cells, connective tissue, and further inflammatory cell accumulation. The inflammatory cells and damaged endothelium promote oxidation of the deposited lipid, which becomes a further source of tissue damage and inflammation. With time the hallmark lesion of atherosclerosis, the raised **atheroma** (athere = porridge), forms in the intima. The atheroma is a plaque with a necrotic core rich in lipid. The deposit is often rich in cholesterol, which can become crystalline. The core is covered by a fibrous cap tissue containing immune and inflammatory cells (often foamy macrophages), smooth muscle cells, and other connective tissue. This lesion is termed a

Low-density lipoprotein (LDL) Plasma protein molecule carrying cholesterol to the tissue.

Foamy macrophages Macrophages carrying lipids.

Atheroma Formation of plaque with a necrotic core rich in lipids.

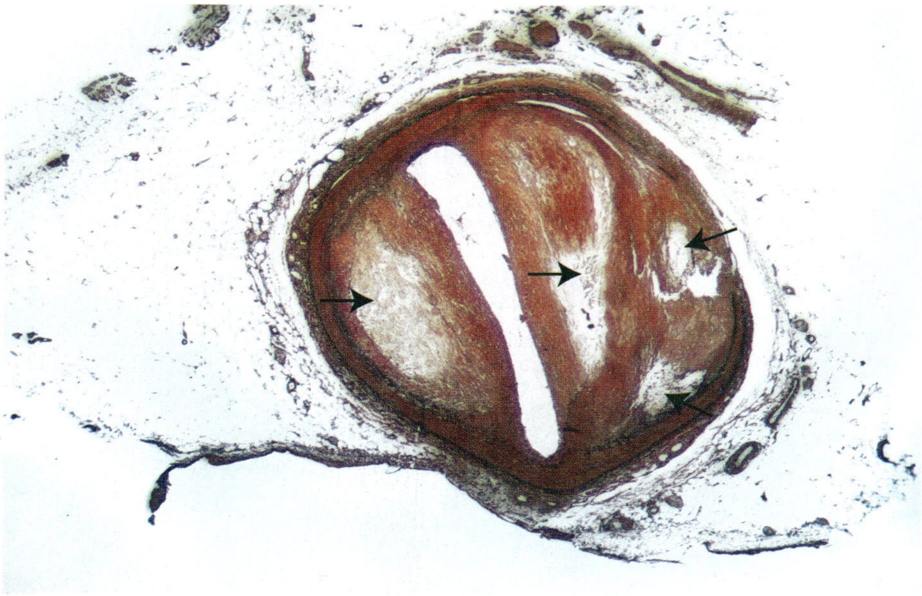

Figure 10-15 Low-magnification microphotograph of a coronary artery in cross section illustrating several atheromatous plaques (*arrows*) surrounded by dense fibrous tissue. Atheromatous deposits reduce the lumen of the artery to a narrow slip (original magnification ×40).

Courtesy of Leonard V. Crowley, MD, Century College.

Stenosis Abnormal narrowing of a passageway.

Thrombotic stroke Reduction in blood flow in the brain due to thrombus.

fibrofatty plaque (**Figure 10-15**). The gradual growth of the atheroma, likely over decades, leads it to protrude into the lumen of the artery where it compromises blood flow. The artery can initially remodel to enlarge the lumen, but this is a limited process that will ultimately result in arterial **stenosis** (narrowing) and reduced blood through the artery and oxygenation of adjacent tissue. As the atheroma enlarges, the surface of the vessel over the atheroma becomes increasingly damaged and fibrotic (termed complicated plaque). Turbulent hemodynamic flow over the stenosed (stiffened) area will result in further endothelial damage with possible ulceration and plaque rupture. The ruptured plaque releases thrombotic lipids and calcified damaged cellular debris into the circulation.

Hemorrhage into the plaque may occur suddenly, increasing its size and totally blocking blood flow. The damaged endothelium over the atheroma becomes increasingly prothrombotic as the endothelium is lost and the fibrous cap is exposed, leading to platelet adhesion and the formation of an adherent thrombus blocking arterial flow. The thrombus may detach and travel in the vessel to a distant site where it lodges as an embolus (**Figure 10-16**).

The clinical consequences of atherosclerosis depend on where it occurs. In coronary arteries, it results in cardiac ischemia. If atherosclerotic plaques narrow the coronary arteries by 50 percent to 75 percent, the arteries may still be able to supply enough blood to the heart muscle if the individual is not very active and no excessive demands are placed on the heart.(**Figure 10-17**). However, the blood supply may become inadequate under exertion when the heart requires more blood to satisfy the increased demands. If the reduction in blood flow is sudden and sufficiently severe, a myocardial infarct (heart attack) will occur. In cerebral vessels, a **thrombotic stroke** leading to brain ischemia will result in damage and death of neural tissue.

The damaged aortic wall may balloon outward as an abdominal aortic aneurysm (often termed an AAA, or "triple A") that can rupture with catastrophic

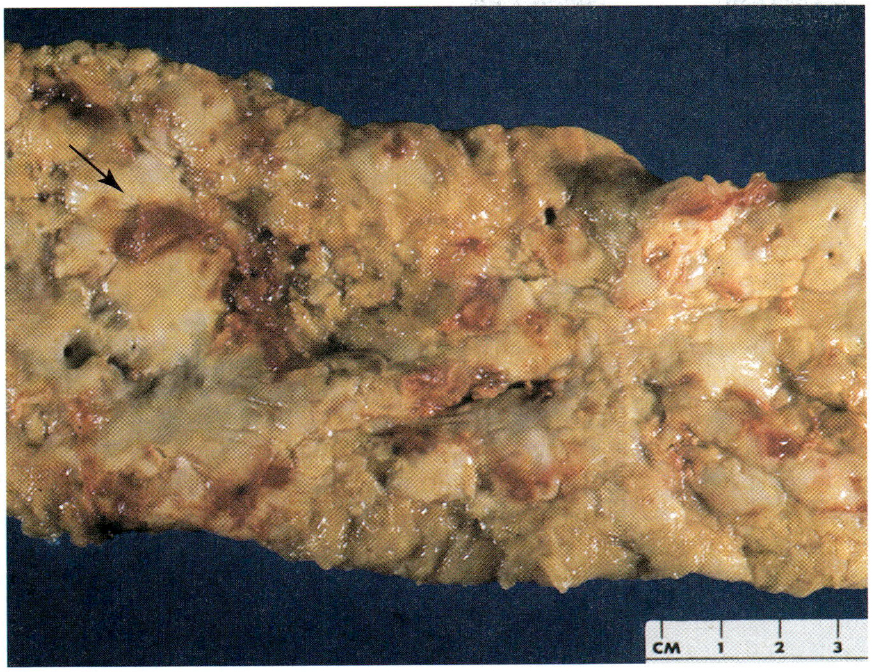

Figure 10-16 Advanced atherosclerosis of aorta. Many plaques are ulcerated and are covered by thrombus material (*arrow*).

Courtesy of Leonard V. Crowley, MD, Century College.

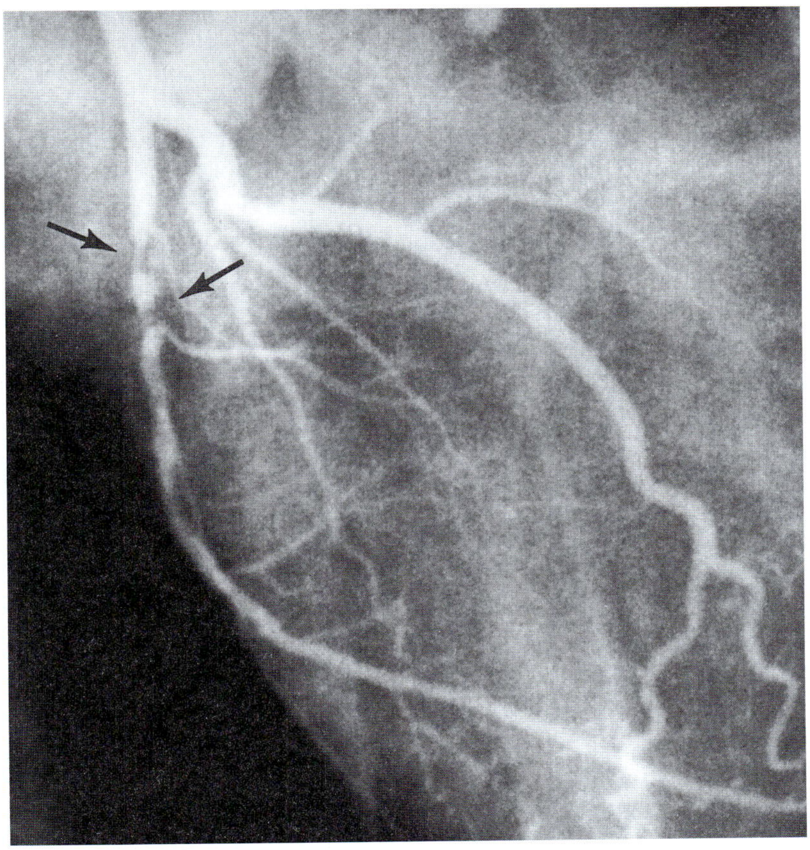

Figure 10-17 A coronary angiogram illustrating several areas of coronary artery narrowing (*arrows*). The individual demonstrated exertional chest pain (angina pectoris) on exercise.

Courtesy of Leonard V. Crowley, MD, Century College.

Vascular claudication
Severe cramping leg pain due to atherosclerosis of arteries in the leg.

Fatty streak lesions
Early sign of atherosclerosis as elongated flat accumulations of foam cells.

results. Atherosclerosis of the arteries supplying the legs results in **vascular claudication** with severe cramping leg pain, impaired mobility, and potentially gangrene of the lower limb. Atherosclerosis of the renal arteries can lead to loss of kidney function; in the mesenteric vessels, atherosclerosis can result in lethal necrosis of the gut.

Natural History of Atherosclerosis

A myocardial infarction (MI) is often a sudden and unexpected event. MI can occur in people under 40, but the incidence increases with age, with men exhibiting an increase after 45 and women after 55. The average age for a first MI in men is 65.5 and for women 72. However, the process of atherosclerosis that precipitated this event began far earlier in the person's life, perhaps as early as the first decade. The first signs of atherosclerosis emerge as precursor lesions detectable in children in their first and second decade. These **fatty streak lesions** consist of accumulations of lipid-rich foam cells within the intima. The lesions often appear elongated (hence the term streak) and parallel to the direction of blood flow. Since they are mostly flat, blood flow remains unaffected. Fatty streaks first appear in the thoracic aorta, but the distribution of these lesions does not mirror the location of atheromas in adults (which are not frequent in this location). Somewhat later in life, fatty streaks begin to appear in coronary vessels in locations where fibrofatty atheromas become more common with increasing age, suggesting the fatty streaks are a precursor lesion of atherosclerosis. With time, fibrofatty atheromas develop, a process that may take decades. This occurs at sites where endothelial injury occurs, a process in which blood flow dynamics plays a role. The atheroma may initially be stable, but as it begins to grow in size, it becomes clinically significant and causes luminal stenosis and reduced blood flow (**Figure 10-18**).

Reduced blood flow may result in some degree of cardiac ischemia when the heart is stressed by exercise or in some other way (Figure 10-17). The cardiac ischemia manifests as cramping chest pain (cardiac angina). This pain can be relieved using vasodilators to increase the luminal diameter of the

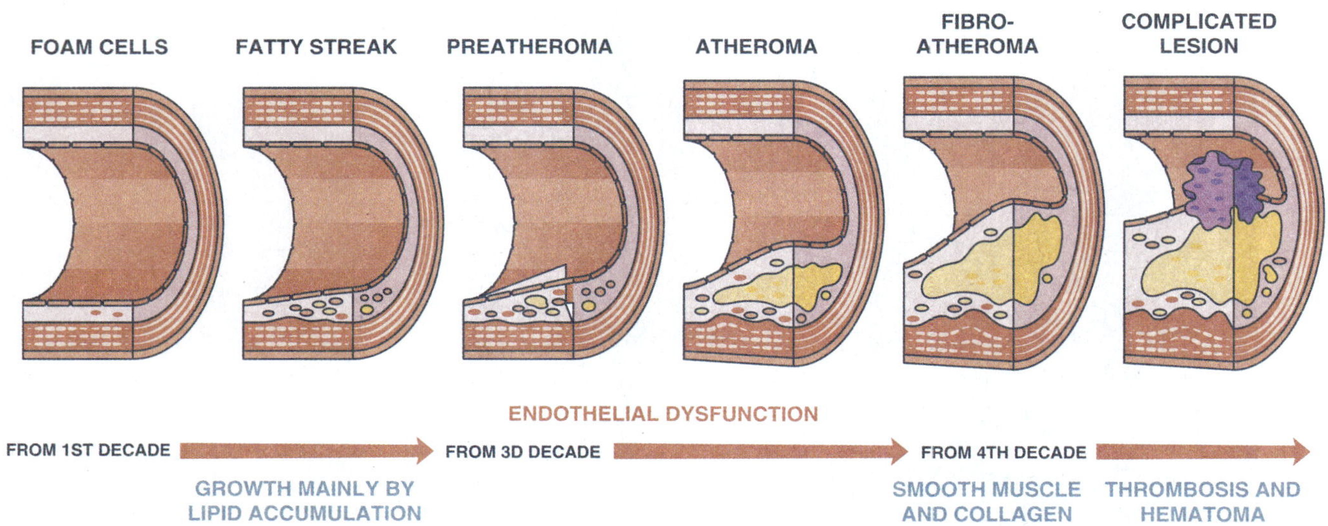

Figure 10-18 Progression of atherosclerosis. Atherosclerosis starts initially as the accumulation of foamy cells near an area of damage. As it progresses the lesion accumulates more fat and becomes more complicated, resulting in the narrowing of the lumen of the arteries.

vessels. As the process continues, changes to the plaque destabilize it and render it prothrombotic. Eventually (frequently in the late sixth or seventh decade), an acute change to a complicated lesion results in clinically evident and possibly catastrophic disease. Hence, atherosclerosis is a chronic, multidecade process. Prevention of atherosclerosis requires modification of risk factors and recognition that some risk factors may not be changed and require positive therapeutic intervention.

Risk Factors for Atherosclerotic Disease: Introduction

A number of modifiable factors are known to increase the risk of developing atherosclerotic vascular disease and its associated complications. The four major risk factors include elevated blood lipids, high blood pressure, cigarette smoking, and diabetes. The most important is elevated blood lipids, **hyperlipidemia**, specifically **hypercholesterolemia**, which even in the absence of other risk factors can promote atheroma development. Most serum cholesterol is associated with low-density lipoprotein (LDL), the plasma protein molecule that carries cholesterol to the tissue where it is metabolized. LDL cholesterol is often termed "bad lipid" and is strongly associated with increased risk. **High-density lipoprotein (HDL)** carries cholesterol from the periphery (and from atheromas) to the liver for excretion as bile and is often termed "good lipid," as higher levels of HDL reduce risk to some degree.

The remaining major modifiable risk factors include high blood pressure, cigarette smoking, and diabetes. If one risk factor is present, the likelihood of coronary heart disease and heart attacks is twice that of an individual lacking risk factors. If two risk factors are present, the risk increases fourfold, and if three factors are present, the risk of heart attack is seven times that for an individual with none.

Other modifiable factors play a less important (or more poorly defined) role. Obesity and a sedentary lifestyle increase the risk of atherosclerotic disease. It is likely these factors interact to promote high blood lipids, elevated blood pressure, and the risk of metabolic syndrome with subsequent type II diabetes, discussed in Chapter 20. Elevated levels of blood **homocysteine**, **homocysteinemia**, present a major risk factor that may have a genetic component. It is uncertain whether dietary therapy using B vitamins and folic acid reduces the incidence of cardiovascular disease. Likewise, an elevated level of the acute phase reactant **C-reactive protein**, associated with inflammation, is an independent risk factor for atherosclerosis; it is uncertain whether modification by drug therapy is effective in reducing this risk. A number of genetic diseases, including familial hypercholesterolemia and homocystinuria, are associated with increased risk for atherosclerosis. Drug therapy using lipid-lowering agents is highly effective for the former. Other major risk factors, such as age and male sex, obviously cannot be modified. Recently an additional blood lipoprotein, Lp(a) (referred to as "lp little a"), has been shown to be a significant independent risk factor for atherosclerotic disease when elevated. The lipoprotein is similar to low-density lipoprotein in carrying cholesterol to tissue. However, the major risk may be related to the protein part of the molecule, which can serve to promote thrombosis by interfering with the dissolution of fibrin (a major component of thrombi),

Hyperlipidemia Elevated blood lipids.

Hypercholesterolemia Elevated blood cholesterol.

High-density lipoprotein (HDL) Plasma protein molecule carrying cholesterol away from the tissue.

Homocysteine/homocysteinemia Sulfur-containing amino acid/excessive levels of homocysteine.

C-reactive protein Acute phase reactant associated with inflammation.

hence promoting thrombosis. Levels of Lp(a) vary and are under genetic control. It is unclear if levels are significantly modified by diet. Drugs currently in use to lower lipids are ineffective with Lp(a), although several new agents are currently undergoing trial.

Blood Lipids

It is abundantly clear that elevated levels of serum cholesterol are associated with atherosclerosis and cardiovascular disease. When assessing cholesterol levels, three forms of cholesterol are usually measured. Free serum cholesterol, LDL-linked cholesterol, and HDL-linked cholesterol. Ideal values and levels change depending upon age and gender at birth. Cholesterol is found in nutrients of animal origin (eggs, meats, and dairy products). Recent analysis of studies looking at dietary cholesterol intake suggests that increased intake of dietary cholesterol can result in increased serum cholesterol levels. However, the effect of dietary cholesterol levels on blood cholesterol is complex, as intrinsic cholesterol production is reduced as dietary levels increase, promoting a balance. Overall, dietary cholesterol does not have as strong an association with heart disease as was once believed. However, a typical Western diet, which importantly includes high levels of saturated fats (as well as significant dietary cholesterol), can lead to increased LDL (bad) cholesterol and elevated risk of heart disease. For most individuals, limitation of saturated fat (and now generally banned trans fats) is most important.

The liver makes cholesterol because it is needed by many processes in the body, including building cell membranes. If dietary cholesterol is inadequate, the liver will increase cholesterol synthesis. Genetics and lifestyle factors influence the liver's production of cholesterol and its carrier proteins as well. Individuals with abnormally high levels of cholesterol need to be on medications to keep their serum cholesterol levels at a heart-healthy level (see the following section). Not subject to controversy are both the ability of trans fats to raise LDL cholesterol and lower HDL cholesterol. Reducing the consumption of trans fats reduces cardiovascular risk. Trans fats were introduced into commercially prepared foods to improve shelf life and baking characteristics. Now more than 40 governments, including the United States, have banned trans fats.

Triglycerides Lipids used to store excess calories in fat cells.

Triglycerides are the lipids used for storage of excess calories in fat cells for future use as an energy source (unlike cholesterol, which is used in cell membrane and hormone synthesis). High levels of triglycerides indicate excess caloric intake over energy needs and are associated with cardiovascular disease (and also obesity, metabolic syndrome, and type II diabetes). Triglyceride levels are best reduced by losing weight, cutting back on calories, and lifestyle modifications.

Several dietary lipids may improve lipid profiles by increasing HDL ("good" cholesterol) and lowering triglycerides. Monounsaturated fats (such as those found in olive oil, avocados, almonds, and dark chocolate) do not raise LDL while raising HDL. Omega-6 polyunsaturated fatty acids (omega-6 PUFA found in seed oils and nuts) and omega-3 polyunsaturated fatty acids (omega-3 PUFA found in fish oils) both have claimed benefits in terms of lipid metabolism (such as decreasing LDL cholesterol and triglycerides and increasing HDL cholesterol). The omega 3 and 6 indicate the position of an unsaturated double bond in the long carbon chain. Currently, the AHA suggests eating at least two portions of oily fish weekly as a source of omega-3 PUFA but recommends a "moderate" amount of omega-6 PUFA. Claims about health benefits of omega-6 PUFA have become contentious because of the finding that an omega-6 PUFA (linoleic acid) might promote the synthesis of a mediator of inflammation (arachidonic acid). Hence, there are claims that seed oils rich in linoleic acid are a significant health risk. Current evidence strongly argues against this supposed health risk and supports the benefit of omega-3 PUFA in nutrition.

Therapeutic Approaches to Hyperlipidemia

The decision to actively lower blood lipid levels, and in particular cholesterol levels, is clinically based on the overall risk of cardiovascular disease. Individuals with known cardiovascular disease or with genetic diseases that elevate cholesterol levels clearly benefit from drug-based therapy using a class of agents termed **statins**. Even individuals without known cardiovascular disease with elevated blood lipid levels can demonstrate reduced risk of developing disease or exacerbation of undiagnosed early disease when their blood lipid levels are treated. Clinicians use risk calculation estimators (one is available online from the American Heart Association) to estimate the risk of a myocardial infarct in the next decade and suggest intervention based on the degree of future risk. Lifestyle modification—including weight loss, exercise, and diet modification—is often suggested in an initial attempt to improve cholesterol levels in individuals without current disease. These interventions provide an overall health benefit, but they have little if any effect on overall mortality from cardiovascular disease. Serum cholesterol levels depend on genetic factors, and once body mass is elevated, those levels respond poorly to dietary modification. For these reasons, the use of drug therapy with statins to lower serum cholesterol levels is clearly of benefit. Statins are a class of agents that inhibit the enzyme HMG-CoA reductase, which is critical to the synthesis of cholesterol by the liver. Potential side effects of statin use include muscle pain and (rarely) serious damage to muscles. The availability of generics has reduced cost significantly. The decision of when to treat otherwise healthy individuals and how aggressively to attempt to lower cholesterol levels is complex and still not fully settled. Clearly, individuals with very low serum cholesterol levels (below 70 mg/dl) would not demonstrate sufficient future risk to warrant therapy, but individuals with higher levels (and other risk factors such as low HDL) would likely benefit from reduced risk. Recent guidelines recommend statin therapy in individuals without cardiovascular risk factors who have levels of 190 mg/dl LDL cholesterol or greater. Individuals who have specific risk factors should consider therapy at a much lower level of 70 mg/dl or greater. Overall, individual risk factors, including age and family history, should be considered.

Statins Drugs effective against the development of atherosclerosis.

There is no controversy regarding the benefit of aggressive attempts to lower serum cholesterol in individuals either with known cardiovascular disease or with very high risk of such (such as young individuals who have familial hypercholesterolemia, a relatively common autosomal dominant disease resulting in much increased levels of LDL cholesterol in childhood).

C-Reactive Protein

C-reactive protein (CRP) is one of several proteins produced by the liver and released into the bloodstream in response to tissue injury or inflammation. The protein is one of the body's nonspecific defenses against infection and provides some protection against the harmful effects of inflammation by neutralizing various products produced by the cells that accumulate at the site of the inflammation. Measurement of CRP has been used for many years to monitor the activity of diseases associated with inflammation, such as rheumatic fever and rheumatoid arthritis.

Recently, very sensitive tests have been developed that can detect slight CRP elevations in people who do not appear to have evidence of an inflammatory or infectious disease. Studies have demonstrated that an elevated CRP level in an otherwise normal person predicts an increased long-term risk of cardiovascular disease, probably because the elevated CRP is detecting the accumulation of macrophages, lymphocytes, lipids, and products of tissue injury within unstable plaques in coronary arteries. The increase in relative risk associated with CRP elevation is similar to (and slightly higher than) the relative risk attributable to hypertension and hyperlipidemia. The CRP test is recommended as an additional screening test to detect people at risk of coronary artery disease, who then can be offered treatment to reduce their risk factors. Although the CRP levels are highly nonspecific, levels of 140 or higher can be the result of numerous causes of inflammation; the AHA suggests levels above 3.0 mg/L are indicative of high risk.

Homocysteine

Homocysteine is a sulfur-containing amino acid formed enzymatically from methionine, an essential amino acid abundant in animal protein. Homocysteine is metabolized by biochemical pathways in which vitamin B_6, vitamin B_{12}, and folic acid are required. Blood concentrations of homocysteine are higher in men than in premenopausal women but increase in women after menopause. Renal function also influences homocysteine blood levels, which are elevated in people with kidney disease.

Abnormal homocysteine metabolism is characteristic of a rare hereditary disease termed homocystinuria. The disease results from a gene mutation leading to an enzyme defect that impairs the normal metabolism of homocysteine. Affected individuals have an extremely high concentration of homocysteine in their blood and excrete the amino acid in their urine. Those affected show evidence of marked vascular disease, which has its onset at a very young age. These manifestations include atherosclerosis of coronary arteries and other major arteries, strokes, and blood clots in arteries and veins.

Clinical studies demonstrated that many people with cardiovascular disease, strokes, and peripheral vascular disease have elevated homocysteine blood levels, and a high homocysteine blood level is a risk factor for atherosclerosis, comparable to the increased risk associated with hypercholesterolemia, smoking, and hypertension. In most people, in whom renal function is normal, the elevated homocysteine level may be related to a deficiency of B vitamins and folic acid; however, it is unclear whether dietary supplementation reduces the risk of cardiovascular disease in individuals who do not have hereditary homocystinuria.

Hypertension and Hypertensive Cardiovascular Disease

Primary Hypertension

Hypertension is a critical and modifiable risk factor for cardiovascular disease, and attempts have been made to define a normal "ideal" blood pressure and set guidelines for therapy to reduce risk should this pressure be exceeded (**Figure 10-19**).

Traditionally, normal blood pressure is considered to be below 120/80 (systolic/diastolic). A pressure consistently higher than 130/90 is termed stage 1

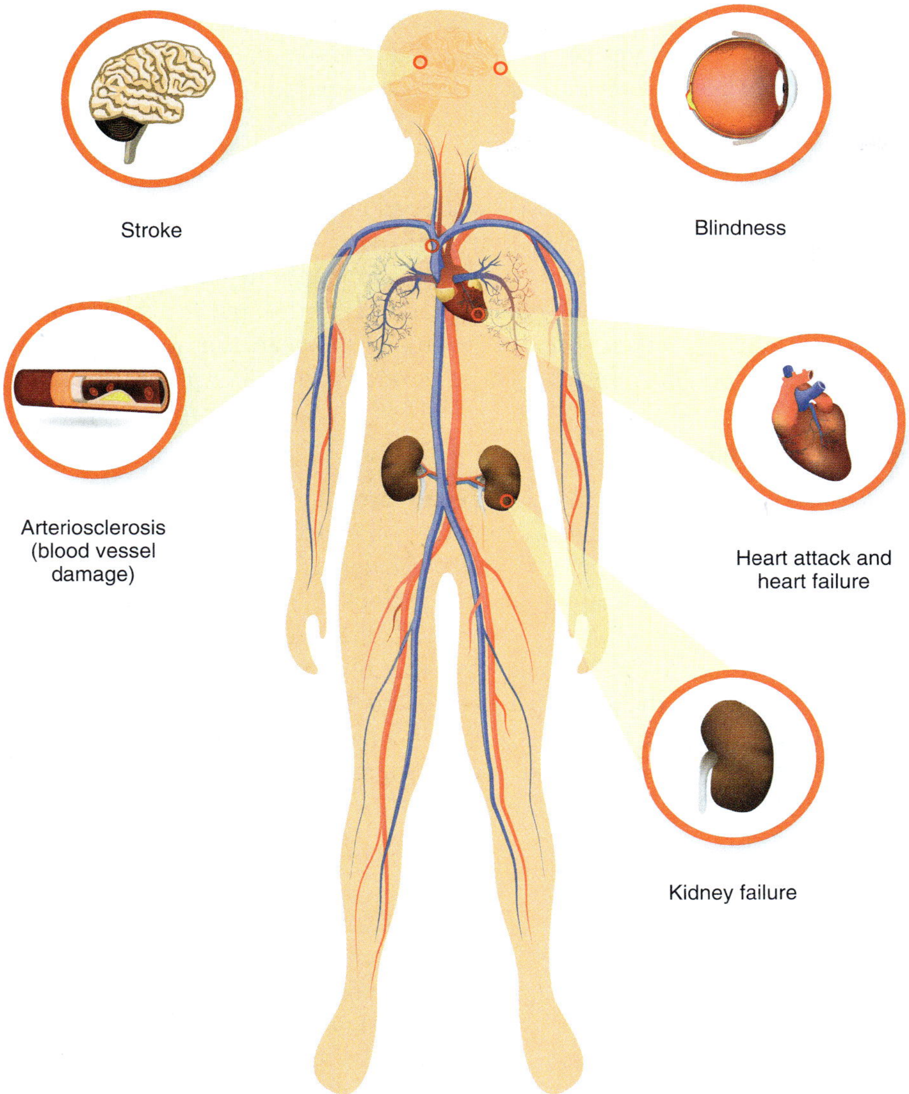

Figure 10-19 The far-reaching effects of hypertension. Hypertension not only affects the cardiovascular system. Other organ systems can undergo pathological changes as the result of unresolved hypertension.

hypertension, whereas in-between values are considered to be elevated and indicate a potential problem. Levels of 140 or higher over 90 or higher are considered as hypertension stage 2. The higher the pressure, the greater its harmful effects. Normal blood pressures are defined on the basis of population studies and vary depending on age and sex among normal individuals. Rather than defining "normal," current guidelines set "blood pressure goals" above which antihypertensive therapy should be considered. Threshold values for an otherwise normal individual are 130/90.

Ninety-five percent of cases of hypertension (so-called **essential hypertension**) have no easily identifiable cause but rather are multifactorial, with genetics, salt intake, and vascular tone all playing a role. In the case of vascular tone, increased sympathetic activity can result in excessive vasoconstriction of the small arterioles throughout the body, which raises the diastolic pressure. Because of the high peripheral resistance, the heart needs to pump more forcefully to overcome the resistance created by the constricted arterioles and supply

Essential hypertension High blood pressure with no identifiable cause.

adequate blood to the tissues, which leads to a compensatory rise in systolic blood pressure. Therefore, both systolic and diastolic pressure rise when the primary problem is excessive arteriolar vasoconstriction.

Cardiac Effects

The heart responds to the increased workload resulting from the high peripheral resistance by becoming enlarged, particularly in the left ventricle, which serves as the pump for systemic circulation. Although the enlarged heart may be able to function effectively for many years, the cardiac pump is being forced to work beyond its "rated capacity." Eventually, the heart can no longer maintain adequate blood flow, and the patient develops symptoms of cardiac failure.

Vascular Effects

Because the blood vessels are not designed to carry blood at such a high pressure, the vessels wear out prematurely. Hypertension accelerates the development of atherosclerosis in the larger arteries and is a major risk factor for cardiovascular disease. The arterioles also are injured; they thicken and undergo degenerative changes, and their lumens become narrowed. This process is termed arteriolosclerosis. Sometimes the walls of the small arterioles become completely necrotic due to the effects of the sustained high blood pressure. Weakened arterioles may rupture, leading to hemorrhage. The brain is particularly vulnerable, and cerebral hemorrhage (hemorrhagic stroke) is a relatively common complication of severe hypertension.

Renal Effects

The narrowing of the renal arterioles decreases the blood supply to the kidneys, which, in turn, leads to injury and degenerative changes in the glomeruli and renal tubules. Severe hypertension may cause severe derangement of renal function and eventually leads to renal failure (**Figure 10-20**).

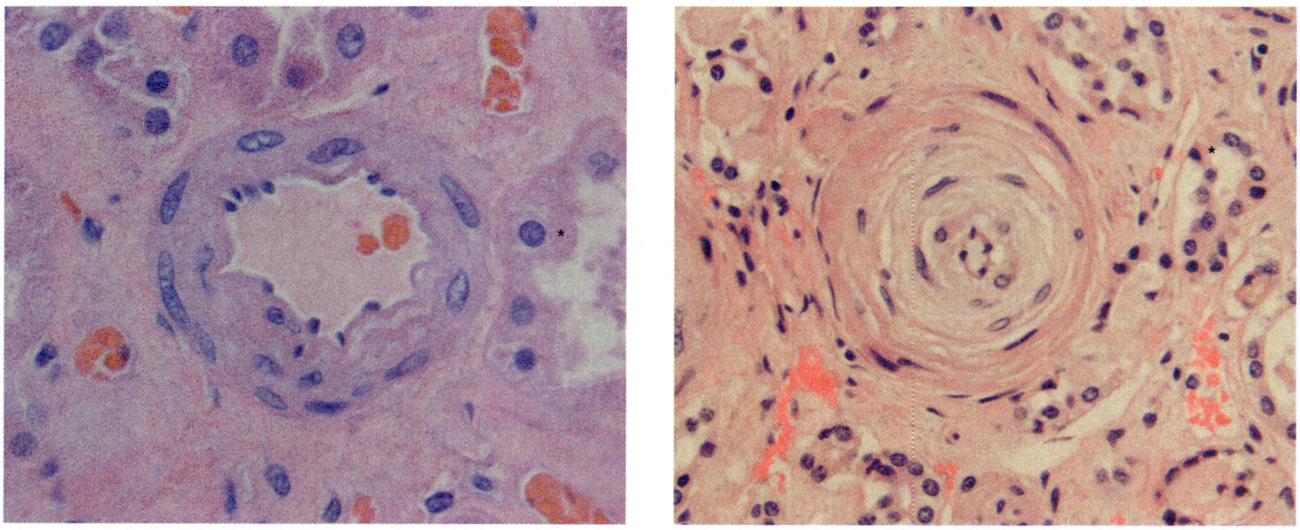

(A) (B)

Figure 10-20 **(A)** Renal arteriole of normal size. Its wall is composed of a few concentric layers of smooth muscle cells. **(B)** Renal arteriole from a patient with long-standing hypertension. The wall is greatly thickened and contains many concentric layers of smooth muscle cells and a marked reduction in the size of the lumen.

Secondary Hypertension

In 5 percent of patients, hypertension results from a known disease or condition such as chronic kidney disease (see Chapter 17), endocrine gland dysfunction such as a pituitary or an adrenal tumor, or a hyperactive thyroid gland (see Chapter 22). The high blood pressure associated with these conditions is termed "secondary hypertension" because the cause of the hypertension is known. In many cases, successful treatment of the underlying condition cures the hypertension.

Treatment of Hypertension

Although the reason for hypertension cannot be determined in most instances, blood pressure can be reduced to more normal levels, thereby lowering the risk of complications of high blood pressure. This is accomplished by administering various drugs that lower the blood pressure using a variety of mechanisms. Commonly used drugs include thiazide-type diuretics that increase the ability of the kidney to remove salt and water from the circulation, thus lessening the "load" the heart must pump against. Calcium channel blockers inhibit the contraction of arteriolar smooth muscle cells, lowering peripheral resistance. ACE inhibitors reduce the production of angiotensin II, which is a potent vasoconstrictor. Several other classes of antihypertensive drugs also can be useful in particular clinical circumstances.

Hypertension and the Aorta: Aneurysms

An aneurysm is a dilatation of the wall of an artery, or an outpouching of a portion of the wall. Most **aneurysms** are acquired as a result of atherosclerosis, which causes weakening of the vessel wall. One type of aneurysm involving the cerebral arteries is the result of a congenital abnormality of the vessel wall and is considered in conjunction with the nervous system (see Chapter 23).

Aneurysm Dilatation of a structure, such as the aorta, a cerebral artery, or a part of the ventricular wall.

Arteriosclerotic Aneurysm

A small artery that undergoes arteriosclerotic change becomes narrowed and may eventually become thrombosed. A large artery, such as the aorta, has a diameter so large that complete obstruction is uncommon. However, atheromatous deposits tend to damage the wall of the aorta, reducing its elasticity and weakening the wall. The aortic wall tends to balloon out under the stress of the high pressure within the vessel, forming an aortic aneurysm. Aortic aneurysms usually develop in the distal part of the abdominal aorta, where the pressure is highest and the atheromatous change is most severe (**Figure 10-21** and **Figure 10-22**). Usually, the interior of the aneurysm becomes covered with a layer of thrombus material, and the wall often becomes partially calcified. Aneurysms also occur in the thoracic aorta, usually in association with a history of tobacco use and hypertension.

Atherosclerosis is the major cause of aortic aneurysms, but there appears to be some genetic predisposition as well, because 15 to 20 percent of patients with an aneurysm also have another affected family member. An aortic aneurysm usually enlarges slowly and does not produce symptoms initially. Because a small aneurysm is difficult to detect by physical examination,

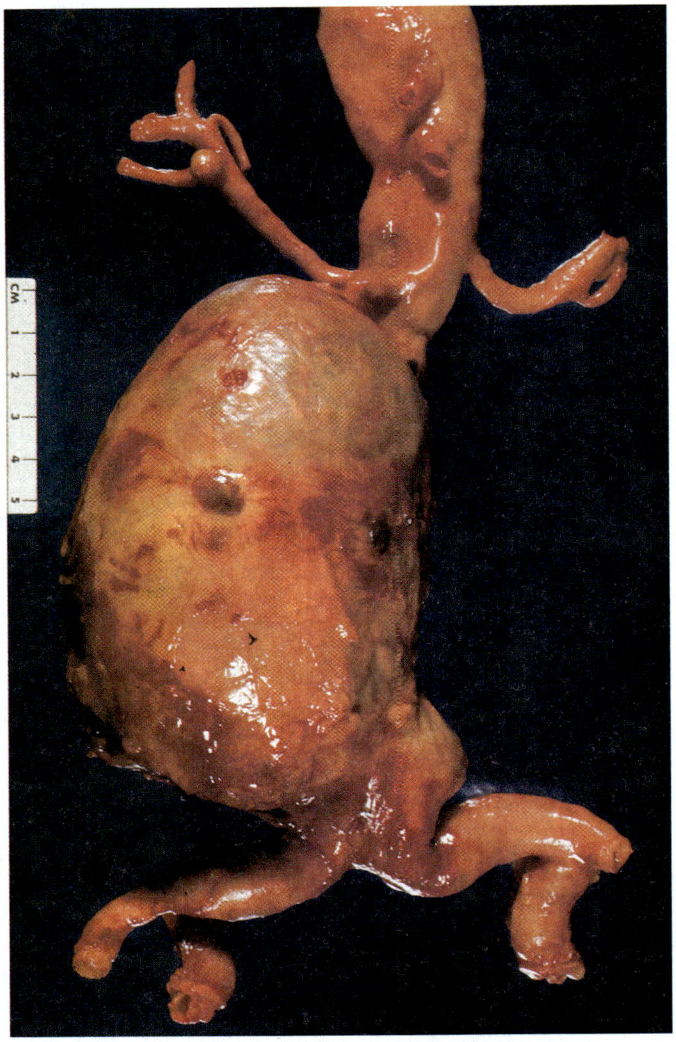

Figure 10-21 Large arteriosclerotic aneurysm extending from renal arteries (*above*) to lilac arteries (*below*).

Courtesy of Leonard V. Crowley, MD, Century College.

current guidelines recommend a routine ultrasound screening examination to identify an asymptomatic aneurysm in any adult older than age 65 who has ever smoked or has other risk factors that predispose them to atherosclerosis, such as a family history of an aortic aneurysm.

Aortic aneurysms are dangerous because they may rupture, leading to massive and often fatal hemorrhage. The normal cross-section diameter of the abdominal aorta is about 2 cm. An aneurysm exceeding about 5 cm in diameter may rupture and should be repaired. In general, the larger the aneurysm, the greater the likelihood of rupture (**Figure 10-23**).

The standard open surgical aneurysm repair procedure consists of opening the aneurysm and sewing a nylon or Dacron graft into the aorta above and below the aneurysmal segment so that the blood flowing through the aorta flows through the graft rather than through the aneurysm. It is not necessary to excise the aneurysm that has been bypassed by the graft, and usually the walls of the aneurysm are wrapped around the graft. This procedure is a well-established, reliable, and highly successful method of treatment, but it is a major surgical procedure and poses significant risks to older patients who may have coronary artery disease and other medical problems.

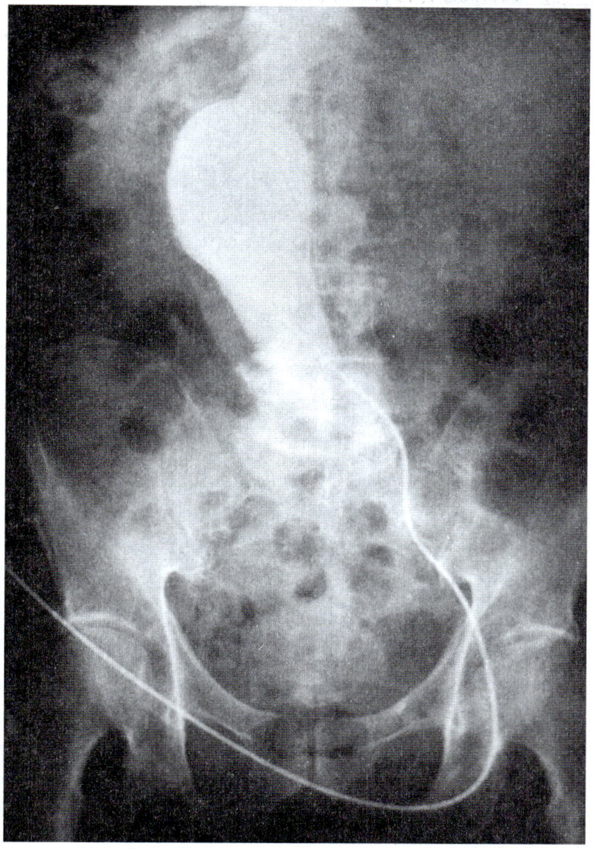

Figure 10-22 An aortic aneurysm demonstrated on X-ray by injection of contrast material into the aorta.

Courtesy of Leonard V. Crowley, MD, Century College.

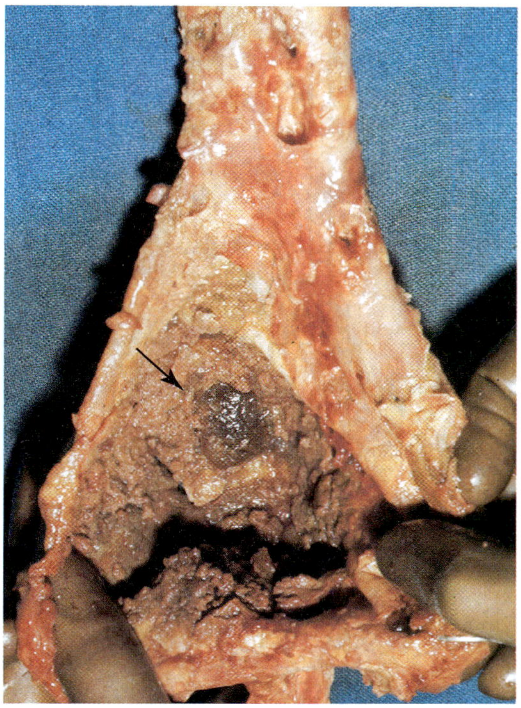

Figure 10-23 Interior of atherosclerotic aneurysm, illustrating marked degenerative change in wall. An extremely thin area in the wall (*arrow*) predisposes it to rupture.

Courtesy of Leonard V. Crowley, MD, Century College.

Dissecting Aneurysm of the Aorta

The thick middle layer of the aorta is termed the "tunica media." It is composed of multiple layers of elastic tissue and muscle bonded together by fibrous connective tissue. Degenerative changes sometimes occur in the tunica media, causing the layers to lose their cohesiveness and separate (**Figure 10-24**). Then the pulsatile force of the blood flowing through the aorta may cause the inner half of the aortic wall to pull away from the outer half in the region where the media has degenerated, and sometimes the inner lining (tunica intima) tears as the media separates. This complication is especially likely to occur in individuals with high blood pressure.

After an intimal tear has developed, blood is forced into the aortic wall. The area of medial degeneration forms a cleavage plane that permits the blood to dissect within the media for a variable distance. This event, a dissecting aneurysm of the aorta, is associated with severe chest and back pain. The term dissecting refers to the splitting (dissection) of the media by the blood, and the somewhat misleading term aneurysm was applied because the affected part of the aorta appears wider than normal. The widening results from the hemorrhage within the aortic wall, but the lumen of the aorta is not dilated.

The intimal tear that starts the dissection is usually either in the ascending aorta just above the aortic valve or in the descending aorta just beyond the origin of the large arteries that arise from the aortic arch (**Figure 10-25**). If the tear is in the ascending aorta, the blood often dissects proximally as well as distally within the aortic wall, extending into the base of the aorta where the aortic valve attaches and the coronary arteries arise, leading to compromise of cardiac function. A dissection in the ascending aorta is often fatal because

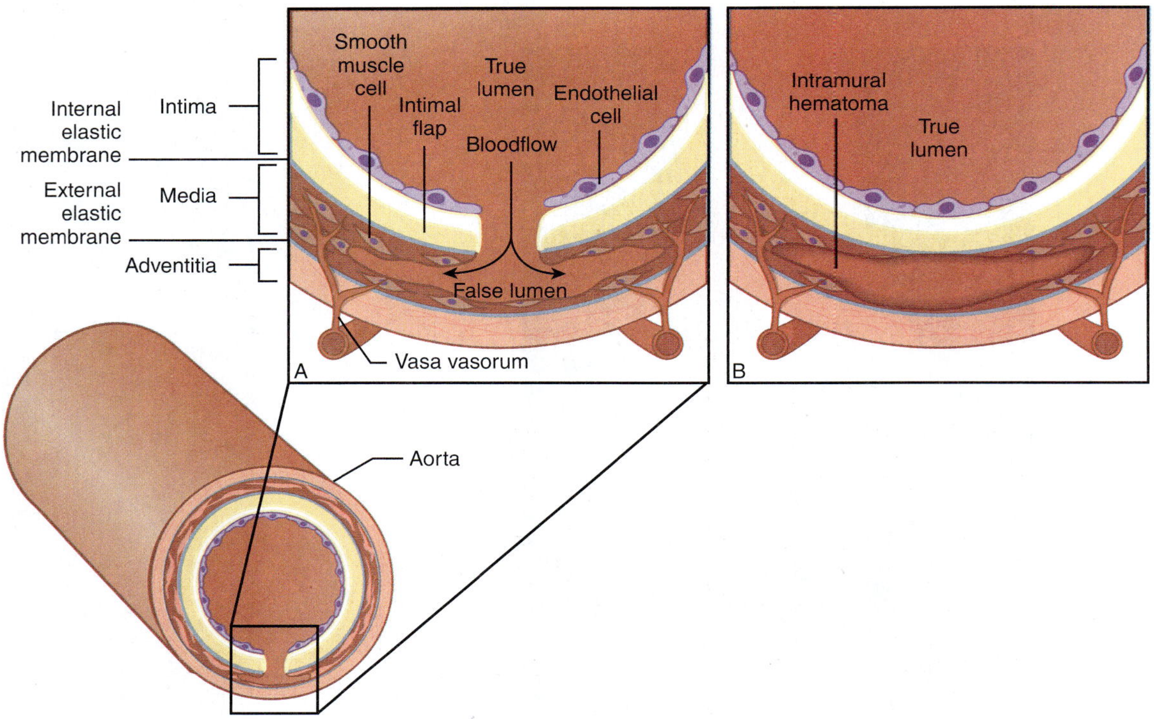

Figure 10-24 Characteristic degenerative changes in the media of the aortic wall (termed cystic medial necrosis) has led to a loss of the cohesion between the inner and outer layers of the aortic wall and allowed blood (bright red wedge) to dissect down the tunica media of the aorta.

Courtesy Dr. Donald Yandow, Department of Radiology, University of Wisconsin School of Medicine.

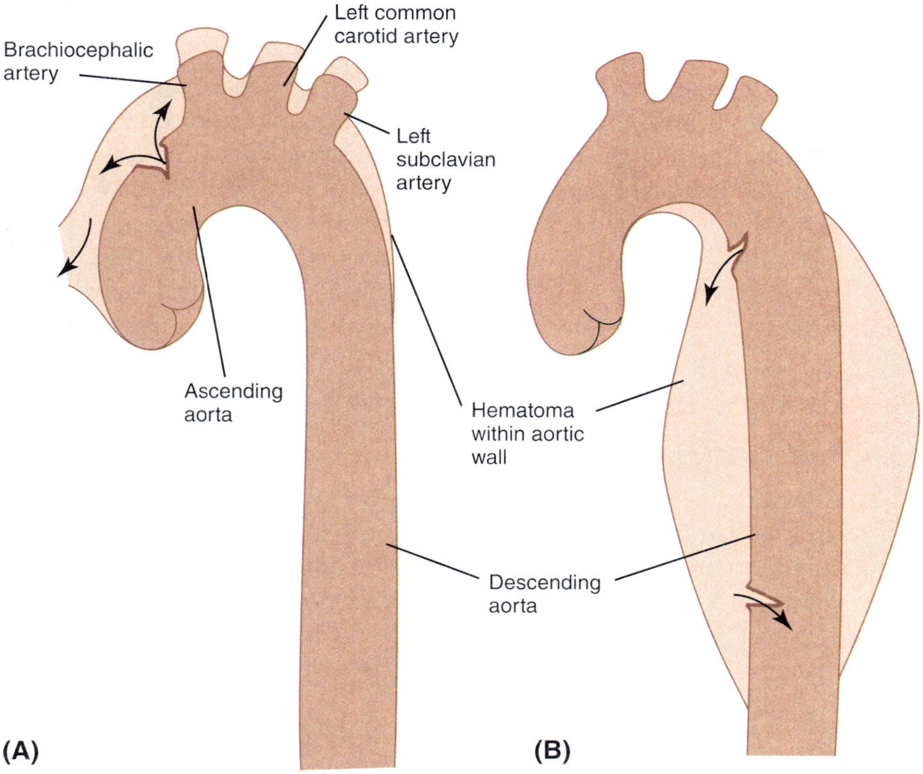

Figure 10-25 Sites of aortic dissection. **(A)** Tear in ascending aorta causes both proximal and distal dissection. **(B)** A tear in the descending aorta may cause extensive distal dissection and may rupture back into the lumen or aorta.

the blood frequently ruptures through the outer wall of the aorta at the base of the heart, leading to extensive hemorrhage into the mediastinum or pericardial sac.

If the intimal tear is in the descending aorta, the blood dissects distally and may extend the entire length of the aorta, leading to impairment of blood flow to the kidneys, the intestines, or other vital organs.

Diagnosis of Coronary Artery Disease

Clinicians can now evaluate the extent of coronary artery disease as well as the exact sites where the main coronary arteries are obstructed. Cardiac catheterization, also known as cardiac cath or heart catheterization, is a medical procedure used to diagnose and treat some heart conditions. Cardiac catheterization can provide an in-depth look at heart pathology, including performing procedures to evaluate heart function. This procedure is often used to diagnose the causes of symptoms such as chest pain or irregular heartbeat. The information gained from a cardiac catheterization procedure, along with results from other testing, can be used to determine a treatment plan for the patient. In some circumstances, the treatment may be enacted while the patient is still undergoing the imaging procedure. During cardiac catheterization, a long, thin, flexible tube called a catheter is threaded into a blood vessel in the arm, groin, upper thigh, or neck. The catheter is then threaded through the blood vessels to the heart. Contrast dye can be injected through the catheter, and the functioning of the heart can be evaluated in real time using imaging technology. The dye can be injected into the coronary arteries to determine whether the arteries are narrowed or blocked.

Cardiac catheterization may also be used instead of some heart surgeries to repair heart defects and replace heart valves. This is accomplished by passing a catheter into the aorta and injecting a radiopaque dye directly into the orifices of the coronary arteries. The filling of the coronary arteries can be observed, along with the location and degree of arterial obstruction (Figure 10-17). Echocardiograms of the heart using ultrasound are also useful in detecting coronary artery disease. Stress tests use exercise or drugs to stimulate the heart, whose function is measured using either ECG or, in some cases, a radiotracer injected into the circulation to measure whether areas of the heart have diminished blood flow (nuclear stress test).

Treatment of Coronary Artery Disease

Medical Treatment

Medical treatment of coronary artery disease consists of administering drugs that reduce myocardial oxygen consumption and improve coronary circulation (antianginal drugs). If the patient exhibits cardiac irregularities, drugs that reduce myocardial irritability also are prescribed (antiarrhythmial drugs). Factors that potentiate coronary artery disease also are controlled or eliminated whenever possible: smoking, hypertension control, improved diet, weight loss, and increased exercise.

Surgical Treatment

Several surgical approaches, termed myocardial revascularization procedures, have been devised to improve blood supply to the heart muscle. Surgery is often recommended for patients who do not respond satisfactorily to medical treatment. The usual surgical method is to bypass the obstructions in the coronary arteries by means of segments of saphenous vein obtained from the patient's legs. The proximal ends of the grafts are sutured to small openings made in the aorta above the normal openings of the coronary arteries, and the distal ends are sutured into the coronary arteries beyond the areas of narrowing (**Figure 10-26**). Myocardial revascularization operations are generally reserved for patients with severe sclerosis of all three major coronary arteries, and usually grafts are used to bypass all three arteries. The operation alleviates or greatly improves symptoms of angina and may also improve survival in some groups of patients. Unfortunately, the high arterial pressure carried by the vein grafts sometimes causes the grafts to undergo progressive intimal thickening, which may lead to complete occlusion of the grafts. Many of the grafts eventually also develop the same type of atherosclerosis that occurred in the coronary arteries.

The internal thoracic arteries, which can be referred to by their older name, internal mammary arteries, also can be used to bypass obstructed coronary arteries. The internal thoracic arteries are paired arteries that arise from the aorta and descend along the undersurface of the thoracic cavity just lateral to the sternum. They can be dissected from their normal location and connected to the coronary arteries, thereby delivering blood directly from the aorta to the coronary arteries beyond the narrowed or blocked areas. Because the arteries are able to carry blood under much higher pressure than veins, artery grafts are less likely to become narrowed or obstructed. In some patients, both vein grafts and internal thoracic arteries are used to restore adequate blood flow to the myocardium.

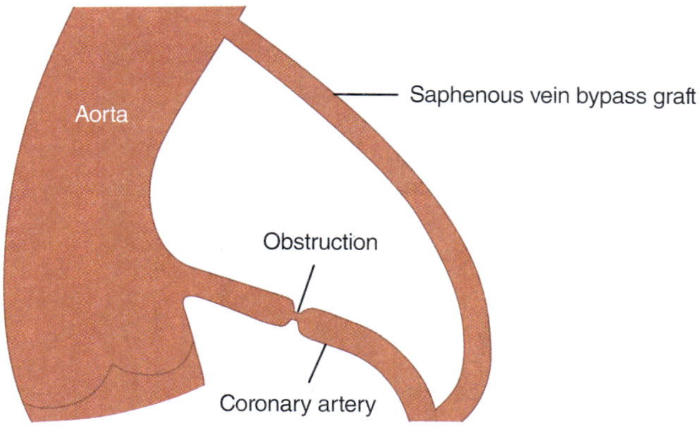

(A)

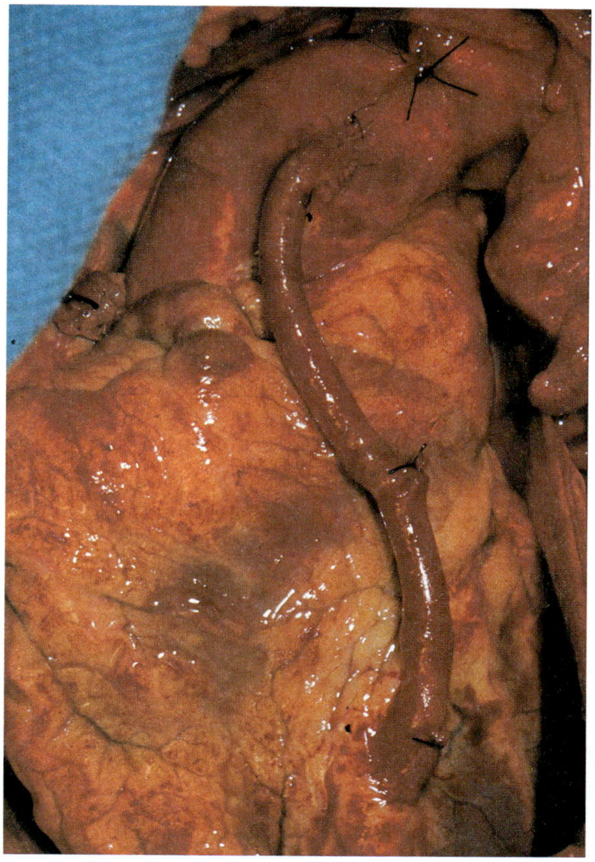

(B)

Figure 10-26 **(A)** Principle of surgical treatment of coronary heart disease by means of saphenous vein grafts that bypass obstructions in coronary arteries. **(B)** Vein graft extending from the aorta above the origin of the coronary arteries to the anterior interventricular (descending) coronary artery distal to the site of arterial narrowing.

(B) Courtesy of Leonard V. Crowley, MD, Century College.

Coronary Angioplasty

Many patients with less extensive coronary artery disease can be treated successfully by dilating narrowed areas in the coronary arteries instead of bypassing them, thereby avoiding major surgery. The procedure is termed coronary angioplasty (angio = vessel + plasty = molding) and is illustrated in **Figure 10-27**. By means of a technique similar to that used to perform a cardiac catheterization, a guiding catheter is introduced through the skin and into a large artery in the arm or leg, threaded into the narrowed coronary artery, and positioned at the site of narrowing. Then the balloon catheter is threaded through the guide catheter until the balloon lies within the narrowed area. After the balloon is properly positioned, it is inflated briefly under high pressure, which smashes the plaque and pushes it into the arterial wall, enlarging the lumen of the artery and improving blood flow to the myocardium.

Successful dilatation of a narrowed coronary artery restores normal blood flow through the artery. Unfortunately, in some successfully treated patients, the stenosis recurs within 6 months after balloon angioplasty and may require redilatation. In an attempt to solve the problem of restenosis, most physicians now perform balloon angioplasty using a **stent**, which is often a short, expandable metal mesh tube that is placed over the balloon catheter with the

Stent Short tube often made of expandable metal mesh used to hold the blood vessel open.

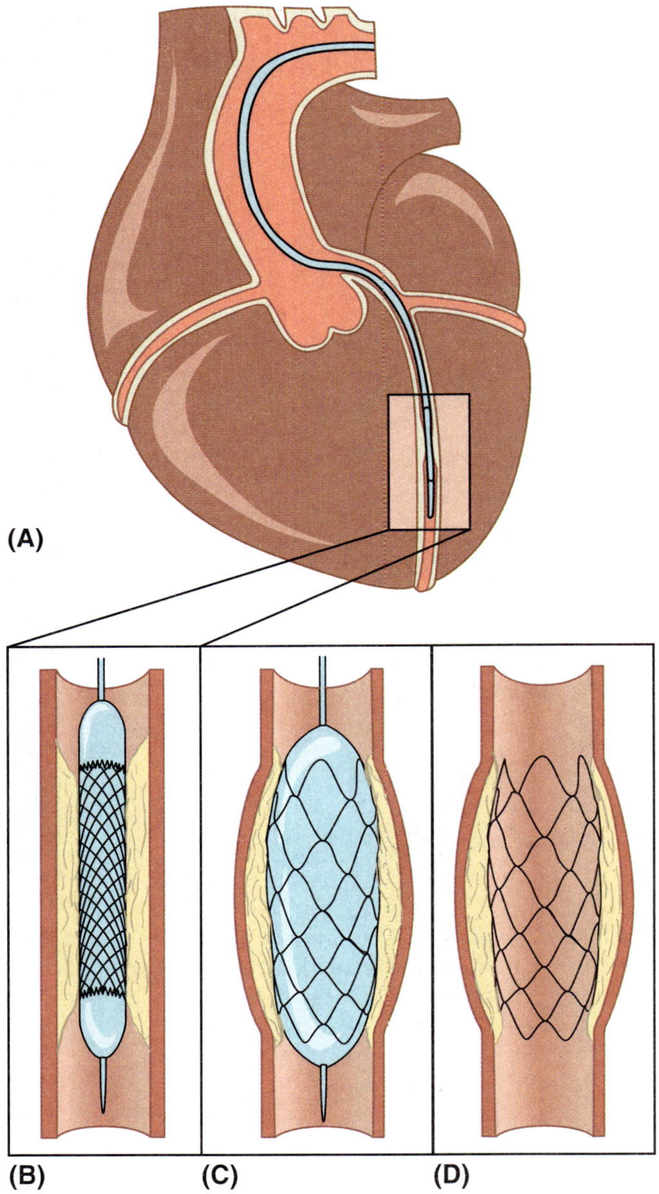

Figure 10-27 Principle of coronary angioplasty. **(A)** An overview illustrating the positioning of the guide catheter at the site of narrowing in the coronary artery. **(B)** A balloon catheter covered by unexpanded stent advanced through a guide catheter and positioned within a narrow segment of artery. **(C)** Balloon inflated, relieving arterial obstruction by smashing plaque and simultaneously expanding the stent. **(D)** Balloon catheter withdrawn, leaving an expanded stent that forms a rigid support to maintain the caliber of the dilated artery.

metal mesh collapsed. The stent expands as the balloon is inflated to enlarge the lumen of the artery and functions as a rigid support to help keep the vessel open (Figure 10-27). Stents may be drug-eluting, releasing agents that prevent reocclusion of the vessel. This procedure is usually supplemented by administration of drugs that prevent accumulation of platelets at the site where the stent was placed. The arterial wall responds to the metal stent by proliferation of connective tissue and smooth muscle cells that grow through the meshes in the stent and cover its inner surface, followed by gradual ingrowth of endothelial cells to provide a smooth interior lining for the stent. Consequently, platelets are less likely to adhere at the site of the stent placement and cause thrombosis of the stented vessel. **Figure 10-28** provides additional information regarding stents and their efficacy.

Although use of stents has been helpful and initially has a high success rate, restenosis of the dilated artery still occurs in about 10 percent of patients, resulting from ingrowth of tissue extending from the inner layers of the stented artery into the lumen of the vessel between the meshes of the stent. As noted, in an attempt to avoid this problem, stents coated with drugs that suppress the cell proliferation responsible for narrowing the stented artery can be used.

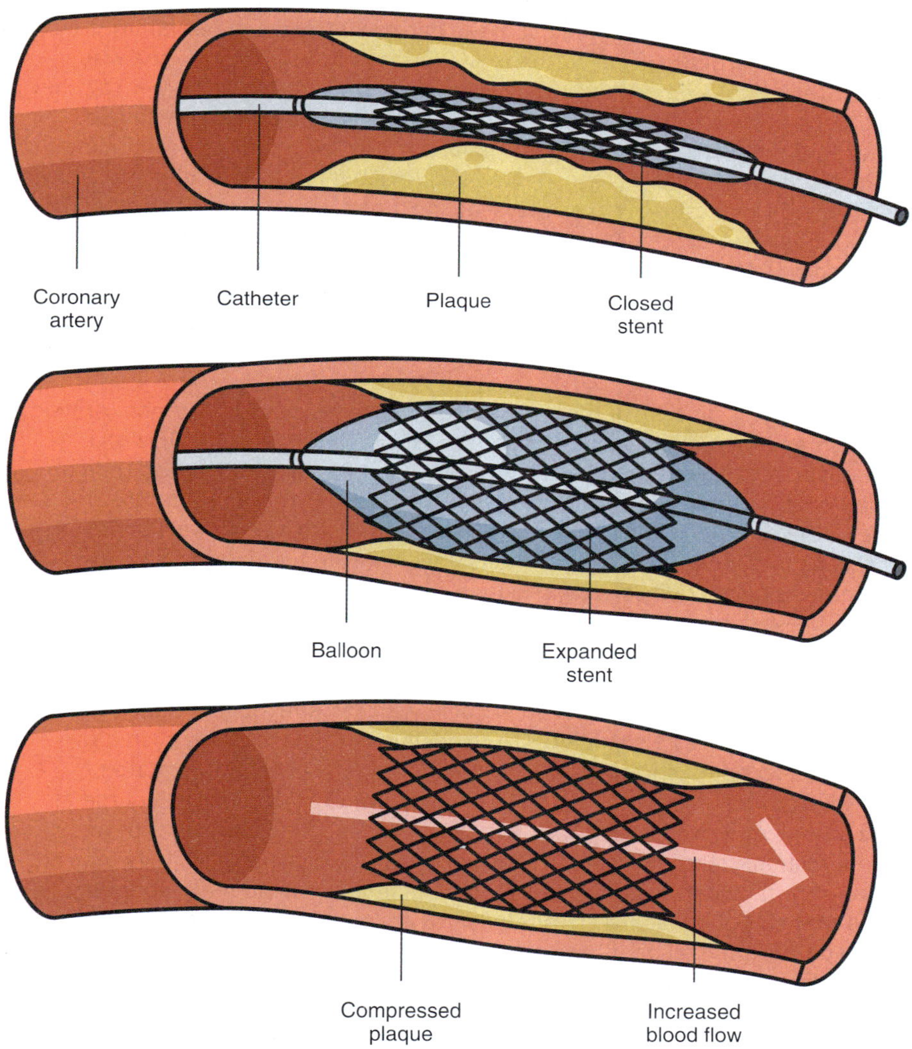

Figure 10-28 Coronary artery stent placement. The use of coronary artery stents to increase blood flow to the coronary arteries, which become restricted due to atherosclerosis, is very common. The procedure is much less invasive than bypass surgery, with the patient recovering more quickly. A meshwork stent is placed inside the blood vessel to keep the lumen open.

Case 10-1

Grace, the 63-year-old matriarch of a large extended family, loved cooking for everyone, including all the holidays and family celebrations when the whole group gathered. Lately she noticed that she seemed to feel tired all of the time. The family gathering today really took it out of her. She felt short of breath while cooking and her back and neck were painful. She took a seat at the kitchen table because she felt nauseous and worried she might vomit, which wouldn't be good with a house full of family. As she was sitting there resting her head on her hands, some of her grandchildren came in. They looked at her right away and knew something was off. When they asked her what's wrong, she explained her symptoms and suggested maybe she was just fighting off one of the "bugs" that seemed to be going around. It did not surprise her because things at work right now were really stressful and she was probably just run down. She told everyone not to worry; she just needed a moment. Her granddaughter, a college student, had just finished an internship in the emergency department of the local hospital and did not feel comfortable just letting things go.

Under grave protest, Grace got in the car and let some of her family drive her to the emergency room. When they explained her symptoms, she was taken back right away. After an ECG, some blood tests, and a chest X-ray, they got some answers. Grace's heart was not functioning as well as it should. They said they were going to admit her and run some more tests, including echocardiograms and more in-depth blood chemistry. Grace protested loudly; she thought that everyone was overreacting, and she just needed to go home and put her feet up. One member of the team said they suspected Grace may have coronary artery disease. After some more tests, they would work with Grace to develop a treatment plan that would help with her symptoms and manage her condition.

Discussion

Cardiovascular disease is the number one cause of death for women. Among women and men, atherosclerotic cardiovascular disease (ASCVD) is on a steady increase, with many men experiencing an event at ages less than 65. For women, symptomatic onset often occurs later. However, in Europe and the United States, the incidence of mortality from ASCVD shows a sharp increase in middle-aged women, ages 45–65. Missed or delayed diagnosis appears to be a significant contributing factor. In general, men receive guideline-recommended preventive measures and therapy sooner and at a much higher rate than women.

The stereotypical risk factors, smoking, obesity, hyperlipidemia, and aging, affect men differently than women, with the effects in men being much more extensively studied. Sex-specific factors, including premature menopause, polycystic ovary syndrome (PCOS), and pregnancy-related complications, contribute to atherosclerosis progression and the course of the pathology in women. Women may also present with symptoms beyond those that are stereotypical for heart disease or a heart attack. They may not present with chest-crushing pain from angina but instead may experience pain in their back, neck, arm, shoulder, or abdomen. In addition, nausea and vomiting and sleep disturbances are reported in women more often than in men. Their symptoms often occur as they are going about their everyday tasks, whereas men often experience symptoms associated with increased exertion or exercise. Women tend to be more sensitive to stressful environments, including those in the workplace or home. Consequently, increased emotional or psychological stress can trigger symptoms in women and contribute to their disease progression.

Grace presented with "atypical" symptoms of cardiovascular disease, whereas "typical" symptoms are associated with what is generally presented by men experiencing a cardiovascular event. Her granddaughter's astute evaluation of the situation and rapid response were exactly what needed to happen to ensure Grace experienced the best possible outcomes. While this case study ends with Grace being admitted to the hospital for more extensive evaluation, for many women the result could have been death if their symptoms were ignored or treated lightly.

Etiology and Pathogenesis

Cardiovascular disease, most likely coronary artery disease (CAD)

Questions

1. What risk factors for cardiovascular disease can be identified in Grace's case study?
2. What tests and other kinds of evaluation would be needed to get the most complete picture of Grace's cardiovascular health?
3. If cardiovascular disease is the number one cause of death for women in the United States, why do you think it doesn't get the same level of attention as other serious illnesses in women?
4. What other information would you want to gather regarding Grace's life and background?
5. How would the social determinants of health affect Grace's prognosis and care plan?

Questions for Review

1. Describe how blood flows through the venous system. What happens when flow is interrupted?
2. What is the difference between a thrombus and an embolus? What is an infarct?
3. What factors predispose to arterial thrombosis?
4. What are the causes and effects of intracardiac thrombi?
5. What conditions predispose to thrombosis by increasing the coagulability of the blood?
6. What genetic factors lead to increased risk of atherosclerosis?
7. What tests are used to diagnose diseases of the circulatory system?
8. What is the usual cause of an aortic aneurysm? How is an aneurysm treated?
9. What is the difference between an arteriosclerotic aneurysm of the aorta and a dissecting aneurysm of the aorta?

References

Lilly LS. *Pathophysiology of Heart Disease: A Collaborative Project of Medical Students and Faculty.* 6th ed. Wolters Kluwer; 2016.

- The area of circulatory disease is so broad (and so detailed) that no set of readings can fully do it justice. This very well regarded text presents a readable and somewhat technical overview aimed at medical and advanced undergraduate students. It is an excellent single source for additional background for diseases of blood circulation. It is particularly strong on therapy and has a good discussion of atherosclerosis.

American Heart Association. *How are women's symptoms different during a heart attack?* September 14, 2023. https://www.youtube.com/watch?v=io4Ovh-Q2IA&t=1s

Rubenfire M. 2018 AHA/ACC Multisociety Guideline on the Management of Blood Cholesterol. Published November 10, 2018. https://www.acc.org/latest-in-cardiology/ten-points-to-remember/2018/11/09/14/28/2018-guideline-on-management-of-blood-cholesterol

- The American College of Cardiology website has much available material, which is updated immediately. The YouTube video from the American Heart Association supports the case study and is very informative.

Find High Blood Pressure Tools and Resources. American Heart Association. https://www.heart.org/en/health-topics/high-blood-pressure/find-high-blood-pressure-tools--resources

- A collection of short and very useful fact sheets on a variety of topics, including high blood pressure.

Yusuf S, Joseph P, Rangarajan S, et al. Modifiable risk factors, cardiovascular disease, and mortality in 155,722 individuals from 21 high-income, middle-income, and low-income countries (PURE): A prospective cohort study. *Lancet.* doi:10.1016/S0140-6736(19)32008-2

- This is a landmark study with extensive important data. For example, overall 70% of cardiovascular disease cases and deaths are attributed to modifiable risk factors. The appended reference list is also of real utility. The interested reader should try and obtain a copy of the full study.

Arnett DK, Blumenthal RS, Albert MA, et al. 2019 ACC/AHA guideline on the Primary Prevention of Cardiovascular Disease. J Am Coll Cardiol. 2019;74(10):1376-1414. http://www.onlinejacc.org/content/74/10/e177

- This summary presents an extensive set of guidelines for healthy cardiac living. It includes "Top 10 Take-Home Messages for the Primary Prevention of Cardiovascular Disease," which should be studied with care while one is still young enough for the recommendations to be of particular use.

Lubrano V, Balzan S. Consolidated and emerging inflammatory markers in coronary artery disease. *World J Exp Med.* 2015;5(1):21-32.

- The reading reviews the evidence that C-reactive protein and other markers of inflammation are independent risk factors for cardiovascular disease and adverse outcomes. The article covers areas not addressed in depth in this chapter.

Huisman MV, Klok FA. How I diagnose acute pulmonary embolism. *Blood.* 2013;121(22):4443-4448. doi:10.1182/blood-2013-03-453050

- Although not the most recent review in the area, this article is notable for the discussion of how the quantitative concepts of epidemiology introduced in the first chapter of this text are coupled with modern medical approaches to render a diagnosis. The authors are both experts in the field who have authored many additional detailed papers in the area of pulmonary embolic disease.

American College of Rheumatology. Vasculitis. https://www.rheumatology.org/I-Am-A/Patient-Caregiver/Diseases-Conditions/Vasculitis

Jennette JC, Falk RJ. Pathogenesis of antineutrophil cytoplasmic autoantibody-mediated disease. *Nat Rev Rheumatol.* 2014;10(8):463-473.

- Vasculitis is an important pathogenetic mechanism not discussed in detail in the chapter but covered in the supplemental readings and in the two above. The first article is a good general overview into the etiology and classification of the vasculitides. ANCA disease discussed in the second article is of particular interest because of the singular mechanisms involved in its pathogenesis. The reading is by two of the world's experts.

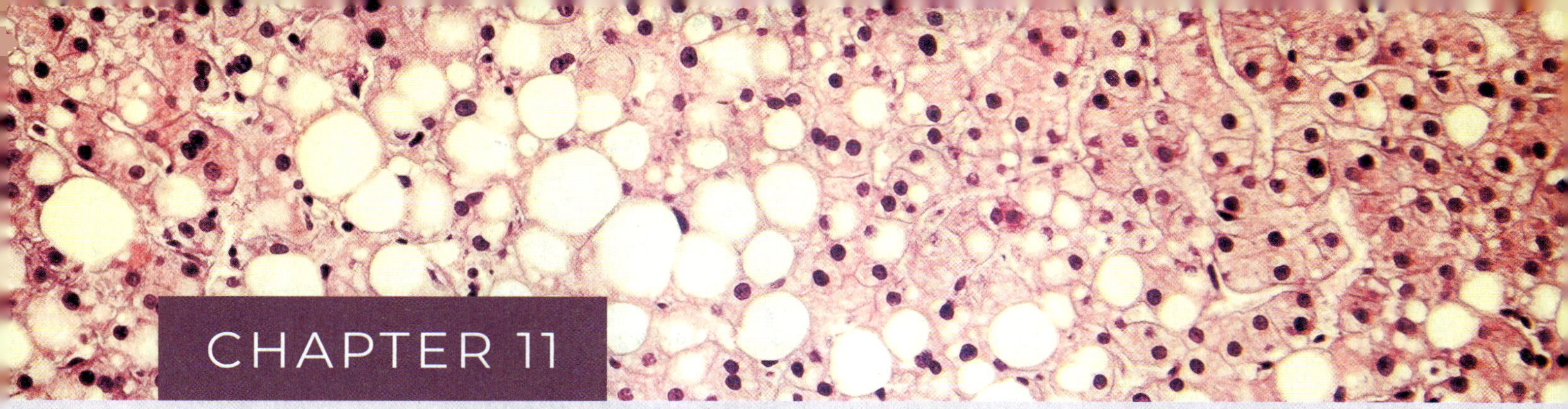

CHAPTER 11

Diseases of the Lymphatic System

LEARNING OBJECTIVES

1. Explain the role of the spleen in protecting the body against infection.
2. Describe the types and causes of leukemia; describe the precursors of leukemia.
3. Compare and contrast leukemia and lymphoma.
4. List the common causes of lymph node enlargement.

The Lymphatic System

The lymphatic system consists of the lymph nodes and spleen, together with various organized masses of lymphoid tissue found elsewhere throughout the body, such as the tonsils, the adenoids, the thymus, and the lymphoid aggregates in the intestinal mucosa, respiratory tract, and bone marrow. The primary function of the lymphatic system is to provide immunologic defenses against foreign material by means of cell-mediated and humoral defense mechanisms. The lymph nodes, which constitute a major part of the system, form an interconnected network linked by lymphatic channels (**Figure 11-1**).

Lymph nodes are small, bean-shaped structures that vary from a few millimeters to as much as 2 cm in diameter. They are interspersed along the course of lymphatic channels, where they create a filtration system. Frequently, they form groups at locations where many lymphatic channels converge, such as around the aorta and inferior vena cava, in the mesentery of the intestine, in the axillae (armpits) and groin, and at the base of the neck. Each node consists of a mass of **lymphocytes** supported by a meshwork of reticular fibers, the reticuloendothelial system. As the lymph flows through the nodes, the phagocytic cells filter out and destroy any microorganisms or other foreign materials that entered the lymphatic channels. The lymphocytes and mononuclear phagocytes within the node also interact with foreign material to initiate an immune response. The functions of the various lymphoid cells and their role in immunity are considered in Chapter 5.

Lymphocyte A mononuclear blood cell produced in lymphoid tissue that takes part in cell-mediated and humoral immunity.

The spleen is specialized to filter blood rather than lymph. Much larger than lymph nodes, it is about the size of a man's fist and is located under the ribs in

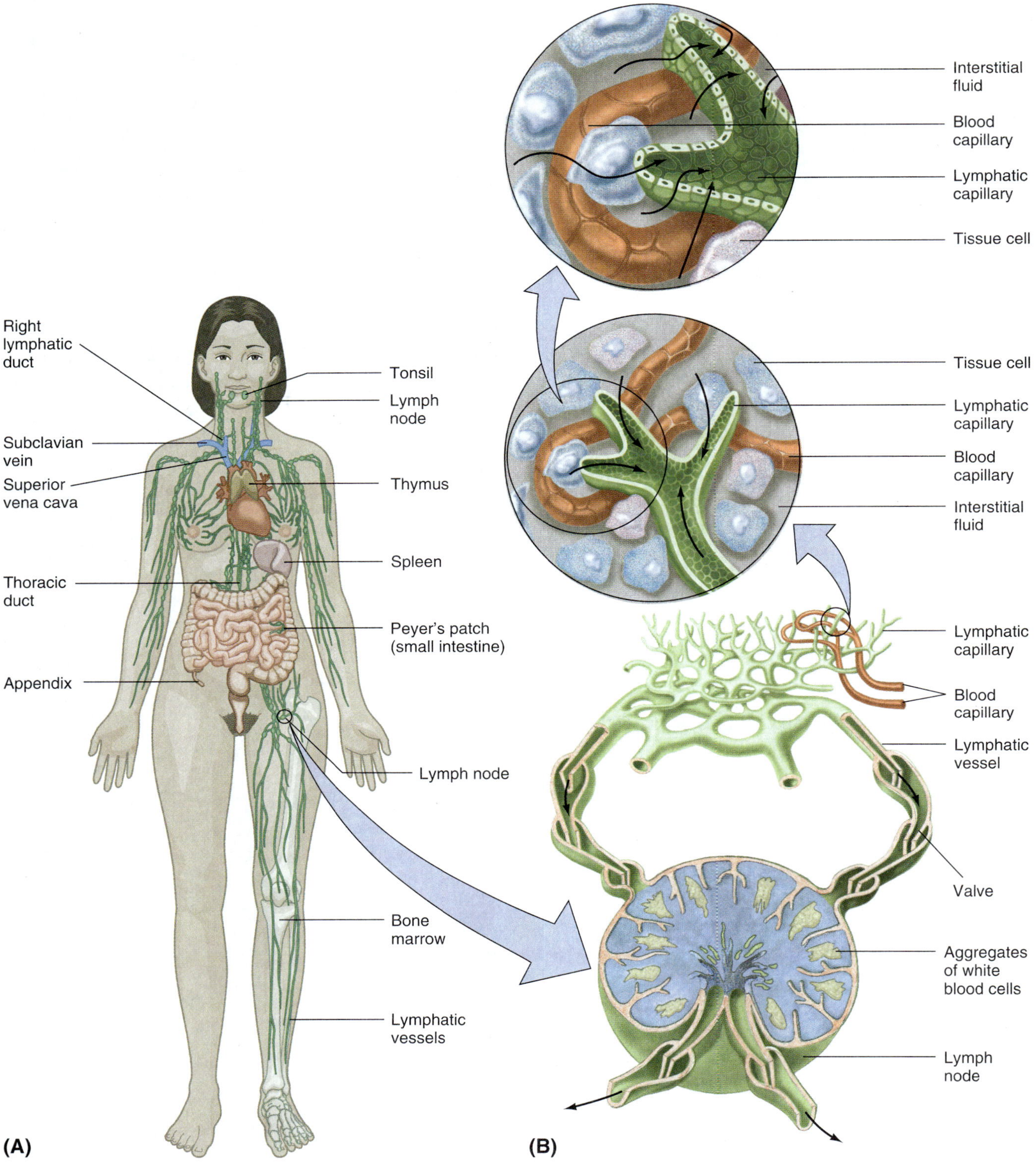

Figure 11-1 The lymphatic system. **(A)** The lymphatic system consists of vessels that transport lymph back to the circulatory system. **(B)** Lymph nodes interspersed along the vessels filter the lymph.

the left upper part of the abdomen. It contains two tissue types: red pulp and white pulp. The white pulp consists of compact masses of organized lymphocytes and phagocytic cells embedded in a network of sinusoids within a supporting framework composed of reticular fibers. The lymphocytes in the white pulp are capable of manufacturing antibodies and activating other immune system cells to facilitate prompt elimination of blood-borne pathogens. As the blood flows through the red pulp of the spleen, worn-out red cells are removed from the circulation by the phagocytic cells, and the iron that they contain is salvaged for reuse. Abnormal red cells, such as those damaged by disease, shaped abnormally, or containing a large amount of an abnormal **hemoglobin**, will also become targets of the splenic phagocytes, accounting for their shortened survival in the circulation. The spleen functions as an efficient blood filtration system eliminating pathogens and foreign materials using phagocytic cells stored there.

Splenectomy, removal of the spleen, may be required to prevent fatal hemorrhage from a trauma-damaged spleen. The procedure is also frequently performed on patients with blood diseases characterized by excessive destruction of blood cells within the spleen, such as thrombocytopenic **purpura** and some types of hereditary hemolytic **anemia** (see Chapter 12).

After a splenectomy, individuals may experience a reduced immune response to pathogens, especially encapsulated bacteria, with pneumococcal disease being of particular concern. Due to their altered immunocompetence, these individuals should receive vaccines, which will help stimulate their immune response. Many healthcare providers also recommend that a splenectomized individual either take prophylactic antibiotics routinely or begin taking antibiotics at the first sign of a respiratory infection or other febrile illness.

The thymus is a bilobed lymphoid organ overlying the base of the heart. It is a large structure during infancy and childhood but gradually undergoes atrophy in adolescence. Only a remnant persists in the adult. The thymus plays an essential role in the prenatal development of the lymphoid system and in the formation of the body's immunologic defense mechanisms. It plays an especially important role in the immune system's ability to distinguish between self and non-self antigens (see Chapter 5).

Leukocytes-White Blood Cells

Leukocytes are much less numerous than red cells (**erythrocytes**), averaging about 7000 per microliter. Leukocytes consist of the following cell type: neutrophils, **eosinophils**, **basophils**, **monocytes**, and lymphocytes. The first three types are collectively called **granulocytes**, because of the characteristic granules in their cytoplasm or **polymorphonuclear leukocytes (PMN)** because of the multiple lobes of their nuclei. The last two cell types are collectively called mononuclear cells since their nuclei do not have multiple lobes. Although all lymphocytes are derived from a bone marrow stem cell, those destined to be B lymphocytes continue to mature further in the bone marrow until released into the circulation. Precursors of T lymphocytes further mature in the thymus prior to entering the circulation (see Chapter 5). Properties of blood cells are summarized in Table 12-1 (For a discussion of hematopoiesis, see Chapter 12). In contrast to the relatively long survival of red cells, most white cells have a short survival time, varying from several hours to several days. They must be replenished continually. In contrast, naïve lymphocytes that are not yet programmed for a specific antigen survive for 1 to 3 months. Lymphocytes that react to a specific antigen may survive for years as memory lymphocytes.

The proportions of the subtypes of leukocytes varies with the age of the individual. In adults, the most numerous are neutrophils, constituting about 70 percent of the total circulating white cells. Neutrophils predominate in acute inflammatory reactions and are actively phagocytic. Lymphocytes are the next most common type of white cell in adults and are the predominant leukocytes in the blood of children. The lymphocytes in the peripheral blood constitute

Hemoglobin An oxygen transport protein within red cells composed of an iron-porphyrin complex (heme) combined with a protein chain (globin).

Purpura Bleeding under the skin or mucus membrane observed as large discolored areas on the skin.

Anemia A decrease in hemoglobin or red cells or both.

Leukocyte Collective term for white cells.

Erythrocyte Commonly known as red blood cells (RBCs), these are the most abundant blood cells, specifically designed to transport oxygen from the lungs to body tissues and carbon dioxide back, using the iron-rich protein hemoglobin.

Eosinophil A cell whose cytoplasm is filled with large, uniform granules that stain intensely red with acid dyes.

Basophil A cell that contains numerous variable-sized granules that stain intensely purple with basic dyes.

Monocyte The largest leukocyte, a phagocytic cell that forms part of the reticuloendothelial system.

Granulocytes Collective name for neutrophils, eosinophils, and basophils.

Polymorphonuclear leukocytes (PMN) A leukocyte having a multilobed nucleus whose cytoplasm is filled with fine granules.

only a small fraction of the total lymphocytes found in the body; most can be located in the lymph nodes, spleen, and other lymphoid tissues discussed in this chapter. Lymphocytes continually recirculate from the bloodstream into lymphoid tissues. Lymphocytes participate in cell-mediated and humoral defense reactions (as discussed in Chapter 5).

Small numbers of eosinophils, basophils, and monocytes also are normally present in the blood. Eosinophils play a role in allergic reactions and in defense against parasites. They increase in allergic diseases, in the presence of worm or other animal-parasite infections, and in a few other conditions. Basophils contain granules of histamine and an anticoagulant called **heparin**. Monocytes are actively phagocytic and important in the response to certain types of chronic and viral infections. Monocytes also contribute to chronic inflammatory responses. Monocytes are the circulating precursors to the macrophages found in the tissues. A monocyte/macrophage–lymphocyte interaction is necessary in the initial phase of the immune response to most foreign antigens. These cells also play a role in the cell-mediated immune reaction (see Chapter 5).

Heparin An anticoagulant produced by the liver.

Infectious mononucleosis A common viral disease, the most common cause of benign lymphocytosis.

Epstein-Barr virus A virus that causes infectious mononucleosis.

Diseases of The Lymphatic System

The principal diseases affecting the lymphatic system are infections and neoplasms.

Benign Lymphocytosis

Benign lymphocytosis, an increase in the number of circulating lymphocytes, is most often a reflection of viral disease. The circulating lymphocytes may be enlarged and atypical-looking. **Infectious mononucleosis** is a common cause of benign lymphocytosis, particularly in children and adolescents. The disease is caused by herpesvirus 4, **Epstein-Barr (EB) virus** (usually EBV). The virus causes an acute, debilitating, febrile illness associated with a diffuse hyperplasia of lymphoid tissue throughout the body, particularly the lymph nodes and spleen, which may double or triple in size. The lymphocytes circulating in the peripheral blood show distinctive morphologic abnormalities (**Figure 11-2**). The atypical lymphocytes are cytotoxic

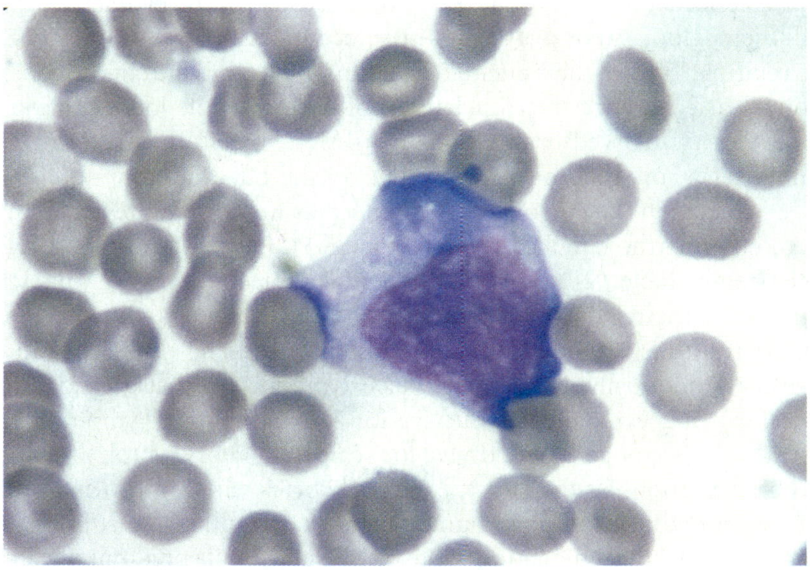

Figure 11-2 Large lymphocyte from an individual with infectious mononucleosis, illustrating characteristic morphologic abnormalities (original magnification × 1000).

Courtesy of Leonard V. Crowley, MD, Century College.

(CD8+) T lymphocytes, which destroy **B cells** infected by EBV. Enlargement and ulceration of lymphoid tissue in the throat is responsible for the sore throat often accompanying the disease.

Disease diagnosis is most often based on clinical symptoms and detection of antibodies using a monospot test. EBV infection results in the production of antibodies directed toward the virus and an unusual class of **heterophile antibodies** that react with unrelated substances (sheep and horse red cells). The monospot test detects such antibodies and is very specific to the disease.

Generally, the disease is self-limited, and no specific treatment is required. However, it may be several weeks before the patient feels well again, and the spleen may be sensitive to trauma while it remains enlarged. Contact sports and any activity which could lead to trauma to the spleen should be avoided until the illness resolves.

B cell A lymphocyte that differentiates into plasma cells and is associated with humoral immunity.

Heterophile antibodies Antibodies that react with substances unrelated to the immunizing antigen.

Lymphadenitis An inflammation of lymph nodes draining a site of infection.

Leukemia A neoplastic proliferation of leukocytes.

Inflammation of the Lymph Nodes (Lymphadenitis)

Lymph nodes draining an area of infection may become enlarged and tender resulting from stimulation of inflammatory and immune responses and the concomitant swelling associated with these processes. This condition is referred to as **lymphadenitis**.

Leukemia

The term **leukemia** refers to a neoplasm of hematopoietic tissue. In contrast to solid tumors, which form discrete deposits, leukemic cells diffusely infiltrate the bone marrow and lymphoid tissues, spill over into the bloodstream, and infiltrate the various organs of the body. The leukemic cells may be mostly mature, arrested at some stage of development, or extremely primitive (**Figure 11-3**). The overproduction of white cells in leukemia may be

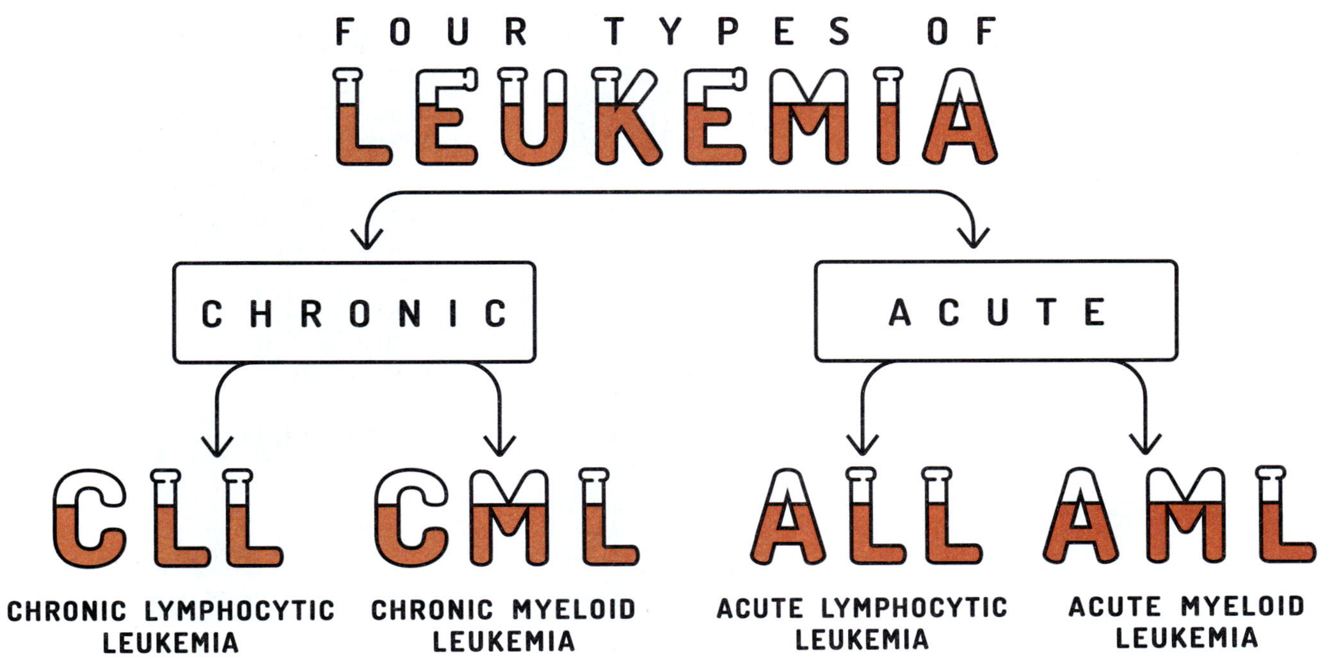

Figure 11-3 Leukemia can be divided into two subcategories: chronic or acute. Those subcategories each contain two types of leukemia.

evident in the peripheral blood exhibiting a very high white blood cell count. In some cases of leukemia, the proliferation of the white cells is largely confined to the bone marrow, and there is no significant increase in the number of white cells in the bloodstream. This disease may present with some degree of overlap with **lymphoma**, where the neoplastic cells are predominantly found in lymph nodes and other lymphoid organs such as the spleen but may also occur in essentially any tissue. Lymphomas can be "leukemia-like" and be found in the blood and bone marrow.

Lymphoma A neoplasm of lymphoid cells limited to lymph nodes and sometimes spleen.

Myeloid leukemia Characterized by rapid growth of abnormal white blood cells that accumulate in the bone marrow and interfere with the production of normal blood cells.

Lymphoid leukemia Neoplasm of B-cell or T-cell lineage involving primarily the bone marrow and peripheral blood.

Classification of Leukemia

Leukemia is classified on the basis of both the cell type and the maturity of the abnormally proliferating cells. Any type of hematopoietic cell can give rise to leukemia, but the most common types are **myeloid leukemia** and **lymphoid leukemia**. Leukemia developing from stem cells that would normally give rise to the leukocytes containing specific granules, granulocytes (neutrophils, eosinophils, and basophils), falls into the myeloid leukemia category. Leukemia developing from precursor cells that give rise to monocytes is called monocytic leukemia (often myelomonocytic leukemia); lymphocytic leukemia is derived from lymphoid precursor cells. Various complex subclassifications have been established within these major groups based on the characteristics of the cell membranes, the enzymes present within the leukemic cells, and genetic changes.

If the leukemia cells are mostly primitive forms, the leukemia is classified as acute leukemia (**Figure 11-4**). Such leukemias have rapid onset, are

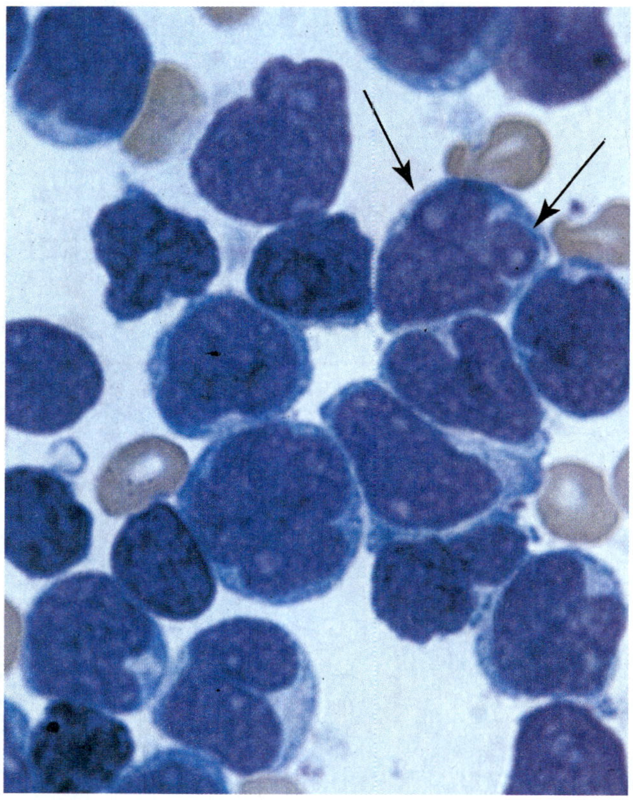

Figure 11-4 A photomicrograph of a blood smear from a patient with acute leukemia. The nuclei of the white cells have the fine chromatin structure and prominent nucleoli indicating immaturity (arrows). Nuclei are irregular in size and configuration.

Courtesy of Leonard V. Crowley, MD, Century College.

clinically aggressive, and are characterized by the presence of blasts (poorly differentiated or immature cells). If the cells are more mature-appearing, the leukemia is classified as chronic leukemia. Chronic leukemias have an insidious onset and are usually less aggressive and may be compatible with relatively long survival.

Myelogenous Leukemias

Chronic myelogenous leukemias are classified as myeloproliferative disorders, of which chronic myelogenous leukemia (CML) and **polycythemia** vera (see Chapter 12) are common examples. Myeloproliferative disorders are characterized by highly cellular bone marrows containing an abundance of precursors for the leukemic cell (myeloid precursors in the case of CML). The elevated number of circulating cells may range from mature granulocytes to immature forms (**Figure 11-5**). Almost all cases of CML are associated with the presence of a **Philadelphia chromosome**, which represents a translocation between two chromosomes (9 and 22). This results in the formation of BCR-ABL fusion protein (kinase) with inappropriately increased activity, which is responsible for the leukemic process (see Chapter 6). Specific drugs such as imatinib are available to inhibit this abnormal enzymatic activity. The drug is initially effective in greater than 90 percent of patients, but resistance occurs with time, requiring either another inhibiting drug or other forms of therapy. With time and failure of drug therapy, CML tends to progress to an acute blast phase, and increased numbers of such cells appear in the bone marrow and blood. Blast cells acquire additional mutations and become resistant to drug therapy. The prognosis for blast phase CML is poor.

Polycythemia An increase of red cells and hemoglobin above normal levels.

Philadelphia chromosome Chromosome translocation common in neoplastic cells of chronic myelogenous leukemia.

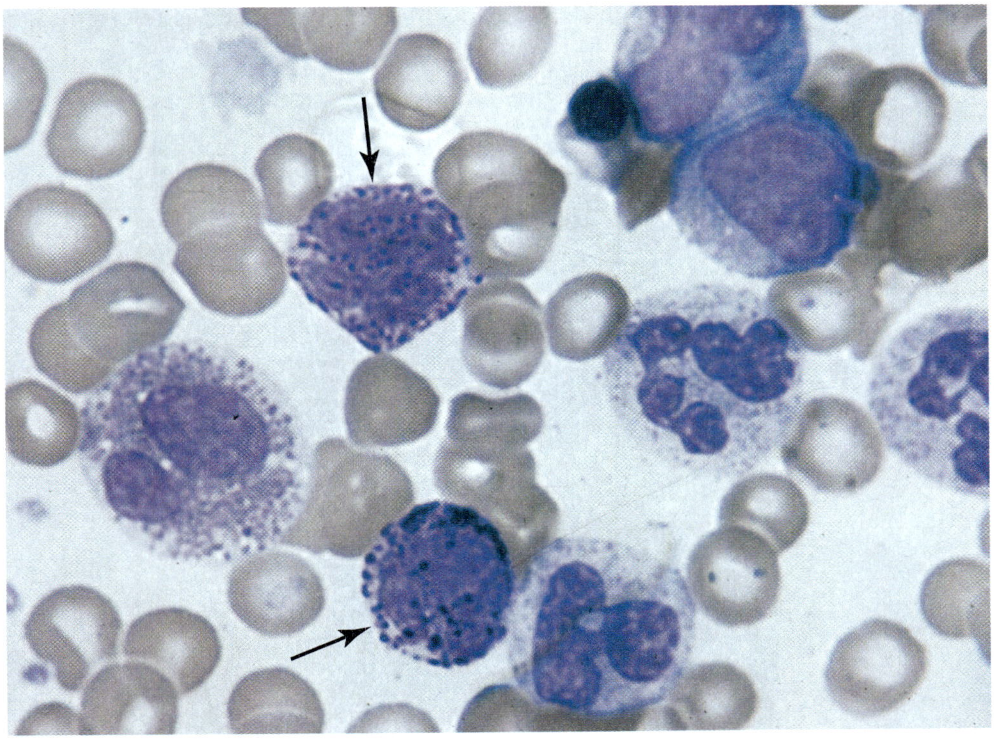

Figure 11-5 Chronic granulocytic leukemia. Most of the cells in the photomicrograph are mature. Note the basophils (*arrows*), the eosinophil (*left of arrows*), and the two neutrophils (*right of arrows*).

Courtesy of Leonard V. Crowley, MD, Century College.

Acute myeloid leukemia (AML) is the most common type of acute leukemia. AML may arise de novo or, less frequently, as a side effect of radiation or chemotherapy. In AML, greater than 20 percent of undifferentiated myeloblasts, immature precursors to granulocytes, are found in the bone marrow, where they crowd out normal hematopoietic cells, resulting in **leukopenia**, **thrombocytopenia**, and anemia. AML cells harbor many mutations. There are many types of AML, and specific forms of chemotherapy are available for several of them.

Leukopenia An abnormally small number of leukocytes in the peripheral blood.
Thrombocytopenia A deficiency of platelets.

Lymphocytic Leukemias

In chronic lymphocytic leukemia (CLL), the circulating cells are mostly small, mature lymphocytes (**Figure 11-6**). The most common type of CLL is mature B cell leukemia, which is equivalent to small-cell lymphocytic lymphoma (SLL). The two differ only in whether the disease is predominantly based in the bone marrow or in the lymph node and blood. B cell CLL/SLL is the most common type of adult leukemia in the Western world. The disease is most commonly indolent and is often discovered as an incidental finding. Patients without symptoms may not require therapy and often survive more than 10 years. However, about 30 percent of patients will experience progression of the disease to other forms of leukemia/lymphoma with worsening symptoms. Patients with CLL may develop hypogammaglobulinemia and susceptibility to infection and autoimmune hemolytic anemia. Although the disease may be kept in check using chemotherapy, it generally cannot be cured.

Acute lymphoblastic leukemia (ALL) (or more specifically, precursor B-cell ALL, often referred to simply as PBC-ALL) is the most common malignancy of childhood. It generally occurs in children between 2 and 5 years of age, with more than half of cases occurring in children younger than 6. At times the disease predominantly involves lymph nodes and is referred to as

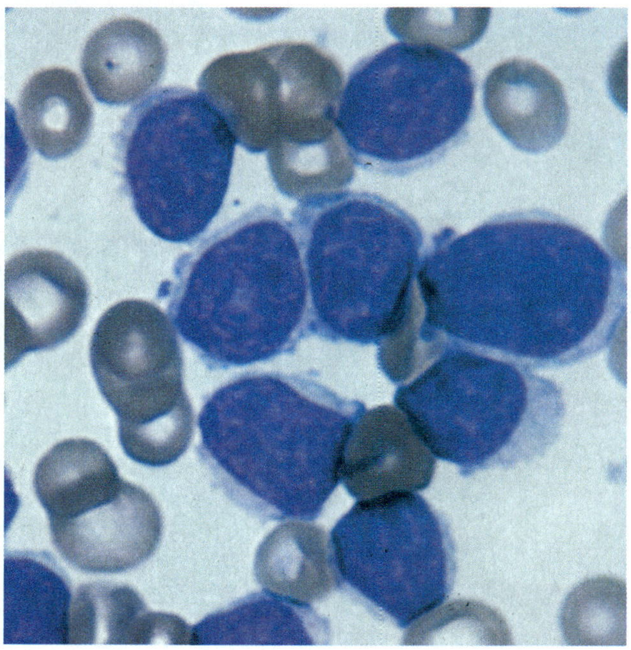

Figure 11-6 Chronic lymphocytic leukemia. The dense nuclear chromatin structure indicates that the lymphocytes are mature (compare with Figure 11-5). The total white count is elevated.

Courtesy of Leonard V. Crowley, MD, Century College.

lymphoblastic lymphoma. Small- to medium-size lymphoblasts, which are similar to very early precursors of mature B cells, replace much of the bone marrow and can be found in the blood. This results in anemia, neutropenia, and thrombocytopenia because precursors for these cell lines are lost from the marrow. (Additional details of childhood precursor B-cell ALL are discussed in Case 11-1). The disease may disseminate into the CNS and other organs. Occasionally, however, the marrow may be crowded with abnormal cells, but the number of white blood cells in the blood is normal or decreased. Many different chromosomal abnormalities can be found in PBC-ALL. Sequencing of the genomes and transcriptomes of the cells helped create a classification and subclassification for the types of ALL. This intense genetic analysis leads to better diagnostic and therapeutic protocols. Therapeutic advances now allow for a 90 percent total remission rate in children. **T cell**–derived disease also occurs, and current 5-year survival rates are similar to PBC-ALL.

Many additional forms of neoplastic diseases of lymphoid cells are characterized depending on the cell type (B cell versus T cell) and stage of maturity of the neoplastic cell involved. As a single example, **multiple myeloma** is a neoplasm of plasma cells, with the highly differentiated B cell responsible for the production of **immunoglobulins**. For this reason, multiple myeloma is often characterized by the production of an M-protein (myeloma protein or monoclonal gammopathy). The uniform immunoglobulin produced by the neoplastic plasma cells, which are monoclonal (derived from a single transformed neoplastic cell), can be detected in the blood. In many ways, multiple myeloma resembles leukemia, but the neoplastic plasma cell proliferation is generally confined to the bone marrow (**Figure 11-7**). The malignant cells produce "punched-out" lytic lesions of the bones, which may lead to bone destruction and fractures characteristic of the disease (**Figure 11-8**). At times an M-protein may be detected in the blood prior to the detection of abnormal plasma cells in the bone marrow. This is termed a monoclonal gammopathy of unknown significance (MGUS). Although an MGUS is not associated with symptomatic disease, it is a precursor lesion that indicates a risk of developing multiple myeloma.

T cell A type of lymphocyte associated with cell-mediated immunity.

Multiple myeloma A neoplasm of plasma cells characterized by production of M-protein.

Immunoglobulins The class of proteins that includes antibodies.

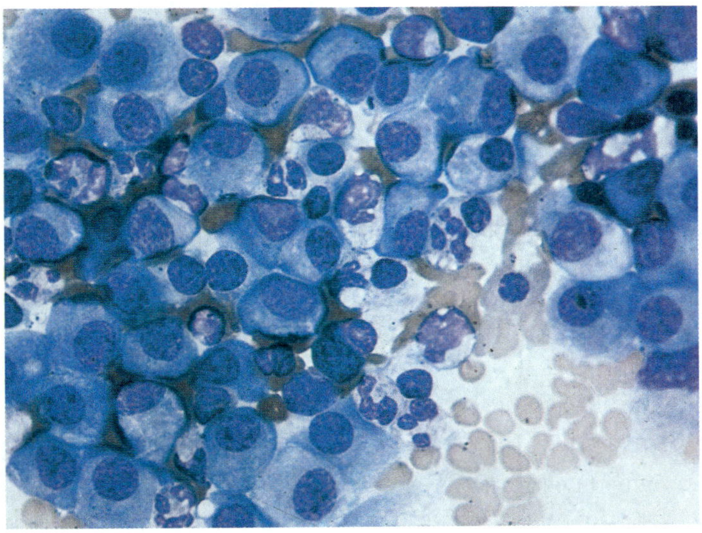

Figure 11-7 Photomicrograph illustrating aspirated bone marrow from a patient with multiple myeloma. Almost all cells are immature plasma cells containing large eccentric nuclei and abundant cytoplasm.

Courtesy of Leonard V. Crowley, MD, Century College.

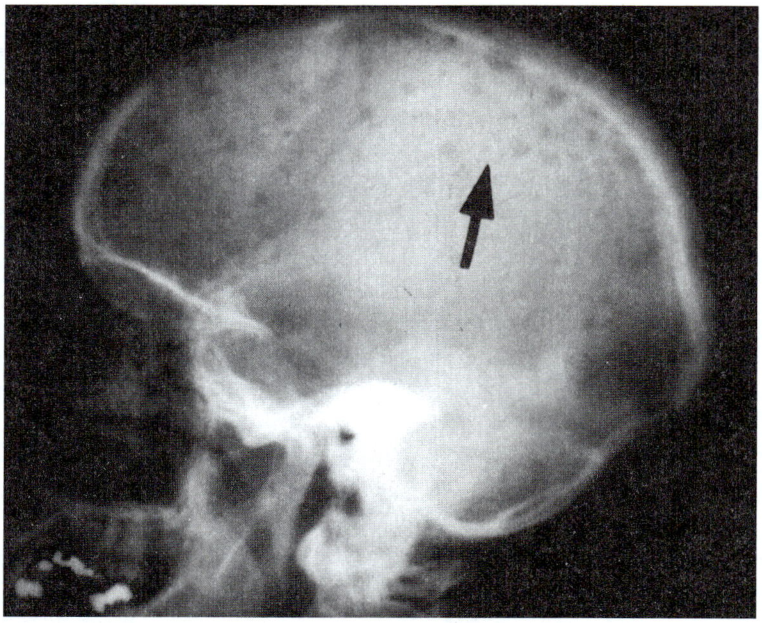

Figure 11-8 A skull X-ray from a patient with multiple myeloma. Multiple punched-out areas in skull bones (*arrow*) result from bone destruction caused by nodular masses of neoplastic plasma cells growing in bone marrow.

Courtesy of Leonard V. Crowley, MD, Century College.

Precursors of Leukemia: The Myelodysplastic Syndromes

Acute leukemia in older patients may not have an abrupt onset but can be preceded by a period lasting from several months to several years. During that time, affected patients have only a refractory anemia, sometimes associated with reduced white cells (leukopenia) and low blood **platelets** (thrombocytopenia). Examination of the bone marrow of these patients reveals variable degrees of disturbed growth and maturation of red cells, white cell precursors, and megakaryocytes, but not leukemia. The condition is termed **myelodysplastic syndrome** (myelo = marrow + dysplasia = disturbed growth). Several different types have been described that differ somewhat in their clinical and hematologic manifestations. In general, the more severe the maturation disturbance in the bone marrow, the greater the likelihood that leukemia will eventually occur. Nearly half of patients with myelodysplastic syndrome will develop AML. Unfortunately, there is no specific treatment available for most patients with these conditions, although some patients with severe "pre-leukemic" changes in their bone marrow have been treated successfully by bone marrow transplantation.

Platelet A component of the blood; a roughly circular or oval disk formed from the plasma membrane of the megakaryocytes found in the bone marrow. Platelets are a key component in blood coagulation.

Myelodysplastic syndrome Marrow disease with features of a "pre-leukemia."

Lymphomas

Neoplasms of lymphoid tissue are called lymphomas, as distinguished from leukemias, which develop in the bone marrow and blood-forming organs (**Figure 11-9**). In some cases there may be overlap between the definitions, with the difference depending on where the seemingly identical neoplastic cells predominate (blood vs. lymph system). Lymphoma includes heterogeneous malignancies that arise from the clonal proliferation of lymphocytes, over 80% of which derive from B cells. Most of the rest come from T cells,

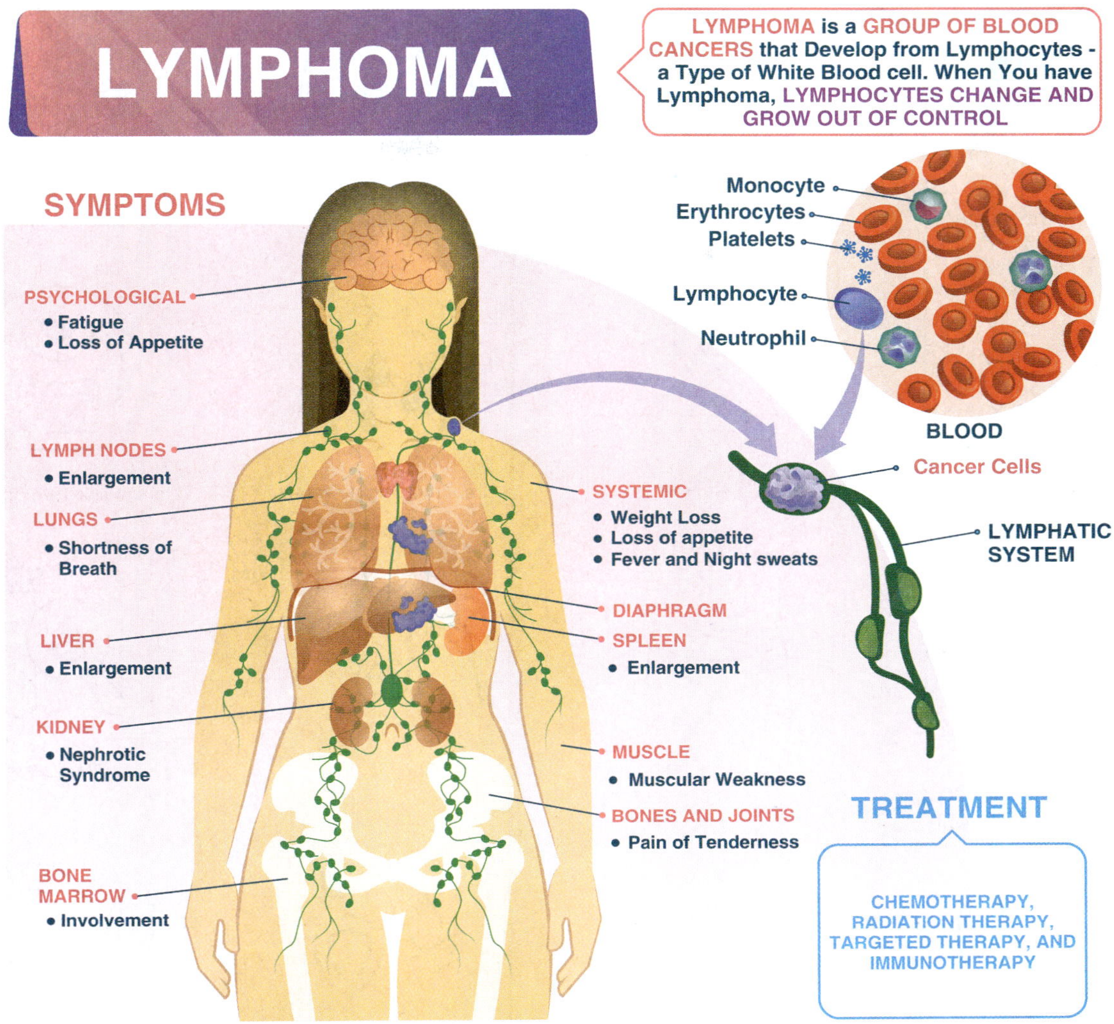

Figure 11-9 Lymphoma could potentially affect many areas of the body since the lymphatic system is found in all parts of the body and the abnormal lymphoma cells could spread via the lymphatic system or the circulatory system.

and a few originate from NK cells (natural killer cells) or histiocytes. The classification of lymphomas is very complex, with at least 60 types recognized, representing approximately 5% of malignancies. The neoplastic cells of lymphomas arise from abnormal proliferations of the cells at different development stages, some relatively mature, others clearly immature. The abnormal proliferation of lymphoid cells often disrupts the normal functions of the immune system, which may impair the body's immune defenses, resulting in increased susceptibility to infections.

Lymphomas are subdivided into two major categories: **Hodgkin's lymphoma (HL)** (**Figure 11-10**), which is the most common, and non Hodgkin lymphoma (non-HL). Non-HL can be further subdivided into over 60 types, including B-cell neoplasms (the most common), and T or NK lymphomas (**Figure 11-11**). HL has several distinctive features and is defined by the presence of pathological Hodgkin Reed-Sternberg (HRS) cells, which are of B-cell origin. HL occurs in young adults (and is the most common cancer in adolescents ages 15–19) but also occurs in people over 60 (the distribution is bimodal). This is in contrast to non-HL, where disease frequency increases with age, with an average age at diagnosis of 67 (although there are some exceptions to this general rule).

Hodgkin's lymphoma (HL) A form of lymphoma that occurs in young adults with Hodgkin and Reed-Sternberg cells mixed with other cell types.

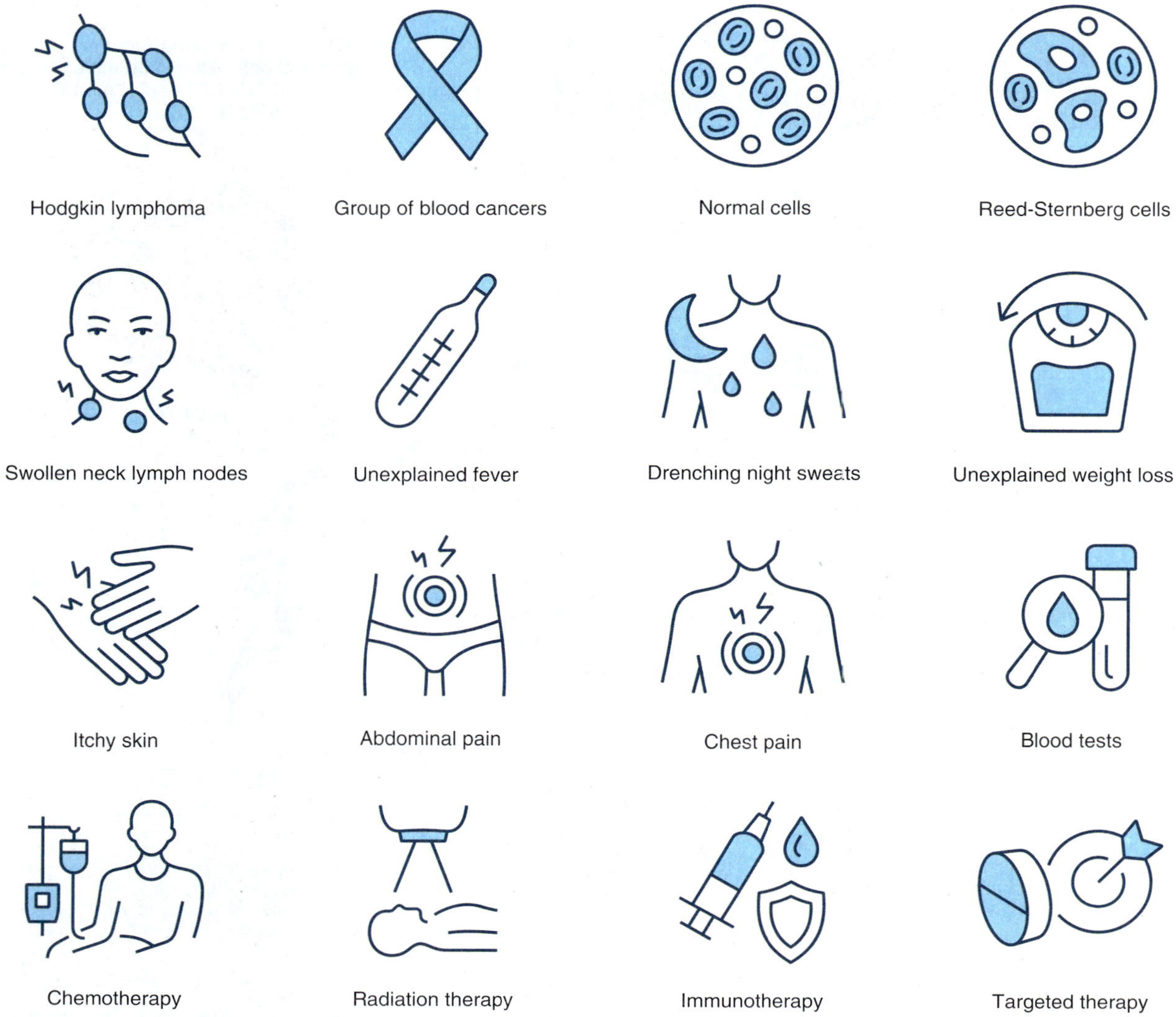
Hodgkin lymphoma
Group of blood cancers
Normal cells
Reed-Sternberg cells
Swollen neck lymph nodes
Unexplained fever
Drenching night sweats
Unexplained weight loss
Itchy skin
Abdominal pain
Chest pain
Blood tests
Chemotherapy
Radiation therapy
Immunotherapy
Targeted therapy

Figure 11-10 There are many things that must be taken into consideration when diagnosing and treating Hodgkin lymphoma. Hodgkin lymphoma is highly treatable and the outcome for most patients is very positive.

Hodgkin cell Abnormal mononucleated lymphocyte.

Reed-Sternberg cell Abnormal multinucleated lymphocyte.

HL often starts in a single lymph node or small group of nodes and then spreads to adjacent nodes before eventually spreading to other parts of the body. HL has a variable histologic appearance, characterized by two possible cell types: **Hodgkin cells** and **Reed-Sternberg cells**, depending on the number of nuclei present (one for Hodgkin cells and two for Reed-Steinberg cells). The Reed-Sternberg cells are intermixed with lymphocytes, plasma cells, eosinophils, and fibrous tissue, the distribution of which define a disease subtype. Although the Reed-Sternberg cells are the neoplastic component responsible for the disease, they make up only a small proportion of the total cells in the affected node. The cytokines they secrete attract the other admixed cells.

For most cases of HL, no underlying cause is defined, but EBV infection and immunodeficiency states such as AIDS may play a role in some forms of the disease.

All other lymphomas, of which there are over 60 types, are grouped together under the general term of non-HL. Most are B-cell lymphomas that are quite variable in their histologic appearance, clinical presentation, and prognosis, depending on the developmental stage, the function of the lymphocyte that

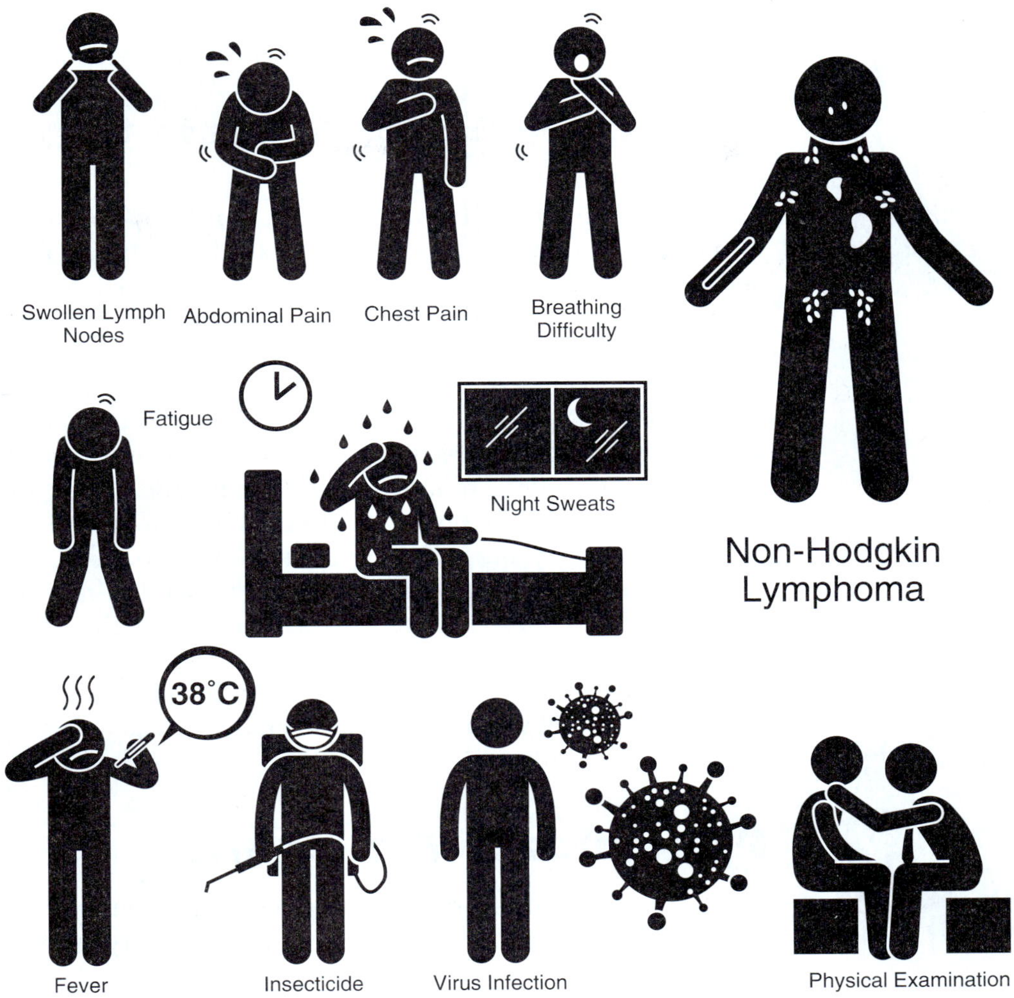

Figure 11-11 Non-Hodgkin lymphoma is a diagnosis of exclusions. Often the symptoms are so nebulous that diagnosis is difficult, making selecting the proper treatment modalities difficult as well.

gave rise to the lymphoma, and the level at which the cells crowd out normal cells. The disease is often widespread by the time the lymphoma is diagnosed.

The variable histologic appearance with its poor correlation with clinical outcomes created difficulties in classifying lymphomas. The most common type (about 30% of all non-HL) is a diffuse large B-cell lymphoma, which is considered aggressive with about a 65% 5-year survival rate. Lymphomas are classified into prognostic groups based on their histologic appearance and, most importantly, the use of sophisticated determination of the cell surface characteristics of the lymphoma cell as measured using immunological tests. The complexity of lymphoma diagnosis requires the expertise of hematologists and hematopathologists to evaluate the tests used to identify the type of non-HL affecting the patient. This determination affects the treatment plan and prognosis for the patient.

Metastatic Tumors in Lymph Nodes

Lymph nodes may be affected by the spread of metastatic cells from malignant tumors arising in the breast, lung, colon, or other sites. The nodes first affected lie in the immediate drainage area of the tumor. The tumor may then spread to other more distant lymph nodes through lymphatic channels and could eventually gain access to the circulatory system through the thoracic duct.

The Enlarged Lymph Node as a Diagnostic Problem

Lymphadenopathy Enlargement of one or more lymph nodes.

The patient who visits a clinician because of **lymphadenopathy** in one or more lymph nodes can present a difficult diagnostic problem. Lymph node enlargement may be a manifestation of a localized infection in the area drained by the node, a systemic infection with initial manifestations in the node, a metastatic tumor in the node, or an early manifestation of leukemia or malignant lymphoma. Often, the etiology of the lymphadenopathy can be determined from the clinical evaluation of the patient in conjunction with laboratory studies, including an examination of the peripheral blood. Testing may include various forms of lymph node biopsy, including excision of the entire lymph node. The tissue is submitted to the pathologist for microscopic and immunological examination. In some cases, the histological pattern of the node can be diagnostically useful. It may be necessary to determine whether lymphocyte proliferation within the lymph node arose from the clonal expansion of a single abnormal lymphocyte, indicating a lymphoid neoplasm, or from many different lymphocytes that formed multiple clones of cells (polyclonal proliferation), characteristic of a benign lymphocyte proliferation.

Principles of Treatment

The goal of the healthcare team treating leukemia or lymphoma is to produce a durable (long-lasting) remission. This (at least in theory) requires destruction of all the neoplastic lymphoid cells that could resume division at some future time and allow the disease to recur. Sometimes the abnormal proliferation of the leukemic cells can be stopped for a variable period of time with the range of treatments available. The patient may then appear to have completely recovered and is said to be in remission. If the disease returns, or relapses, other treatment modalities will need to be considered. The type of therapy is dependent on many clinical variables, including the age of the patient, the severity of the disease when diagnosed, the specific type of leukemia or lymphoma, and which, if any, genetic markers are present. For example, ALL in children was nearly uniformly fatal in the mid-1960s with an overall cure rate of less than 10 percent. By the mid-1980s, following advances in the treatment of CNS disease associated with ALL, cure rates approached 50 percent. Currently, modern chemotherapy protocols lead to a cure rate of 90 percent (see the chapter case study for more details). A similar increase in survival has occurred with Hodgkin lymphoma; cure rates now approach 98 percent with the use of chemotherapy, often combined with limited X-ray therapy. Specific drugs that target the abnormal gene product directly responsible for the neoplastic disease are already in use, but only limited agents are available to deal with relapse when the neoplasm has become resistant to the drug used for treatment. Another concern with chemotherapy is that treatment may result in secondary cancers years after successful therapy for the primary disease. Many forms of leukemia and lymphoma may be resistant to therapy or relapse after initially successful therapy, but sometimes they can be treated by hematopoietic stem cell transplantation.

Hematopoietc Stem Cell Therapy (Bone Marrow Transplantation)

Hematopoietic stem cells (HSC) for transplantation may be obtained from several sources. The best known is bone marrow, although cord blood harvested at delivery provides a very rich source of HSC. Increasingly, HSC may be harvested from peripheral blood taken from donors using sophisticated apheresis machines, which can "sort out" circulating HSC based on their cell surface properties and return the unneeded cells to the donor. It is now also possible to use cell sorting to harvest normal cells from the patient and use those for the transplant, autologous cell transplantation (described later). This technique allows processing of a large volume of blood from a donor with little or no side effects. Each source of HSC has advantages and disadvantages associated with it, and the choice depends on available donor material and the needs of the patient.

A major concern in HSC transplantation involves the need for the transplanted cells to be accepted by the host (patient) and likewise, that the transplanted (grafted) cells do not trigger an overly severe **graft versus host disease** (GVH). GVH occurs because the donor lymphocytes in the transplant are immunologically active and can recognize the patient's cells as antigenically different. The transplanted cells' attempt to destroy host tissue leads to various clinical manifestations, including skin rash, liver injury, gastrointestinal symptoms, and, in severe cases, death. This is the reverse of the usual situation in which the patient's immune system tries to reject the transplant. Although the healthcare team tries to control the level of GVH, the condition can prove beneficial in that the transplanted cells are effective in destroying the remaining neoplastic cells in the host. Thus, there occurs a delicate balance where the beneficial effects of GVH outweigh the detrimental ones.

Graft versus host disease Condition where a graft of immunologically active cells mounts a response to the host.

Allogeneic/syngeneic/autologous Terms used to classify the relationship of donor cells to the patient: not from self/from an identical twin/from self.

In some cases, HSC may be obtained from the patient (autologous transplant). In this scenario, the patient receives chemotherapy to induce remission. Bone marrow or peripheral blood HSC is harvested from the patient. Healthy HSC cells are identified and collected. They are grown in the laboratory until there is a sufficient number to repopulate a bone marrow transplant. As part of the bone marrow transplant procedure, the patient receives a high-dose chemotherapy, with the intent of removing any lingering cancer cells, which could be present. The bone marrow is destroyed and then repopulated with health cells from the patient that are grown in the lab. This type of HSC therapy uses the patient's own cells and, therefore, GVH is not a concern.

Transplants that are not **autologous** come from either a related or unrelated donor. Such transplants are termed **allogeneic** (not from self). One fortuitous special case is when a patient (host) has an identical twin. Such donors are termed **syngeneic** and are antigenically identical to the patient. The transplant will not be rejected, and any GVH is relatively mild. In the likely absence of an identical twin, the next best source of donors is a sibling (full brother or sister). Matching is done by testing for antigens controlled by the HLA gene complex, which controls the synthesis of those cell surface proteins (antigens) most critical in telling the immune system what is self and what is foreign. Three sets of HLA antigens (HLA-A, HLA-B, and HLA-DRB1) are most critical in determining how compatible transplanted tissue will be. The three sets of antigens are (almost always) inherited as blocks, and the antigens inherited from the maternal and paternal chromosomes are both expressed on tissue. Because siblings inherit one set of antigens from the mother and one from the father, there is a 25 percent chance that any two full siblings will inherit the exact same set of six antigens from their parents. This is called a six-antigen match (HLA-A, HLA-B, and HLA-DRB1 are identical from both parents) and provides the best, most histocompatible match and best results in HSC transplants. However, many other factors (antigens) not likely to be identical in siblings are also important in determining **histocompatibility**. For this reason, even when a six-antigen sibling donor is available, patients must be prepared (primed) before transplantation using potent immunosuppressive drugs to prevent graft rejection because some degree of GVH is likely to occur.

Histocompatibility The degree of being compatible between tissues of different individuals, such as donor and recipient, controlled by the HLA gene.

In the absence of a six-antigen sibling match, large data banks of volunteer, previously HLA-typed, unrelated donors may be searched to find identical donors. These donors are not as effective as matched siblings and are more likely to be rejected. Sometimes unmatched or partially matched siblings may also be considered as donors. Banks of stored cord bloods are also available, but the number of HSC available from these is a major limitation in use to transplant adults.

Five-year survival rates following sibling donor HSC transplantation depend on the particular leukemia or lymphoma being treated and the clinical status of the patient. Although marrow/HSC transplantation is an important advance, it is not always successful. Patients may develop life-threatening infections related to the immunosuppression required to maintain the transplant, and in some patients, the leukemia recurs, arising from the patient's surviving leukemic cells that were not destroyed by the prior chemotherapy and radiation.

Case 11-1

Chelsea is a 4-year-old female who has been feeling poorly for the past several weeks. She has complained of bone pain and has started to limp while playing outside. Her mother notes that she tires easily, appears pale, and comes in to take naps. Chelsea now spikes a moderate fever in the evening (38.5°C, 101.3°F oral). More alarming, Chelsea experiences repeated nose bleeds (epistaxis) and developed small purple spots (**petechiae**) on her arms and legs. Concerned that Chelsea may have a "summer virus," her mother brings her to the family pediatrician.

Petechia Small pinpoint hemorrhage or larger hemorrhage caused by decreased platelets, abnormal platelet function, or capillary defect.

On physical examination, the pediatrician finds enlarged lymph nodes and possibly an enlarged spleen. Noting the patient's pallor and signs of a bleeding tendency and fatigue, the pediatrician suspects disease involving the blood and bone marrow, including anemia, idiopathic thrombocytopenic purpura (ITP, possibly postviral), or a leukemia. An in-office CBC (complete blood count) reveals a very elevated white cell count with low red cell and platelet counts. A peripheral blood smear discloses multiple abnormal cells with very little cytoplasm, which the pediatrician believes are lymphoblasts (**Case Figure 11-1A**). The pediatrician refers Chelsea to a pediatric hematologist for further evaluation.

The hematologist suspects that Chelsea suffers from acute lymphoblastic leukemia of childhood and orders several additional tests. These include a bone marrow aspiration (**Case Figures 11-1B** and **11-1C**). Chelsea's bone marrow biopsy reveals a predominance of lymphoblastic cells and a great reduction of the other cell lineages (developing granulocytes, thrombocytes, and red blood cells) in the marrow. A normal marrow is provided for comparison. A lumbar puncture is performed to evaluate whether leukemic cells are present in cerebrospinal fluid. No such cells are found. A chest X-ray shows no abnormality. Immunological studies of Chelsea's leukemic cells indicate they are of B-cell origin and have cell surface antigens characteristic of immature cells. A karyotypic analysis of the leukemic cells shows the cells are hyperdiploid, having greater than the normal 46 chromosomes.

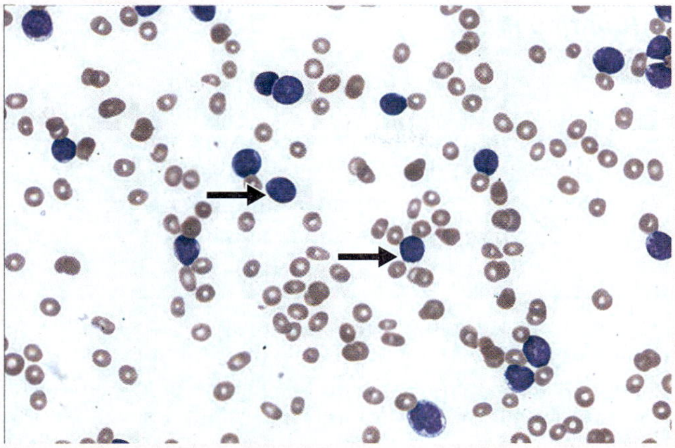

(A)

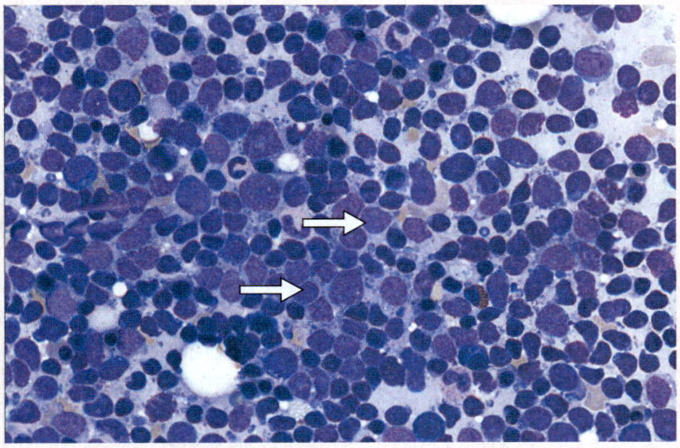

(B)

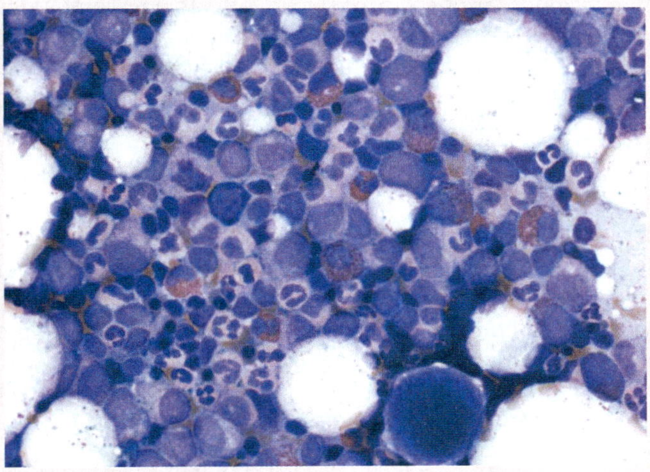

(C)

Case Figure 11-1 **(A)** Peripheral blood smear from patient. Two examples of lymphoblastic cells are indicated (*arrows*). **(B)** Bone marrow sample from patient. The majority of marrow cells are lymphoblasts (*arrows*). **(C)** Normal bone marrow demonstrating multiple lineages of developing cells. The clear spaces are fat found in normal marrow.

Courtesy of Department of Pathology and Laboratory Medicine, University of North Carolina at Chapel Hill.

(continues)

Case 11-1 *(Continued)*

Chelsea begins a long course of chemotherapy. Her initial evaluation (based on age, cell number, cell type, and chromosome number) would place her in a standard (not high-risk) group. Although therapy will continue for a long while, Chelsea has an excellent chance of a cure. The 5-year survival rate with no evidence of further relapse is 95 percent for similar patients, and overall a cure rate of greater than 80 percent is expected.

Discussion

The evaluation of childhood leukemia and therapy of the disease is complex and depends on several variables, including the age of the patient, the severity of the disease at diagnosis, and the nature of the leukemic cell and the molecular abnormalities present in those cells. A small percentage of children with ALL have a Philadelphia chromosome and a BCR-ABL fusion gene, as discussed under chronic myelogenous leukemia. These patients have a worse prognosis, but treatment with kinase inhibitors has much improved survival.

Chemotherapy for childhood ALL is a multistep process. Initial therapy (remission induction) usually takes place for about 4 weeks, with some time initially in a hospital setting, and involves the use of several chemotherapeutic agents in combination. Almost all (95 percent) patients have success in achieving remission initially. This is followed by the consolidation phase, with the aim of eliminating any residual disease, which involves continuing outpatient chemotherapy for as long as 6 to 9 months. This is followed by a prolonged maintenance phase with continuing less intense chemotherapy. In addition, therapy against leukemia in the CNS is always included and is started during remission induction. This includes intrathecal medication (administration of drugs within the membranes of the spinal cord) to ensure the drug enters the cerebrospinal fluid. Up to 20 percent of patients will suffer a relapse, which is often treated by redoing the initial remission induction therapy. All of the drugs used have toxic side effects.

Some children treated with these agents will get a secondary cancer (AML). A number of other chronic long-term effects, including impairment of fertility, learning problems, and heart and lung disease, may also occur. For this reason, long-term follow-up of childhood cancer survivors is critical.

Etiology and Pathogenesis

B-cell acute lymphoblastic leukemia of childhood.

Questions

1. Are there known predisposing environmental or genetic factors for acute lymphoblastic leukemia?
2. What are some of the potential risks and side effects of the chemotherapy used in the treatment of acute lymphoblastic leukemia?
3. No evidence of leukemic cells was found in Chelsea's cerebrospinal fluid. Nevertheless, therapy for CNS disease was performed. Why is such therapy always done in these cases?
4. What psychosocial effects might Chelsea's illness have on both her and her family?
5. Can you estimate the economic cost of Chelsea's therapy? What would happen if Chelsea were not covered by medical insurance?

Questions for Review

1. What is the lymphatic system? How is it organized?
2. What are the major cells of the lymphatic system?
3. What are the major functions of the lymphatic system?
4. What are the functions of the spleen? What are the adverse effects of splenectomy?
5. What is the EBV ? What is its relationship to infectious mononucleosis?
6. What are the clinical manifestations of infectious mononucleosis?
7. How is the disease treated? What are some possible complications of the infection?

References

Hayashi H, Makimoto A, Yuza Y. Treatment of pediatric acute lymphoblastic leukemia: A historical perspective. *Cancers*. 2024;16(4):723. doi:10.3390/cancers16040723

- This article provides a good historical perspective on the history of treatment of pediatric acute lymphoblastic leukemia and helps the reader understand how treatment has evolved in the last few decades.

Del Giudice I, Raponi S, Della Starza I, et al. Minimal residual disease in chronic lymphocytic leukemia: A new goal? *Front Oncol*. 2019;9:689.

- An interesting article that discusses an important concept in chronic disease therapy. How do you tell how good therapy really is? What percentage of neoplastic cells have you eradicated? How good is "good enough"? Of particular interest to the budding molecular biologist.

Xavier AC, Attarbaschi A, Gratzinger D, Balagué O. Dedicated diagnostic approaches for mature B-cell non-Hodgkin lymphomas occurring in children, adolescents, and young adults. *Histopathology*. 2025;86(1):17-37. doi:10.1111/his.15362

Moore T. Bone Marrow Transplantation. Medscape. Updated January 20, 2017. Accessed May 29, 2025. Archived May 11, 2017 at https://web.archive.org/web/20170511060525/https://emedicine.medscape.com/article/1014514-overview

Shadman M. Diagnosis and Treatment of Chronic Lymphocytic Leukemia: A Review. *JAMA*. 2023;329(11):918-932. doi:10.1001/jama.2023.1946

Jamil A, Mukkamalla SKR. Lymphoma. StatPearls [Internet]. Last updated July 17, 2023. https://www.ncbi.nlm.nih.gov/books/NBK560826/

- A collection of recent and useful articles on lymphoma and leukemia diagnostics, trends, and treatments.

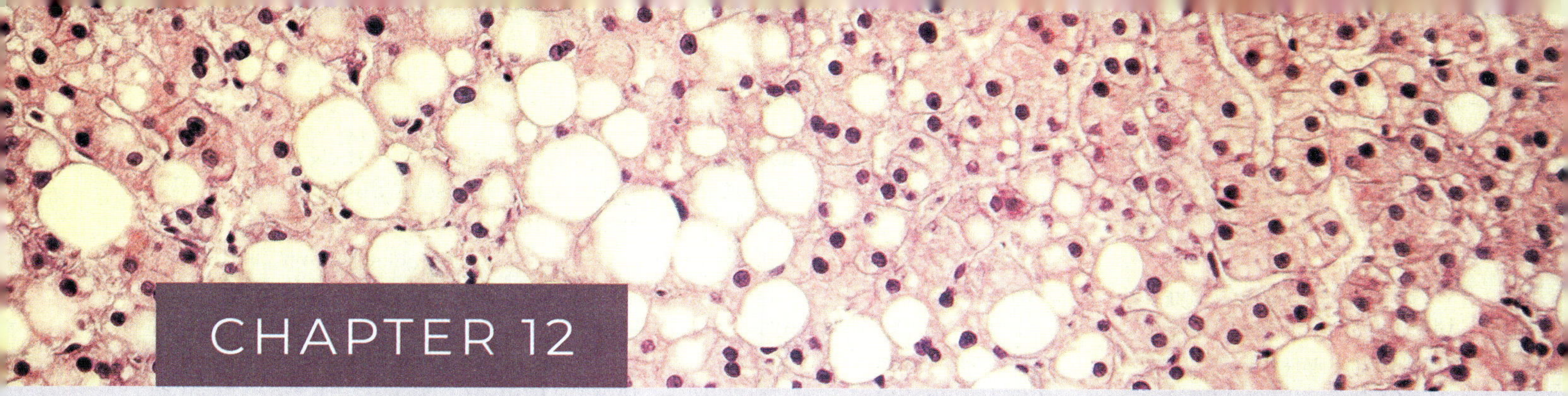

CHAPTER 12

Diseases of Red Blood Cells, Thrombocytes, and Hemostasis

LEARNING OBJECTIVES

1. Describe the composition of the blood and explain the function of each component.
2. Outline the process whereby blood cells are produced.
3. Describe the function and structure of hemoglobin.
4. Categorize the causes of anemia and explain how anemic blood cells may be described.
5. Explain how the treatment of anemia corresponds with its categorization.
6. List and describe the inheritance and effects of abnormal hemoglobin molecules such as sickle cell disease and thalassemia.
7. Describe the causes and effects of polycythemia and thrombocytopenia.
8. Delineate the functions of blood vessels and platelets in controlling bleeding.
9. Explain primary hemostasis and secondary hemostasis and list the coagulation factors involved.
10. Describe how the extrinsic and intrinsic clotting pathways contribute to hemostasis.
11. List the most common clinically significant disturbances of hemostasis and describe their clinical manifestations and therapy.
12. Explain how laboratory tests contribute to evaluating hemostasis.
13. Describe the processes and problems involved in hematopoietic stem cell therapy.
14. Compare and contrast hemorrhage with thrombosis.

The Hematopoietic System

Composition and Function of Human Blood

Blood contains both fluid and cellular components. Plasma, the fluid component of blood, contains proteins, nutrients, waste products, vitamins, and inorganic salts. Plasma also serves to transport the cellular components of the blood—red cells (erythrocytes), white cells (leukocytes), and platelets (thrombocytes)—to all parts of the body via the circulatory system. Erythrocytes transport oxygen (O_2) to tissues and carbon dioxide (CO_2) to the lungs. About 10 percent of CO_2

Hemostasis The body's biological processes to stop bleeding and prevent hemorrhage, including vasoconstriction, platelet plugging, and coagulation.
Fibrinogen A precursor in plasma converted into fibrin by thrombin during blood coagulation.
Fibrin The meshwork of protein threads that form during the clotting of blood.

is dissolved in the plasma and tissue fluids: 5 to 7 percent of the CO_2 dissolved in the plasma and the remainder dissolved in the tissue fluids. Erythrocytes carry the balance of CO_2, which is approximately 90 percent. Leukocytes provide critical host defenses (Chapters 5 and 11). Platelets, also known as thrombocytes, play a critical role in **hemostasis**, the termination of bleeding. The proteins carried by plasma serve a variety of functions. The protein present in greatest concentration is albumin, providing the colloid osmotic pressure (oncotic pressure) that helps retain fluid within the blood vessels. Albumin also is a carrier for a variety of substances, including hormones and drugs. Immunoglobulins (antibodies) are critical in the adaptive immune response. **Fibrinogen**, which becomes **fibrin** when activated, forms the framework for the hemostatic plug (clot) that stops bleeding. The volume of blood, which varies with the size of the individual, is about 5 liters (about 5 and one-third quarts) in the average-sized man.

Almost half of the blood volume consists of cellular elements (**Figure 12-1**). All blood cells arise from a common precursor cell within the bone marrow called the pluripotential hemopoietic stem cell. Those cells undergo further differentiation in the marrow to form a lymphoid stem cell, the source of lymphocytes critical in the immune response. A series of progenitor cells also arises, which in turn differentiate to form the precursors of red cells, which will eventually mature into erythrocytes, nonlymphoid white cells, and thrombocytes. The numbers of circulating red cells, white cells, and platelets are expressed as the number per microliter (µL) of blood (1 mL = 1,000 µL). This same quantity can also be expressed as the number per milliliter (mL) of blood.

Red cells are the most numerous cells, averaging about 5 million per microliter of blood. A mature red blood cell (RBC) is an extremely flexible biconcave disk measuring about 7 micrometers (microns) in cross-section diameter. This biconcave configuration contributes to the characteristic central pallor with a more intensely stained periphery observed in a stained blood smear. The biconcave configuration also contributes to the large surface area/volume ratio important for optimal gas exchange. The red cell shape contributes to its extreme flexibility, which allows red cells to squeeze through small blood capillaries less than half the diameter of the red cells. Red cells normally survive for about 4 months (120 days) in circulation.

Blood thrombocytes, also known as platelets, are actually pieces of the cell membrane of a precursor cell found in the bone marrow, the megakaryocyte. Platelets are essential for normal blood coagulation. Platelets have a short survival time, comparable to that of most leukocytes.

Properties of blood cells are summarized in **Table 12-1**. In contrast to the relatively long survival of red cells, approximately 120 days, most leukocytes have a relatively short survival time (For a more detailed discussion of leukocytes, see Chapter 11).

Normal Hematopoiesis

The bone marrow replenishes the blood cells that are continually worn out and removed from the circulation. It also responds to stressors such as infection or, in the case of red cells, bleeding or low oxygen levels, by increasing the number of appropriate cells released into the circulation. The rate of release of blood cells from the marrow is controlled by circulating cytokines that can stimulate blood cell production. Efficient production of blood cells requires a sufficient supply of the pluripotent stem cells and the materials necessary for the cell

(A)

(B)

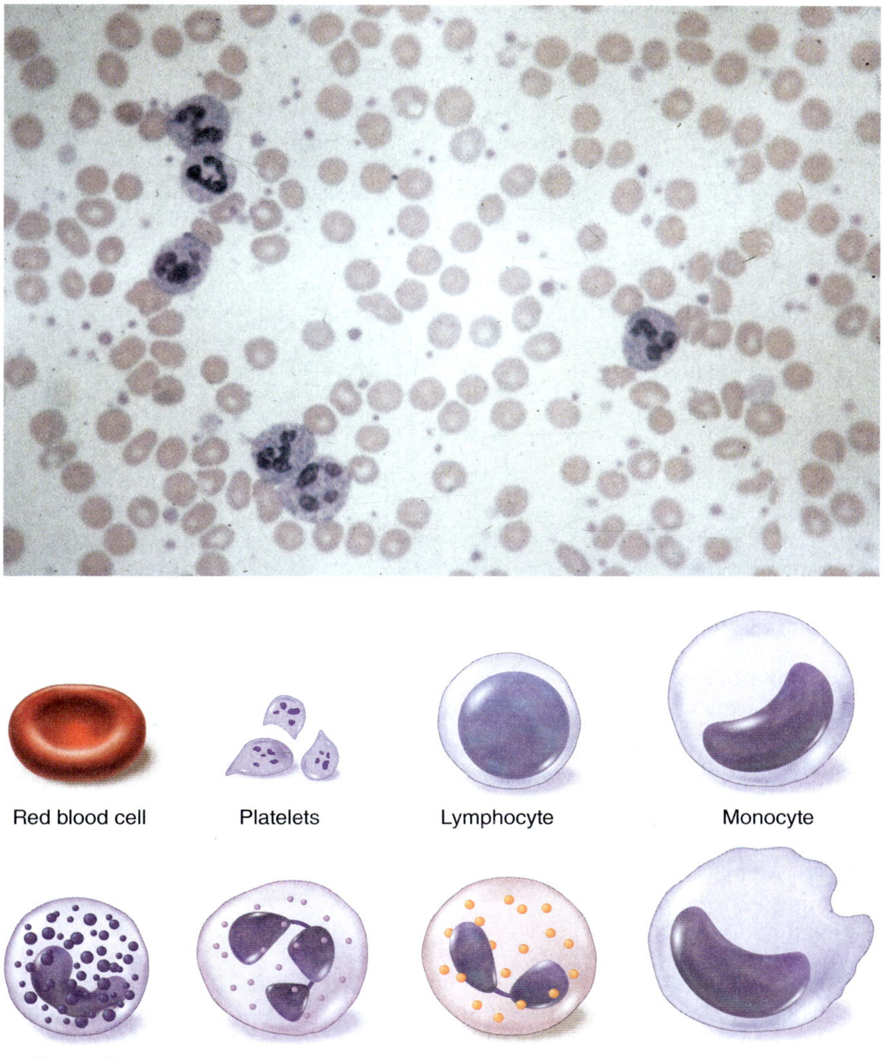

Figure 12-1 **(A)** Stained blood film. Red cells appear as biconcave disks. Several neutrophils can be identified (*dark staining cells with multilobed nuclei*). Small dark structures are platelets. **(B)** Identifying cells on a stained laboratory blood smear can be difficult. These sketches illustrate the general characteristics that help differentiate the cell types.

(A) Courtesy of Leonard V. Crowley, MD, Century College; **(B)** © Dee-sign/Shutterstock

division. Lack of these cells results in bone marrow failure and decreased levels of all circulating blood cells (pancytopenia). Important materials for erythropoiesis (RBC production) (**Figure 12-2**) include vitamin B_1 and folic acid, required for DNA synthesis in the dividing and maturing red cell precursors, and iron, required for the synthesis of the heme portion of hemoglobin. Extreme protein deficiency can result in decreased levels of blood cell production.

Red cells develop from large precursor cells in the bone marrow that are termed proerythroblasts (pro = before + erythro = red + blast = a primitive cell). As the red cell precursors mature, the cells go through different stages during which the nucleus shrinks and increasing amounts of hemoglobin are synthesized. Finally, when about 80 percent of the hemoglobin has been synthesized, the immature red cells lose their nucleus but retain their ability to produce proteins in the cytoplasm. At this stage, the reticulocytes leave the marrow and travel into the circulation. Reticulocytes may sometimes be detectable

Table 12-1 Summary of Blood Cells

Name	Light Micrograph	Description	Concentration (Number of cells/mm³)	Life Span	Function
Red blood cells (RBCs)	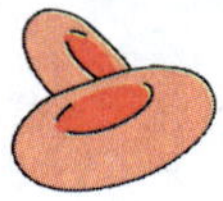	Biconcave disk; no nucleus	4 million to 6 million	120 days	Transports oxygen and carbon dioxide
White blood cells (WBCs) Neutrophil	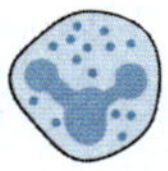	Approximately twice the size of RBCs; multilobed nucleus; clear-staining cytoplasm	3,000 to 7,000	6 hours to a few days	Phagocytizes bacteria
Eosinophil	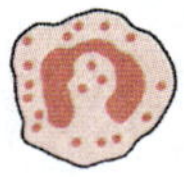	Approximately the same size as a neutrophil; large pink-staining granules; bilobed nucleus	100 to 400	8 to 12 days	Phagocytizes antigen–antibody complex; attacks parasites
Basophil	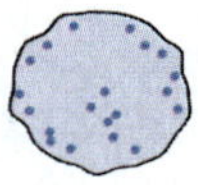	Slightly smaller than a neutrophil; contains large, purple cytoplasmic granules; bilobed nucleus	20 to 50	Few hours to a few days	Releases histamine during inflammation
Monocyte	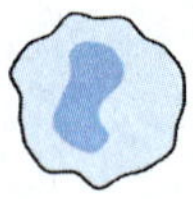	Larger than neutrophil; cytoplasm grayish-blue; no cytoplasmic granules; U- or kidney-shaped nucleus	100 to 700	Lasts many months	Phagocytizes bacteria, dead cells, and cellular debris
Lymphocyte	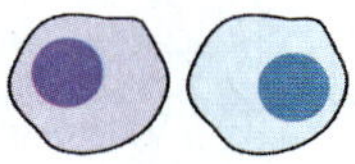	Slightly smaller than neutrophil; large, relatively round nucleus that fills the cell	1,500 to 3,000	Can persist many years	Involved in immune protection, either attacking cells directly or producing antibodies
Platelets	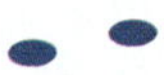	Fragments of megakaryocytes; appear as small dark-staining granules	250,000	5 to 10 days	Play several key roles in blood clotting

in circulation and are distinguished using special stains that detect residual RNA and DNA. They appear slightly larger and more blue than a mature red cell. A high reticulocyte count is an indicator that the bone marrow is being strongly stimulated to produce red cells. This situation may occur in cases of extreme blood loss. Normally reticulocytes rapidly complete differentiation into erythrocytes, losing their ability to synthesize proteins.

Erythrocyte production is regulated by the oxygen content of arterial blood. A decreased oxygen supply to the tissues stimulates the kidney to secrete the hormone erythropoietin. Erythropoietin stimulates the bone marrow precursor cells to increase production of erythrocytes. Kidney disease may result in a low level of red cells being synthesized and reduced RBC levels in the blood, anemia.

Because the RBC lacks a nucleus, it cannot synthesize new enzyme molecules to replace those that gradually wear out. After about 4 months (120 days), the cell is no longer able to function. The worn-out red cell is removed by the

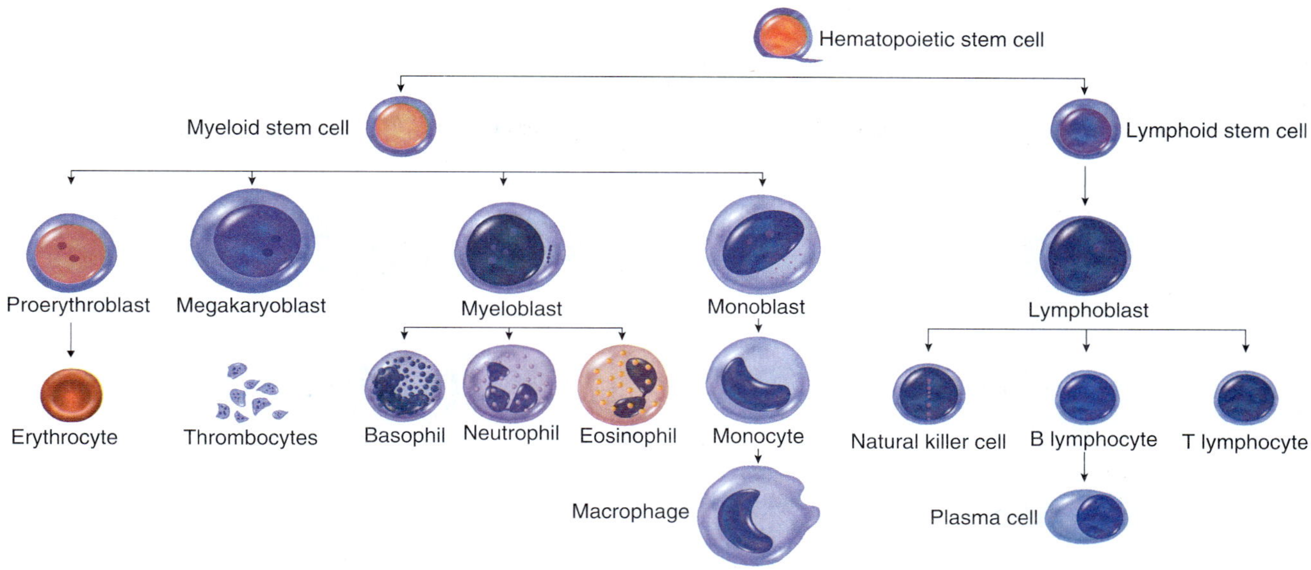

Figure 12-2 All blood cells arise in the bone marrow from pluripotent hematopoietic stem cells. As the precursor cells differentiate further, the progenitor cells become multipotent and more specialized, finally differentiating into the blood cells, which will eventually circulate.

mononuclear phagocyte system, primarily in the spleen, and its hemoglobin degraded. The globin chains are broken down, and their component amino acids recycled to make other proteins. The iron is extracted and saved to make new hemoglobin. The porphyrin ring, however, cannot be salvaged. It is degraded, and the breakdown products are excreted by the liver as bile pigment.

The factors regulating the production of white blood cells and their delivery into the circulation are complex. Inflammation and physiologic processes such as exercise and stress can increase the number of white cells in the blood. The mechanism may involve either increased marrow synthesis or the release of preformed pools of cells stored in the marrow. A number of protein cytokines and growth factors are responsible for regulating these processes.

Structure and Function of Hemoglobin

Hemoglobin, the oxygen-carrying protein formed by the developing red cells, is composed of four separate protein subunits termed globins, which in turn fit together to form a four-chain molecule called a tetramer (tetra = four). Each subunit consists of two parts: the globin chain and a heme group. Heme is a complex nitrogen-containing ring structure (called a porphyrin ring) containing an iron atom. The heme and globin components that make up normal hemoglobin are synthesized separately within the erythroblast. The steps in porphyrin ring synthesis occur both in the cytoplasm and mitochondria. Iron is brought to the cell by an iron transport protein, transferrin, which binds to transferrin receptors on the cell surface. The receptor transferrin complex is internalized, the iron released, and inserted into the porphyrin molecule (**Figure 12-3**).

Several types of globin chains, differing in their amino acid composition, can contribute to the hemoglobin molecule. Different types of hemoglobin with different proportions are synthesized depending on developmental stage. The different globin chains are designated by lower case Greek letters—alpha (α), beta (β), gamma (γ), delta (δ), epsilon (ε), and zeta (ζ). Hemoglobin contains

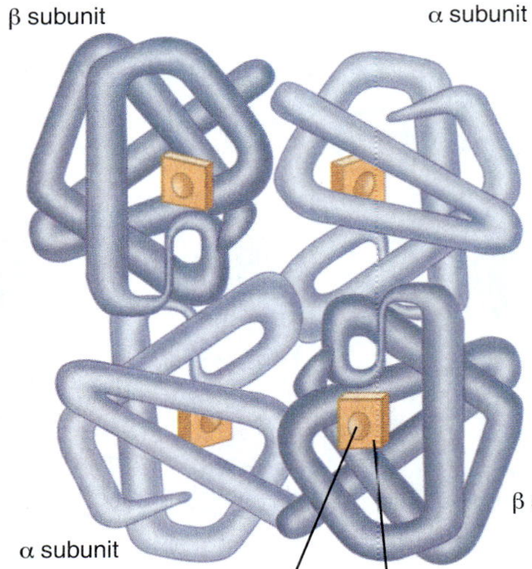

Figure 12-3 The hemoglobin molecule. The heme groups containing the porphyrin ring are shown as squares.

four globin chains creating a tetramer made of two different globin pairs. For example, in the normal adult, about 98 percent of hemoglobin is called hemoglobin A, consisting of two alpha chains and two beta chains. This hemoglobin can also be designated by the shorthand notation $\alpha_2\beta_2$. The remaining 2 percent is called hemoglobin A_2, a tetramer composed of two alpha and two delta chains ($\alpha_2\delta_2$), where the delta chains substitute for beta chains. Embryonic red cells are produced in the fetal yolk sac. This type of hemoglobin uses alpha-like zeta chains (ζ) and beta-like epsilon chains (ε). During fetal development, red cell synthesis shifts to the liver. Zeta and epsilon chain synthesis slows, and alpha chain (α) and gamma chain (γ) synthesis increases to form HbF, fetal hemoglobin (or hemoglobin F). Fetal hemoglobin absorbs and releases oxygen more efficiently than adult hemoglobin when oxygen partial pressure is lower, which is to be expected in the fetal environment. Late in pregnancy, fetal production of beta chains replaces gamma chains, and adult hemoglobin (HbA) begins to replace fetal hemoglobin in the red cells.

The hemoglobin of a newborn infant contains 50 to 95 percent fetal hemoglobin, the rest being the adult type. Normally, no significant fetal hemoglobin synthesis occurs after birth. As new red cells are produced by the infant, the new "replacement" red cells contain essentially only hemoglobin A. Consequently, the concentration of hemoglobin A rises in the infant's blood as hemoglobin F falls. By about 6 months of age, the hemoglobin is almost entirely hemoglobin A.

Oxygen Transport by Hemoglobin

The heme group gives hemoglobin the ability to reversibly combine with oxygen. For hemoglobin to transport and release oxygen effectively, the iron must be in the ferrous (Fe^{2+}) state, and its binding site must be available to pick up and release oxygen. In the lungs, where the oxygen partial pressure is high, hemoglobin combines with oxygen to form oxyhemoglobin. In the tissues, where oxygen partial pressure is much lower, the oxygen leaves the heme group and diffuses into the surrounding tissue fluid. Two important conditions impair the ability of hemoglobin to transport oxygen: (1) oxidation of the iron to form a different type of hemoglobin called methemoglobin, and (2) attachment of carbon monoxide to the heme iron to form carboxyhemoglobin.

Iron Metabolism and Hematopoiesis

The body contains about 4 g of iron, 75 percent of which is contained in hemoglobin. Most of the rest is held as a reserve supply stored in the liver, bone marrow, and spleen. In storage it combines with an iron-binding protein, apoferritin, forming an iron–protein complex, ferritin. A small amount of iron also circulates in the blood bound to a protein called transferrin. Iron transport around the body occurs with iron bound to transferrin.

The average daily iron intake from foods is 10–20 mg, but men absorb about 1 mg of iron per day, and women and children absorb slightly more. Rates of iron deficiency vary by race and other sociodemographic factors. Six percent of White and Black toddlers and 12% of Hispanic toddlers aged 1 to 3 years in the United States are iron-deficient. Deficiency most often occurs in children and adolescents in food-insecure households. Iron deficiency anemia may initially not be noticed but with time can lead to fatigue, headaches, irritability, pica (a craving for non-food substances), and a variety of other symptoms. Additional iron is also required during pregnancy to supply the needs of the developing fetus. Children require greater amounts of iron to synthesize more hemoglobin during periods of rapid growth when the blood volume is increasing. During pregnancy and in children, iron deficiency anemia can result in problems with brain development and long-term neurological and developmental consequences.

Because there is no mechanism for iron elimination other than blood loss during menstruation in women, and excessive iron is toxic; iron uptake, which occurs predominantly via the mucosal cells in the duodenum, is carefully regulated. Hepcidin is a protein synthesized by the liver that blocks dietary iron uptake by the duodenal cells and interferes with the transport of iron to developing erythrocytes. In the case of sufficient iron stores, hepcidin levels are increased. Synthesis of hepcidin is decreased when iron stores are low. From the duodenal mucosa, the iron is transported by transferring to the bone marrow for hemoglobin synthesis and to the liver and other storage sites where it is available for later use. **Figure 12-4** summarizes how iron is handled in the body.

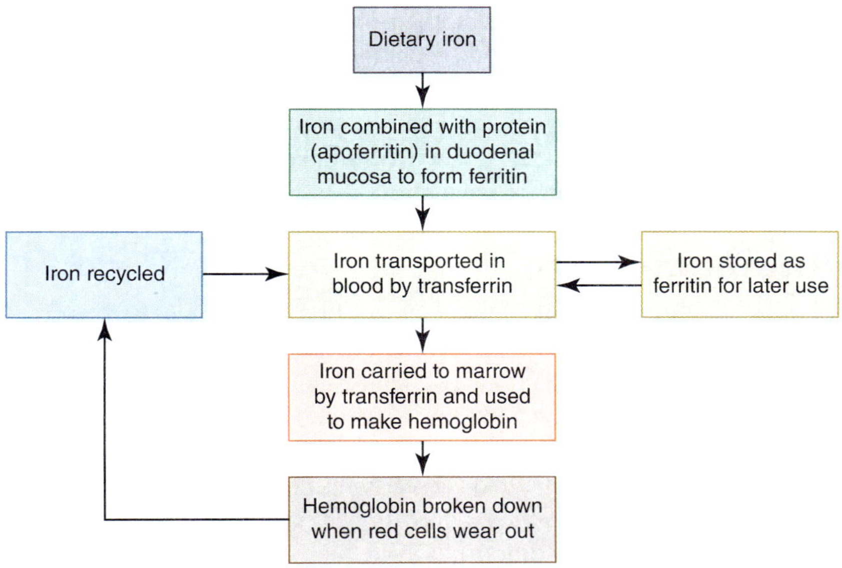

Figure 12-4 Iron uptake, transport, storage, and utilization for hemoglobin synthesis. Most of the iron used for hemoglobin synthesis is recycled from worn-out red cells. Chronic blood loss removes iron-containing cells from the circulation, and the iron contained in the red cells can no longer be recycled to make hemoglobin, which leads to iron deficiency anemia.

As red cells wear out and are destroyed, the iron from the hemoglobin is recycled through transportation by transferrin back to the bone marrow, where it is reused to make new hemoglobin. If sufficient recycled iron is not available for hemoglobin synthesis, additional iron is mobilized from storage sites.

Iron Overload: Hemochromatosis

The human body contains no iron excretory pathways. Consequently, any excess iron entering the body cannot be eliminated, creating an overload of iron, which accumulates in the body's tissues and organs. Eventually, the accumulation leads to organ damage, followed by scarring, leading to permanent derangement in the functions of the affected organs.

The usual cause of iron overload stems from a genetic disease, hemochromatosis, which is transmitted as an autosomal recessive trait. The disease may result from mutations in several genes controlling iron metabolism, but classic type 1 hemochromatosis is by far the most common. It results from mutations in a gene called HFE (which stands for high Fe, or high iron). The mutated HEF gene occurs in about 10 percent of the White population. Manifestations of the disease take years to develop as iron accumulates in the body and causes organ damage. Patients with untreated hemochromatosis often have characteristic manifestations of iron accumulation: tan to brown skin tone caused by iron accumulation in the skin; diabetes caused by damage to the insulin-producing cells of the pancreas; diffuse scarring of the liver (cirrhosis), which interferes with blood flow through the liver (discussed in Chapter 19); and heart failure caused by heart muscle damage and associated scarring resulting from the iron deposits.

Early recognition and treatment prevent progression of the disease and arrest organ damage. Treatment consists of repeated withdrawal of blood (phlebotomy) to remove iron, often combined with drugs that bind (chelate) iron to remove it from the body.

The excessive iron absorption and storage characteristic of hemochromatosis can be identified by the same type of laboratory tests used to measure iron storage and transport in subjects with iron deficiency anemia: serum ferritin, serum iron, and serum iron–binding capacity. When the body is overloaded with iron, serum ferritin is very high, reflecting the greatly increased iron stores that can be as much as 15 to 20 g or more instead of the normal amount of about 1 g. Serum iron is also much higher than normal, and the iron-binding protein transferrin is completely loaded (saturated) with iron. These tests all point to increased uptake and storage of iron.

Methemoglobin

If the iron in the heme of hemoglobin oxidizes from the normal ferrous (Fe^{2+}) to the ferric (Fe^{3+}), the hemoglobin is converted to methemoglobin and is no longer able to carry oxygen. A small amount of hemoglobin is oxidized to methemoglobin continuously, but the concentration is less than 1 percent of the total hemoglobin. Red blood cells have an enzyme (methemoglobin reductase) that converts methemoglobin back to normal oxygen-carrying hemoglobin which keeps methemoglobin levels low. Methemoglobin cannot transport oxygen; consequently, methemoglobinemia, the condition in which high levels of methemoglobin are produced, presents with symptoms related to **ischemia**. Methemoglobin appears as a dark red-brown "chocolate" color. A 15 to 20 percent concentration in the blood changes the color of the skin. Higher levels will result in headache, confusion, delirium, cardiovascular symptoms, and ultimately (at levels above 70 percent) death. Methemoglobinemia can be caused by hereditary diseases that result

Ischemia Poor blood supply to cells of tissues that may lead to injury or death.

in a type of hemoglobin (hemoglobin M) particularly susceptible to the formation of methemoglobin or to defects in the methemoglobin reductase enzyme. Unfortunately, many different drugs and chemicals can oxidize hemoglobin to methemoglobin. The list includes nitrates and nitrites, some frequently used local anesthetics, such as benzocaine, contained in topical anesthetics, and several nonprescription drugs. The preferred treatment of severe methemoglobinemia involves intravenous administration of the compound methylene blue. The methylene blue increases the activity of the RBC methemoglobin reductase enzyme, speeding the conversion of methemoglobin (Fe^{3+}) back to normal hemoglobin (Fe^{2+}).

Carboxyhemoglobin

Outside of the body, in the presence of adequate oxygen, combustion converts carbon-containing compounds to carbon dioxide and water. However, incomplete combustion from inadequate oxygen levels during burning forms carbon monoxide. When carbon monoxide enters the blood, it binds hemoglobin with a 200–300 times greater affinity than oxygen. Consequently, carbon monoxide combines preferentially with hemoglobin to form carboxyhemoglobin. Carboxyhemoglobin remains in the blood since carbon monoxide dissociates very slowly from hemoglobin. Carboxyhemoglobin cannot transport oxygen. Hence, exposure to even a low concentration of carbon monoxide for a long time is harmful. As progressively larger quantities of hemoglobin are converted to carboxyhemoglobin, the levels of oxygen available to the tissues continue to decrease, and death may result. If a person exposed to a sublethal concentration of carbon monoxide is removed from the source of the exposure, the carbon monoxide dissociates slowly from its combination with hemoglobin, and the oxygen-carrying capacity of the blood slowly returns to normal.

Manifestations of carbon monoxide exposure depend upon the concentration to which the person has been exposed. A concentration of 3 percent or higher in a nonsmoker, and 10 percent or more in smokers indicates significant exposure. Smokers become exposed to carbon monoxide in cigarette smoke, so many already demonstrate the presence of carboxyhemoglobin on an everyday basis. A high concentration of carboxyhemoglobin in the blood may lead to serious long-term cardiovascular and neurologic problems resulting from the exposure and, if exposure is acute and not corrected, death. An affected person should be removed from the source of exposure and given a high concentration of oxygen by mask to help replace the carbon monoxide with oxygen. If necessary, the oxygen may need to be delivered in a hyperbaric chamber at 2–3 atmospheres.

It is easier to prevent carbon monoxide poisoning than to treat it. Many communities now require carbon monoxide detectors in private homes to call attention to any undetected malfunction of the home heating system. Indoor kerosene heaters or poorly vented open fires used as heat sources present a continuing problem, especially in situations where housing is not well regulated. Auto exhaust fumes in nonventilated spaces such as garages with the doors closed also may result in high levels of carbon monoxide exposure. Both types of exposure commonly result in deaths, both accidental and suicidal.

Anemia

Anemia, literally "without blood," refers to a decrease in red blood cell numbers or to subnormal hemoglobin levels in circulating red cells. Anemia is classified either by etiology or by cell morphology, the size and appearance of the red blood cells, as determined by available testing.

Etiologic Classification of Anemia

Anemia can occur due to inadequate production of red cells, excessive RBC loss, or destruction of the cells (**Figure 12-5**). Inadequate production may result from an insufficiency of stem cells. Stem cells containing genetic abnormalities, experiencing damage from bone marrow trauma, or becoming crowded out by other abnormal stem cells could contribute to inadequate production of stem cells. Insufficient levels of factors required for RBC differentiation and development, such as iron and vitamins, can also impede cell maturation. Excessive loss of red cells may be caused either by external or internal blood loss or by accelerated destruction of the cells in the circulation. **Table 12-2** presents a classification of the various causes of anemia.

When describing the appearance of the RBC, anemias may be normocytic, macrocytic, or microcytic, referring to red blood cells that are normal-sized, larger than, or smaller than normally sized cells, respectively. If microcytic cells also contain a reduced hemoglobin content, they appear pale in color in a blood smear, and the term *hypochromic* (reduced color) *microcytic* (small cell) *anemia* applies. The appearance of the cells provides a clue to the etiology. Iron deficiency anemia is a hypochromic microcytic anemia. Anemia caused by vitamin B_1 or folic acid deficiency is a macrocytic anemia. Most other types of anemia are normocytic. Changes in cell shape may also offer clues to the etiology of the anemia.

Iron Deficiency Anemia

Iron deficiency anemia is the most common anemia worldwide. It presents often in children, women of childbearing age, and cases of chronic blood loss. Iron deficiency anemia may result from either insufficient intake of dietary iron,

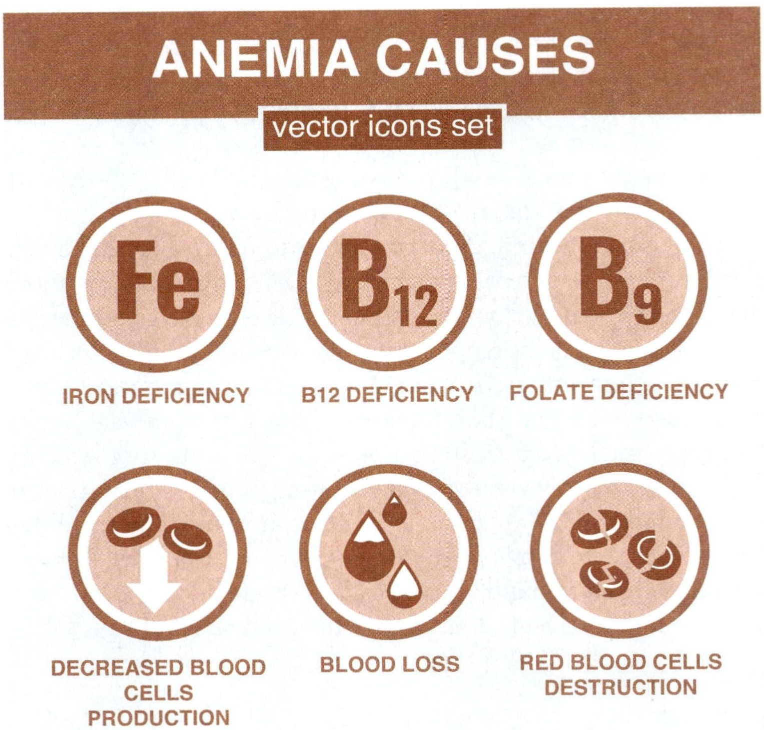

Figure 12-5 The etiology of anemia often involves lack of building materials, improper construction of the red blood cells, or pathological destruction of the red blood cells.

Table 12-2 Etiologic Classification of Anemia

Inadequate Production of Red Cells
Caused by inadequate "raw materials"
Iron deficiency
Vitamin B_{12} deficiency
Folic acid deficiency
Caused by impaired function of the bone marrow factory
Anemia of chronic disease
Bone marrow damaged or destroyed (aplastic anemia)
Bone marrow replaced by foreign or abnormal cells (bone marrow replacement anemia)
Excessive Loss of Red Cells
Caused by external blood loss (hemorrhage)
Caused by shortened survival of red cells in the circulation
Defective red cells (hereditary hemolytic anemia)
Abnormal red cell shape
Abnormal hemoglobin within red cells
Defective hemoglobin synthesis within red cells
Deficient red cell enzymes
"Hostile environment"
Anti-red cell antibodies
Mechanical trauma to circulating red cells

failure to absorb iron from the diet, **hemorrhage**, or chronic blood loss sometimes associated with undiagnosed gastrointestinal cancer (**Figure 12-6**).

Hemorrhage Release of blood into surrounding tissue.

Iron deficiency caused by inadequate dietary intake may occur in infants during periods of rapid growth. A normal, full-term infant possesses a reserve supply of iron that was transferred to the fetus during the last part of pregnancy. Consequently, the newborn infant generally has an adequate short-term supply of iron available during the neonatal period when the production of red blood cells accelerates to supply the needs of an increasing blood volume generated by the rapid growth of the neonate. A premature infant, however, may not obtain its full component of iron stores, and consequently, the reserve supply may be inadequate. Even in full-term infants, the reserve supply of iron is limited and must be supplemented. Breast milk contains very little iron, although the amount available is usually well absorbed. Breast-fed neonates may be placed on supplemental iron drops. Once the infant diet progresses toward weaning, cereals, fruits, vegetables, and other foods containing iron will add to increasing the iron stores. For this reason, many health care providers gradually add supplementary foods containing additional sources of iron to infants' diets. Rapidly growing adolescents and pregnant or lactating people also require increased iron. Individuals facing food insecurity or those living with an inadequate or poorly balanced diet may develop iron deficiency anemia as well.

Approximately 25 percent of people worldwide have anemia. Iron deficiency, the most common cause, is responsible for 50 percent of all anemias. The prevalence of iron deficiency anemia in the United States is lower than in most developing countries. However, it still affects approximately 10% of women of childbearing age and about 9% of children. Since each milliliter of blood contains 0.5 mg of iron, a loss of 500 ml of blood represents a loss of 250 mg of iron, equivalent to one-fourth of the body's entire iron reserves. Acute blood loss as well as chronic blood loss also contribute to iron deficiency anemia. Unless dietary intake of iron is extremely liberal, iron stores soon become exhausted and iron deficiency anemia develops.

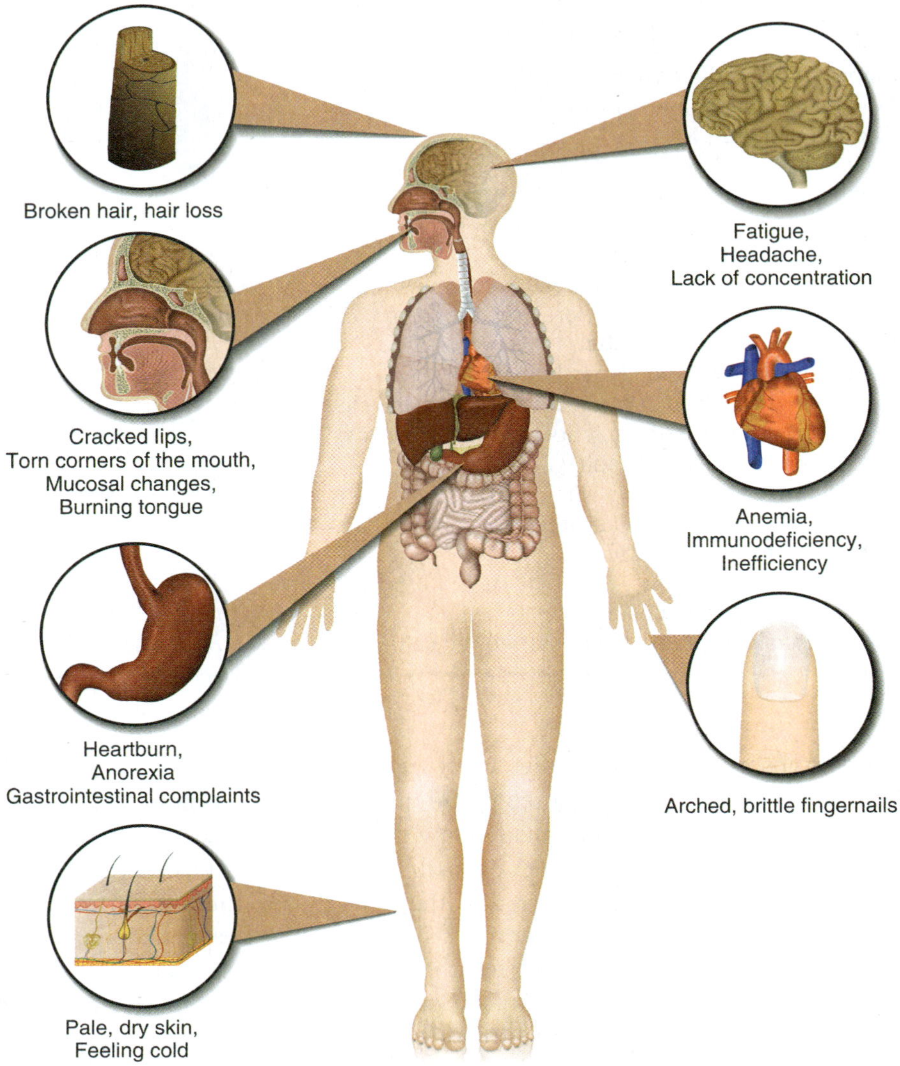

Figure 12-6 Anything that affects the blood will affect other parts of the body. An, example is iron deficiency, which can manifest in various ways.

Iron deficiency anemia is a hypochromic microcytic anemia (**Figure 12-7**). The cells appear pale because they contain less hemoglobin than normal. Their size is reduced as well.

Laboratory Tests to Evaluate Iron Metabolism in Iron Deficiency Anemia

Laboratory tests that measure iron stores, iron transport, and iron metabolism can be used as diagnostic tests in patients with suspected iron deficiency anemia. These include measurements of serum ferritin, serum iron, and total serum iron-binding capacity.

A very small amount of ferritin (about 100 µg per liter) is normally present in blood serum. The serum level is often proportional to the total ferritin stored in the body. Consequently, measurement of serum ferritin can be used to estimate total body iron stores. In iron deficiency anemia, body iron stores become depleted, resulting in low serum ferritin levels. However, the total iron-binding capacity in the serum is much higher than normal. Consequently, the characteristic laboratory profile of iron deficiency anemia is low serum ferritin and

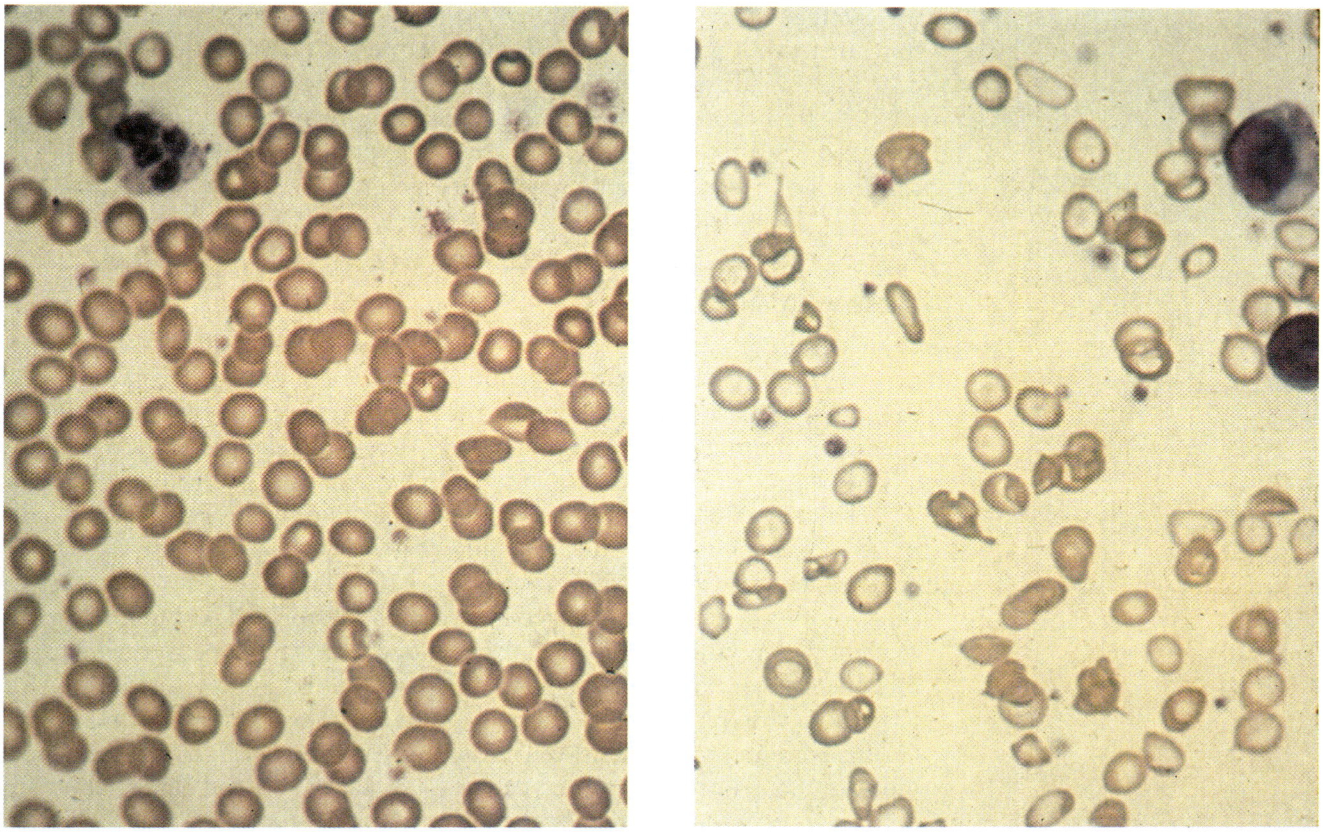

(A) (B)

Figure 12-7 **(A)** Normal red cells. **(B)** Cells showing hypochromic microcytic anemia caused by chronic iron deficiency (original magnification ×400).

Courtesy of Leonard V. Crowley, MD, Century College.

serum iron. The serum will demonstrate a much higher than normal serum iron-binding capacity, and the transferrin measurement will demonstrate a much lower than normal percentage of iron saturation level.

Evaluation and Treatment of Iron Deficiency Anemia

To treat a patient with iron deficiency anemia, the etiology of the anemia must be determined, with the goal of therapy directed toward alleviating the cause rather than the symptoms. In someone with a history of a very poor diet, the cause may be obvious. If an adult experiences anemia as a result of cryptic blood loss, the source of the bleeding must be found. For example, blood loss may be caused by a bleeding ulcer or an ulcerated carcinoma of the colon. In women, excessive menstrual bleeding can lead to iron deficiency anemia. When the cause of the blood loss has been determined, proper treatment of the underlying cause can be instituted. In addition, the patient will probably be given supplementary iron to replenish the body's depleted iron stores.

Anemia of Chronic Disease

People who endure chronic diseases, depending upon the nature of the disease, may experience hypochromic microcytic anemia. Chronic inflammatory conditions such as an ongoing infection, certain immune diseases, and malignant neoplasms, which result in increased RBC destruction or poor iron absorption and transport, put people at an increased level of risk.

Stimulated by the inflammatory cytokine IL-6, hepcidin levels become upregulated. As previously noted, increased levels of hepcidin correlate with decreased circulatory levels of iron.

This IL-6–hepcidin interaction is believed to be part of the innate immune response (Chapter 5) and may add additional protection from pathogens such as species of malaria and streptococcus, which require iron for infectivity.

Suppression of Bone Marrow Stem Cell Function/ Aplastic Anemia

Many conditions can depress bone marrow function, including chronic infection or suppression of marrow stem cells. As noted previously, chronic diseases may impair erythropoiesis and lead to mild or moderate anemia (the anemia of chronic disease). White blood cell and platelet production are usually not disturbed.

The anemia of chronic disease usually causes only a relatively mild suppression of bone marrow function and improves when the underlying disease is identified and treated. Unfortunately, destruction of the bone marrow stem cells or other irreversible damage to the bone marrow leads to poor or nonexistent erythropoiesis and overall hematopoiesis. This type of anemia falls into the category of aplastic anemia (a = without + plasia = growth). This term is not strictly accurate because the stem cell damage may lead to leukopenia and thrombocytopenia as well as anemia. This anemia is classified as a normocytic anemia because the red cells are normal in size and shape, although inadequate in number. Many agents can induce aplastic anemia. Radiation, anticancer chemotherapy drugs, and various toxic chemicals (benzene being a prime example) may cause severe marrow damage. Other drugs, including some antibiotics, anti-inflammatory drugs, and anticonvulsant drugs, may damage marrow stem cells in susceptible individuals. In many cases, however, aplastic anemia becomes a manifestation of an autoimmune response in which the body's own cytotoxic T cells attack and destroy the marrow stem cells. A type of viral disease (parvovirus B19 infection, responsible for fifth disease in children) can rarely result in pure red cell aplasia in individuals with underlying hematologic disease.

Aplastic anemia is treated initially by blood and platelet transfusions to maintain an adequate volume of circulating blood cells while diagnosing the cause of the bone marrow failure. If the marrow damage resulted from a toxic drug or chemical and is not too severe, marrow function may recover. However, in severe aplastic anemia, other methods of treatment need to be undertaken to restore marrow function. Many patients respond to immunosuppressive agents that act against the destructive (cytotoxic) T lymphocytes responsible for stem cell destruction. Hematopoietic stem cell transplantation using bone marrow, cord blood, or stem cells isolated from the circulation may be required.

Vitamin B_{12} and Folic Acid Deficiency Anemias

DNA synthesis requires vitamins B_{12} and B_9. "Folate" refers to naturally occurring vitamin B_9, while "folic acid" refers to the man-made version. In the absence of either vitamin, DNA synthesis is impaired, and the developing red blood cells in the bone marrow exhibit characteristic disturbances of cell maturation. Impaired DNA synthesis delays nuclear development while allowing for normal cytoplasmic development. Therefore, abnormally large cells develop that do not survive normally in the circulation. These immature, large-developing red blood cells, megaloblasts, are the hallmark of megaloblastic erythropoiesis. The mature red cells derived from the abnormal maturation are larger than normal, vary in size, and some may have an oval shape. When classified morphologically, this anemia is referred to as macrocytic anemia. The development of white cell precursors and megakaryocytes is also abnormal. Consequently, patients with megaloblastic anemia usually also have leukopenia (low white cell count) and **thrombocytopenia** (low platelet count) as well as macrocytic anemia. Vitamin B_{12} is found in meat, milk, liver, and other foods rich in animal protein, but not in vegetable products. Strict vegetarians who do not eat meat or dairy products must rely on vitamin B_{12}-fortified cereals or other nonprotein vitamin B_{12}-fortified foods as their source of the vitamin. However, normal body stores of vitamin B_{12} take years to be depleted. A person who suddenly converts to a vegan diet will not develop vitamin B_{12} deficiency rapidly (if at all). Folic acid is widely distributed in nature, being found in abundance in green leafy vegetables as well as in many foods of animal origin. Both are tied to neurological function. Folic acid deficiency before and during pregnancy can lead to the development of neural tube defects (Chapter 16).

Thrombocytopenia
A deficiency of platelets.

Anemia as a Result of Folic Acid Deficiency

The body stores limited amounts of folic acid, which will rapidly become depleted if not replenished continually. Since 1998, the United States implemented mandatory folic acid supplementation for all foodstuffs containing wheat flour. People who exist on food sources that may not be supplemented can be expected to have a higher level of folic acid deficiency and the concomitant anemia. This cohort would include those with gluten intolerance who avoid wheat-based products, cultures where the major grain flour is cornmeal, and those with food insufficiency. Those who have impaired folic acid absorption would be at risk as well. People with chronic physical and mental conditions that either limit their diet or result in deficient diets are also at risk for folic acid insufficiency. Pregnant and lactating people also are at risk because pregnancy greatly increases folic acid requirements. Folic acid deficiency anemia in pregnancy can be avoided with the use of prenatal vitamins since most prenatal vitamins contain higher levels of folic acid. Several drugs, including methotrexate (an antimetabolite used in the treatment of cancer and rheumatoid arthritis) and the antiepileptic agent phenytoin, can interfere with the action of folic acid.

Anemia as a Result of Vitamin B_{12} Deficiency/Pernicious Anemia

Efficient absorption of vitamin B_{12} ingested in food requires a protein called intrinsic factor, secreted by gastric mucosal cells. After the intrinsic factor combines with the vitamin B_{12}, the B_{12}–intrinsic factor complex is absorbed from the distal small intestine. The absorbed vitamin is stored in the liver and made available to the bone marrow and other tissues as required for cell growth and maturation. A common cause of vitamin B_{12} deficiency, pernicious anemia, involves atrophy of the gastric mucosa. This autoimmune condition results in antibodies directed against gastric mucosal cells and intrinsic factor. Atrophic gastric mucosa fails to secrete intrinsic factor, acid, and needed digestive enzymes, so consequently, vitamin B_{12} is not absorbed. The vitamin B_{12} deficiency causes impaired erythropoiesis as well as various neurologic disturbances. Due to the impaired erythropoiesis, vitamin B_{12} deficiency anemia results.

Pernicious anemia is not the only cause of vitamin B_{12} deficiency. People who have large gastric resections or a gastric bypass procedure to control obesity may not be able to secrete enough intrinsic factor or absorb enough vitamin B_{12}–intrinsic factor complexes sufficient to supply their needs. Similarly, an individual with chronic intestinal disease affecting the vitamin B_{12}–absorbing area (such as Crohn's disease) may also be unable to absorb the vitamin adequately.

Pernicious anemia and other vitamin B_{12} deficiency anemias must be treated with intramuscular administration of vitamin B_{12}. Parenteral administration avoids the problem of poor absorption of the vitamin.

Acute Blood Loss

Normocytic anemia may result from an episode of acute blood loss, as from a massive hemorrhage. Provided that iron stores are adequate, the lost blood is rapidly replaced by the stem cells in the bone marrow, and the newly formed red cells are normal. This is in contrast with the anemia of chronic blood loss, in which the red cells are hypochromic and microcytic because prolonged bleeding has depleted the body's iron stores.

Accelerated Blood Destruction

Normal red cells survive for about 120 days, but their survival can be considerably shortened by various diseases and conditions. If the regenerative capacity of the marrow is not sufficient to keep up with the accelerated destruction, anemia results. The resulting anemia is called hemolytic anemia. It may be a result of either an intrinsic defect in red blood cells or an extrinsic condition that shortens the circulating life of cells. Hemolytic anemias caused by an inherited genetic defect in red cell structure are referred to as hereditary hemolytic anemias. Those resulting from damage to normal red cells by antibodies or other injurious agents are called acquired hemolytic anemias.

Hereditary Hemolytic Anemias

The genetically determined abnormalities of red cells that may shorten their survival fall into four major groups: abnormally shaped cells, abnormal hemoglobins, defective hemoglobin synthesis, or enzyme deficiencies (**Table 12-3**).

Shape Abnormalities. The most common genetic hemolytic anemia in Caucasians is hereditary spherocytosis with two distinct genetic forms (dominant and recessive), the dominant form being most common. The disease is

Table 12-3 Inheritance and Manifestations of Some Hereditary Hemolytic Anemias

Anemia	Inheritance	Characteristics of Red Cells	Manifestations
Hereditary spherocytosis	Dominant or recessive	Spherocytic	Mild-to-moderate chronic hemolytic anemia Rarely life-threatening (every form)
Hereditary ovalocytosis (elliptocytosis)	Dominant	Oval	Usually asymptomatic; may have mild anemia
Sickle cell anemia	Recessive (see the following discussion) (abnormal hemoglobins/ sickle cell disease)	Normocytic; cells sickle under reduced oxygen tension	Marked anemia
Hemoglobin C disease	Recessive	Normocytic	Mild-to-moderate anemia

Anemia	Inheritance	Characteristics of Red Cells	Manifestations
Sickle cell hemoglobin C disease	Codominant	Normocytic; cells sickle under reduced oxygen tension	Moderate anemia
β thalassemia minor	Recessive (carrier) (heterozygous)	Hypochromic microcytic; total number of red cells usually increased	Mild anemia
β thalassemia major	Recessive (homozygous)	Hypochromic microcytic	Severe anemia; usually fatal in childhood
α thalassemia	Complex genetics	Microcytic	Mild to lethal in utero
Glucose-6-phosphate dehydrogenase deficiency	X-linked recessive	Normocytic; enzyme-deficient cells	Episodes of acute hemolytic anemia precipitated by drugs or infections

most frequently found in people with Northern European and North American ancestry but can be found in people with various ethnic backgrounds or mixed ancestry. Hereditary deficiency of RBC membrane proteins (mostly spectrin) results in defective linkage of the RBC inner membrane cytoskeleton to its outer lipid bilayer. Consequently, the membrane loses stability with progressive loss of the lipid bilayer. New red cells produced by the bone marrow and released into the circulation exhibit a normal biconcave disk configuration, but as bits of their unstable cell membranes become detached from the cell lipid bilayer, the surface area of the red cell membrane is progressively reduced. The red blood cell membrane morphs into a spherical shape, accommodating their reduced surface area relative to their cell volume (**Figure 12-8**). This change in the surface area/volume ratio alters the physiological properties

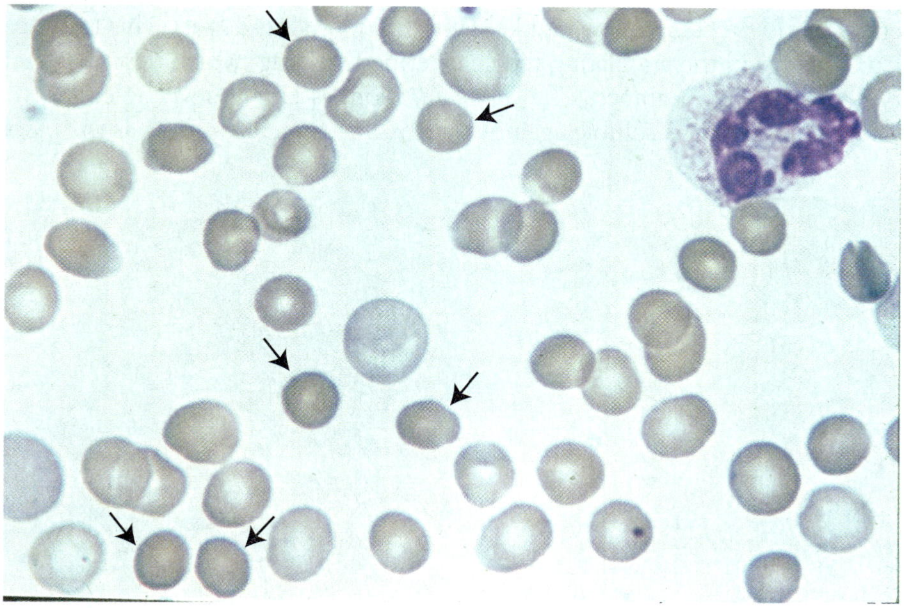

Figure 12-8 A stained blood film from a person with hereditary spherocytosis. The many small dark cells with little or no central pallor are spherocytes (*arrows*). The larger, more normal-appearing red cells are young red cells that have the same cell membrane defect but have not been circulating long enough to acquire a spherical shape. The relatively large, faintly blue-staining red cell in the center of the field is a reticulocyte.

of the cells. As blood flows through the spleen, normal, flexible disk-shaped red cells can progress through the splenic pulp and into the thin-walled veins (sinusoids) that carry the blood out of the spleen. Spherocytes are not thin enough or flexible enough to get through the spleen. They become trapped in the spleen and destroyed by the phagocytic cells in the splenic pulp, resulting in a chronic moderate hemolytic anemia. The bone marrow increases red cell production in response to the decreased oxygen-carrying capacity of the blood. Splenectomy cures the anemia by removing the main site of red cell destruction, but it has no effect on the basic red cell defect. Rarely, the anemia may suddenly become worse, necessitating transfusion (aplastic crisis). This is often the result of parvovirus B19 infection.

A somewhat similar condition, which is transmitted as an inherited dominant trait, is called hereditary elliptocytosis. As the name indicates, the red cells are oval rather than round. Most affected individuals are not inconvenienced by the abnormality, but some have a mild hemolytic anemia that can be cured by splenectomy.

Abnormal Hemoglobins/Sickle Cell Disease. If a gene coding for the globin chain of hemoglobin is abnormal, the amino acids forming the globin chains will be altered, leading to the formation of an abnormal hemoglobin. Genes directing the synthesis of the various types of hemoglobin are effectively codominant. However, expression of clinical disease most often appears recessive, in that disease generally does not occur in the heterozygous carrier. Many different abnormal hemoglobins can be identified and characterized by various laboratory tests. Some of the structurally abnormal hemoglobins function normally, but others have unusual properties that impair their function.

Hemoglobin S (sickle hemoglobin) is one of the more important abnormal hemoglobins. Its formation results from a point mutation changing a single amino acid in the beta chain of hemoglobin. When the oxygen tension of the blood falls, as in venous blood, the hemoglobin S molecules aggregate and form rigid fibers, a process somewhat like crystallization (Figure 12-9). This leads to a shape change in the circulating red cells termed sickling, which describes their comma-shaped appearance. The "crystallization" is largely reversible, and the hemoglobin becomes soluble again when the oxygen tension rises as the blood

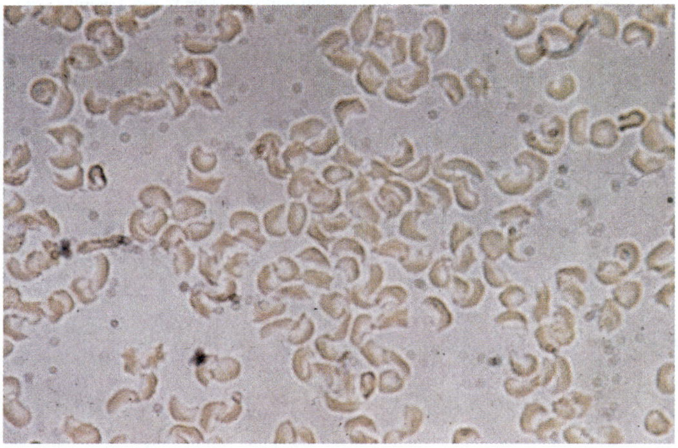

(A)

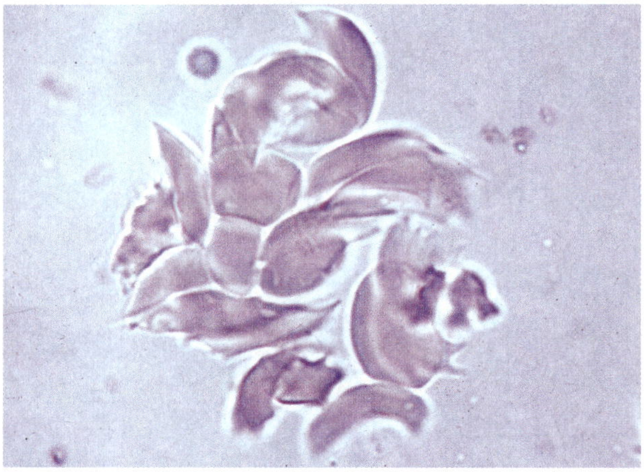

(B)

Figure 12-9 Distortion of red cells containing sickle hemoglobin when incubated under reduced oxygen tension. **(A)** Overview of cells under low magnification (×100). **(B)** Higher magnification view of red cell distortion caused by sickle hemoglobin.

Courtesy of Leonard V. Crowley, MD, Century College.

is oxygenated in the lungs. The hemoglobin S gene is common in parts of the world where the blood parasitic *P. falciparum* malaria is (or was) common. The sickle cell trait affects the parasite's growth and reproduction within red cells. Furthermore, infected red cells are rapidly eliminated from the blood, reducing parasite proliferation. The low oxygen level within red cells from carriers also inhibits parasite growth. Consequently, the parasite doesn't grow well inside the heterozygotes red blood cells, conveying a relative form of resistance to malaria in sickle cell heterozygotes. Homozygotes carrying two hemoglobin S genes experience a range of clinical symptoms, and until the twentieth century, their overall prognosis for attaining adulthood was poor. Geographically the gene can be found in populations originating from sub-Saharan Africa, West Africa, the Middle East, and the Indian subcontinent. In Europe, the gene is found in populations living around the Mediterranean region (**Figure 12-10**). The United States Center for Disease Control and Prevention (CDC) estimates that approximately 100,000 Americans have sickle cell disease (SCD). The CDC also estimates that 1 in 13 babies (about 8%) born to African-American parents possesses sickle cell trait, and 1 in 365 African-Americans babies is born with SCD.

The homozygous state of SCD is a serious disease. The cells of affected individuals contain no hemoglobin A, and they become sickled within the capillaries where the oxygen partial pressure is lower than in arterial blood. The clumps of sickled red cells occlude blood vessels, obstruct blood flow, and cause progressive damage to the heart, kidneys, spleen, and other organs due to impaired circulation. Anemia develops because the cells containing sickle hemoglobin have a shortened survival time in circulation. Consequently, the bone marrow greatly increases its production of red cells (demonstrated by an elevated peripheral blood reticulocyte count) to compensate for the shortened red cell survival.

Newborn infants with sickle cell anemia do not have problems initially because their red cells also contain a large amount of fetal hemoglobin. This fetal hemoglobin "dilutes" the concentration of sickle hemoglobin in the red cells, allowing these cells to function more like the red cells of a person with sickle cell trait. Symptoms usually do not appear until the infant is about 6 months old, when the red cells containing both fetal and sickle hemoglobin have been replaced by red cells containing almost entirely sickle hemoglobin.

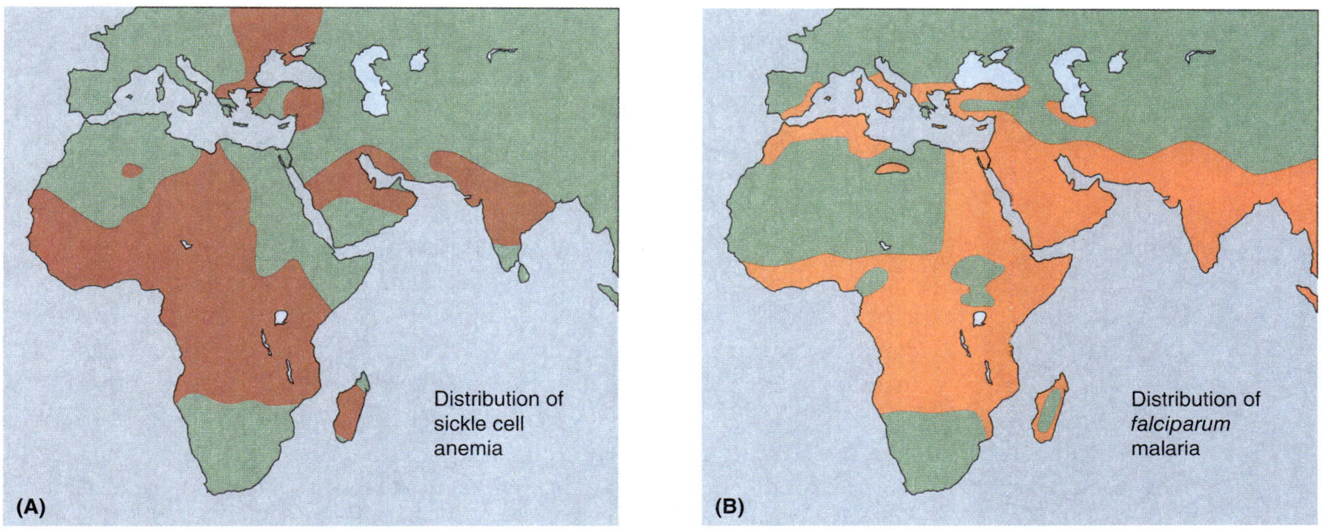

Figure 12-10 **(A)** Geographic distribution of sickle cell anemia. **(B)** *Falciparum* malaria in the 1920s before extensive malaria control programs were launched.

A serious consequence of sickle cell disease is the occurrence of a vaso-occlusive crisis. Such episodes occur periodically in about half of patients and are characterized by severe and debilitating pain that may occur in many different areas, including the bones and abdomen. Vaso-occlusive crises may lead to infarction and damage to many organs, including the liver, kidney, and spleen. Eventually, destruction of the spleen is associated with serious bacterial infections. There are many triggers for such episodes, including low oxygenation of the blood and changes in body core temperature (related to fever or environmental heat or cold). Even outside of crisis, individuals often suffer from chronic bone and joint pain. Anemia is always present but is generally compensated, although individuals may lack stamina. An aplastic crisis may occur following parvovirus B19 infection. Splenic sequestration can result in life-threatening anemia in which the spleen becomes enlarged rapidly and the blood cell count drops rapidly. There are many other serious and potentially life-threatening effects of the disease, including central nervous system involvement and stroke, which may affect as many as 30 percent of children. Currently, individuals with SCD have about a twenty-year reduction in life expectancy to 50–60 years with a much reduced quality of life.

The RBCs of people with the sickle cell trait (heterozygotic for the hemoglobin S gene) typically appear normal at resting conditions. However, under extreme oxidative stress, their RBCs can sickle and undergo polymerization. Over time, some cells will remain in the sickled shape even after they are reoxygenated. Participation in intense physical activity or spending time in low-oxygen environments, such as higher altitudes or those experiencing decreased lung function, can be triggers of a potential sickling crisis. Severe dehydration also may induce or aggravate sickling. Although rare, there is a risk of sudden death if clumps of sickled red cells block coronary arteries. Screening for the sickle cell trait is suggested prior to many high-stress athletic endeavors and other activities. In the United States, the National Collegiate Athletic Association (NCAA) requires athletes from all divisions to be tested for sickle cell trait or provide proof of previous testing. Athletes testing positive are not barred from competition but may be more closely monitored during training and competition. It is important to remember that carriers of the trait do *not* have sickle cell disease and are very unlikely to suffer ill effects from their carrier status. They may, however, transmit the gene to their offspring who, with two carrier parents, have a 25 percent chance of developing sickle cell disease and a 50 percent chance of having sickle cell trait.

Although currently there is no generally accessible cure for sickle cell disease, advances in treatment have improved survival, and many affected persons now live 60 years or greater. SCD disease treatment includes several different types of therapies. Pharmaceutical agents can manage symptoms and control pain. Hydroxyurea can be given to stimulate the bone marrow to produce fetal hemoglobin, which lowers the concentration of sickle hemoglobin in the red cells and thereby reduces the severity of the disease manifestations. Defibrotide, a drug used to treat severe veno-occlusive disease by protecting the liver from damage, can prevent sickle red blood cells from adhesion. Other medicines, including over-the-counter pain meds, can also contribute to improving the patient's daily life. Antibiotics can be prescribed to lower the risks of bacterial infections. Blood transfusions address the complications resulting from anemia. Blood and bone marrow transplants potentially replace the hematopoietic stem cells with donor cells free of the genetic mutation. A major limitation is the availability of suitable donors whose marrow or stem cells will not be rejected. A more exciting approach is to use the patient's own (autologous) stem cells, which have been modified outside the body, to produce normal hemoglobin when reinfused into the patient. Two successful approaches are in advanced trials. One approach (Lyfgenia) adds copies of normal hemoglobin beta genes to the patient's own stem cells to produce non-sickling HbA in the patient. The other approach (Casgevy) also modifies the patient's hemopoietic stem cells but in this case uses gene editing technology to turn off the gene that "tells" the cell to stop making fetal hemoglobin (HbF) after birth. After reinfusion, the patient's modified blood now has high enough levels of HbF to prevent or reduce the effects of SCD. Both techniques have proven successful in eliminating veno-occlusive disease in patients and appear to last at least multiple months. It should be noted that both approaches involve complex and potentially risky treatment, which can only be undertaken in specialized medical centers at very high cost. Hence, currently neither approach is likely to be widely used.

Simple, readily available tests can detect sickle cell trait in affected individuals, and genetic counseling is recommended for couples who are at risk of having a child with sickle cell anemia. DNA analysis of fetal cells can determine whether the fetus carries the sickle cell gene and, if present, whether the fetus is homozygous or heterozygous for the gene. Screening for sickle cell trait is mandatory for newborns in the United States.

Another common abnormal hemoglobin, termed hemoglobin C, is the result of a point mutation different from that of hemoglobin S. Hemoglobin C can also be protective in malaria infection; consequently, it makes sense that this mutation has a high prevalence in Atlantic West Africa and Southeast Asia. Hemoglobin C is also found in a diverse population in Africa, South and Central America, and Southern Europe. Heterozygous individuals, whose cells contain both hemoglobin A and hemoglobin C, are normal clinically. People homozygous for the hemoglobin C gene have a mild hemolytic anemia.

Some people possess genes for two abnormal hemoglobins. This may occur, for example, if one parent carries the hemoglobin S gene and the other carries the hemoglobin C gene, and each parent transmits the abnormal gene. In this case, the red cells of the affected person contain both abnormal hemoglobins in approximately equal amounts, and a hemolytic anemia results.

Defective Hemoglobin Synthesis/Thalassemia. Thalassemia (Mediterranean anemia) constitutes inherited anemias in which reduced amounts of otherwise normal hemoglobin chains are synthesized. Thalassemia reflects a complex group of inherited blood disorders commonly found in people of Italian, Greek, Middle Eastern, Southern Asian, and African descent.

This genetically determined condition is transmitted as a Mendelian-dominant trait, although heterozygous carriers are only mildly affected and may be asymptomatic (hence, some authorities consider the disease to be clinically recessive!). The defective synthesis may be of either the alpha chains (alpha thalassemia) or the beta chains (beta thalassemia). The frequency of the two forms of thalassemia differs greatly in different populations. Beta thalassemia is relatively common in people of Greek and Italian ancestry but is also common in the Middle East and areas of Asia and Africa. The term "thalassemia" comes from the Greek word "thalassa," meaning "sea," and derives from the high incidence of the condition in people who live in regions surrounding the Mediterranean. Alpha thalassemia is considered to be the most common single-gene defect in the world. Either silent carriers or mildly affected individuals are common among individuals of African descent. (There is about a 15 percent rate of silent carriers among American Blacks, although severe disease is rare.) Alpha thalassemia is also common in Southeast Asian (and less frequently in Mediterranean populations) where it occurs in a more severe or even lethal form. Both thalassemias provide some degree of protection from malaria in the heterozygous state, which explains the distribution of the disease (similar to that of sickle cell anemia).

Beta-thalassemia is an inherited disorder resulting from various mutations (over 200 disease-causing mutations have been identified) or, rarely, deletions of the beta-globin gene (HbB) on chromosome 11. These mutations are primarily point mutations that affect transcriptional control, translation, and splicing of the Hb Beta gene and gene product. In beta thalassemia, the production of beta chains is reduced; however, alpha chain production is not, so the synthesis of the two types of chains is unbalanced. An excess of alpha chains accumulates and precipitates within the red cells, shortening their survival. Because hemoglobin synthesis is reduced, the red cells appear hypochromic and microcytic, somewhat like the appearance of the cells in iron deficiency anemia. In thalassemia, however, the hypochromia is the result of deficient hemoglobin production because of inadequate beta chain synthesis rather than deficient production caused by iron deficiency. Usually, the cells also contain an increased amount of hemoglobin A_2, which does not contain beta chains, to compensate in part for the reduced synthesis of hemoglobin A. The level of residual fetal hemoglobin (having a gamma rather than a beta chain) varies from patient to patient, and those with high levels of fetal hemoglobin have milder disease.

If a person is heterozygous for beta thalassemia, the anemia is mild, and the condition is called thalassemia minor. The red cells are hypochromic and microcytic, but there is no additional morbidity or mortality associated with the disease. The homozygous condition, which is called beta thalassemia major, occurs if both parents have thalassemia minor and each transmits the abnormal gene. The affected individual has a severe chronic hemolytic anemia associated with excess compensatory erythropoiesis sometimes outside of the marrow (extramedullary hematopoiesis). Iron overload related to both excess absorption and required transfusion therapy leads to iron deposition in tissues and associated liver disease. Chelation therapy to remove excess iron is critical, and splenectomy may be helpful.

The inheritance of alpha thalassemia is more complex because two functional alpha chain genes are present in tandem on the normal chromosome. A normal individual has four (rather than two) alpha chain genes. Silent alpha thalassemia results when a single alpha chain gene on one chromosome is deleted (or defective), leaving three functioning genes. This condition is asymptomatic and very difficult to diagnosis. Alpha thalassemia trait results when there is loss of two alpha chain genes (and two functional chains remain). This can occur in two forms. Both genes may be lost from a single chromosome (a cis configuration), or one gene may be defective on each chromosome (a trans configuration). In either case, the clinical condition is the same. There is a mild microcytic anemia and a somewhat elevated red blood cell count, but patients are clinically normal. However, a mating between two people having the cis configuration can result in offspring with no functional alpha chain genes, a condition termed homozygous alpha thalassemia (also called hydrops fetalis and alpha thalassemia major). Hydrops fetalis patients die at birth or soon after from heart failure and have a very enlarged liver related to severe anemia. Most of their hemoglobin is termed hemoglobin Bart's (Hb Barts) and consists of four gamma chains. This form of hemoglobin does not efficiently deliver oxygen to tissues. Since it has such a high affinity for oxygen, the oxygen does not diffuse off the molecule into the tissues. Hemoglobin H disease results when there is a single functioning alpha chain gene, and it is named for the presence of the four-beta-chain-containing hemoglobin seen in such patients. Disease symptoms range from very mild in some patients to those who have severe microcytic and hemolytic anemia and require repeated transfusions. Iron overload from repeated hemolysis and therapeutic transfusions may occur with increasing age.

Red Cell Enzyme Deficiencies. Red cells derive energy by metabolizing glucose in a series of biochemical reactions catalyzed by various enzyme systems. These same energy-producing reactions also indirectly help prevent oxidation of the hemoglobin, including exposure to the potentially harmful effects of oxidizing drugs or other damaging agents. This protective function becomes compromised if certain red blood cell enzymes are deficient. In those situations, exposing the red blood cells to an oxidizing agent causes denaturation and precipitation of the protein chains of hemoglobin and the cell-membrane proteins.

One of the most common red cell enzyme defects involves a deficiency of the enzyme glucose-6-phosphate dehydrogenase (G6PD). This condition, transmitted as an X-linked recessive trait, leads to instability of the enzyme resulting in abnormal functioning. Because the mutant gene is carried on the X chromosome, affected males do not produce any normal enzyme, and all red blood cells are subject to hemolysis. Females who carry the mutant gene on one of their X chromosomes are also at risk of drug-induced hemolysis, because of random inactivation of one of the X chromosomes in females. The normal red cells and enzyme-deficient red cells are present in approximately equal proportions, resulting in less intense hemolysis. G6PD deficiency is the most common human enzyme defect, affecting over 400 million people worldwide, affecting more men than women as a result of X-linked inheritance. Geographically, tropical and subtropical areas record a higher occurrence rate. Data from in vitro studies demonstrate impaired growth of *P. falciparum* parasites in G6PD-deficient erythrocytes. Attempts to confirm that G6PD deficiency is protective in field studies of malaria have yielded conflicting results, but recent results from large case-control studies conducted in East and West Africa provide strong evidence that the most common African G6PD deficiency variant, G6PD A-, is associated with a significant reduction in the risk of severe malaria for both G6PD female heterozygotes and male hemizygotes. The protective mechanism for G6PD deficiency and malaria is still being investigated. With regards to ethnicity, G6PD deficiency is more common in people of African, Mediterranean, or Asian descent. It is estimated that about 10% of Black males in the United States are affected. The enzyme-deficient cells become injured by drugs that do not affect normal red cells and by various bacterial and viral infections. More than 40 drugs are known to induce an acute hemolytic anemia in susceptible individuals, including such commonly used drugs as sulfonamides, aspirin, some diuretics, some antibiotics, and some vitamins. The resulting anemia is also known as favism because it can be triggered by ingestion of fava beans (a common part of the Mediterranean and Middle Eastern diet) resulting in hemolysis in affected individuals. Hemolysis begins soon after exposure to the drug or infectious agent and continues for about a week. Considerable red cell destruction results, followed by red cell regeneration and return of red cell levels to normal in about 4 or 5 weeks.

Acquired Hemolytic Anemia. Sometimes the red blood cells form normally but are unable to survive because they are released into a "hostile environment." For example, antibodies that attack and destroy the red cells may be present in the circulation. Some of the autoimmune diseases, such as lupus erythematosus, and diseases of the lymphatic system may be associated with a hemolytic anemia caused by autoantibodies.

Drugs can cause hemolytic anemia by inducing formation of antibodies that damage red cells. Three different immunologic mechanisms have been identified. The most common mechanism results from the effect of the drug on the body's immune system, leading to the formation of an autoantibody directed against the red cell membrane. Other mechanisms include the formation of drug–protein complexes. The drug combines with a plasma protein, forming an antigenic drug–protein complex that induces antibody formation. The antigen and antibody complexes attach to the red cells, leading to their destruction. In other cases, the drug binds to the red cell membrane, forming an antigenic drug–membrane complex, which spurs the development of an antibody that attacks the cell membrane and damages the red cells.

Red blood cells may be destroyed by mechanical trauma. Some diseases are characterized by significant enlargement of the spleen. Red cells passing through a greatly enlarged spleen can become subject to considerable mechanical trauma, accelerating their destruction. Occasionally, a hemolytic anemia may follow insertion of an artificial heart valve, leading to the destruction or injury of the cell due to contact with some part of the artificial valve. In thrombotic microangiopathic hemolytic anemia, red cells are damaged by contact with fibrin deposited as microthrombi within small vessels. Disseminated intravascular coagulation is frequently associated with this type of anemia. Fragmented blood cells (schistocytes) appear in blood smears from such patients (see also the case in this chapter).

Diagnostic Evaluation of Anemia

The evaluation of a patient with anemia consists of a careful medical history and physical examination along with a complete blood analysis to assess the degree of anemia and determine whether leukopenia and thrombocytopenia also are present. Microscopic examination of a blood smear or use of automated instrumentation should determine whether the anemia is hypochromic microcytic, normocytic, or macrocytic. The rate of production of new red cells can be estimated by determining the percentage of reticulocytes in circulation. An increased percentage of reticulocytes indicates rapid regeneration of red cells. In some patients, tests that measure iron stores, iron transport, and iron metabolism may be informative (see Laboratory Tests to Evaluate Iron Metabolism in Iron Deficiency Anemia). A bone marrow biopsy may lead to useful information. In this procedure, a small amount of bone marrow is removed from the pelvic bone, sternum, or other site and examined microscopically. Characteristic abnormalities in the maturation of the marrow cells are seen in pernicious anemia and in anemia caused by folic acid deficiency. Bone marrow examination also detects interference with bone marrow functions secondary to infiltration by leukemic cells or metastatic tumor cells. If chronic blood loss from the gastrointestinal tract is suspected, stools are examined for blood, and studies of the gastrointestinal tract are performed to localize a site of bleeding.

Polycythemia

An increase of red cells and hemoglobin above normal levels, termed polycythemia (**Figure 12-11**), is usually secondary to an underlying disease that produces decreased arterial oxygen saturation (secondary polycythemia), or less

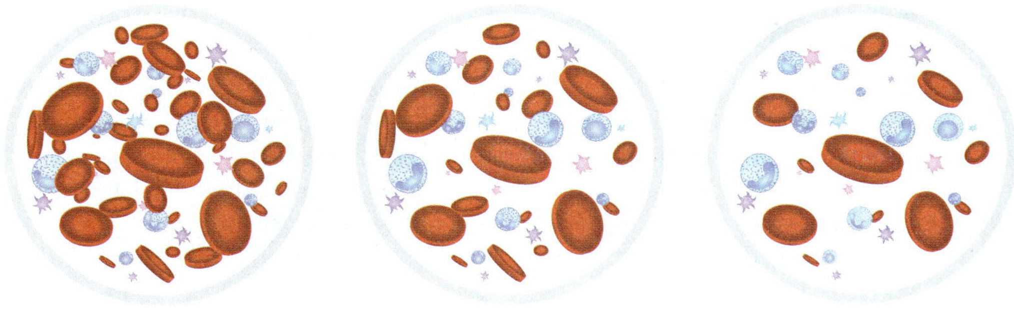

Figure 12-11 Polycythemia occurs when the amount of RBC/volume has greatly increased. The extra cells lead to difficulties with blood flow, clot formation, and eventually iron deposits within the skin and other organs.

frequently may represent a manifestation of a leukemia-like overproduction of red cells for no apparent reason (primary polycythemia).

Primary Polycythemia

Primary polycythemia, polycythemia vera (true polycythemia), manifests due to diffuse hyperplasia of the bone marrow, almost always related to a particular somatic mutation of the JAK2 gene. Clonal growth of cells with the mutation overcomes normal cells. As the erythroid progenitor cells with this mutation mature, they no longer require erythropoietin for growth. Polycythemia vera is characterized by overproduction, predominantly of precursors to red cells but also of white blood cells and platelet precursors. However, the peripheral blood shows only a mild to moderate increase in white cells and platelets. The disease exhibits many features of a neoplastic process and is classified as a myelodysplastic syndrome. It has been considered "pre-leukemia" because some patients with polycythemia vera eventually develop acute myelogenous (granulocytic) leukemia. Rarely, mutations in the erythropoietin receptor gene are responsible for a congenital form of primary polycythemia.

Secondary Polycythemia

Any condition associated with a reduced amount of oxygen transported in the bloodstream (low arterial PO_2; see Chapter 13) leads to increased erythropoietin production by the kidney and to increased numbers of circulating red cells. The condition may accompany pulmonary emphysema, pulmonary fibrosis, or some other type of chronic lung disease that impairs the oxygenation of the blood. Rarely, polycythemia may be the result of overproduction of erythropoietin by a renal tumor or other tumor.

Complications and Treatment of Polycythemia

The symptoms of polycythemia are related to the increased blood volume and increased blood viscosity. Many patients with polycythemia develop thromboses because of the increased blood viscosity and elevated platelet levels. Polycythemia vera is usually treated by drugs that suppress the bone marrow overactivity. Secondary polycythemia is sometimes treated by periodic removal of excess blood.

Thrombocytopenia

Petechiae Small pinpoint hemorrhages caused by decreased platelets, abnormal platelet function, or capillary defect.

Purpura Bleeding under the skin or mucus membrane observed as large discolored areas on the skin.

Blood platelets arise from the cytoplasm of megakaryocytes in the bone marrow. These small cell fragments serve a hemostatic function, sealing small breaks in capillaries and interacting with plasma factors in the initial stages of blood clotting. A significant reduction in the numbers of circulating platelets leads to numerous small, pinpoint hemorrhages derived from blood leaking from the capillaries in the skin and mucous membranes, termed **petechiae**, and to larger areas of hemorrhage called ecchymoses. This type of skin and mucous membrane bleeding is termed "**purpura**," and the disease is referred to as "thrombocytopenic purpura" (**Figure 12-12**). The number of platelets may be reduced by bone marrow disease or by accelerated destruction of platelets in the circulation.

Many cases of thrombocytopenic purpura develop when drugs, chemicals, or other substances damage the bone marrow. Others develop when the bone marrow becomes infiltrated by leukemic cells or metastatic carcinoma. These conditions are referred to as secondary thrombocytopenic purpura because the purpura results from an underlying disease of the bone marrow. Sometimes the bone marrow produces platelets normally, but the platelets are rapidly destroyed in the circulation. Autoantibodies directed against platelets can often be detected in the blood of affected individuals. Cases of this type, in which no underlying disease can be detected, are called idiopathic (from an obscure or unknown cause) thrombocytopenic purpura. All cases of idiopathic thrombocytopenia involve the productions of autoantibodies IgG directed against the thrombocytes. The disease is now referred to as immune thrombocytopenia purpura (ITP). ITP can be found in children

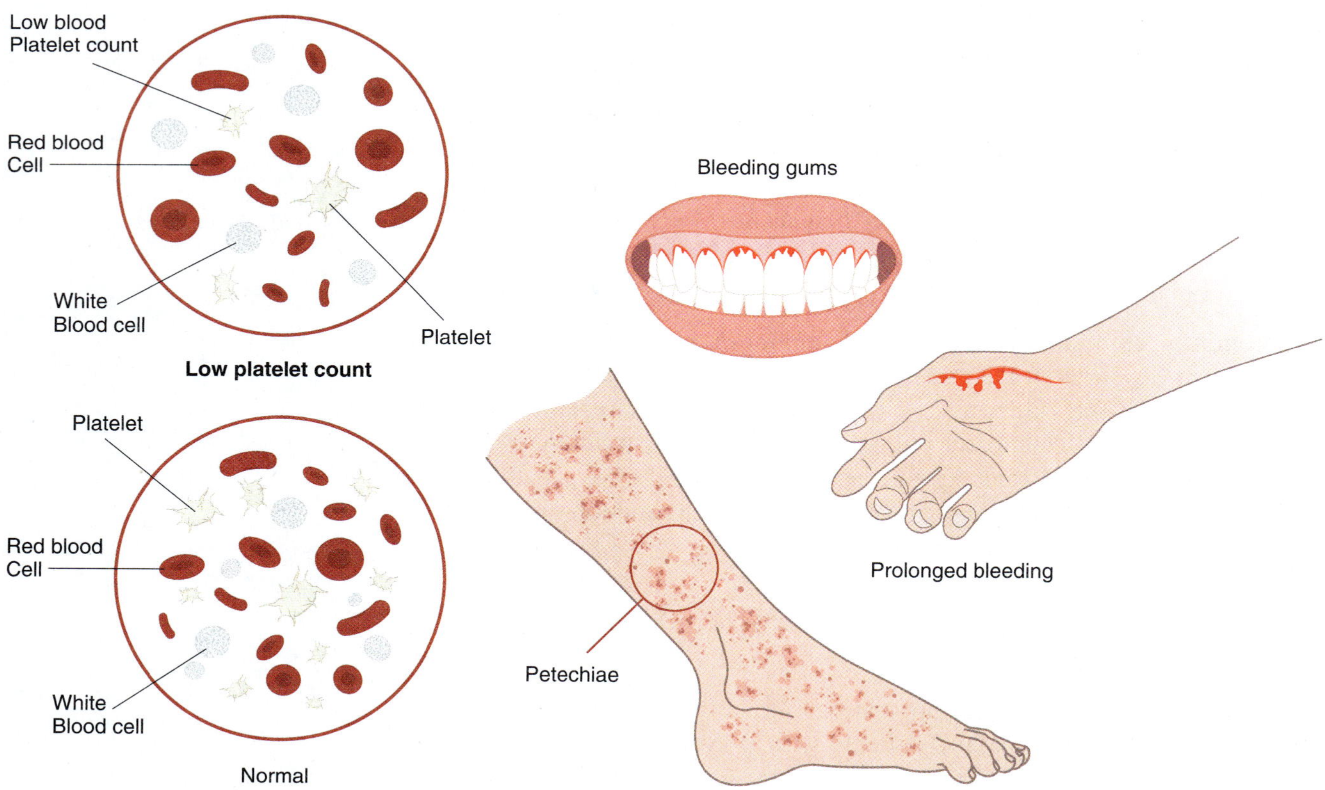

Figure 12-12 Decreased platelet counts can result in reddish purple spots, nose bleeds, and a prolonged bleeding time.

often following a mild viral disease. In children the condition subsides within a relatively short amount of time with very limited treatment. Most children experience spontaneous recovery within 3 months. Approximately 25 percent of the affected children will develop chronic ITP. Adults are more likely to present with chronic ITP and will rarely spontaneously resolve. Treatment regimens closely follow platelet counts and reports of bleeding to determine the best course for chronic ITP. If the platelet count is so low that the patient is at risk of severe life-threatening bleeding, the decreased number of thrombocytes needs to be addressed.

Description of Hemostasis

Hemostasis (blood clotting) is central to the body's response to injury. Rupture of larger veins and arteries, and other vascular injury, can result from trauma, inflammation, neoplastic damage, erosion of a vessel wall, or congenital malformations of the vasculature. All may lead to hemorrhage, the uncontrolled movement of blood into tissues, body spaces, and the gastrointestinal or urinary tracts. **Hemorrhagic diathesis** refers to a variety of clinical disorders, some inherited, some acquired, in which a usually insignificant or even unnoticed injury leads to unusual bleeding (**Figure 12-13**).

Hemorrhagic diathesis
Variety of clinical disorders in which small injuries lead to unusual bleeding.

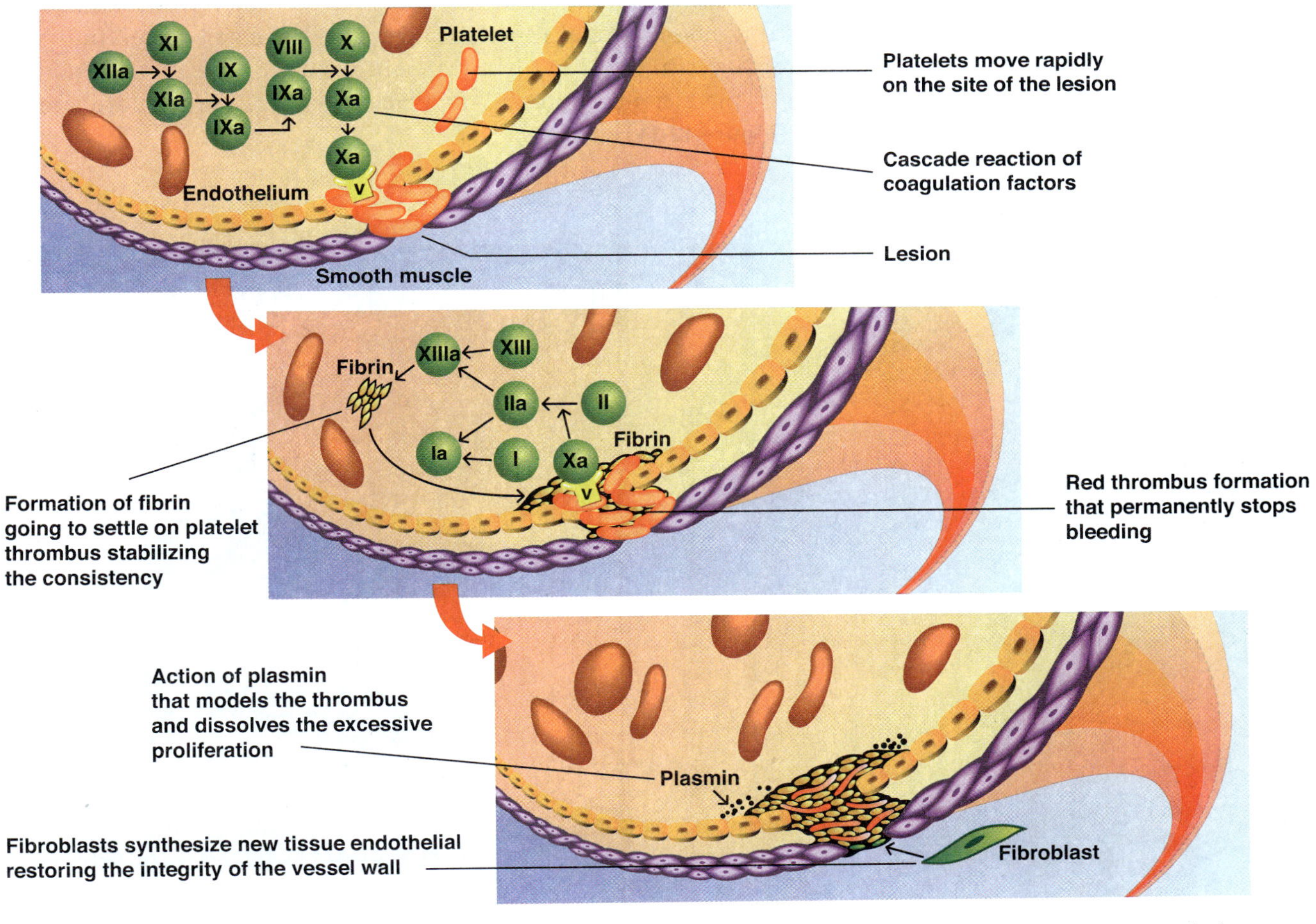

Figure 12-13 Hemostasis refers to maintaining a relatively stable blood volume with methods such as coagulation control and methods to maintain blood volume.

Thrombus Clot within a blood vessel.
Thrombosis The formation of blood clots (thrombi plural, thrombus singular) within the vascular system.
Hematoma Accumulation of blood within tissue.
Ecchymosis Bruise.
Hemarthrosis Arthritic condition caused by bleeding into the joint.
Hemothorax Hematoma within the chest.
Hemopericardium Hematoma between the heart and its pericardial lining.

Normal hemostasis must accomplish two seemingly contradictory functions: maintenance of blood in a fluid, **thrombus**-free state in normal vessels while maintaining the ability to form a localized hemostatic plug at the site of an injury. Thrombi refers to plugs within blood vessels, with clots occurring outside the blood vessels. The overall process is usually referred to as blood clotting or coagulation. **Thrombosis**, the opposite of hemorrhage, entails blood coagulation inside the body that blocks blood flow. The proper functioning of the hemostasis system depends on the integrated functioning of four major components. These include the integrity of the small blood vessels and their endothelium, adequate numbers of structurally and functionally normal thrombocytes (platelets), and normal levels of circulation coagulation factors balanced with normal levels of coagulation inhibitors, which control, localize, and terminate the hemostatic process, preventing pathogenic thrombosis. Adequate concentrations of calcium ions in the blood are also necessary for appropriate hemostasis (although hypocalcemia is not commonly associated with hemorrhagic symptoms).

Some specialized terminology is associated with the description of hemorrhagic processes. A **hematoma** is the accumulation of blood within tissue. It may be insignificant, such as a bruise (**ecchymosis**) on a limb, or life-threatening should it occur within the skull. A large accumulation of blood within a body space is named based on the space: **hemarthrosis** (within joints), **hemothorax** (within the chest), and **hemopericardium** (between the heart and its pericardial lining). Such accumulations usually lead to compromised normal function. Petechiae are small 1 to 2 mm pinpoint hemorrhages in the skin, mucous membrane, or serosa, often indicating failure of platelet function and capillary bleeding. Purpura are similar but larger (**Figure 12-14**).

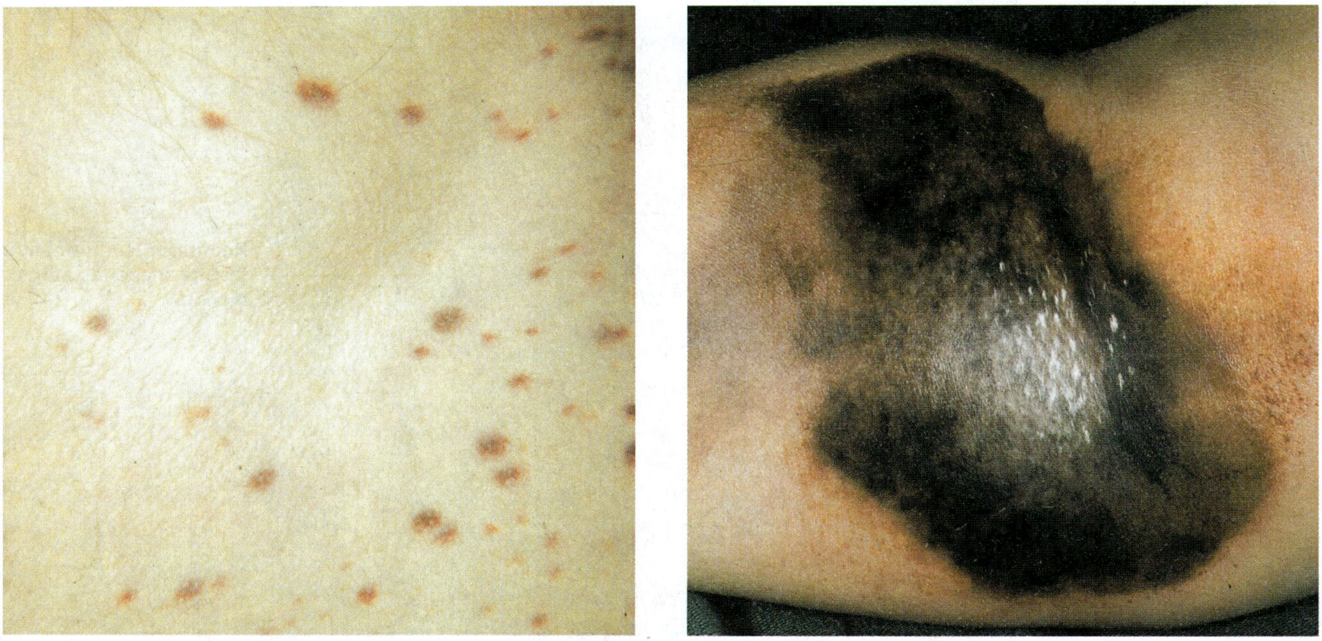

(A) (B)

Figure 12-14 Characteristics in bleeding in patients with disturbed hemostatic function. **(A)** Petechial hemorrhages indicative of thrombocytopenia or defective platelet function. **(B)** A large hemorrhage (hematoma) associated with deficiency of plasma coagulation factors.

Courtesy of Leonard V. Crowley, MD, Century College.

Blood Vessels and Their Endothelial Lining

In hemostasis, the small blood vessels are the body's first line of defense. If a vein or artery is injured, it automatically vasoconstricts, facilitating closure of the vessel by a blood clot. In a normal vessel, the endothelia, the cells that line blood vessels, act as an anticoagulant surface by secreting a variety of molecules that prevent the adherence and activation of platelets. In addition, the surface of uninjured endothelium is rich in coagulation inhibitors. Injury to a vessel leads to disruption of the endothelium, exposing the underlying connective tissue. Thrombocytes accumulate and adhere to the subendothelial tissue at the site of injury. They plug the defect in the vessel wall, liberate vasoconstrictors and compounds that cause further platelet aggregation, and release phospholipids that initiate the process of blood coagulation (**Figure 12-15**).

Abnormalities of the Vessel Wall and Endothelial Cells

In addition to physical damage, other forms of injury to either the vessel or the endothelium can lead to hemorrhage and activation of hemostasis. An uncommon autosomal dominant genetic disorder, **Osler-Weber-Rendu disease (OWRD)** (also called **hereditary hemorrhagic telangiectasia [HHT]**), leads to defects in blood vessels in the body expressed as telangiectases, spider veins in the skin and mucous membrane, and venous and arterial malformations occurring in any body system. The result is the occurrence of severe spontaneous nosebleeds (epistaxis), gastrointestinal bleeding, and a variety of arteriovenous defects in the liver and lung. The disease tends to progress with age.

After injury, the normally anticoagulant endothelial cells promote coagulation at the injured area. The cells may express **tissue factor**, a protein that is a major trigger for coagulation, and secrete **von Willebrand factor (vWF)**, a very large protein that acts as a "glue" to promote platelet adhesions to collagen in the subendothelial layer. Lack of functional vWF, known as von Willebrand disease (vWD), is most commonly inherited as an autosomal dominant condition with symptoms that range from a mild to a severe hemorrhagic condition similar to hemophilia. VWD in its mildest form is perhaps the most commonly observed genetic disease associated with bleeding. Females may experience heavy bleeding during their menstrual cycle or complications

Osler-Weber-Rendu disease (OWRD)/hereditary hemorrhagic telangiectasia (HHT) Disease caused by hereditary defects in blood vessels leading to spontaneous bleeding.

Tissue factor Protein that is a trigger for extrinsic coagulation.

von Willebrand factor (vWF) A large protein that acts to adhere platelets to collagen.

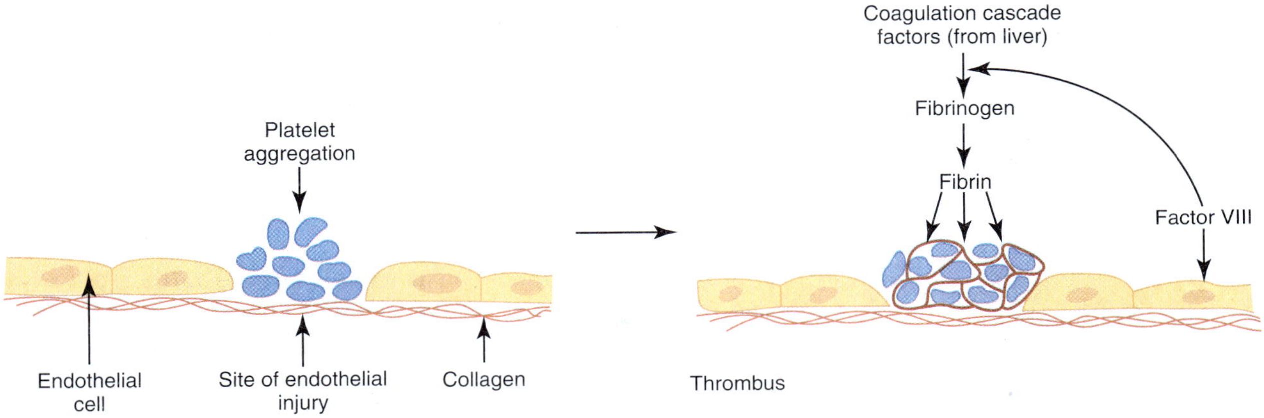

Figure 12-15 Platelets aggregate and stick to collagen at the site of endothelial injury.

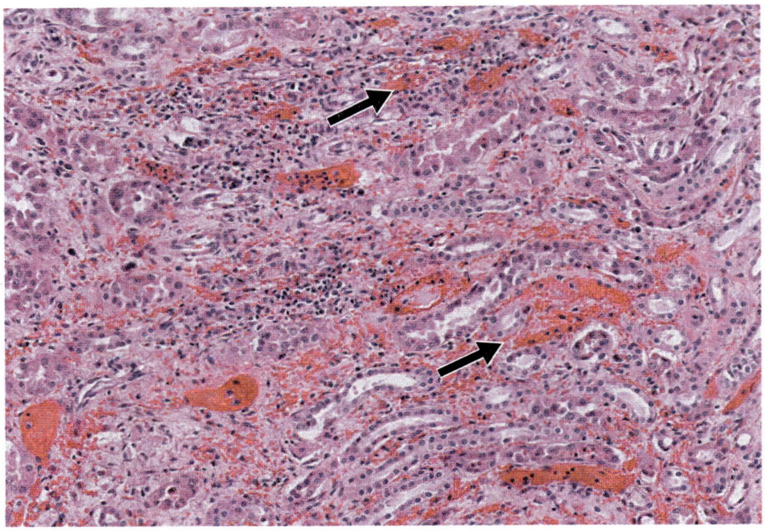

Figure 12-16 Kidney from a patient who died of Rocky Mountain spotted fever. There are multiple areas of hemorrhage from damaged vasculature into the renal parenchyma (*arrows*).

Courtesy of Department of Pathology and Laboratory Medicine, University of North Carolina at Chapel Hill.

Rocky Mountain spotted fever Disease caused by rickettsial infection of endothelial cells.

Disseminated intravascular coagulation (DIC) A rare but serious condition that causes blood clotting within the blood vessel and can be life threatening.

Platelet activation Release of active clotting components after adhesion of platelets.

Platelet agonists Substances promoting platelet function.

during pregnancy and childbirth. Disorders in endothelial function may also be acquired as a result of scurvy (vitamin C deficiency), vasculitis, and infectious diseases such as **Rocky Mountain spotted fever**. The disease is caused by bacteria, rickettsia, which infect and damage the endothelial cells lining the small blood vessels throughout the body (**Figure 12-16**). The rash and severe headache characteristic of the disease result from loss of normal endothelial function and leakage of blood outside of the capillaries.

Hemorrhagic fever viruses (such as Ebola) produce systemic hemorrhagic effects and subsequent shock by damaging the endothelium. Release of a number of substances into the circulation can lead to widespread, seemingly random intravascular coagulation. A life-threatening condition, **disseminated intravascular coagulation (DIC)**, results in paradoxical bleeding because of consumption of available coagulation factors by the plethora of small clots found in DIC, leaving insufficient amounts of factors available to control hemostasis.

Blood Vessels and Platelets

Platelets, or thrombocytes, play an essential role in blood coagulation. They are very small anucleate fragments of cell membrane derived from the megakaryocytes found in the bone marrow. Their survival in circulation lasts about 7-10 days. Damaged platelets and old platelets are removed by macrophages in the spleen. Platelets contain contractile proteins and two types of granules storing a variety of bioactive mediators of coagulation essential for normal functions. Immediately after vessel injury, platelets adhere to the wall of the injured vessel, forming a temporary "patch" at the site of injury. VWF is critical in this process. Initial adhesion of platelets provokes further **platelet activation** and the secretion of a number of active molecules, such as serotonin. Serotonin (a histamine-like substance) causes vasoconstriction and promotes blood clotting. In addition, several **platelet agonists**, including ADP and thromboxane A2 (a lipid-derived prostaglandin-like substance), are released. These substances promote platelet–platelet aggregation and recruit additional platelets from the circulation. Platelets undergo a shape change greatly increasing their surface area. This mass of aggregated platelets, the **primary hemostatic plug**, initially controls bleeding but can be reversed or washed away. The formation of the primary hemostatic plug defines **primary hemostasis**, that part of the hemostatic process that does not involve the humoral (circulating) coagulation factors.

Aggregated platelets express negatively charged phospholipids on their surface. Such phospholipids provide critical surfaces on which **secondary hemostasis** is carried out. This process involves the plasma coagulation factors, a series of inactive enzymes and cofactors that assemble in the presence of the phospholipid surface and calcium ions to produce active enzymes. Early in this process, the enzyme **thrombin** is produced from its inactive precursor, **prothrombin**. Thrombin plays a critical role in secondary hemostasis. However, some of the earliest thrombin produced binds to a specific receptor on the aggregated platelets, resulting in platelet contraction and formation of an irreversible fusion of platelets and fibrinogen. This mass forms the stable **secondary hemostatic plug**, with platelets and a fibrin meshwork derived from fibrinogen constituting the major components of the mature thrombus. The development of a mature thrombus also requires the interactions of many circulating coagulation factors.

Primary hemostatic plug Mass of aggregated platelets at site of injury.
Primary hemostasis Part of hemostatic process that is mostly platelet-dependent.
Secondary hemostasis Process involving plasma coagulation factors.
Thrombin A coagulation factor formed by activation of prothrombin in the process of blood coagulation.
Prothrombin Clotting factor activated by factor X to release thrombin/F.IIa.
Secondary hemostatic plug Formation of mature thrombus along with fibrin.
Iatrogenic Disease resulting from a medical examination or treatment.

Abnormalities of Platelet Numbers or Function

Thrombocytopenia (thrombus = T clot + cyte = cell + penia = deficiency), a decrease in the number of thrombocytes (platelets), may be a result of injury or disease of the bone marrow resulting in damage to the megakaryocytes. Thrombocytopenia may also occur because the bone marrow became infiltrated by leukemic cells or by metastatic cancer cells that spread to the skeletal system, crowding out the megakaryocytes. Antiplatelet autoantibodies may destroy the platelets in the peripheral blood. The most common cause of thrombocytopenia is **iatrogenic** (medically caused), often the result of cytotoxic therapy used in cancer treatment, which damaged the bone marrow. Non-steroidal anti-inflammatory drugs (such as aspirin) block the synthesis of thromboxane and interfere with platelet function. Sometimes platelets appear normal in quantity but abnormal in function and therefore cannot initiate the clotting process. Bleeding associated with defective or inadequate platelets is generally manifested by small petechial hemorrhages rather than by large areas of hemorrhage; however, a major diminution of platelet number and function can result in severe hemorrhage and may be treated by platelet transfusions.

Platelets from patients with Bernard-Soulier syndrome lack a functional receptor (GP1b) required for binding to vWF, preventing the platelets from binding at sites of endothelial injury. The platelets from patients with Glanzmann thrombasthenia lack a functional receptor (GP IIb-IIIa) required for binding fibrinogen and cannot form a stable thrombus that prevents bleeding. Both conditions are uncommon autosomal recessive diseases associated with severe bleeding.

Plasma Coagulation Factors

The blood plasma contains a number of different proteins collectively called coagulation factors, designated by Roman numerals (and occasionally by historical names). The process of blood coagulation is often referred to as a clotting cascade. Each component of the cascade is formed from an inactive precursor circulating in the blood, with each activated component in turn activating the next member of the cascade. Critical to the process is the presence of a negatively charged cell membrane phospholipid surface on which the reactions take place. Calcium ions anchor certain factors to that surface. The humoral coagulation process (that which depends on blood protein clotting factors) can be initiated from two pathways of activation that come together into a common pathway. This scheme is presented in a simplified and abbreviated manner. Coagulation can be activated via either an **extrinsic pathway** (so named because it was believed to need substances outside the vascular system for activation) or an **intrinsic pathway** (because all the substances necessary for activation were felt to be "intrinsic" to the vessels). Activation of the extrinsic pathway is now considered to be the key step in triggering circulatory coagulation (Figure 12-17).

Extrinsic pathway Clotting process needing substances outside the vascular system for activation.

Intrinsic pathway Clotting process needing only substances within the blood vessels.

Factor VII (F.VII) is normally present in plasma as an inactive enzyme. However, in the presence of tissue factor (TF) (normally present in the tissue surrounding the blood vessel or turned on in a damaged endothelial cell), F.VII becomes active and in turn activates another proenzyme, F.X, to an active enzyme, F.Xa. F.Xa in turn activates prothrombin (also called F.II) to release the critical enzyme thrombin (sometimes called F.IIa). This is the same thrombin molecule described earlier in relation to its role in platelet activation, but the protease has several other critical functions. Thrombin removes small peptides

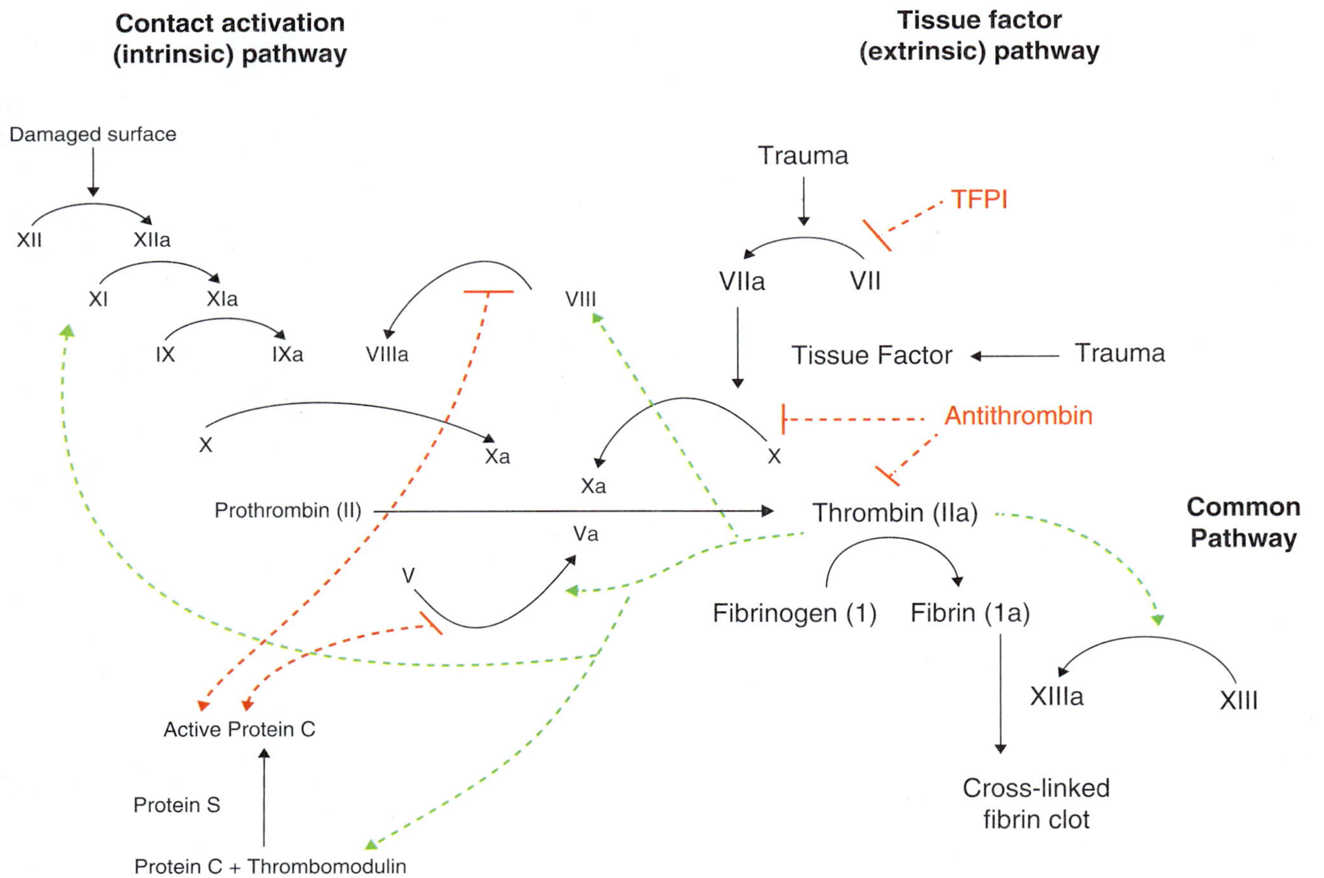

Figure 12-17 The clotting cascade can be initiated in one of two ways: through contact, the intrinsic pathway, or by active tissue factors.

from the fibrinogen molecule (a soluble protein synthesized in the liver), converting it into the insoluble fibrous protein fibrin, which, as noted previously, forms the bulk of the mature clot. Plasma F.XIII, which must be activated by thrombin, acts on the fibrin clot by forming bonds between the fibrin molecules, increasing the strength and stability of the clot. Another critical function of thrombin is to activate two non-protease "cofactors" critical in humoral coagulation, F.V and F.VIII (antihemophilic factor). When activated by thrombin, the cofactors speed up the coagulation process by many thousandfold. For example, active F.V (F.Va) "orients" F.Xa and prothrombin on the phospholipid surface in the presence of the calcium ion, which speeds up the enzymatic reaction producing thrombin.

The intrinsic pathway is an alternative (and critical) second method of generating F.Xa (thrombin). The exact steps in intrinsic pathway activation are complex, but basically the inactive protease F.XII becomes active F.XIIa in the presence of collagen and other surfaces. F.XIIa activates F.XI to F.XIa, which in turn activates the protease F.IX to F.IXa. In a manner analogous to F.Xa activating prothrombin (in the presence of F.Va), F.IXa activates F.X to F.Xa in the presence of the cofactor F.VIIIa. Once again, the cofactor F.VIIIa is critical to speed up the reaction. This part of the intrinsic pathway is associated with two relatively common serious hemorrhagic diseases. Lack of active F.VIII causes **hemophilia A**, sometimes referred to as classic hemophilia; lack of active F.IX causes **hemophilia B**.

Hemophilia A Bleeding disease caused by lack of active F.VIII.

Hemophilia B Bleeding disease caused by lack of active F.IX.

Plasminogen Precursor compound of plasmin in the blood.

Plasmin Blood enzyme that degrades blood plasma proteins, including fibrin clots.

Fibrinolytic system Process of breaking down clots.

Coagulation Inhibitors and Fibrinolysis

Coagulation factors are counterbalanced by various coagulation inhibitors that restrict the clotting process. Coagulation inhibitors protein C and protein S function together to inactivate two coagulation factors, Va and VIIIa. Another important member of this group is antithrombin III, which inhibits not only thrombin but also several other activated coagulation factors.

An equally important control system is one that digests fibrin after it has formed. Fibrin provides the framework for mature clots. Biological clot dissolution requires that this framework become disrupted. An inactive precursor compound in blood plasma, **plasminogen**, is activated to form **plasmin**, which dissolves fibrin in blood clots. The **fibrinolytic system** becomes activated at the same time that the coagulation process is initiated, with thrombin activating this system while continuing the clotting cascade. Another important plasminogen activator is a substance called tissue plasminogen activator (TPA), which is released from endothelial cells in the region where the clot is forming. In clinical situations where blood clots need to be dissolved, tissue plasminogen activator or another plasminogen activator, streptokinase, is administered intravenously to dissolve blood clots in the coronary arteries of patients who have had a recent heart attack (see Chapter 9). Administration of one of these plasminogen activators within a few hours after onset of symptoms dissolves the clot and restores flow through the artery, minimizing heart muscle damage resulting from the blockage.

Calcium and Blood Coagulation

Adequate amounts of calcium ions (Ca^{2+}) are required in all phases of blood coagulation. However, calcium levels sufficiently low to affect blood coagulation are most often incompatible with life.

Deficiency of Plasma Coagulation Factors

Deficiencies of coagulation factors usually result from genetic abnormalities and are relatively rare. Only three hereditary bleeding diseases occur with any frequency.

Hemophilia A (F.VIII deficiency) and B (F.IX deficiency) result from X-linked gene mutations. As a result, these diseases primarily affect males, while females are affected only if both of their X chromosomes carry the gene mutation. Clinically, the diseases present with episodes of crippling hemorrhage in joints and internal organs even after minor injury and, at times, life-threatening intracerebral bleeds. Both hemophilia A and B exhibit the same clinical manifestations. Serious symptoms occur in patients when the levels of the affected proteins fall below 5 percent of normal. The most common, hemophilia A (HA) or classic hemophilia, is characterized by a decrease in coagulation F.VIII (also called antihemophilic factor). The less common form of hemophilia, hemophilia B (HB), or Christmas disease, results from a deficiency of F.IX, which is also called Christmas factor (named after an affected patient, not the holiday). Factor IX is synthesized by hepatocytes within the liver. F.VIII is synthesized in several organs but predominantly in the liver by a population of endothelial cells. HA, with a prevalence of one in every 5000 live births, is more common than HB, which affects one in every 30,000 live births.

The third one, vWD, a previously mentioned hereditary bleeding disease, affects both males and females. The dysfunctional vWF protein is important in both primary and secondary hemostasis. When severe, it may also result in excessive bleeding after a minor injury. The difference, though, is that the bleeding is not in the joints, like hemophilia. The vWF is synthesized in endothelial cells and released into the bloodstream, where it forms a complex in the circulation with F.VIII and is required to maintain a normal level of F.VIII in the blood. For this reason, the level of F.VIII is often low in patients with von Willebrand disease, although synthesis of F.VIII is normal (**Figure 12-18**).

Patients with hemophilia A, hemophilia B, and von Willebrand disease with bleeding episodes can be treated by administration of factor concentrates prepared from human blood plasma or currently using recombinant DNA technology. Adequate continuing treatment of hemophilia A & B is critical to prevent serious (or even fatal) bleeding in severe disease. However, even in the absence of trauma, bleeding into joint spaces leads to severe inflammation and ultimate joint destruction. For this reason, appropriate routine therapy must be undertaken to prevent crippling disease. Frequent IV infusions of the factor may be necessary to adequately treat the patient because of the short biological half-life of the infused factors. The recent development of several modified EHL (extended half-life) factors has dramatically reduced the need for constant therapy. Ultimately, molecular therapy may provide a cure for the hemophilias, much as is beginning to happen with sickle cell disease. Successful long-lasting molecular therapy has recently been reported for hemophilia B, and much work is being undertaken to extend this to the more common hemophilia A.

Vitamin K–dependent factors, including F.II, VII, IX, and X and the inhibitor of coagulation protein C, are produced in the liver. Vitamin K is required for a secondary, postsynthetic modification of certain glutamic acid residues (gamma carboxylation) in these factors, which is necessary for calcium ion

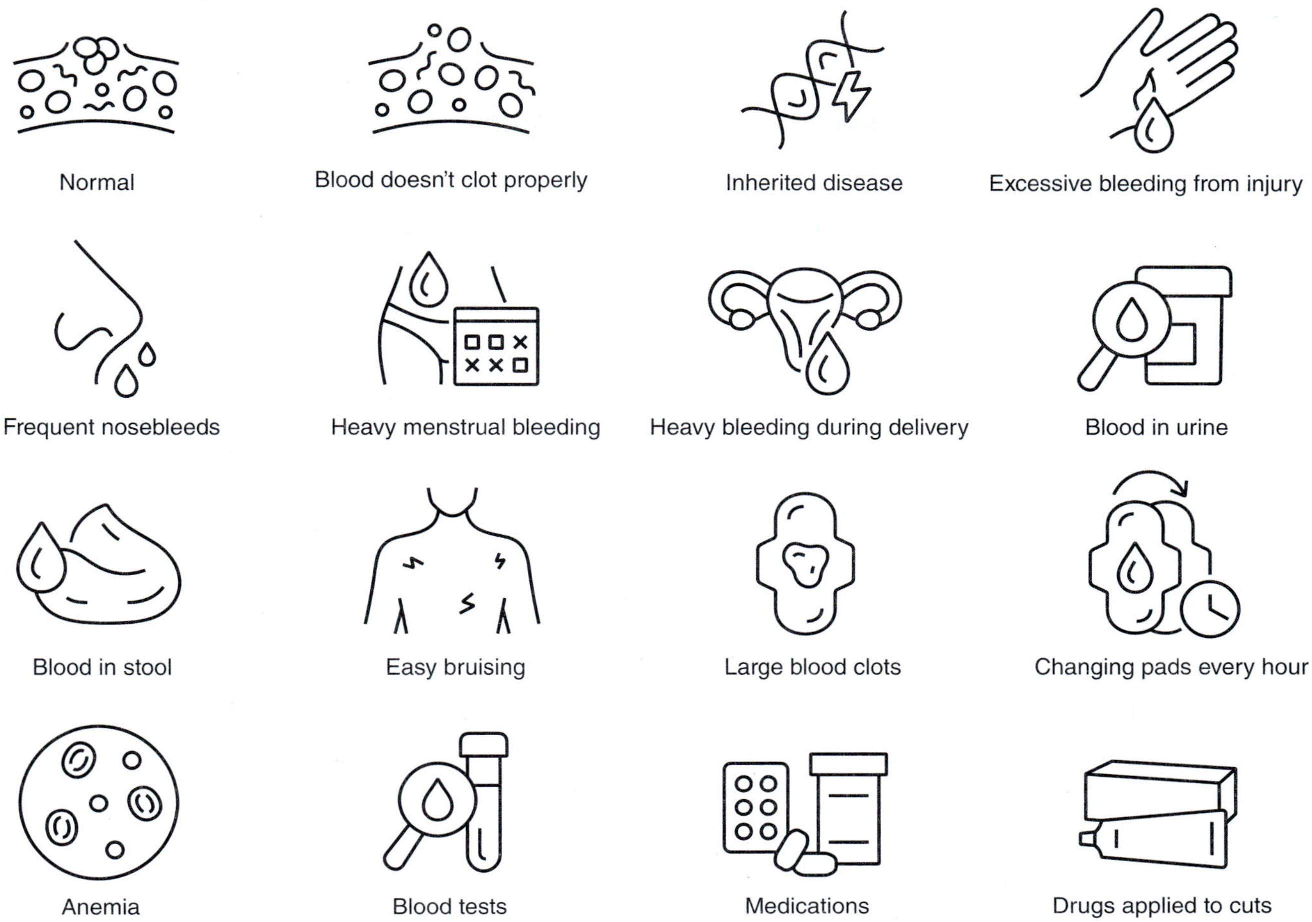

Figure 12-18 There are several types of vWD of varying degrees of severity. Women are often troubled by severe menstrual bleeding, and hemorrhage may occur during childbirth.

binding. The lack or deficiency in this vitamin can result in the synthesis of inactive factors and bleeding disease. Vitamin K is synthesized by intestinal bacteria and also can be obtained from foods, especially green leafy vegetables. As a fat-soluble vitamin, vitamin K requires bile for its absorption. Inadequate synthesis of vitamin K may occur if the intestinal bacteria have been eradicated by prolonged antibiotic therapy. Another vitamin K–deficient group is newborn infants, who lack the intestinal bacteria to make the vitamin and are not yet eating foods that contain the vitamin. They are at risk for serious bleeding called hemorrhagic disease of the newborn. To prevent this condition, newborn infants routinely receive a vitamin K injection to prevent spontaneous bleeding.

Patients with severe liver diseases may also exhibit a bleeding tendency because their badly damaged liver can no longer synthesize adequate amounts of coagulation factors.

Anticoagulant drugs are sometimes used to treat patients with an increased tendency to develop blood clots due to disease processes or a sedentary lifestyle. Post-operative patients may be given anti-coagulants to prevent clot formation post-surgery or during times of limited activity. Anti-coagulants may be given to patients with some types of heart disease in which blood clots tend to form within the cardiac chambers or to patients with some types of artificial heart valves to prevent clot formation within these valves. The type of anticoagulant prescribed for a patient will depend on many factors, including the mechanism of action of the anticoagulant.

Heparin, a sulfated glycosaminoglycan, is also a commonly used antithrombotic drug that functions by complexing with the inhibitor protein antithrombin III, promoting its ability to inhibit F.X and thrombin. A major drawback is that heparin must be injected and may be associated with serious thrombotic side effects. Warfarin-like drugs such as Coumadin can be taken orally and block the effect of vitamin K on the vitamin K–dependent factors. A number of other anticoagulant drugs are available that may have advantages over warfarin-like drugs in specific clinical situations. Some popular anticoagulant drugs act by interfering with thrombin or factor X in the humoral phase of blood coagulation. Such anticoagulants can be given as a standard daily dose without requiring laboratory tests, which simplifies the patient's treatment.

Liberation of Procoagulant Material into the Circulation

In some diseases associated with bacterial shock, high levels of tissue necrosis and the release of other substances, such as postpartum amniotic fluid and procoagulant materials into the circulation result in widespread intravascular coagulation of the blood (**Figure 12-19**). Because clotting uses platelets and the various plasma (humoral) coagulation factors, the levels of these components in the blood drop precipitously, resulting in a hemorrhagic state. Fibrin thrombi form in and may occlude small blood vessels.

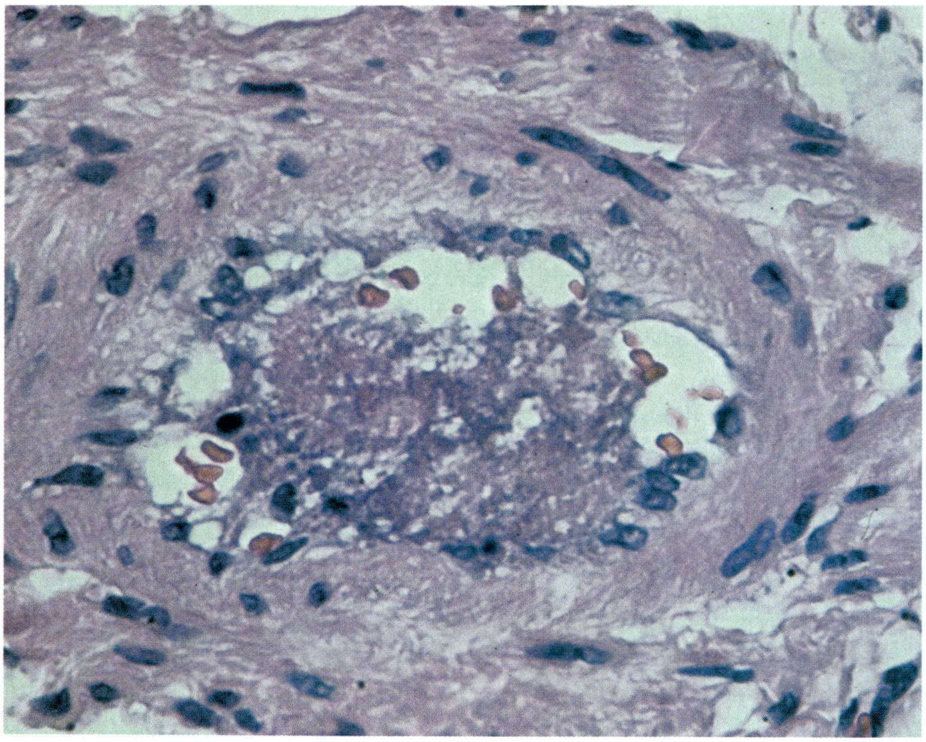

Figure 12-19 Fibrin thrombus in small blood vessel of a patient with disseminated intravascular coagulation syndrome (original magnification ×400).

Courtesy of Leonard V. Crowley, MD, Century College.

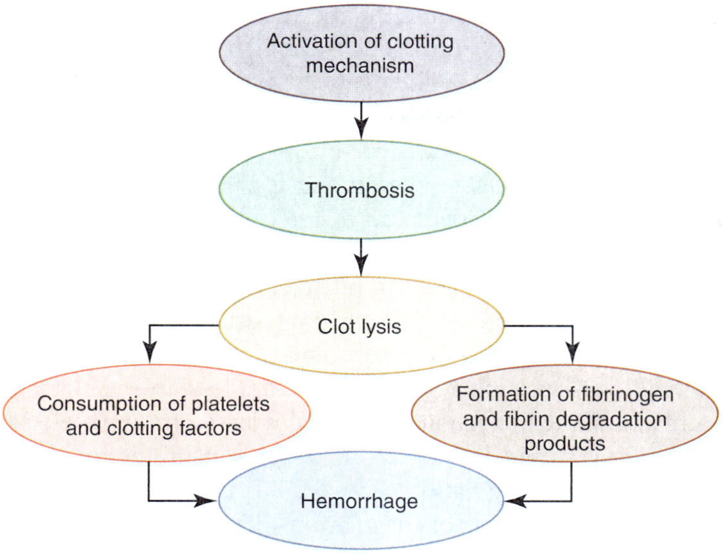

Figure 12-20 Pathogenesis of disseminated intravascular coagulation syndrome.

In response to widespread intravascular clotting, the body activates the fibrinolytic system, which dissolves fibrin-containing clots and reduces the potential for obstruction of the circulatory system. The breakdown products produced during degradation of the fibrin (fibrinopeptides) act as additional inhibitors of the clotting process. This abnormal bleeding state is called disseminated intravascular coagulation syndrome, or **consumption coagulopathy**. The latter term alludes to consumption of the clotting factors as a result of the pathogenic coagulation process. **Figure 12-20** summarizes the pathogenesis of this bleeding syndrome. Although expressed as a hemorrhagic state, the inciting cause is the widespread intravascular triggering of thrombosis. D-dimer is a fibrinopeptide that is derived only from the breakdown of fibrin (not the breakdown of fibrinogen). Immunoassays for the measurement of D-dimer in blood are very sensitive for detecting thrombosis and are much elevated in disseminated intravascular coagulation (see also the chapter case).

Consumption coagulopathy A disturbance of blood coagulation within the blood vessel as a result of the uncontrolled activation of the coagulation mechanism.

Bleeding time Time needed for a small standardized skin incision to stop bleeding.

Laboratory Tests to Evaluate Hemostasis

Several laboratory tests can evaluate the overall efficiency of the coagulation process, detect the presence of inhibitors of coagulation, and estimate the number and function of the platelets.

The number of platelets in the blood can be estimated by examining the blood smear, and more precise data can be obtained by using automated blood cell counting devices. Special tests (platelet aggregometry) also are available to evaluate the ability of platelets to aggregate in the presence of agonists such as thromboxane and thrombin. The function of both capillaries and vWF in the hemostatic process is sometimes evaluated by measuring the time it takes for a small, standardized skin incision to stop bleeding, a test termed the **bleeding time**. Both platelet function tests and the bleeding time are extremely sensitive to the use of NSAIDs (such as aspirin), and patients must refrain from their use for a period of time prior to testing.

Several tests are used to evaluate coagulation factor function and to monitor the efficacy of anticoagulant therapy when using warfarin-like drugs such

Partial thromboplastin time (PTT) test A test that measures the overall efficiency of the blood coagulation process. Detects defects in intrinsic coagulation and is used to monitor heparin therapy.

Prothrombin time (PT) test A test that detects defects in extrinsic coagulation and is used to monitor warfarin-like anticoagulant therapy.

Thrombin time test A laboratory test measurement that determines the concentration of fibrinogen in the blood by determining the clotting time of the blood plasma after addition of thrombin.

as Coumadin. The tests, performed in the laboratory from plasma obtained from blood collected in tubes containing the anticoagulant citrate, which binds calcium ions, include the **partial thromboplastin time (PTT) test**, or more often the activated partial thromboplastin time (aPTT), the **prothrombin time (PT) test**, and the **thrombin time test**. Each test measures a different part of the coagulation process. When the tests are used together, the location of the coagulation factor deficiency can be identified if any of the tests yield an abnormal result. The tests are now done using automated equipment to measure how long it takes for a plasma sample to clot after the addition of calcium.

The activated partial thromboplastin time test measures the time it takes for blood plasma to clot after a lipid substance and an activating agent such as silica are added to the plasma along with calcium to start the clotting process. The lipid added is similar to the lipid material released from platelets to initiate secondary hemostasis, and the activating agent substitutes for the activation that occurs in intrinsic coagulation. The aPTT is most often used to measure defects in the intrinsic pathway of coagulation (F.IX and F.VIII deficiency in particular) and to monitor the effect of heparin anticoagulation, but the test is also sensitive to defects in the common part of the pathways (F.X, F.V, prothrombin, and fibrinogen).

The prothrombin time test measures the time it takes for blood plasma to clot after adding a commercially available preparation (thromboplastin) along with calcium to start the coagulation. The thromboplastin added mimics the tissue factor and platelet-derived lipid, which triggers the extrinsic pathway of coagulation. A prolonged PT is indicative of a defect in F.VII or the previously mentioned factors in the common pathway. However, the real utility of the PT test is measuring the effect of warfarin-like anticoagulants such as Coumadin. The PT test is designed by manufacturers for this purpose and is used to determine the INR (international normalized ratio), a standardized test to evaluate how long it takes blood to clot compared to a standardized average. This test is often used to adjust drug dosages for patients on blood thinners such as warfarin.

The thrombin time test determines the clotting time of plasma after the addition of thrombin. Therefore, the test measures the level of fibrinogen and its ability to clot in the presence of thrombin, which may be deficient in some conditions. The level of fibrinogen (irrespective of its ability to clot) can be measured directly by other tests, and one can also test for fibrin degradation products, which are increased if fibrinolysis is excessive and thrombosis is occurring, such as in DIC as mentioned previously. A variety of tests can be used to measure the activity of specific coagulation factors. For example, the plasma of patients suspected of having hemophilia with an abnormally prolonged PTT can be tested for specific levels of F.VIII and F.IX to determine whether they have hemophilia A or B, an important distinction for choosing appropriate therapy. Uncommonly, some individuals (such as hemophiliacs lacking a particular coagulation factor and occasionally otherwise normal individuals) may produce antibodies (termed inhibitors) against the therapeutically infused replacement factor (or as part of an autoimmune response to an endogenous coagulation factor). Laboratory tests for such inhibitors involve mixing patient and normal plasma prior to aPTT testing to determine whether the patient plasma will reduce the activity of coagulation factors in the normal plasma.

Case 12-1

John is a 4-year-old child who goes with his family on a trip to visit a farm. During the trip, he drinks a glass of raw (unpasteurized) milk fresh from the cow. His father objects, but his mother, noting that the farm is "organic," encourages him to drink. Late the next day, John complains to his mother that he feels warm. She notes an oral temperature of 102°F (38.9°C) and treats him with acetaminophen. John develops diarrhea and complains of stomach pain. His pediatrician diagnoses gastroenteritis (believing it to be reovirus, which was currently affecting children in John's daycare) and suggests food restriction, fluid replacement, and alternating ibuprofen and acetaminophen for fever control.

John's parents become increasingly concerned. There are traces of blood in the child's stool, and he is becoming lethargic. On day 4 of John's illness, his parents note that he is pale, his face has become puffy, and he seems to be urinating very little, if at all (is becoming anuric). Alarmed, John's pediatrician has him admitted to a local hospital.

At the local hospital, John is found to be hypertensive, and tests of kidney function disclose acute renal failure with elevated levels of serum creatinine. Blood studies are abnormal, with a low platelet count, decreased levels of several coagulation factors including fibrinogen, and elevated levels of fibrin degradation products. A peripheral blood smear shows that several percent of the red cells are schistocytes (fragmented irregular cells). Stool culture shows *E. coli* O157:H7. John remains hospitalized for several days, and his blood electrolyte levels, renal function, and platelet count are carefully monitored. His hydration status is checked to maintain normal fluid volume. He is treated with an antihypertensive drug, a calcium channel blocker. Renal dialysis is considered, but John slowly begins to recover renal function. He is discharged with frequent follow-up visits to monitor his continuing renal function.

Discussion

The case is a classic presentation of Shiga toxin–producing E. coli–induced hemolytic uremic syndrome (STEC-HUS), predominantly a pediatric disease usually occurring in children between 1 and 4 years of age. This is most frequently caused by *E. coli* O157:H7, an enterohemorrhagic strain of the bacteria that produces an enterotoxin (a bacterially secreted toxin that targets the gastrointestinal tract). A similar toxin is produced by the *Shigella* species of bacteria responsible for types of bacterial dysentery (hence the term Shiga toxin). The bacteria *E. coli* O157:H7 is very resistant and may contaminate the environment for months. Most cases of STEC-HUS are related to meat or milk products contaminated with animal waste, and cattle are the major reservoir. Contaminated raw milk would be a likely source in this case. About 10 percent of children infected with *E. coli* O157:H7 will develop STEC-HUS. The disease presents three sets of abnormalities: (1) microangiopathic anemia, a type of anemia related to mechanical damage of red cells as they pass through thrombosed or otherwise damaged small blood vessels, (2) thrombocytopenia, and (3) acute renal failure.

The abnormalities are all related to the effect of the Shiga toxins produced by the bacteria. The toxin is produced by bacteria that adhere to the gut wall and is absorbed from the inflamed colon. Subsequently, the toxin binds to vascular endothelial cells, predominantly in the gut and kidney. The toxin-damaged endothelial cells become prothrombotic, leading to platelet adhesion and aggregation and the formation of microthrombi within the vasculature of the kidney. The damaged endothelium and adherent fibrin thrombi shear red cells as they flow through, resulting in the microangiopathic

(continues)

Case 12-1 *(Continued)*

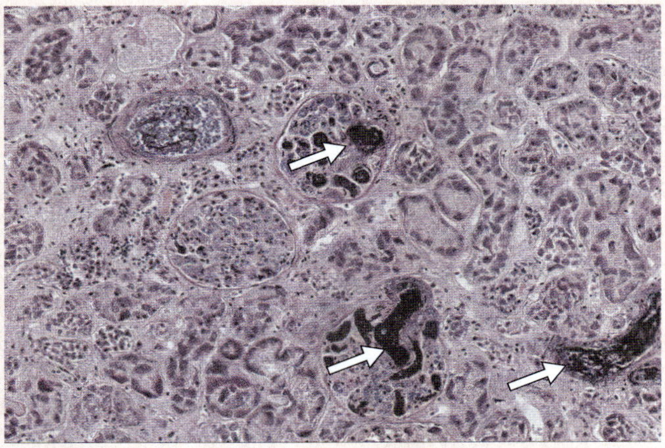

Case Figure 12-1 Kidney from a patient suffering from bacterial hemolytic uremic syndrome. A special stain to highlight fibrin has been used. Thrombi are visible in renal (glomerular) capillaries and small vessels (*arrows*).

Courtesy of Department of Pathology and Laboratory Medicine, University of North Carolina at Chapel Hill.

anemia characterized by the presence of damaged red cells (schistocytes). The disseminated intrarenal thrombosis leads to consumption of platelets (hence thrombocytopenia) and also of coagulation factors. Fibrinolysis of the microthrombi leads to the presence of fibrin degradation products. The vascular damage to the kidney results in acute renal failure (**Case Figure 12-1**).

Etiology and Pathogenesis

Infection with a Shiga toxin–producing strain of bacteria, *E. coli* O157:H7, resulting in STEC hemolytic uremic syndrome. STEC-HUS can be seen as a renal-/gut-limited form of disseminated intravascular coagulation.

Questions

1. What preventative measures should be undertaken to prevent infection by foodborne enteropathic bacteria?
2. Some advocates suggest that the production of antibiotic-free beef will lower the incidence of *E. coli* O157:H7 infections. Do you believe there is any potential validity to the claim?
3. STEC-HUS may be seen as a localized form of DIC. Support this contention.
4. STEC-HUS initially can be diagnosed using a simple blood-based test that can be done in many doctors' offices. What is the test, and how is it used to make the diagnosis?

Questions for Review

1. What types of cells are found in the circulating blood, and what are their major functions?
2. What is anemia?
3. What is iron deficiency anemia? How does it arise? How is it treated? What is the morphologic appearance of the red cells?
4. What is the effect of vitamin B_{12} and folic acid on blood cell maturation? What type of anemia results from deficiency of these vitamins?
5. What is the difference between an aplastic anemia and a hemolytic anemia? What is the difference between polycythemia and

thrombocytopenia? What is hemochromatosis? What are its manifestations? How is hemochromatosis diagnosed and treated?

6. What are the key components of the blood clotting mechanism?
7. What are some of the common disturbances of blood coagulation?
8. What is thrombocytopenia? What type of bleeding is produced when platelets are markedly reduced? What types of diseases are associated with thrombocytopenia?
9. What is primary hemostasis?
10. What types of diseases produce abnormalities in primary hemostasis?
11. What is the consequence of liberation of procoagulant material into the circulation?
12. What laboratory tests are used to evaluate the coagulation of blood?

References

Valdez R, Zutter MM, Li S, et al. Hematopathology. In: Rubin E, Reisner HM, eds. *Principles of Rubin's Pathology*. 7th ed. Wolters Kluwer; 2019:587-646.

- It is difficult to provide pertinent and useful supplementary readings for the introductory reader in the area of hematology because it encompasses an extremely wide range of physiological processes and diseases. Many recent changes in the classification of and suggested therapies for hematological disease are based on an increased understanding of the molecular basis of these diseases. This chapter in a recent pathology textbook aimed at medical education is a good place to start. Additional readings provide recent in-depth reviews of selected topics.

Education. American Society of Hematology. Accessed May 29, 2025. https://www.hematology.org/education

- This website has an excellent collection of material (including images and videos) that is aimed at educators. The images of blood smears are particularly useful, as is a comprehensive image bank.

Maakaron JE. Anemia. Medscape. Updated June 2, 2025. Accessed May 29, 2025. https://emedicine.medscape.com/article/198475-overview

- Although aimed at clinicians, this overview is easy to read and has information on diagnosis and therapy.

Carbon Monoxide Poisoning Basics. Centers for Disease Control and Prevention. Updated April 17, 2024. Accessed May 29, 2025. https://www.cdc.gov/carbon-monoxide/about/index.html

- An informative website on the pathogenesis, manifestations, and treatment of this condition, which is often called the "silent killer," also containing links to other resources. The prevalence tends to increase when economic difficulties prevent families from having safe and effective means of providing heat during the winter. Therapeutic approaches under a variety of conditions are summarized.

ACSM and NCAA Joint Statement on Sickle Cell Trait and Exercise. Last updated February 8, 2023. Archived April 20, 2024, at https://web.archive.org/web/20240410172512/https://www.ncaa.org/sports/2013/12/18/acsm-and-ncaa-joint-statement-sickle-cell-trait-and-exercise.aspx

Sickle cell disease (SCD). Centers for Disease Control and Prevention. Accessed May 29, 2025. https://www.cdc.gov/ncbddd/sicklecell/index.html

Mangla A, Agarwal N, Maruvada S, et al. Sickle Cell Anemia. StatPearls [Internet]. Last updated September 4, 2023. https://www.ncbi.nlm.nih.gov/books/NBK482164/

- The first is the link to the NCAA policy on athletes with sickle cell disease and sickle cell trait. It provides good basic information for student athletes, coaches, and parents. The second provides information on several levels from the health professional to the person concerned about the genetics of sickle cell disease. The third resource from StatPearls covers the pathophysiology, epidemiology, and management of sickle cell anemia.

Needs T, Gonzalez-Mosquera LF, Lynch DT. Beta Thalassemia. StatPearls [Internet]. Updated May 1, 2023. https://www.ncbi.nlm.nih.gov/books/NBK531481/

Harewood J, Azevedo AM. Alpha Thalassemia. StatPearls [Internet]. Updated September 4, 2023. https://www.ncbi.nlm.nih.gov/books/NBK441826/

- For the reader interested in more specific detailed information on the thalassemias, these references clearly and concisely explain the important aspects of the different variations of the disease.

Porter JL, Rawla P. Hemochromatosis. StatPearls [Internet]. Updated October 5, 2024. https://www.ncbi.nlm.nih.gov/books/NBK430862/

Warner MJ, Kamran MT. Iron Deficiency Anemia. StatPearls [Internet]. Updated August 7, 2023. https://www.ncbi.nlm.nih.gov/books/NBK448065/

Chambers K, Ashraf MA, Sharma S. Physiology, Hepcidin. StatPearls [Internet]. Updated April 17, 2023. https://www.ncbi.nlm.nih.gov/books/NBK538257

Zamora EA, Schaefer CA. Hereditary Spherocytosis. StatPearls [Internet]. Updated July 4, 2023. https://www.ncbi.nlm.nih.gov/books/NBK539797/

Chaudhry R, Killeen RB, Babiker HM. Physiology, Coagulation Pathways. StatPearls [Internet]. Updated June 2, 2025. https://www.ncbi.nlm.nih.gov/books/NBK482253/

- These StatPearls articles provide additional details on various conditions and mechanisms covered in the chapter.

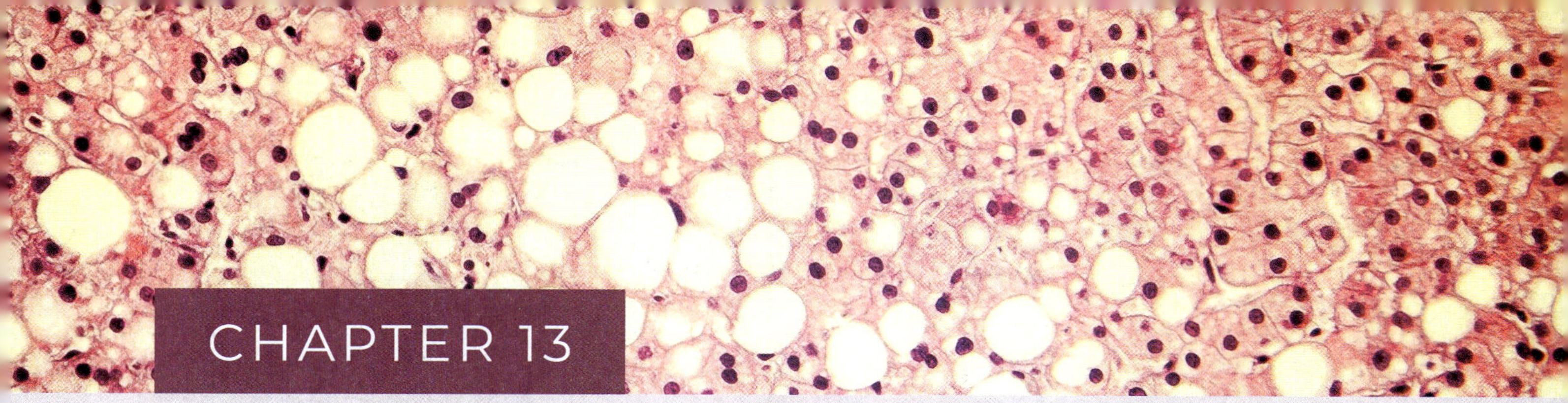

CHAPTER 13

The Respiratory System

LEARNING OBJECTIVES

1. Explain the anatomic and physiologic principles of ventilation and gas exchange.
2. Describe the physiological basis and use of pulmonary function tests.
3. Describe the causes, clinical effects, complications, and treatment of pneumothorax and atelectasis.
4. Describe the clinical symptoms, complications, and treatment of pneumonia.
5. Describe the histologic characteristics of a tuberculosis infection. Explain the possible outcome of the infection. Describe methods of diagnosis and treatment.
6. Differentiate between bronchitis and bronchiectasis.
7. List the anatomic and physiologic derangements in chronic obstructive lung disease. Explain its pathogenesis. Describe the clinical manifestations and methods of treatment.
8. Describe the pathogenesis and manifestations of bronchial asthma and respiratory distress syndrome.
9. Explain the causes and effects of pulmonary fibrosis. Describe the special problems associated with asbestosis.
10. List the major types of lung carcinoma. Describe the clinical manifestations of lung carcinoma and explain the principles of treatment.

Oxygen Delivery: A Cooperative Effort

Normal life processes require that an adequate supply of oxygen be delivered to the tissues and that the volatile waste products of cell metabolism be removed. These functions are carried out by a cooperative effort of the respiratory and circulatory systems. The respiratory system oxygenates the blood and removes carbon dioxide. The circulatory system transports these gases in the bloodstream.

Structure and Function of the Lungs

The lungs consist of three distinct components: a system of tubes whose chief function is to conduct air into and out of the lungs; the **alveoli (singular, alveolus)**, where oxygen and carbon dioxide are exchanged between air; and the pulmonary vasculature, notably the pulmonary capillaries, the targets of gas exchange. Just as a tree branches progressively and ends in a foliage of leaves, so the conducting tubes branch repeatedly and terminate in clusters of pulmonary alveoli. The lung is divided into several large segments called lobes.

Alveoli/alveolus One of the terminal air sacs of the lung.

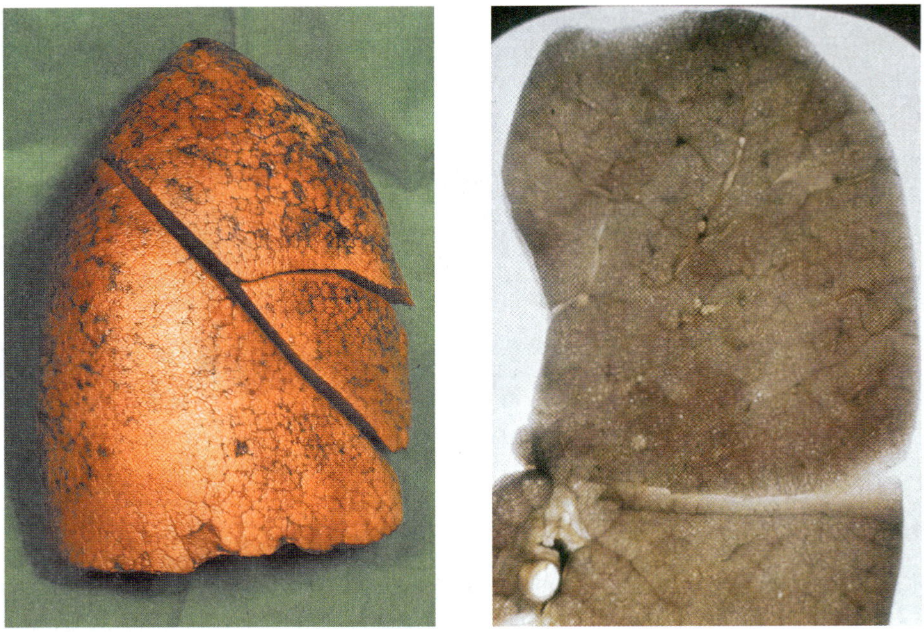

(A) (B)

Figure 13-1 Normal lung that has been inflated and air-dried so that the structure of the lobes and lobules can be visualized and the fine structure of the alveoli can be studied. **(A)** External surface illustrating lobes and fissures. The faint cobblestone-like pattern of the pleural surface defines the individual lung lobules. **(B)** A backlighted section of lung illustrating the fine, spongelike pattern produced by the respiratory units where gas exchange occurs.

Courtesy of Leonard V. Crowley, MD, Century College.

Each lobe in turn consists of a large number of smaller units called lobules. The architecture and structural features of a normal lung can be studied to the best advantage when the lung is inflated and air dried (**Figure 13-1A**). The individual lobes, fissures, and pleural surfaces are well defined. The poorly defined cobblestone-like pattern of the pleural surface defines the location of the individual **lung lobules**, which frequently are accentuated by environmental carbon pigment deposited in the alveolar macrophages, ultimately residing in the connective tissue that surrounds and circumscribes the individual lobules, a process termed **anthracosis**. When sections of normal air-dried lung are examined against an illuminated background, the spongelike, fine structure of a normal lung, which is essential for normal gas exchange, can be examined (**Figure 13-1B**).

Lung lobule A small group of terminal bronchioles and their subdivisions.

Anthracosis Carbon pigment deposited in the connective tissue around the individual lobules of lung.

Bronchi/bronchus One of the large subdivisions of the trachea.

Bronchiole One of the small terminal subdivisions of the branched bronchial tree.

Bronchi, Bronchioles, and Alveoli

The largest conducting tubes are called **bronchi** (singular, bronchus). Tubes less than one mm in diameter are called **bronchioles** (little bronchi), and the smallest bronchioles, which function only for conduction of air, are called terminal bronchioles. The tubes distal to the terminal bronchioles are called respiratory bronchioles because they have alveoli in their walls and not only transport air but also participate in gas exchange. Each terminal bronchiole gives rise to several respiratory bronchioles, which branch to form alveolar ducts. The alveolar ducts in turn subdivide into alveolar sacs, and multiple alveoli open into each alveolar sac (**Figure 13-2**).

Each alveolus is a small air space surrounded by a thin wall, the alveolar septum, which consists of thin-walled capillaries supported by a few connective

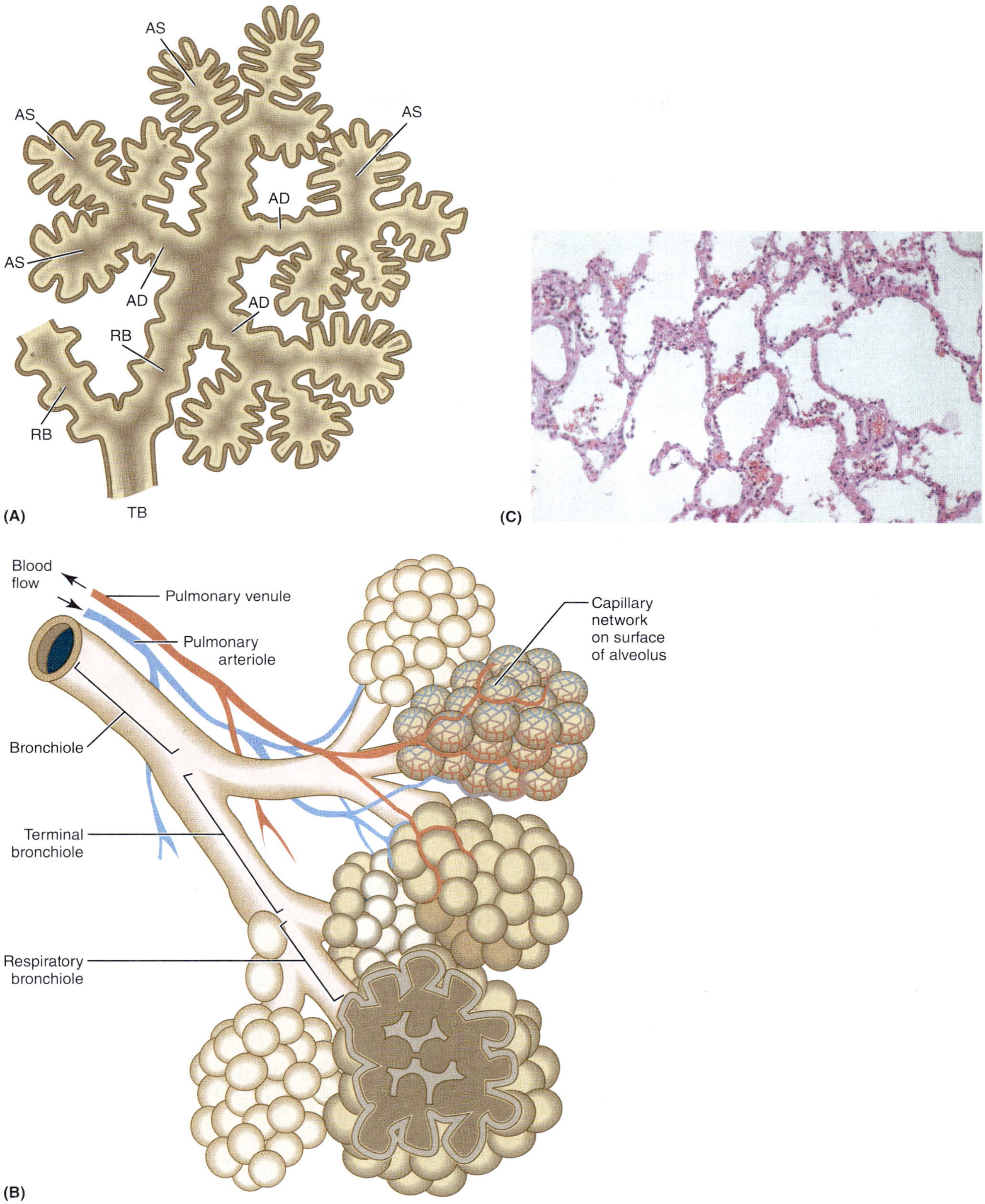

Figure 13-2 **(A)** Structure of a respiratory unit. A representative terminal bronchiole is designated TB. A respiratory bronchiole (RB) has alveolar sacs projecting from the wall of the bronchiole. Alveolar ducts are designated AD, and alveolar sacs are designated AS. Multiple alveoli (not labeled) open into each alveolar sac. **(B)** Structure of terminal air passages. The interior of one alveolar duct is illustrated in cutaway view. **(C)** Histologic structure of the lung illustrating alveoli and thin alveolar septa containing pulmonary capillaries (original magnification ×100).

(C) Courtesy of Leonard V. Crowley, MD, Century College.

tissue fibers and lined by a layer of epithelial cells (Figure 13-2C). Hence, the air in the alveolus is closely apposed to the circulation by a single layer of cells lining the alveolus, a basement membrane, and the endothelial cells lining the capillary. Each alveolus contains a relatively small volume of air surrounded by a large network of capillaries, conditions that promote rapid diffusion of oxygen and carbon dioxide between alveolar air and pulmonary capillaries as the blood flows through the lung. Any condition that enlarges the pulmonary alveoli or reduces the number of pulmonary capillaries impedes the efficiency of pulmonary ventilation. Under normal conditions, the connective tissue supporting the alveolar capillaries is insignificant; however, in some diseases, this interstitial connective tissue may become prominent and interfere with gas exchange—for example, in **interstitial pneumonia** or idiopathic pulmonary fibrosis. Diseases in which increased fibrosis leads to reduced functional lung volume and decreased pulmonary compliance (distensibility or "stretch") are termed *restrictive* lung disorders. Diseases that interfere with airflow to the alveoli are termed *obstructive* lung disorders, common examples of which are chronic bronchitis, asthma, and **emphysema**. The distinction between the two classifications is not always clear cut. Pulmonary diseases are also classified by anatomical location. Pulmonary vascular diseases (discussed in Chapters 9 and 10) include such conditions as pulmonary emboli and pulmonary hypertension.

Interstitial pneumonia Characterized by the thickening of supporting tissues between the air sacs of the lungs.

Emphysema Disease in which the air spaces in the lung are enlarged and their walls destroyed.

Type I pneumocytes/type II pneumocytes Cells lining the alveoli.

Surfactant Substance which reduces the surface tension of a liquid, such as water. In the lungs, a lipid material secreted by type II pneumocytes that facilitates respiration by decreasing the surface tension of the fluid lining the pulmonary alveoli.

Respiratory unit A functional unit of the lung consisting of a cluster of respiratory bronchioles, alveolar ducts, and alveoli derived from a single terminal bronchiole. Another term for acinus.

Pleura The mesothelial covering of the lung (visceral pleura) and chest wall (parietal pleura).

Two types of cells line the alveoli. Most are flat squamous cells termed **type I pneumocytes**, which are important in gas exchange. A few are larger cuboidal **type II pneumocytes**, secretory cells that produce a lipid material termed **surfactant** that reduces surface tension. Surface tension is the attraction between molecules of a fluid that causes the fluid to aggregate into droplets instead of spreading as a thin film. The surface tension of the molecules in the fluid lining the alveoli would normally tend to pull the alveolar walls together. This effect would hinder expansion of the lungs during inspiration and would cause the alveoli to collapse during expiration because of the cohesive force of the water molecules. Surfactants act somewhat like a detergent, lowering the surface tension of the fluid and thereby facilitating respiration. In case of damage to type I pneumocytes, type II can divide and produce additional type I cells.

The functional unit of the lung is termed a "**respiratory unit**." It is formed by the cluster of respiratory bronchioles, alveolar ducts and sacs, and alveoli derived from a single terminal bronchiole. A lung lobule consists of a small group of terminal bronchioles and the respiratory units that arise from them. Lobules are partially circumscribed by connective tissue septa and are easiest to identify just beneath the **pleura**, where the connective tissue septa defining the lobules can be easily seen (Figure 13-1A).

Respiration has two functions corresponding to the two structural components of the lungs: ventilation and gas exchange. Both ventilation and gas exchange must function normally if respiration is to be effective.

Ventilation

Air is moved into and out of the lungs by the bellows action of the thoracic cage. During inspiration, the ribs become more horizontal because of the action of the intercostal muscles, and the diaphragm descends. Consequently, the volume of the thoracic cage increases. The lungs expand to fill the larger intrathoracic space, and air is drawn into the lungs through the trachea and bronchi. During expiration, the ribs become more vertical and the diaphragm rises.

The volume of the thoracic cage is reduced. The lungs, which conform to the size of the thorax, also decrease in volume, and air is expelled.

Normal respiratory movements require that respiratory muscles, innervation of the muscles, and mobility of the thoracic cage are normal. Ventilation is impaired if the nerve supply to the respiratory muscles is damaged by disease, as in poliomyelitis, or if the respiratory muscles undergo atrophy and degeneration. Ventilation is also impaired if the thoracic cage is immobile. For example, a person buried in sand up to his neck will suffocate because he is unable to move his thoracic cage and therefore cannot move air into and out of his lungs.

Gas Exchange

Oxygen and carbon dioxide, along with nitrogen and water vapor, are in the atmospheric air that we breathe, in the air within the pulmonary alveoli, and in the blood. At sea level, the atmospheric pressure exerted by the mixture of all the gases is 760 mm Hg. Each gas exerts a proportionate part of the total atmospheric pressure, depending on its concentration in the mixture of gases. For example, the concentration of oxygen in atmospheric air is 20 percent. Therefore, the pressure exerted by oxygen is 20 percent of the total pressure exerted by all the gases (0.20×760 mm Hg $=$ 152 mm Hg). The part of the total atmospheric pressure exerted by a gas is called the partial pressure of the gas. Partial pressure is usually expressed by the letter "P" preceding the chemical symbol for the gas—for example, PO_2 152 mm Hg.

Gases diffuse between blood, tissues, and pulmonary alveoli because of differences in their partial pressures. Venous blood returning from the tissues is low in oxygen (PO_2 40 mm Hg) and high in carbon dioxide (PCO_2 47 mm Hg). This blood is pumped through the pulmonary capillaries, where it comes into contact with the air in the pulmonary alveoli. Alveolar air has a much higher concentration of oxygen (PO_2 105 mm Hg) but a lower concentration of carbon dioxide (PCO_2 35 mm Hg). Therefore, oxygen diffuses from alveolar air into pulmonary capillaries, and carbon dioxide diffuses from pulmonary capillaries into the alveoli. The situation is reversed in the tissues. The tissue oxygen concentration is much lower (PO_2 about 20 mm Hg), and the carbon dioxide concentration is much higher (PCO_2 about 60 mm Hg); so oxygen diffuses into the tissues from the blood, and carbon dioxide diffuses in the opposite direction.

When carbon dioxide is dissolved in aqueous solution, there is an equilibrium between free carbon dioxide and carbonic acid. Hyperventilation lowers the alveolar carbon dioxide partial pressure (PCO_2) and leads to a rapid decrease in the concentration of carbon dioxide and carbonic acid in the plasma. Decreased or inadequate pulmonary ventilation results in elevation of alveolar PCO_2, which in turn raises plasma carbon dioxide and carbonic acid as described in Chapter 17.

Exchange of gases between alveolar and pulmonary capillaries is accomplished by diffusion across the alveolar membrane (**Figure 13-3**). Efficient gas exchange requires (1) a large capillary surface area in contact with alveolar air, (2) unimpeded diffusion of gases across the alveolar membrane, (3) normal pulmonary blood flow, and (4) normal pulmonary alveoli. The spongy structure of the lungs, in which each tiny air sac is surrounded by a large network of capillaries, provides the large surface area required for efficient gas exchange. In general, changes to the surface area to volume ratio (SA/V) will alter the diffusion of gases across the alveolar membranes. (**Figure 13-4A**). Destruction of alveolar septa leads to coalescence of alveoli and a reduction in the size of the capillary network surrounding the alveoli, resulting in less efficient gas exchange (**Figure 13-4B**).

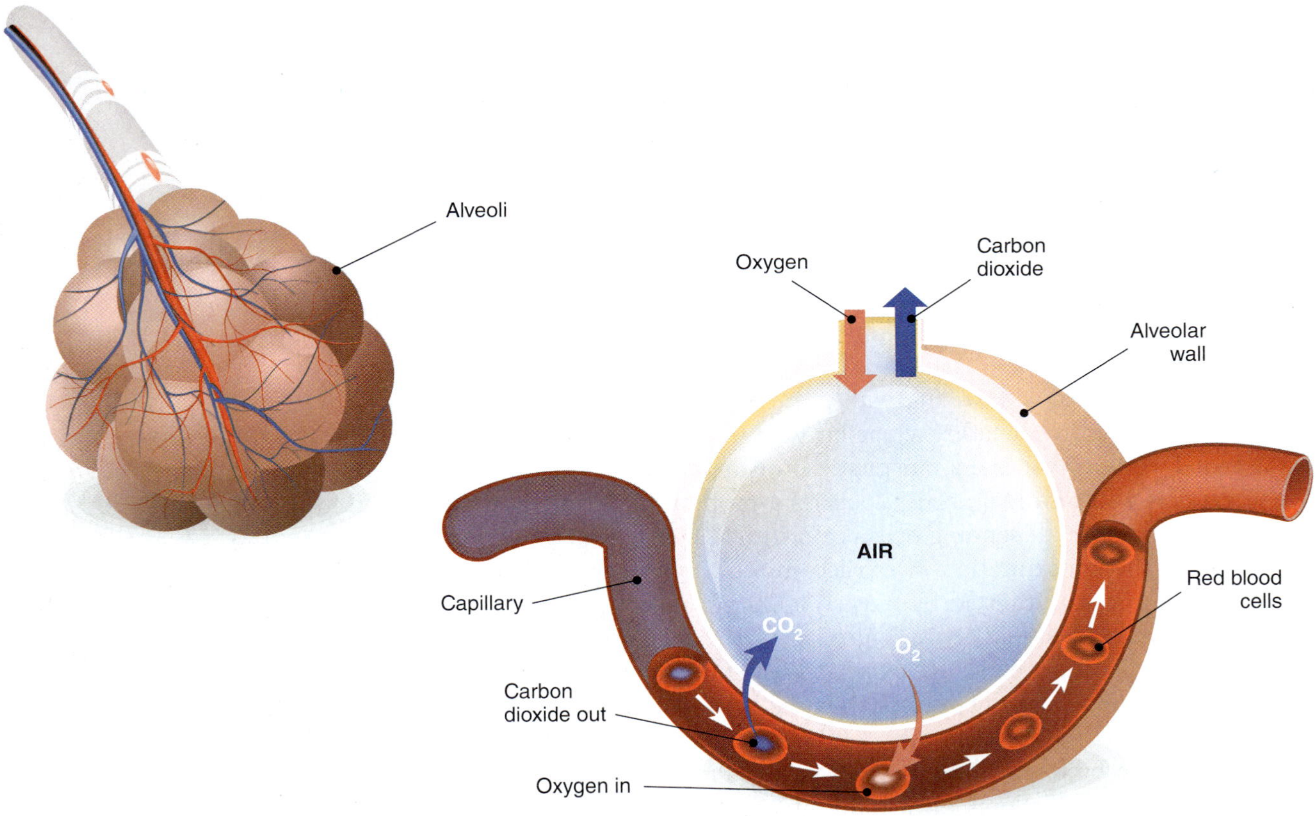

Figure 13-3 Exchanges of gases between alveolar and pulmonary capillaries.

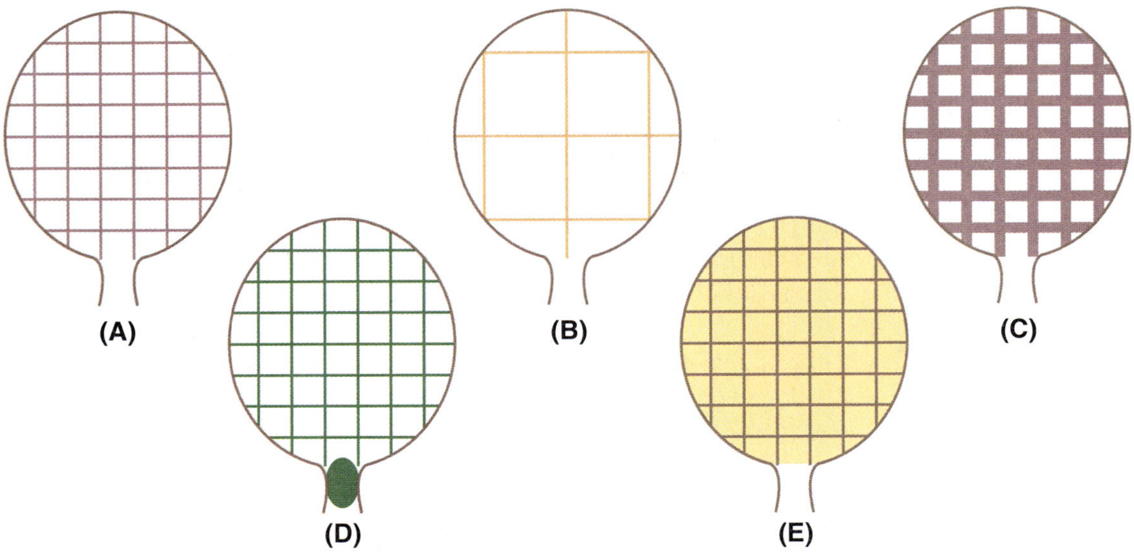

Figure 13-4 Types of structural and functional abnormalities that adversely affect pulmonary gas exchange. **(A)** Normal alveoli and pulmonary blood flow. **(B)** Destruction of alveolar septa leading to coarsening of alveolar structure with a corresponding reduction in size of the pulmonary capillary bed. **(C)** Fibrous thickening and scarring of alveolar septa, impeding diffusion of gases across alveolar membrane. **(D)** Obstruction of pulmonary blood flow to a part of the lung. **(E)** Alveoli filled with fluid or inflammatory exudate.

If the alveolar septa are thickened and scarred, the diffusion of gases across the thickened alveolar membranes is impeded (**Figure 13-4C**). Gas exchange is also impaired if pulmonary blood flow to a portion of the lung is obstructed, as might be caused by a pulmonary embolus obstructing a large pulmonary artery or by blockage of pulmonary capillaries by fat emboli or foreign material (**Figure 13-4D**). If the pulmonary alveoli become filled with fluid or inflammatory exudate, inspired air cannot enter the diseased alveoli, and pulmonary gas exchange is impeded (**Figure 13-4E**).

The Pleural Cavity

The lungs are covered by a thin membrane called the pleura, which also extends over the internal surface of the chest wall. Because the lungs fill the thoracic cavity, the two pleural surfaces are in contact. The potential space between the lung and the chest wall is the pleural cavity. Normally, the opposing pleural surfaces move smoothly over one another. In disease, however, the pleural surfaces may become roughened because of inflammation and may become adherent. Inflammatory exudate may accumulate in the pleural cavity and separate the two pleural surfaces.

The lungs are held in an expanded position within the pleural cavity because the pressure within the pleural cavity (intrapleural pressure) is less than the pressure of the air within the lungs (intrapulmonary pressure). The pressure differences develop when the thoracic cavity enlarges after birth. When respirations are initiated, the size of the thoracic cavity increases, creating a partial vacuum. The lungs become filled with air at atmospheric pressure and expand to fill the enlarged thoracic cavity, stretching the elastic tissue within the lungs. The tendency of the stretched lung to pull away from the chest wall and return to its original contracted state creates a slight vacuum within the pleural cavity. Because the intrapleural pressure is slightly less than atmospheric pressure, it is often called "negative pressure."

Pulmonary Function Tests

Pulmonary function tests can be used to evaluate the efficiency of pulmonary ventilation and pulmonary gas exchange. Pulmonary ventilation is usually tested by measuring the volume of air that can be moved into and out of the lung under standard conditions. Two commonly used measurements are **vital capacity**, which measures the maximum volume of air that can be expelled after a deep inspiration, and the **one-second forced expiratory volume (FEV_1)**, which measures the maximum volume of air that can be expelled in one second. If the bronchioles are narrowed by inflammation or spasm, impeding the movement of air out of the lungs, FEV_1 is often reduced. Specialized tests can measure the total volume of air in the lungs and the volume of air remaining in the lungs after a maximum expiration.

Vital capacity The maximum volume of air that can be forcefully expelled after a maximum inspiration.

One-second forced expiratory volume (FEV_1) The maximum volume of air that can be expelled from the lungs in one second.

The concentrations of oxygen and carbon dioxide (O_2 and CO_2) in the patient's arterial blood can also be measured to determine the efficiency of gas exchange in the lungs. In chronic pulmonary disease, oxygenation of the blood is inefficient. Oxygen concentration is reduced, and arterial oxygen saturation is decreased correspondingly. Often, the arterial PCO_2 also is higher than normal because carbon dioxide is inefficiently eliminated by the lungs. Arterial blood for analysis is usually collected by inserting a small needle into the radial artery in the wrist and withdrawing a small amount of blood.

One can also determine how effectively the lungs are oxygenating the blood (arterial oxygen saturation) using a device called a pulse oximeter. A fingertip is inserted into the device, which measures photoelectrically the changes in light absorption of the hemoglobin in the fingertip capillaries at various wavelengths during systole and diastole. Then the data are used to automatically calculate the oxygen saturation of the blood (the percentage of blood that is carrying oxygen; normal values are usually over 90%), and the result will be displayed promptly.

Pneumothorax

Pneumothorax
Accumulation of air in the pleural cavity.

Because the intrapleural pressure is below that of the atmosphere, air flows into the pleural space if the lung or chest wall is punctured. When this occurs, the negative pressure that holds the lung in the expanded position is lost, and the lung collapses because the elastic tissue within the lung contracts. This condition, which is termed a **pneumothorax** (pneumo = air), may follow any type of lung injury or pulmonary disease that allows air to escape from the lungs into the pleural space. It also may result from a stab wound or some other penetrating injury to the chest wall that permits atmospheric air to enter the pleural space (**Figure 13-5**).

Occasionally, pneumothorax occurs without apparent cause. This is termed *spontaneous* pneumothorax. Most cases occur in young, healthy people, usually as a result of rupture of a small, air-filled, subpleural bleb at the apex of the lung.

The sudden escape of air into the pleural cavity that is associated with any type of pneumothorax usually causes chest pain and often some shortness of breath. The breath sounds, which normally can be heard with a stethoscope when the air moves in and out of the lung during respiration, are diminished on the affected side. A chest X-ray reveals partial or complete collapse of the lung and the presence of air in the pleural cavity (**Figure 13-6**).

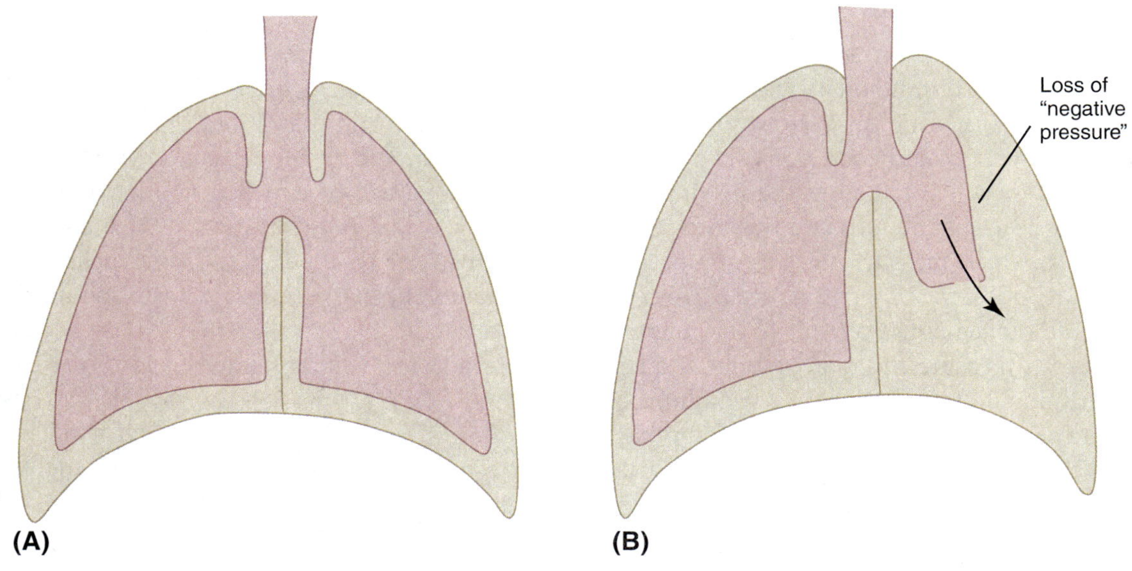

Figure 13-5 **(A)** Normal relation of lung to chest wall. Pleural space is exaggerated, and surfaces are normally in contact. "Negative pressure" is primarily a result of the tendency of the stretched lung to pull away from the chest wall. **(B)** Pneumothorax caused by a perforating injury of the lung, allowing the air under atmospheric pressure to escape into the pleural cavity.

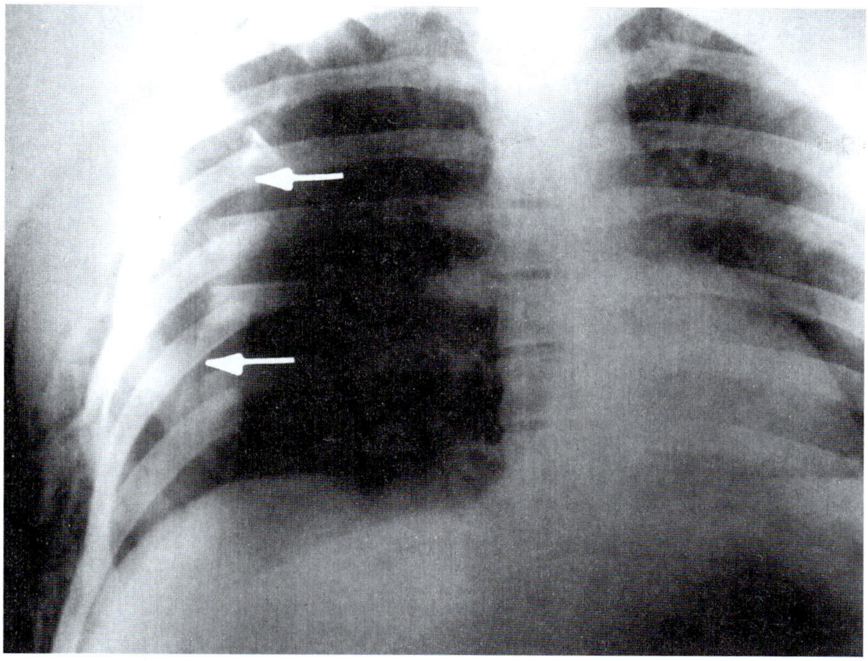

Figure 13-6 X-ray illustrating pneumothorax secondary to multiple rib fractures in which broken ends of fractured ribs have torn through the pleura and the underlying lung. The surface of the lungs is no longer in contact with chest wall (*arrows*).
Courtesy of Leonard V. Crowley, MD, Century College.

The development of a positive (higher than atmospheric) pressure in the pleural cavity, called tension pneumothorax, may accompany any type of pneumothorax. This dangerous complication may occur if the lung has been perforated in such a way that the pleural tear acts as a one-way valve (**Figure 13-7**). With each inspiration, more air enters the pleural cavity but cannot escape.

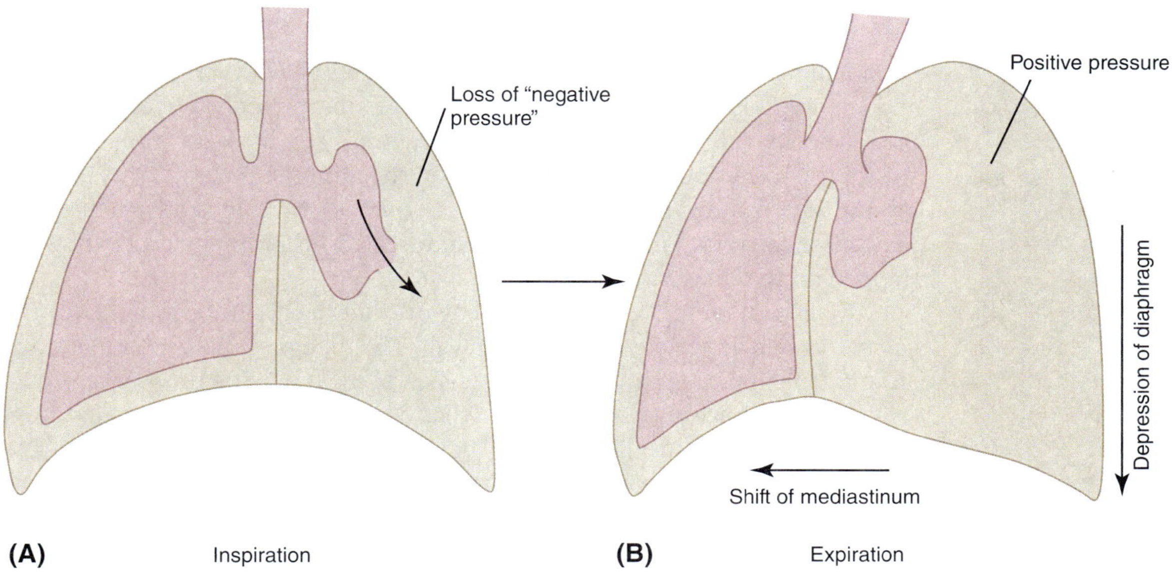

Figure 13-7 Pathogenesis of tension pneumothorax. **(A)** Air enters the pleural cavity during inspiration as intrapleural pressure falls. **(B)** Rising intrapleural pressure on expiration closes the pleural tear, trapping air within the pleural space. The diaphragm on the affected side is displaced downward. The trachea and mediastinal structures are shifted away from the side of pneumothorax and encroach on the opposite pleural cavity.

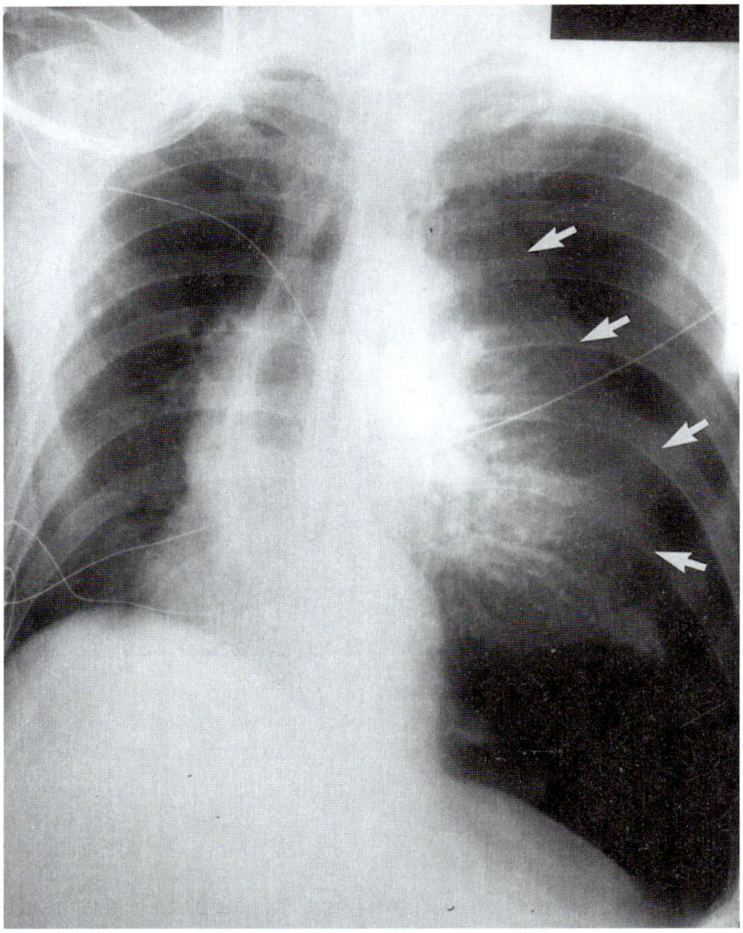

Figure 13-8 An X-ray on tension pneumothorax showing the surface of the collapsed lung (*arrows*). Note the low diaphragm on the affected side and displacement of mediastinal structures.

Eventually, the pleural cavity becomes overdistended with air under pressure, and the affected lung collapses completely. As the pressure builds up in the pleural cavity, the heart and mediastinal structures are displaced away from the side of the pneumothorax and encroach on the opposite pleural cavity, impairing the expansion of the opposite lung (**Figure 13-8**). A tension pneumothorax can be fatal if it is not recognized and treated promptly by evacuating the trapped air to relieve the pressure.

A pneumothorax is usually treated by inserting a chest tube into the pleural cavity through an incision in the chest wall. The tube prevents accumulation of air in the pleural cavity and aids reexpansion of the lung. The tube is connected to an apparatus with a one-way valve that permits the air to be expelled from the pleural cavity during expiration but prevents the air from being sucked back into the pleural cavity during inspiration. The tube is left in place until the tear in the lung heals and no more air escapes. Any air remaining in the pleural cavity is gradually reabsorbed into the bloodstream, and the lung reexpands as the air is absorbed. Sometimes a slight vacuum is applied to the tube to evacuate the air more rapidly and hasten reexpansion of the lung.

Atelectasis

Atelectasis literally means incomplete expansion of the lung (ateles = incomplete + ectasia = expansion). It refers to a collapse of parts of the lung. There are two types of atelectasis: obstructive and compression. A special form of atelectasis may occur in neonates that have not synthesized sufficient surfactant to allow for lung expansion. This may result in a condition termed *neonatal respiratory distress syndrome*.

Atelectasis Collapse of the lung, either caused by bronchial obstruction (obstructive atelectasis) or external compression (compression atelectasis).

Obstructive Atelectasis

Complete blockage of a bronchus by thick mucus secretions, by a tumor, or by an aspirated foreign object prevents air from entering or leaving the alveoli supplied by the blocked bronchus, and the air already present is gradually absorbed into the blood flowing through the lungs. As a result, the part of the lung supplied by the blocked bronchus gradually collapses as the air is absorbed. The volume of the affected pleural cavity also decreases correspondingly, causing the mediastinal structures to shift toward the side of the atelectasis and the diaphragm to elevate on the affected side (**Figure 13-9** and **Figure 13-10**). If the bronchial obstruction is relieved promptly, the lung reexpands normally.

Atelectasis sometimes develops as a postoperative complication. Because of postoperative pain, the patient does not cough or breathe deeply, and mucous secretions accumulate in the bronchi. To prevent this problem, the healthcare providers encourage the postoperative patient to breathe deeply and cough frequently to keep the respiratory passages clear of secretions. A device called an incentive spirometer allows the patient to monitor his breathing and work to prevent the problem.

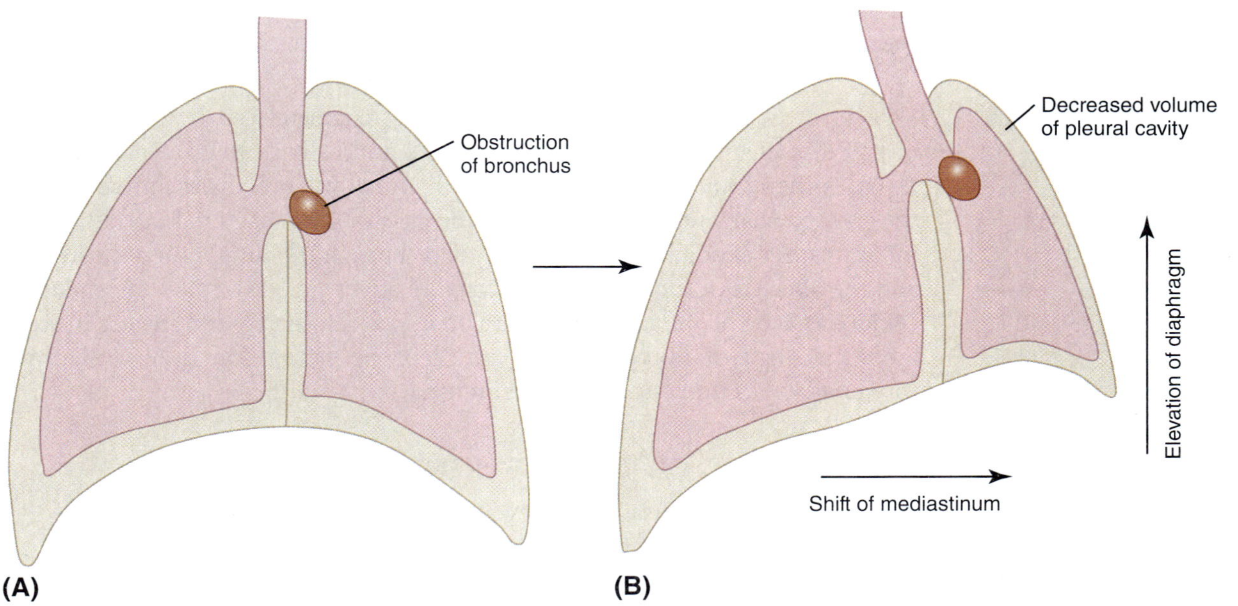

Figure 13-9 Atelectasis caused by bronchial obstruction. **(A)** Blockage of the bronchus prevents aeration of the lung supplied by the obstructed bronchus. **(B)** Absorption of air caused collapse of the lung and a corresponding reduction in size of the pleural cavity. The diaphragm rises, and the mediastinum shifts toward the affected side.

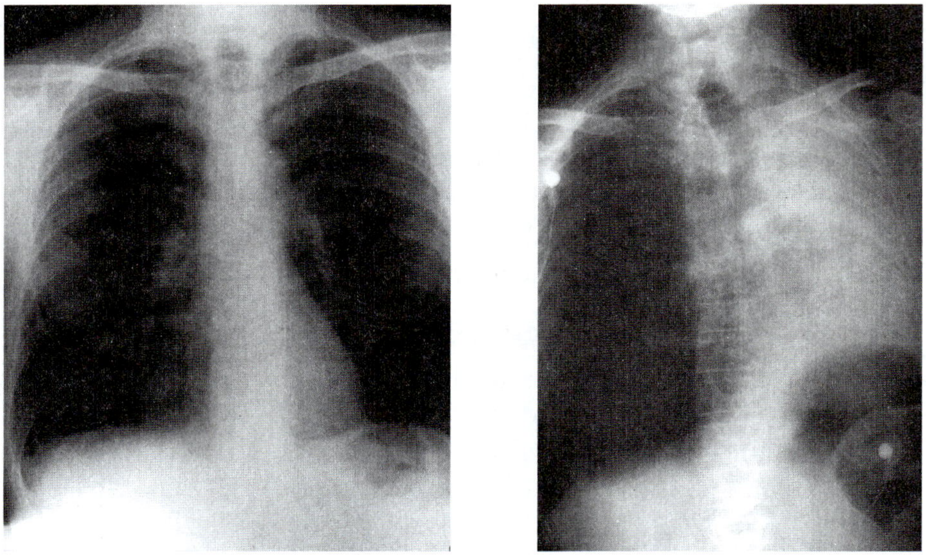

(A) (B)

Figure 13-10 Complete atelectasis of the left lung caused by obstruction of the left, main bronchus. **(A)** Chest X-ray before development of atelectasis. **(B)** Atelectasis of the entire left lung. The collapsed lung appears dense because the air has been absorbed. The left half of the diaphragm is elevated. The trachea and mediastinal structures are shifted toward the side of the collapse.

Compression Atelectasis

Compression atelectasis results when fluid, blood, or air accumulates in the pleural cavity, reducing its volume and thereby preventing full expansion of the lung.

Pneumonia

Pneumonia Inflammation of the lung.

Pneumonia is an inflammation of the lung characterized by the same type of vascular changes and exudation of fluid and cells as that of inflammation in any other location. However, the inflammatory process is influenced by the spongy character of the lungs. In the case of most bacterial infections, the inflammatory exudate spreads unimpeded through the lung, filling the alveoli, and the affected portions of lung become relatively solid (termed *consolidation*) (**Figure 13-11**). The inflammatory exudate may reach the pleural surface in some areas, causing irritation and inflammation of the pleura; sometimes inflammatory exudate accumulates in the pleural space.

Classification of Pneumonia

Pneumonia may be classified in several ways, including etiology, anatomic distribution, or predisposing factors.

The etiologic classification is the most important because it serves as a guide to treatment. Pneumonia may be caused by bacteria, chlamydiae, mycoplasmas, rickettsiae, viruses, or fungi. Whenever possible, the pneumonia is classified in greater detail by designating the exact organism responsible for the infection, such as the pneumococcus, staphylococcus, mycoplasma, or coronavirus. The most common type of bacterial pneumonia is caused by infection with *Streptococcus pneumoniae*. Pneumonia as a result of infection by this

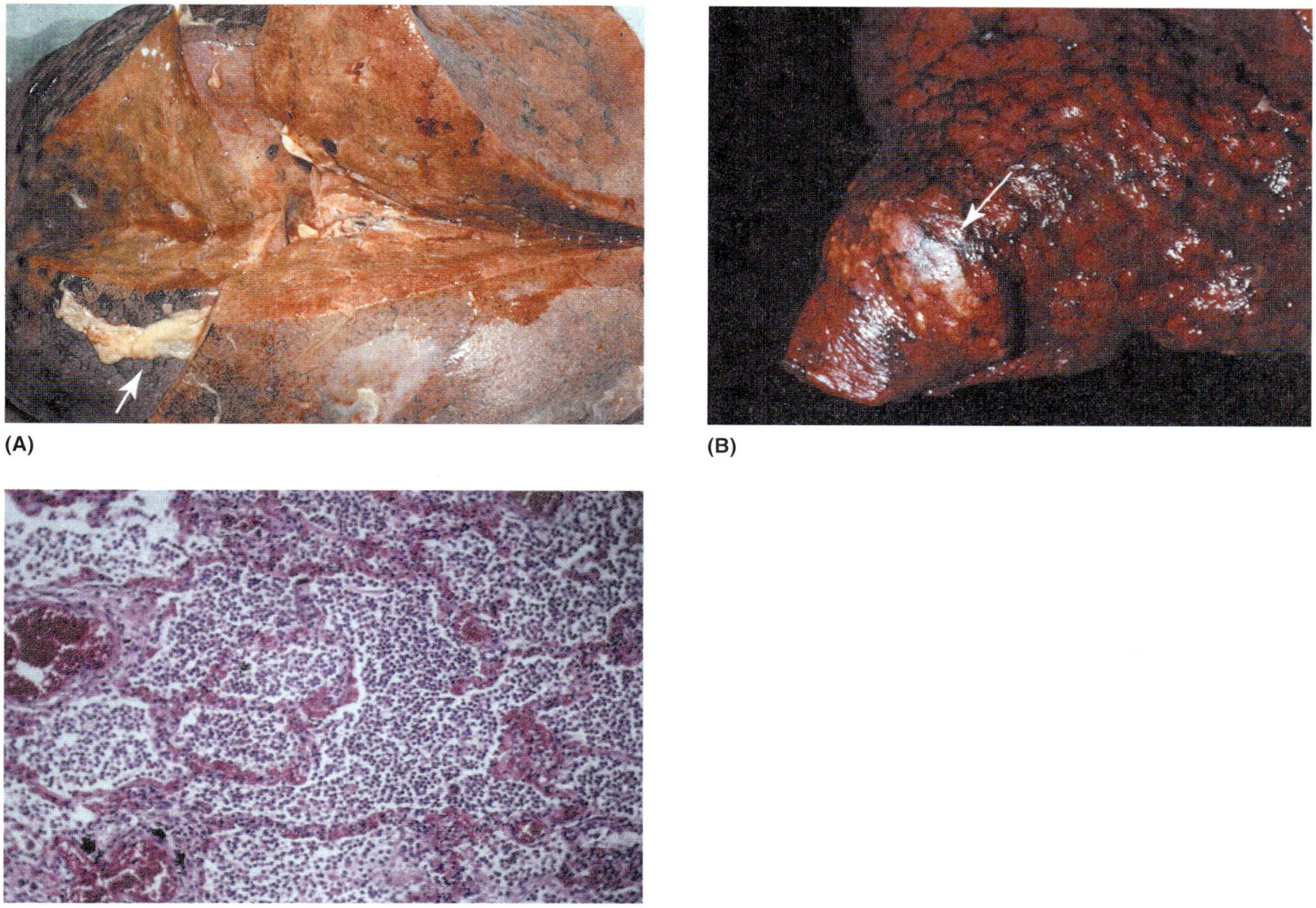

(A) (B) (C)

Figure 13-11 **(A)** Consolidation of lung lobe caused by lobar pneumonia. The lung has been incised, and cut surfaces are exposed. There is a deposit of fibrin (*arrow*) on pleura. **(B)** Bronchopneumonia. Inflammation involved lung lobules rather than an entire lobe. The most severely involved lobules (*arrow*) are shown. **(C)** Histologic appearance of pneumonia. Alveoli are filled with neutrophils, and no air can enter the affected alveoli (original magnification ×100).

Courtesy of Leonard V. Crowley, MD, Century College.

organism is a common cause of death in debilitated elderly individuals. A variety of bacteria can cause community-acquired pneumonia, including *Haemophilus influenzae* and *Staphylococcus aureus*, the latter most commonly following a viral infection. Pneumococcal pneumonia generally occurs in adolescent to middle-aged individuals, often following an infection of the upper respiratory tract such as influenza when host defense barriers are compromised. Antibiotic-resistant strains of microbes are a serious problem in hospitalized patients or those likely to have recurrent pneumonias. Chapter 7 provides additional details on pathogenic microorganisms.

The anatomic classification describes what part of the lung is involved (Figure 13-11). Lobar pneumonia refers to an infection of the entire lung lobe. Bronchopneumonia describes an infection involving only parts of one or more lobes (lung lobules) adjacent to the bronchi. Lobar pneumonia and bronchopneumonia are infections caused by pathogenic bacteria. The classic example of lobar pneumonia is that caused by *Streptococcus pneumoniae*; however, with antibiotic therapy, many cases are expressed as bronchopneumonias. A third anatomic classification is interstitial pneumonia, or primary atypical pneumonia, and is usually caused by a virus or commonly, mycoplasma (*Mycoplasma pneumoniae*). This type of pulmonary infection involves the pulmonary alveolar septa rather than the alveoli, and the inflammatory cells infiltrating the septa are primarily lymphocytes, monocytes, and plasma cells rather than neutrophils.

Classification of pneumonia by predisposing factors is common. Any condition associated with poor lung ventilation and retention of bronchial secretions predisposes an individual to the development of pneumonia. Postoperative pneumonia is a pulmonary inflammation that develops in the postsurgical patient who is unable to cough or breathe deeply; the resultant poor ventilation and retention of secretions predispose to atelectasis of lung lobules, which is followed by secondary bacterial invasion leading to bronchopneumonia. Aspiration pneumonia occurs when a foreign body, food, vomit, or other irritating substance is aspirated into the lung. Obstructive pneumonia develops in the lung distal to an area where the bronchus is narrowed or obstructed. Blockage of a bronchus by a tumor or foreign body leads to poor aeration and retention of bronchial secretions in the obstructed part of the lung, which predisposes to infection.

Clinical Features of Pneumonia

The signs and symptoms of pneumonia are those of any systemic infection. The patient is ill and has an elevated temperature, and the number of white blood cells in the peripheral blood is frequently higher than normal. Bronchial inflammation is evident, manifested by cough and purulent sputum. If the inflammatory process involves the pleura, the patient experiences pain on respiration because the inflamed pleural surfaces rub against each other. The patient may also have symptoms related to partial loss of lung function caused by consolidation of part of the lung, resulting from the accumulation of inflammatory cells within the alveoli. Oxygenation of the blood is impaired, and the patient may become quite short of breath. Pneumonia is treated by correcting any predisposing factors that contributed to the development of the pulmonary infection and administering antibiotic therapy when appropriate.

Legionnaires' disease
A type of pneumonia caused by an airborne bacterium called *Legionella pneumophila*.

Legionnaires' disease is a type of pneumonia caused by a gram-negative, rod-shaped bacterium called *Legionella pneumophila* that is widely distributed in the environment: in the soil and in freshwater ponds, lakes, and streams. The organism thrives in moist environments, such as air-conditioning ducts, shower heads, humidifiers, and hot tubs. People become infected by inhaling airborne organisms in aerosolized water droplets. The infection is not transmitted directly from person to person. The disease was first recognized in 1976 among people attending an American Legion convention in Philadelphia. After the infectious agent was identified, it was determined in retrospect that this same organism had in the past caused other outbreaks of pneumonia, but the infectious agent was not identified at the time. Clinically, the disease is characterized by the usual symptoms of a pulmonary infection and often abdominal pain. The chest X-ray reveals characteristic evidence of pneumonia. The infection responds to appropriate antibiotics. Pontiac fever is a related, milder form of the disease with flu-like symptoms that is not associated with pneumonia.

Additional Lung Infections: SARS, MERS, and COVID-19

These conditions, severe acute respiratory syndrome (SARS), Middle Eastern respiratory syndrome (MERS), and COVID-19, are highly communicable, serious pulmonary infections caused by unusual beta coronaviruses that have spread rapidly through several countries since each was first identified (SARS in late 2002, MERS in 2012, and COVID-19 in late 2019 to early 2020). SARS was last reported in 2004; MERS infections are still occurring in 2025. COVID-19 is currently considered to be endemic, with cases occurring in essentially every country in the world. During the COVID-19 pandemic there were at least 705 million cases worldwide and seven million deaths. In the United States there were over 111 million cases and one million deaths, with hundreds of cases still occurring weekly. Several antiviral drugs (Paxlovid, for example) are currently available for mild to moderate disease and can prevent severe illness and death.

Coronaviruses are ribonucleic acid (RNA) viruses that received their name from the crownlike spikes projecting from the viruses as seen by electron microscopy (corona = crown). There are many groups of coronaviruses that cause disease in animals and humans. Previously, most of the infections in humans caused by coronaviruses were common colds, not lower respiratory tract infections. The SARS-, MERS-, and COVID-19 (SARS-COV-2)–associated viruses, however, are unique in that they are the first ones known to cause severe, potentially lethal disease in people. Precautions to prevent infection when dealing with patients include personal protective equipment such as gloves, gowns, masks, and eye protection.

The illnesses begin with chills and fever, sometimes mild respiratory symptoms, and occasionally diarrhea. After 3 to 7 days, manifestations of lower respiratory tract infection appear: cough, shortness of breath, and evidence of pneumonia demonstrated by chest X-ray examination. The severity of the illness varies with the causative virus, with about one-third of the cases being fatal in MERS infections. The fatality rate in COVID-19 is variable and has declined since early in the pandemic. Initial estimates were from under 1 percent to over 2 percent but were strongly dependent on the age and health status of the patient. Currently the overall fatality rate in the United States is about 0.6%. The lungs of severely affected patients show the characteristic features of adult respiratory distress syndrome, and patients require mechanical ventilation using an increased oxygen concentration to improve the diffusion of oxygen across the thickened edematous alveolar septa, as well as other measures to improve pulmonary function. Most cases of COVID-19 are mild (80 percent), but about 5 percent are critical and require pulmonary support. Although current cases in the recent outbreak of MERS are a result of human-to-human spread, dromedary camels are reservoirs for the virus. The disease started in the Middle East, with cases reported worldwide (including a major outbreak in Korea). All cases have been linked to or occur in the Middle East (predominantly Saudi Arabia). To date, two cases have been imported into the United States.

Unlike SARS, which was spread predominantly in hospital settings, the great majority of COVID-19 cases are the result of person-to-person respiratory droplet spread. COVID-19 is transmitted predominantly by inhaled aerosol droplets (although the eyes, surfaces, and other portals of entry can play a role in spread). For this reason, effective surgical masks and other forms of aerosol protection have been suggested to minimize spread between infected persons and others. Vaccination is partially effective in preventing severe disease but appears to require occasional boosters to account for waning immunity and new coronavirus variants.

Respiratory Syncytial Virus (RSV)

RSV is a common, predominantly seasonal, viral disease that generally produces mild, cold-like symptoms. However, RSV can cause severe illness in infants and the elderly and is a leading cause of infant hospitalization.

The disease can cause infections of the bronchioles and pneumonia in severe cases. RSV spreads by aerosols and contaminated surfaces, much like COVID-19 and other common respiratory diseases. There is an effective vaccine recommended for the elderly and for pregnant mothers.

Pneumocystis Pneumonia

Humans harbor *Pneumocystis jirovecii*, a small yeast-like fungus of low pathogenicity in immunocompetent individuals. The fungus does not affect healthy people but may cause serious pulmonary infections in susceptible individuals. Those at risk include adults whose immune defenses have been impaired by communicable disease, such as AIDS, or by administration of immunosuppressive drugs, and premature infants in whom immune defenses are poorly developed.

The fungi, intermixed in the alveolar exudate, can be demonstrated by special staining procedures (**Figure 13-12**).

Clinically, pneumocystis pneumonia is characterized by progressive shortness of breath and cough in a person whose immunologic defenses are impaired and who is at high risk of developing the disease. The infection is always very

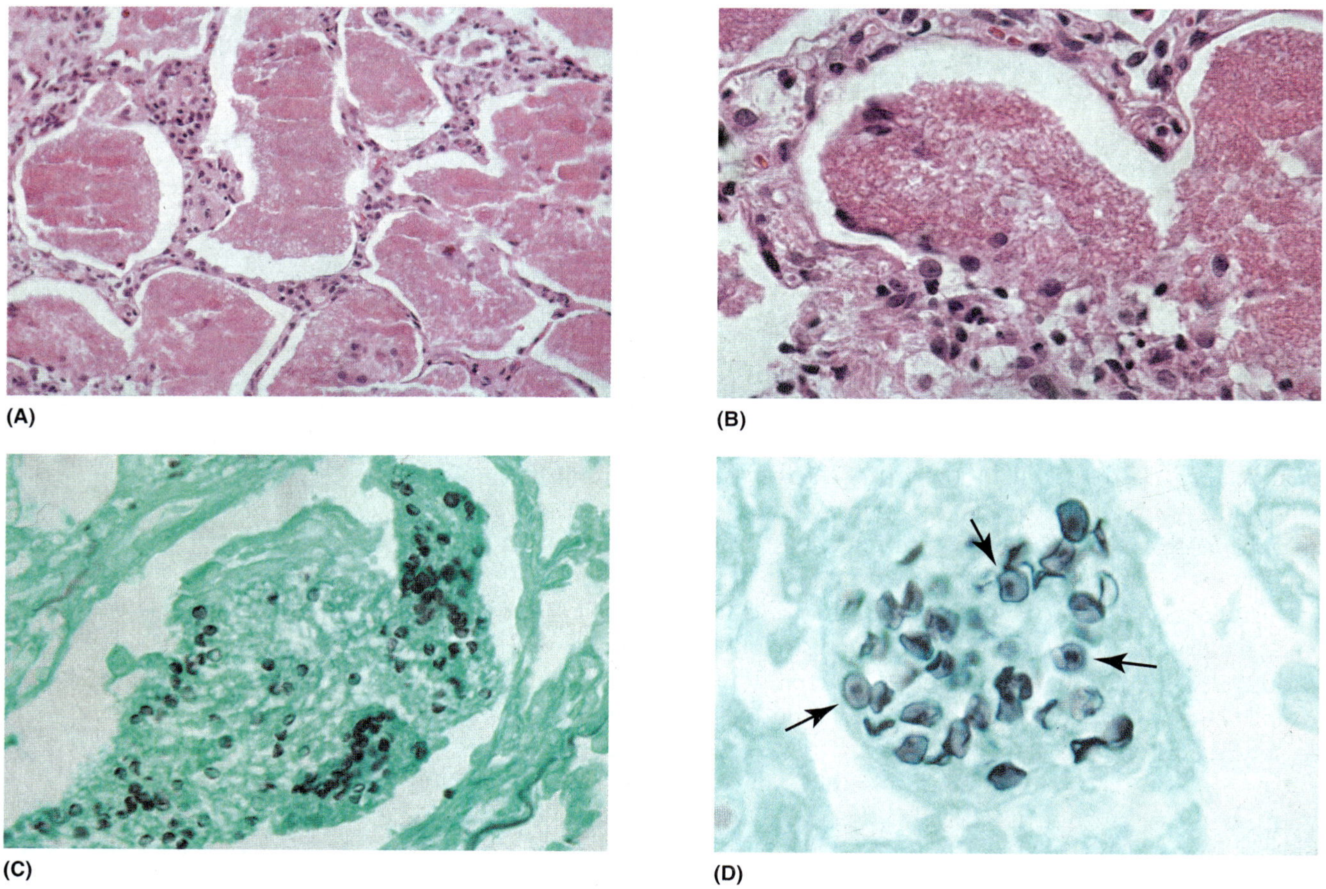

Figure 13-12 Pneumocystis pneumonia. **(A)** Pulmonary alveoli filled with dense protein exudate (original magnification ×100). **(B)** Higher magnification, illustrating the foamy, "soap-bubble" appearance of the alveolar exudate. The clear areas in the alveolar exudate are *Pneumocystis* organisms that are not stained by routine stains (original magnification ×400). **(C)** Demonstration of *Pneumocystis jirovecii* cysts within the alveolar exudate by means of silver-containing stains (original magnification ×400). **(D)** High-magnification view of the organisms demonstrated by silver stains. Central dark dots within the cysts are clusters of sporozoites (original magnification ×1000).

Courtesy of Leonard V. Crowley, MD, Century College.

serious and may be life-threatening because it affects people whose ability to respond to infection is greatly impaired. Once common in AIDS patients, effective antiretroviral therapy and drug treatment have reduced the frequency of cases.

Tuberculosis

Pulmonary tuberculosis (TB) is a distinctive type of pneumonia caused by an acid-fast bacterium, the tubercle bacillus *Mycobacterium tuberculosis*. Because the tubercle bacillus has a capsule composed of waxes and fatty substances, it is more resistant to destruction than many other organisms. The body's response to the tubercle bacillus also differs from the usual acute inflammatory reaction. **Epithelioid macrophages**, characterized by their flat, epithelial appearance, accumulate around the bacteria; many of them fuse, often forming large, multinucleated cells called giant cells. Lymphocytes and plasma cells accumulate, and fibrous tissue proliferates around the central cluster of epithelioid macrophages and giant cells. The central portion of the cellular aggregation usually becomes necrotic. Because of its anatomically gross appearance, the necrotic center is described as **caseous** (derived from the German word for cheese). This characteristic nodular mass of cells with central necrosis is called a caseating granuloma, and the inflammatory process is called a granulomatous inflammation (**Figure 13-13**). The granulomatous response to the tubercle bacillus and the necrosis within the granulomas indicate the development of cell-mediated immunity against the organism, which is the primary immune defense against the tubercle bacillus. Caseating granulomas (sometimes called tubercules) are highly characteristic of tuberculosis infection. Other disease processes can result in granulomatous inflammation, but in those cases the granulomas do not have caseating centers.

Epithelioid macrophages Activated macrophages that resemble the appearance of epithelial cells.

Caseous Necrotic center of nodule characteristic of tuberculosis.

Primary tuberculosis Initial infection of tuberculosis.

Course of a Tuberculous Infection

The initial infection (**primary tuberculosis**) is acquired from organisms inhaled in airborne droplets that have been coughed or sneezed into the air by a person with active tuberculosis who is discharging organisms into the

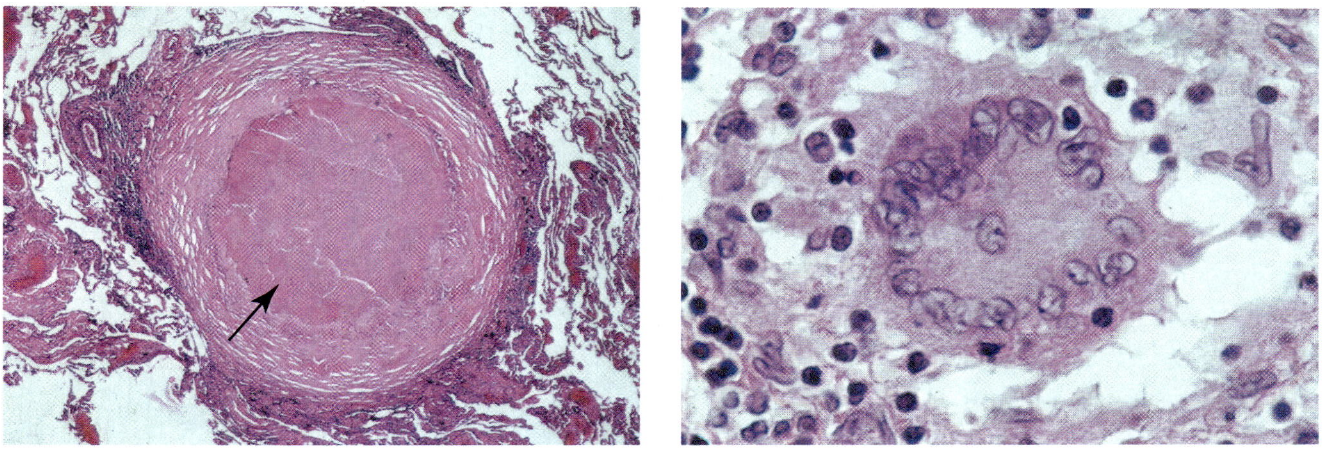

(A) (B)

Figure 13-13 **(A)** Granuloma as a result of tuberculosis. The central part (*arrow*) consists of necrotic tissue (original magnification ×40). **(B)** Multinucleated giant cell characteristic of tuberculosis infection (original magnification ×400).

Courtesy of Leonard V. Crowley, MD, Century College.

environment. The organisms lodge within the pulmonary alveoli, where they proceed to multiply. Initially, the organisms introduced into the lungs do not elicit a marked inflammatory reaction because they do not produce any toxins or destructive enzymes that damage the tissues. Macrophages phagocytose the bacteria but are unable to destroy them; they may even carry the organisms to other parts of the lung and into the regional lymph nodes. After several weeks, however, a cell-mediated immunity develops. Sensitized lymphocytes attract and activate macrophages, which acquire a greatly enhanced phagocytic and destructive capability. The activated macrophages attack and destroy many of the organisms, forming characteristic granulomas containing areas of necrosis surrounded by a rim of fibrous tissue. In the majority of cases, the infection is arrested; the granulomas in the lung and regional lymph nodes heal with scarring and calcification, often followed by development into inactive lesions called **Ghon complexes** (**Figure 13-14**). In most cases, the infection does not cause any symptoms, and the person may be unaware of the infection. Sometimes the granuloma in the lung is large enough to be identified in a chest X-ray, but often the area of infection is too small to be detected. A positive skin test (Mantoux or tine test) reveals a hypersensitivity to the proteins of the tubercle bacillus and may be the only evidence of recent infection.

Ghon complexes Inactive tubercular lesions.

Latent tuberculosis Arrested tuberculosis infection containing viable organisms.

Progressive primary tuberculosis Initial tubercular infection that does not go into remission.

Cell-mediated immunity generally controls the infection, and the arrested infection may never cause any further problems. This condition is **latent tuberculosis** because the healed granulomas contain small numbers of viable organisms. Although these individuals are not infectious, the disease may become reactivated, leading to secondary (cavitary) progressive pulmonary tuberculosis if the body's cell-mediated immunity declines.

Not all primary infections respond as favorably. If a large number of organisms are inhaled or if the body's defenses are inadequate, as in patients with AIDS, the inflammation may progress, a condition termed **progressive primary tuberculosis**, which occurs in less than 10 percent of primary TB exposures. In these cases, there is extensive destruction of lung tissue

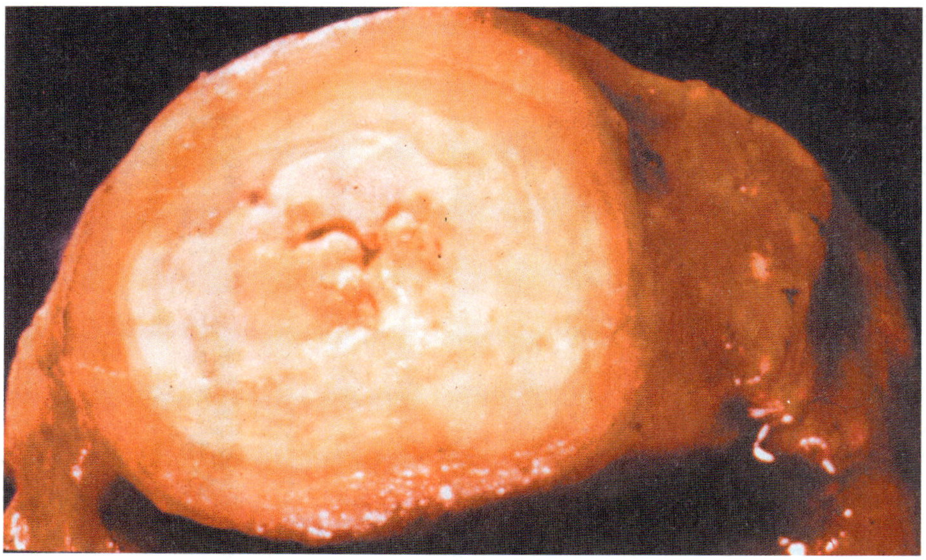

Figure 13-14 Ghon complex from a healed pulmonary granuloma as a result of primary tuberculosis. The central part consists of necrotic tissue containing calcium deposits surrounded by a rim of dense fibrous tissue.

Courtesy of Leonard V. Crowley, MD, Century College.

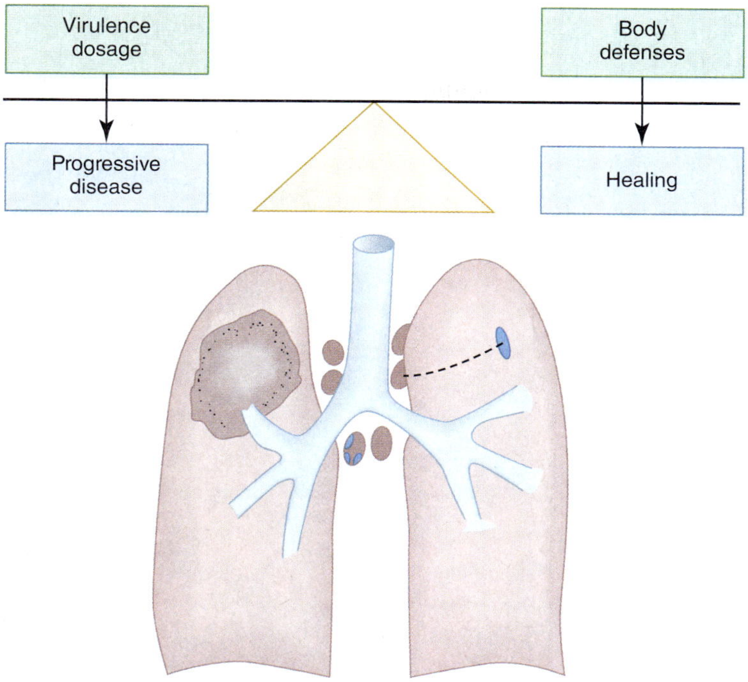

Figure 13-15 Possible outcome of a tuberculosis infection in relation to virulence and dosage of the organism and resistance of the body. The frequent involvement of the regional lymph nodes is indicated. *Left*, a progressive disease with the formation of a cavity within the lung, caused by infection by a large number of organisms or inadequate body defenses. *Right*, healing with scarring as a result of small numbers of organisms or a high degree of resistance to infection.

(**Figure 13-15**) and potential spread of the infection throughout the body. Organisms are often carried in lymphatic channels from the lung into the peribronchial lymph nodes, leading to tuberculous inflammation in the regional lymph nodes. Systemic spread of disease is associated with the formation of multiple small granulomas in many organs, a condition termed **miliary tuberculosis** (because of the resemblance of the small granulomas to millet seeds).

Miliary tuberculosis Multiple foci of tuberculosis throughout the body as a result of bloodstream dissemination of tubercle bacilli from a primary focus in the lung or peribronchial lymph nodes.

Ninety percent of cases of active progressive pulmonary tuberculosis do not result from the initial infection but rather reactivation of latent TB leading to active progressive disease or occasionally reinfection. If the immune competency of the individual is lowered due to pathological processes, by treatment with adrenal corticosteroids, or by other factors, an apparently healed focus of tuberculosis may flare up and lead to active progressive tuberculosis. In these cases, the granulomatous inflammatory process makes contact with a bronchus, and the necrotic inflammatory tissue is discharged into it. A cavity then forms within the lung, surrounded by granulomatous inflammatory tissue containing masses of tubercle bacilli (**Figure 13-16**). People who have active progressive tuberculosis with a tuberculous cavity can infect others because they discharge large numbers of tubercle bacilli in their sputum, which can lead to additional cases of both primary and secondary TB.

Extrapulmonary Tuberculosis

Sometimes tuberculosis develops in the kidneys, bones (particularly the spine, where it is termed *Pott's disease*), adrenal glands, uterus, fallopian tubes, or other extrapulmonary locations. The infection results from hematogenous spread of tubercle bacilli from a focus of tuberculosis in the lung. Sometimes,

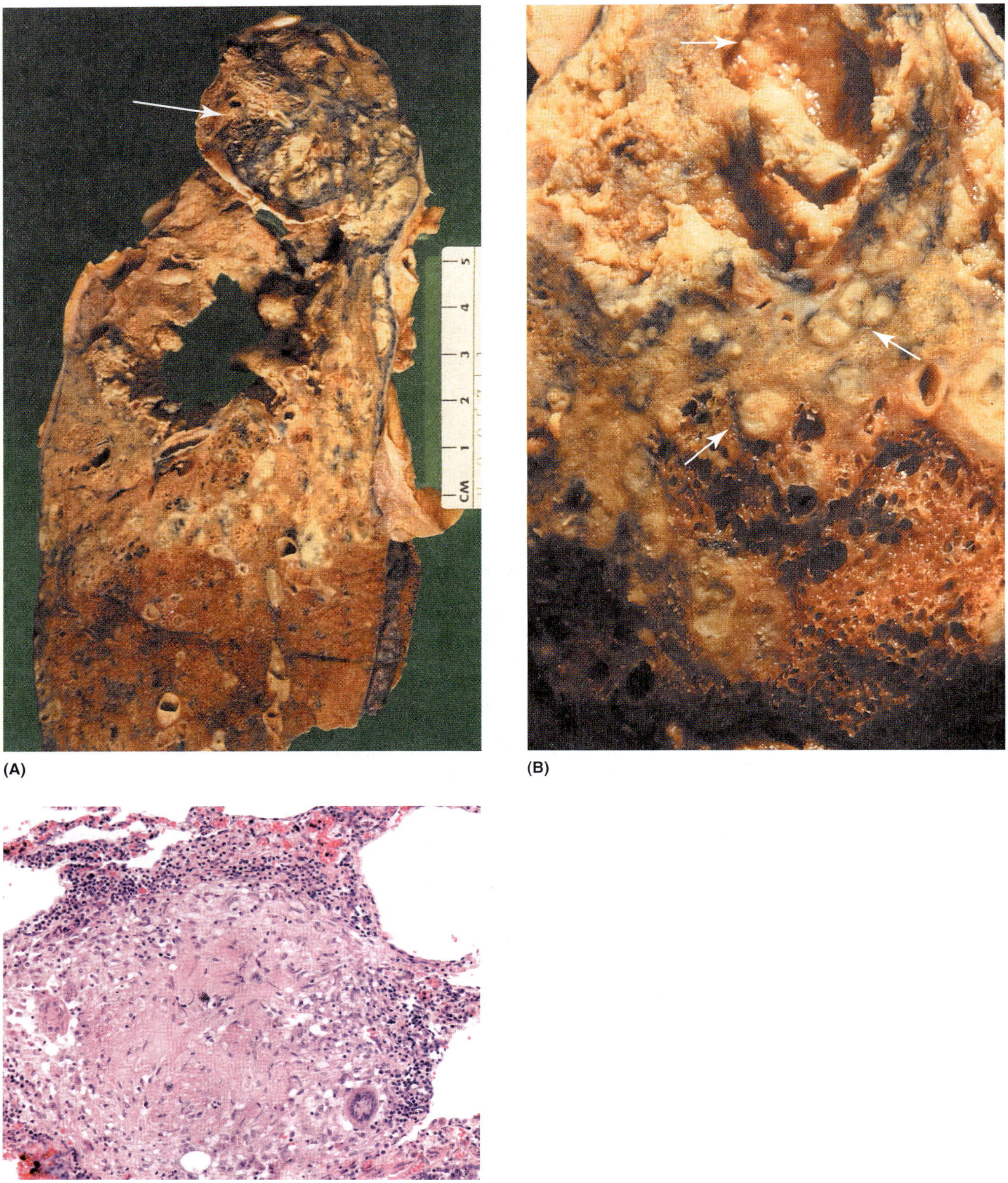

(A)

(B)

(C)

Figure 13-16 Far-advanced pulmonary tuberculosis. **(A)** The upper lobe (*arrow*) has been completely destroyed by tuberculosis, and there is extensive tuberculosis in the lower lobe with a large cavity in the lung that communicated with a bronchus. Only the lower part of the lobe is free of disease (*extreme bottom*). **(B)** A closer view of tuberculosis. A large cavity (*upper arrow*) surrounded by nodular and diffuse granulomatous inflammation. Several discrete granulomas (*lower arrows*) can be seen below the cavity. **(C)** Granuloma of tuberculosis in a human lung showing a central fibrosis surrounded by a chronic infiltrate in giant cells.

(A, B) Courtesy of Leonard V. Crowley, MD, Century College; **(C)** © Jose Luis Calvo/Shutterstock the secondary focus of infection may progress even though the pulmonary infection has healed, leading to an active extrapulmonary tuberculous infection without clinically apparent pulmonary tuberculosis.

Diagnosis and Treatment of Tuberculosis

Tuberculous infection is associated with the development of hypersensitivity to proteins in the tubercle bacillus, as discussed in Chapter 5, Immunity, Hypersensitivity, Allergy, and Autoimmune Diseases. A positive skin test indicates that the person was at one time infected with the tubercle bacillus; it does not necessarily indicate an active infection. In some areas, immunization to TB (BCG immunization) is common and will result in "false positive" skin tests. Hence, clinical examinations, including chest radiographs and bacteriological examination of specimens such as sputum and urine, are critical. Additional nucleic acid–based tests can also be used to detect the organism and predict resistance to forms of drug therapy as discussed shortly.

At present, the recommendation is that individuals who develop an infection with the tubercle bacillus, as manifested by conversion of a negative into a positive skin test reaction, be treated with antituberculosis drugs. Treatment is also recommended for patients with inactive tuberculosis who have an increased risk of developing a reactivation of an old, apparently healed tuberculous infection.

The incidence of TB in the United States has continued to rise since 2003 and is currently at its highest level since 2011. Much of the rise is related to international travel and migration with 75% of cases found in the foreign-born patients. Such individuals may come from areas where the prevalence of tuberculosis is much higher. Many of these unfortunate people with active tuberculosis or latent disease do not receive adequate ongoing medical care; they also may not be motivated to complete the full course of treatment needed to arrest the disease. Failure to complete treatment leads to treatment failure, and premature cessation of treatment promotes the emergence of drug-resistant strains of the organism. Large, localized outbreaks of TB have occurred in the United States, including a recent major outbreak in Kansas City.

Drug-Resistant Tuberculosis

Effective drug treatment of tuberculosis has transformed the infection from a potentially fatal chronic disease to one that could be treated effectively by a number of antibiotics and chemotherapeutic agents. Unfortunately, drug-resistant tuberculosis is becoming a major problem. Tuberculosis caused by organisms resistant to at least two of the most commonly used antituberculosis drugs is designated as multiple drug–resistant tuberculosis (MDR-TB), which is more difficult to treat. Currently the rate of MDR-TB is low in the United States (less than 1.5 percent, with most cases occurring in the foreign-born). However, rates may be as high as 20 percent in some parts of the world. The drug-resistance problem has become even more concerning. Some strains no longer respond to a large number of antituberculosis drugs, and an infection by these organisms is designated extremely drug-resistant tuberculosis (XDR-TB). Although XDR-TB is very uncommon in the United States, with less than 70 cases reported to date, it is a major public health risk. Several countries have reported XDR-TB resistant to all currently available drugs. People with XDR-TB need to obtain treatment at a facility accustomed to dealing with these resistant organisms, and the patients' activities need to be restricted so they cannot spread the infection. The World Health Organization has become increasingly concerned about the spread of XDR-TB cases. Most have been concentrated in Eastern Europe, South Africa, and Asia, but as noted, cases do appear in the United States, and control measures to prevent further spread are considered essential.

Bronchitis and Bronchiectasis

Bronchiectasis Dilatation of bronchi caused by a weakened airway wall as a result of infection.

Chronic obstructive pulmonary disease (COPD) Combination of emphysema and chronic bronchitis.

Acute inflammation of the tracheobronchial mucosa is common in many upper respiratory infections. The raw throat and cough associated with many respiratory infections are a result of the associated acute bronchitis. Chronic bronchitis also is common; often, it results from constant irritation of the respiratory mucosa by smoking cigarettes or breathing air containing large amounts of atmospheric pollution.

Sometimes the bronchial walls in parts of the lung become weakened as a result of severe inflammation or other factors, and the affected bronchi become markedly dilated. This condition is termed **bronchiectasis** (ectasis = dilation). The distended bronchi tend to retain secretions. Consequently, patients with bronchiectasis frequently have a chronic cough associated with the production of large amounts of purulent sputum. Often, they suffer repeated bouts of pulmonary infection. Bronchiectasis is not curable, but symptoms may respond to drug and exercise therapy. Oxygen therapy may be required in severe disease. Bronchiectasis can be recognized by means of lung function tests and radiography.

Chronic Obstructive Pulmonary Disease (COPD)

COPD is a chronic inflammatory lung disease that causes obstructed airflow. Emphysema and chronic bronchitis are the two common conditions that exemplify the disease. COPD affects nearly 16 million adults; it is a major cause of disability, and it was the sixth leading cause of death in the United States in 2021, according to the CDC. Exposure to irritant gases, most commonly cigarette smoke, is by far the most common cause of COPD; other factors, such as occupational exposure, air pollution, and α-1 antitrypsin deficiency also play a role. The main clinical manifestations of COPD are dyspnea and cyanosis. Dyspnea is a sensation of shortness of breath. Cyanosis is a blue tinge of the skin and mucous membrane that results from excessively reduced hemoglobin in the blood. Blood with reduced hemoglobin is dark purplish red, in contrast with normally oxygenated blood, which is bright red.

In emphysema, the normally fine alveolar structure of the lung is destroyed, and large, cystic air spaces form throughout the lung (**Figure 13-17**). The destructive process usually begins in the upper lobes but eventually may affect all lobes of both lungs. The chief symptom of emphysema is shortness of breath. A characteristic "barrel chest" is usually associated with emphysema. Initially, this is noted only on exertion, but later it may be present even at rest. The patient usually also has a chronic cough with purulent sputum, owing to the associated chronic bronchitis. Eventually, severely affected patients may die because they lack enough functionally normal lung tissue to sustain life or because of a superimposed pulmonary infection. Emphysema is also a frequent cause of respiratory acidosis, one of the common disturbances of acid–base balance presented in Chapter 17.

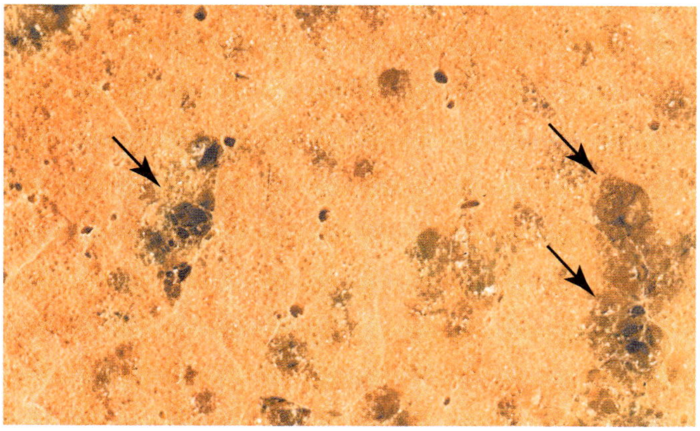

(A)

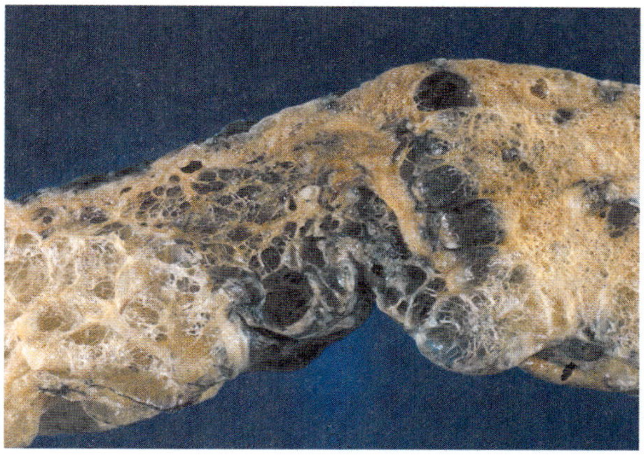

(B)

Figure 13-17 Sections of air-dried lung preparations illustrating the gross appearance of emphysema. **(A)** Mild emphysema. Beginning breakdown of lung tissue to form cystic spaces (*arrows*). Most of the alveoli appear normal. **(B)** Advanced emphysema with multiple confluent cystic spaces within lung. Very little normal lung tissue remains. The dark color is a result of accumulation of carbon pigment in the emphysematous lung from inhaling "dirty" air.

Courtesy of Leonard V. Crowley, MD, Century College.

A chronic cough with sputum production is commonly associated with chronic bronchitis. The patient finds it hard to breathe and becomes more susceptible to secondary infection due to the mucus accumulation.

The three main anatomic derangements in chronic obstructive pulmonary disease are (1) inflammation and narrowing of the terminal bronchioles, (2) dilatation and coalescence of pulmonary air spaces, and (3) loss of lung elasticity. These derangements in turn cause severe disturbances in pulmonary function.

Derangements of Pulmonary Structure and Function in Emphysema

Chronic inflammation of the bronchioles probably initiates the destructive process. Chronic inflammation causes swelling of the bronchial mucosa, which reduces the caliber of the bronchi and bronchioles and stimulates increased bronchial secretions. Because a tube's resistance to air flow varies inversely with the fourth power of its radius, a slight reduction in the caliber of the bronchioles greatly restricts the flow of air. Normally, the bronchi and bronchioles dilate slightly during inspiration to facilitate airflow into the lungs and narrow down during expiration. In patients with emphysema, however, inflammation in the bronchioles causes air to become trapped in the lungs during expiration. This prevents the lung from fully emptying, leading to chronic overinflation. As a result, the capacity to take additional air during a deep breath is compromised, limiting the person's ability to increase ventilation in response to greater respiratory demand.

The bronchiolar obstruction due to inflammation also disturbs pulmonary function by causing unequal air flow to various parts of the lung. Some alveoli are overventilated; others are inadequately supplied, reducing the overall efficiency of pulmonary ventilation. The excess air supplying the overventilated alveoli is "wasted" because more is provided than is needed to completely oxygenate the blood flowing through the surrounding pulmonary capillaries. Conversely, the blood flowing to the poorly ventilated alveoli does not become fully oxygenated. When it mixes with normally oxygenated blood flowing from other parts of the lungs, the oxygen content of the blood delivered to the tissues is reduced.

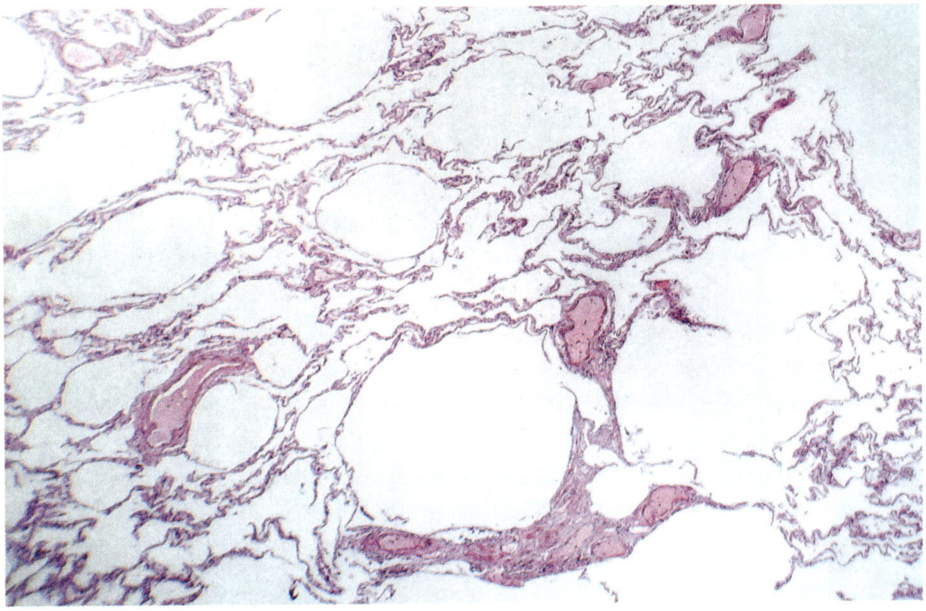

Figure 13-18 Photomicrograph of emphysematous lung. Note the large cystic airspaces that have resulted from the destruction of the alveolar walls.

The destruction of the alveolar septa leads to enlargement of the air spaces and at the same time reduces the number of pulmonary capillaries available for gas exchange. Diffusion of gases is much less efficient from large cystic spaces because the spaces contain a much larger volume of air than does a normal alveolus and are surrounded by a relatively sparse network of capillaries. Moreover, the movement of air into and out of the enlarged spaces is impeded by the bronchiolar obstruction caused by inflammation (**Figure 13-18**).

Destruction of the alveolar septa also leads to loss of the elastic tissue in the septa that forms the structural framework of the lungs, and so the lungs no longer "recoil" normally after they have been stretched during inspiration. Expiration is no longer a passive process. The air must be actively forced out of the lungs by contraction of the intercostal muscles. Breathing takes more effort and in turn requires greater oxygen consumption. The pressure required to actively force air out of the lungs during expiration also raises the intrapleural pressure and compresses the lungs, which causes further problems with pulmonary ventilation. The bronchi and bronchioles have lost their normal structural support because of loss of lung elasticity and tend to collapse during expiration, obstructing the outflow of air and trapping more air within the lungs.

Pathogenesis of Chronic Obstructive Pulmonary Disease

Cigarette smoking is by far the major factor responsible for COPD in the United States. In developing countries, women exposed to fumes produced by cooking with biomass fuels (wood, crop wastage, etc.) are also at increased risk. Exactly how the destructive effect on the lung occurs is not completely understood. **Figure 13-19** summarizes one concept of the pathogenesis of this serious and disabling disease. Smoking and lung irritants expose the bronchial mucosa to chronic irritation, eventually producing chronic bronchitis associated with a chronic cough and increased bronchial secretions. The inflammatory swelling

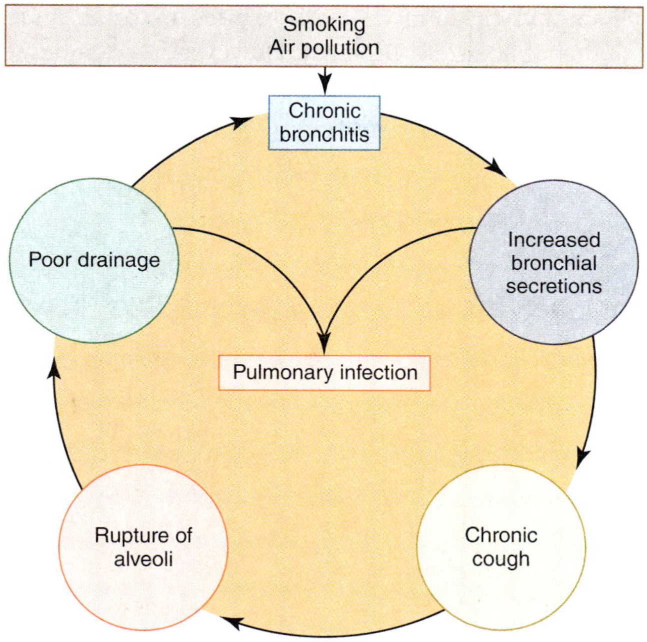

Figure 13-19 A concept of the pathogenesis of chronic obstructive pulmonary disease.

of the mucosa narrows the smaller bronchioles, increasing their resistance to expiration and causing air to be trapped within the lung.

The leukocytes that accumulate in the bronchioles and alveoli contribute to the lung damage by releasing proteolytic (protein-digesting) enzymes, principally elastase, that attack the elastic fibers making up part of the lung's structural framework. The body produces an intrinsic anti-elastase (alpha$_1$ antitrypsin), but the inflammatory infiltrate due to heavy smoking overwhelms this natural defense mechanism. The association of emphysema with a genetic lack of alpha$_1$ antitrypsin (see the following discussion) emphasizes the central role that inflammation-associated release of proteolytic enzymes plays in the generation of emphysema. In addition to furthering pulmonary damage and inflammation, cigarette smoke chemically inactivates alpha$_1$ antitrypsin, increasing damage to the alveolar walls by the proteolytic enzyme released by leukocytes.

Repeated bouts of coughing, with consequent extreme elevations in intrabronchial pressure, cause the alveolar septa to rupture, gradually converting the alveoli into large, cystic air spaces. The lungs become overdistended and lose their normal elasticity. The patient cannot expel air normally from the overdistended lungs because lung elasticity is lost and the bronchioles are obstructed; difficulty expectorating the excessive bronchial secretions also is apparent. Retention of secretions and poor drainage of secretions from the bronchi tend to perpetuate chronic bronchitis, and a vicious circle is created. The diseased lungs are also more susceptible to infection because of impaired pulmonary ventilation, bronchial inflammation, bronchiolar obstruction, and excessive bronchial secretions. Therefore, patients with COPD frequently have repeated bouts of pneumonia, further damaging the lung tissue.

Prevention and Treatment

For the most part, COPD can be prevented by refraining from smoking and avoiding inhalation of other substances known to be injurious to the lungs. Atmospheric air pollution and secondhand smoke contribute to the increasing incidence of emphysema, and various measures are being undertaken to control this serious public health problem. However, after emphysema has developed, the damaged lungs cannot be restored to normal. Several measures can be employed to promote the drainage of bronchial secretions, to improve pulmonary ventilation, and to decrease the frequency of superimposed pulmonary infections. These measures, along with cessation of smoking, will retard or arrest further progression of the disease.

Emphysema as a Result of Alpha$_1$ Antitrypsin Deficiency

Blood and other body fluids contain a serum protein called alpha$_1$ antitrypsin, a normally occurring antineutrophil elastase, and its concentration in the blood is genetically determined. Most individuals produce normal amounts of this molecule, others are severely deficient, and a third group has subnormal levels of this protein.

Individuals with severe antitrypsin deficiency are prone to develop an uncommon type of progressive pulmonary emphysema that usually becomes manifest in adolescence or early adulthood and tends to affect chiefly the lower lobes of the lungs. People with only moderately reduced antitrypsin levels do not develop severe emphysema at an early age but are quite susceptible to lung damage from cigarette smoking, atmospheric air pollution, or respiratory infections.

Bronchial Asthma

Bronchial asthma is characterized by periodic recurring bronchial hyperresponsiveness and recurring bronchoconstriction of the smooth muscle in the walls of the smaller bronchi and bronchioles in response to a number of different agents. It is also associated with increased secretions by the bronchial mucous glands. Asthmatic attacks cause shortness of breath and wheezing respirations occur, caused by restricted movement of air through the tightly constricted air passages. The physiologic derangements in asthma resulting from narrowing of the bronchioles are similar to those in patients with COPD. Bronchiolar spasm exerts a greater effect on expiration than on inspiration because the caliber of the bronchioles varies with the phase of respiration. Consequently, air flow is impeded more on expiration than on inspiration, which leads to air being trapped in the lungs and overinflation of the lungs. The disease is most commonly diagnosed in the young (most before the age of 18) and often becomes milder (or disappears) with increasing age.

Many cases of asthma have an allergic basis, although other factors such as cold and exercise may contribute to the disease. The attacks are precipitated by inhalation of dust, pollens, animal dander, or other allergens, which interact with mast cells coated with IgE antibody. This leads to release of chemical mediators that induce bronchospasm. Acute attacks are treated by administering drugs such as epinephrine or short-acting beta-2 adrenergic agonists such as albuterol, which relaxes the bronchospasm, combined with an antisecretory drug. Often, attacks can be prevented by administering drugs that block the release of mediators from mast cells, such as cromolyn sodium and other drugs, including corticosteroids; long-acting theophylline is also used often. Therapy is complex and generally undertaken by a specialist in the disease, often an allergist. (Allergic diseases are considered in Chapter 5.)

Respiratory Distress Syndrome

Neonatal respiratory distress is discussed in detail in Chapter 16.

Adult Respiratory Distress Syndrome

Adult respiratory distress syndrome (ARDS) is referred to as **diffuse alveolar damage (DAD)** by pathologists and is sometimes called "shock lung" because shock may be associated with the syndrome. ARDS may result from any process that disturbs the alveolar capillary permeability with resultant movement of fluid into the alveolar space. Damage to either the capillary endothelium or the alveolar epithelium may be involved. The most common risk factors are sepsis and related septic shock, bacterial infection, trauma, burns, fractures, near drowning, inhalation of toxic agents, and aspiration of vomitus; sometimes no cause is evident. In many instances, reduced blood flow to the lung (shock) may occur and result in alveolar damage.

Adult respiratory distress syndrome (ARDS)/diffuse alveolar damage (DAD) A life threatening lung injury that causes fluid accumulating into the lungs.

Whatever the predisposing cause of the alveolar damage, the pathophysiologic derangements are damage to alveolar capillaries and alveolar lining cells, impaired formation of surfactant, leakage of protein-rich fluid from the injured capillaries into the alveolar septa with formation of intra-alveolar hyaline membranes, and impaired diffusion of oxygen across the swollen, thickened alveolar septa. Later in the course of the disease, fibrosis of the damaged lung tissue may occur and further compromise respiration (**Figure 13-20**).

Treatment is directed toward correcting the shock, treating the underlying condition that initiated the respiratory distress, and improving the oxygenation of the blood by means of a ventilator capable of delivering an increased concentration of oxygen to the lungs under slightly increased pressure, thereby

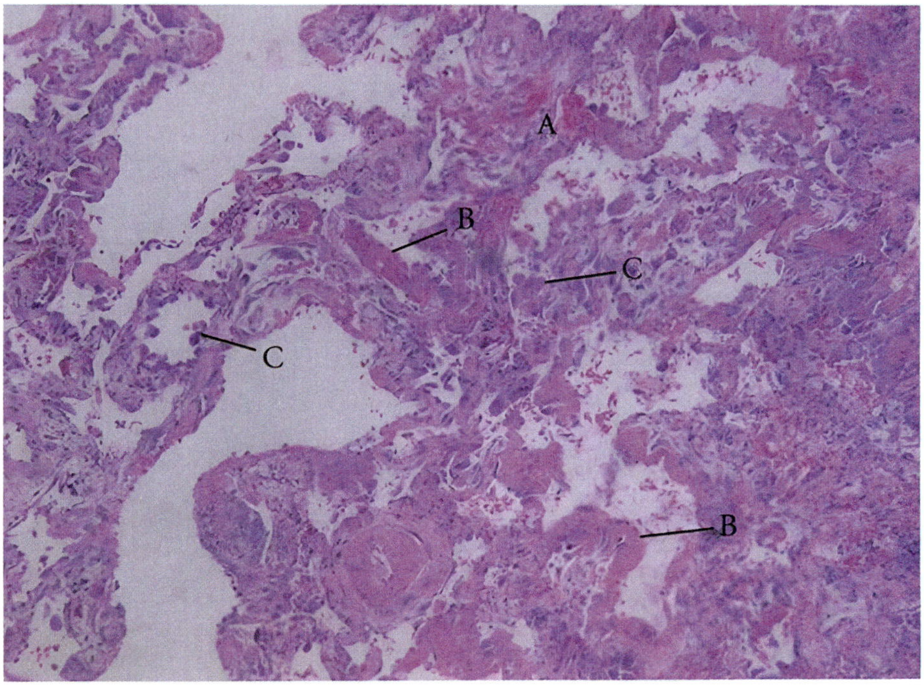

Figure 13-20 Histopathology showed late diffused alveolar damage (DAD). Interstitial edema and hemorrhage **(A)**, formation of hyaline membranes **(B)**, and pneumocyte hyperplasia **(C)**.

Bruminhent J, Yassir S, Pippim J. Acute interstitial pneumonia (hamman-rich syndrome) as a cause of idiopathic acute respiratory distress syndrome. Case Rep Med. 2011;2011:628743. doi:10.1155/2011/628743. Epub 2011 May 29.

facilitating diffusion of oxygen across the swollen alveolar septa. Extracorporeal membrane oxygenation (ECMO) has been used as a temporary last-resort therapy. In ECMO a device artificially oxygenates and removes CO_2 from blood outside the body until ARDS subsides, with very limited success. Even with therapy, ARDS has a mortality rate of 30 to 40 percent.

Pulmonary Fibrosis

The lungs are continually exposed to a number of injurious substances, such as irritant gases discharged into the atmosphere and many kinds of airborne organic and inorganic particles. As noted previously, severe pulmonary injury and ARDS may lead to pulmonary fibrosis. Fibrous thickening of alveolar septa makes the lungs increasingly rigid, restricting normal respiratory excursions. Diffusion of oxygen and carbon dioxide between alveolar air and pulmonary capillaries also is hampered because of the increased thickness of the alveolar septa. Pulmonary fibrosis (PF) causes progressive respiratory disability similar to that encountered in pulmonary emphysema (**Table 13-1**).Some types of diseases characterized by injury to connective tissue may have as their major manifestation injury to the connective tissue framework of the lung, leading to pulmonary fibrosis. A variety of interstitial pneumonias associated with fibrosis are classified as idiopathic and are of uncertain etiology. These conditions are marked by patchy collagen deposition, dense scarring, and areas of fibroblast proliferation. The most common of these, usual interstitial pneumonia (UIP)/idiopathic pulmonary fibrosis, may in some cases be viral, in other cases genetically related, and about 20 percent of the time associated with autoimmune diseases that affect connective tissue, such as rheumatoid arthritis. Unlike pneumonias of bacterial origin, which are susceptible to antibiotic therapy, UIP is slowly progressive with loss of pulmonary function over several years, and lung transplantation may be the only therapeutic option.

Pneumoconiosis An occupational lung disease caused by inhalation of injurious substances.

Certain occupational diseases are recognized as being caused by inhalation of injurious substances. The general term **pneumoconiosis** (pneumo = lung + konis = dust + osis = condition) is used to refer to lung injury

Table 13-1 **Common Causes of Pulmonary Fibrosis**

Type of Pulmonary Fibrosis	Clues that Doctors Use
Drug-induced	Prior or current use of amiodarone, nitrofurantoin, chemotherapy, methotrexate, or other drugs known to affect the lungs
Radiation-induced	Prior or current radiation treatment to the chest
Environmental (called hypersensitivity pneumonitis)	Exposure to mold, animals, or other triggers
Autoimmune (called connective tissue disease–related)	Joint inflammation, skin changes (particularly on the fingers and face), dry eyes or mouth, and/or? abnormal blood tests
Occupational (called pneumoconiosis)	Prior or current exposure to dusts, fibers, fumes, or vapors that can cause PF (such as asbestos, coal, silica, and others)
Idiopathic	When no cause can be identified

Reproduced with permission from Pulmonary Fibrosis Foundation. Pneumoconiosis Occupational Pulmonary Fibrosis. Accessed at, https://www.pulmonaryfibrosis.org/understanding-pff/types-of-pulmonary-fibrosis/occupationalpf

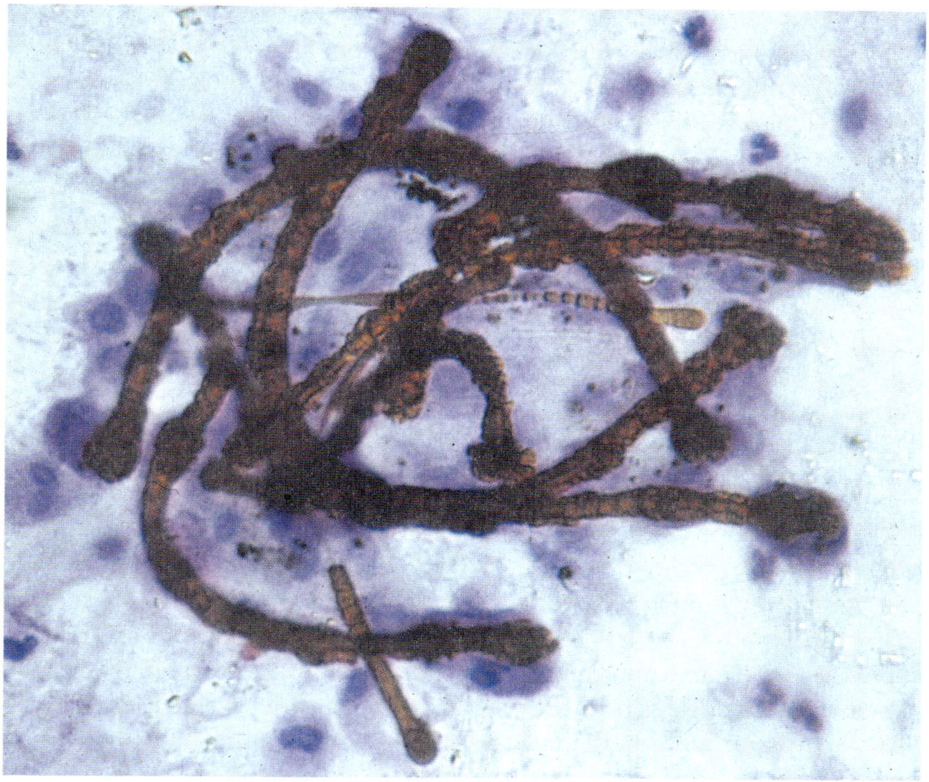

Figure 13-21 Cluster of asbestos bodies in septum (original magnification ×1000)
Courtesy of Leonard V. Crowley, MD, Century College.

produced by inhalation of injurious dust or other particulate material. The best known of the pneumoconioses are **silicosis** and **asbestosis**. Silicosis is a type of progressive nodular pulmonary fibrosis caused by inhalation of rock dust and other materials containing silica. Recent cases have occurred in workers installing silica-containing kitchen countertops. Asbestosis is a diffuse pulmonary fibrosis caused by inhalation of asbestos fibers. Within the body, the fibers become coated with a protein having a high content of iron to form characteristic structures called asbestos bodies. Sometimes these can be identified in the sputum of patients with asbestosis (**Figure 13-21**). Inhalation of coal dust, cotton fibers, certain types of fungus spores, and many other substances associated with certain occupations also may cause pulmonary fibrosis.

Silicosis A type of occupational lung disease caused by inhalation of silica-rich rock dust.

Asbestosis A type of pneumoconiosis caused by inhalation of asbestos fibers.

Patients with asbestosis have other problems as well because asbestos fibers appear to be carcinogenic. These patients have a higher incidence of lung carcinoma than the general population, and some develop an unusual type of malignant tumor (malignant mesothelioma) arising from pleural mesothelial cells.

Vaping- (E-Cigarette-) Induced Lung Injury

E-cigarettes were first made available in 2003 as a safer alternative to cigarettes for nicotine delivery. The devices are battery-powered vaporizers that use a heating element to vaporize (aerosolize) an "e-liquid," which is inhaled by the user. Because the device does not pyrolyze tobacco and paper as in a cigarette, e-cigarettes supposedly allow nicotine dosing without the risk of exposure to carcinogenic products. Currently, e-cigarettes use commercially made or home-assembled cartridges available from regulated or nonregulated and potentially illicit sources. E-liquids initially contained nicotine in a suspending liquid, such as propylene glycol or glycerin, and flavorings. Although sold as a device to curtail cigarette addiction, e-cigarettes are most often used as recreational devices, particularly among adolescents. Use of e-cigarettes (vaping) as a mechanism to deliver THC (tetrahydrocannabinol), the major psychoactive metabolite of marijuana, has been increasing.

Starting in mid-year of 2019, a series of emergency department visits characterized by symptoms of acute severe respiratory distress, including cough, chest pain, and shortness of breath, accompanied by gastrointestinal symptoms, were noted among individuals who vaped, in some cases leading to severe chronic lung disease. The syndrome was named e-cigarette- or vaping-associated lung injury (EVALI or VAPI). As of the end of 2019, 2500 cases have been reported from all 50 states, with over 50 deaths. After reaching a peak in 2020, EVALI cases have much declined but are still occasionally reported.

Currently, the oily (fat-soluble) compound vitamin E acetate is suspected to be responsible for EVALI. Although the compound is found in many foods and used as a dietary supplement and cosmetic ingredient with no toxicity, the use of the substance as a thickening agent in many THC-containing vaping fluids appears to cause lung injury when inhaled as an aerosol. Although the findings should still be considered preliminary, there is precedent for inhaled oils causing a severe lung injury termed *exogenous lipoid pneumonia*, which has some similarities to EVALI. Cases of EVALI have shown ARDS/diffuse alveolar damage and "organizing pneumonia" characterized by hyaline membranes, fibrin-containing exudates, and proliferating fibroblasts. Interestingly, macrophages with ingested oils were not present, suggesting that EVALI is not simply a response to inhaled oily material.

Lung Carcinoma

Lung carcinoma is another important disease related to cigarette smoking. Lung carcinoma was once uncommon. Now lung cancer is the chief cause of cancer deaths, which kills 125,000 people annually. It is a common malignant tumor in men, and the mortality in women caused by lung carcinoma now exceeds that of breast carcinoma. The tumor is uncommon in nonsmokers. Because the neoplasm often arises from the bronchial mucosa, the term *bronchogenic carcinoma* is often used when referring to lung cancer. There are several different histologic types. Squamous cell carcinoma and adenocarcinoma are two of the more common (**Figure 13-22**). A third type composed of large, bizarre epithelial cells is referred to as large cell carcinoma. A fourth type is composed of small, irregular dark cells with scanty cytoplasm that look somewhat like lymphocytes. This small cell carcinoma carries a very poor prognosis (**Figure 13-23**). Until recently it was sufficient for the pathologist to classify lung cancer as being of small cell type or "other non–small cell lung cancer (NSCLC)" because disseminated small cell lung cancer, although having a very poor long-term prognosis (7 percent 5-year survival, all stages combined), is susceptible to chemotherapy and radiation, which provide short-term relief. Currently, a number of adenocarcinomas of the lung have been characterized as having defined somatic mutations of the EGFR and ALK genes, which can be treated with drugs that block the kinase activity of the mutated

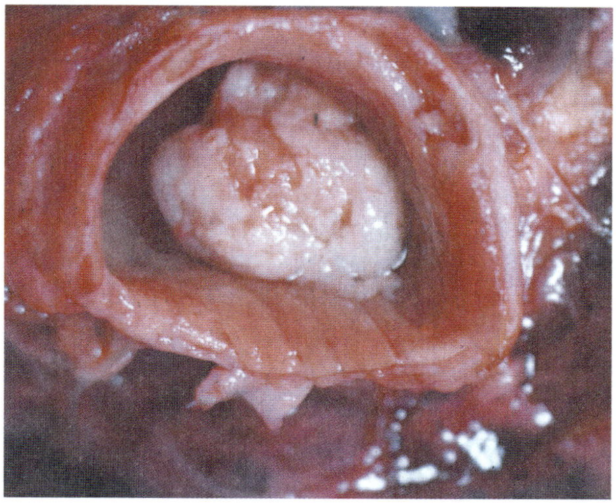

(A)

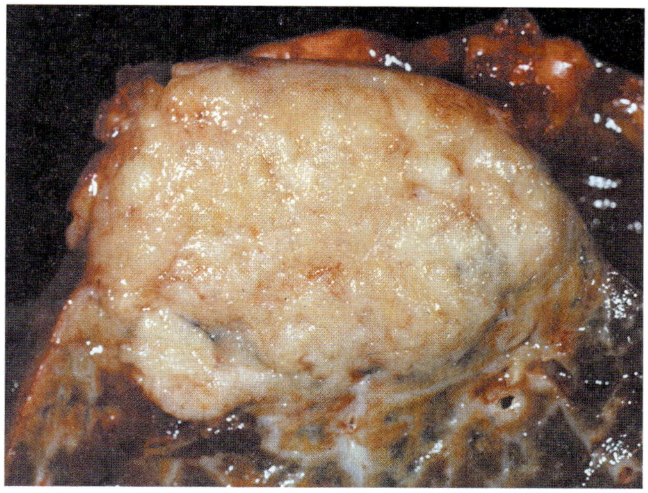

(B)

Figure 13-22 Gross appearance of lung carcinoma. **(A)** A squamous cell carcinoma partially obstructing a major bronchus. **(B)** An adenocarcinoma arising from smaller bronchus at the periphery of the lung.

Courtesy of Leonard V. Crowley, MD, Century College.

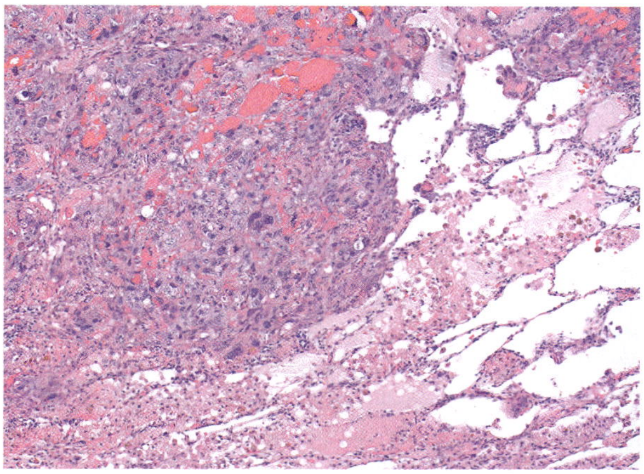

(A)

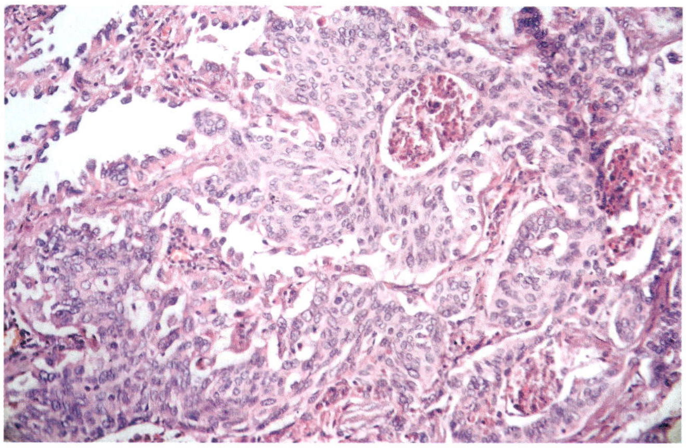

(B)

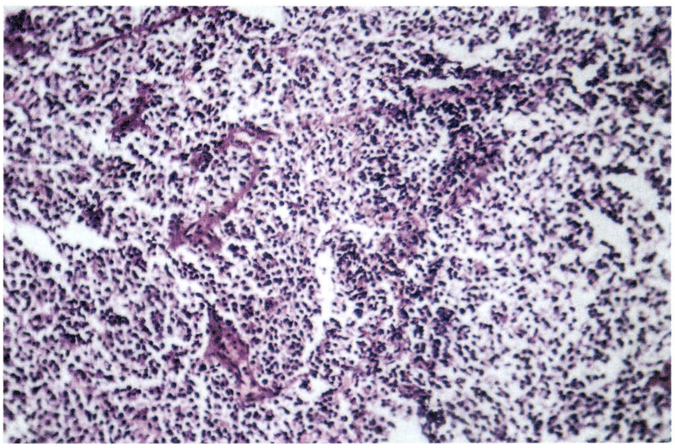

(C)

Figure 13-23 Histologic appearance of three common types of lung carcinoma. **(A)** Squamous cell carcinoma of the lung (left half of image) replacing normal healthy lung tissue (right side) with tumor cells undergoing mitotic division. **(B)** Adenocarcinoma showing malignant glandular cell formation. **(C)** Small cell carcinoma revealing densely packed malignant cells, characteristic of an aggressive lung malignancy.

genes (oncogenes), as discussed in Chapter 6. Although only a limited number of adenocarcinoma patients have the "drugable" mutation (predominantly Asiatic, female nonsmokers), this targeted form of chemotherapy may slightly prolong life (at best providing several months of disease-progress-free survival). Recently, inhibitors of immune checkpoint proteins (see Chapter 6) have been increasingly used in the treatment of both NSCLC and SCLC.

Because of the rich lymphatic and vascular network in the lung, the neoplasm readily gains access to lymphatic channels and pulmonary blood vessels and soon spreads to regional lymph nodes and distant sites. Treatment usually consists of surgical resection of one or more lobes of the lung. Radiation therapy in combination with anticancer chemotherapy rather than surgery is used to treat small cell carcinoma and is also used to treat tumors that are too far advanced for surgical resection. Results of treatment are disappointing because the disease is often widespread by the time it is recognized.

Chest X-rays for lung carcinoma have not been very effective in reducing lung carcinoma mortality because, often, the detected tumor has already spread beyond the lungs and is no longer curable. Specialized CT examinations can pick up tumors earlier, which provides a better chance of survival, but repeated CT procedures for screening are expensive and expose the individual to significantly more radiation than chest X-ray exams. A specialized form of CT (low, dose spiral CT) does reduce mortality in people with high risk (a minimum 20 pack-year smoking history).

Because 87 percent of lung cancers are caused by smoking, many physicians believe that the longer-term goal should be to eliminate the cause of most lung cancers by not smoking.

Case 13-1

Wilber is a 5-year-old male child of two upper-middle-class parents who live in Spotless Dell Community in a recently built home. Wilber has previously been healthy with only an occasional upper respiratory tract infection. About a month ago, Wilber complained of facial pain along with a case of the "sniffles." He began to cough at night (generally in the early morning) and also when he played outside with other children. Because the coughing was mild and tended to stop on its own and was not accompanied by production of sputum (was "nonproductive"), Wilber's parents were not concerned and assumed he had a "cold." About 2 weeks ago, Wilber's parents purchased a robotic vacuum cleaner (a Roomba). Wilber enjoyed following it around his bedroom but started to complain about feeling "funny" in his chest. His mother noticed that he made an odd "whistling" sound as he breathed out (expired). Wilber's complaints were occasional but tended to occur when the vacuum cleaner was being used or when Wilber's mother fluffed up the duvet or changed the sheets on Wilber's bed. Concerned that Wilber might be developing an "allergy," his parents brought Wilber to see his pediatrician.

Wilber's pediatrician was concerned that the child's symptoms might indicate very mild pediatric asthma. Wilber did report some facial pain when pressure was applied to his maxillary area, and the pediatrician noted that his conjunctivae were slightly inflamed, suggesting the possibility of mild allergic rhinitis. His physical examination was otherwise normal. Still concerned, the pediatrician asked Wilber to imagine trying to "blow out birthday candles as hard as possible." With forced expiration, she noticed a distinct wheeze (whistling sound due to air turbulence on expiration, suggesting some degree of pulmonary obstruction). Because the symptoms were mild, the pediatrician elected to forgo additional testing and suggested that Wilber's parents should not use the vacuum cleaner in Wilber's presence and that they buy special impermeable bed covers for his room. The pediatrician also prescribed a rapid-acting beta-2 agonist as an inhaler (albuterol). The drug causes smooth muscle relaxation in the respiratory system, acting as a bronchodilator. The pediatrician instructed Wilber's parents to use the drug when episodes of wheezing occur. His parents were also instructed to keep track of how frequently wheezing occurs and to immediately report back if symptoms worsen or if the wheezing is not relieved.

The medication initially controls Wilber's wheezing attacks, but after a time they appear to increase in frequency. Wilber complains of increased chest discomfort and interacts less with his playmates. Wilber's pediatrician is now more concerned about the presence of asthma and prescribes the use of an inhaled corticosteroid (beclomethasone), which both acts as an inhibitor of and relaxer for bronchoconstriction and as an anti-inflammatory, reducing the sensitivity of the airway to agents inducing the asthma attacks. She instructs the parents to use the albuterol inhaler only when Wilber suffers from sudden discomfort. Wilber does much better on the inhaled corticosteroid for several months, and his parents decide to taper the medication, noting no change in Wilber's health.

Wilber and his parents decide to visit his grandparents who live in a 120-year-old house on a ranch in Dusty Gulch. Wilber's parents pack the albuterol inhaler because they are somewhat concerned about the presence of "dust and germs" triggering an attack. At his grandparents' house, Wilber sleeps in a room with heavy hand-woven carpets on the floor and antique loomed fabrics on the walls. He wakes up in the early morning and calls his parents, complaining of difficulty breathing. He says his chest feels tight, and his parents note a very loud wheeze as Wilber attempts to exhale. They note that his chest muscles seem to be "working hard" as he attempts to breathe. They have Wilber use the albuterol inhaler, but it has little effect. Panicked, they rush Wilber to the local hospital's urgent care center. At the center, the on-call resident notes that Wilber has a very increased respiratory rate (over 30 breaths per minute), an increased heart rate (130 beats per minute), and a markedly reduced oxyhemoglobin saturation (determined using a pulse oximeter to be 92 percent saturation). Concerned with the inability of a moderate dose of a rapid-acting bronchodilator to afford relief, the resident increases the dose of this drug and begins IV therapy with corticosteroids. He also has Wilber inhale oxygen via a face mask. After an hour, Wilber's oxyhemoglobin saturation begins to climb, and after 6 hours, Wilber is feeling much better with improved breathing and lack of wheezing. He is scheduled for an intensive workup by a pediatric allergist in the next few days.

Discussion

Asthma is a complex chronic disease in which symptoms result from an obstruction of air flow, which is often periodic and triggered by an inciting agent. The most common inciting agent is an environmental allergen that triggers immune-mediated bronchospasm, mucosal edema, and excess mucus production, which plugs the airways. With time this leads to structural changes in the airway that include the continued presence of inflammatory cells (often eosinophils), basement membrane thickening, mucous gland hyperplasia, and mucoid plugging of airways (**Case Figure 13-1**). The immunology of asthma is complex and discussed in Chapter 5. In brief, IgE has a high affinity to mast cells. Binding allergens to IgE antibodies triggers the mast cells to release a number of inflammatory mediators, including histamine, which causes bronchoconstriction. Other immune cells, such as eosinophils, are also involved in this process and promote additional airway damage.

Many environmental allergens can trigger allergic asthma. At the top of the list are dust mites, other household insects such as roaches, and animal dander. The **hygiene hypothesis** suggests that current increases in the rate of childhood asthma are a result of child-rearing in an excessively

(continues)

Hygiene hypothesis
Hypothesis that lack of early childhood exposure to infectious agents, symbiotic microorganisms (such as the gut flora or probiotics), and parasites increases susceptibility to allergic reaction or response by suppressing the natural development of the immune system.

Case 13-1 (Continued)

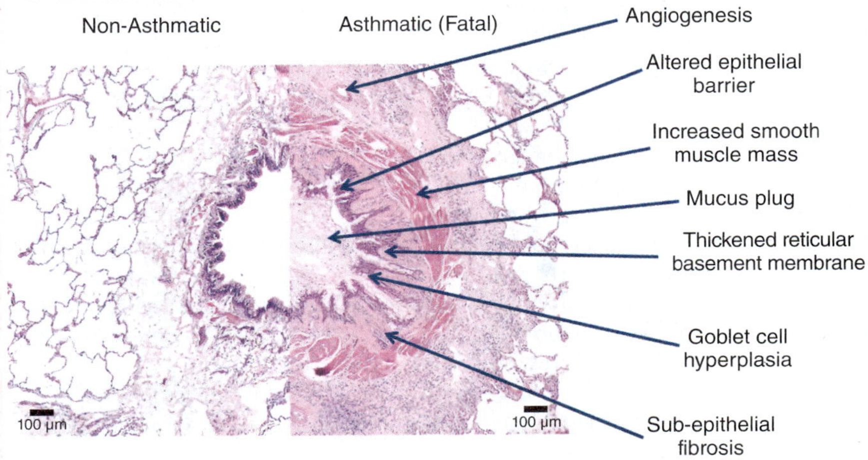

Case Figure 13-1 Histopathology of respiratory tissue from a case of fatal asthmatic individual demonstrates many of the classic pathologic changes (compared to the non-asthmatic tissue), including mucus plug, epithelial basement membrane thickening, and smooth muscle hyperplasia.

Reproduced from Hsieh A, Assadinia N, Hackett TL. Airway remodeling heterogeneity in asthma and its relationship to disease outcomes. Frontiers in Physiology. 2023;14. doi:https://doi.org/10.3389/fphys.2023.1113100

clean environment. Studies have suggested that children raised in farm environments have fewer cases of asthma than those raised in nonrural environments. In Wilber's case, the association of symptoms with exposure to vacuuming, disturbed bedding, and textiles suggests that household dust mites are a likely trigger.

The treatment of asthma is complex and far more extensive than discussed in the case. Treatment involves pulmonary function tests, determination of the allergic trigger, and evaluation of multiple potential therapeutic interventions. However, it is important to understand that asthma is a serious disease affecting at least 10 percent of the population. There has been a surprising increase in incidence (some accounts report increases of over 75 percent in recent years). Asthma is the most common reason for admission to pediatric hospitals and accounts for more school absences than any other chronic disease. In addition, unrelieved asthma (status asthmaticus) results in 5000 deaths per year. Case Figure 13-1 is taken from such a lethal case.

Etiology and Pathogenesis

Allergic asthma is triggered by the presence of environmental allergens, possibly dust mites, resulting in inflammation of the respiratory tree, airway hypersensitivity, bronchospasm, excess mucus production, and inflammation-induced changes in the respiratory tree.

Questions

1. In addition to dust mites, insects, and animal dander, what are other common triggers for allergic asthma?
2. What are common nonallergic triggers for asthma?
3. Can you think of any additional studies that would help to prove (or disprove) the hygiene hypothesis of asthma susceptibility?
4. Allergic asthma is an example of type 1 hypersensitivity. What are the major characteristics of this type of hypersensitivity reaction?
5. How could Wilber's parents alter their household environment to prevent additional asthmatic attacks in Wilber?
6. How can the allergen(s) responsible be identified?

Questions for Review

1. How do the lungs function? What is the difference between ventilation and gas exchange? How is pulmonary function disturbed if the alveolar septa are thickened and scarred?
2. What is pneumothorax? How does it develop? What is its effect on pulmonary function?
3. What is pneumonia? How is pneumonia classified? What are its major clinical features?
4. How does the tubercle bacillus differ in its staining reaction from other bacteria? What type of inflammatory reaction does it cause? What factors determine the outcome of a tuberculous infection? How does a cavity develop in lungs infected with tuberculosis? Is a person with a tuberculous cavity infectious to other people? What is miliary tuberculosis?
5. A patient has tuberculosis of the kidney, but no evidence of pulmonary tuberculosis is detected by means of a chest X-ray. How did this happen?
6. What is meant by the term *inactive tuberculosis*? Under what circumstances may an old inactive tuberculous infection become activated? What type of patients are susceptible to reactivation of a tuberculous infection?
7. What is the difference between bronchitis and bronchiectasis?
8. What is pulmonary emphysema? What factors predispose to its development? How may it be prevented? What is the difference between pulmonary emphysema and pulmonary fibrosis?
9. What is the relationship between carcinoma of the lung and cigarette smoking? How is lung carcinoma treated?

References

Funkhouser WK. Pulmonary pathology. In: Reisner HM, ed. *Pathology: A Modern Case Study*. 2nd ed. McGraw-Hill Lange; 2020.

- A brief introduction to the pathology of pulmonary disease that is strong on overviews and case studies. It covers additional important diseases of the lung not included in this chapter.

Daley BJ. Pneumothorax Medscape. Updated January 22, 2024. Accessed May 2, 2025. https://emedicine.medscape.com/article/424547-overview

Atelectasis. American Lung Association. Accessed May 2, 2025. https://www.lung.org/lung-health-diseases/lung-disease-lookup/atelectasis

- The first website presents an overview of the physiology, pathology, and therapy of pneumothorax. The second website is a brief overview of the causes of atelectasis with links to additional details.

Tuberculosis (TB). Centers for Disease Control and Prevention. Accessed May 2, 2025. http://www.cdc.gov/tb/

Treating Tuberculosis. Centers for Disease Control and Prevention. Updated April 17, 2025. Accessed May 2, 2025. https://www.cdc.gov/tb/treatment/index.html

About Middle East Respiratory Syndrome (MERS). Centers for Disease Control and Prevention. Updated December 4, 2024. Accessed May 2, 2025. https://www.cdc.gov/mers/about/

- The first two websites present an up-to-date overview of the status of TB infection in the United States and the treatment of latent TB. The final reference provides the latest information on the MERS outbreak in the Middle East. The site is updated frequently.

Gamache J. Bacterial Pneumonia. Medscape. Updated July 3, 2024. Accessed May 2, 2025. https://emedicine.medscape.com/article/300157-overview

Mosenifar Z. Viral Pneumonia. Medscape. Updated July 21, 2024. Accessed May 2, 2025. https://emedicine.medscape.com/article/300455-overview

- The amount of material on bacterial and viral pneumonia is enormous and highly specialized. These two e-medicine references do a very nice job of summarizing these important areas and provide many additional resources for those interested.

Sharma GD. Pediatric asthma. Medscape. Updated May 24, 2024. Accessed May 2, 2025. https://emedicine.medscape.com/article/1000997-overview

Azzam W. Status Asthmaticus. Medscape. Updated November 18, 2024. Accessed May 2, 2025. http://emedicine.medscape.com/article/2129484-overview

- These two references were most helpful in the construction of the case. They provide an overview of the diagnosis, pathophysiology, and therapy of asthma.

American Thoracic Society. Acute Respiratory Distress Syndrome. Accessed May 2, 2025. https://site.thoracic.org/advocacy-patients/patient-resources/acute-respiratory-distress-syndrome

- Acute respiratory distress syndrome (diffuse alveolar damage to the pathologist) is a major cause of acute respiratory failure and mortality associated with many forms of injury to the lung. This brief patient-oriented review covers definition, risk factors, and therapy of what is an often misunderstood condition.

Brandsma CA, Van den Berge M, Hackett TL, Brusselle G, Timens W. Recent advances in chronic obstructive pulmonary disease pathogenesis: From disease mechanisms to precision medicine. *J Pathol*. 2020;250(5):624-635. Accessed May 2, 2025. doi:10.1002/path.5364

What is COPD? COPD Foundation. Updated September 23, 2024. Accessed May 2, 2025. https://www.copdfoundation.org/What-is-COPD/Understanding-COPD/What-is-COPD.aspx

Silverman EK. Genetics of COPD. *Annu Rev Physiol*. 2020;82:413-431. doi:10.1146/annurev-physiol-021317-121224

- The set of three references covers the pathology associated with smoking: emphysema, COPD, and other forms of lung damage. The third article provides accurate information on the genetics and alpha$_1$ antitrypsin deficiency, a condition that synergizes with smoking to promote early onset emphysema.

Health Effects of Vaping. Centers for Disease Control and Prevention. Updated January 31, 2025. Accessed May 2, 2025. https://www.cdc.gov/tobacco/e-cigarettes/health-effects.html

Zulfiqar H, Sankari A, Rahman O. Vaping-Associated Pulmonary Injury. StatPearls [Internet]. Updated June 25, 2023. https://www.ncbi.nlm.nih.gov/books/NBK560656/

E-cigarette or Vaping Use-Associated Lung Injury (EVALI). American Lung Association. Accessed May 2, 2025. https://www.lung.org/lung-health-diseases/lung-disease-lookup/evali

Navon L, Jones CM, Ghinai I, et al. Risk factors for e-cigarette or vaping product use–associated lung injury (EVALI) among adults who use e-cigarette, or vaping, products—Illinois, July–October 2019. *MMWR Morb Mortal Wkly Rep*. 2019;68(45):1034-1039.

Blount BC, Karwowski MP, Shields PG, et al. Vitamin E acetate in bronchoalveolar-lavage fluid associated with EVALI. *N Engl J Med*. 2020;382(8):697-705.

Mukhopadhyay S, Mehrad M, Dammert P, et al. Lung biopsy findings in severe pulmonary illness associated with e-cigarette use (vaping). *Am J Clin Pathol*. 2020;153(1):30-39.

- This set of references provides an overview of what is currently known about lung injury and vaping. The last reference is the best description of the lung injury associated with EVALI to date and conflicts with some of the earlier reports. Note that lung pathology diagnosis is extremely complex.

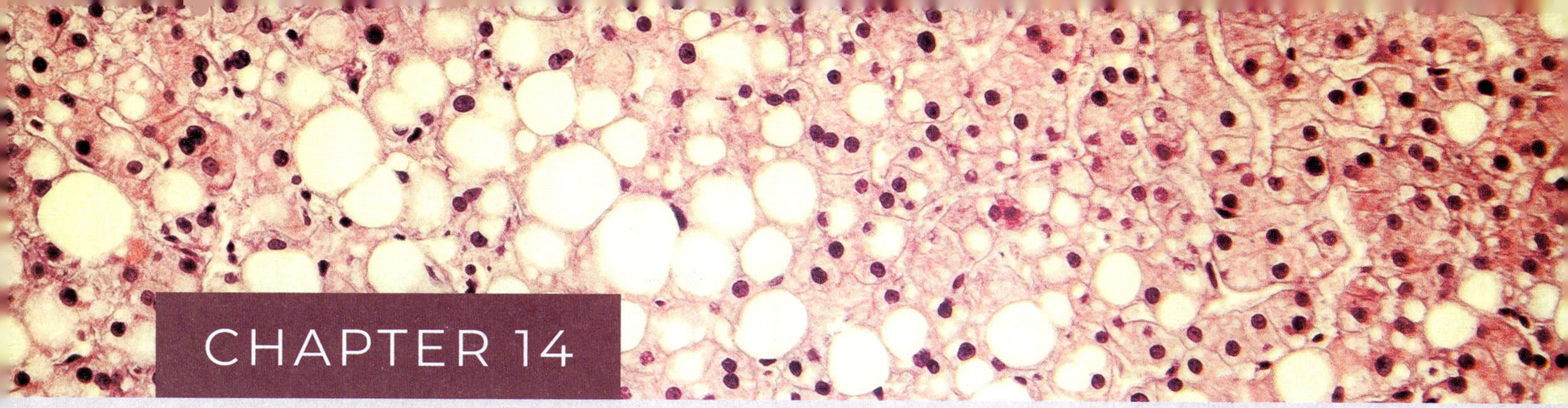

CHAPTER 14

The Breast

LEARNING OBJECTIVES

1. Describe the normal structure and physiology of the breast. List and define the common developmental abnormalities.
2. List the three common breast diseases that present as a lump in the breast and explain how they are differentiated.
3. Describe the clinical manifestations of breast carcinoma. Explain the methods of diagnosis and treatment.
4. Explain the role of heredity in the pathogenesis of breast carcinoma.
5. Explain the classification and staging of breast carcinomas and the implications from prognosis.
6. Explain the applications and limitations of mammography in the diagnosis and treatment of breast disease.
7. Explain the current treatment regimens and the influence of cancer stage and size.

Structure and Physiology of the Breast

The female breasts are each composed of about 20 lobes of glandular tissue embedded in fibrous and adipose tissue (**Figure 14-1**). The lobes are arranged circumferentially, much like petals on a flower. Each lobe consists of clusters of glands (terminal ductules or acini) in which milk is made during pregnancy, a series of intralobular ducts connecting the acini, and embedded stromal tissue. Taken together, these three components are called the **terminal duct lobular unit (TDLU)**. The ducts of the TDLU converge to form large ducts that extend to the nipple. The ductules and ducts of the lobular system are bilayered. The luminal epithelial cells lining the ducts serve as the source of milk during lactation and contribute to much of the breast pathology, the most important being carcinoma. The outer layer is myoepithelial in nature and characteristically is lost in invasive breast cancer (**Figure 14-2**). Preservation versus loss of the bilayered nature of the lobular system is an important diagnostic criterion in separating benign from malignant breast disease.

Terminal duct lobular unit (TDLU) Lobe of the female breast, including the cluster of milk gland ducts and stromal tissue.

The breasts represent modified sweat glands specialized to secrete milk. Before puberty, breast tissue in both sexes consists only of branching ducts and fibrous tissue without glandular tissue or fat. In the female, the breasts enlarge at puberty in response to estrogen and progesterone produced by the ovaries, whereas the unstimulated male breasts retain their prepubertal form. Postpubertal

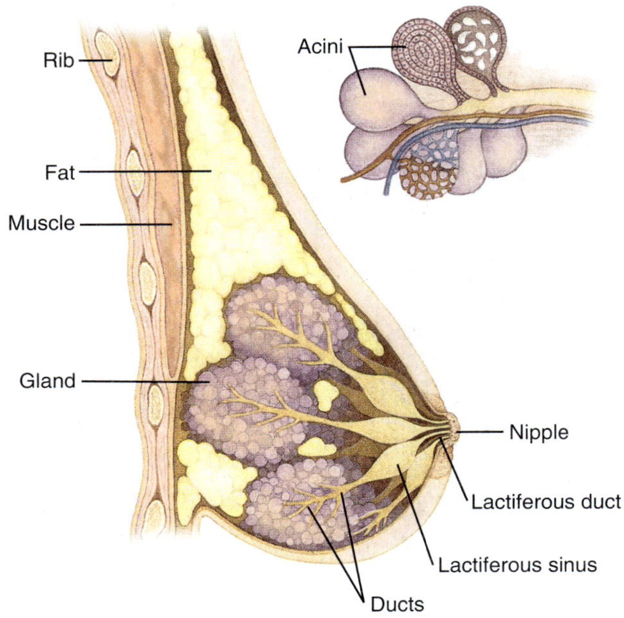

Figure 14-1 Anatomy of the breast ducts and lobules.

changes in the female include proliferation of glandular and fibrous tissue and accumulation of adipose tissue within the breasts. Variations in the size of the postpubertal breasts of nonpregnant women are primarily the result of variations in the amount of fat and fibrous tissue in the breasts rather than differences in the amount of glandular tissue.

Suspensory ligaments anchor the breast tissue to the breast wall. They extend from the skin of the breast to the connective tissue covering the muscles of the chest wall. The breasts receive an abundant blood supply and exhibit rich lymphatic drainage. Lymphatic channels drain from each breast into groups of lymph nodes located in the armpit or axilla (axillary lymph nodes), above the clavicle (supraclavicular lymph nodes), and beneath the sternum (mediastinal lymph nodes).

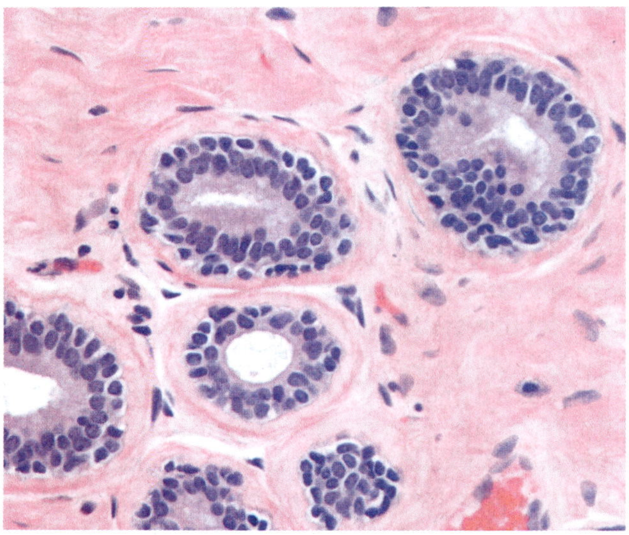

Figure 14-2 Breast glands. Each gland is lined by two layers of cells: an inner epithelial layer and an outer layer of myoepithelial cells.

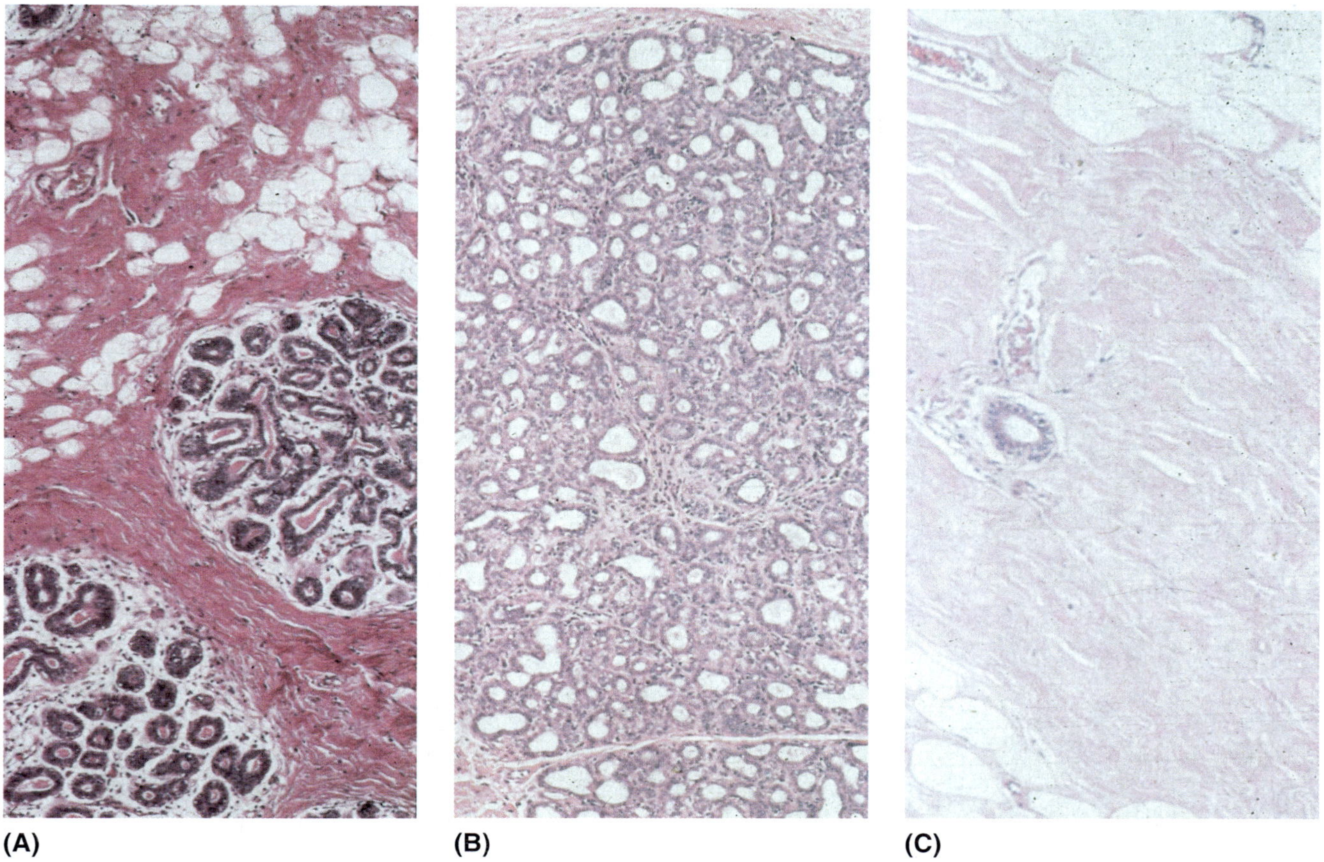

Figure 14-3 Photomicrographs illustrating the appearance of breasts under varying hormonal conditions (original magnification ×40). **(A)** Normal nonpregnant breast. Two lobules of glandular tissue appear in the lower half of the photograph. **(B)** Glandular hyperplasia in pregnancy. **(C)** Postmenopausal atrophy.

The breasts are extremely responsive to hormonal stimulation. Mild cyclic hyperplasia followed by involution of breast tissue occurs normally during each menstrual cycle. The glandular and ductal tissues of the breast become markedly hypertrophic under the hormonal stimulus of pregnancy and lactation, and the breast undergoes regression in the postpartum period. After menopause, sex hormone levels decline, and the breasts gradually decrease in size. **Figure 14-3** illustrates the histologic appearance of breast tissue under varying hormonal conditions.

Abnormalities of Breast Development

Accessory Breasts and Nipples

Embryologically, the breasts develop from columns of cells called **mammary ridges**, which extend along the anterior body wall from the armpits to the upper thighs. Most of the ridges disappear in the course of prenatal development except for the parts in the midthoracic region, which give rise to the breasts and nipples. Sometimes people have extra breasts or nipples. These can most commonly be found in the armpits or on the lower chest below and medial to the normal breasts, but they may appear anywhere along the course of the embryonic mammary ridges (the milk line). Extra nipples and breast

Mammary ridges
Location of embryonic cells that develop into breasts.

tissue may be a source of embarrassment to the individual, but usually they do not cause other problems.

Unequal Development of the Breasts

The fully developed breasts are usually similar in size and shape but not identical. Occasionally, one breast may fail to develop as much as its counterpart and may be significantly smaller than the opposite breast. Moreover, any condition that causes the breasts to enlarge may accentuate the disproportion.

Breast Hypertrophy

At puberty, one or commonly both female breasts may overrespond to hormonal stimulation and enlarge excessively. True breast hypertrophy is primarily caused by overgrowth of fibrous tissue, not glandular tissue or fat. The person may experience considerable back and shoulder discomfort caused by the excessive weight of the breasts. If symptoms are severe, the excessive breast tissue may be surgically resected, after which the breasts may be reconstructed.

Gynecomastia

Gynecomastia Excessive development of the male breast.

Fibrocystic change (FCC) Common benign cystic change in breast tissue.

Occasionally, at puberty, the ductal and fibrous tissue of the adolescent male breast begins to proliferate, forming a distinct nodule of breast tissue under the nipple. This condition, called **gynecomastia** (gyne = woman + mastos = breast), may affect one or both breasts. It appears to result from a temporary physiological imbalance of male and female hormones that sometimes occurs in the male at puberty. Normally, the male secretes both male and female hormones, but male hormones predominate and "cancel out" the effects of the female hormones. Gynecomastia results when there is a temporary increase in estrogen relative to male hormones. The condition, while not clinically serious, may cause considerable emotional distress to the affected youth. Nonphysiological gynecomastia may occur in males who use certain drugs, experience liver or kidney failure, or develop hormone-producing tumors of the testes. Unilateral breast masses or enlargement in males must be examined to rule out cancer, which does occur in males.

Inflammatory Lesions of the Breast

Acute mastitis occurs as an inflammatory response to a bacterial infection, most often with *Staphylococcus aureus*. Damage to the nipple during breastfeeding allows penetration of bacteria into the breast tissue, resulting in infection and inflammation. Treatment generally includes antibiotics. Subareolar abscesses may become chronic. Occurrence can be associated with manipulations of the nipple area such as piercing but also with cigarette smoking. In severe cases, fistulas may form, necessitating a surgical repair.

Nonproliferative Fibrocystic Change in the Breast

Nonproliferative (benign) cystic changes in breast tissue, often called benign cystic disease or benign **fibrocystic change (FCC)**, commonly occurs and bears no increased risk for development of cancer. About one-third of women from the age of 20 to the menopausal period experience FCC, after which the condition recedes. It is characterized by focal areas of proliferation of glandular and fibrous tissue in the breast associated with localized dilatation of

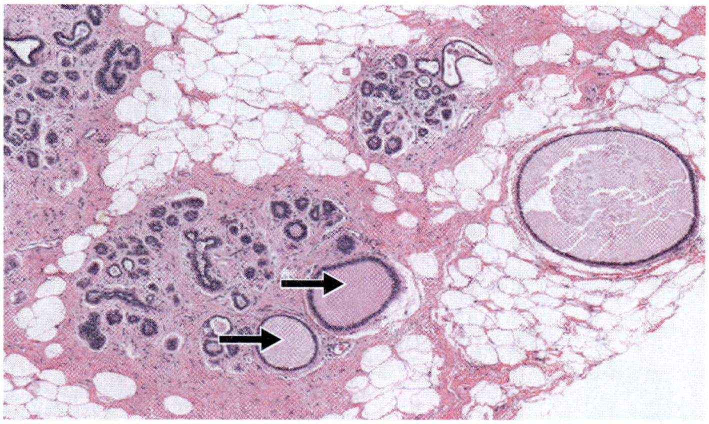

Figure 14-4 Nonproliferative cystic change in a breast. The biopsy demonstrates multiple localized dilated ducts forming cysts varying in size (*arrows*).
Courtesy of Department of Pathology and Laboratory Medicine, University of North Carolina at Chapel Hill.

ducts, resulting in the formation of various-sized cysts within the breast. Cystic change appears to be caused by irregularities in the response of the breast tissue to the normal cyclic variations of each menstrual cycle. Clinically, a breast cyst may feel very firm and may appear to be a solid tumor. Ultrasound examination of the breast can distinguish a cyst from a solid mass in the breast (**Figure 14-4**). Often, if the clinician believes the mass to be a cyst rather than a solid tumor, an attempt is made to aspirate the cyst. A needle is introduced into the breast under local anesthesia. If a cyst is present, the fluid is aspirated and the mass disappears. If no fluid can be obtained, surgical excision is performed. Fibrocystic change associated with nonproliferative changes in the ducts bears no increased risk for subsequent development of cancer. At times the ducts may show varying degrees of proliferative fibrocystic changes, which present a slightly increased risk of cancer development.

Fibroadenoma

Fibroadenoma is the most common benign tumor of the female breast. It occurs most frequently in the third and fourth decades but also may present in a juvenile (adolescent) form. The tumors contain both an epithelial (glandular) and surrounding stromal component. They are painless, well circumscribed, and slow growing, but may increase in size during pregnancy. These tumors are usually solitary and often detected during routine **mammography**. Although the tumor is benign, it may, in some cases, be excised to distinguish it from a potentially malignant tumor (phyllodes tumor), which is similar in appearance but generally larger and more rapid in growth (**Figure 14-5**).

Mammography
Technique used to create an X-ray image of the breast that helps to detect tumors and other abnormalities within the breast.

Carcinoma of the Breast

Breast carcinoma occurs in both sexes. It is a rare tumor in men (2800 new cases in 2025) whose breast tissue is not subjected to stimulation by ovarian hormones. In women, it is the most frequently diagnosed cancer and ranks second as a cause of cancer deaths (exceeded only by lung cancer), with about 317,000 new cases of invasive disease diagnosed in 2025. This number comes from Cancer.gov, using statistical models for analysis, which were age-adjusted calculated rates for new female breast cancer. The numbers of cases have been rising on average 0.6% each year

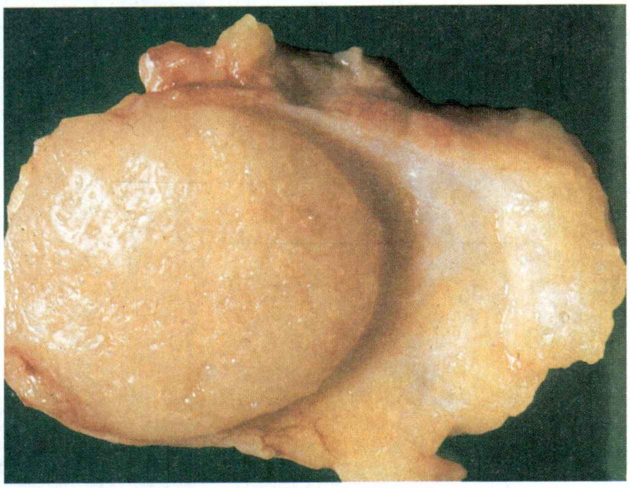

(A)

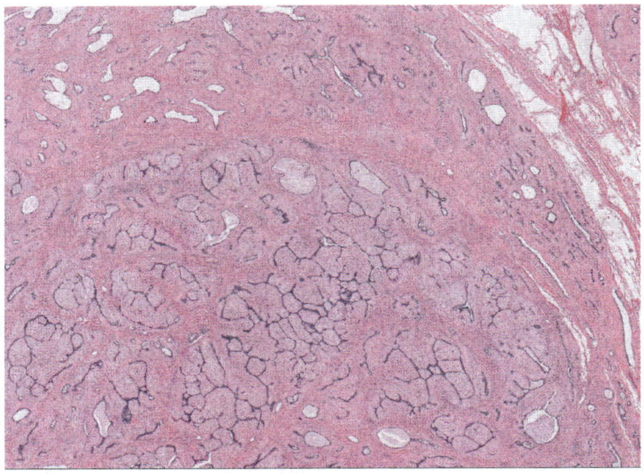

(B)

Figure 14-5 Benign fibroadenoma of the breast. The tumor is well circumscribed and readily separates from the breast. **(A)** Gross specimen. **(B)** Photomicrograph (low power); the fibrous stromal component and compressed glands and ducts are visible.

(A) Courtesy of Leonard V. Crowley, MD, Century College; **(B)** Courtesy of Department of Pathology and Laboratory Medicine, University of North Carolina at Chapel Hill.

Menarche Onset of menses.

***Ductal carcinoma in situ* (DCIS)** The precursor lesion to most breast cancer.

over 2013–2022. On the other hand, age-adjusted death rates have been falling on average 1.2% each year over 2014–2023. Modifiable risk factors include being overweight, being physically inactive, consuming alcohol, or being a heavy smoker. Hormonal factors also influence the risk of breast carcinoma. Women who never bore children or had their first child after age 30 are at increased risk, as are women who have had early onset of menses (**menarche**), or late menopause (implying a long menstrual history). High breast tissue density (increased glandular relative to fat tissue) measured by mammography may also indicate increased risk. However, this may be due in part to the difficulty of early detection in such breasts rather than to heightened risk. A tendency for breast carcinoma to run in families occurs to some extent. A woman experiences a higher than normal risk if her mother or sister had a breast carcinoma. Inherited mutations can lead to striking increases in breast cancer susceptibility. Two genes, BRCA1 and BRCA2, although rare in the population (less than 1 percent), account for up to 10 percent of all female breast cancer victims and up to 20 percent of breast cancers that occur in families. In summary, the etiology of breast cancer is multifactorial and involves genetic background, hormonal status, and poorly defined environmental factors. Significant differences in breast cancer frequencies can be noted in different populations and socioeconomic groups. Mammography has highlighted that breast cancer originates as *in situ* disease, restricted to the ducts and lobular system and at that point not (yet) capable of metastasis. **Ductal carcinoma *in situ* (DCIS)**, the precursor lesion to most breast cancers, is now diagnosed with fivefold greater frequency as a result of screening mammography. With time, DCIS can lead to populations of neoplastic cells that traverse the ductal basement membrane, invade the surrounding tissue, and metastasize to distant sites. Because it is unclear which cases of DCIS will progress invasively, they are treated aggressively with excision and radiation, sometimes followed by hormonal therapy. The process of progression is accompanied by loss of the myoepithelial cell layer surrounding the ducts and lobules of the TDLU (**Figure 14-6**).

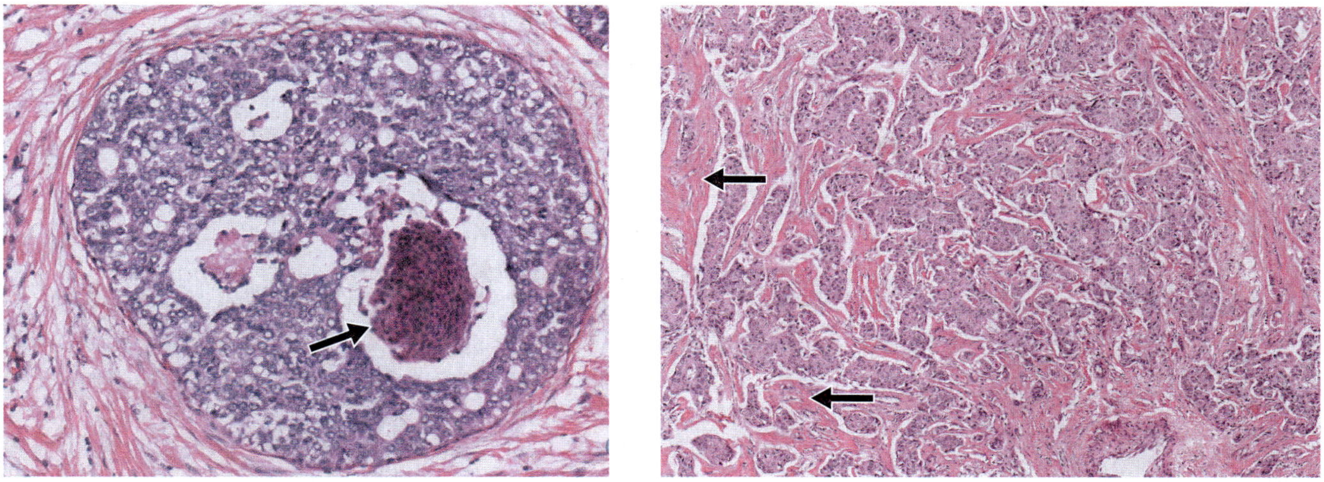

(A) (B)

Figure 14-6 Ductal carcinoma. **(A)** Ductal carcinoma *in situ* (DCIS). This high-grade lesion demonstrates intraductal necrosis (*arrow*) characteristic of the lesion. The lesion is confined by the basement membrane. **(B)** Invasive ductal carcinoma infiltrates breast tissue and is associated with a fibrotic reaction of surrounding tissue (*arrows*).

Courtesy of Department of Pathology and Laboratory Medicine, University of North Carolina at Chapel Hill.

Breast Carcinoma Susceptibility Genes

A small proportion of breast carcinomas are hereditary and can be traced to inheritance of mutant breast cancer susceptibility genes as mentioned previously. The two most important susceptibility genes, BRCA1 and BRCA2, both involve the process of DNA repair. The BRCA1 gene is very large, and a high number of different mutations have been described. A woman who inherits a mutant BRCA1 gene has between a 40 to 80 percent chance of developing breast carcinoma during her lifetime. In addition, her lifetime risk for ovarian cancer becomes approximately 20 to 40 percent. A woman who inherits a mutant BRCA2 gene faces a 30 to 60 percent lifetime risk for breast carcinoma, but the lifetime risk of ovarian carcinoma lowers to about 10 to 20 percent, significantly lower than the risk associated with a BRCA1 mutation. (The role of tumor suppressor genes is covered in Chapter 6.) Although the frequency of BRCA1/BRCA2 mutations remains relatively low in the general population (0.2 percent or less), the frequency is up to 10-fold higher in some populations (notably those of Ashkenazi Jewish background). Individuals descended from families with higher incidences of breast cancer, those who have early onset or bilateral breast cancer, and those of Ashkenazi Jewish background should consider genetic testing for mutations in BRCA1/BRCA2. There is no simple way to reduce the risk of breast, ovarian, and several other cancers in these genetic carrier individuals. Hence, intensive screening tests every 6 months are recommended to identify and treat any newly detected carcinomas in this high-risk group. Unfortunately, early-stage carcinomas detected by screening tests do not guarantee a successful response to treatment. It is difficult to detect an ovarian carcinoma in its early stage, and many breast carcinomas in affected women are aggressive, rapidly growing tumors that may already have spread by the time they are detected. Consequently, many high-risk women carrying BRCA1 or BRCA2 mutations may consider removing their fallopian tubes and ovaries or undergo a bilateral mastectomy. Often both procedures are performed to avoid the risks of both breast and ovarian carcinoma. BRCA mutations also increase the risk of breast cancer (and cancer of the prostate and other sites) in males.

Classification of Breast Carcinoma

Breast cancers are classified according to the site of origin, the presence or absence of invasion, the degree of differentiation, and more recently, the molecular characteristics (nature of genes expressed) of the tumor cells. More than 90 percent of carcinomas are **ductal carcinomas** and they arise from the epithelium of the ducts. The rest arise from the lobules and are designated **lobular carcinomas**. As previously noted, a precursor *in situ* lesion for ductal carcinoma (DCIS) has been defined. Lobular carcinoma *in situ* (LCIS) occurs but is usually not considered an *in situ* carcinoma that requires surgical excision. However, certain specific types of LCIS may be an *in situ* precursor for forms of lobular carcinoma and require excisional therapy.

The therapy and prognosis for invasive breast carcinoma depend on many variables, but current practice focuses in part on the molecular characteristics of the carcinoma cells, which differ from case to case. The characteristics examined include the presence of several cell surface receptors, including **estrogen receptors (ER)** and **progesterone receptors (PR)**, which are almost always present or absent together, and the **human epidermal growth factor receptor 2 (HER-2)**. ER-positivity is a favorable prognostic indicator and suggests that the cancer cells may still respond to hormonal stimulation. Patients with these cancers prove excellent candidates for drugs that block the effects of estrogens (such as tamoxifen) and slow the growth of the cancer cells. Some breast carcinomas overexpress (make excessive amounts of) the HER-2 protein and other genes associated with HER-2. These carcinomas behave aggressively with a poor prognosis. However, they do become candidates for therapy using antibodies that target the HER-2 receptor or for a drug that blocks the pathway stimulated by HER-2, which includes tyrosine kinase inhibition. Tests that determine the **gene expression profile** of breast carcinomas provide additional information. These tests determine which sets of proteins can be produced by the carcinomas and divide the disease into subtypes with particular prognostic characteristics. **Luminal A** carcinomas make up about 50 percent of cases and are most like the normal (non-neoplastic) breast epithelial cells, making them low grade. Generally, they express ER. Individuals with these carcinomas benefit from an excellent prognosis, and treatment involves hormonal therapy. **Luminal B** tumors (15 percent to 20 percent of cases) have a higher grade than Luminal A tumors but usually still express some level of ER. Individuals with these carcinomas have a poorer prognosis and are treated with both hormonal and other forms of chemotherapy. Individuals with **basal-like tumors** (15 percent to 20 percent of cases) sustain a poor prognosis. Their pattern of gene expression is most similar to the myoepithelial cells that line breast TDLUs. These **triple-negative** tumors commonly lack ER, PR, and HER-2. Most tumors in BRCA1-positive individuals are of this type. Although the tumors are sensitive to chemotherapy, patients experience a high relapse rate, and the tumors tend to metastasize to the viscera and brain. HER-2-positive tumors (10 percent of cases) are extremely aggressive. These tumors contain multiple copies of the gene responsible for the HER-2 protein, expressing large amounts of the HER-2 receptor on their surface. Like basal-cell-type tumors, they undergo high rates of cell division but can be treated using anti-HER-2 therapy. Another important factor in deciding on the likely prognosis of breast carcinoma (and choosing a therapy) is the stage of the tumor at the time of detection.

Ductal carcinoma Tumor arising from the epithelium of the ducts.

Lobular carcinoma Tumor of the breast arising from the lobules.

Estrogen receptors (ER)/progesterone receptors (PR) A protein on the surface of certain cells, which binds estrogen or progesterone. The presence or absence of the receptors is an important aspect of cancer diagnosis and treatment.

Human epidermal growth factor receptor 2 (HER-2) A protein on the surface of breast cells that can bind to the human epidermal growth factor.

Gene expression profile List of proteins synthesized by the cells, often used for diagnosis of cancer.

Luminal A/Luminal B Specific types of gene expression profiles found in breast cancer cells.

Basal-like tumors Type of breast cancer cell demonstrating a specific gene expression profile with tumor cells look similar to the epithelial cells of the basal layer of the breast's milk ducts.

Triple-negative Breast cancer cell lacking ER, PR, and HER-2.

Pathogenesis of Breast Carcinoma

In its early stages, a breast carcinoma is too small to be detected by breast examination but can often be visualized by mammography (**mammogram**), sometimes as early as 2 years before it becomes large enough to form a palpable lump within the breast. Frequently, focal areas of necrosis occur within the proliferating tumor cells, and calcium salts diffuse from the bloodstream into the areas of necrosis (**Figure 14-7**). These small focal calcium deposits often can be identified in mammograms, which raises a suspicion of calcium deposits within a ductal carcinoma. Calcium deposits are not conclusive evidence of breast carcinoma. Calcium deposits also accumulate in some benign breast lesions.

Mammogram An X-ray image of the breast that helps to detect tumors and other abnormalities within the breast.

Many breast carcinomas induce fibrosis in the surrounding normal breast tissue that is being invaded by the tumor cells (see Figure 14-6B). Consequently, many breast cancers feel very firm and exhibit a puckered, scarred appearance with irregular margins that blend into the surrounding breast tissue. This appearance is caused more by the proliferation of fibrous tissue in response to the tumor than by the tumor cells themselves. Nevertheless, this appearance is quite characteristic of many breast cancers and aids in identifying a carcinoma by mammography. Not all breast carcinomas display such a characteristic appearance. In many instances, the mammogram identifies an abnormal or suspicious area within the breast that could be an early carcinoma but is not conclusive, and a biopsy is necessary to establish the exact diagnosis. As a breast tumor continues to grow, it infiltrates the breast tissues more extensively and, left untreated, eventually metastasizes to regional lymph nodes and distant sites. Hence, early diagnosis allows prompt treatment and much improves the cure rate. For this reason, routine screening mammography is recommended for all women.

Mammography

A mammogram is a special type of low-dose X-ray examination that allows the clinician to visualize the internal structure of the breast and recognize abnormalities that may not be detected by clinical examination. There are two main types of mammography: 2D digital mammography and 3D mammography—also called digital breast tomosynthesis, digital tomosynthesis, or just tomosynthesis—used

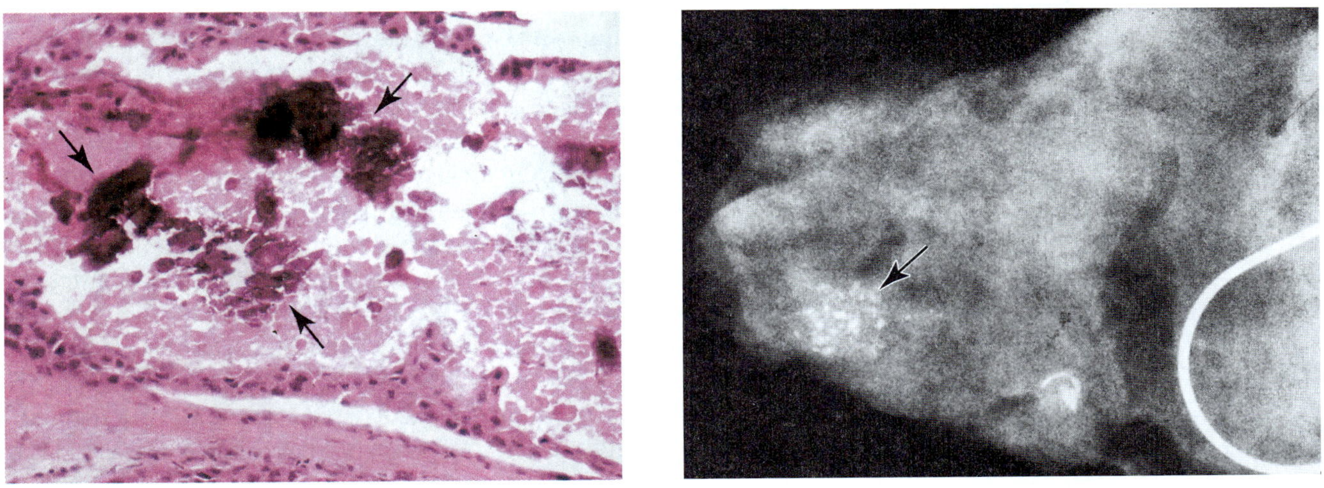

(A) **(B)**

Figure 14-7 **(A)** Ductal carcinoma of the breast, showing necrosis and calcification (*arrows*) within the tumor. **(B)** Characteristic appearance of stippled calcification within the tumor (*arrow*) that can be identified by mammograms.

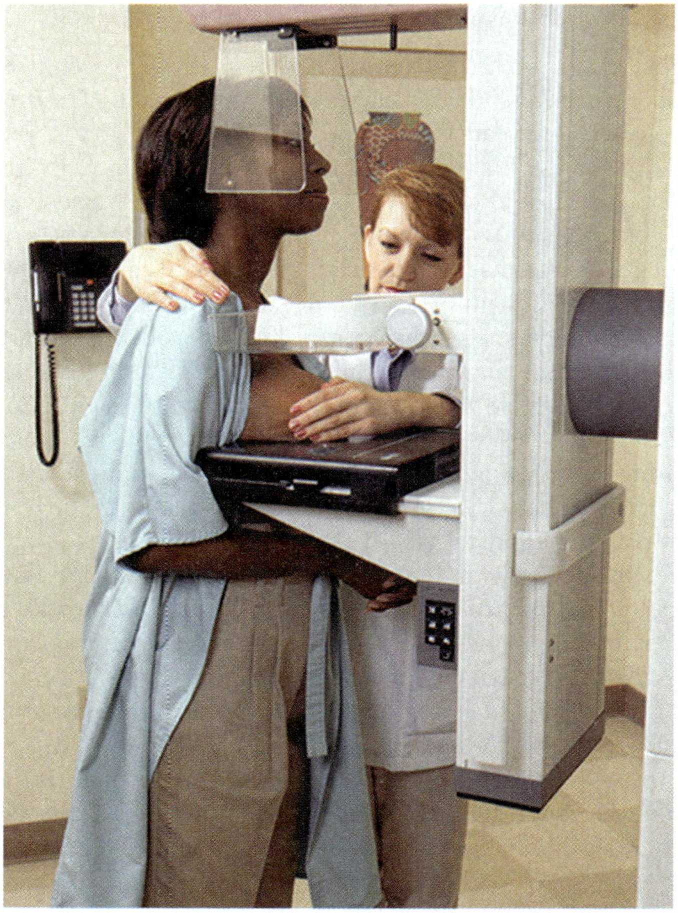

Figure 14-8 Technique of mammography. During the examination the breast will be compressed by the clear plastic paddle positioned over the breast.

in special circumstances. During a mammogram, a paddle compresses, allowing the breast tissue to be spread out and facilitate better visualization (**Figure 14-8**).

The fibrous and glandular tissue of the breast appears as interlacing white strands. The less-dense fatty tissue, which transmits X-rays readily, appears dark (**Figure 14-9** and **Figure 14-10**). Cysts and tumors within the breast appear as dense white masses surrounded by the less-dense dark tissue of the adjacent normal breast. Cysts and benign tumors appear well circumscribed, whereas malignant tumors often have irregular margins that indicate infiltration of the tumor into the surrounding breast tissue. These same criteria distinguish between benign and malignant tumors on gross examination when a biopsy specimen is examined. Malignant tumors also frequently contain fine flecks of calcium that indicate calcification within the carcinoma. This is another feature suggestive of malignancy when seen on the mammogram.

Mammography can pick up small tumors before they can be detected by breast examination; the procedure yields both false-positive and false-negative results. About 10 percent of women screened have an abnormal mammogram, although only about 5 percent of this group have cancer. The procedure may not always identify a small carcinoma in the dense breast tissue, which obscures the tumor. Screening has reduced breast cancer mortality 20 percent to 30 percent in women 50 to 69 years of age, and slightly less in women 40 to 49 years of age, probably because those women present with denser breast tissue and faster growing tumors. Mammography is sensitive in detecting

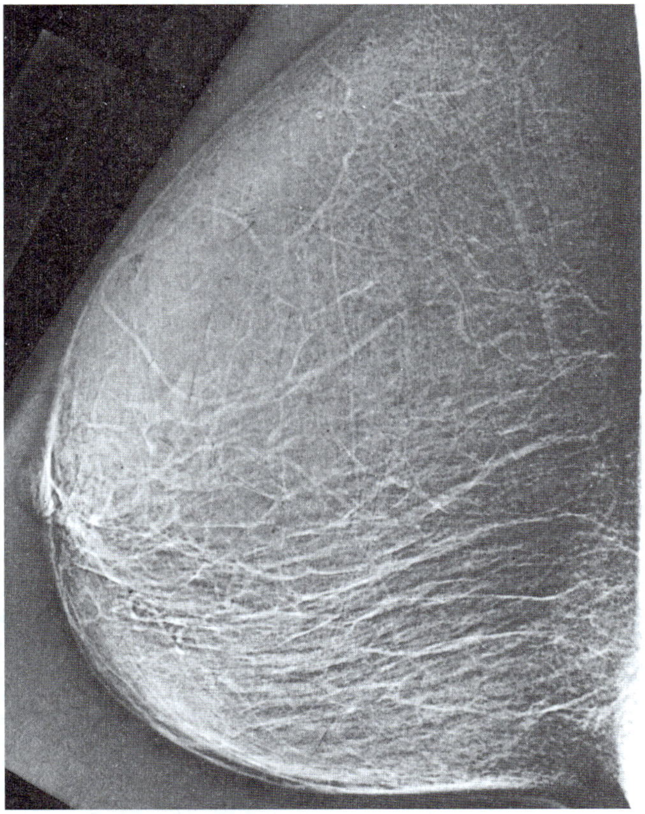

Figure 14-9 A normal mammogram.
Courtesy of Leonard V. Crowley, MD, Century College.

changes, so routine examination carefully comparing prior and current results is of critical importance in detecting breast cancer in its earliest state. Digital breast tomography (3D mammography) and MRI imaging techniques for breast examination are available. They are not currently recommended as screening techniques but are currently seeing increasing use.

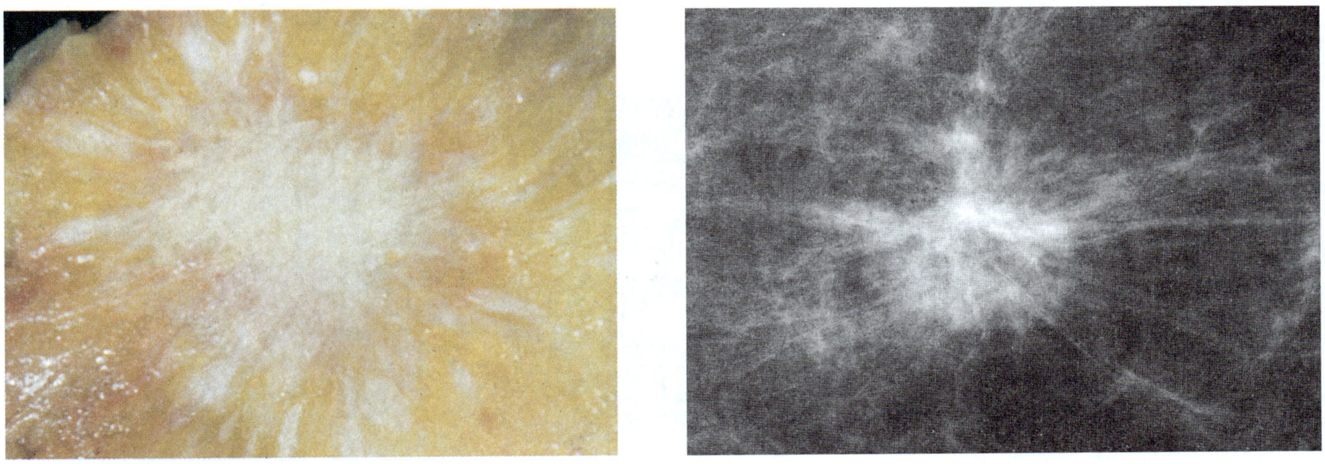

(A) **(B)**

Figure 14-10 Breast carcinoma. **(A)** Cross section of breast biopsy. The tumor appears as a firm, poorly circumscribed mass that infiltrates the surrounding fatty breast tissue. **(B)** The appearance of breast carcinoma in a mammogram. The tumor appears as a white area with infiltrating margins. Note that the same criteria used to identify breast carcinoma on gross examination are used to recognize malignancy in the mammogram.
Courtesy of Leonard V. Crowley, MD, Century College.

The American Cancer Society (ACS) recommends annual mammographic breast screening with an option to start at age 40 and continuing with yearly mammograms between the ages of 45 and 54. Women 55 and older should get mammograms yearly or biannually, continuing as long as they have a life expectancy of at least 10 years. Women at high risk based on family history, genetic testing (such as for BRCA), or other factors should get a yearly mammogram and breast MRI starting at age 30. Breast MRIs should not substitute for mammograms. An MRI examination is more likely to detect cancer but may miss some lesions best detected by mammography. Women with very dense breasts on a mammography might consider a supplemental MRI examination but as yet there is no firm recommendation from the ACS. Breast self-examination to detect early changes in the breast has not proven effective in detecting cancer, yet some health care providers suggest it as a potentially useful adjunct to mammography.

Clinical Manifestations

The most common initial manifestation of breast carcinoma is a lump in the breast. It may be detected by the patient or by a routine mammogram. A more advanced carcinoma may cause secondary changes in the overlying skin or the nipple. The neoplasm may infiltrate the suspensory ligaments, exerting traction on the ligaments and causing them to shorten. Because the ligaments attach to the skin of the breast, the shortening of the ligaments causes the overlying skin to retract as well. Consequently, skin or nipple retraction generally indicates the presence of an infiltrating carcinoma deeper within the breast.

If the tumor infiltrates and plugs the lymphatic vessels that drain lymph from the skin, the overlying skin may become edematous. Skin edema produces a rather characteristic appearance in which the normal cutaneous hair follicles stand out sharply as multiple small depressions within the edematous skin. The appearance has been compared with the skin of an orange and is usually called the orange-peel (peau d'orange) sign (**Figure 14-11**). Unfortunately, this finding indicates an advanced carcinoma that has already invaded lymphatic vessels and probably also metastasized to regional lymph nodes. The likelihood of curing the cancer is much reduced at this stage. A type of breast cancer termed Paget disease may present with changes to the nipple, including retraction, scaling, and itching and is often associated with invasive disease.

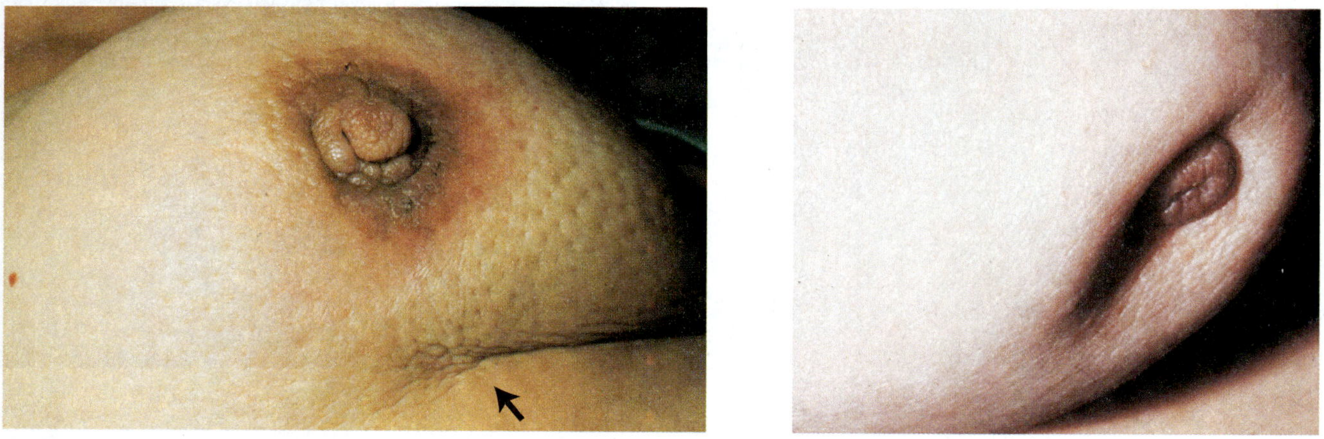

(A) (B)

Figure 14-11 Changes in the breast caused by advanced carcinoma. **(A)** Skin reaction (*arrow*) and orange-peel appearance of the skin. **(B)** Nipple retraction.

Courtesy of Leonard V. Crowley, MD, Century College.

If the patient delays in consulting her health care provider and a breast cancer is not treated, the tumor will eventually infiltrate the entire breast and will become fixed to the chest wall. The tumor will also metastasize widely. Although a far-advanced cancer often can be controlled for a time by various methods of treatment, there is no longer a possibility of cure.

Treatment

There are several ways to treat breast carcinoma, including surgery, radiation, and/or drug therapy, depending on the stage, prognostic characteristics, and desire of the patient. Decisions will be guided by the grade (often considering disease subtype based on gene expression profiles), receptor status, and stage of the disease at the time of diagnosis.

The TNM scores (see the following section) are grouped to determine the stage. Similar stages tend to have the same prognosis. Although the grading system is complicated, the higher the stage, the poorer the prognosis. For example, stage I disease is characterized by small tumors and either no or very minimal spread to lymph nodes; stage IV disease is defined by having distant metastases. Stage I disease has a 100 percent 5-year survival rate; at initial diagnosis, 60 percent of women have stage I disease. Stage IV disease has a 22 percent 5-year survival rate, emphasizing the importance of early detection (**Table 14-1**).

Table 14-1 Breast Cancer Stage Groupings and Corresponding Survival Rates

Stage	Simplified Description	5-Year Survival
Stage 0	Carcinoma *in situ* (ductal carcinoma *in situ*, DCIS)	100%
Stage IA	Tumor less than 2 cm	99% Survival rates also depend on age, overall health
Stage IB	Tumor less than 2 cm, with microscopic foci* of cancer in lymph nodes	Data not available
Stage IIA	Tumor less than 2 cm with spread to 1–3 axillary lymph nodes** OR Tumor between 2 and 5 cm without spread to lymph nodes	93% (for all scenarios)
Stage IIB	Tumor between 2 and 5 cm with spread to 1–3 axillary lymph nodes OR Tumor larger than 5 cm without extension to lymph nodes	Data not available
Stage IIIA	Tumor no more than 5 cm, with spread to 4–9 axillary lymph nodes or enlarged internal thoracic lymph nodes, OR Tumor larger than 5 cm with spread to up to 9 axillary lymph nodes	72% (for all scenarios))
Stage IIIB	Tumor of any size that has grown into chest wall or skin, with or without nodal spread	Data not available
Stage IIIC	Tumor of any size that has spread to 10 or more axillary lymph nodes, to axillary and internal thoracic lymph nodes, or to infra- or supraclavicular lymph nodes	Data not available
Stage IV	Cancer of any size with any degree of lymph node involvement, with spread to distant sites	22%

*Microscopic foci are tumor deposits less than 2 mm in diameter.

**Regional lymph nodes include both axillary and internal thoracic lymph nodes. Axillary lymph nodes are easily accessible to the surgeon, but internal thoracic (mammary) ones are usually sampled only when they are highlighted by the sentinel lymph node procedure. Involvement of internal thoracic lymph nodes imparts a slightly worse prognosis than involvement of axillary lymph nodes. Survival rates depend on other factors such as the hormone and growth factor expression by the tumor as well as patient age and overall health.

Staging of Breast Cancer: The TNM System

Sentinel lymph node The lymph node that is located closest to a malignant tumor, which is examined to determine whether the tumor has spread to the node. If the sentinel node is not involved, additional lymph node dissection is not required.

Breast cancer staging is determined using the TNM system. "T" represents the tumor size and whether the tumor is localized to the breast or spread into adjacent tissue. In the TNM system, "N" represents nearby lymph nodes. This too is evaluated by the surgeon, most often guided by a technique called **sentinel lymph node** analysis. The invasion of nearby lymph nodes by cancer cells negatively affects prognosis and depends on the number of nodes involved (and in some cases, how many cancer cells have invaded the node). Finally, the "M" represents invasion of distant sites by cancer cells (metastases), which has serious impact on the likelihood of 5-year survival. M is determined using both physical examination and a number of radiographic procedures (such as CT).

Staging of Breast Cancer: The Role of the Sentinel Node

Although cancer that invaded lymph nodes may be detectable based on node size and texture, small numbers of cancer cells are detected through microscopic analysis of the node by a pathologist. Many lymph nodes, primarily in the axillary area, drain the lymphatic channels of the breast. If one or more axillary lymph nodes contain metastatic carcinoma, the tumor has already spread beyond the breast; the greater the number of involved lymph nodes, the less favorable the prognosis.

When cancer is found in the sentinel node, more extensive analysis of additional nodes is necessary (**Figure 14-12** and **Figure 14-13**).

Surgical and Other Techniques in Breast Cancer Therapy

There are many variables, including the cancer stage and the nature of the particular tumor, that are taken into account in deciding on the nature of the surgery to be used. The clinician (oncologist specializing in breast cancer),

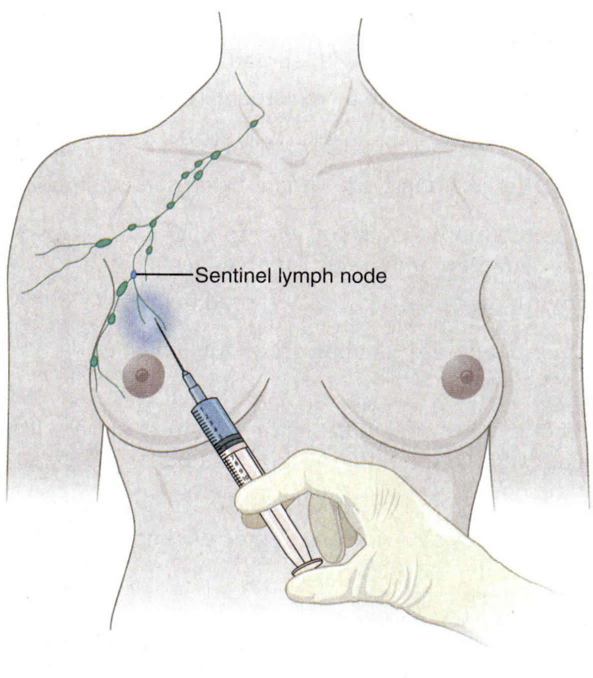

Figure 14-12 Schematic diagram of a sentinel lymph node biopsy.

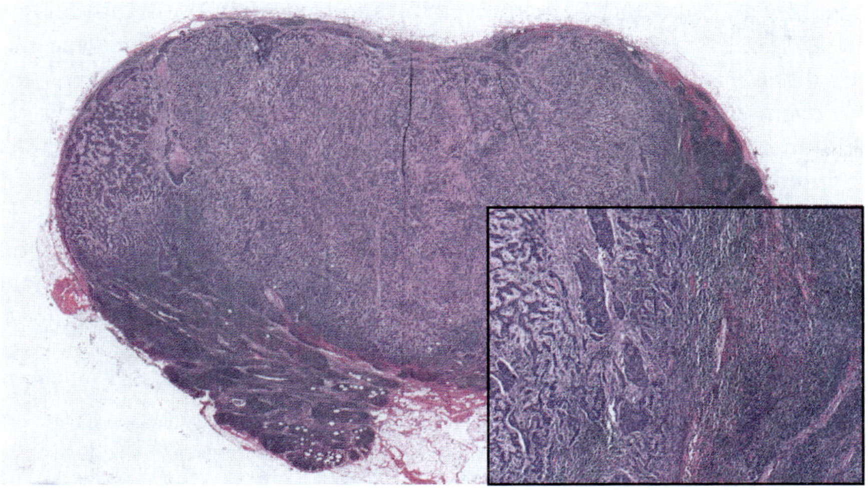

Figure 14-13 Axillary lymph node with metastatic tumor. Inset: Breast tumor cells on the right are effacing the normal lymphatic tissue on the left (high power).
Courtesy of Department of Pathology and Laboratory Medicine, University of North Carolina at Chapel Hill.

the pathologist who evaluated the surgical specimen, and most certainly the patient will decide on their preference. Surgical treatment of breast cancer can be divided into two general approaches. The first, **breast-conserving surgery**, sometimes called a "lumpectomy," attempts to remove the minimal amount of breast tissue while still removing all of the cancer and nearby tissue. The degree of tissue removed will depend on the size and location of the lesion. The surgeon, working closely with the pathologist, examines the removed tissue during surgery to ensure that the cancer is removed with adequate margins of healthy tissue on all sides of the removed tissue. In DCIS, breast-conserving surgery accompanied by radiation therapy results in as good a prognosis as a mastectomy. DCIS patients sometimes decide against radiation therapy (for example, in cases of pregnancy). DCIS patients may also elect mastectomy (particularly in cases where DCIS is extensive). Generally, radiation therapy is not needed, and breast reconstructive surgery can be done quickly. Stage I disease without lymph node involvement may be treated much as described for DCIS. Systemic hormonal therapy will likely be used if the tumor is hormone receptor–positive (ER- or PR-positive). Larger tumors may also be treated with systemic chemotherapy, particularly in tumors likely to be fast-growing.

Breast-conserving surgery Surgery designed to remove the minimal amount of breast tissue.

When the cancer is large or has spread (higher stage cancers), total mastectomy may be required. The choice between more limited (sparing skin and some lymph nodes) and more extensive procedures is complex and depends both on the nature of the cancer and patient preferences.

Overall Breast Cancer Therapy

Overall breast cancer therapy describes both surgical and other treatment techniques and may be applied locally or systemically.

Systemic Therapy

The decision to use neoadjuvant chemotherapy (chemotherapy prior to surgery) and the details of drugs and regimens are complex and depend on the perceived benefit versus risk of therapy. The decision to use systemic chemotherapy depends on the tumor type and the details of tumor biology. In general, those types of breast cancer with higher risk of recurrence and metastatic disease, such as HER-2-positive and triple negative breast cancer, benefit from chemotherapy. Triple negative disease may benefit from the addition of platinum-containing drugs to the standard two-drug therapy but at the cost of significant added toxicity.

Luminal type A and B tumors that are HER-2 negative remain the most commonly diagnosed type. A and B can be difficult to distinguish, and the decision to use **neoadjuvant therapy**, commonly using two different anticancer drugs, depends on the perceived likelihood of relapse in 10 years. Commercial multigene assays provide useful information on the likelihood of recurrence. Patients with high or intermediate risk clearly benefit from neoadjuvant chemotherapy, while low-risk patients likely do not.

Neoadjuvant therapy Therapy used before primary cancer treatment.

Aromatase inhibitor A drug that inhibits the conversion of adrenal androgenic steroids to estrogens, used to treat postmenopausal women with estrogen receptor-positive breast carcinoma.

Very early luminal breast cancer cells express an estrogen receptor and also, most frequently, a progesterone receptor on their surfaces. Tamoxifen is a selective estrogen-receptor modulator (SERM) that acts to inhibit the division of the cancer cells (but not kill them) by binding to the estrogen receptor. For this reason, tamoxifen continues to be taken by the patient for many years. In postmenopausal women, estrogen is produced in tissues other than the breast. **Aromatase inhibitors** prevent the conversion of estrogen precursors (androgens) into estrogen by blocking the enzyme aromatase in peripheral tissues such as the adrenal gland. In postmenopausal patients, both tamoxifen and aromatase inhibitors may be used, but current data suggests that the latter may be more effective and may be taken for at least 5 years, although its use is associated with potentially serious side effects.

Those with HER-2-positive breast cancer clearly benefit from the addition of monoclonal antibody therapy in addition to chemotherapy for up to 1 year. The monoclonal antibody binds to the HER-2 receptor and slows down cancer cell growth. Rarely, serious cardiac complications are associated with its use. The addition of a second anti-HER-2 antibody to therapy is of clear benefit even in patients with metastatic disease.

Metastatic Breast Cancer Therapy

Although metastatic breast disease must be considered incurable, with therapy it may become a chronic disease. Progression-free survival of patients and even overall survival may be prolonged by therapy. Metastases may differ in their biology from the primary tumor, so it is important to confirm the continued presence of estrogen and progesterone receptors and HER-2 when such are found in the primary lesion. Bone-modifying drugs, such as bisphosphonates and others, used in postmenopausal patients stabilize bone loss related to anti-estrogen therapy but also reduce the recurrence of bone metastasis and prolong survival. Anti-estrogen therapies may prolong survival in ER-positive disease. In the case of HER-2-positive disease, monoclonal antibody therapy directed against the HER-2 protein, sometimes conjugated to a chemotherapeutic drug, is used. A large number of chemotherapeutic agents are available for use in the treatment of metastatic disease, and the selection of the most appropriate is complex and often involves the combination of multiple drugs. Work on more effective chemotherapeutic regimens and additional targeted therapies is ongoing, with new agents being announced frequently.

Case 14-1

Jane is a 33-year-old concerned about the possibility of breast disease. A maternal aunt was diagnosed with invasive breast cancer at the age of 48. Jane's mother (age 62) has been biopsied on several occasions for suspicious breast lesions that were diagnosed as benign cysts and twice as fibroadenomas. Because of her concern, Jane is careful to practice breast self-examination and has elected to have yearly mammography starting at age 30. Jane paid to be tested for BRCA1 and BRCA2 and was found to be negative. She has been diagnosed as having mild fibrocystic formations in her breast tissue but otherwise had a normal mammogram 6 months ago. On self-examination, Jane now notes a single hard mass in the upper inner quadrant of her left breast. The mass appeared to be adherent to the skin. Jane's physician confirmed a 3-cm mass that was tender to firm on palpation. The physician noted a slight skin retraction over the mass and was concerned about the possibility of a rapidly growing carcinoma. Mammography revealed an irregular mass with some architectural distortion and calcification, supporting the concern for malignancy. Because of this concern, Jane elected to have an excisional biopsy in which the entire mass was removed. The surgeon noted the mass was yellow in color, appeared to be fibrotic with areas of calcification, and had several small cystic regions. Microscopic analysis of the tissue (**Case Figure 14-1**) demonstrated a process consistent with **fat necrosis** (also called **enzymatic fat necrosis**) of the breast. This is a specific form of necrosis associated with damage to areas of the body rich in lipid-containing cells. Fat necrosis in the breast is a benign process that requires no therapy. However, the process may be difficult to differentiate from cancer and requires biopsy for diagnosis. A much-relieved Jane reflected upon possible trauma to her breast. About three months before noting the mass, Jane remembers that she came to a very sudden stop while driving. She noted some bruising and pain along the area of her breast crossed by the seatbelt.

Fat necrosis A specific form of inflammation that occurs after trauma (or other damage) to areas of the body rich in lipid.
Enzymatic fat necrosis See fat necrosis.

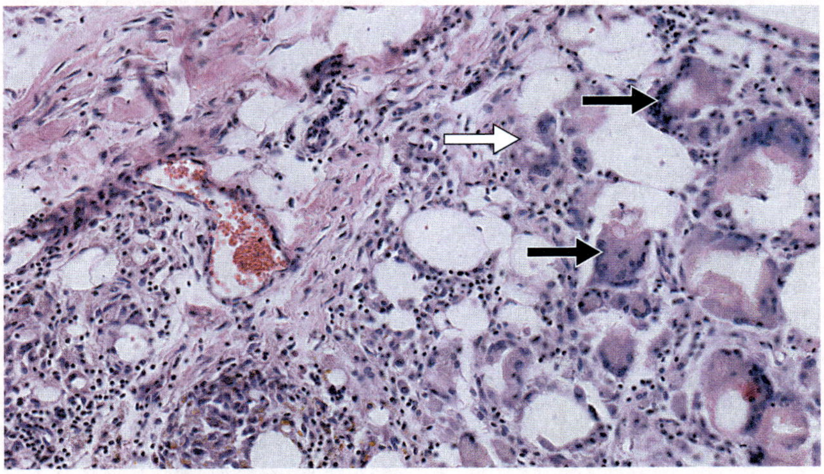

Case Figure 14-1 Excisional biopsy of breast demonstrating fat necrosis (photomicrograph). Examples of giant cells (*black arrows*) and lipid-filled (foamy) macrophages (*white arrow*). Lymphocytes and numerous small oil cysts are scattered through the tissues. Fibrosis is present on the upper left margin.
Courtesy of Department of Pathology and Laboratory Medicine, University of North Carolina at Chapel Hill.

(continues)

Case 14-1 *(Continued)*

Discussion

Fat necrosis is a form of inflammation that occurs after trauma (or other damage) to areas of the body rich in lipid. In fat necrosis, lipid released from damaged fat cells is saponified by tissue lipases in the presence of calcium. The lipid may form cysts in the tissue and provokes a chronic inflammatory response. Macrophages ingest the lipid (foamy macrophages) and fuse to form giant cells in response to the irritant material. Ultimately, healing occurs accompanied by fibrosis (scarring), deposition of calcium in the tissue, and potentially residual lipid cysts. Pathologists usually think about the area around the pancreas when they consider fat necrosis because it is common in this region in response to pancreatitis. (In this setting fat necrosis has serious medical consequences.) However, fat necrosis is not uncommon in the breast and buttocks. Fat necrosis accounts for about 3 percent of benign breast lesions. Seatbelt-induced injury and trauma related to breast surgery are common causes. Most cases of fat necrosis in the breast are easy to diagnosis based on the presence of radiolucent cysts (using mammography often combined with ultrasound) and may not require a biopsy. With time, continuing inflammation, fibrosis, and calcification may present in a manner similar to cancer and require a biopsy. For this reason, a careful patient history that discloses possible breast trauma is important in the clinical decision-making process. Although it was understandable for Jane to be concerned about breast cancer given her history, it is important to realize that the majority of breast lesions biopsied are not cancer (**Case Figure 14-2**).

Etiology and Pathogenesis

Fat necrosis of the breast as a result of seatbelt-induced tissue trauma.

Question

1. Given Jane's family history, were her concerns about early onset breast cancer justified?
2. The American Cancer Society suggests routine mammography begin at age 40. Other expert opinions suggest starting later. What drawbacks would there be to recommending routine mammography very early (at age 20 or 30, for example)?
3. Suppose Jane's mammogram disclosed a cystic area. Do you believe she would have been wise to proceed to a biopsy?

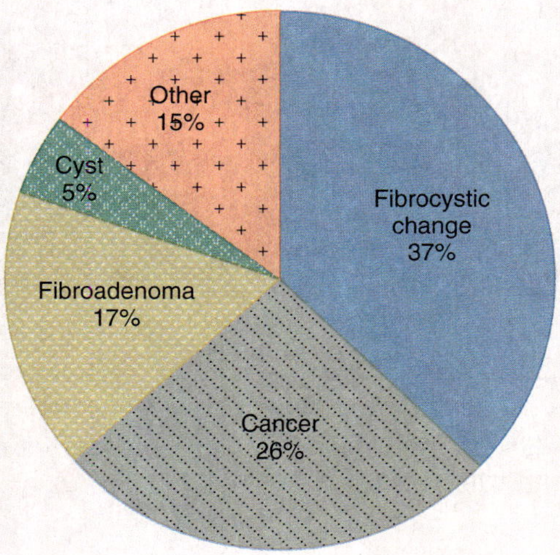

Case Figure 14-2 Relative frequency of lesions of the breast that are biopsied out of concern for cancer.

Questions for Review

1. What are the common diseases of the breast that may be manifested as a lump in the breast? How are they distinguished from one another by a physician?
2. What is a mammogram? How is it used by a physician?
3. What are estrogen receptors in tumor cells? How is estrogen receptor analysis used in management of patients with breast carcinoma?
4. What is gynecomastia?
5. What methods are used to treat breast carcinoma?
6. What is an aromatase inhibitor, and how is it used?

References

Livasy C, Calhoun BC. Breast pathology. In: Reisner H, ed. *Pathology: A Modern Case Study*. 2nd ed. McGraw-Hill Lange; 2020:Chapter 17.

Breast Cancer. American Cancer Society. Accessed May 2, 2025. https://www.cancer.org/cancer/types/breast-cancer.html

Breast Cancer—Patient Version. NIH National Cancer Institute. Accessed May 2, 2025. http://www.cancer.gov/cancertopics/types/breast

Breast Cancer Screening (PDQ®)—Patient Version. NIH National Cancer Institute. Accessed May 2, 2025. https://www.cancer.gov/types/breast/patient/breast-screening-pdq

Breast Cancer Screening Guidelines. American Cancer Society. Accessed May 2, 2025. https://www.cancer.org/health-care-professionals/american-cancer-society-prevention-early-detection-guidelines/breast-cancer-screening-guidelines.html

- The literature about breast cancer is immense and at times controversial. This set of five articles has been selected as an overview. The first reference provides a brief review of the pathology of breast cancer aimed at undergraduate medical students. It presents a readable and case-rich introduction to the area for anyone interested in the background to the diagnosis of breast disease, including infection and inflammation, not covered in detail in this chapter. References two and three provide excellent overviews and additional references to breast cancer screening and therapy. Many of the clinical guidelines in this chapter are those given by the American Cancer Society. The last two references cover the area of screening, including potential risks.

BRCA Gene Changes: Cancer Risk and Genetic Testing. NIH National Cancer Institute. https://www.cancer.gov/about-cancer/causes-prevention/genetics/brca-fact-sheet#:~:text=Testing%20for%20inherited%20harmful%20changes%20in%20BRCA1%20and%20BRCA2%20may,with%20a%20particular%20targeted%20therapy

- A recent overview of the characteristics of this inherited form of breast cancer. Not dated.

Khattab A, Kashyap S, Monga DK. Male Breast Cancer. StatPearls [Internet]. Updated September 10, 2024. https://www.ncbi.nlm.nih.gov/books/NBK526036/

- Although uncommon, male breast cancer has a very poor prognosis and is often ignored.

Tan PH, Lai LM, Carrington EV, et al. Fat necrosis of the breast: A review. *Breast*. 2006;15(3):313–318.

- All breast disease is not cancer. This review was useful in constructing the case. The condition is becoming increasingly frequent in cases of breast reconstruction and aesthetic modification.

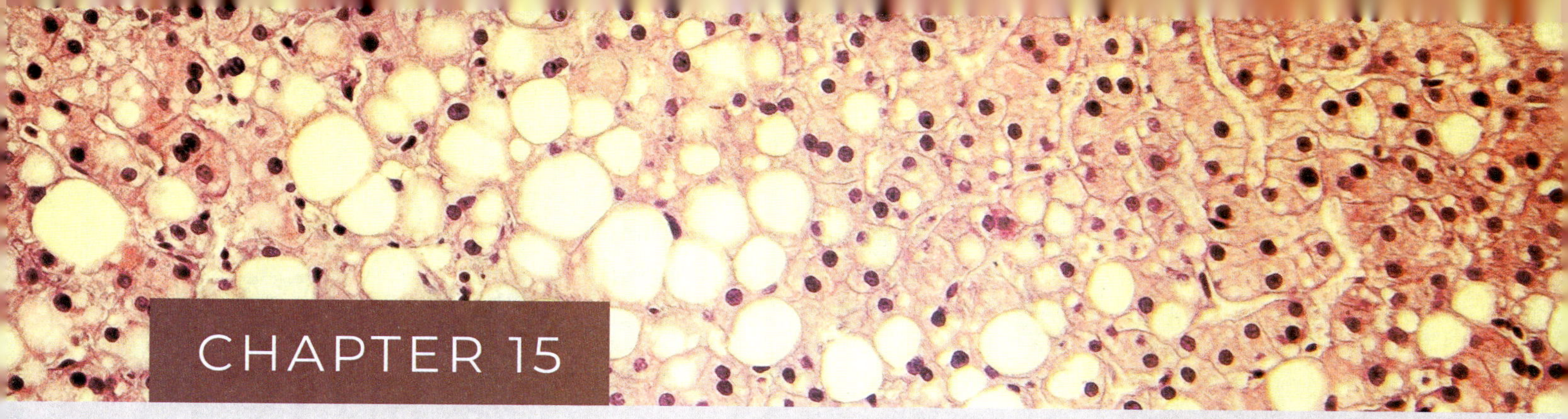

CHAPTER 15

Pregnancy and Infertility

LEARNING OBJECTIVES

1. Explain the causes and effects of spontaneous abortion and ectopic pregnancy.
2. Describe commonly used prenatal screening and genetic testing procedures.
3. Describe the mechanism and clinical manifestations of the problems associated with abnormal attachment of the placenta within the uterus and abnormal attachment of the umbilical cord.
4. Differentiate between identical and fraternal twins. Describe how zygosity can be determined from examination of the placenta.
5. Classify the types of gestational trophoblast disease. Explain their prognoses, and describe the methods of treatment.
6. Explain the pathogenesis, clinical manifestations, diagnostic criteria, and methods used to treat hemolytic disease of the newborn.
7. Understand the causes and effects of gestational diabetes and pregnancy-associated toxemia.
8. Define the two types of infertility.
9. Explain potential treatments for infertility.

Pregnancy

Duration of Pregnancy

The total duration of pregnancy from **fertilization** to delivery is termed the period of **gestation**, approximately 38 weeks when dated from the time of ovulation. Usually, however, the actual date of ovulation is not known, and the length of gestation is calculated from the beginning of the last normal menstrual period. Expressed in this way, the duration of pregnancy is 40 weeks because the first day of the calculation is actually about 2 weeks before the date of conception. The gestation calculated in this way may also be expressed as 280 days, as 10 lunar (28-day) months, or as 9 calendar (31-day) months. Often the 9 calendar months are subdivided into three periods termed trimesters, each of 3 months' duration. Pregnancy brings many physical and physiological changes to the pregnant person. Some can be considered mild and/or tolerable, while others will need medical management. **Figure 15-1** illustrates many of them. Some will be covered in more detail in this chapter.

Fertilization Penetration of the ovum by the sperm.

Gestation Duration of pregnancy from fertilization to delivery.

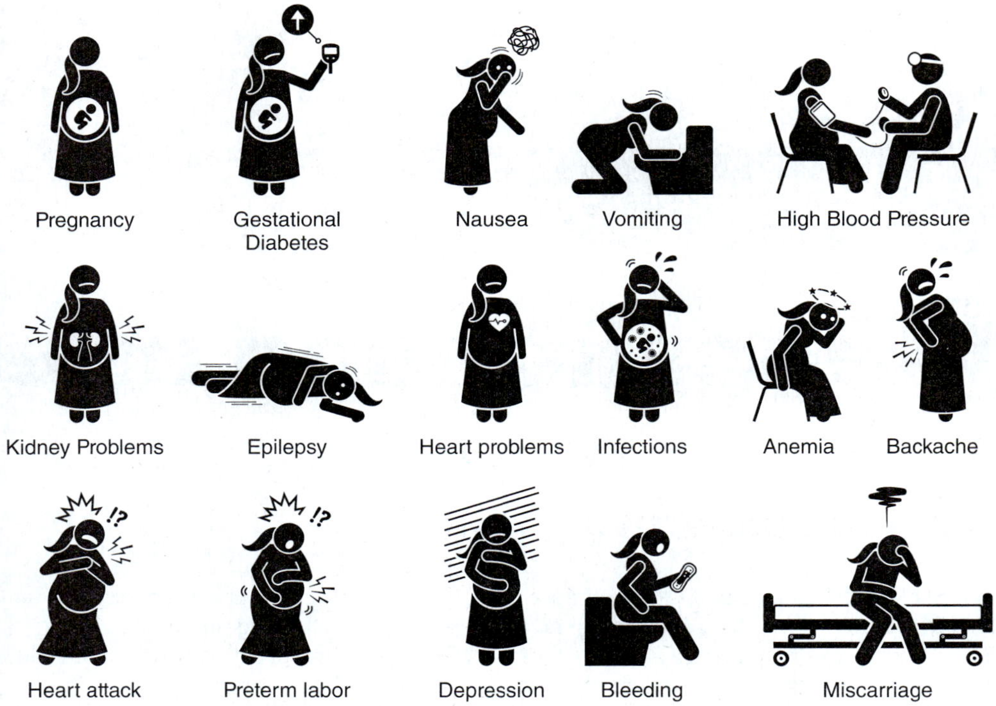

Figure 15-1 Pregnancy complications. In addition to the most frequently seen pregnancy complications in this figure, other pregnancy complications may still arise.

Decidua The endometrium of pregnancy.

Embryo Developing organism from fertilization until organogenesis. A human embryo is from conception until the beginning of the ninth week of gestation.

Chorion The layer of trophoblast and associated mesoderm that surrounds the developing embryo.

Chorionic villi Fingerlike columns of cells extending from the chorion that anchor the chorionic vesicle in the endometrium.

Placenta Flat, disk-shaped structure that maintains the developing organism within the uterus.

Body stalk The structure connecting the embryo to the chorion. Eventually develops into the umbilical cord.

Decidua, Fetal Membranes, and Placenta

The Decidua—The Pregnant Endometrium

The endometrium of pregnancy is termed the **decidua**. **Figure 15-2** demonstrates the relationship of the **embryo** to the surrounding amniotic sac and **chorion** about 7 weeks after fertilization. **Figure 15-3** diagrammatically illustrates these relationships in both early and late pregnancy.

The Chorion and Chorionic Villi

The chorion contains the fetal blood vessels that extend into the **chorionic villi**. The villi arising from the deeper portion of the chorion are actively proliferative. These villi project into the large blood-filled spaces within the maternal part of the **placenta** (the decidua basalis) through which the maternal blood flows. Some of the villi also function as anchoring villi, which attach the chorion to the maternal tissues. Blood vessels that form within the villi as they grow become connected with blood vessels in the chorion and the **body stalk**, as well as within the body of the embryo. As soon as the embryo's heart begins to beat, blood begins to flow through this developing network of vessels.

The Amniotic Sac

The amniotic sac is enclosed within the chorion. At first the sac is much smaller than the chorionic cavity (see Figure 15-2); as the pregnancy progresses the enlarging sac expands into the chorionic cavity. Eventually the amniotic

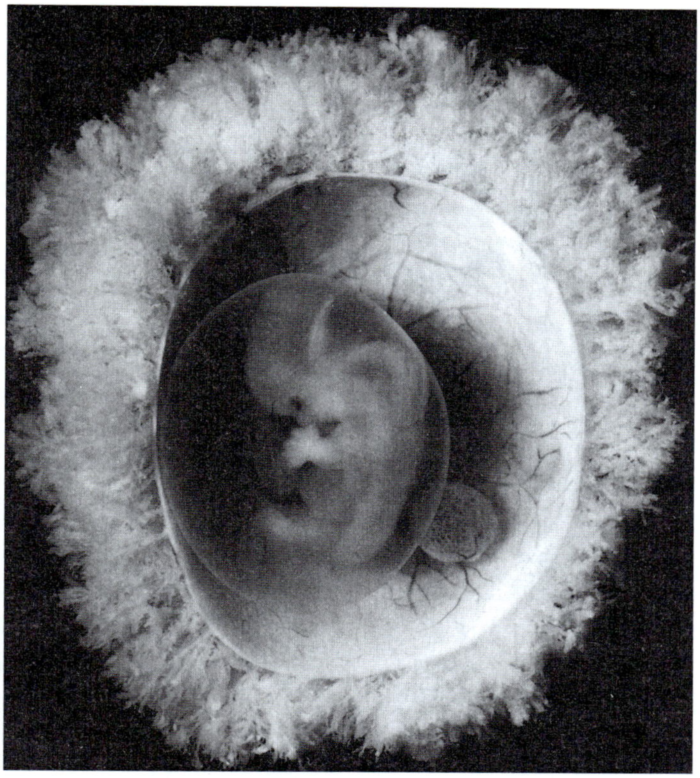

Figure 15-2 Relationship of the embryo to the amniotic sac, yolk sac, and chorionic cavity at about 7 weeks after contraception. The chorionic sac has been bisected. At this stage, villi still arise from the entire periphery of the chorion, and the amniotic sac surrounding the embryo does not completely fill the chorionic cavity. The embryo is attached to the chorion by the umbilical cord (not shown). The yolk sac is located to the right of the amniotic sac, between the amniotic sac and the chorion.
Courtesy of Carnegie Science.

sac completely fills the chorionic cavity, and the amniotic membrane lies against the chorion. The sac functions as a buoyant, temperature-controlled environment that protects the **fetus** throughout pregnancy and contributes to processes that open the cervix during childbirth.

Fetus A precursor in plasma converted into fibrin by thrombin during blood coagulation.

Yolk sac A sac formed that will contribute to the gastrointestinal tract and other important embryonic structures.

The Yolk Sac

In the human being, the **yolk sac** never contains yolk but performs other important functions, serving as the source of hematopoietic cells and the primordial germ cells that eventually form sperm and eggs in the developing gonads. Part of the yolk sac becomes incorporated into the body of the embryo to form the intestinal tract. The part that is not included within the embryo persists for a time but usually atrophies. In a small number of adults, a remnant persists as a Meckel diverticulum (discussed further in Chapter 16).

The Placenta

The placenta is a flattened, disk-shaped structure weighing about 500 g. It has a dual origin, both fetal and maternal (**Figure 15-4**). The amnion and chorion extend from the margins of the placenta to form the fluid-filled sac that encloses the fetus and ruptures at the time of delivery. The fetus is connected to the placenta by the umbilical cord, which contains two arteries. On the surface of the placenta, the artery divides into multiple branches, each supplying an

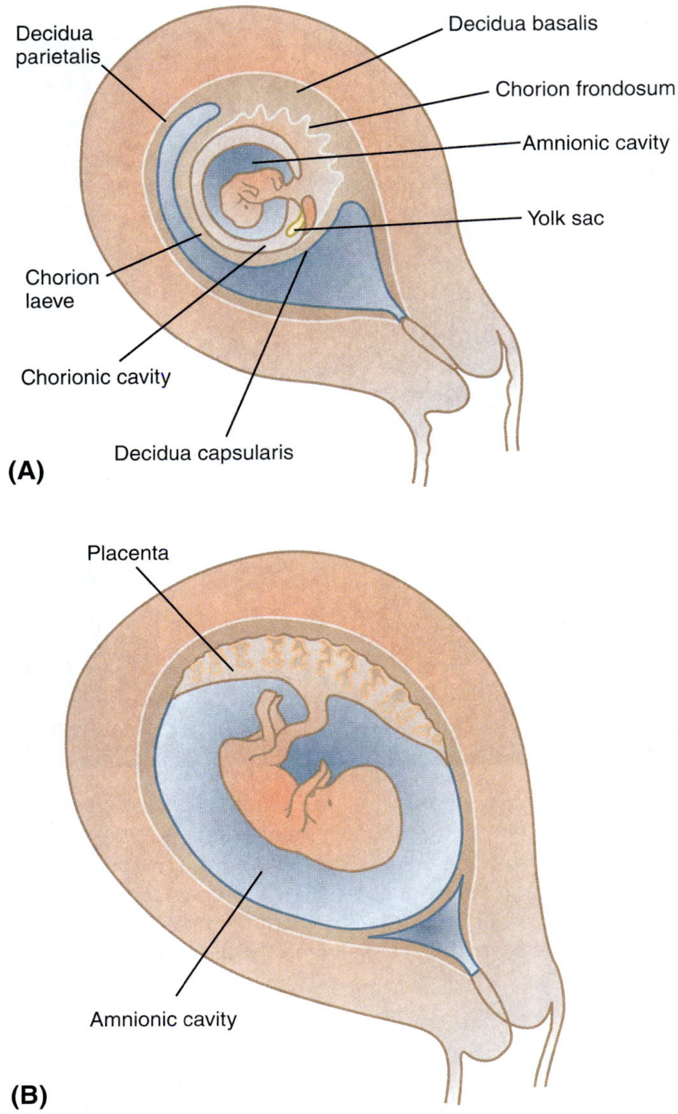

Figure 15-3 **(A)** Relationship of the fetus to the decidua, fetal membranes, and chorion in early pregnancy. The part of the yolk sac not incorporated within the fetus lies between the amniotic sac and the chorion. **(B)** Relationship in late pregnancy. The amniotic sac envelops the fetus and now completely fills the chorionic cavity. The amniotic membrane lies against the chorion. The decidua capsularis has fused with the chorion laeve and has become adherent to the decidua parietalis on the opposite wall of the uterus.

individual cluster of villi separated by a partition termed a cotyledon. Blood returning from the cotyledons is collected into large veins on the surface of the placenta to form the umbilical vein, which returns the blood to the fetus.

Circulation of Blood in the Placenta

The placenta has a dual circulation of blood (**Figure 15-5**). The fetoplacental circulation delivers arterial blood low in oxygen from the fetus to the chorionic villi through the umbilical artery and returns oxygenated blood to the fetus through the single umbilical vein. The uteroplacental circulation delivers oxygenated arterial blood from the mother into the large placental blood spaces located between the villi, termed the intervillous spaces. The blood

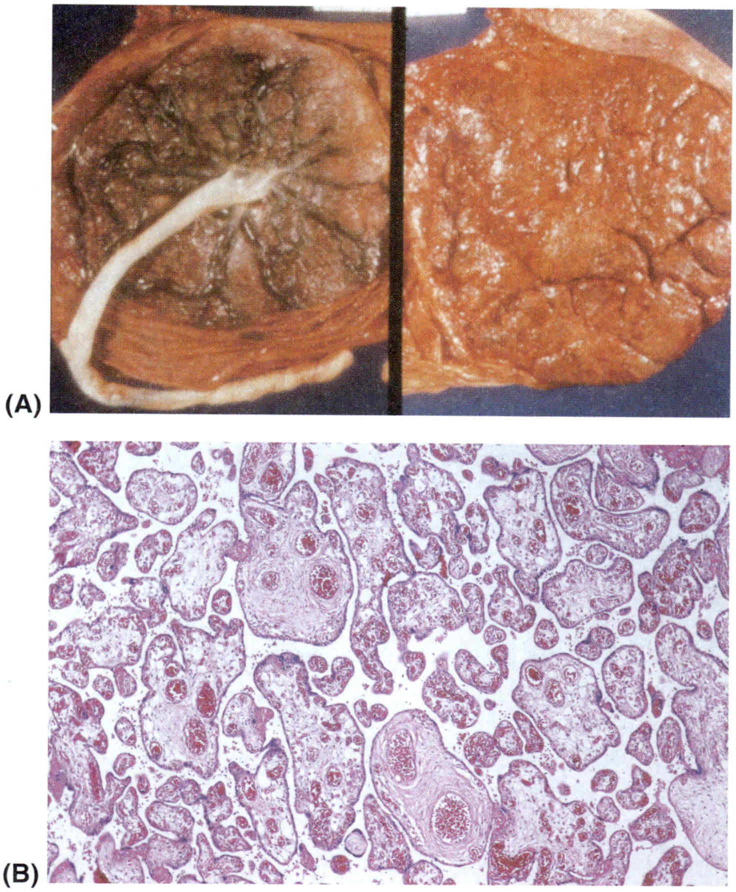

Figure 15-4 **(A)** Normal placenta. The fetal surface (*left side*) shows the umbilical cord and cord vessels that subdivide on the placental surface to supply chorionic villi. The cobblestone appearance of the material surface of the placenta (*right side*) is caused by the cotyledons, which are clusters of villi separated by partitions extending between the villi. **(B)** Histologic section of placenta revealing chorionic villi viewed in cross section. Blood vessels in villi contain fetal cells. When the placenta is within the uterus, the spaces between the villi are filled with maternal blood (original magnification ×100).

Courtesy of Leonard V. Crowley, MD, Century College.

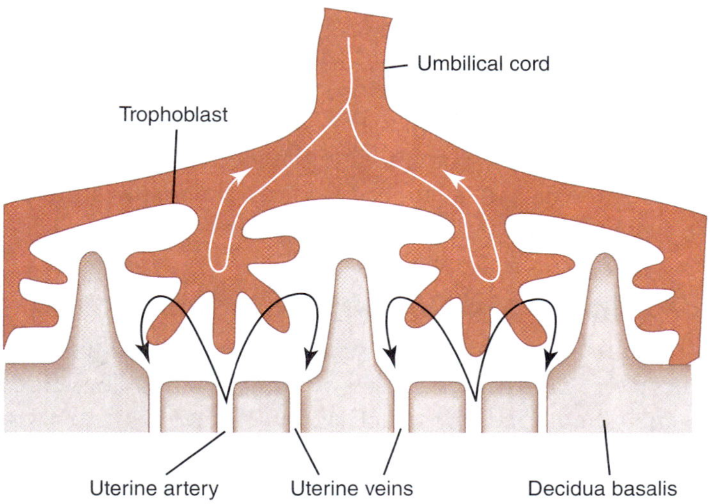

Figure 15-5 Dual circulation of blood in the placenta. Fetal blood circulates through the villi, and maternal blood flows around the villi, but circulations do not intermix.

flows into the intervillous spaces from the many uterine arteries that penetrate the basal portion of the placenta. Blood flows back into the maternal circulation through veins that penetrate the basal part of the placenta. The arrangement of the two circulations in the placenta brings the maternal and fetal blood into close approximation. In this way, oxygen and nutrients can be exchanged between the maternal and fetal circulations, but there is no actual intermixing of fetal and maternal blood, although very small amounts of fetal blood sometimes enter maternal circulation through small defects in the placental membrane. Fetal DNA can be found in the maternal circulation due to migration of fetal cells and, in large part, the release of DNA from apoptotic cells in the placenta. Hence, most "fetal DNA" in the maternal circulation is better termed placental DNA.

Endocrine Function of the Placenta

The placenta synthesizes two steroid hormones, estrogen and progesterone, and two protein hormones, termed **human chorionic somatomammotropin (hCS)** (also termed human placental lactogen) and **human chorionic gonadotropin (hCG)**. HCS stimulates maternal metabolic processes by acting as an anti-insulin, increasing maternal glucose levels. hCG is quite similar to the gonadotropic hormones produced by the pituitary gland that suppresses the onset of menstruation. Pregnancy tests detect hCG. The newer, more sensitive tests performed on blood or urine become positive as early as 10 to 12 days after fertilization, even before the first missed menstrual cycle.

Human chorionic somatomammotropin (hCS) One of the hormones produced by the placenta that has properties similar to the pituitary growth hormone. Also termed human placental lactogen.

Human chorionic gonadotropin (hCG) A hormone made by the placenta in pregnancy with actions similar to pituitary gonadotropins. Same hormone is made by neoplastic cells in some types of malignant testicular tumors.

Polyhydramnios An excess of amnionic fluid.

Anencephaly A congenital malformation considered to be a neural tube defect where parts of the brain, cranium and scalp may be missing.

Oligohydramnios An insufficient quantity of amnionic fluid.

Amniotic Fluid

The quantity of amniotic fluid, produced both by filtration and by excretion, varies with the stage of pregnancy. During the early part of pregnancy, the amniotic fluid is formed chiefly by filtration of fluid into the amniotic sac from maternal blood as it passes through the uterus and from fetal blood passing through the placenta. Additional fluid diffuses directly through the fetal skin prior to its maturation and keratin formation from the fetal respiratory tract. Later, when the fetal kidneys begin to function at about the eleventh week, the fetus urinates into the amniotic cavity, and fetal urine becomes the major source of amniotic fluid. By late pregnancy, 500 ml of urine is contributed by the fetus. Both filtration and fetal urine continually add to the volume of fluid, but the additions are counterbalanced by losses of amniotic fluid into the fetal gastrointestinal tract. Normally, the fetus swallows as much as 400 ml of fluid per day. This fluid is absorbed from the fetal intestinal tract into the fetal circulation, transferred across the placenta into the mother's circulation, and eventually excreted by the mother in her urine. Excess fluid also contributes to fetal urine and is recirculated into the amniotic fluid.

Polyhydramnios and Oligohydramnios

Polyhydramnios is a condition in which the volume of amniotic fluid is markedly increased. This can be caused by congenital maldevelopment of the fetal brain, including conditions such as **anencephaly** (see Chapter 16), which disturbs the normal swallowing mechanism so that the fetus is unable to swallow amniotic fluid, or a congenital obstruction of the fetal upper intestinal tract that blocks the entry of swallowed fluid into the small intestine where it can be absorbed. **Oligohydramnios** is a marked reduction in the volume of amniotic fluid that occurs either because the fetal kidneys have failed to develop and no urine is formed or because a congenital obstruction blocks the urethra so that urine cannot be excreted. When preterm rupture of membranes occurs too early to allow for immediate delivery, those neonates who survive suffer from oligohydramnios and developmental abnormalities associated with it (as discussed in **Case 15-1**) and have a high incidence of intrauterine infection.

Hormone-Related Conditions Associated with Pregnancy

The hormones produced by a woman's endocrine glands and by her placenta during pregnancy maintain the pregnancy and sustain the fetus, but some have undesirable effects on the pregnant woman. Nausea and vomiting during early pregnancy are related to the rapidly increasing levels of estrogen. Since nausea and vomiting often occur in the morning, the term morning sickness arose to describe this condition. However, nausea and vomiting associated with early pregnancy can occur at any time during the day. This condition usually subsides by the end of the first trimester. **Hyperemesis gravidarum** literally means excessive vomiting of pregnancy; it probably results from the same hormonal basis as morning sickness but is more prolonged and severe. Weight loss and dehydration may require treatment with intravenous fluids.

Hyperemesis gravidarum Excess vomiting associated with pregnancy.

Prenatal Screening and Genetic Testing

In general, prenatal testing during pregnancy takes different approaches. Screening tests look at the growth and development of the fetus to ensure that the fetus is attaining well-documented milestones. Genetic testing seeks to examine DNA from the fetus to look for chromosomal or other genetic abnormalities.

Screening Tests

As part of routine health care for pregnancy, ultrasound examinations measure the growth of the fetus. Serial ultrasound testing may begin around 8 to 10 weeks of pregnancy. With a normally progressing pregnancy, the first screening ultrasound usually occurs between 10 and 13 weeks of pregnancy. At this time, the number of fetuses, the speed of the fetal heart rate, and the size of the fetus can be established. In pregnancies further along than 11 weeks, a nuchal translucency test may be part of the ultrasound finding. By measuring the thickness of the fetus' neck and determining if a buildup of fluid is present, some genetic conditions, such as Down syndrome or other genetic disorders, may be suggested, or a possibility which would warrant additional more directed follow-up.

The second screening ultrasound usually occurs around 20 weeks' gestation. It can be referred to as the anatomy scan. It checks the developing organs as well as looks for abnormal levels of fluid in the amniotic sac or placenta. While not 100 percent accurate, a normal scan does offer a measure of reassurance during the pregnancy, and an abnormal scan will lead to follow-up testing. Usually during this scan, the sex of the baby can be determined with a 95% accuracy rate for those wishing to know that information prior to birth.

Ultrasounds may be ordered during the third trimester to assess both fetal and maternal health in preparation for delivery. Ordering a third trimester ultrasound is up to the discretion of the healthcare provider and the pregnant person.

Metabolic marker testing and numerous other blood tests occur throughout pregnancy to assess the course of the pregnancy and the potential effects of the pregnancy on the health of the pregnant person.

Genetic Testing

Cell-Free (cfDNA) Testing

Parents may find it desirable to undertake testing that looks at the genetic make-up of the fetus. CfDNA (cell-free DNA) testing takes a sample of blood from the pregnant person and looks for small pieces of fetal DNA that may be circulating as a normal part of the pregnancy. This type of testing finds chromosomal abnormalities such as trisomy 21 (Down syndrome) or other chromosomal disorders mostly linked to one of the common chromosomal trisomy arrangements and can also detect the sex of the fetus. CfDNA testing is currently not used to detect individual gene mutations or variations. However, such testing is becoming increasingly feasible when such mutations are suspected based on family history.

Chorionic Villus Sampling (CVS)

The chorionic villi are part of the placenta contributed by the fetus and therefore contain fetal DNA. Using guidance from ultrasound, the healthcare provider biopsies a chorionic villus from the placenta. The cells are cultured, and DNA is extracted for a more thorough analysis. Generally, the procedure can be performed between 10 and 13 weeks' gestation. Like any invasive procedure, there are associated risks, including potential fetal loss, infection, and bleeding. For this reason cfDNA testing is preferable when such is feasible.

Amniocentesis

Amniocentesis is removal of amniotic fluid, also referred to as an aspiration biopsy, from the amniotic sac after 14 weeks' gestation. The fluid contains fetal cells as well as other proteins and substances. The fetal cells can be used for genetic screening, and the other substances in the fluid can be diagnosed as signs of fetal disease or distress. As an invasive procedure, there are risks to the pregnancy similar to those for CVS. In addition, leakage of amniotic fluid may occur.

Spontaneous Abortion

Most spontaneous abortions (miscarriages) occur early in pregnancy, generally within the first 12 weeks. As the duration of the pregnancy increases, the incidence of spontaneous abortion decreases. In most cases, the cause of spontaneous abortion in early pregnancy cannot be determined, but it is likely to result from lethal chromosomal abnormalities. Many embryos recovered from spontaneous abortions show a variety of serious developmental defects.

As many as 50 to 75 percent of pregnancies end before getting a positive result on a pregnancy test. Most people will never know that they were pregnant, though some may suspect that they were because of pregnancy loss symptoms. By week 5 the overall chance of losing a pregnancy is about 20%. By weeks 14 to 20, the chance of experiencing a miscarriage is less than 1 percent. Beyond week 20, a pregnancy loss is termed a **stillbirth**, and this may cause a person to

Stillbirth Spontaneous abortion after twenty weeks' gestation.

go into labor. Stillbirth is relatively rare and is getting rarer because very young babies may be able to survive outside the uterus, thanks to modern technology.

If a dead fetus is retained for some time within the uterine cavity, the breakdown products of the fetal tissue can diffuse into the maternal circulation. These substances possess thromboplastic activity and may induce a hemorrhagic disease in the mother by depleting maternal blood coagulation factors. A retained dead fetus is one cause of **disseminated intravascular coagulation (DIC)** syndrome, which is discussed in Chapter 12.

Disseminated intravascular coagulation (DIC) A rare but serious condition that causes blood clotting within the blood vessel and can be life threatening.

Ectopic Pregnancy

An ectopic pregnancy (ecto = outside) is the development of an embryo outside the uterine cavity. Most ectopic pregnancies occur in the uterine tubes, but on rare occasions a fertilized ovum develops in the ovary or abdominal cavity (**Figure 15-6**). Implantation can take place in the uterine tube if transport of the ovum is delayed. A previous infection may cause failure of the tubal muscle contractions and can predispose a pregnancy to this condition. Uterine tube infections often can be followed by scarring and fusion of tubal folds, retarding the passage of the fertilized egg through the tube. Frequently, the conditions that predispose to a tubal pregnancy affect both fallopian tubes. Because of the potential life-threatening risk of a ruptured tubal pregnancy, a healthcare provider always considers the possibility of ectopic pregnancy for any woman of reproductive age who exhibits suggestive symptoms. Both surgical and nonsurgical approaches are used to remove the ectopic fetus. A single oral dose of an antimetabolite drug termed methotrexate can terminate the tubal pregnancy, eliminating the need for a surgical procedure in which the tube is incised and the pregnancy is evacuated.

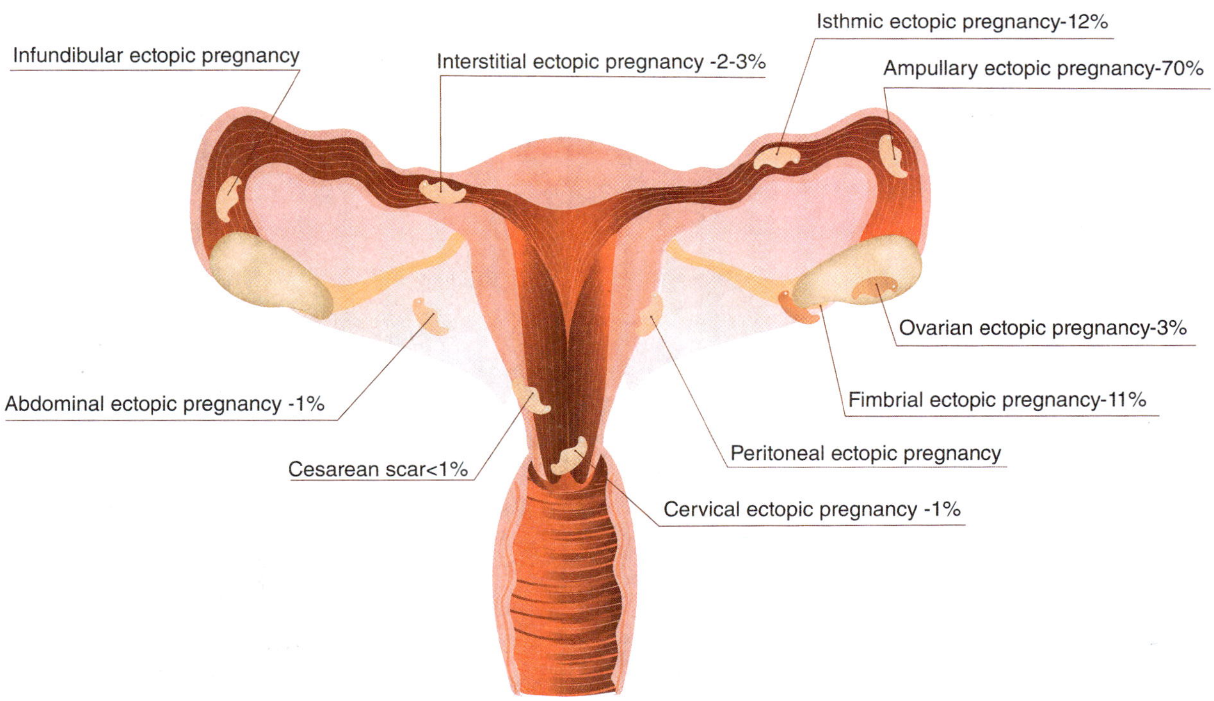

Figure 15-6 Potential sites for ectopic pregnancy. A developing embryo that does not implant in the uterus can implant in other places, including outside of the reproductive tract.

Abnormal Attachment of the Umbilical Cord and Placenta

Velamentous Insertion of the Umbilical Cord

Velamentous insertion of umbilical cord Attachment of the umbilical cord to the fetal membranes rather than to the placenta.

If the umbilical cord vessels are not gathered together normally, the cord attaches to the membranes attached to the placenta (fetal membranes) rather than to the placenta itself. When this occurs, the umbilical vessels must travel for a distance within the fetal membranes before reaching the placenta (**Figure 15-7**). This is termed a **velamentous insertion of umbilical cord** (velum = veil). The abnormality may be hazardous to the fetus if the vessels become located in the membranes that extend over the cervix since these vessels may be compressed or ruptured in the course of labor or delivery. If one of the vessels ruptures, the circulation between the fetus and placenta is disrupted, and the fetus bleeds to death through the ruptured vessel. Because the maternal and fetal circulations are not interconnected, however, the flow of maternal blood through the intervillous space is not disturbed, and the mother does not suffer any adverse effects. Even if the vessels crossing the cervix do not rupture, they may be compressed by the fetal head during delivery, causing fetal death by shutting off the circulation through the umbilical vessels.

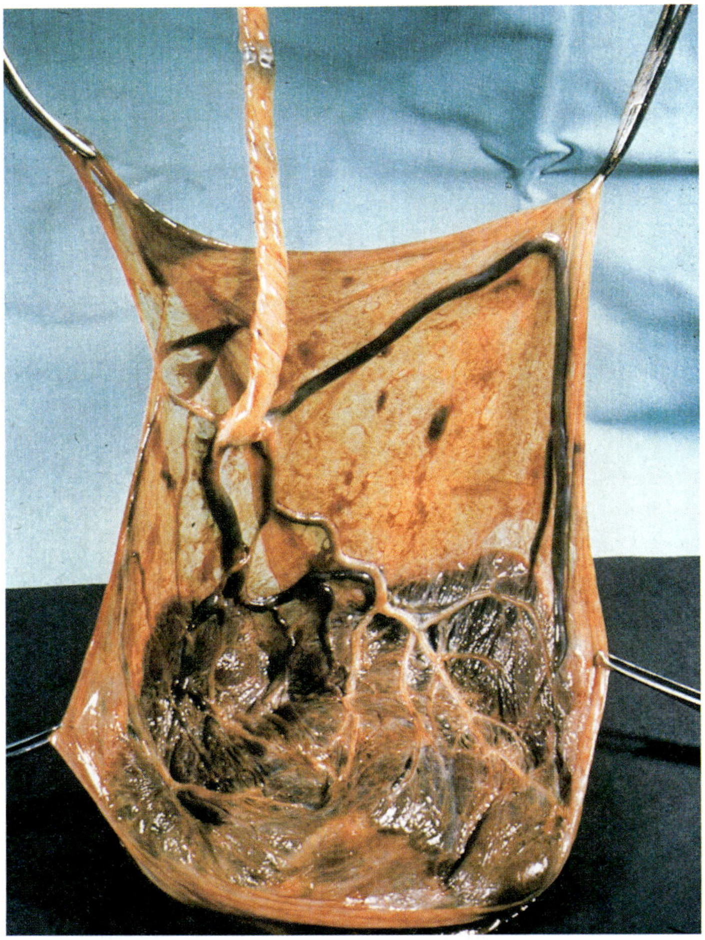

Figure 15-7 Velamentous insertion of umbilical cord. Note the vessels traversing the membranes to reach the placenta.

Courtesy of Leonard V. Crowley, MD, Century College.

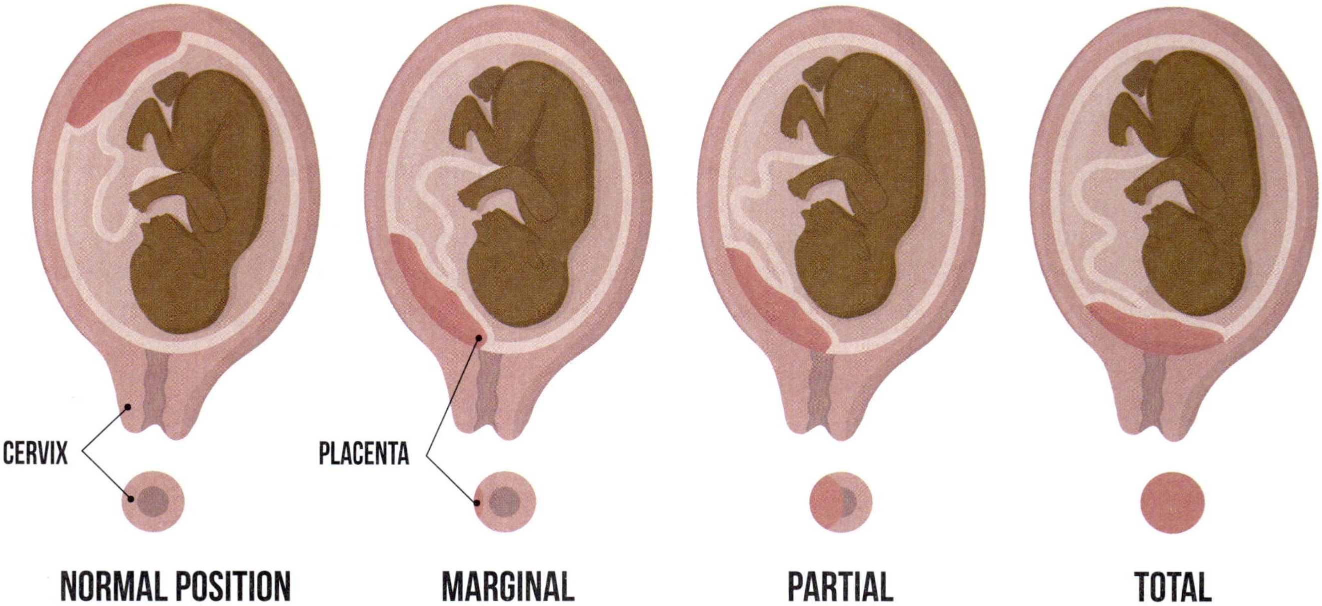

Figure 15-8 Placental placement. The first diagram illustrates normal placental placement. As the placenta implants closer to the cervix, the potential for a placental rupture and placenta previa increases significantly.

Placenta Previa

Normally, the placenta attaches high on the anterior or posterior uterine wall. If the placenta becomes attached in the lower part of the uterus, it may cover the cervix. This is termed a **placenta previa** (**Figure 15-8**). The term means a placenta blocking the exit from the uterus (pre = before + via = pathway). The patient with a placenta previa experiences episodes of bleeding during the last part of pregnancy because of partial separation of the placenta from the uterine wall. Normally, the lower part of the uterus undergoes gradual dilatation during the last part of pregnancy in preparation for childbirth. The abnormally located placenta is unable to stretch to conform to the contour of the expanding lower part of the uterus, and parts of the placenta tear loose. The tearing disrupts the large uterine vessels that penetrate the basal part of the placenta to supply the intervillous spaces (see Figure 15-3). In contrast with a velamentous insertion of the cord, which places only the infant in jeopardy, a placenta previa is hazardous to the mother as well. The mother may bleed to death if a large part of the placenta is torn from the uterine wall. Large areas of placental disruption may also prevent proper oxygenation of fetal blood passing through the placenta, leading to the death of the fetus. Because the placenta blocks the cervix, vaginal delivery is not possible without the risk of severe hemorrhage and injury to the cervix. Delivery is generally accomplished by cesarean section.

Placenta previa
Attachment of the placenta in the uterus such that it partially or completely covers the cervix.

Twins and Multiple Pregnancies

Currently, about 3.4 percent of all pregnancies are twins. Twins may be either identical (monozygotic) or fraternal (dizygotic). Approximately 0.01 percent of pregnancies are triplets or greater in number; however, quadruplets, quintuplets, and sextuplets are extremely rare. The incidence of all types of multiple pregnancies is higher than normal with the use of fertility-enhancing technology and assisted reproduction techniques.

Dizygotic (Fraternal) Twins

Seventy percent of twins are fraternal, resulting from fertilization of two separate ova by two different sperm. Fraternal twins are no more alike than any other siblings, but they share a family resemblance because they are born of the same parents. Each fertilized ovum implants separately, and each twin forms its own placenta and fetal membranes. Frequently, the margins of the two placentas grow together and fuse, but each fetus remains enclosed within its own amnion and chorion. A fused placenta of this type is termed a diamniotic dichorionic placenta.

Monozygotic (Identical) Twins

Thirty percent of twins are identical and result from the splitting of a single fertilized ovum. Splitting may occur at various times after fertilization, as illustrated in **Figure 15-9**. In about 30 percent of monozygotic twin pregnancies, the fertilized ovum splits before the **inner cell mass** forms, which is on the third day after fertilization. Each half of the **zygote** implants separately, forms a complete embryo, and develops its own placenta. The two placentas may remain separated or may become fused to form a diamniotic dichorionic placenta in the same manner as that for fraternal twins (**Figure 15-10**).

Inner cell mass A group of cells derived from the fertilized ovum that is destined to form the embryo.
Zygote The fertilized ovum.

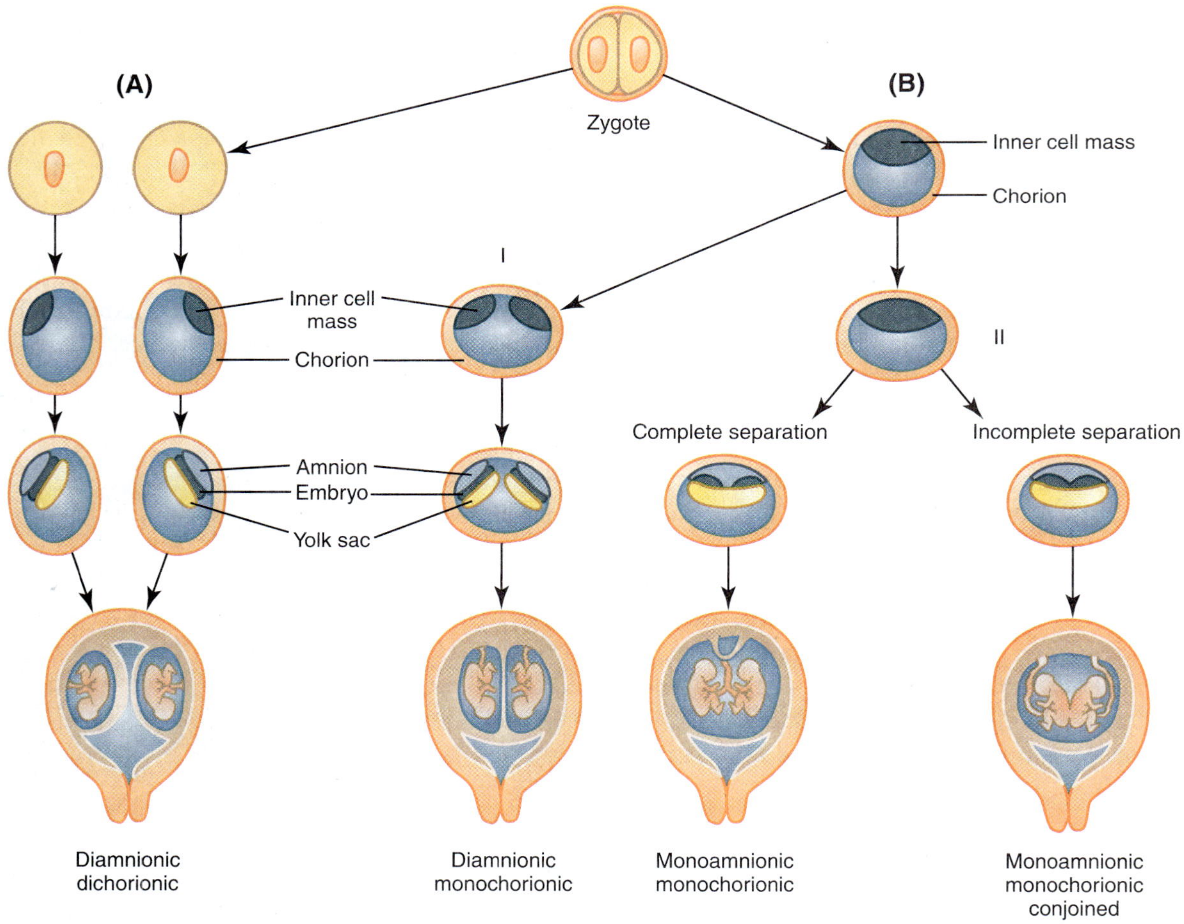

Figure 15-9 Stages at which formation of identical twins can occur, and types of placenta associated with each stage of twinning. **(A)** Early splitting of fertilized ovum, forming two separate zygotes that develop and implant separately. **(B I)** Inner cell mass splits, giving rise to two embryos within single chorionic cavity. **(B II)** Later splitting of inner cell mass after the amniotic sac has formed. Complete separation of the inner cell mass gives rise to two embryos within a single amniotic sac. Incomplete separation gives rise to conjoined twins.

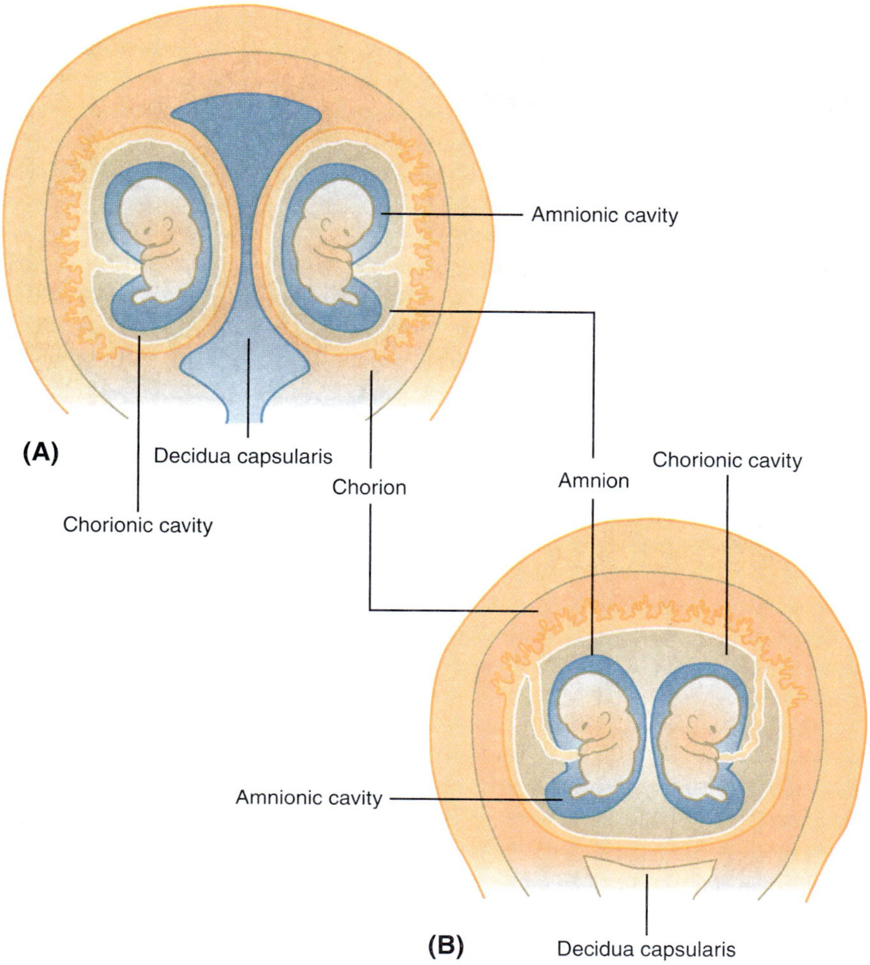

Figure 15-10 A comparison of the formation of the placentas and fetal membranes in twins. **(A)** Separate implantations leading to the formation of a dichorionic placenta. **(B)** Twins developing in a single chorionic cavity and forming a monochorionic placenta. A dichorionic placenta can be encountered in either fraternal or identical twins. A monochorionic placenta occurs only in identical twins.

More commonly (in almost 70 percent of monozygotic twin pregnancies), the inner cell mass divides after the **blastocyst** forms but before implantation takes place. In this instance, each half of the inner cell mass forms a complete embryo and develops its own amnion and yolk sac, but both develop within a single chorionic cavity. This gives rise to a diamniotic monochorionic placenta.

Rarely, the inner cell mass divides after the amniotic sac has already formed. When this occurs, the two embryos develop within a single amniotic cavity and form a monoamniotic monochorionic placenta. If the division of the inner cell mass is incomplete, **conjoined twins** (Siamese twins) are formed.

Blastocyst A stage of development of the fertilized ovum (zygote) in which a central cavity forms within the cluster of developing cells.

Conjoined twins Identical twins, historically known as Siamese twins, that are joined to one another and often share organs in common.

Twin Transfusion Syndrome

The placental circulations of monochorionic identical twins are connected by multiple vascular anastomoses (interconnecting blood vessels) up to 15 percent of the time, leading to intermixing of blood from the two fetuses in the placentas (**Figure 15-11**). Sometimes the placental anastomoses are such that an excess of blood from the fetoplacental circulation from one infant (termed the donor twin) flows into the circulation of the second twin (termed

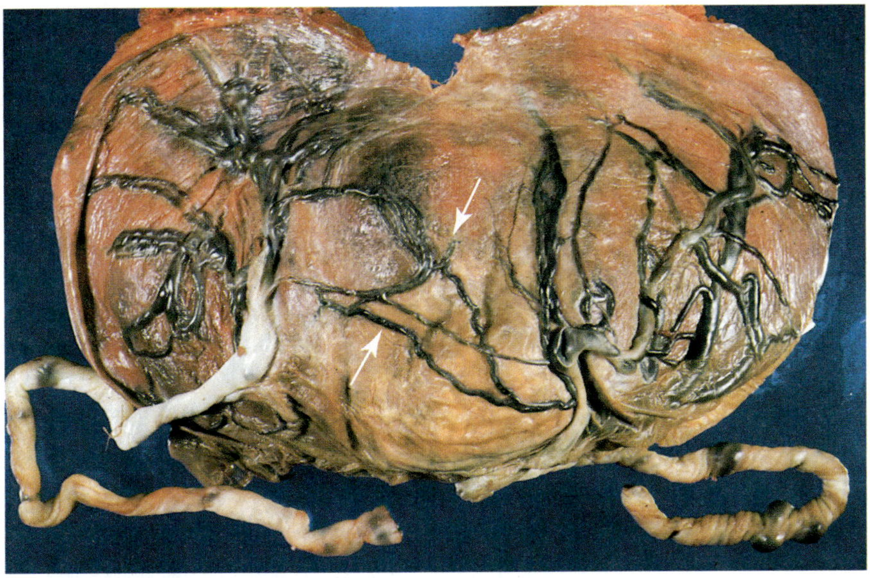

Figure 15-11 Placenta of identical twins with amnions removed revealing interconnecting blood vessels (*arrows*).

Courtesy of Leonard V. Crowley, MD, Century College.

the recipient). If this occurs, the donor twin may become anemic and the recipient twin may become overloaded with blood (polycythemic). Minor differences in the blood volumes of the two twins can be tolerated, but large disproportions are harmful to both twins. The severe anemia may be fatal to the donor twin, and the circulation of the recipient twin may become so overloaded by the great excess of blood that the polycythemic twin dies of heart failure. Fetoscopic laser destruction of anastomoses is used in severe cases to terminate the transfer of blood between the fetuses.

Vanishing Twins and Blighted Twins

Sometimes one twin of a twin pregnancy fails to develop and dies early in pregnancy. Ultrasound studies of first trimester pregnancies reveal that many more pregnancies start out as twins than survive to term. The twin that fails to survive may be a vanishing twin that is completely absorbed, leaving no trace, or may persist as a blighted twin, which is a degenerated embryo or fetus that is retained within the uterus until the surviving fetus is delivered at term.

Conjoined Twins

Incomplete separation of the inner cell mass leads to a variable degree of union between conjoined twins. The twins may be joined at the head, thorax, abdomen, or pelvis, the union being face-to-face, side-to-side, or back-to-back. The extent of union is variable but often quite considerable, with the twins sharing common internal organs to such a degree that it is not possible to separate them surgically. The conjoined twins are generally equal in size and are often well formed except for their failure to separate.

Disadvantages of Twin Pregnancies

Twins are at a disadvantage compared with singletons. Because they are overcrowded in the uterus, a twin is always smaller than a single infant at a comparable stage of gestation. Overdistention of the uterus frequently promotes preterm onset of labor, leading to delivery of preterm infants with a reduced chance of survival. Congenital malformations occur twice as often in twins as in singletons, and vascular anastomosis within the placental circulation may lead to a twin transfusion syndrome.

Toxemia of Pregnancy: Preeclampsia and Eclampsia

Mild **preeclampsia** is a pregnancy-associated hypertension with an elevated blood pressure exceeding 140/90 in a previously normotensive patient (or in the case of a known hypertensive, an increase in systolic blood pressure by 15). Preeclampsia can present with signs and symptoms, including but not limited to, elevated blood pressure. **Figure 15-12** highlights some of the other indicators. A daily dose of aspirin is sometimes initiated for pregnant people deemed to be at risk for developing preeclampsia. Severe preeclampsia is accompanied by protein in the urine, any time from the 20th week of gestation to the end of the pregnancy, along with pulmonary edema, reduced urine output, and other symptoms. Preeclampsia occurs in up to 6 percent of the pregnancies and is more common with first pregnancies in older women, in twin pregnancies, and in obese women who have had preeclampsia in a previous pregnancy or have a family history. According to the CDC, preeclampsia is estimated to

Preeclampsia A pregnancy-related complication characterized by hypertension and proteinuria that usually occurs after the twentieth week of gestation, thought to be caused by placental dysfunction.

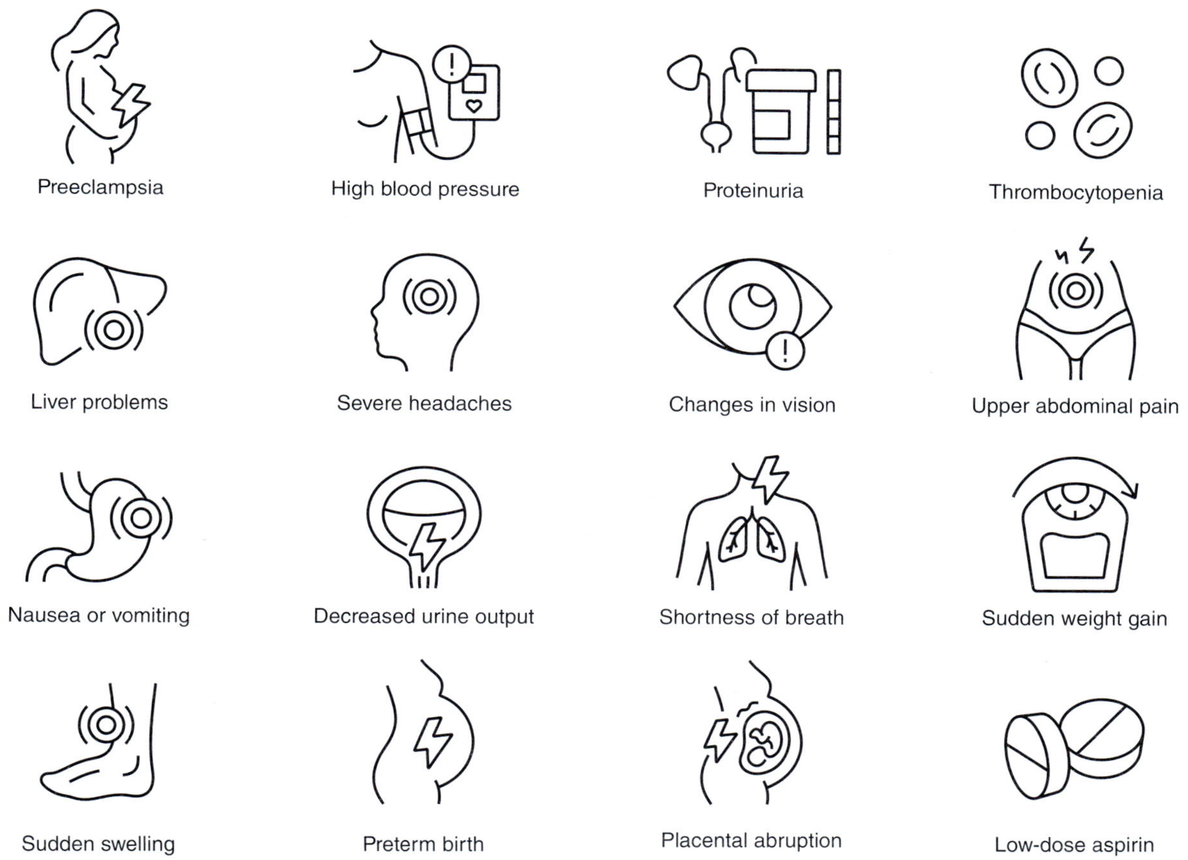

Figure 15-12 Preeclampsia can present with many different symptoms. A pregnant person suffering from preeclampsia may present with only one symptom or several. High blood pressure generally serves as a red flag for this condition.

occur in 5 to 7 percent of all pregnancies and is one of the leading causes of maternal difficulties during pregnancy. Worldwide, the annual rate for deaths caused by preeclampsia is over 70,000 maternal deaths and 500,000 fetal deaths. In the United States, Black women experience a preeclampsia rate that is 60 percent higher than in White women. Not only are Black women more likely to develop preeclampsia, but they are more likely to experience adverse outcomes associated with the condition, such as kidney damage and death. In all likelihood, these poorer outcomes are related to an array of factors collectively termed the social determinants of health, which will be covered later as they relate to fetal and maternal health.

There are a number of genetic factors associated with the risk for preeclampsia. Genes implicated in the control of blood pressure or placental development are associated with risk for the condition. In severe cases, the condition may be associated with convulsions and is then referred to as **eclampsia**.

Eclampsia One or more convulsions in a pregnant woman with preeclampsia.

Trophoblast Cell derived from the fertilized ovum that gives rise to the fetal membranes and contributes to the formation of the placenta.

Hydatidiform mole A neoplastic proliferation of trophoblast associated with the formation of large cystic villi.

Invasive hydatidiform mole An aggressive hydatidiform mole that invades the uterine wall.

Choriocarcinoma A malignant proliferation of trophoblastic tissue.

The disease is likely to be caused by inadequate blood flow to the placenta, leading to placental ischemia with subsequent release of cytokines that produce systemic effects. Constriction of blood vessels and increased vascular resistance lead to hypertension, endothelial damage, and specifically, damage to the glomeruli of maternal kidneys. This may progress to proteinuria and the presence of intravascular thrombi. Extremely severe cases can lead to partial separation of the placenta from the uterine wall and also may be complicated by a disseminated intravascular coagulation syndrome (described in Chapter 12). This is termed HELLP syndrome and is characterized by hemolytic anemia, liver damage, and low platelet count. Infant mortality can exceed 50 percent in severe disease, with a risk of maternal death.

Mild cases of preeclampsia can be managed by bed rest and close observation while delaying preterm delivery as long as possible without endangering the pregnant person's health. Severe cases are hazardous to both the pregnant person and fetus. Treatment consists of trying to control the hypertension and vascular damage until the fetus is mature enough for preterm delivery even as early as 20 weeks' gestation, but preferably delaying until 24 weeks' gestation if possible. A number of drugs are used to control the hypertension and hopefully prevent convulsions. The condition usually relents when the placenta (which appears to be the cause of the problem) is expelled after delivery. Unfortunately, for some individuals, the hypertension and other issues may continue into at least the first 72 hours postpartum.

Hydatidiform Mole and Choriocarcinoma

Sometimes, when a pregnancy does not develop normally, the embryo either fails to form or dies and is absorbed, but the trophoblastic cells covering the villi continue to grow at an excessive rate. The proliferating **trophoblast** produces a much larger number of chorionic gonadotropins (hCG) than are encountered in a normal pregnancy. Serial determinations of hCG levels are used to monitor the course of disease. Masses of abnormal proliferating trophoblastic tissue may invade the uterus, spread into the vagina, and even metastasize to distant sites. Three different degrees of abnormal trophoblastic activity (gestational trophoblast disease) are recognized: **hydatidiform mole**, **invasive hydatidiform mole**, and **choriocarcinoma**.

The hydatidiform mole, the most common type, which occurs in about 80 percent of affected patients, is a relatively benign trophoblast proliferation.

The invasive mole, a more aggressive and destructive proliferative process, occurs in about 15 percent of patients. Choriocarcinoma describes a malignant growth of trophoblastic tissue that occurs in only a small percentage of patients. This aggressive trophoblastic neoplasm can metastasize widely and kill the patient unless controlled by proper treatment.

Hydatidiform Mole

In a hydatidiform mole, the villi that are covered by proliferating trophoblast become converted into large cystic structures resembling masses of grapes (**Figure 15-13**). The unusual name given to this condition is derived from its outward appearance. A hydatid is a fluid-filled vesicle, and a mole is a shapeless mass of tissue.

Most hydatidiform moles result from fertilization of an abnormal ovum lacking maternal chromosomes. The abnormal ovum is usually fertilized by a single sperm bearing an X chromosome, which then duplicates its chromosomes so that all 46 chromosomes in the fertilized egg are derived from the father. No embryo develops, and the chorionic villi become cystic structures covered by actively proliferating trophoblastic tissue. This is the most common type of mole, termed a complete mole.

Less commonly, a hydatidiform mole results from fertilization of a normal ovum by two sperm, resulting in a fertilized ovum containing three sets of chromosomes, 1 maternal and 2 paternal, for a total of 69 chromosomes, and the trophoblastic tissue consists of a mixture of normal and cystic villi. This type of mole, which does not exhibit aggressive growth, is termed a partial mole.

A hydatidiform mole is a relatively common complication of pregnancy occurring about once in 1500 pregnancies in the United States and Canada but is encountered 10 times more frequently in women from the Far East and Southeast Asia. It occurs more frequently in girls under 15 years of age. Risk then increases for women over age 40.

Because of the increased volume of the placenta caused by the multiple cystic villi, the patient with a mole experiences an enlargement of the uterus that is much greater than would be expected in relationship to the duration of the pregnancy. Erosion of maternal blood vessels by the mole may cause irregular

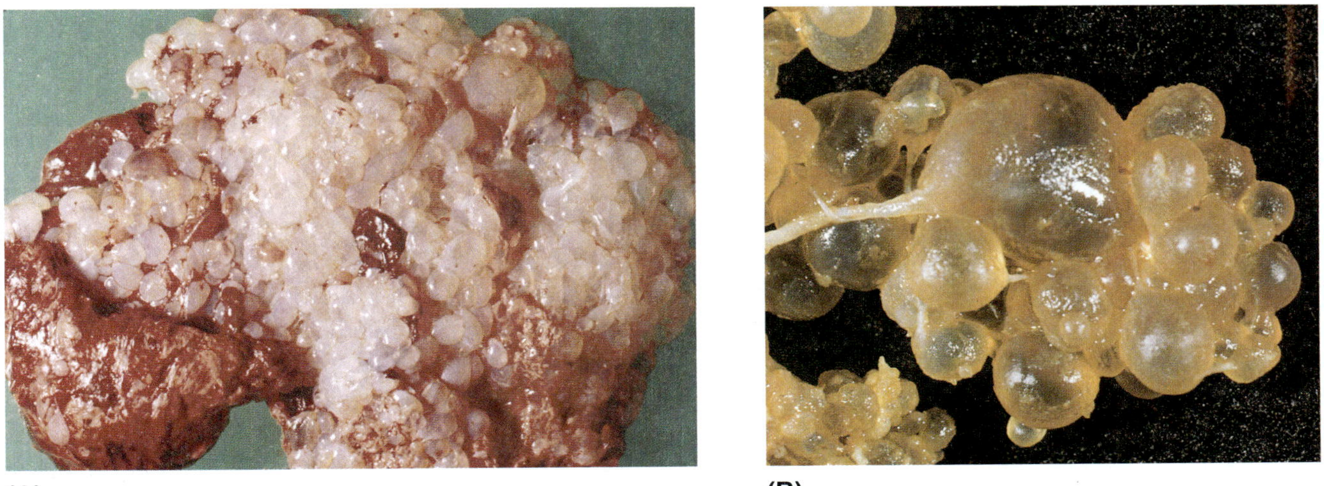

(A) **(B)**

Figure 15-13 Hydatidiform mole. **(A)** Placenta converted into a large mass of cystic villi. **(B)** Closer view of cystic villi.

uterine bleeding. The overdistension of the uterus caused by the mole may precipitate uterine contractions, leading to expulsion of pieces of the mole.

Diagnosis of a mole is based on the clinical features of the pregnancy, by identifying cystic villi covered by proliferating trophoblast expelled from the uterus, or by ultrasound examination, which reveals a characteristic appearance caused by the cystic villi that fill the uterine cavity. Because complete moles occasionally progress to choriocarcinoma, chemotherapy is required if hCG levels do not normalize after removal of the mole. Disseminated disease rarely occurs after therapy.

An invasive mole resembles a complete hydatidiform mole but exhibits a much more marked trophoblastic proliferation and a much more aggressive behavior. Although trophoblastic tissue may invade deeply into the uterine wall and cause considerable bleeding, it does not metastasize.

Choriocarcinoma

Choriocarcinoma is the most aggressive form of **gestational trophoblast disease** and behaves like a malignant tumor. Masses of abnormally actively proliferating trophoblast may extend into the vagina and may metastasize to the lungs, brain, and other distant sites. Unless treated, the tumor may eventually kill the patient. Choriocarcinoma is usually treated vigorously by several courses of anticancer chemotherapy, generally leading to a cure even in metastatic disease. Therapy is monitored by serial determination of hCG levels.

Gestational trophoblast disease A general term for all diseases characterized by abnormal trophoblast proliferation. Includes both hydatidiform mole and choriocarcinoma.

Gestational diabetes Elevated blood glucose caused by insulin resistance resulting from elevated hormones related to pregnancy. Blood glucose returns to normal postpartum, but the woman has an increased risk of diabetes later in life.

Gestational Diabetes

Effects of Hyperglycemia on Pregnancy

In all pregnancies during the second trimester and later, higher placental hormone levels cause the body to become less responsive to insulin, inducing some degree of insulin resistance. Consequently, the potential exists for increased blood glucose levels, hyperglycemia (**Figure 15-14**). In most cases, rising insulin levels lead to compensation to a normal blood glucose level; however, about 8% of mothers will be diagnosed with **gestational diabetes**.

Gestational hyperglycemia harms the fetus during organ system development. See Chapter 16 for a timeline of embryonic and fetal organ development and discussion of specific congenital malformations. The increased glucose may contribute to congenital malformations or even lead to fetal death. Later in the pregnancy, the extra glucose crosses the placenta, promoting fetal growth. Consequently, the fetus grows larger than average size with larger fetal kidneys secreting more urine, increasing the volume of amniotic fluid. Delivery of the larger fetus may be more difficult, possibly requiring a cesarean section. After delivery, the infant's blood glucose may fall precipitously (hypoglycemia). Post-delivery, the newborn's pancreatic insulin secretion needs to adjust to much lower glucose levels. The infant also faces neonatal respiratory distress problems caused by inadequate surfactant, as described in Chapter 16.

Some previously non-diabetic women, upon becoming pregnant, may not produce enough insulin to maintain a normal glucose concentration. That condition is termed gestational diabetes since the blood glucose is likely to return to normal after the pregnancy. Women with gestational diabetes may be at higher risk of developing type 2 diabetes in later years. Gestational diabetes occurs in as many as 8 percent of pregnancies, with a high incidence in older women, obese women, and women from ethnic groups presenting with a high frequency of diabetes.

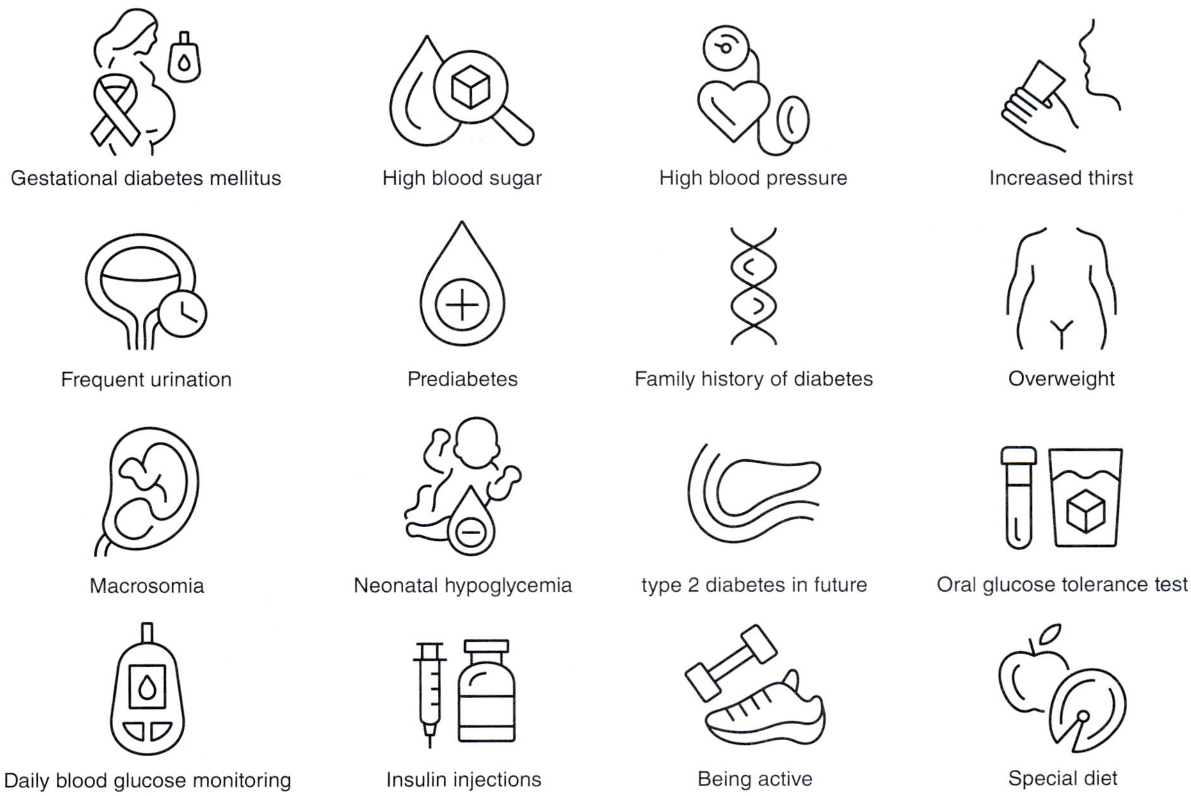
Gestational diabetes mellitus
High blood sugar
High blood pressure
Increased thirst
Frequent urination
Prediabetes
Family history of diabetes
Overweight
Macrosomia
Neonatal hypoglycemia
type 2 diabetes in future
Oral glucose tolerance test
Daily blood glucose monitoring
Insulin injections
Being active
Special diet

Figure 15-14 Gestational diabetes affects the pregnant person and the fetus, with the potential for severe complications for both. The fetus may develop macrosomia or experience neonatal hypoglycemia.

Hemolytic Disease of the Newborn (Erythroblastosis Fetalis)

Hemolytic disease of the newborn is a hemolytic anemia in the newborn infant resulting from sensitization of the mother to a "foreign" blood group antigen present in the red cells of the fetus but lacking in the maternal cells. Although most cases of severe hemolytic disease result from Rh incompatibility between an Rh D antigen–negative mother and her Rh D antigen–positive fetus, mother–fetus blood group incompatibility involving other blood group systems also rarely causes hemolytic disease. The mother reacts by forming antibodies directed against the fetal cells that cross the placenta, generally at the time of birth. Although disease usually does not occur with the first "incompatible" pregnancy, in subsequent incompatible pregnancies, maternal antibodies cross the placenta and damage the fetal red cells, leading to a severe anemia in the affected fetus. The other name for this disease, erythroblastosis fetalis, comes from the large numbers of nucleated red blood cells (erythroblasts) produced in the blood of severely affected anemic infants to compensate for the rapid destruction of red blood cells by maternal antibodies (**Figure 15-15**).

The severely affected infant is extremely anemic and very edematous, a condition termed hydrops fetalis. The edema is the result of heart failure and impaired hepatic plasma–protein synthesis, caused by the severe anemia. If the hemolytic process is less intense, the infant may be born alive but will be moderately or severely anemic. Infants with mild disease may appear normal at birth but become anemic and jaundiced soon afterward.

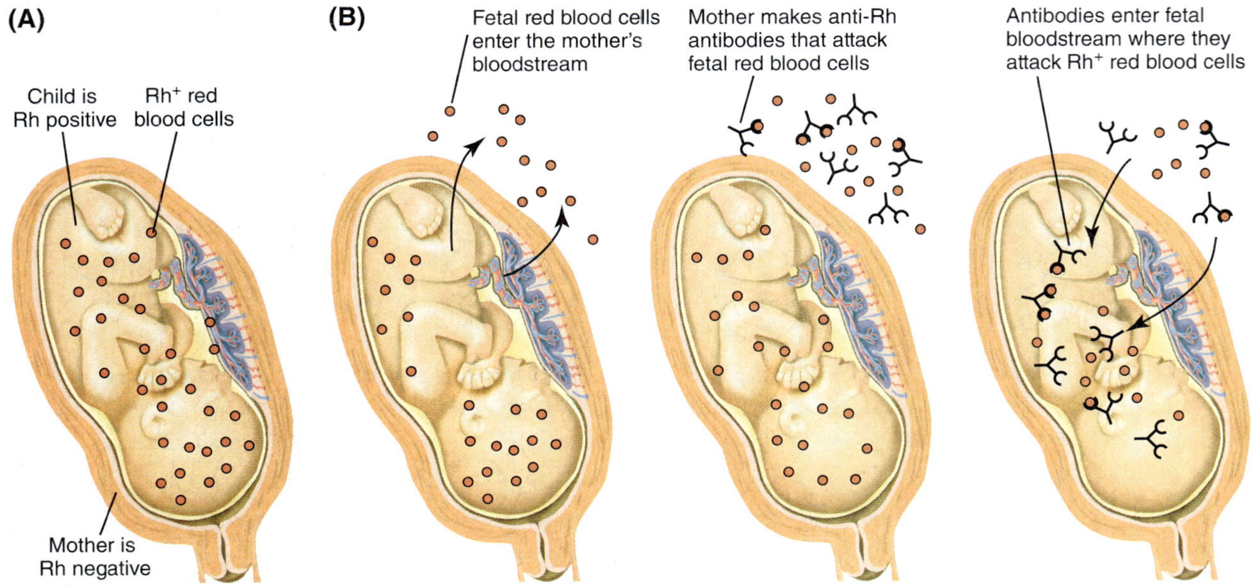

Figure 15-15 The Rh factor and pregnancy. **(A)** Rh-positive cells from the fetus enter the mother's blood at birth. If the mother is Rh-negative, her immune system responds by producing antibodies to the Rh-positive RBCs and destroying them. **(B)** Problems arise if the mother becomes pregnant again and has another Rh-positive baby. If the mother was not treated the first time, antibodies to the Rh-positive RBCs cross the placenta and destroy the fetal RBCs.

Anemia invariably develops or increases in severity after delivery; jaundice also develops rapidly. **Figure 15-16** illustrates the typical changes in hemoglobin and bilirubin levels after delivery in an infant with hemolytic disease. In the uterus, hematopoiesis is stimulated by both the increased blood destruction and the low oxygen tension in the fetal blood. After delivery, respiration is established, the arterial oxygen tension in the infant's blood rises, and the rate of compensatory hematopoiesis declines. However, blood destruction continues at the same rate.

The accelerated blood destruction in hemolytic disease also causes jaundice. The high rate of red cell breakdown leads to production of large amounts

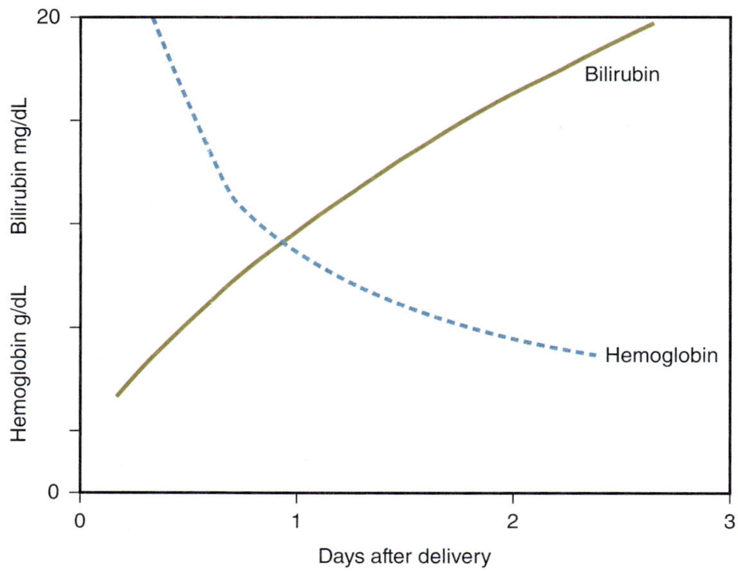

Figure 15-16 Changes in the hemoglobin and bilirubin concentration that take place after delivery in infants with hemolytic disease.

of bile pigment. Before delivery, the bile pigment crosses the placenta into the maternal circulation and is excreted by the mother. After delivery, the infant's liver is still relatively inefficient in conjugating and excreting bilirubin. As a result, the level of unconjugated bilirubin in the infant's blood rises rapidly, resulting in **hyperbilirubinemia** (hyper = elevated + bilirubin + heme = blood), which is hazardous to the infant. The high level of unconjugated bilirubin is toxic to the nervous system, where it causes bile staining and degeneration of basal ganglia (basal nuclei) and damage to other parts of the brain as well, leaving the infant with cerebral palsy, mental retardation, and hearing loss. This condition is termed **kernicterus** (kern = kernel, referring to brain basal nuclei + icterus = jaundice) or **bilirubin encephalopathy**.

Hyperbilirubinemia High levels of unconjugated bilirubin in the newborn.

Kernicterus/bilirubin encephalopathy Severe brain damage caused by high levels of unconjugated bilirubin in the infant.

Exchange transfusion Partial replacement of the patients blood with blood from another source in hemolytic disease of the newborn.

Prevention of Rh Hemolytic Disease With Rh Immune Globulin

Postpartum Administration

As previously stated, the first Rh-positive infant born to an Rh-negative mother is usually normal because Rh antibodies are rarely formed during the first pregnancy. Although a few Rh-positive cells may periodically enter the mother's circulation during pregnancy, their numbers are not sufficient to induce sensitization. The greater numbers of Rh-positive cells required to sensitize the mother usually do not enter the maternal circulation until during delivery. When the placenta begins to separate from the uterus and is eventually expelled, the barrier separating the maternal and fetal circulations is disrupted, and some of the Rh-positive fetal cells within the villi may be expressed into the uterine blood vessels and may enter the mother's circulation. After maternal sensitization has occurred, Rh hemolytic disease will develop in any subsequent pregnancy in which the fetus is Rh-positive.

Rh hemolytic disease now occurs rarely. The formation of Rh antibodies by an Rh-negative mother can be prevented by treating the mother with RhoGAM, an immunoglobulin preparation containing a high concentration of human anti Rh D antibodies. The first dose is usually given at 28 to 30 weeks antepartum and repeated at birth. RhoGAM is also given to Rh-negative mothers following an abortion or miscarriage. Such therapy is extremely successful in preventing hemolytic disease of the newborn and is routinely offered to all pregnant Rh D–negative women. Combined antepartum and postpartum administration reduces the incidence of sensitization to about 0.5 percent.

When administered to an unsensitized Rh-negative pregnant person, the anti-Rh D antibody in the immunoglobulin coats the Rh antigen sites on the surface of any fetal red cells. The antibody-coated cells are rapidly removed. This treatment is of no value if anti-Rh D antibodies are already present. A very small number of Rh-negative women form Rh antibodies in their first pregnancy, apparently because of prior contact with Rh antigen from an unrecognized abortion, transfusion of Rh-positive blood, or another cause.

Treatment of Hemolytic Disease

Although hemolytic disease caused by Rh incompatibility was formerly a more common problem than it is now, it still does occasionally occur because of poor prenatal care. In these cases, an **exchange transfusion** may be undertaken to provide the infant with a population of cells that will not be destroyed by the antibody. In the case of hemolytic disease caused by Rh incompatibility, a transfusion of Rh-negative blood is given. At the same time, exchange transfusion provides the infant with bilirubin-free plasma to replace the jaundiced plasma, thereby helping to prevent severe elevation of potentially toxic unconjugated bilirubin. It should be emphasized that the exchange transfusion has no effect on the infant's own blood type.

The elevated level of unconjugated bilirubin that causes kernicterus can also be somewhat reduced by exposing the unclothed jaundiced infant to ultraviolet light continuously for several days. The light exposure acts by converting the toxic unconjugated bilirubin into less toxic compounds that are not as hazardous to the infant. This procedure, termed **phototherapy**, has reduced the need for exchange transfusions. The level of unconjugated serum bilirubin normally rises after delivery even in normal infants, usually reaching a peak of about 6 mg/dl or sometimes even higher within the first few days after delivery, and then falls toward normal. In hemolytic disease, unconjugated bilirubin levels rise faster, and levels are often much higher than in a normal newborn. Levels exceeding 20 mg/dl are potentially hazardous, put the infant at risk of kernicterus, and require treatment to lower the serum bilirubin level. Phototherapy is sometimes used in neonates who have high levels of unconjugated bilirubin because of delays in liver maturation rather than immune destruction of red cells.

Phototherapy Fluorescent light treatment of jaundiced babies to reduce the concentration of unconjugated bilirubin in their blood.

ABO hemolytic disease A mild hemolytic disease in group A or B infants and group O mothers as a result of maternal anti-A and anti-B antibodies.

ABO Hemolytic Disease

With the decline in the frequency of Rh hemolytic disease, most cases of hemolytic disease result from ABO blood group differences between the pregnant person and infant. In this condition, termed **ABO hemolytic disease**, the pregnant person is group O (and has anti-A and anti-B antibodies in their system), and the infant is either group A or group B. In many women, the A or B fetal antigens stimulate the production of IgG maternal ABO antibodies, which can cross the placenta. The disease occurs in a first ABO-incompatible pregnancy because it is caused by preexisting anti-A and anti-B antibodies in the mother. ABO hemolytic disease is a much less severe disease than Rh incompatibility and is generally only detected antepartum when hyperbilirubinemia occurs.

Social Determinants of Health in Pregnant Individuals

U.S. Centers of Disease Control and Prevention (CDC) reports that the maternal mortality rate in 2023 was 18.6 deaths per 100,000 live births, which was a decrease from 22.3 in 2022. These rates are not representative of pregnant people from all backgrounds. Black persons, who had 15.6 percent of all live births, had maternal mortality rates of 49.5 and 50.3 deaths per 100,000 live births in 2022 and 2023, respectively. Pregnant individuals of color in the United States, regardless of educational status or economic means, remain 3.5 times more likely to die from pregnancy-related causes than White pregnant persons. Pregnant individuals from economically disadvantaged groups and those who reside in underserved rural populations, as well as pregnancies where the pregnant person identifies with a gender minority group, also encounter larger risk estimates.

While many factors contribute to these outcomes, a few broad ideas can be considered. Genetic factors, such as gene polymorphisms, may contribute to increased levels of preeclampsia and preterm birth within some groups, but genetic factors alone do not account for the range and magnitude of the disparities. The social determinants of health (SDOH) (**Figure 15-17**) clearly impact outcomes for the individual and groups within a society.

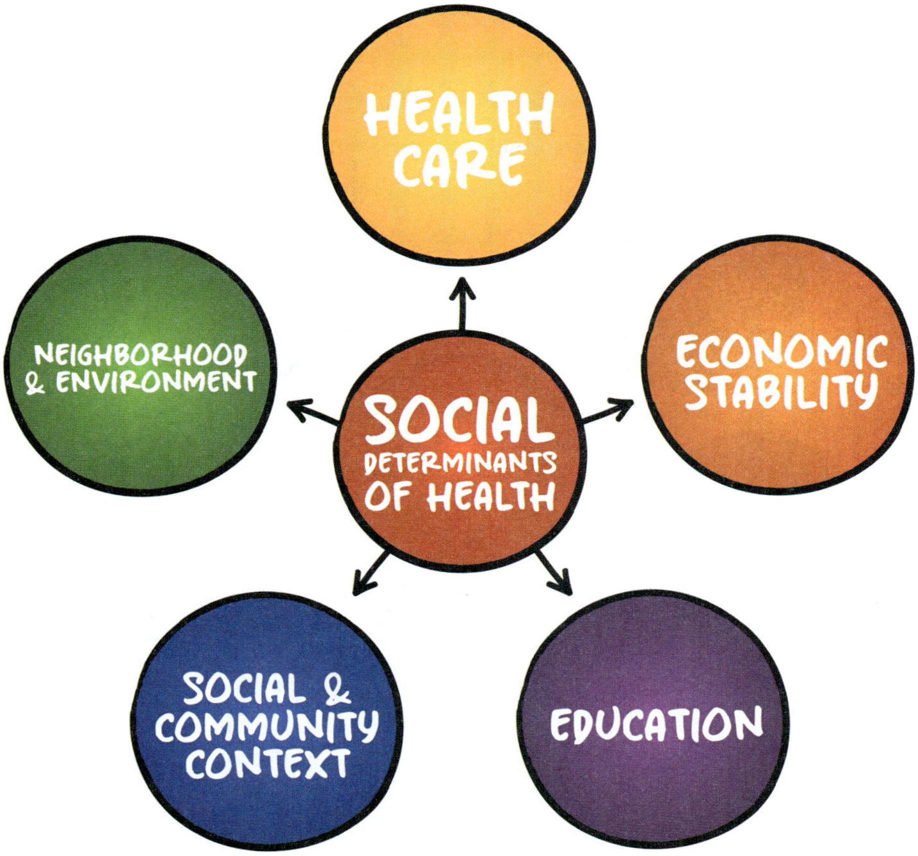
HEALTH CARE
NEIGHBORHOOD & ENVIRONMENT
SOCIAL DETERMINANTS OF HEALTH
ECONOMIC STABILITY
SOCIAL & COMMUNITY CONTEXT
EDUCATION

Figure 15-17 Social determinants of health. An individual's personal health is influenced by many things, including their genetic make-up and personal decisions. In addition, other factors outside of their control contribute to how well their health and health care are managed.

Paternal Influences on Pregnancy

The fertilizing sperm contributes half of the zygote's DNA. For a long time, many considered that the only paternal contribution during pregnancy. Recent studies in laboratory models now suggest that paternal physiologic and other stressors contribute to epigenetic changes in sperm, which can result in changes in placentation affecting the growth and development of the embryo and fetus.

Infertility

Infertility is a disease of either the male or female reproductive system. The clinical definition of infertility is failure to achieve a pregnancy after 12 months of unprotected sex. In both sexes, lifestyle issues, such as alcohol and tobacco use, and obesity contribute to reproductive difficulties. Additionally, exposure to environmental toxins and pollutants can damage the development of either eggs or sperm. Male-derived infertility usually arises from two general issues. First, difficulties with ejecting semen, or second, sperm abnormalities. These abnormalities may include low numbers of sperm, issues with sperm motility, and abnormal sperm morphology (**Figure 15-18**).

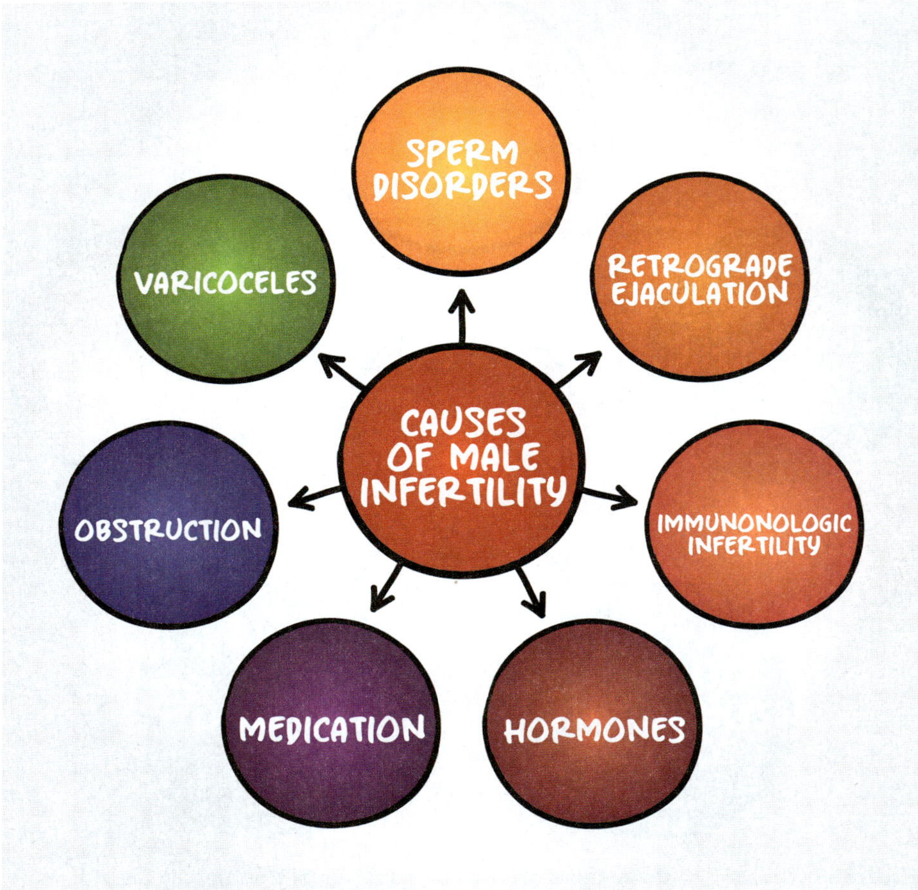

Figure 15-18 Etiology of male infertility. While any one of the factors illustrated in this figure can lead to male infertility, it is also possible that there is more than one contributing factor.

In the female reproductive system, difficulties may arise with the production and maturation of ova. Physical changes, including prevention of passage of the egg or zygote through the uterine tube or difficulty for implantation to occur in the uterus, also contribute to failure to achieve a full-term pregnancy. The inability to maintain a pregnancy for 40 weeks, which may stem from several causes, contributes to female infertility as well.

Primary infertility means that no pregnancy was ever achieved by the person. Infertility is referred to as secondary when at least one prior pregnancy occurred. Some estimates suggest that one in six people experience infertility at some point in their reproductive life. Care for infertility includes prevention, diagnosis, and treatment. Many, especially those in middle- and low-income groups, find it financially difficult to obtain the necessary care. Worldwide, equitable treatment and access to services continue to be issues. Generally, infertility care is not considered during the development of national healthcare plans and policy.

Male Reproductive System Infertility

Disorders of ejection of semen can result from multiple pathologies (**Figure 15-19**). One or more of the tubes carrying sperm and semen may be obstructed, often from injuries or infections of the genital tract. Endocrine

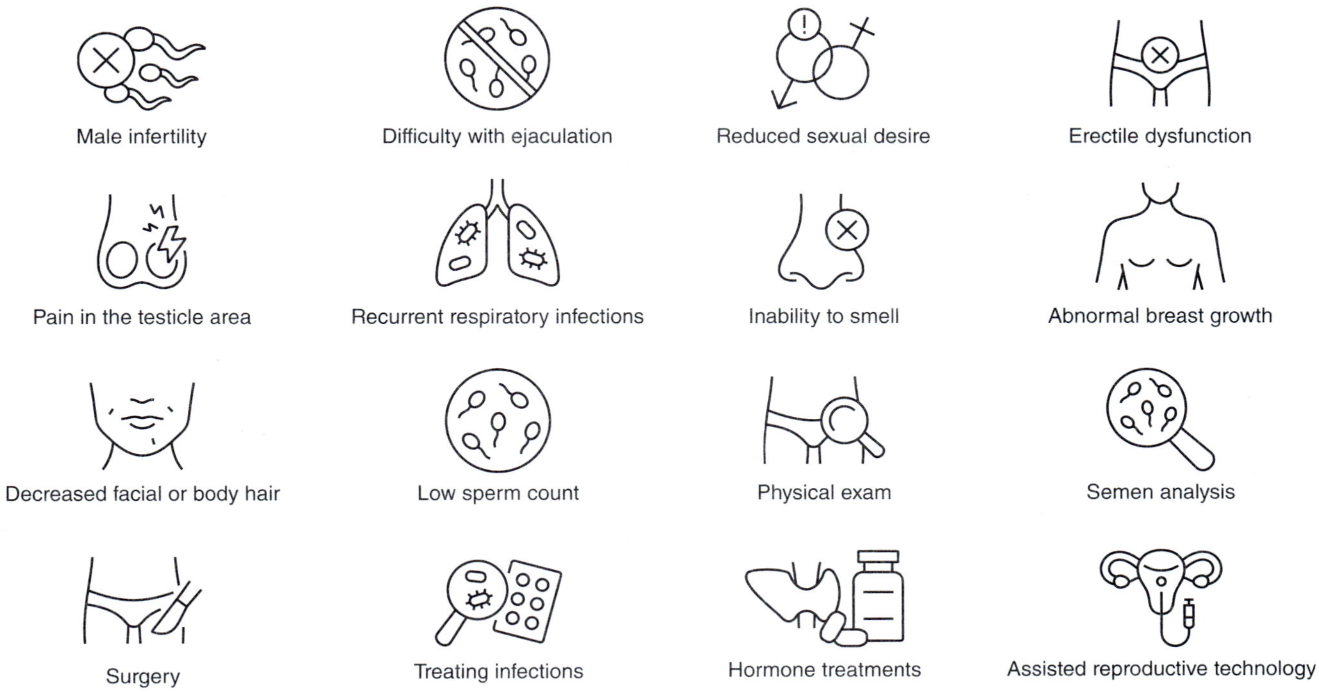

Figure 15-19 Other manifestations of male infertility and potential solutions.

hormone disorders of either the hypothalamus, pituitary, or testicular cells, which contribute to sperm production, can lead to low sperm counts. Testicular or pituitary cancers can also lead to hormonal imbalances. Abnormal sperm production (**Figure 15-20**) may result from anatomical abnormalities, such as varicoceles, or chemical interactions, such as chemotherapy or anabolic steroid use.

Female Reproductive System Infertility

The female reproductive system can present with obstructed uterine tubes (**Figure 15-21**), the etiology of which may include untreated sexually transmitted infections, abdominopelvic surgery, postpartum (after childbirth) infection or sepsis, and complications from an unsafe abortion. Uterine disorders

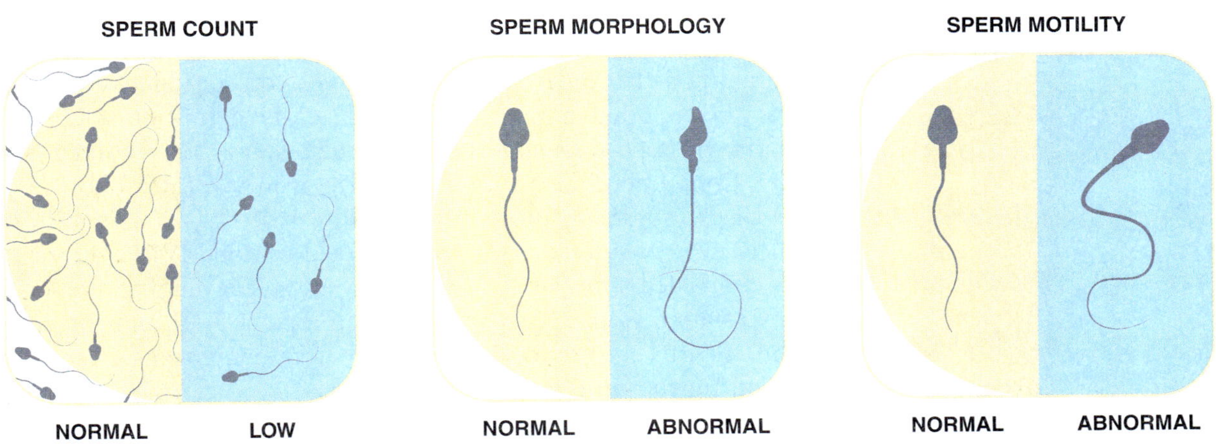

Figure 15-20 Semen analysis examines not only the number of available sperm but also their potential to function.

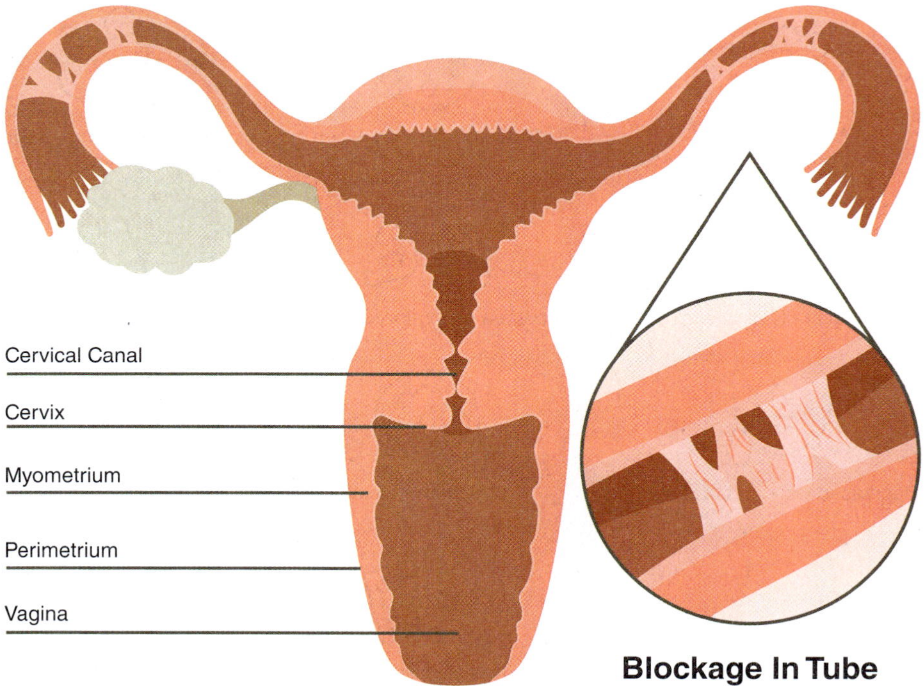

Figure 15-21 Uterine tube blockage. Conception is not possible if the uterine tube does not permit passage of the egg or of sperm.

contributing to infertility can include endometriosis or other inflammatory responses, fibroids, or congenital uterine defects. Polycystic ovarian syndrome and other disorders of follicular maturation impair ova maturation and release. Endocrine hormone disorders affecting either the hypothalamus or pituitary glands will impact egg release and development as well as the uterus's ability to establish and maintain a pregnancy. The etiology of female infertility will vary by country and region. The background prevalence of STDs and the availability of treatment will vary from country to country as well as within countries. Access to female reproductive care, or lack thereof, also contributes to overall female infertility rates.

Assisted Reproductive Technology (ART)

In Vitro Fertilization

Depending upon the underlying etiology, assisted reproductive technology (ART) may be included in the treatment choices. By definition, ART includes any fertility-related treatment that manipulates eggs or embryos outside the body. Consequently, any kind of sperm manipulation followed by *in vivo* use of the sperm or ovarian stimulation that does not require ovum retrieval is not considered ART. In vitro fertilization (IVF) (**Figure 15-22**) involves controlled stimulation of the ovary and retrieval of several oocytes. The oocytes are mixed with spermatozoa in a petri dish, and the embryos are maintained in culture for 3 to 5 days before being transferred into the uterus. During the time in culture, embryos can be examined for genetic analysis or other testing. Viable embryos that were not transferred can be

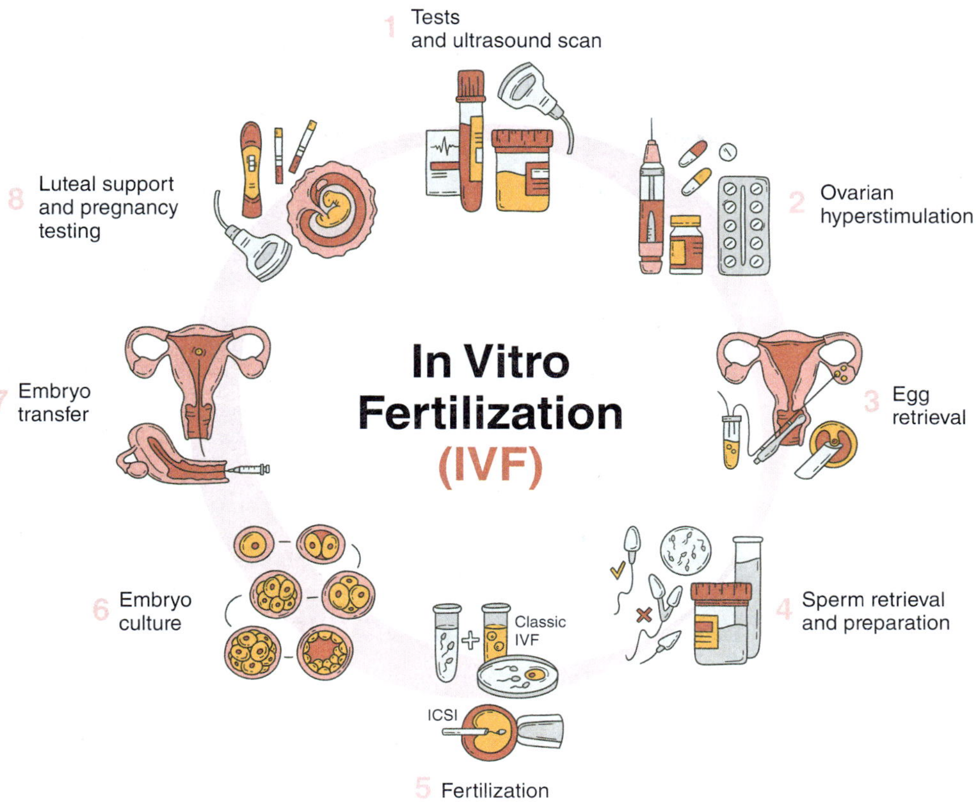

Figure 15-22 IVF sequence. IVF and other forms of assisted reproduction can be a complicated solution to infertility. There can be many steps in the process leading to significant investments in time, emotional capital, and finances.

cryopreserved for future transfer if necessary. IVF mitigates uterine tube blockage as well as other infertility etiologies such as male factor infertility, diminished ovarian reserve, ovarian failure (with donor eggs), ovulatory dysfunction, and unexplained infertility.

Intracytoplasmic Sperm Injection

Intracytoplasmic sperm injection (ICSI) involves using a micropipette to inject a single sperm into the cytoplasm of the egg (**Figure 15-23**). The resulting embryo is still maintained in tissue culture until it is transferred to the uterus on day 5. This procedure is frequently used when male infertility issues are present, or gametes underwent cryopreservation prior to a procedure.

Uterine Transplantation

Another developing technology in cases of uterine factor infertility includes uterine transplantation. Uterus transplantation is a recent, still experimental medical innovation that can make pregnancy possible for people with absolute uterine factor infertility (AUFI).

The procedure requires a uterus donor. Uterus donors can be living or deceased. Attempt for pregnancy can occur only after the uterine transplant is well established.

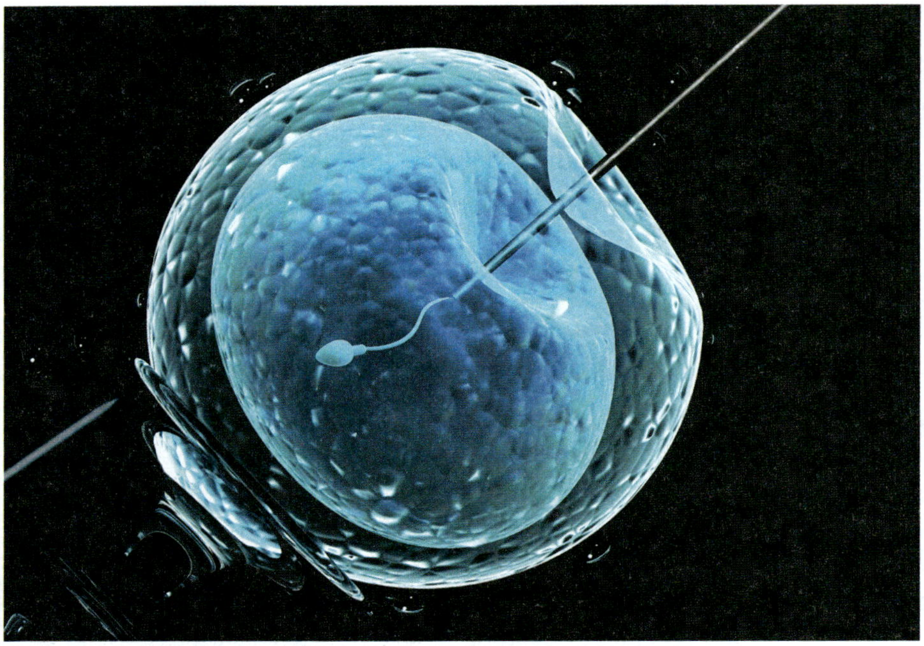

Figure 15-23 Direct sperm injection. Using a very fine glass needle, it is possible to inject a single sperm into the ovum, which increases the potential for conception.

Case 15-1

Sarah and Sidney had one child, a healthy 2-year-old female. The couple was delighted when Sarah became pregnant with a male child. Unfortunately, the pregnancy did not turn out well. An ultrasound of the developing fetus at 18 weeks' gestation detected a possible abnormality of the child's urinary system, and Sarah's developing fetus was now subject to frequent careful examination. At 24 weeks, an MRI study of the developing fetus disclosed definite swelling of the fetal bladder, ureters (hydroureter), and swelling and abnormalities of the developing kidneys (hydronephrosis). Continued monitoring of fetal development confirmed the problem. The fetal abnormalities were accompanied by a reduced amount of amniotic fluid (oligohydramnios).

Sarah and Sidney discussed the findings with their obstetrician. They were told that the chances of the child surviving to birth were low. Even if the fetus survived, death soon after birth was extremely likely. Although many parents in such circumstances would elect to undergo a therapeutic abortion, Sarah and Sidney elected to continue the pregnancy. At 32 weeks, the child was found to be in an abnormal position (breech), and a uterine infection was suspected. The child was delivered by C-section but expired shortly after birth. Heartbroken, the couple agreed to a complete autopsy in an attempt to understand what went wrong with the pregnancy and to help them understand the risk of such an event occurring in a subsequent pregnancy.

Autopsy Results

At birth, the child had an abnormal facial appearance (facies). The facial features (nose, chin, and forehead) appeared to be compressed and flattened as if they had developed pressed against the uterine wall. One leg was malrotated (a clubfoot). Internal examination disclosed severe pulmonary hypoplasia. The two lungs together weighed 6 g; normal lungs would have weighed about 37 g (**Case Figure 15-1**). The lungs were collapsed and could

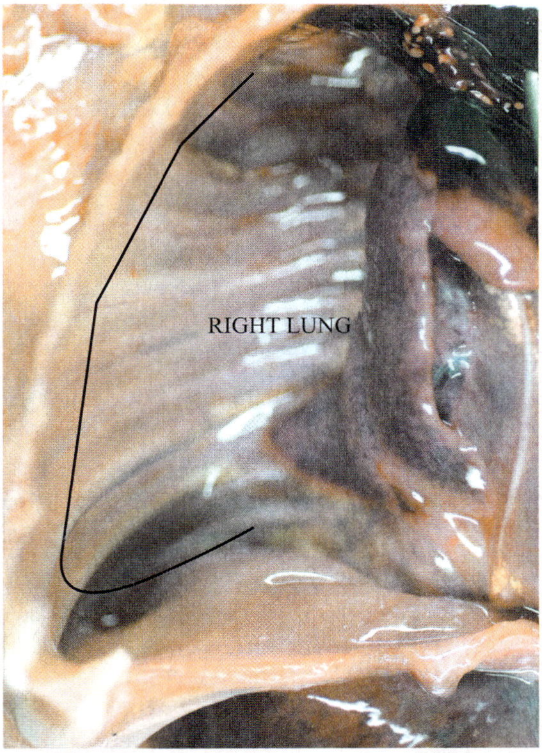

Case Figure 15-1 Hypoplastic right lung in a case of Potter sequence. The line indicates the expected extent of a normal lung.

Courtesy of Vincent Moylan Jr. MS PA (ASCP), Department of Pathology and Laboratory Medicine, University of North Carolina at Chapel Hill.

not function to provide oxygen at birth. The kidneys were fluid-filled and had cysts the pathologist described as being consistent with an obstruction in the urinary system (obstructive nephropathy). The ureters were fluid-filled and dilated, as was the bladder. Examination showed that the outlet from the bladder was defective, and the urethra (which normally would carry urine from the bladder to the opening in the penis) was malformed. This lack of a urinary outlet caused fetal urine to "back up" into the bladder, ureters, and kidney. The pathologist diagnosed Potter sequence.

Discussion

Potter sequence is also termed Potter syndrome, but sequence is the more accurate term. A syndrome is often defined as a group of signs and symptoms that occur together and are characteristic of a disease. The term sequence is used by healthcare providers who study developmental abnormalities to define the secondary consequences of a defect in development. The defect could be the result of dysplasia (an intrinsic disruption of the proper development of an organ such as might be caused by a genetic defect), of a disruption (an environmental disruption of proper development not intrinsic to the fetus), of a deformation (a secondary defect of development related to some other primary cause), or, as in the case of Potter sequence, of a combination of all three.

At the heart of Potter sequence is the oligohydramnios, a lack of the proper amount of amniotic fluid. Why should this occur? The simplest explanation is early disruption of fetal membranes causing chronic physical leakage. Usually, however, the cause of oligohydramnios is more complex. Starting at about 16 weeks' gestation, the source of the bulk of amniotic fluid is fetal urine. The fetus swallows the amniotic fluid (mostly fetal urine) and recycles it through the kidneys. Any interruption in this cycle will result in oligohydramnios.

(continues)

Case 15-1 *(Continued)*

Dysplasia Localized areas of dysregulated growth.

One common cause is failure of the fetal kidneys to develop (bilateral renal **dysplasia**), which is invariably fatal. With no kidneys, no fetal urine is produced. A second cause is a blockage in the urinary tract, which may happen at the level of the urethra (urethral valves, a blockage within the lumen of the urethra) or because of more complex failures of development of the urinary tract (as was the case here). If there is no outlet for urine into the amniotic fluid, the urine backs up, swelling the bladder and the ureters and leading to pressure damage to the developing kidneys. The lack of amniotic fluid has other serious consequences. Pulmonary development in the fetus requires the breathing in of amniotic fluid into the developing lung. If this does not occur, pulmonary hypoplasia results. Finally, amniotic fluid protects and cushions the developing fetus. When the protective fluid is absent, the fetus tends to be pressed against the uterine wall, which results in "flattened" facial features and malpositioned and malrotated limbs. Thus, many of the seemingly unconnected defects in Potter sequence are related to the lack of amniotic fluid, which may be caused by a number of mechanisms. Because of the multiple potential causes, the exact frequency of Potter sequence is unclear. Although about 1 in 5000 births have Potter sequence related to renal agenesis (sometimes termed classic Potter), the overall frequency is perhaps five times higher. Risk is higher in males. Many mutations are associated with renal agenesis, but in the absence of a family history or the occurrence of multiple affected pregnancies, the risk of recurrence is low.

Etiology and Pathogenesis

Potter sequence is caused by complex maldevelopment of the lower urinary tract leading to total urinary obstruction.

Questions

1. Certain types of Potter sequence might be amenable to intrauterine therapy. Which causes of Potter sequence might be corrected? For which causes would this be unlikely?
2. Injection of fluid into the uterus has been suggested as a potential intervention for Potter sequence. What are some potential problems with this approach?
3. What other developmental abnormalities are frequently detected using fetal ultrasound?
4. Fetal DNA can be recovered from maternal circulation and sequenced to detect mutations. Would this approach aid in the early diagnosis of Potter sequence?
5. Potter sequence is a consequence of a combination of dysplasia, disruption, and deformation. How are each of these related to the findings in the case?

Questions for Review

1. Why do spontaneous abortions occur? What are the consequences of prolonged retention of a dead fetus within the uterine cavity?
2. What is an ectopic pregnancy? What factors predispose to development of an ectopic pregnancy in the fallopian tube? What are the consequences of a tubal pregnancy?
3. What is the difference between a hydatidiform mole and a choriocarcinoma?
4. In infants with hemolytic disease, why does jaundice increase after delivery? Why does anemia become more severe after delivery?
5. How is hemolytic disease diagnosed? How is the disease treated?

6. What structures contribute to the formation of the placenta? What are the main functions of the placenta?
7. Describe some of the important abnormalities of the placenta and umbilical cord that may have an unfavorable effect on pregnancy.
8. What is the source of amniotic fluid? What factors regulate the total volume of amniotic fluid?
9. What are the possible causes and the significance of polyhydramnios? Of oligohydramnios?'
10. How might epigenetic factors influence pregnancy and fetal development?
11. How do healthcare disparities contribute to increases in poor maternal and fetal outcomes?
12. In what circumstances might donor sperm contribute to a positive outcome in infertility treatment?
13. How is infertility treatment associated with basic human rights?

References

Chiras DD. Human development and aging. In: *Human Biology*. 9th ed. Jones & Bartlett Learning; 2019:421-440.

Torchia MG, Persaud TVN. *The Developing Human: Clinically Oriented Embryology*. 12th ed. Elsevier; 2024.

- Human development and pregnancy is a complex and well-documented area. Those seeking additional details should start with the chapter listed in the first reference, which provides an excellent overview of the area. The figures are of particular use. The second reference is a recent text much used in medical education that provides clinically relevant details.

Birth Data. National Center for Health Statistics. Updated January 28, 2025. Accessed May 2, 2025. https://www.cdc.gov/nchs/nvss/births.htm

- A portal for extensive statistical data relating to all births in the United States. The "What's New" list is of particular interest.

What are Possible Causes of Stillbirth? National Institute of Child Health and Human Development, National Institutes of Health. Reviewed August 25, 2023. Accessed May 2, 2025. https://www.nichd.nih.gov/health/topics/stillbirth/topicinfo/causes

- This site looks at causes of stillbirth and racial disparities of stillbirth. This is a must-read for those interested in the social aspects of prenatal care.

Prince MK, Daley SF, Ayers D. Substance Use in Pregnancy. StatPearls. Updated July 21, 2023. Accessed May 2, 2025. https://www.ncbi.nlm.nih.gov/books/NBK542330/

- Illicit drug use during pregnancy presents a serious risk to both mother and fetus. This is a brief informative review with references.

Wagle S. Hemolytic Disease of the Newborn. Medscape. Updated June 3, 2024. Accessed May 2, 2025. https://emedicine.medscape.com/article/974349-overview

- Although less of a problem in the United States, hemolytic disease of the fetus and newborn still occurs. This article is a good overview that is strong on the immune (serological) aspects of the problem.

Bisson C, Dautel S, Patel E, Suresh S, Dauer P, Rana S. Preeclampsia pathophysiology and adverse outcomes during pregnancy and postpartum. *Front Med (Lausanne)*. doi:10.3389/fmed.2023.1144170

- This reference is a recent review covering physiological aspects of a condition that is still a major contributor to morbidity in pregnancy.

Grijseels EW, van-Hornstra PT, Govaerts LC, et al. Outcome of pregnancies complicated by oligohydramnios or anhydramnios of renal origin. *Prenat Diagn*. 2011;31(11):1039-1045.

Gupta S. Potter Syndrome. Medscape. Updated June 6, 2024. Accessed May 7, 2025. http://emedicine.medscape.com/article/983477-overview

- These two sources were used in constructing Case 15-1.

Villines Z. What are the average miscarriages rates by week? Medically reviewed by Stacy A. Henigsman, DO. *Medical News Today*. Updated on April 17, 2023. Accessed May 2, 2025. https://www.medicalnewstoday.com/newsletter?utm_source=medicalnewstoday.com&utm_medium=househead&utm_campaign=newsletter_signup&utm_term=IAB&utm_content=728X9.0

- This article provides a timeline for when pregnancies are most likely to end in spontaneous abortion. It also underscores that more pregnancy losses may occur very early in pregnancy.

What Is the Typical Pregnancy Ultrasound Schedule? UPMC Magee-Womens. May 8, 2023. Accessed May 2, 2025. https://share.upmc.com/2023/05/pregnancy-ultrasound-schedule/

- Sonography has become a routine part of obstetrical care with a typical schedule. This article explains what information could be available from an ultrasound at what stages in gestation.

Cell-Free DNA Prenatal Screening Testing. American College of Obstetricians & Gynecologists. Accessed May 2, 2025. https://www.acog.org/womens-health/infographics/cell-free-dna-prenatal-screening-test

- CfDNA testing is becoming more popular and embraced by caregivers and pregnant people. This article explains what type of information can actually be obtained through cfDNA testing.

Navaratnam K, Alfirevic Z; the Royal College of Obstetricians and Gynaecologists. Amniocentesis and chorionic villus sampling: Green-top Guideline No. 8. *BJOG*. 2022;129(1):e1-e15. doi:10.1111/1471-0528.16821

- DNA testing procedures involve risks, which are clearly outlined here. The article explains the use and timing of each test.

Girardi G, Longo M, Bremer AA. Social determinants of health in pregnant individuals from underrepresented, understudied, and underreported populations in the United States. *Int J Equity Health*. 2023;22(1):186. doi:10.1186/s12939-023-01963-x

- Overview of factors that contribute to increased adverse outcomes in pregnancies associated with marginalized groups.

Bhadsavle SS, Golding MC. Paternal epigenetic influences on placental health and their impacts on offspring development and disease. *Front Genet*. 2022;13:1068408. doi:10.3389/fgene.2022.1068408 PMID: 36468017; PMCID: PMC9716072.

- This article discusses sperm contribution to placentation and pregnancy outcome and introduces potential epigenetic changes in sperm and their potential outcomes for generations.

Infertility. World Health Organization. Updated May 22, 2024. Accessed May 2, 2025. https://www.who.int/news-room/fact-sheets/detail/infertility

- This site provides general information on infertility and a global perspective on how infertility affects human rights.

Jain M, Singh M. Assisted Reproductive Technology (ART) Techniques. StatPearls [Internet]. Updated June 7, 2023. https://www.ncbi.nlm.nih.gov/books/NBK576409/

- This article provides an overview of most-often-used ART procedures and contains links to more in-depth discussions.

Običan SG, Leavitt K, Scialli AR. Do Assisted Reproductive Techniques Increase the Risk of Birth Defects? Society for Birth Defects Research & Prevention. Accessed May 2, 2025. https://www.birthdefectsresearch.org/primer/reproductive-techniques.asp

- This site provides an overview of birth defect rates associated with ART and includes a discussion of what needs to be considered when talking about birth defect rates associated with these procedures.

American Pregnancy Association. Symptoms & Signs of Miscarriage. http://americanpregnancy.org/pregnancy-complications/miscarriage/

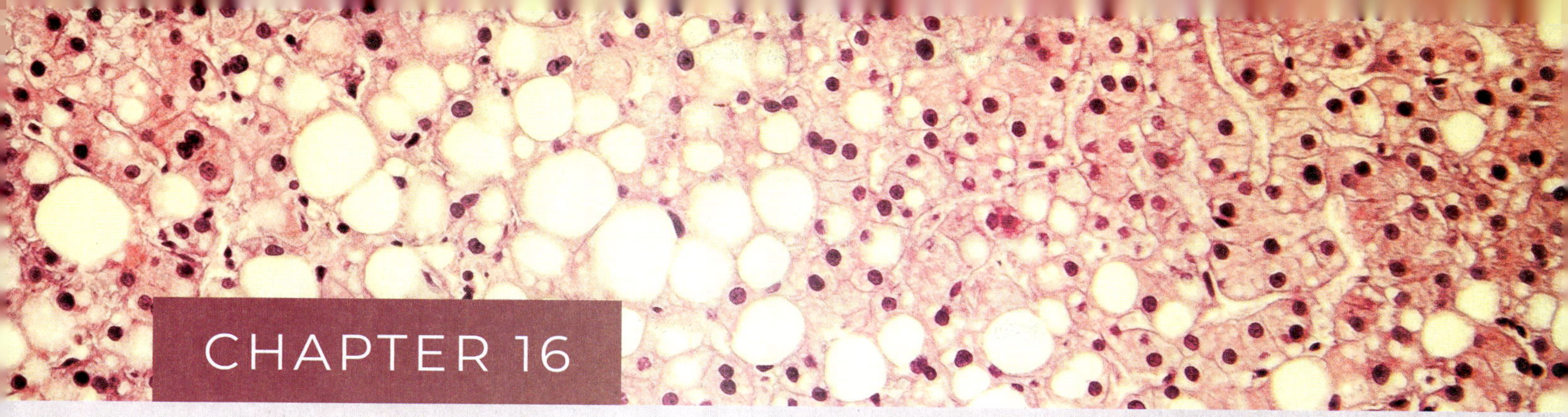

CHAPTER 16

Congenital and Developmental Diseases

LEARNING OBJECTIVES

1. Describe some of the more important malformations resulting from intrauterine injury.
2. List the common causes of congenital malformations and their approximate incidence.
3. Explain the concept of multifactorial origin. Give an example of a multifactorial congenital anomaly and describe factors which may have contributed to this condition.

Congenital Disease

The term **congenital** anomaly or congenital disease (birth defect) refers to structural or functional abnormalities that were initiated during gestation. Many researchers prefer to use the term anomaly rather than abnormality or birth defect to define an intrinsic defect in development that may be genetic, environmental, or of mixed origin. Such anomalies may be associated with structural disorders (and are often termed **malformations**) or may be functional and developmental disorders in nature. Many major congenital anomalies are of medical or social concern and are likely to require intervention.

Congenital Present at birth.

Malformation Defect in development.

Diagnosis of congenital disease can occur prenatally, neonatally (at the time around birth) or any other time later in life. Congenital anomalies are often incompatible with intrauterine development or extrauterine life. Chromosomal abnormalities contribute significantly to fetal loss and stillbirth. At least 50 percent of known early pregnancy loss in the first trimester is associated with chromosomal abnormalities. Functional abnormalities (and some structural abnormalities) may not be recognized until the child enters school or even later. Approximately 1 of 33 infants will be diagnosed with a structural defect within the first year of life, which can contribute to the infant mortality rate and is the second leading cause of infant death after preterm birth.

The distinction between the results of structural and functional defects can be difficult to define. Disabilities resulting from functional abnormalities include intellectual disabilities such as learning disorders and autism spectrum disorders. (These types of disabilities are often labelled as neurodivergent, a term that is poorly defined, is not a medical term, and does not in and of itself indicate a functional congenital abnormality.) For example, autism in its severe forms clearly has a genetic component, and in that sense, can be considered a functional defect, presumably a reflection of a structural defect in neurological development and organization.

Gene mutation Change in the DNA sequence of the gene.

Fetal lung dysplasia Abnormal development of the lungs in a fetus.

About half of congenital anomalies cannot be linked to a specific cause. Approximately 15–25% of all recognized congenital diseases can be attributed to chromosomal abnormalities and single **gene mutations** or variations (discussed in Chapter 3). External environmental factors, including infectious disease and exposure to chemicals, drugs, or other agents, contribute to 1 in 20, or about 6–8%, of reported congenital diseases. The remaining diagnosed structural or congenital anomalies most likely result from a mixture of various genetic and environmental factors (are multifactorial). The Center for Disease Control (CDC) website indicates that approximately 1 in 33 (roughly 3%) of babies in the United States are born with a birth defect. However, the data is limited because the United States does not have a national birth registry and birth anomaly tracking system. A majority of states do track some selected birth defects, but that varies by state. The CDC tracking network collects state-based results and provides data on a number of common birth defects believed to be associated with environmental risk (**Table 16-1**).

Special terminology is used in the clinical description of congenital anomalies. Anomalies in which there is a defect in the organization of cells resulting in tissue defects are termed *dysplasias*. Abnormalities of bone development can, for example, result in a variety of skeletal defects (skeletal dysplasias). A lack of amniotic fluid (oligohydramnios) can disrupt pulmonary development resulting in **fetal lung dysplasia**.

Table 16-1 Frequency of Birth Defects in the United States

Specific Defect	Occurrence/Births	Approximate Annual Rate	Type of Defect
Anencephaly	1/5246	700	Brain/Spine
Encephalocele	1/10,365	354	Brain/Spine
Spina Bifida no anencephaly	1/2875	1278	Brain/ Spine
Atrioventricular septal defect	1/1712	2145	Heart
Coarctation of the aorta	1/1712	2146	Heart
Truncus arteriosus	1/15,984	230	Heart
Double outlet right ventricle	1/4237	867	Heart
Pulmonary valve atresia	1/6708	548	Heart
Tetralogy of Fallot	1/2077	1768	Heart
Transposition of the great arteries	1/3348	1097	Heart
Cleft lip with and without cleft palate	1/1032	3560	Mouth and Face
Club foot	1/536	6850	Muscle and Bones
Diaphragmatic hernia	1/3214	1143	Muscle and Bones
Limb deficiencies	1/2064	1779	Muscle and Bones

Data from Centers for Disease Control and Prevention. (2024, November 19). Data and statistics on birth defects. Birth Defects. https://www.cdc.gov/birth-defects/data-research/facts-stats/index.html

Minor congenital malformations may be predominantly of cosmetic significance (such as partial fusion of several toes, extra nipples, or abnormal scalp hair whorls), and they occur in more than 10 percent of live births. A single example of a minor abnormality in an individual may be considered part of normal human variation rather than an anomaly. However, the co-occurrence of multiple minor or major defects in an individual in a repeated pattern is likely to indicate the presence of a congenital **syndrome**, a potentially more serious defect characterized by a common set of abnormalities related to a single cause. Related to syndromes are development sequences in which a single causative agent affects growth and development in multiple areas, all of which were initiated by the original causative agent or event.

Syndrome Signs and symptoms often collectively associated with a disease or pathogenic process.

Fetal deformation Misshapen fetus caused by compression or mispositioning during fetal development.

Fetal disruption Structural changes noted at birth.

Although the majority of congenital abnormalities are intrinsic defects of development, there are also anomalies resulting from extrinsic forces such as maternal uterine tumors. The previously mentioned oligohydramnios can also result in **fetal deformation** due to compression or mispositioning during intrauterine development. An example would be a misshapen or asymmetric skull. Somewhat related to deformations are developmental **fetal disruptions**, which result from mechanical or vascular events that interfere with otherwise normal development. This most commonly occurs when fibrous bands present in the amniotic fluid encircle and trap part of the developing fetus, leading to amputation of a developing limb.

External stresses on the pregnant person, such as poverty, famine, armed conflicts, and poor access to prenatal health care, contribute to increased congenital abnormalities or disease.

Figure 16-1 highlights some of the personal and demographic factors that may contribute to an increase in infants born with congenital abnormalities.

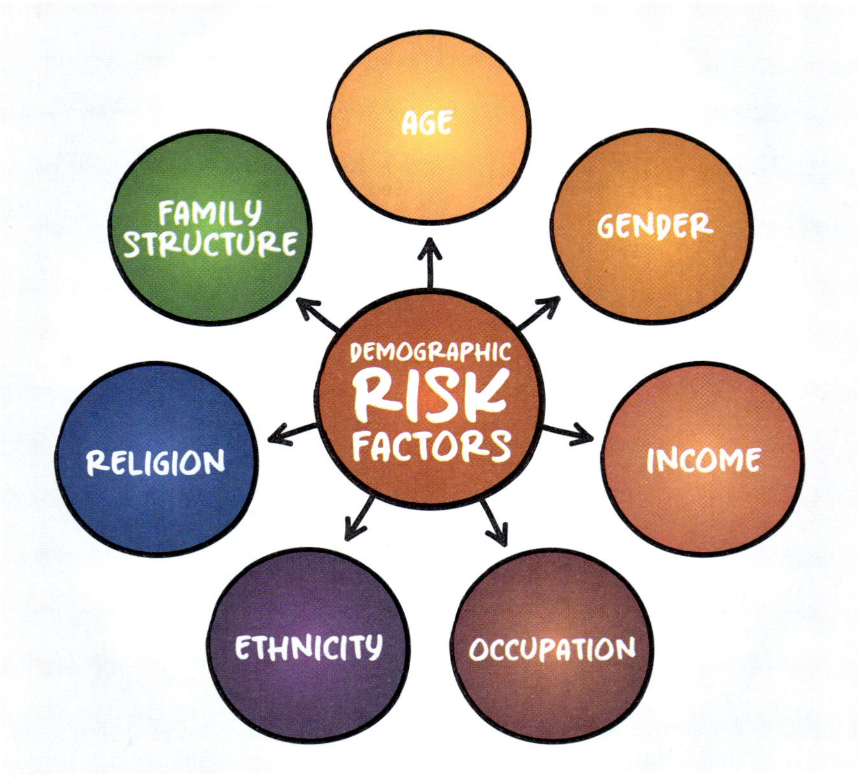
DEMOGRAPHIC
RISK
FACTORS
AGE
GENDER
INCOME
OCCUPATION
ETHNICITY
RELIGION
FAMILY STRUCTURE

Figure 16-1 Demographic risk factors that can contribute to congenital abnormalities.

Harmful Drugs and Chemicals

Today we know that many drugs, chemicals, and pharmaceutical agents can potentially harm the developing embryo and fetus. Such agents are termed *teratogens*. The outcome of the teratogenic exposure varies based upon the intensity of the exposure and the timing of the exposure during development. **Figure 16-2** presents a timeline for when a developing organ system would be most vulnerable to external and internal influences which could result in congenital anomalies.

Phocomelia A congenital reduction deformity where the limbs do not develop properly and the hands and/or feet are abnormally close to the trunk.

The online TERIS database has current information on the teratogenic risk of over 1700 drug exposures during pregnancy. The drugs are sometimes used clinically. Until the mid-20th century, most thought that the placenta provided protection during pregnancy and that the intrauterine environment was a protected space. Unfortunately, a drug marketed worldwide in the late 1950s and early 1960s disproved that hypothesis. Thalidomide, originally developed as a sedative with very little side effects, was also found to alleviate the symptoms of early pregnancy nausea and vomiting (morning sickness) and sleep disturbances. The drug never gained FDA approval in the United States but was highly sampled by pharmaceutical representatives to physicians' offices. The drug produced highly characteristic malformations, including **phocomelia**, in which the proximal bones of the extremities were highly reduced or absent, with the hands or feet arising from the trunk in a flipper-like pattern. The location and severity of the malformations varied depending upon the time of exposure during early pregnancy. The drug also caused malformations of the heart, gastrointestinal tract, eyes, and ears. At the time developmental toxicology testing involved laboratory rodents. Rodent placentas do not metabolize thalidomide like human placentas, and consequently, the drug was not initially detected as a teratogen. Despite the hazard of thalidomide to the fetus, the

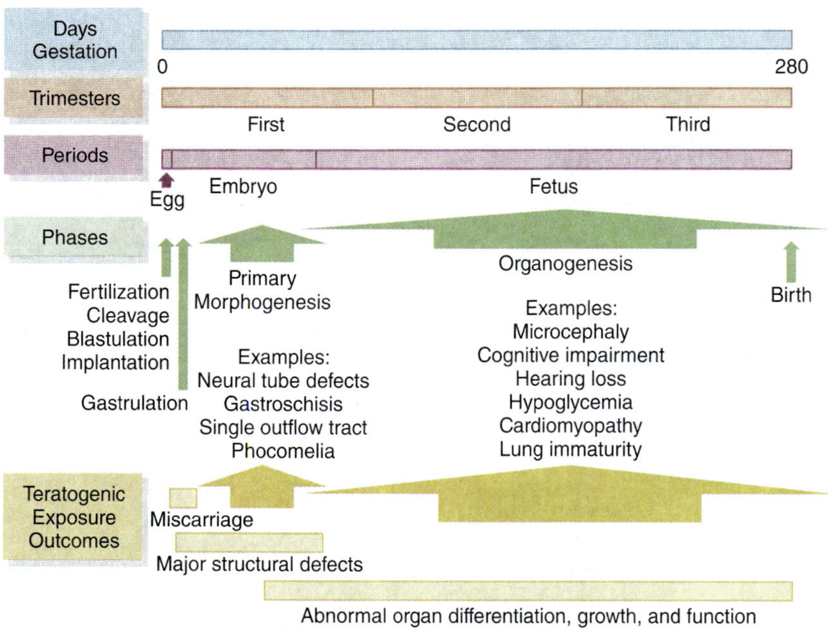

Figure 16-2 Timeline of embryo and fetal vulnerability. Organs and organ systems develop at different times and with different rates during growth in utero. This figure shows the general developmental timeline and when particular organ systems may be the most vulnerable.

Reproduced from Hales, B., Scialli, A., & Tassinari, M. (Eds.). (2018). Teratology Primer, 3rd Edition. Society for Birth Defects Research and Prevention. https://www.birthdefectsresearch.org/primer/

drug is still used for treating some diseases, including leprosy and multiple myeloma, a form of lymphoid cell cancer. Because of the extreme hazard of the drug on fetal development, healthcare providers prescribing the drug are required to take great precautions to be certain that the patient is not pregnant and will not become pregnant while taking the drug.

Other drugs in current use can cause congenital malformations. For example, the drug isotretinoin (formerly Accutane)—although useful in treating severe cystic acne—is a potent teratogen. As many as 30 percent of infants exposed in utero during the first trimester show some degree of craniofacial, neurological, or other defects. Because of the risk, women with childbearing potential must agree to using two effective forms of birth control while using the drug. The drug is a derivative and metabolite of vitamin A that interferes with normal fetal pattern development. Because of this, there is continuing concern about the use of excessive vitamin A during pregnancy.

Currently, all drugs used in the United States are rated in five categories by the FDA according to the degree of possible risk to the fetus balanced against the drug's potential benefit to the patient (**Table 16-2**). Ratings range from "A" for drugs that are generally considered safe for use in pregnancy to "D" for drugs that may injure the fetus but are of enough benefit to the patient that their use may outweigh the risk to the fetus. "X"-rated drugs are contraindicated in pregnancy because the severe risk to the fetus outweighs any possible benefit to the patient.

Cigarette smoking and consumption of alcoholic beverages during pregnancy can contribute to congenital disease as well. Cigarette smoking leads to intrauterine growth retardation (IUG) resulting in the birth of smaller than normal infants and preterm delivery. Maternal smoking is a risk factor for both sudden infant death syndrome (SIDS) and sudden intrauterine unexplained death syndrome (SIUD). **Sudden infant death syndrome (SIDS)**, an otherwise unexplained death of a child under the age of 1 year, can be related to maternal smoking during pregnancy, with a 3 times higher rate in infants exposed during pregnancy. The infant's sleep position can also be correlated with SIDS, making it another multifactorial congenital disease. Alcohol consumption during pregnancy, prenatal alcohol exposure (PAS), can result in a characteristic pattern of developmental abnormalities termed fetal alcohol syndrome disorders (FASD). There is no defined safe amount of consumption during pregnancy. **Fetal alcohol syndrome** (FAS) presents with recognizable

Sudden infant death syndrome (SIDS) Unexplained death of child under the age of one year.

Fetal alcohol syndrome Developmental abnormalities related to heavy alcohol consumption during pregnancy.

Table 16-2 Five Categories of All Drugs Used in the United States Rated by the FDA According to Degree of Possible Risk to the Fetus

	Category Interpretation
A	No risk to fetus demonstrated in well-controlled studies in humans.
B	No evidence of risk to fetus. Either animal studies show risk but human studies do not, or there are no adequate human studies but animal studies do not indicate risk.
C	Risk to fetus cannot be ruled out. No human studies available to assess risk. Animal studies either are not available or indicate possible risk.
D	Positive evidence of risk to fetus; however, drug is needed to treat patients, and no safer alternative drug is available. Potential benefit to patients outweighs risk to fetus.
X	Absolutely contraindicated in pregnancy. Severe risk to fetus greatly outweighs any possible benefit to patients.

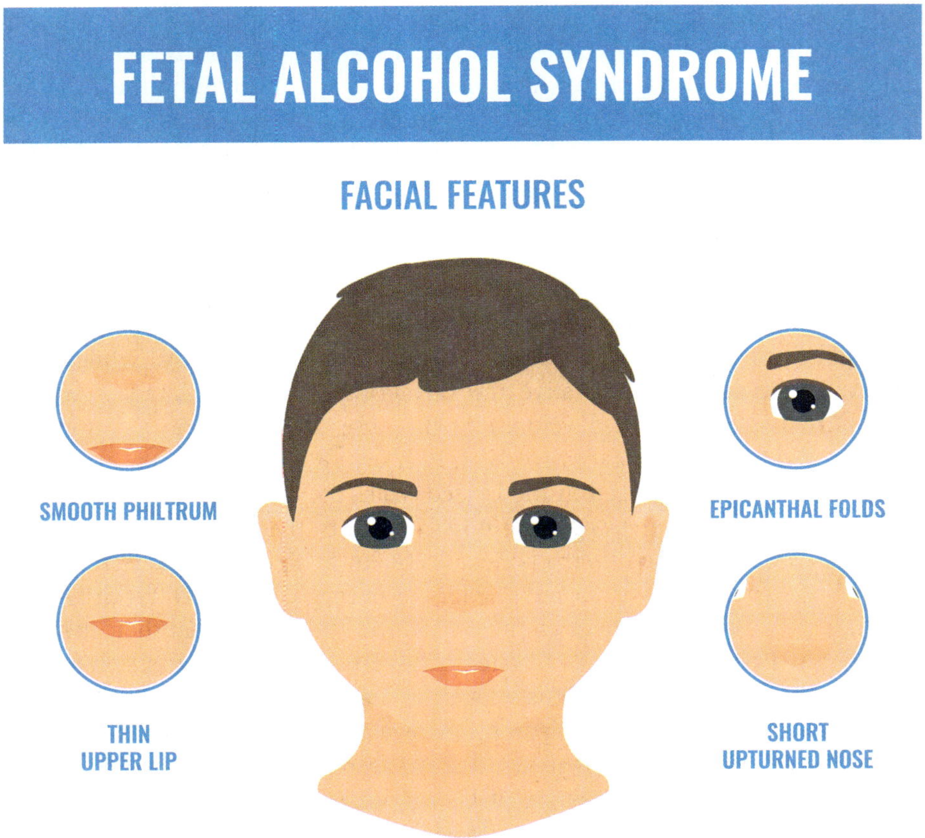

Figure 16-3 Fetal alcohol syndrome facial signs. Fetal alcohol syndrome can be manifest in changes to facial structure. At first, it was believed it caused mostly structural defects. Later research indicated cognitive and behavioral effects.

structural abnormalities to the brain, including cognitive and developmental abnormalities, and is often seen with abnormal cranial and facial development (**Figure 16-3**), as well as other structural malformations. FASD encompasses a broader range of effects, including cognitive and behavioral disorders without any physical abnormalities.

Drugs, such as heroin, methadone, and cocaine, impair fetal growth and development and may lead to congenital malformation. In addition, the infant may be drug-dependent at birth. Maternal cocaine use may also disturb blood flow through the placenta, leading to intrauterine fetal death.

Many new drugs and antibiotics are not recommended for use in pregnancy, especially during the early part of pregnancy when the embryo is especially vulnerable (see Figure 16-2) because the possible effects of the drugs on the developing embryo are not known. This is particularly true of drugs of abuse, whose composition are often unknown.

Radiation

Exposure to radiation during pregnancy may harm the fetus and contribute to subsequent childhood diseases, including childhood leukemia. As little as two to three abdominal CTs may be associated with increased risk; consequently, a risk-to-benefit analysis must be undertaken prior to X-ray examinations or diagnostic tests using radioactive materials during pregnancy. This is particularly true during the first 15 weeks of fetal development, perhaps even more so during the 14 days post-conception when pregnancy may not have been detected.

Maternal Infections

Some infections acquired during pregnancy may injure the developing fetus. Even infectious agents that produce either asymptomatic disease or only mild symptoms in the mother can result in serious damage to the developing fetus. Infection with **Zika virus**, a flavivirus related to the yellow fever virus, is transmitted by the bite of an *Aedes* species mosquito and may proceed unnoticed in the infected person or result in a generally mild disease characterized by fever, rash, headache, conjunctivitis, and other constitutional symptoms (**Figure 16-4**). However, the virus can infect the developing fetus, resulting in a variety of severe fetal brain defects, characteristically including **microcephaly**. Surviving children are seriously compromised and may require continuous specialized care. In the United States, 15% of pregnancies confirmed to have Zika infection in the first trimester resulted in the birth of infants exhibiting a set of birth defects, termed congenital Zika syndrome. The syndrome includes severe neurological damage to the developing fetus, including microcephaly (small head, sometimes with collapse of skull) (**Figure 16-5**), decreased brain tissue, and damage to the developing eye, joints, and muscle tone. In addition, many other developmental defects may be noted during the first 2 years of growth. A major outbreak of disease occurred during 2015–2016 in South America (notably Brazil).

Zika virus An *Aedes* mosquito-borne flavivirus which can cause severe neurological damage in the developing fetus of an infected mother.

Microcephaly Condition in which an infant's head circumference is smaller than normal, often due to failure of the brain to develop normally.

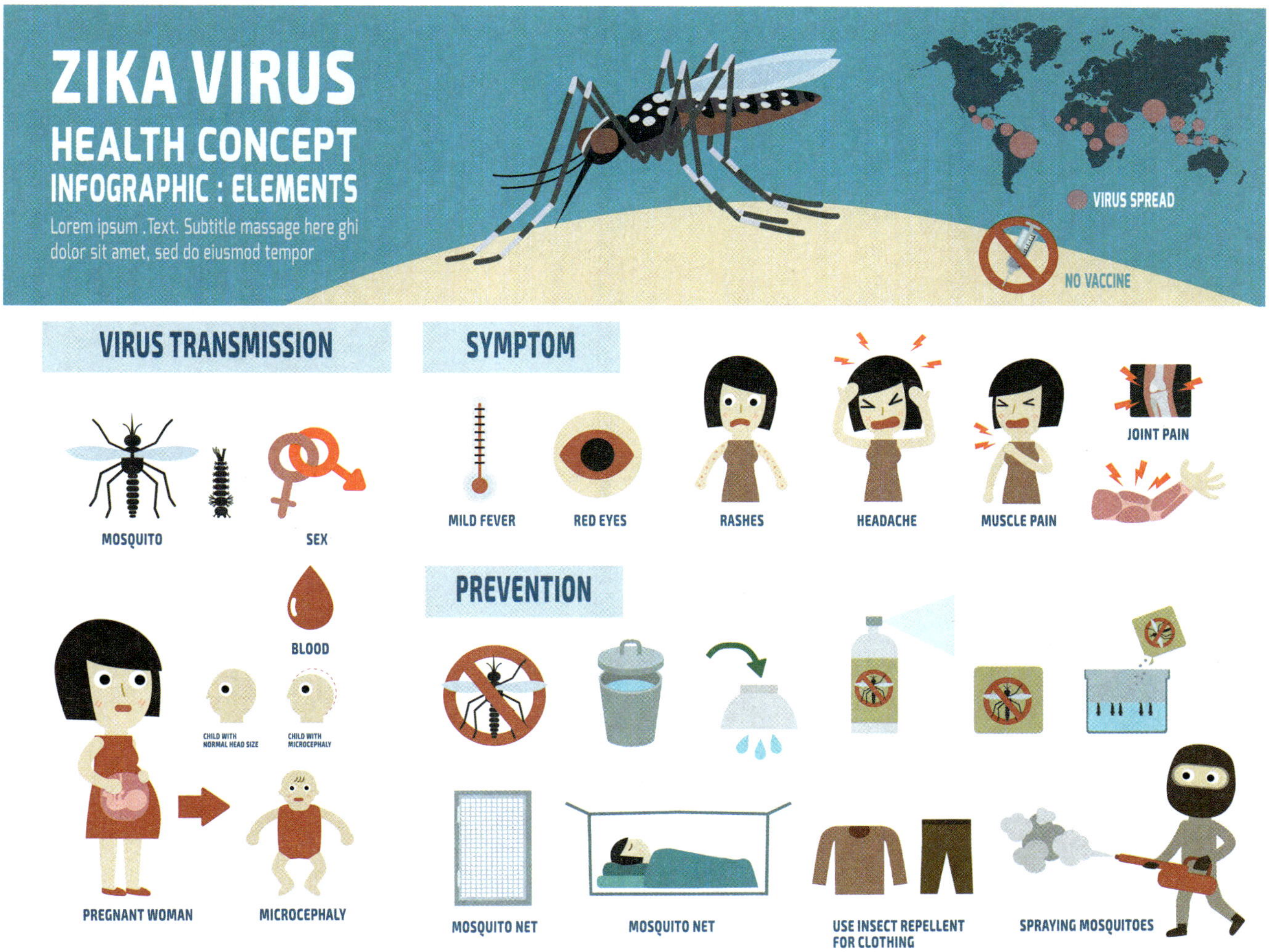

Figure 16-4 Zika virus symptoms and ways to control exposure to mosquitos.

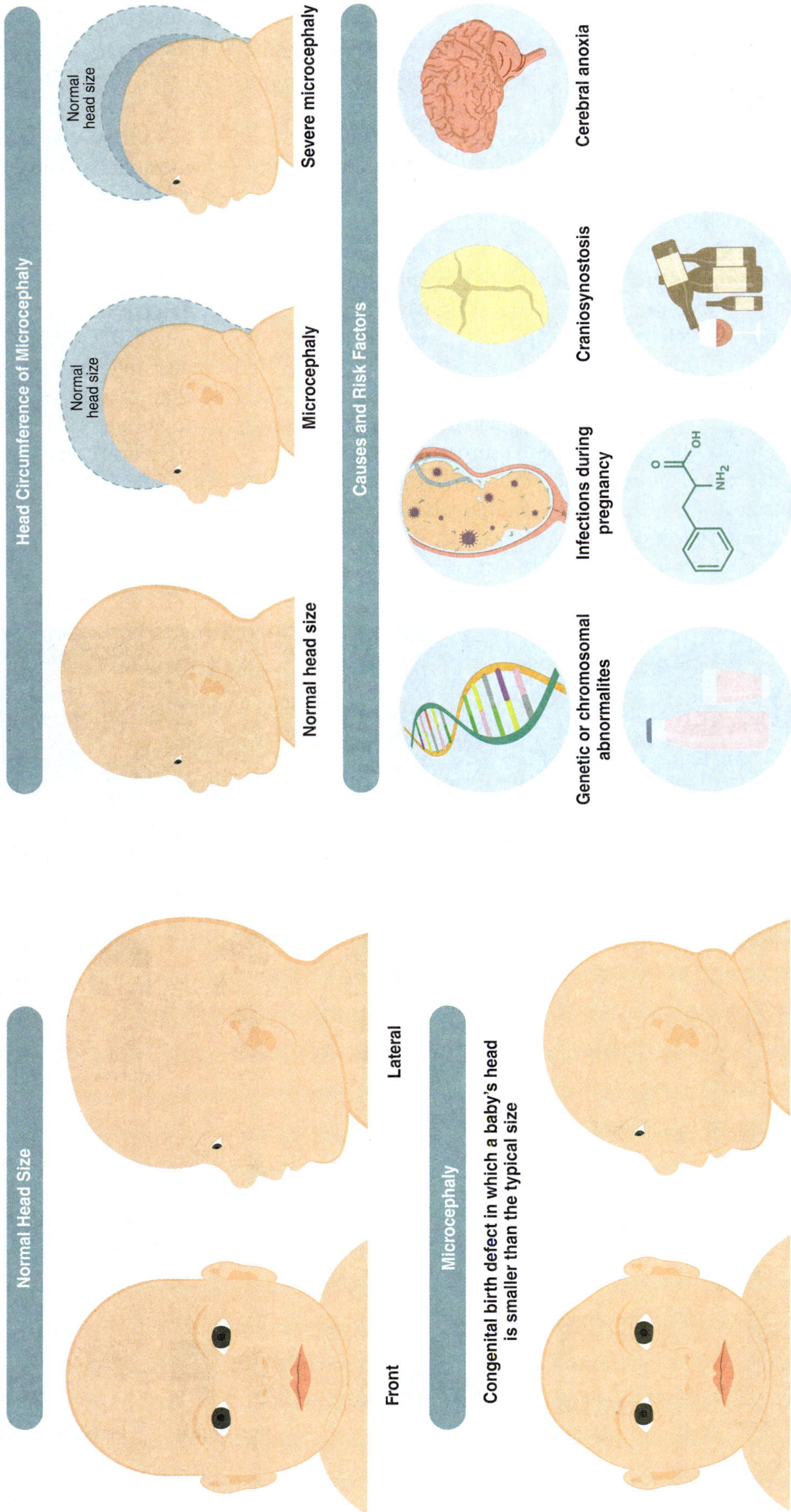

Figure 16-5 Microcephaly can be one manifestation of fetal Zika virus infection. Microcephaly is not limited to Zika virus infection and is considered a nervous system neural tube anomaly.

Currently Zika virus transmission is found in many countries in the Americas, Africa, and other locations. As well as being transmitted by mosquitoes, Zika virus can be transmitted through sexual intercourse. By 2018, over 4800 pregnancies occurred in women with Zika infections. About 14 percent of babies resulting from such pregnancies showed signs of congenital Zika syndrome. Local transmission was reported in the United States (in Florida and Texas) in 2017; however, aggressive mosquito control appears to have currently alleviated insect-borne transmission in the continental United States. Pregnant people are advised to check with the CDC prior to travel to areas where Zika has formerly been reported, including tropical Africa, South America, Southeast Asia, and the Pacific Islands. Currently over 3000 cases have been reported in the Americas, including Puerto Rico.

A group of agents commonly termed the **TORCH complex** produce characteristic injuries to the developing fetus. The term TORCH refers to **T** toxoplasmosis, infection with the parasite *Toxoplasma gondii*; **R** rubella (German measles); **C** cytomegalovirus (CMV); **H** herpes simplex virus; and **O** other, including HIV, parvovirus, syphilis, and several other agents. Rubella virus, cytomegalovirus, toxoplasma, and occasionally herpes cause a similar type of infection in the fetus. A clinical diagnosis of the infectious agent can be identified by histologic examination, cell culture, or serologic or molecular methods. For this reason, the maternal medical history, including exposure and immunization history, as well as physical findings in the newborn is critical in the diagnosis of the specific agent. Of these, CMV transmission in utero is the most common. Up to 4% of pregnant women have primary CMV (a first infection) and are at risk of transmitting it to the fetus.

TORCH complex
Mnemonic for organisms causing maternal infections injurious to the developing fetus.

Rubella

Rubella is a mild illness that is usually acquired in childhood; 90 percent of women of childbearing age have had the disease or have been immunized. The CDC reports that in addition to leading to miscarriage and fetal death, thirty-three percent of the infants infected with congenital rubella die within the first year of life. In surviving pregnancies, fetal exposure to rubella, especially earlier in pregnancy, 12 to 16 weeks' gestation, resulted in 20 percent of children presenting with defects, including congenital cataracts, cardiac malformations, deafness, and neurologic disturbances (**Figure 16-6**). In rare situations, children with congenital rubella can develop progressive rubella panencephalitis, resulting in progressive neurological disease presumably related to viral reactivation often in adolescence. Because of near—universal immunization, congenital rubella has almost been eliminated in the United States.

Cytomegalic Inclusion Disease

Cytomegalovirus derives its name from the enlargement of the cells it infects. The infected cells contain characteristic large, basophilic, intranuclear inclusions, resulting in virus-infected cells' characteristic histologic appearance (**Figure 16-7**). CMV infection is very common and usually asymptomatic, but once the body is infected, the virus can stay within it and become reactivated. The fetus may become infected either from a new maternal infection acquired during pregnancy or from reactivation of a prior maternal infection. A newly acquired (primary) maternal infection poses the greatest risk to the fetus, with a 30 percent to 40 percent risk of transmission; however, only about 10 percent of infected fetuses show symptoms. The virus may

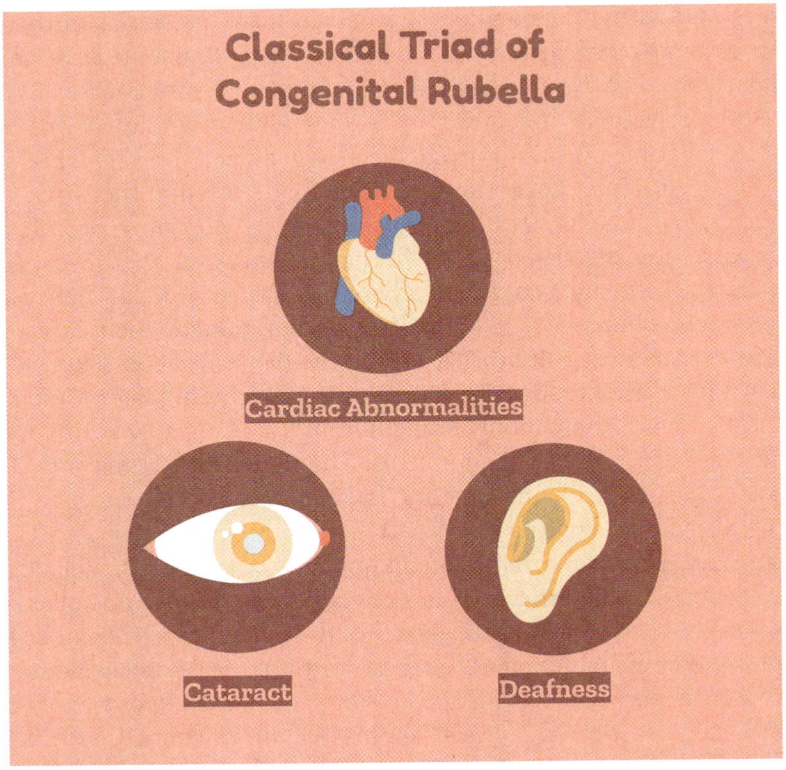

Figure 16-6 Congenital rubella exposure. Exposure to rubella in utero often results in anomalies referred to as the rubella triad.

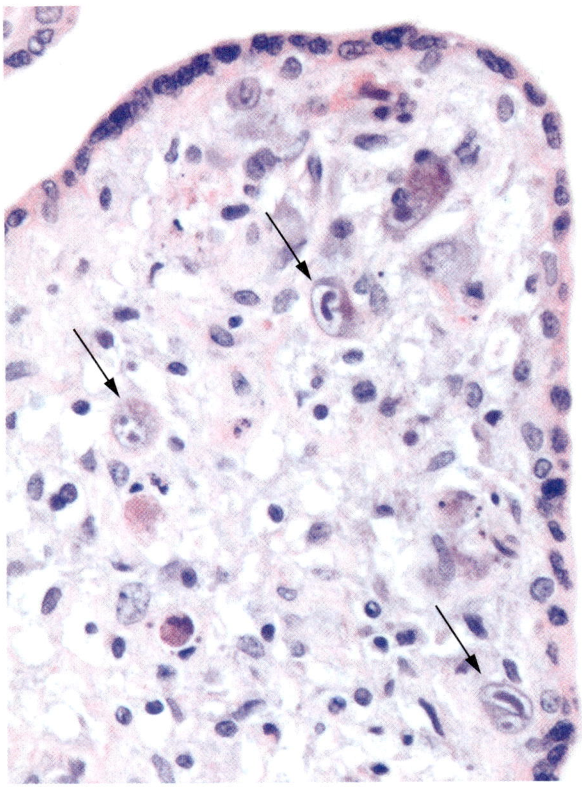

Figure 16-7 Cytomegalovirus. Three large cells with irregular nuclei (*arrows*) each have oddly shaped inclusions in a placental villus. The fetus died in utero of overwhelming cytomegalovirus infection involving the lungs and brain.

cause severe fetal damage, characterized by injury to the brain and eyes, leading to failure of the brain to develop normally (microcephaly), poor cognitive development, and blindness. Infection results in death of 30 percent of infants with severe disease. The cytomegalovirus may also cause a chronic systemic infection of the fetus, similar to that caused by the rubella virus, and the virus can be identified in the tissues of the infected infant. Disease may also be contracted at the time of birth from genital secretions or breastmilk. Asymptomatic neonates may develop hearing loss, retinal disease, and developmental delay within the first 2 years.

HIV

Vertical transmission of HIV from the infected mother to the child can occur before birth; however, infection usually occurs at the time of birth or soon thereafter by ingestion of infected breastmilk. Transmission from the mother is responsible for about 80 percent of all pediatric HIV infection. The risk of transmission by an infected mother depends on the level of HIV in the blood and the degree of contact between the neonate and maternal blood and genital secretions. With appropriate maternal drug therapy, vertical transmission (from mother to fetus) of HIV can be prevented. Most HIV medicines do not increase the risk of birth defects.

Other Virus Diseases in Pregnancy

The herpes simplex virus, the same virus that causes fever blisters, may at times cause intrauterine and neonatal infections. Intrauterine infection is uncommon and results in skin and eye lesions and microcephaly; 90 percent of infections result from passage through an infected genital tract. Neonatal herpes (herpes neonatorum) may be localized to the eye, skin, or mucous membrane or result in severe disseminated disease involving the nervous system, liver, and lung with a very high mortality rate. For this reason, offspring of infected mothers may be treated prophylactically with antiviral therapy.

Some other viruses may occasionally be transmitted to the fetus and cause disease in the fetus. Parvovirus B19 (responsible for "fifth disease," a mild rash-associated disease in children) may be responsible for more than 10 percent of intrauterine fetal death, fetal anemia, and in some cases hydrops fetalis.

Toxoplasmosis

Toxoplasma gondii is a small, ovoid, intracellular parasite. Adults acquire the infection by eating raw or partially cooked meat that is infected with the parasite or by contact with infected cats, which excrete an infectious form of the organism (oocyte) in their feces. As with cytomegalovirus infection, more than 50 percent of women of childbearing age have had a previous inapparent infection and have formed antibodies to the parasite.

Toxoplasmosis infection acquired during pregnancy can result in severe consequences for the fetus, including injury to the brain and eyes, causing microcephaly, obstruction of the ventricles of the brain resulting in hydrocephalus (discussed later), as well as visual disturbances or blindness. Many cases of fetal infection result in death. Primary infection during pregnancy is a major risk factor. Young women show low rates of immunity (≤ 20 percent) and hence are at greatest risk. Although the risk of infection in such women is under 1 percent, pregnant women should avoid eating undercooked meat and should exercise caution in contact with cats and, in particular, cat litter boxes.

A Systemic Overview of Congenital Malformations

Cardiovascular System

Congenital Heart Disease

Cardiac Development and Prenatal Blood Flow. The heart undergoes a complex developmental progression. It is formed from a tube that undergoes considerable growth and change in configuration. The tube folds back on itself and eventually the individual chambers, valves, and large arteries develop.

In utero, the blood flow through the fetal heart differs from its final postdelivery flow pattern. Much of the blood flow in the pulmonary artery is diverted away from the lungs, since the fetus does not breathe air and the artery is used instead to supply other fetal tissues (**Figure 16-8**). One bypass vessel, the ductus arteriosus, connects the pulmonary artery with the aorta, shunting much of the blood pumped into the pulmonary artery directly into the aorta. At birth, when the infant takes its first breath, the lungs expand, constricting the ductus arteriosus and blocking blood flow. Consequently, blood from the pulmonary artery can flow only into the newly expanded lungs. The nonfunctional ductus eventually becomes converted into a fibrous cord, the ligamentum arteriosum. The other fetal bypass, an opening in the atrial septum, the foramen ovale, maintains blood flow between the two atria. Blood flow across the foramen

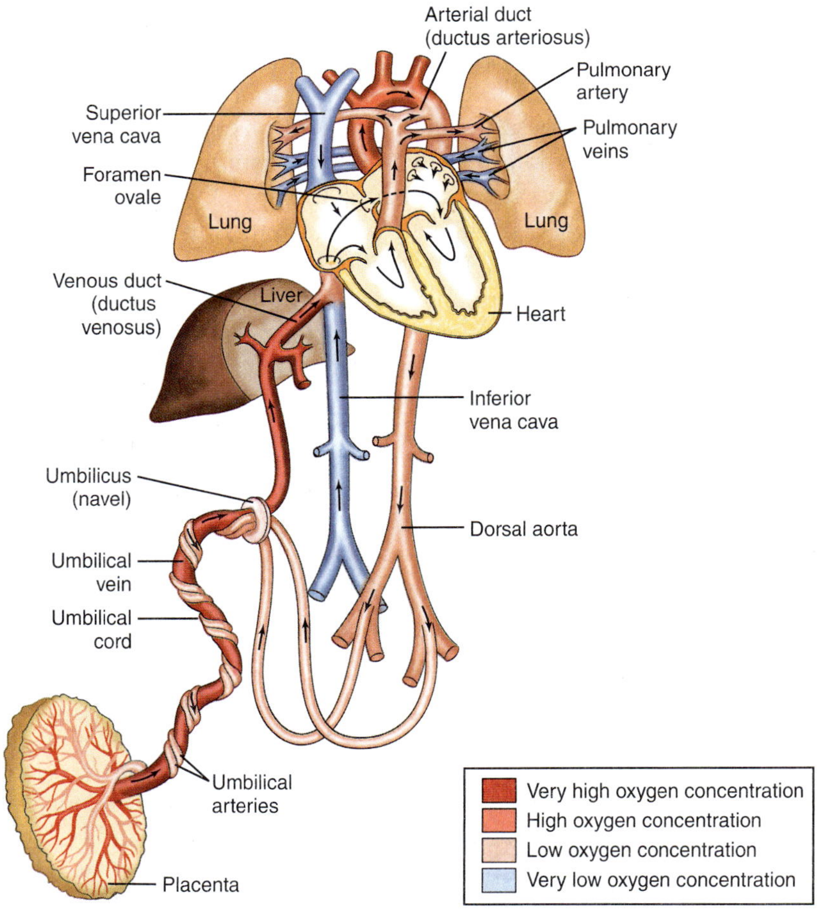

Figure 16-8 General pattern of fetal circulation.

ovale is controlled by a flap of atrial tissue on the left atrial side of the septum that covers (overlaps) the opening in the foramen ovale. The flap functions as a one-way valve allowing blood to flow from the right atrium into the left atrium only. The right-to-left flow is determined by pressure differences between the two chambers. In the fetus, the blood pressure is higher in the right atrium than in the left atrium because only a relatively small volume of blood flows through the lungs. Most is directed into the aorta through the ductus arteriosus. After birth, the left atrial pressure rises when the lungs expand, allowing a large volume of blood to flow through the lungs and into the left atrium. The higher left atrial pressure presses the flap valve against the left atrial surface of the septum, closing the communication between the atria. Usually, the tissue flap fuses with the atrial septum to form a solid partition between the two atria. Sometimes, the fusion is incomplete.

Pathogenesis and Manifestations of Congenital Heart Disease. Sometimes the heart fails to develop normally. Partitions between cardiac chambers may be defective, the cardiac valves may be malformed, or the large vessels entering and leaving the heart may not communicate appropriately with the atrium or ventricle. Some viral infections, such as rubella (German measles), as well as other maternal illnesses during the early phases of pregnancy, may cause improper development of the heart as well as other organs. Some chromosomal abnormalities, such as **Down syndrome** (**trisomy** 21), can result in abnormal cardiac development (**Figure 16-9**). Often the reason for a cardiac abnormality is unknown.

Down syndrome Condition resulting from trisomy for chromosome 21.

Trisomy The presence of an extra chromosome within a cell; having three of a given chromosome instead of the usual pair.

The effects of cardiac structural abnormalities depend on the nature of the defects and how blood circulation becomes disrupted. Many people with congenital heart abnormalities present with a heart murmur caused by turbulence of flowing blood within the heart, secondary to some cardiac malformation.

When fetal shunting mechanisms remain open after birth, blood from the left heart (system circulation) mixes with blood from the right heart (pulmonary circulation). The amount of blood shunted depends on the size of the septal defect, and the direction of the shunt depends on the blood pressure difference between the chambers. A small defect shunts very little blood and has no significant effect on cardiovascular function. A large septal defect can shunt a significant volume of blood, which puts an additional burden on the right ventricle, overfilling it by the shunted blood. The larger volume of blood pumped into the lungs raises the pulmonary blood pressure, eventually damaging the lungs by triggering thickening and narrowing of the pulmonary blood vessels. As the pulmonary vascular damage progresses and the pulmonary artery pressure continues to rise, the right ventricle must overcome the increasing resistance to blood flow through the lungs. The higher right ventricular pressure also causes the right atrial pressure to rise, reducing the pressure differences between the left and right atria. Consequently, the amount of blood shunted from the left to the right atrium also falls. Little or no blood shunting occurs when left and right atrial pressures equalize. If the right atrial pressure exceeds left atrial pressure, blood moves between the atria in the opposite direction, resulting in deoxygenated blood entering the circulation (a right-to-left shunt). This is termed Eisenmenger syndrome and has serious consequences. Right-to-left shunts mix poorly oxygenated blood from the right cardiac chambers with normally oxygenated blood contained in the left cardiac chambers, which reduces the oxygen content of the blood pumped by the left ventricle to supply the body. The affected person's activities usually become severely restricted due to the low oxygen content of the arterial blood.

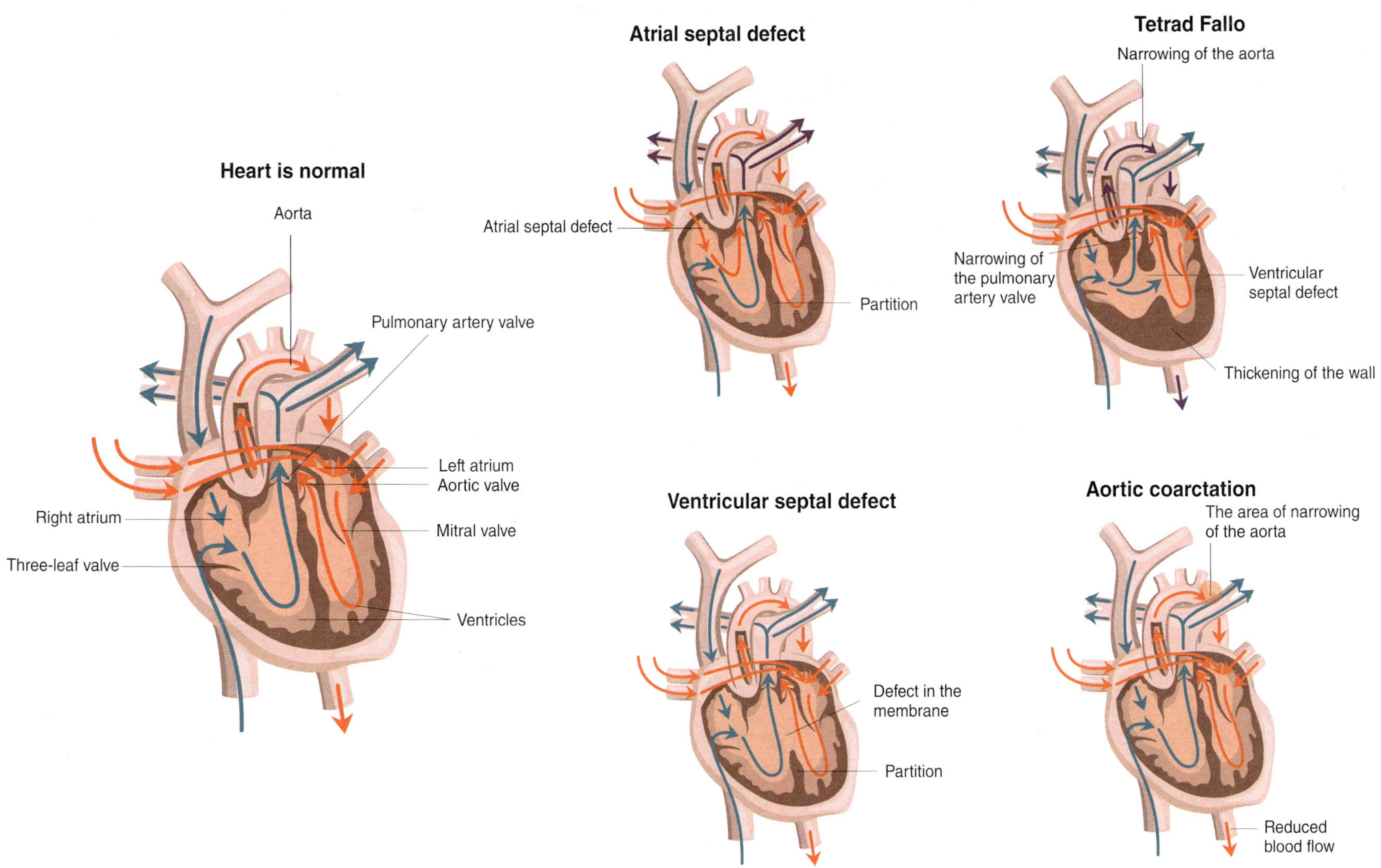

Figure 16-9 Forms of congenital heart disease. Congenital heart disease can be manifested in many different forms. This figure illustrates normal heart development with the abnormalities that could arise.

When the oxygen saturation of the arterial blood becomes low, the skin and mucous membranes acquire a blue color termed cyanosis. Congenital cardiovascular abnormalities associated with cyanosis are grouped together under the general term cyanotic congenital heart disease.

Common Cardiovascular Abnormalities

The more common and important cardiovascular abnormalities fall into four major groups: failure of the normal fetal bypass channels to close; defects in the formation of the atrial and ventral septa; abnormalities that obstruct blood flow through the heart, pulmonary artery, or aorta; and malformations of the aorta and pulmonary artery or abnormal connection of the arteries to the appropriate ventricles.

Patent Ductus Arteriosus. Normally the ductus closes spontaneously soon after birth in full-term infants, in part due to falling levels of prostaglandins. A large open patent ductus shunts blood from the aorta into the pulmonary artery and causes the same clinical manifestations and complications as an intracardiac left-to-right shunt. Treatment includes the use of prostaglandin synthesis inhibitors (such as indomethacin) or, if necessary, surgical closure of the ductus.

Atrial and Ventricular Septal Defects. Usually, an atrial septal defect results from defective development of the partitions that divide the atria with the defect located in the middle of the septum at the site usually occupied by the foramen ovale. Small defects in children often close spontaneously and are often asymptomatic. Larger defects should be closed, which usually can be accomplished using a device inserted into the heart through a peripheral vein. Sometimes an open surgical procedure is required to place a patch over the defect.

A common type of atrial septal defect is patent foramen ovale. The foramen ovale normally becomes nonfunctional after birth, caused by the rapid postdelivery changes in atrial pressures. In newborn infants, the foramen ovale may remain patent and functional in infants with congenital cardiac abnormalities associated with a high right atrial pressure, forcing right-to-left blood flow through the foramen ovale. In about 25 percent of adults, the flap valve does not fuse completely, but the foramen ovale remains nonfunctional as long as the left atrial pressure remains higher than the right atrial pressure.

Ventricular septal defects are also very common. Many are less than three mm in diameter and often close spontaneously, but larger defects require surgical closure. Generally, all large septal defects need to be closed. Atrial septal defects are often corrected by endoscopic procedures using cardiac catheterization, obviating the need for open heart surgery. Ventricular defects can also sometimes be repaired using this technique.

Pulmonary or Aortic Valve Stenosis Caused by Semilunar Valve Maldevelopment. Abnormal development of the semilunar valve leaflets narrows the valve opening, which can vary from 2 to 10 mm in diameter. The degree of obstruction depends on the diameter of the orifice. Pulmonary stenosis obstructs outflow from the right ventricle, and aortic stenosis impedes outflow from the left ventricle. Treatment consists of dilating the valve opening by inserting a balloon-like device into the narrow opening.

Coarctation of the Aorta. Coarctation is a Latin word meaning "narrowing" that describes a localized narrowing of the proximal aorta restricting blood flow into the distal aorta. Usually, the constriction is located distal to the origin of the large arteries arising from the arch of the aorta. The blood pressure in the aorta and its branches proximal to the coarctation is much higher than normal because of the increased resistance created by the narrowed section of the aorta, potentially leading to left ventricular disease. The pressure and volume of blood flowing into the aorta distal to the coarctation are both lower than normal, and collateral circulation develops to bypass the obstruction. An individual with a coarctation may appear normal except for high blood pressure identified when measuring pressure in the brachial arteries but lower-than-normal blood pressure in the arteries of the lower extremities. Usually, the narrowed segment of aorta is relatively short and can be treated by resecting the constricting segment and reconnecting the aorta so that its caliber is normal throughout its entire length. Alternatively, in balloon angioplasty, an intravascular device is used to dilate the aortic constriction, and a stent is inserted to maintain the diameter of the aorta.

The Tetralogy of Fallot and Transposition of the Great Arteries. Both conditions result from abnormal division of a single channel termed the truncus arteriosus, which extends from the developing ventricles and will be divided by a partition to form the aorta and the pulmonary artery. The partition takes a spiral course as it divides the truncus arteriosus, which is why the aorta and the pulmonary artery spiral around each other as they attach to their respective ventricles. The two abnormalities caused by abnormal division of the truncus arteriosus are relatively common, and both cause intermixing of deoxygenated blood with oxygenated blood, leading to marked cyanosis and related problems.

The tetralogy of Fallot results when the dividing septum in the truncus is misplaced and divides unequally. The results become the hallmark abnormalities that define the tetralogy of Fallot: ventricular septal defect, pulmonary stenosis, an enlarged aorta that overrides the septal defect, and right ventricular hypertrophy developing as a consequence of pulmonary stenosis. In this condition, poorly oxygenated blood in the right ventricle flows through the septal defect to mix with blood from the left ventricle flowing into the aorta. Treatment consists of enlarging the opening of the narrowed pulmonary artery and closing the septal defect.

Transposition of the great arteries results if the septum that divides the truncus arteriosus does not follow its normal spiral course when it divides the truncus into the aorta and pulmonary artery. Consequently, the aorta and pulmonary artery develop parallel to each other instead of spiraling around each other. The aorta becomes located to the right of the pulmonary artery instead of behind and to the left of the pulmonary artery. The aorta becomes connected to the right ventricle, and the pulmonary artery attaches to the left ventricle, severely disrupting blood flow in both the pulmonary and systemic circulations.

Consequently, poorly oxygenated blood enters into systemic circulation and the flow of oxygenated blood remains confined to the pulmonary circuit, where it serves no useful purpose. After birth, the condition is not compatible with life unless there is a communication that permits some intermixing of blood between the pulmonary and systemic circulations, such as a patent foramen ovale, atrial septal defect, or ventricular septal defect. Generally, such communications do not provide enough oxygenated blood to supply the infant's needs.

The current treatment of this condition is termed the arterial switch operation; the aorta is connected to the left ventricle, and the pulmonary artery is attached to

Table 16-3 Features of Common Congenital Cardiovascular Abnormalities

Abnormality	Physiologic Disturbance	Complications	Treatment
Patent ductus arteriosus	Aorta to pulmonary artery shunt	Pulmonary hypertension	Ligate or excise ductus
Patent foramen ovale	Right-to-left atrial shunt	Usually nonfunctional as long as left atrial pressure exceeds right atrial pressure	Usually no treatment required
Atrial, ventricular, and combined septal defects	Left-to-right shunt	Pulmonary hypertension damages lungs. Right ventricular hypertrophy	Close defect
Pulmonary stenosis	Obstructed outflow from right ventricle	Right ventricular hypertrophy	Dilate narrowed valve opening
Aortic stenosis	Obstructed outflow from left ventricle	Left ventricular hypertrophy	Dilate narrowed valve opening
Aortic coarctation	Obstructed flow into aorta distal to coarctation	Hypertension in arteries supplying head and upper limbs	Excise coarctation and reconnect aorta
Tetralogy of Fallot	Right-to-left shunt Ventricular septal defect straddled by enlarged aorta Pulmonary stenosis Right ventricular hypertrophy	Cyanosis Polycythemia Clubbing of fingers and toes	Enlarge pulmonary artery opening Close septal defect
Transposition of great arteries	Aorta attached to right ventricle and pulmonary artery attached to left ventricle	Only communication between systemic and pulmonary circulations is through ductus arteriosus and foramen ovale	Reattach aorta and pulmonary artery to proper ventricles Reposition coronary arteries

the right ventricle. It is also necessary to reposition the coronary arteries so they are connected properly to the artery supplying blood to the left ventricle.

Table 16-3 summarizes the principal features of the congenital cardiovascular malformations described in this section.

Congenital Hydrocephalus

Congenital hydrocephalus, usually caused by a congenital abnormality in the ventricular system, is most commonly either a congenital obstruction, an abnormal formation of the cerebral aqueduct of Sylvius (the narrow channel connecting the third and fourth ventricles), or failure of the openings in the roof and lateral walls of the fourth ventricle to form normally; the obstruction blocks escape of cerebrospinal fluid into the subarachnoid space. An aqueduct obstruction leads to distention of the lateral and third ventricles. An obstruction of the outlet channels in the fourth ventricle leads to distention of all four ventricles.

A complex congenital condition termed the **Arnold-Chiari malformation** results in spinal cord defects (including **meningomyelocele**) and compression of the brain stem and cerebellum downward, sometimes causing a kinking of the lower medulla. The structural defect leads to stenosis of the aqueduct and hydrocephalus. Because in congenital defects the distention can develop before the skull bones have fused, the head may enlarge greatly; the brain undergoes pronounced atrophy secondary to compression by the dilated ventricles. If

Arnold-Chiari malformation Congenital condition with spinal cord defects and compression of the brain stem and cerebellum downward.

Meningomyelocele A type of spina bifida characterized by protrusion of meninges and cord through the defect in the vertebral arches.

hydrocephalus develops in the fetus prior to birth, the head may become so large that it is unable to enter the maternal pelvis during labor. More often, the hydrocephalus develops insidiously after birth, depending on the severity of the defect.

Respiratory Distress Syndrome of Newborn Infants

Respiratory distress syndrome of newborn infants is characterized by progressive respiratory distress that occurs soon after birth, leading to serious problems in oxygenation of the blood. This condition occurs most often in preterm infants, infants delivered by cesarean section, and infants born to mothers with diabetes. The basic cause is an inadequate production of surfactant in the lungs. As a result, the alveoli do not expand normally during inspiration and tend to collapse during expiration. The permeability of the pulmonary capillaries also is increased, and fluid leaks from the pulmonary capillaries into the air passages. The fluid, which is rich in fibrinogen, tends to clot and form adherent membranes that line the air passages. These membranes contribute to respiratory distress by impeding the diffusion of gases between the air passages and the pulmonary capillaries. These prominent acellular red-staining membranes lining the alveoli became the basis for the older name given to this condition, hyaline membrane disease (**Figure 16-10**).

When delivery of a preterm infant with immature lungs is necessary due to medical reasons, administering adrenal corticosteroid hormones to the mother prior to anticipated delivery will stimulate increased production of surfactant by the fetal lungs, thereby reducing the risk of respiratory distress syndrome. Infants who have developed respiratory distress syndrome after delivery are treated with supplementary oxygen and instillation of a

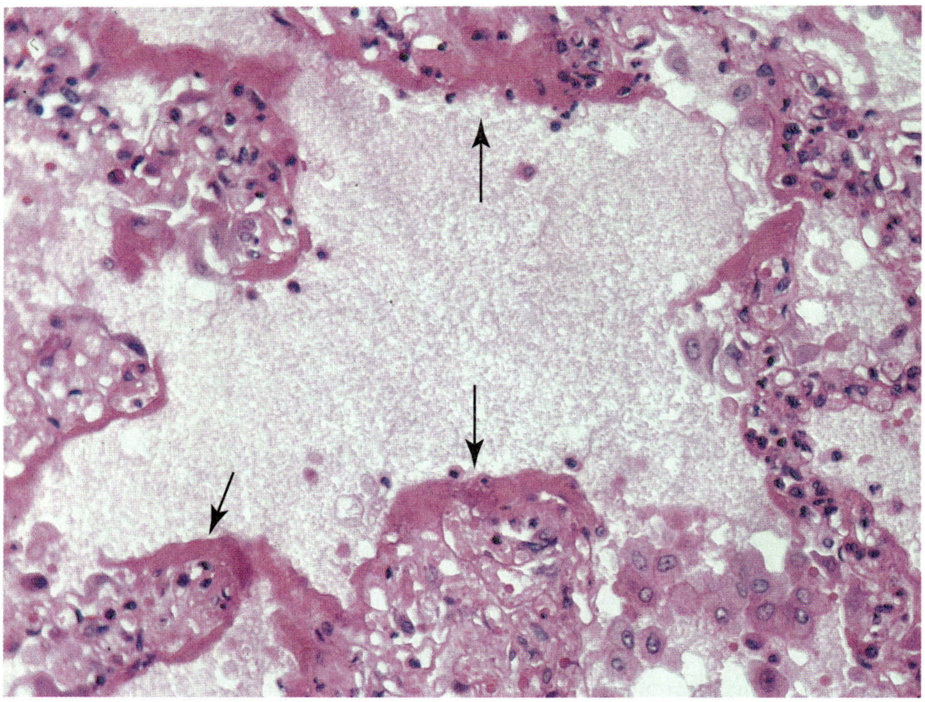

Figure 16-10 Neonatal respiratory distress syndrome. Eosinophilic hyaline membranes (*arrows*) composed of coagulated protein cover alveolar septa, impeding gas exchange between alveoli and pulmonary capillaries.

Courtesy of Leonard V. Crowley, MD, Century College.

Table 16-4 Comparison of Neonatal and Adult Respiratory Distress Syndrome

	Neonatal	Adult
Groups affected	Premature infants Delivery by cesarean section* Infant born to diabetic mother**	Adults who have sustained direct or indirect lung damage
Pathogenesis	Inadequate surfactant	Direct damage: Lung trauma, aspiration, irritant or toxic gases Indirect damage: Reduced pulmonary blood flow caused by shock or sepsis Associated condition: Surfactant production reduced
Treatment	Corticosteroids to mother before delivery Endotracheal surfactant Oxygen	Support circulation and respiration Endotracheal tube and respirator Positive pressure oxygen

*Labor increases surfactant synthesis, which may not have occurred in cesarean delivery.
**High-insulin blood level in the fetus of a mother with diabetes suppresses surfactant.

surfactant-type material that resembles natural surfactant. The material is instilled by means of a tube inserted into the infant's trachea (endotracheal tube), and the surfactant treatments are continued for several days after delivery. **Table 16-4** compares respiratory distress syndrome in infants with a somewhat similar condition in adults, which has a different pathogenesis and method of treatment, although the histologic changes in both conditions are quite similar (see also Chapter 13).

Developmental Disturbances of the Urinary System

The urinary system develops from several different components. The kidneys form from masses of primitive connective tissue (mesoderm) located along the back-body wall of the embryo. The bladder develops as an offshoot of the lower end of the intestinal tract. The ureters, renal pelves, renal collecting tubules, and renal calyces (the urinary drainage system) derive from paired tubular structures termed ureteric buds. Each bud grows upward from the developing bladder and connects with the kidney that is forming on the corresponding side. The kidneys begin their development within the pelvis. Later, as the embryo grows, the kidneys and their excretory ducts occupy a higher location until eventually they ascend to reach their final positions in the upper lumbar region (**Figure 16-11A**).

Sometimes this developmental process is disturbed, and congenital malformations result. Three of the more common developmental abnormalities are failure of one or both kidneys to develop (renal agenesis), formation of extra ureters and renal pelves, or malpositioning of one or both kidneys. Renal agenesis (a = without + genesis = formation) may affect one or both kidneys, but bilateral renal agenesis is uncommon. Bilateral agenesis, which often accompanies other congenital malformations, is incompatible with postnatal life. In contrast, unilateral renal agenesis (**Figure 16-11B**) is a relatively common condition with an incidence of about 1 in 1000, about the same frequency as cleft palate. When one kidney is absent, the other kidney enlarges and can

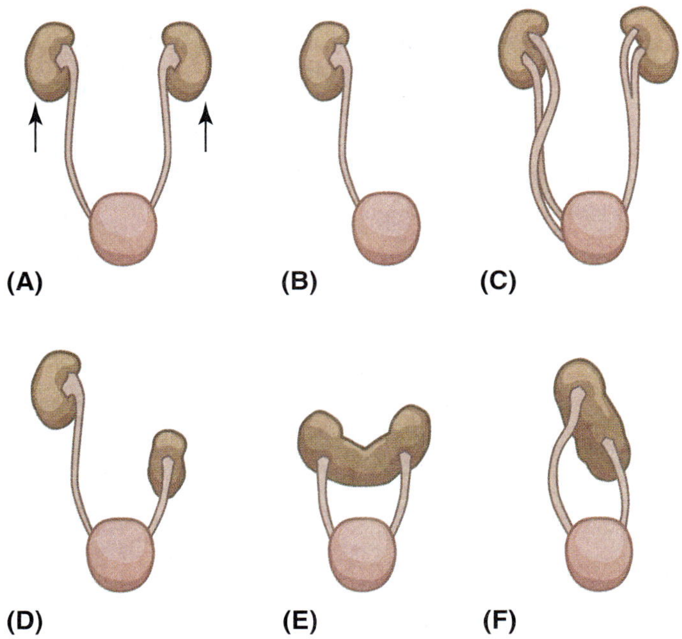

Figure 16-11 Common congenital abnormalities of kidneys and urinary tract. **(A)** Normal ascent of kidneys. **(B)** Unilateral renal agenesis. **(C)** Various types of duplications of ureters and renal pelves resulting from formation of an extra ureteric bud (*left*) or premature splitting of a single ureteric bud (*right*). **(D)** Failure of one kidney to ascend to normal position. **(E)** Horseshoe kidney resulting from fusion of lower poles of kidneys. **(F)** Fusion of the lower pole of one kidney to the upper pole of the opposite kidney, which has failed to ascend normally.

carry out the functions of the missing kidney. The recognition of this condition, however, is of great importance to the clinician who is treating an individual with kidney disease because one can never assume that the patient has two kidneys. Before a surgeon performs a kidney operation, diagnostic studies must be performed to ascertain that the patient has two kidneys. In addition to renal agenesis, various degrees of renal dysplasia result in abnormal structural development of renal tubules, ducts, and glomeruli. These may be genetically related or result from defects in renal differentiation.

Duplications of the urinary tract may be unilateral or bilateral. Sometimes a kidney has an extra renal pelvis and ureter that drains separately into the bladder (complete duplication). Sometimes double ureters draining the kidney unite to form a single ureter just before entering the bladder (partial duplication). Duplications result from abnormal prenatal development of the ureteric buds. A complete duplication results when an extra ureteric bud develops and gives rise to a separate excretory system draining the kidney on the affected side. If the ureteric bud branches after it has formed, only the upper part of the excretory system is duplicated; the lower part of the ureter is not duplicated and enters the bladder normally (**Figure 16-11C**).

Abnormalities of position and fusion of the kidneys may occur if both kidneys remain in the pelvis where they begin their development or if they ascend only part of the way (**Figure 16-11D**). Kidneys that fail to ascend normally are in very close approximation as they develop and may become fused. One of the more common fusion abnormalities is a union of the lower poles of the two kidneys to form a U-shaped mass of renal tissue termed a horseshoe kidney (**Figure 16-11E**). In other cases, when the kidneys ascend abnormally, the upper pole of one kidney may become fused to the lower pole of the other (**Figure 16-11F**).

Renal duplications, malpositioning, and fusions often are of little clinical significance. At times, however, drainage of urine may be impeded by the abnormalities, causing the urine to stagnate and predisposing the patient to urinary infections.

There are a number of inherited renal diseases which result in cystic disease. **Autosomal dominant polycystic kidney disease** is the most common in which the kidney is characterized by a large number of cysts varying in size. In affected individuals, cysts may also occur in the liver, and abnormalities in cerebral vasculature may result in intracranial hemorrhage and death. The disease is characterized by hypertension and often is not recognized until the patient is an adult. Mutations in either of two genes (PKD1 and PKD2) are responsible. There are several additional congenital cystic diseases, including a recessive form (autosomal recessive polycystic kidney disease) in which about 25% of those affected die in utero or show the early onset of progressive renal failure.

Autosomal dominant polycystic kidney disease Autosomal dominant disease characterized by the formation of multiple cysts throughout both kidneys.

Congenital Disorders of the Urethra

Obstructions to the lower urinary tract are common developmental abnormalities in neonatal males. Posterior urethral valves (PUV) are the most frequent obstruction, occurring in about 1 in 8000 male births. The defect occurs when an embryological structure that normally recedes during male development leaves a remnant in the prostatic urethra, termed the verumontanum, which then partially or completely blocks the fetal urethra. The consequence of this can be failure of normal development of the fetal kidney. Early detection and repair via cystoscopy is indicated. Severe cases may lead to total renal dysplasia, failure of pulmonary development (dependent on fetal renal function, Potter sequence), and death in utero or shortly after birth.

Male Reproductive System

Abnormalities of Sexual Differentiation

Abnormalities of sexual differentiation occur at several levels. Chromosomal abnormalities (discussed in Chapter 3) impact with varying degrees on sexual differentiation and fertility. A number of very uncommon single gene defects can result in forms of male pseudohermaphroditism. Individuals having XY chromosomes but with defects in the androgen receptor gene do not respond to male hormones (androgens) during development and have external female genitalia or a mixture of male and female genitalia. Internal sex organs are male but may show abnormalities, and individuals most often are infertile. Severe forms of the disease have occasionally resulted in such individuals being raised as females.

The previously mentioned cases of androgen insensitivity raise the issue of development and sexual differentiation's role in establishing psychosocial sexual orientation. Similar to those conditions termed neurodivergent, defining normal sexual behavior is controversial and fraught. Transgendered individuals have no known abnormality in reproductive development, (i.e., sex chromosomes or anatomic development) although some transgendered individuals may attempt to alter their appearance chemically or surgically. The variables that inform gendered behavior in relation to genetic and anatomic development (broadly speaking, "sex") remain obscure.

Congenital Disorders of Penile Development

Hypospadias (**Figure 16-12**), a congenital abnormality of penile development, occurs when the urethral opening is located on the ventral side of the penis rather than at the tip of the glans. The abnormal location of the urethra may occur near the tip (leading to an abnormal urethral meatus) or further down the shaft (more proximal) near the scrotum. The defect results from abnormal fusion of the genital folds, which occurs during the 12th to 16th week of gestation. At the time they form the shaft of the penis and labioscrotal folds, which fuse to form the scrotum. In epispadias the urethral meatus is on the dorsal (upper) side of the penis, or the entire length of the penile urethra may be open. The condition is most often associated with serious malformations of the bladder (exstrophy, eversion of part of the bladder onto the abdominal wall).

Phimosis, the inability to retract the prepuce (foreskin) over the glans of the penis, is a physiologic condition that normally occurs in newborn males. The condition is the result of adhesion between the epithelium of the foreskin and the glans and usually disappears with continued retraction and erection. The condition may persist in a small percentage of males over the age of 16 and occasionally requires corrective surgery, usually circumcision. Infection of the prepuce and head of the penis (balanitis) can also result in a secondary form of phimosis.

Cryptorchidism

Cryptorchidism (crypto = hidden + orchis = testis), failure of one or both testes to descend into the scrotum, occurs in about 5 percent of term infants at birth and persists through the first year in 20 percent of these infants (**Figure 16-13**). Most commonly, the undescended testes are located in the inguinal or upper scrotal region. Surgical repair of the condition (orchiopexy) is critical because the condition is associated with oligospermia (a low sperm count) if one testis is affected and complete lack of sperm (azoospermia) if both testes are undescended. Early repair (between 6 months and 1 year) is recommended. In addition to infertility, a 20- to 40-fold increase in the rate of testicular cancer is associated with cryptorchidism. Surprisingly,

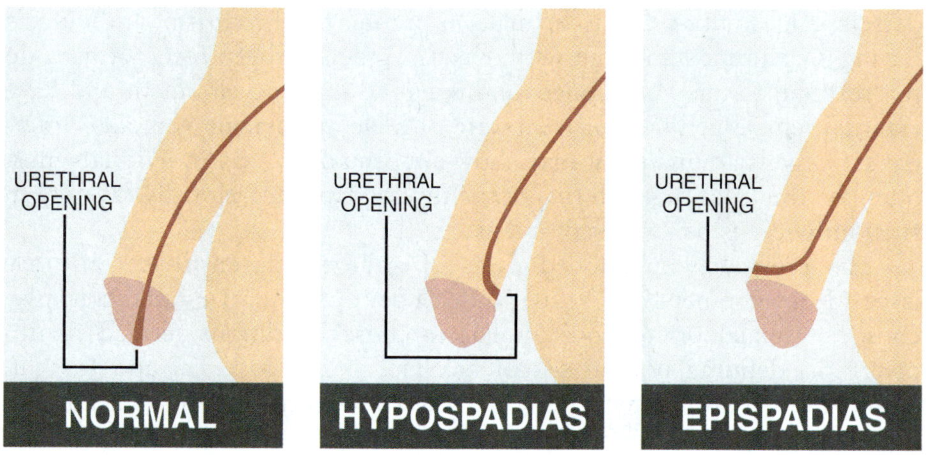

Figure 16-12 Penile congenital anomalies. The placement of the urethral opening leads to abnormal penile development.

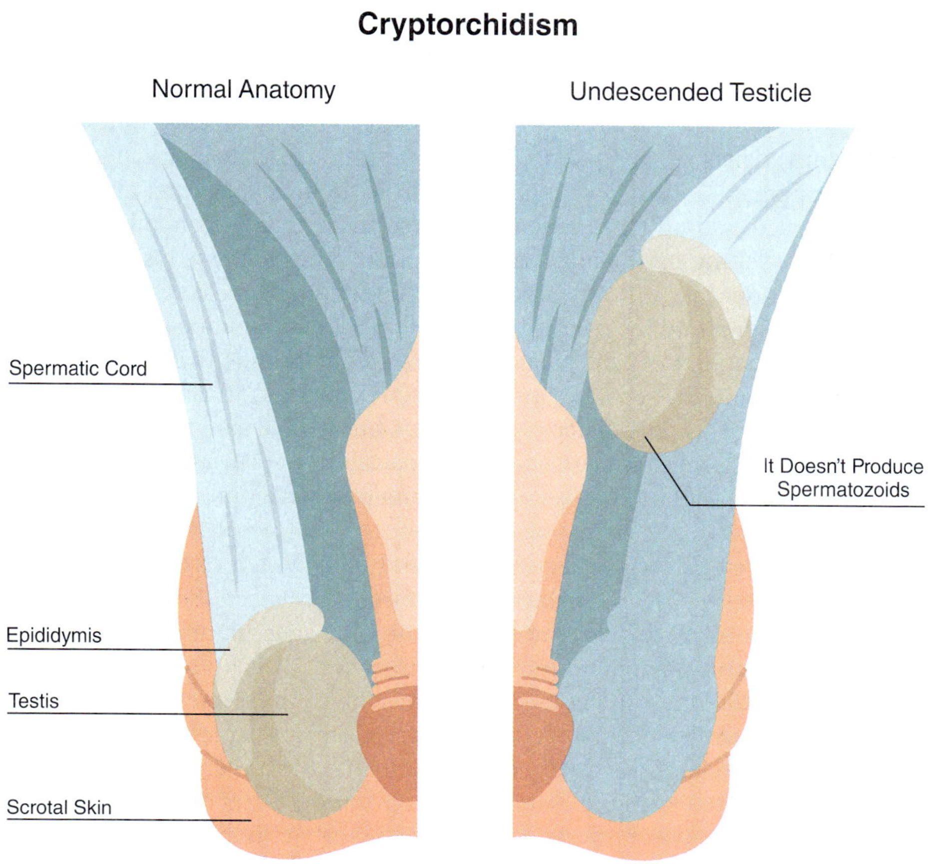

Figure 16-13 Cryptorchidism.

in males where the other testis descended normally, a fourfold increased risk of testicular cancer occurs. Early surgical repair reduces but does not remove the risk of developing cancer later in life.

Abnormalities of the Oral Cavity

Cleft Lip and Cleft Palate

Embryologically, the face and palate are formed by the coalescence of masses of cells that merge to form the facial structures and to separate the nasal cavity from the mouth. In the upper part of the face, the areas of coalescence are located on either side of the midline, a line that passes through the upper lip and jaw and extends into each nostril. The palate is formed by two shelf-like masses of tissue that grow medially and fuse in the midline to close the communication between nose and mouth. If these developmental processes are disturbed, defects may result in the upper lip and jaw (cleft lip) or in the palate (cleft palate).

Cleft lip and cleft palate are common abnormalities that frequently occur in combination. The incidence of these abnormalities is about 1 per 700 births. Both cleft lip and cleft palate follow a **multifactorial pattern of inheritance**. Cleft lip with or without cleft palate and cleft palate alone have different epidemiology and risk factors. The incidence of cleft lip with or without cleft palate is much higher among the children of parents who previously gave birth

Multifactorial pattern of inheritance Transmission of a trait, condition, or congenital anomaly that involves the likely interaction of multiple gene loci as well as probable environmental interactions. The inheritance pattern does not follow Mendelian genetic patterns.

to an infant with cleft lip (but not one with only a cleft palate). The incidence of cleft palate is higher among parents who themselves have a cleft palate (but not with a cleft lip or cleft lip and palate).

Cleft lip may be unilateral or bilateral and range in severity from a relatively minor defect in the mucosa of the lip to a large cleft extending deeply into the upper jaw. Even very minor defects in the muscular ring around the oral cavity detected only on radiography present an increased familial risk for more severe clefting. In the most severe deformity, the cleft extends completely through the upper jaw into the floor of the nose (complete cleft) and may also extend posteriorly into the palate. Large bilateral clefts extending into the palate completely separate the hard palate from the midline tissue that forms part of the upper jaw, and the separated tissue is often displaced forward. Midline cleft palate may occur as an isolated abnormality, but it is usually associated with unilateral or bilateral cleft lip. Cleft lip and palate may occur as isolated defects or, much less frequently, as part of developmental syndromes associated with other defects.

There are several potential risks to a child born with a cleft. Aspiration of milk may occur because of an abnormal connection between the oral and nasal cavity. Airway obstruction may occur because of tongue placement, and feeding difficulties and regurgitation are likely to occur. Cleft lip usually does not cause major difficulties in feeding but might with more severe clefts. Cleft lip and palate frequently occur together but are corrected surgically at different times. Generally, cleft lip is repaired very soon after birth. Repair of cleft palate is generally deferred until the child is between 1 and 2 years old. After the cleft palate is repaired, speech therapy will begin in early childhood to correct the nasal quality that often results from abnormal palatal function.

Abnormalities of Tooth Development

The teeth are specialized structures developed in the tissues of the jaws. Each tooth consists of a solid portion dentine, which forms the bulk of the tooth; an enamel crown covering the exposed surface of the tooth; and a central pulp cavity containing nerve fibers, lymphatics, and blood vessels. The root of the tooth, which is embedded in the jaw, is covered by a thin layer of bonelike tissue cementum, and the tooth is anchored in the jaw by dense connective tissue fibers. There are two sets of teeth. The first set, the temporary or deciduous teeth, consists of a total of 20 teeth (10 in each jaw) that erupt in childhood. Hyperdontia, extra teeth, sometimes occurs. Eventually, the temporary teeth are replaced by a second, permanent set of 32 teeth. When the permanent teeth begin to grow, they press against the roots of the temporary teeth. This causes resorption of the roots and loosening of the temporary teeth, which eventually fall out and are replaced by permanent teeth.

Each deciduous and permanent tooth develops from a separate tooth bud. Development of the tooth requires the interaction of the odontoblasts, the mesenchymal-derived cells that form the dentin, and the epithelial-derived ameloblasts that form the tooth enamel. Calcium is deposited in the dentine and enamel of the tooth as it is being formed. The deciduous teeth are formed before birth and erupt during childhood. The permanent teeth do not begin to develop until after birth and erupt at various times in late childhood and adolescence.

The absence of one or more teeth is relatively common and is often a familial trait that follows a multifactorial pattern of inheritance resulting from the failure of one or more tooth buds to develop. Sometimes, as noted, an extra tooth bud forms, resulting in an extra tooth. Enamel forms within the developing teeth at specific times. If the antibiotic tetracycline is administered while enamel is being formed in the teeth, the antibiotic is deposited with calcium in the enamel and causes permanent yellow-gray to brown discoloration in the crowns and may disturb enamel formation. Therefore, tetracycline (and similar antibiotics such as doxycycline) should not be given to pregnant women or to infants and children up to about the age of 8 years. Excess fluoride ingestion, as might occur by concurrent use of fluoridated water and excess use of fluoridated dental products during tooth development, can result in tooth discoloration (fluorosis), a cosmetic problem.

Congenital Disorders of the Small and Large Intestine

Meckel Diverticulum

A number of congenital disorders of the small intestine may occur. These include atresia and stenosis (complete and partial blockage of the lumen, respectively). The most common is Meckel diverticulum, an abnormal retention of the vitelline duct (vitellus = yolk) that connects the yolk sac to the developing embryo during embryogenesis. Normally, the duct disappears prior to birth, and no trace persists. In about 2 percent of people, however, a remnant termed the Meckel diverticulum remains as a small tubular outpouching from the distal ileum (**Figure 16-14**). Most Meckel diverticula are asymptomatic, but sometimes the diverticulum becomes infected, causing the same symptoms and complications as an acute appendicitis. If a Meckel diverticulum contains misplaced (ectopic) gastric mucosa, the acidic "gastric juice" secreted by the diverticulum may cause a peptic ulcer of the diverticulum, which is at times complicated by bleeding or perforation. Hence, the surgeon searches for a Meckel diverticulum in cases of suspected appendicitis or other abdominal surgery.

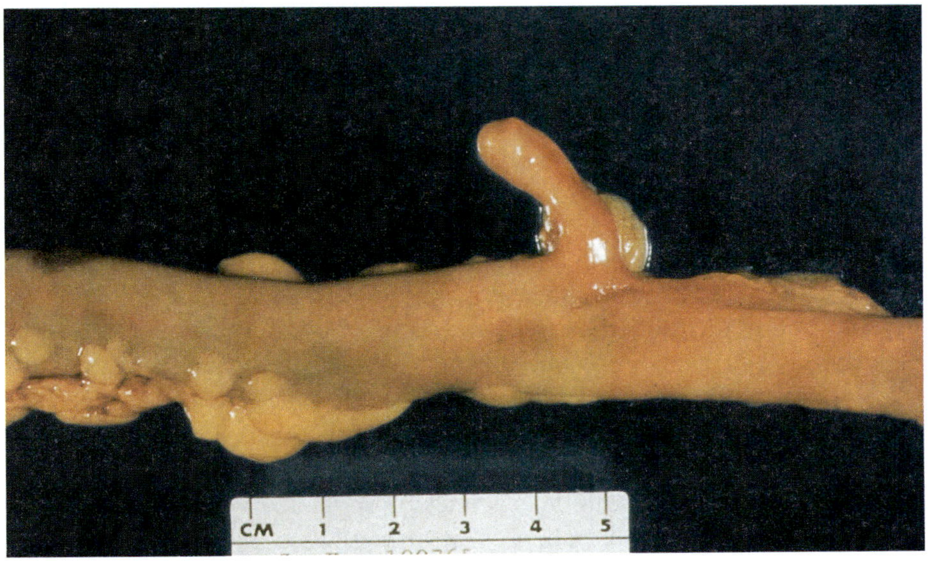

Figure 16-14 Meckel diverticulum of ileum.

Courtesy of Leonard V. Crowley, MD, Century College.

Hirschsprung Disease

Hirschsprung disease is the most common cause of congenital intestinal obstruction, which, if severe, can require surgery. It often becomes apparent proximate to birth. It results from the absence of intestinal ganglion cells between the internal anal sphincter and extending a variable distance into the rectum and left colon. Most cases are sporadic, but some familial occurrences are linked to specific mutations.

Imperforate Anus

Imperforate anus is an uncommon congenital abnormality in which the colon fails to acquire a normal anal opening. It occurs in about 1 in 5000 live births. There are two major types. In one type, the rectum and anus are normally formed and extend to the level of the skin, but no anal orifice is present. Often a small tract (fistula) extends from the blind end of the anal canal to terminate in the urethra, in the vagina, or on the surface of the skin. Usually, this type of imperforate anus can be easily treated by excising the tissue covering the anal opening. In the second type of imperforate anus, the entire distal rectum fails to develop; this condition is often associated with abnormalities of the urogenital tract and skeletal system. Surgical repair of this type of abnormality is much more difficult, and results are less satisfactory.

Nervous System

Development of the Nervous System

In the embryo, the central nervous system first appears as a thickened band of surface cells (ectoderm), the neural plate. Its lateral margins become elevated to form neural folds, which fuse to form a hollow tube, the neural tube. Fusion begins in the middle of the developing tube in the area that will become the future hindbrain (next) and progresses toward both ends until a completely closed tube is formed by the fourth week of embryonic development. Three expansions, the forebrain, midbrain, and hindbrain, develop from one end of the neural tube. The other end remains narrow and becomes the spinal cord. The cerebral hemispheres develop as lateral outgrowths from the forebrain. The hindbrain forms the medulla and cerebellum.

Neural Tube Defects

Failure of either end of the neural tube to close properly leads to serious congenital malformations collectively termed neural tube defects (NTD) that involve the nervous system and the surrounding tissues as well. A closure defect involving the end of the tube destined to form the cerebral hemispheres (the cephalic end) leads to **anencephaly** (ana = without + encephalon = brain). If the opposite end of the tube (the caudal end) is involved, **spina bifida** results. A deficiency of folic acid during the early part of pregnancy when the neural tube is forming plays an important role in causing neural tube defects. The incidence of infants born with NTD decreased approximately 35 prcent since folic acid fortification was mandated in United States food manufacturing of cereals and grains. Using data from birth defects tracking systems, researchers found that since folic acid fortification, about 1300 babies are born each year without an NTD who might otherwise have been affected. Folic acid fortification is an important way to help prevent NTDs. Unfortunately, even with folic acid fortification, not all women of reproductive age are getting the recommended

Anencephaly A congenital malformation considered to be a neural tube defect where parts of the brain, cranium and scalp may be missing.

Spina bifida Incomplete closure of vertebral arches over the spinal cord, sometimes associated with protrusion of meninges and neural tissue through the defect (cystic spina bifida).

amount of folic acid. This puts them at risk for a pregnancy affected by an NTD. Additional public health interventions targeting these women could help reduce the number of babies born with an NTD each year. Hispanic women who have a somewhat elevated risk for NTDs have lower levels of folate in their blood compared to non-Hispanic White women. This may be explained by nutritional differences (folic acid fortification mandates do not include corn masa flour, which is a popular staple item in Hispanic and Latino cultures). The frequency of genetic variants of the *MTHFR* gene (MTHFR C677T in particular) involved in folate metabolism have also been suggested as playing a role.

Anencephaly

Anencephaly occurs most commonly in female infants. Because the cephalic end of the neural tube fails to close, the exposed neural tissue undergoes secondary degenerative changes that convert it into a mass of vascular connective tissue intermixed with masses of degenerated brain and choroid plexus. The anencephalic infant has a striking appearance. The brain is greatly reduced, as are the soft tissues of the scalp and the bones making up the vertex of the skull. The exposed base of the skull is covered only by a vascular membrane. The base of the cranial cavity is abnormally formed, and the orbits are shallow, causing the eyes to bulge outward and be fused and single. The trunk is short, the shoulders are broad, and the neck is not normal; the head arises directly from the trunk and cannot be flexed. As has been noted, anencephaly can be a severe consequence of Zika virus infection during pregnancy. Often the closure defect affects not only the brain but also the part of the neural tube that forms the upper part of the spinal cord. When this occurs, the vertebral arches are absent, as well as the vertex of the skull, and the unclosed spinal cord lies exposed within the wide-open spinal canal, a condition referred to as rachischisis.

Spina Bifida

Malformations of the caudal end of the neural tube and related vertebral arches are generally considered together as spina bifida, which literally means "split spine" and refers to the characteristic failure of fusion of the vertebral arches common to all types of spina bifida (**Figure 16-15**). Occult spina bifida refers to failure of fusion of vertebral arches in the lower lumbar region, which occurs as an isolated abnormality, but it produces no clinical symptoms. This condition is common and may occur in as much as 10 percent of the population, being discovered only after spine imaging for unrelated reasons. The more severe types of spina bifida are characterized by a saclike protrusion of meninges or both meninges and nerve tissue through the defect in the vertebral arches. The malformation is termed a meningocele if the protrusion consists only of meninges and is termed a meningomyelocele (myelo = cord) if parts of the spinal cord or nerve roots also are included in the sac.

In a meningomyelocele, there is often a severe neurologic deficit below the level of the sac because the nerve tissue is incorporated into the wall of the sac and is disorganized so that the conduction of nerve impulses is impaired or completely interrupted. In the most severe (and fortunately rare) form of spina bifida, the caudal end of the neural tube completely fails to close. The distal end of the spinal cord is represented by a flattened mass of nerve tissue that is continuous with the adjacent skin. The larger meningomyelocele sacs often are covered not by skin but merely by a thin, easily ruptured membrane composed only of meninges.

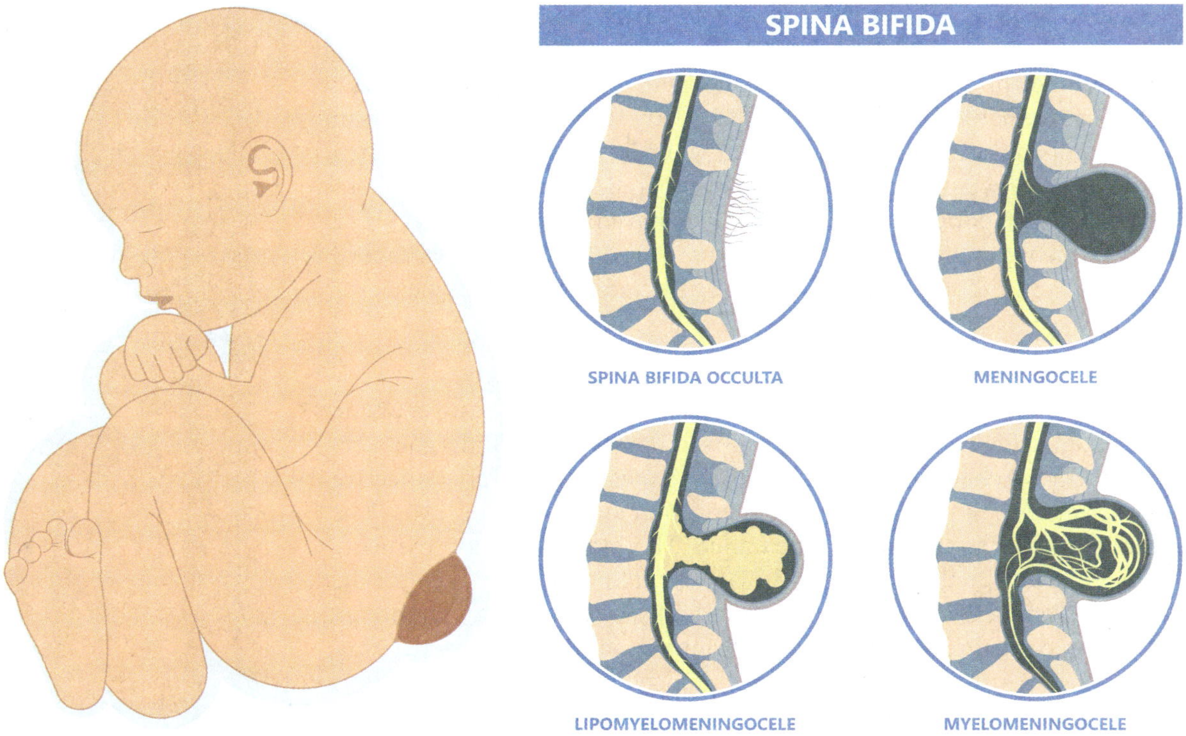

Figure 16-15 Spina bifida manifests in several different structural variations. This figure illustrates how each affects the spinal cord and related peripheral nerves.

Treatment of Spina Bifida

Occult spina bifida is asymptomatic, and no treatment is required. A meningocele usually can be repaired without difficulty with satisfactory results by excising the sac and closing the spinal dura because the meninges are the only component involved in the defect. Unfortunately, a large meningomyelocele is much more difficult to treat, with much less satisfactory results. The condition may be complicated by hydrocephalus. Because spinal cord and nerve roots are often incorporated in the sac, there is frequently some loss of sensation and motor power in the lower extremities. Bowel and bladder function also may be impaired, leading to stasis of urine in the bladder, predisposing to urinary tract infections.

Prenatal Detection of Neural Tube Defects

Alpha-fetoprotein (AFP) Protein produced by fetal liver early in gestation. Sometimes produced by tumor cells. Level is elevated in amnionic fluid when fetus has a neural tube defect resulting in abnormally high levels in the maternal serum.

Alpha-fetoprotein (AFP) levels in maternal blood can be elevated for many reasons, including twins or a multiple pregnancy. About 80 percent of the time, they are elevated if the fetus possesses an open neural tube defect such as anencephaly or spina bifida. AFP levels provide a reliable early screen for neural tube defects. Approximately 90% of neural tube defects can be detected through ultrasound imaging of the developing fetus between 18 and 20 weeks' gestation.

Hydrocephalus

Cerebrospinal Fluid Circulation

The brain contains four ventricles, which are filled with cerebrospinal fluid (CSF). The fluid serves as a protective cushion around the brain and spinal cord. The fluid, secreted by the choroid plexuses of the ventricles, flows from the lateral ventricles into the third ventricle, through the cerebral aqueduct (aqueduct of Sylvius) into the fourth ventricle, and then out into the subarachnoid space through three small openings in the roof of the fourth ventricle. The fluid circulates around the cord and over the convexity of the brain and is resorbed into the large venous sinuses in the dura mater. Secretion of cerebrospinal fluid continues even if the flow of fluid through the ventricular system is blocked. Obstruction to the normal circulation of spinal fluid distends the ventricles proximal to the site of obstruction, with associated compression atrophy of brain tissue around the dilated ventricles. When blockage occurs within the ventricular system, the condition is termed obstructive (or noncommunicating) hydrocephalus, which may be congenital or acquired. Hydrocephalus can result from blockage of the cerebral aqueduct of Sylvius and cause CSF to build up, thinning the cortex and causing severe brain damage.

Congenital Hydrocephalus

Congenital hydrocephalus, usually caused by a congenital abnormality in the ventricular system, is most commonly either a congenital obstruction, an abnormal formation of the cerebral aqueduct of Sylvius (the narrow channel connecting the third and fourth ventricles), or failure of the openings in the roof and lateral walls of the fourth ventricle to form normally; the obstruction blocks escape of cerebrospinal fluid into the subarachnoid space. An aqueduct obstruction leads to distention of the lateral and third ventricles. An obstruction of the outlet channels in the fourth ventricle leads to distention of all four ventricles. A complex congenital condition termed the Arnold-Chiari malformation results in spinal cord defects (including meningomyelocele) and compression of the brain stem and cerebellum downward, sometimes causing a kinking of the lower medulla. The structural defect leads to stenosis of the aqueduct and hydrocephalus. Because in congenital defects the distention can develop before the skull bones have fused, the head may enlarge greatly; the brain undergoes pronounced atrophy secondary to compression by the dilated ventricles. If hydrocephalus develops in the fetus prior to birth, the head may become so large that it is unable to enter the maternal pelvis during labor. More often, the hydrocephalus develops insidiously after birth, depending on the severity of the defect.

Congenital Malformations of the Skeletal System

Malformation of Fingers and Toes

Abnormalities of the fingers and toes are relatively common and, generally, can be corrected surgically. The fingers and toes may fail to separate normally during development (syndactyly), leading to the formation of spade-like hands and feet, a very common defect occurring in about 1 in 2500 births. It may be simple (not involving the bones) or complex (involving the bones and/or nails). Syndactyly is often part of a number of syndromes that show additional and far more serious effects. In other instances, extra digits are formed (polydactyly), sometimes in combination with syndactyly.

Congenital Clubfoot (Talipes)

Clubfoot is a relatively common congenital abnormality, having an incidence of about 1 in 1000 infants. Most cases are of unknown cause and may have a multifactorial pattern of inheritance. The malformation is characterized by an abnormal position of the foot that prevents normal weight-bearing; the affected

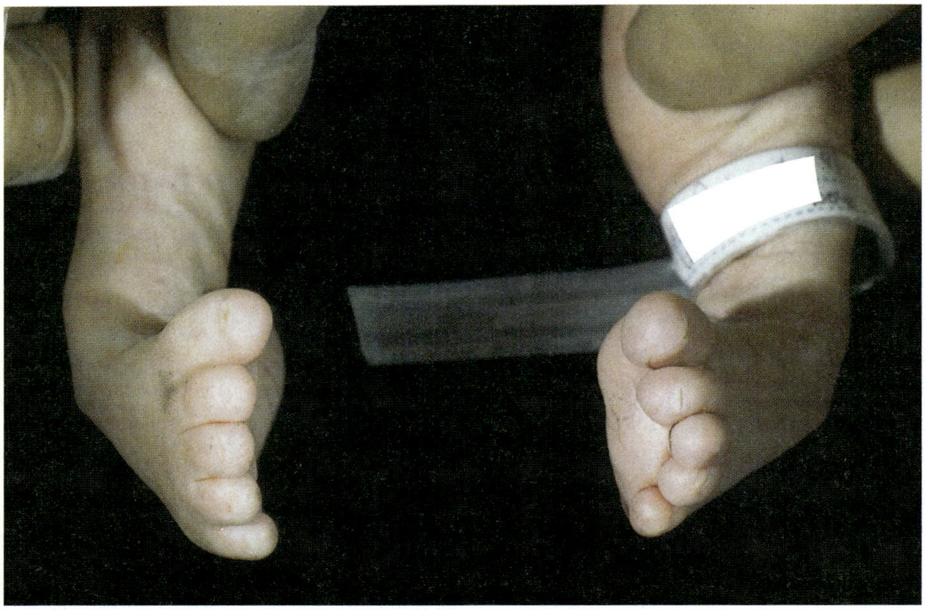

Figure 16-16 Common type of congenital clubfoot (*talipes equinovarus*) in newborn infant.

Courtesy of Leonard V. Crowley, MD, Century College.

individual tends to walk on the ankle rather than on the sole of the foot (talus = ankle + pes = foot). **Figure 16-16** illustrates the most common type of clubfoot deformity, *talipes equinovarus*, in which the foot is turned inward at the ankle (varus position) and fixed in tiptoe (equinus) position. Less commonly, the foot is rotated outward (valgus position) and fixed so that the weight is born on the heel (calcaneus position). Any intrauterine fetal position that causes the foot to assume an abnormal position may cause the foot to develop abnormally if the fetus is genetically predisposed to this malformation. Talipes is treated by manipulating the foot into a normal position and maintaining the corrected position with casts or splints; surgical release of the malrotated limb may be required in some cases.

Congenital Dislocation of the Hip (Hip Dysplasia)

Congenital dislocation of the hip has an incidence of about 1 in 1500 infants, occurring most commonly in females. In this malformation, the hip-joint socket (acetabulum) on the affected side is shallow, its upper rim is less well developed than normal, and the ligaments holding the head of the femur in the socket are relatively lax. As a consequence, the head of the femur fails to maintain its normal position and becomes displaced upward and backward out of the shallow socket (**Figure 16-17**). Like clubfoot, congenital hip dislocation results from the interaction of genetic factors in conjunction with an abnormal intrauterine fetal position. The depth of the hip socket and the laxity of the ligaments are genetically determined. Ligamentous laxity is also related to the sex of the infant, being greater in female infants (which accounts for the more frequent occurrence of congenital hip dislocation in females). If, in addition, the fetus assumes a position that causes the foot and leg to be rotated externally, the thigh also is rotated externally, which tends to displace the head of the femur out of its socket. Some types of breech positions (fetal buttocks rather than head in the

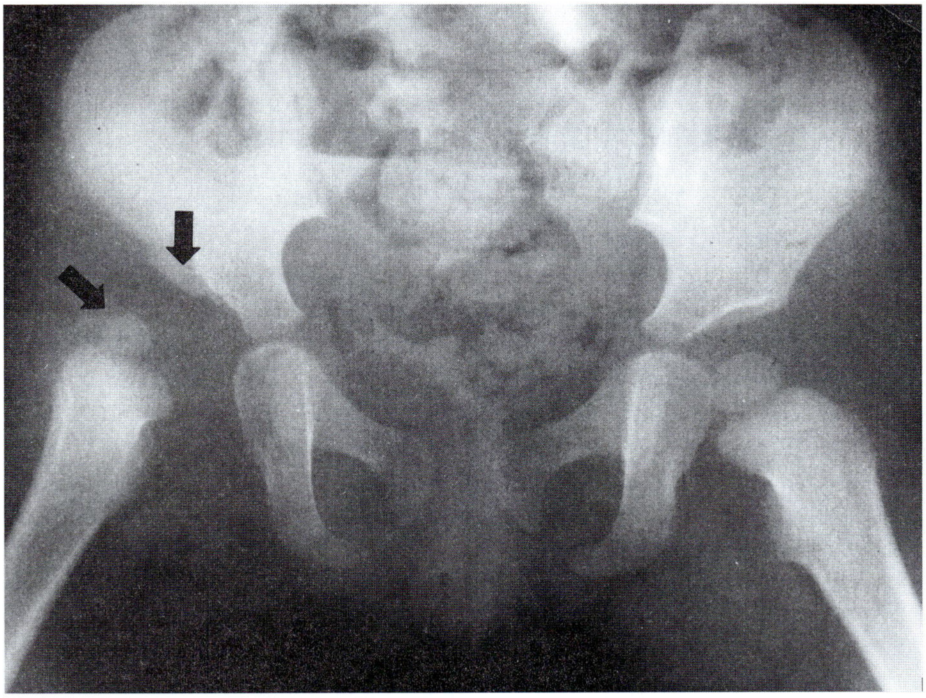

Figure 16-17 A congenital dislocation of the right hip in an 18-month-old child. Radiograph shows that right hip socket (*left*) is shallow, and its upper end (*upper arrow*) is less well developed than normal, permitting the head of the femur (*lower arrow*) to be displaced upward out of the hip-joint socket. The dislocated head is also less well developed than normal.

Courtesy of Leonard V. Crowley, MD, Century College.

lower part of the uterus and the lower extremities with knees extended pressed against the fetal abdomen and chest) predispose to hip dislocation in a genetically susceptible infant.

Congenital dislocation of the hip can frequently be treated effectively by manipulating the displaced femoral head into the acetabulum and maintaining the head within the socket by means of some device that maintains the leg and thigh in proper position, such as a splint or plaster cast.

Case 16-1

The patient was an infant girl born after 36 weeks' gestation. A low birth weight for gestational age and small neonatal size with microcephaly were noted. The skin was covered with numerous small hemorrhages (**petechiae**) and appeared yellow (was jaundiced), indicating liver disease. The abdomen was markedly distended because of extreme enlargement of both the liver and the spleen (**Case Figure 16-1**). A CT scan of the head disclosed multiple defects, with enlargement of the fluid-filled spaces (ventricles) of the brain and abnormal deposits of calcium. The infant was moderately anemic, and the platelet count was reduced, which accounted for the widespread hemorrhages in the skin. Elevation of liver-specific enzymes in the infant's blood suggested serious liver disease. The infant was considered to be seriously ill as a result of a prenatal infection acquired from the mother. Diagnostic possibilities considered were congenital rubella, cytomegalic inclusion disease, systemic herpes virus infection, or toxoplasmosis. The infant died from widespread

(continues)

Petechiae Small hemorrhages.

Case 16-1 *(Continued)*

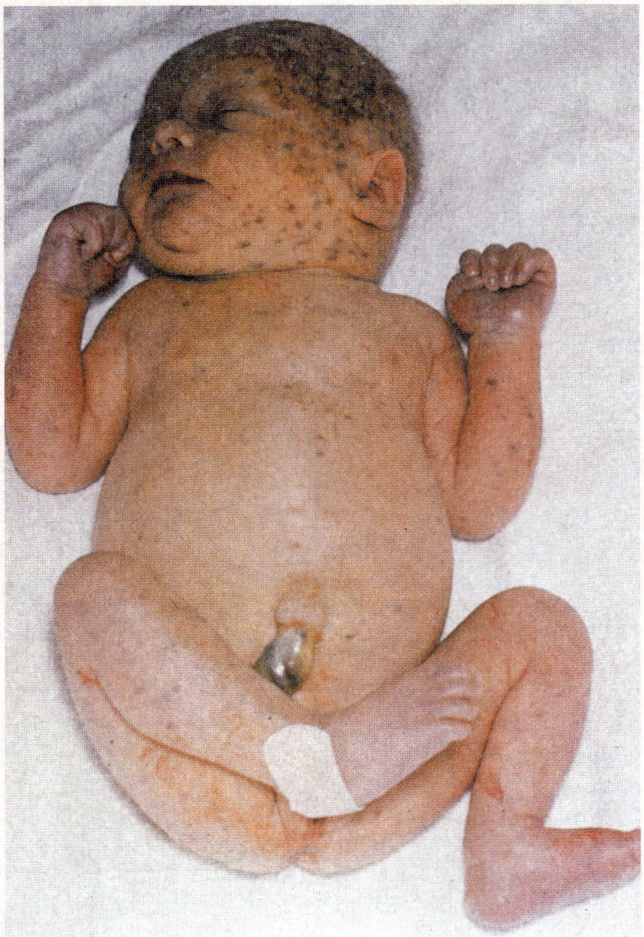

Case Figure 16-1 Severe systematic disease in a newborn infant caused by an inapparent infection of the mother during pregnancy, as described in Case 16-1.
Courtesy of Leonard V. Crowley, MD, Century College.

infection about 5 hours after examination before further diagnostic studies could be undertaken. The autopsy revealed the infection was caused by the cytomegalovirus. Pneumonia was detected, and characteristic cytomegalovirus inclusions were found in the lung. The diagnosis of congenital CMV infection was confirmed by additional laboratory tests (**Case Figure 16-2**).

Discussion

Cytomegalovirus infection (CMV) is the most common congenital infection, infecting between 0.6 percent and 1.0 percent of all births in the developing and developed world. CMV is a herpes virus that usually leads to asymptomatic disease in adults and children with normal immune systems. In developing countries, nearly 100 percent of people have been infected and have acquired antibodies to the virus (are **seropositive**) early in life. The number of seropositive people in developed countries reaches only about 50 percent in young adults. Although the risk of congenital CMV is greatest when the mother is first infected during pregnancy (and in particular during the first half), having antibodies to the virus does not rule out potential infection in utero. In a population in which more than 95 percent of pregnant women are seropositive, 1 percent of neonates are infected at birth, and almost all are born of mothers who were seropositive prior to pregnancy.

Seropositive Having antibodies to a pathogen.

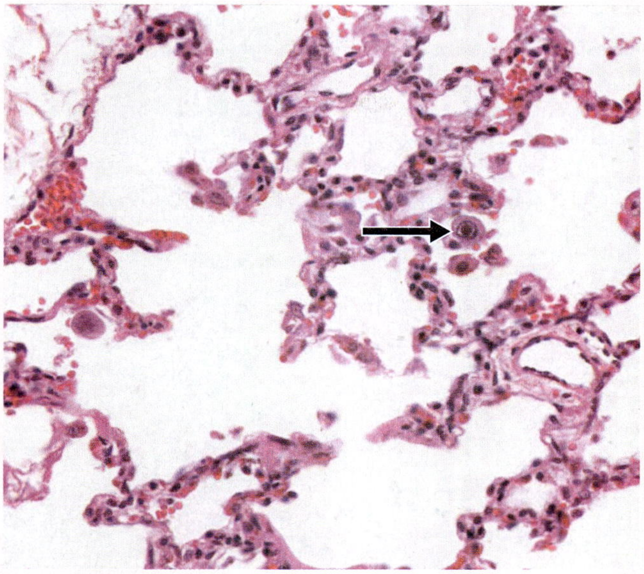

Case Figure 16-2 Characteristic CMV inclusions (*arrow*) in the lung of a newborn with congenital cytomegalovirus disease.

Only 10 percent of CMV-infected neonates show signs of disease at birth, although this group is almost always born to mothers who have had their first CMV infection during pregnancy. Such neonates are most frequently severely affected (as described in this case). The 90 percent of CMV-infected neonates who do not show disease at birth have a 10 percent to 20 percent risk of developing sequelae during childhood, most commonly hearing loss. Antiviral therapy may be considered in children with severe disease, but this is associated with significant side effects.

Etiology and Pathogenesis

The etiology is CMV infection in utero followed by multiorgan damage as a result of viral infection.

Questions

1. Why is it difficult to pinpoint cause and effect for many different birth defects and congenital syndromes?
2. What maternal infections are likely to cause difficulties during the development of the embryo and fetus?
3. What precautionary measures could a pregnant person undertake to ensure the best possible outcomes for their pregnancy and child?
4. Describe in detail one birth defect from each of the main organ systems.

References

Hartl, DL, Cochrane BJ. *Genetics: Analysis of Genes and Genomes*. 9th ed. Jones & Bartlett Learning; 2019.

- The study of congenital and hereditary disease is based on an understanding of modern genetics. An excellent general introduction to the area (with additional details of human disease) may be found here. Chapters 6 and 7 are of particular interest.

An Online Catalog of Human Genes and Genetic Disorders. Online Mendelian Inheritance in Man. http://omim.org

- This is one of the most comprehensive and authoritative sources for genetic disease and genetic medicine. Although complex to use, it is a source that anyone interested in human genetics should consult.

Birth Defects. Center for Disease Control and Prevention (CDC). http://www.cdc.gov/ncbddd/birthdefects/index.html

- An additional online source of authoritative information is the CDC. This URL provides information on birth defects.

Centers for Disease Control and Prevention. Public Health Genomics at CDC. Last updated July 8, 2024. https://www.cdc.gov/genomics/php/about/index.html

- The CDC Public Health Genomics Site has an exhaustive list of current specific references.

Schleiss M. Pediatric Cytomegalovirus Infection. Medscape. Updated April 28, 2023. http://emedicine.medscape.com/article/963090-overview

- Additional information relating to the CMV case may be found in this review.

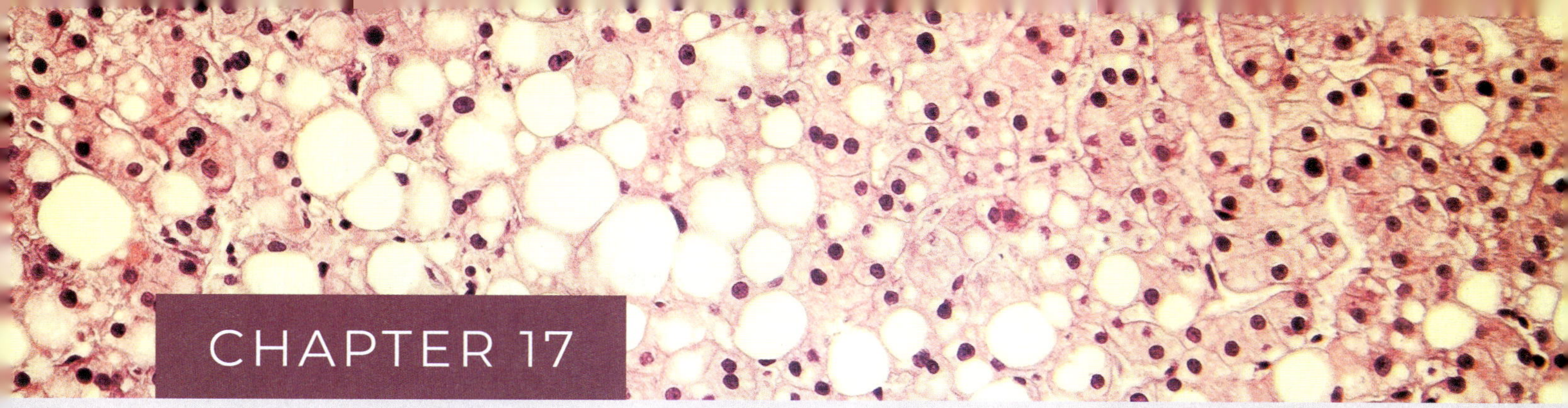

CHAPTER 17

The Urinary System and Fluid Homeostasis

LEARNING OBJECTIVES

1. Describe the role of the kidneys in maintaining water and electrolyte balance in the body.
2. Describe the role of the kidneys in regulation of water volume, osmolality, and blood pH.
3. Describe the normal structures of the kidneys and their functions, with special emphasis on the nephron.
4. Describe chronic kidney disease and its most common causes.
5. Explain the pathogenesis of glomerulonephritis, nephrosis, and nephrosclerosis. Describe the clinical manifestations of each of these disorders.
6. Describe acute tubular injury and tubulointerstitial nephritis.
7. Describe the clinical manifestations and complications of urinary tract infections.
8. Explain the mechanism for formation of urinary tract calculi. Describe the complications of stone formation. Explain the manifestations of urinary tract obstruction.
9. Differentiate the major forms of cystic disease of the kidney and their prognoses.
10. Name the more common kinds of tumors affecting the urinary tract.
11. Describe the causes, clinical manifestations, and treatment of renal failure.
12. Describe the principles and techniques of hemodialysis and renal transplantation.
13. Describe the techniques used to evaluate kidney disease.

Control of Overall Extracellular Water Volume and Osmolality

Control of overall body water volume and plasma osmolality (essentially equivalent to plasma sodium concentration) is complex. Somewhat surprisingly, both osmolality and fluid volume are controlled by two almost totally independent regulatory systems in which the kidneys play a key role. Osmoregulation is controlled by water intake and excretion, which in turn controls sodium concentration in the extracellular fluids. Volume regulation is primarily controlled by sodium retention and excretion. These two systems have different sensors, effector mechanisms, and effects, which will be discussed in this chapter. Simple examples include the following:

Osmoregulation: You are exercising and sweating profusely, your extracellular fluid compartment shrinks, and the concentration of sodium (but NOT the sodium amount) in your extracellular fluids (including plasma) goes up. The change in plasma osmolality is sensed in the hypothalamus, resulting in thirst and suppression of urinary water loss. You drink and now increase the level of extracellular water and decrease the extracellular sodium concentration (plasma osmolality). Lacking a source of water, the hypernatremia (high sodium concentration) could result in cell shrinkage and a variety of neurological problems.

Volume regulation: You suffer from severe bacterial gastroenteritis ("food poisoning") and vomit excessively. This leads to hypovolemia, a decrease in plasma volume that results in a decrease in tissue perfusion and loss of blood pressure. The decrease in perfusion is sensed (at several different anatomic sites), resulting in retention of urinary sodium and subsequent movement of fluid into the vasculature and restoration of circulating fluid volume and blood pressure. Had sodium retention been insufficient, the fall in blood pressure could ultimately have resulted in shock and death.

Although the two regulatory mechanisms are independent, aspects of each are involved in renal physiology—that is, how the physiology of the kidney maintains sodium and water homeostasis.

Body Water Content

Sixty percent of the lean body weight of a male is water containing dissolved solutes such as salts. Females have a slightly lower proportion of water (50 percent). Body water is distributed into several compartments bounded by membranes. Two-thirds of body water is intracellular (contained within the cell membrane), and the remaining one-third is extracellular. The extracellular fluid can be further subdivided into plasma (the liquid within the circulatory system) and the interstitial fluid of the tissue that surrounds the cells.

The body water contains dissolved salts (**electrolytes**) that dissociate in solution, yielding positively charged ions (**cations**) and negatively charged ions (**anions**). The fluid within the cells is separated from the interstitial fluid by the cell membrane, which is freely permeable to water but relatively impermeable to sodium and potassium ions. The principal extracellular ions are sodium (Na^+), chloride (Cl^-), and bicarbonate (HCO_3^-), whereas the principal intracellular ions are potassium (K^+), magnesium (Mg^{2+}), and phosphate (PO_4^{3-}).

The overall electrical charge in each fluid compartment is neutral. The quantity of a specific ion in body fluids is most often measured as **milliequivalents (mEq)**, which is equal to the **millimolar** concentration of the ion times the charge of the ion. This is convenient because concentration in mEq of cations will balance the charge of an equal concentration in mEq of anions.

Electrolyte Substance that can conduct electricity through the movement of ions, but not through the movement of electrons. They include many soluble salts, acids, and bases dissolved in a polar solvent like water.

Cations Positively charged ions.

Anions Negatively charged ions.

Milliequivalents (mEq) Measurement of the amount of an ion in body fluids.

Millimolar Concentration of one thousandth of a mole per liter of solvent.

Regulation of Plasma pH

Control of plasma pH depends critically on the role of the kidneys in regulating bicarbonate levels and on the level of dissolved carbon dioxide (controlled by respiratory rate).

The kidneys play two important roles in regulating the pH of the blood. Under normal circumstances, the kidneys reabsorb almost all of the bicarbonate that otherwise would be lost in the urine and excrete the acids that are the products of cellular metabolism. The kidneys regulate bicarbonate concentration in the plasma by selectively reabsorbing filtered bicarbonate (in the proximal renal tubules) as necessary to meet the body's requirements. In addition, the kidneys can manufacture bicarbonate in the distal renal tubules to replace the amounts lost in buffering acids produced as a consequence of normal metabolic processes.

The relative degree of acidity/alkalinity of the blood is measured in terms of pH units (a measure of the concentration of hydrogen ions) and is normally under careful regulation to fall between pH 7.37 and 7.42. The pH scale is a base 10 logarithmic scale, so the change of one whole unit signifies a 10-fold change in hydrogen ion concentration. Very minimal changes in the pH number can indicate biologically important changes in ion concentrations. A pH of 7.0 is neutral (neither acid nor alkaline). Hence, blood is normally slightly alkaline (**Figure 17-1**).

Regulation of the pH of body extracellular fluid is critical for all metabolic functions in the organism. Enzymes function best over a very narrow range of pH, as the number of available hydrogen ions affects the three-dimensional shape of proteins. Variation of plasma pH much above or below the optimum of pH 7.4 will influence protein structure and enzyme functioning.

The major mechanism for the control of plasma pH is the sodium bicarbonate–carbonic acid buffer system. A buffer system is a solution containing a weak acid and its conjugate base that resists a change in pH. The concentration of carbonic acid (dissolved carbon dioxide), the weak acid, is controlled by the lungs, and the concentration of bicarbonate (the conjugate base) is controlled by the kidneys. Respiratory control of pH is rapid, whereas renal control is relatively slow and may occur over days.

Metabolic Acidosis and Alkalosis

Failure of the kidneys to excrete acidic products of metabolism or produce sufficient bicarbonate results in **metabolic acidosis**.

Metabolic acidosis
Condition with decreased plasma pH resulting from a decrease in serum bicarbonate, often associated with loss of acidic gastric contents, overuse of certain diuretics, or endocrine disease.

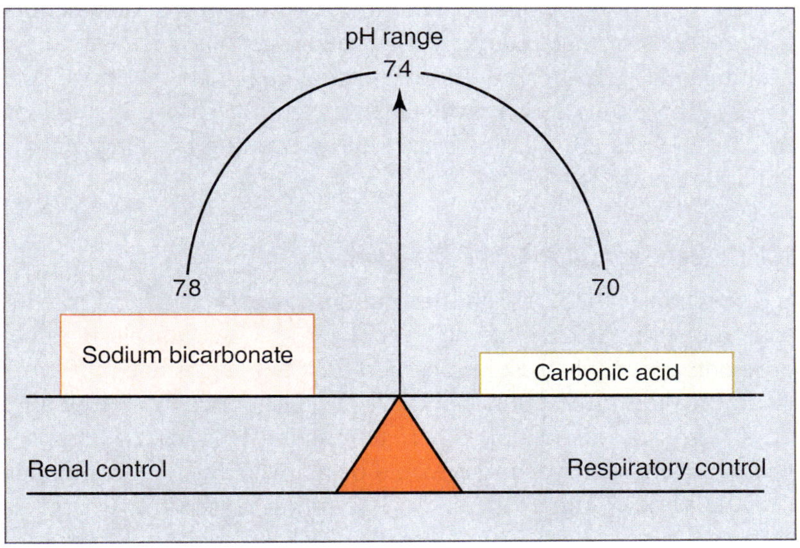

Figure 17-1 "Board-and-fulcrum" concept of normal bicarbonate–carbonic acid relationships.

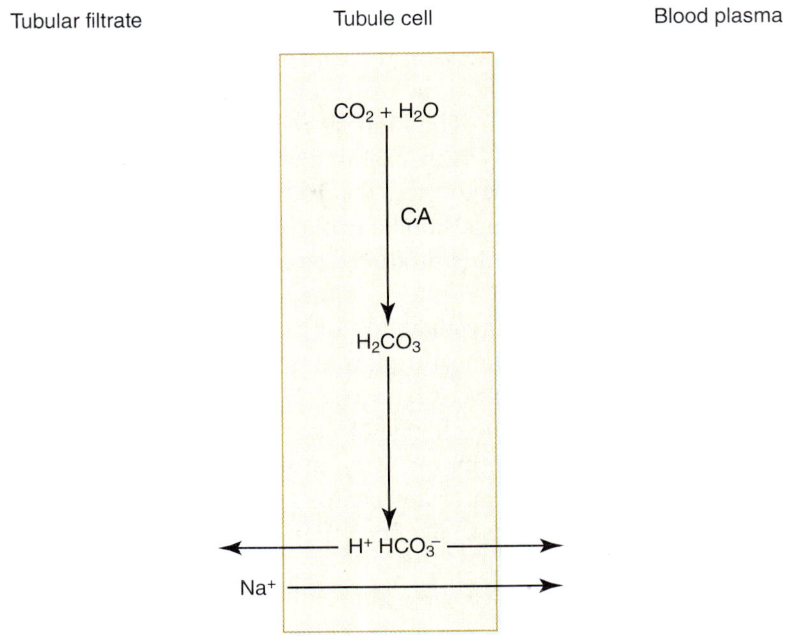

Figure 17-2 Formation and excretion of hydrogen ions by renal tubular epithelial cells in exchange for sodium. CA indicates carbonic anhydrase.

Metabolic alkalosis Condition with elevated plasma pH resulting from increased bicarbonate level due to diseases in the endocrine system or loss of hydrogen ions.

Respiratory alkalosis Elevated blood pH resulting from increased excretion of CO_2.

Metabolic alkalosis can result from disease of the endocrine system, loss of chloride ions, and several other causes. These two (lung/kidney) bicarbonate-regulating functions depend on the secretion of hydrogen ions by the renal tubules in exchange for sodium ions that are simultaneously reabsorbed from the tubular filtrate into the circulation as illustrated in **Figure 17-2**. Under the influence of the enzyme carbonic anhydrase, carbonic acid (H_2CO_3) is formed from carbon dioxide (CO_2) and water (H_2O) within the tubular epithelial cells and dissociates into hydrogen (H^+) and bicarbonate (HCO_3–) ions. The hydrogen ions enter the tubular filtrate in exchange for sodium ions (Na^+). The bicarbonate ions enter the bloodstream along with the sodium ions that have been absorbed from the filtrate.

A special type of metabolic acidosis (anion gap metabolic acidosis) is so named because it results from the addition of "unexpected" acids either produced by the body or ingested. Examples of endogenous acids would be lactic acid resulting in lactic acidosis or those resulting from diabetic ketoacidosis (see Chapter 22). Exogenous agents producing this type of acidosis include ingested methanol or ethylene glycol (antifreeze) and poisoning by salicylates (aspirin and similar compounds).

Respiratory Control of pH

As noted previously, the lungs and respiratory rate play a critical role in regulating plasma pH by controlling the level of carbonic acid in plasma. Carbonic acid represents physically dissolved carbon dioxide. This is in equilibrium with the carbon dioxide in the pulmonary alveoli. (The concentration of a gas in a mixture is expressed in terms of its partial pressure. This is a hypothetical measure of what the pressure of the gas would be if it were the only component and occupied the same volume.) Increased respiration lowers the alveolar carbon dioxide partial pressure (PCO_2) and leads to a rapid decrease in the concentration of carbon dioxide and carbonic acid in plasma. This makes the blood more alkaline (less acid) and is termed **respiratory alkalosis**. Decreased or

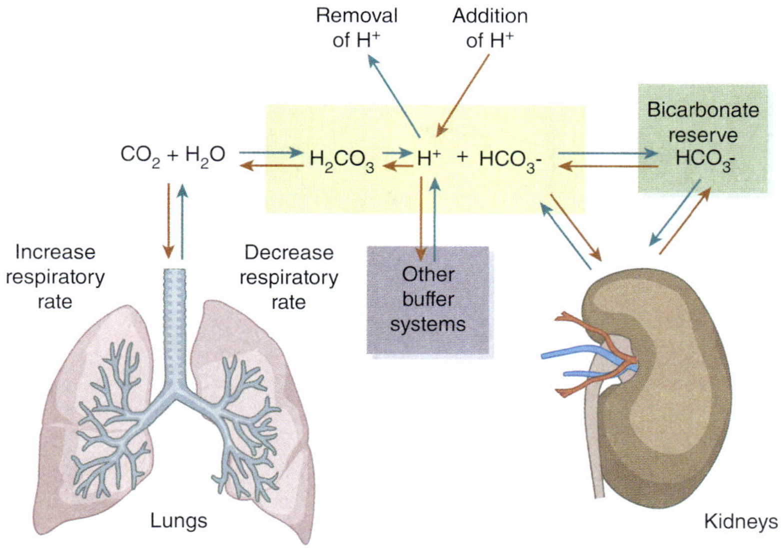

Figure 17-3 A summary of metabolic and respiratory control of plasma pH.

inadequate pulmonary ventilation results in elevation of alveolar PCO_2, which in turn raises plasma carbon dioxide and carbonic acid. This makes the blood more acidic and is termed **respiratory acidosis** (**Figure 17-3**).

Table 17-1 and Figure 17-3 compare metabolic and respiratory causes of acidosis and alkalosis and how the body compensates for them to restore homeostasis.

Respiratory acidosis Decreased plasma pH due to insufficient excretion of CO_2.

Structure of the Urinary System

The urinary system (**Figure 17-4A**) consists of the kidneys, a transport system for the urine, the bladder, and the urethra. An overview of its structure—particularly the structure of the kidney's functional unit, the nephron—is critical to understanding its many functions.

Table 17-1 Comparison of Common Acid–Base Disturbances

Disturbance	Primary Abnormality	Compensation	Usual Causes
Metabolic acidosis	Excess endogenous acid depletes bicarbonate.	Decreased plasma PCO_2 resulting from increased ventilation. Kidney excretes more hydrogen ions and forms more bicarbonate.	Renal failure; ketosis; overproduction of lactic acid, loss from the GI tract
Respiratory acidosis	Inefficient excretion of carbon dioxide by lungs.	Formation of additional bicarbonate or decreased excretion by kidneys.	Chronic pulmonary disease
Metabolic alkalosis	Excess plasma bicarbonate.	Increased plasma PCO_2 resulting from decreased ventilation.	Loss of gastric juice; chloride depletion, excess corticosteroid hormones, ingestion of excessive bicarbonate or other antacids, failure of kidneys to excrete excess bicarbonate
Respiratory alkalosis	Hyperventilation lowers PCO_2.	Increased excretion of bicarbonate by kidneys.	Severe anxiety with hyperventilation; stimulation of the respiratory center by drugs; central nervous system disease

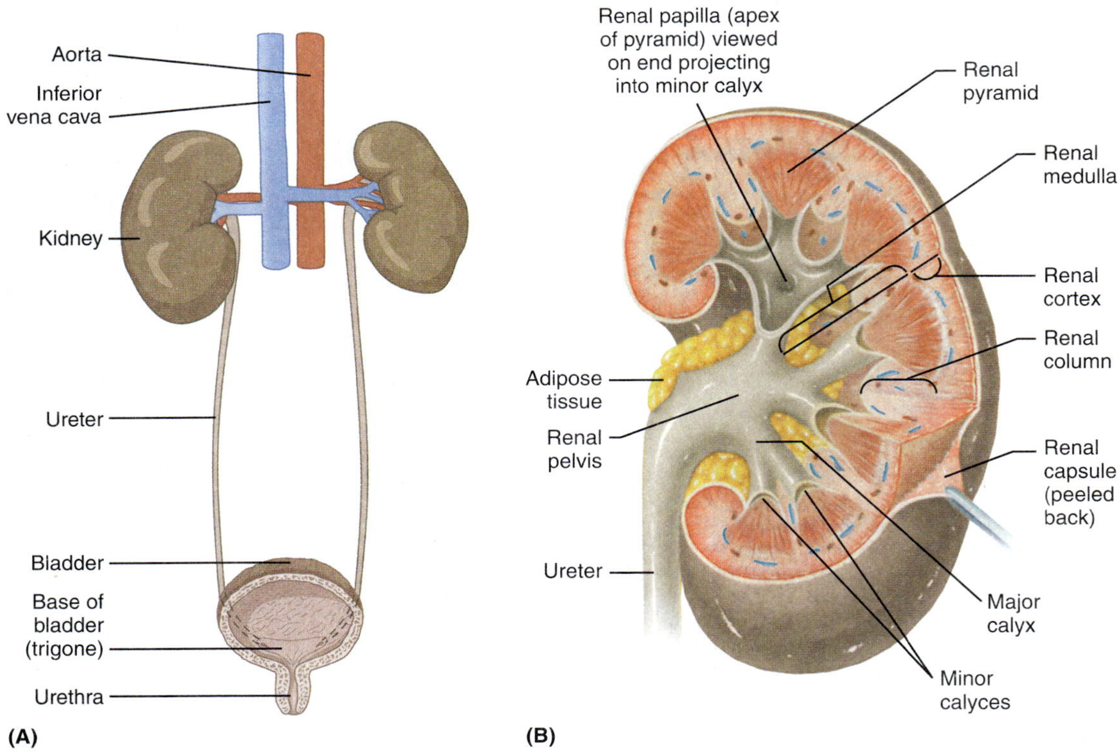

Figure 17-4 **(A)** Components of the urinary system. **(B)** Structure of the kidney in longitudinal section.

The Kidneys

Hilus A depression in an organ from where the blood vessels enter or leave.
Renal pelvis/major calyces Expanded upper end of the ureter and divisions of the renal pelvis.
Cortex Outer layer of an organ.
Medulla Inner part of an organ.
Trigone Triangular area at the base of the bladder.
Urea A normal byproduct of protein metabolism excreted in the urine.

The kidneys are paired, bean-shaped organs located along the dorsal body wall below the diaphragm and adjacent to the vertebral column. Their structure is illustrated in **Figure 17-4B**. The region where the blood vessels enter and leave and where the ureter exits to descend to the bladder is termed the **hilus** of the kidney. The expanded upper end of the ureter is the **renal pelvis**, which divides into several large branches termed the **major calyces** (singular, calyx). Further subdivision forms the minor calyces. The renal substance is divided into an outer **cortex** and an inner **medulla**. The cone-shaped masses of renal tissue in the medulla that project into the minor calyces are termed the renal pyramids, with the renal papilla at the tip facing the renal pelvis. Columns of cortical tissue that extend into the medulla between the pyramids are termed the renal columns.

The calyces and pelves convey the urine into the ureters, which extend downward to enter the posterior wall of the bladder near its base in an area termed the **trigone** (illustrated in Figure 17-4A). Each ureter enters the bladder at an angle; when the bladder contracts, its muscular wall compresses the ureters as they run obliquely through it, somewhat like a one-way valve. This prevents backflow of urine into the ureters during voiding (urination). The ureteral openings into the bladder also appear to have a valvular function preventing backflow.

Function of the Kidney

The kidney is both an excretory organ via the production of urine for the removal of metabolic wastes such as creatinine and **urea** and the organ that maintains homeostasis within the organism by selectively excreting or retaining water and electrolytes as required to maintain a uniform composition of body fluids. Water lost from perspiration, respiration, the GI tract, and in urine must be in balance with water intake; likewise, loss of electrolytes must be balanced with intake, and plasma pH must be kept within narrow limits by regulating hydrogen ion concentration. In a sense, the environment of the body is determined not by what a person ingests but rather by what the kidneys retain.

The kidney also has a critical role in secreting hormones and hormone-like substances that are important in the maintenance of homeostasis (in part by regulating both renal and systemic blood flow and pressure). Erythropoietin produced by interstitial fibroblasts in the kidney is critical for increased red cell synthesis in the bone marrow under hypoxic conditions.

The Ureters

The ureters are muscular tubes that propel the urine into the bladder by wavelike contractions of their muscular walls (**peristalsis**). Urine is discharged into the bladder in spurts and does not drain by gravity.

The Bladder and Urethra

The urinary bladder is the distensible reservoir for urine lined by transitional epithelium (also known as urothelium) continuous with the lining of the remainder of the urinary tract. The opening of the urethra is located at the base of the bladder, with the ureteral openings on either side and behind the urethral opening. The triangular area at the base of the bladder, bounded by the two ureteral orifices posteriorly and the urethral orifice anteriorly, is termed the trigone of the bladder (tri = three).

The Nephron

The basic structural and functional unit of the kidney is the nephron, with about one million nephrons in each kidney. Each nephron consists of a glomerulus, a renal tubule with its draining collecting ducts, and the associated vasculature (**Figure 17-5**). The glomerulus is a tuft of capillaries supplied by an afferent glomerular arteriole. The capillaries of the glomerulus then recombine into an efferent glomerular arteriole, which in turn breaks up into a network of capillaries that supplies the renal tubules, which ultimately conduct urine to the renal calyces. Damage to the vasculature of the nephron (for example, by hypertension, high blood pressure) is likely to affect all of the components of the nephron (glomerulus, tubules, and ducts). The site where the afferent arteriole enters the glomerulus and the efferent arteriole exits is termed the **vascular pole** of the glomerulus.

The histologic structure of the glomerulus and related structures is illustrated schematically in **Figure 17-6**. The expanded proximal end of the tubule is termed **Bowman's capsule**. The tuft of capillaries that make up the glomerulus is pushed into Bowman's capsule much as one would push a fist into a balloon. The layer of Bowman's capsule cells, which is pushed in (invaginated), becomes closely applied to the capillaries of the glomerulus and is termed the visceral layer of Bowman's capsule, or simply the **glomerular epithelium**. The cells of this layer have long, footlike cytoplasmic processes and are usually termed **podocytes** (podos = foot). The outer layer of Bowman's capsule is termed the parietal layer of Bowman's capsule, or simply the **capsular epithelium**. The space between the two layers, into which the urine filters, is termed Bowman's space.

Peristalsis The wavelike contractions of the wall of a tubular anatomic structure such as the alimentary tract or ureter, which propel luminal contents forward.

Vascular pole Site where the afferent arteriole enters the glomerulus and the efferent arteriole exits.

Bowman's capsule The cuplike expanded end of the nephron that surrounds the tuft of glomerular capillaries.

Glomerular epithelium Layer of Bowman's cells closely applied to the capillaries. It is also termed the visceral layer of Bowman's capsule.

Podocytes Cells with highly branched cytoplasmic processes covering the glomerular capillaries of the kidneys.

Capsular epithelium Outer layer of cells of Bowman's capsule. It is also termed the parietal layer of Bowman's capsule.

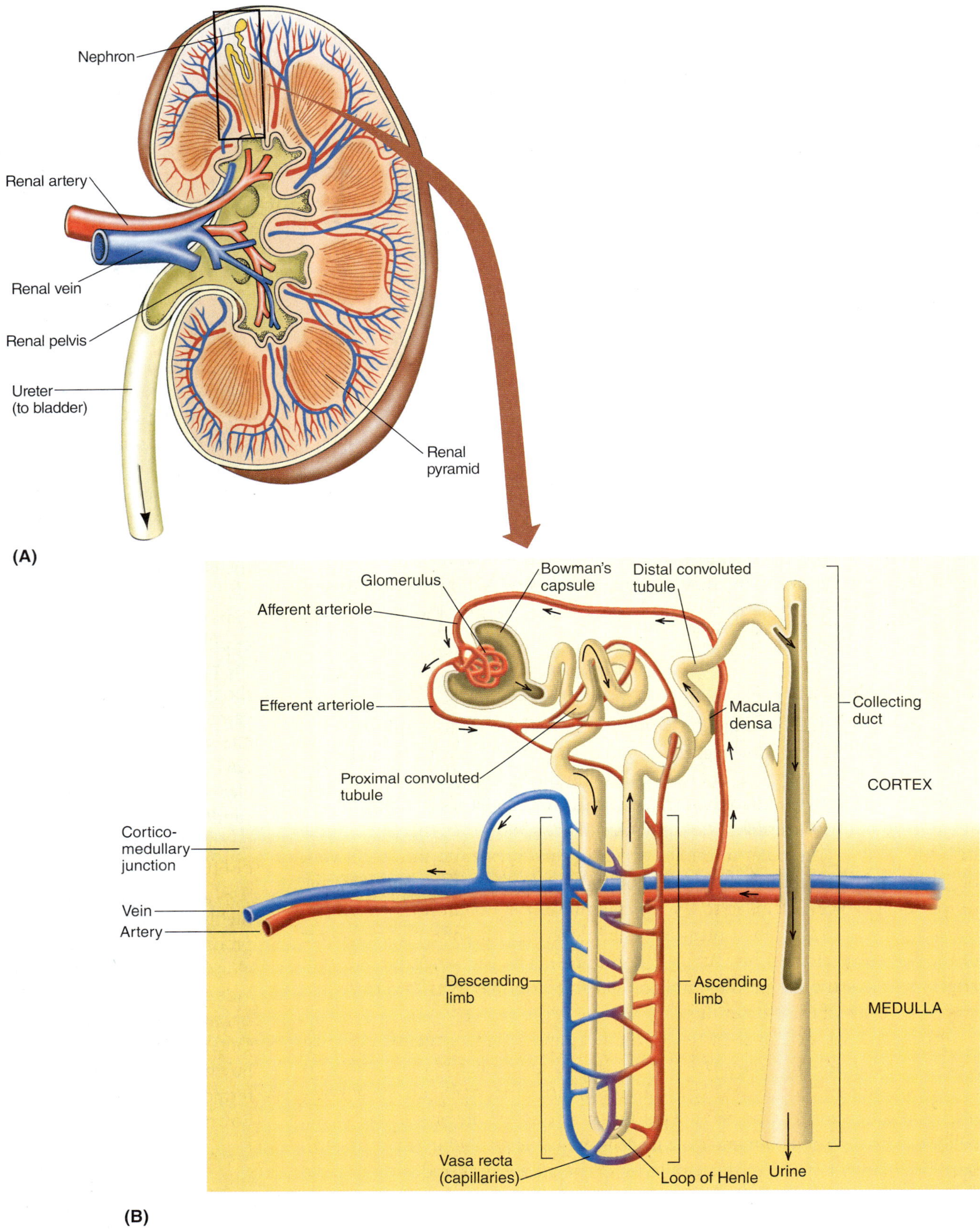

Figure 17-5 The structure of a nephron, including the glomerulus, tubules, collecting ducts, and associated vasculature.

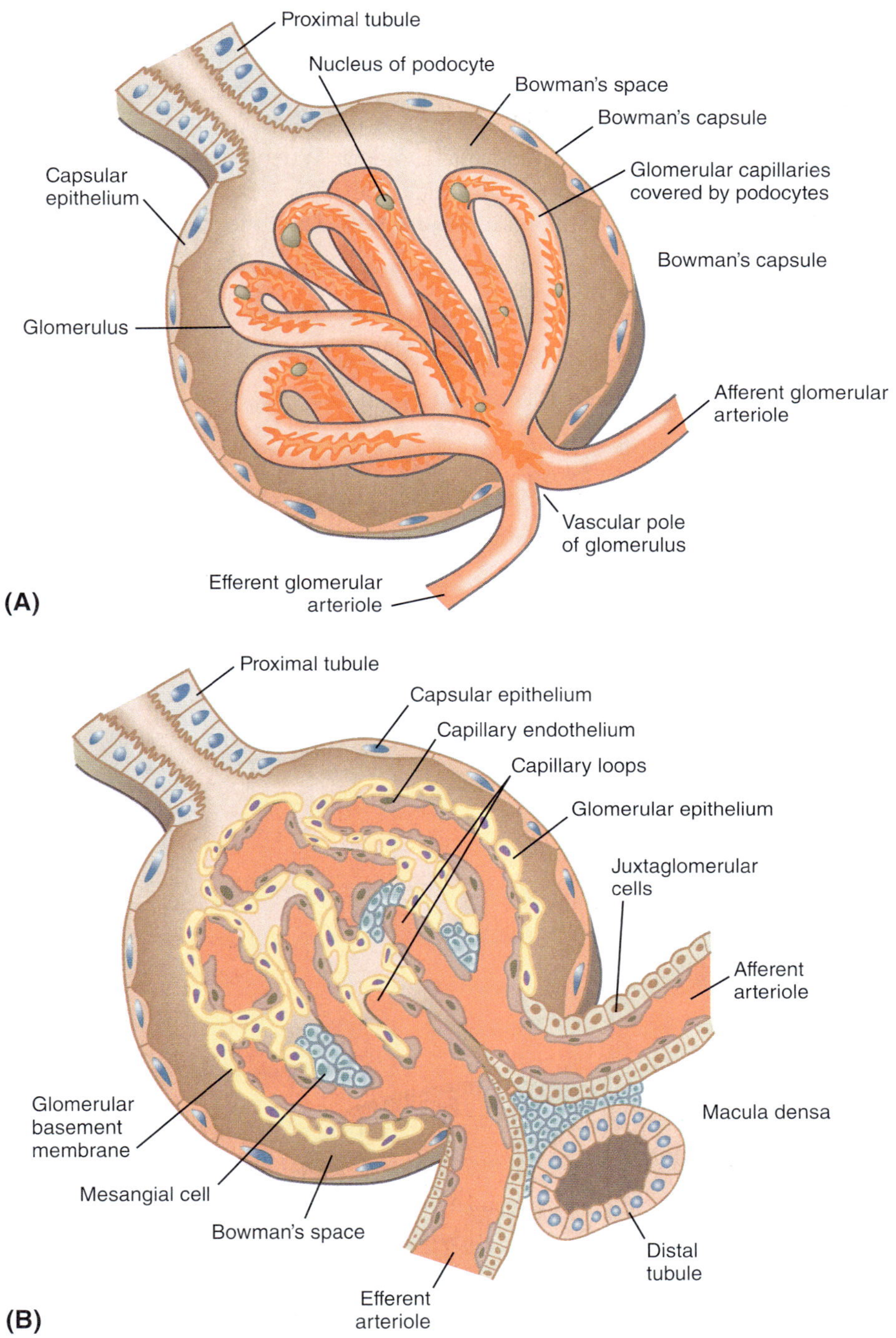

Figure 17-6 The structure of the glomerulus and Bowman's capsule. **(A)** Anterior half of Bowman's capsule removed to reveal capillary tuft covered by podocytes (schematic). **(B)** Cross section through glomerulus to reveal structure of glomerular filter and juxtaglomerular apparatus.

The capillary tuft is held together and supported by groups of highly specialized cells termed mesangial cells (meso = middle + angio = vessel). In addition to their support function, they are also contractile cells that play a role in regulating glomerular filtration by varying the caliber of the capillaries, and they are also phagocytic cells. Also located at the vascular pole is a compact collection of epithelial cells termed the macula densa containing a specialized cluster of cells termed the **juxtaglomerular apparatus** (juxta = near to), which

Juxtaglomerular apparatus A specialized group of cells at the vascular pole of the glomerulus that regulates blood flow through the glomerulus of the kidneys.

Renin An enzyme secreted by the kidneys in response to a fall in blood pressure, blood volume, or sodium concentration.

regulates blood flow through the glomerulus (Figure 17-6B). It also plays a role in regulating blood pressure by producing **renin**.

Water and soluble materials are small enough to filter from the blood through the glomerular capillaries into Bowman's space. Proteins (notably albumin) are retained within the normal capillary. When visualized by electron microscopy, the membrane through which the filtrate passes can be seen to consist of three layers, as depicted in **Figure 17-7**. The inner layer is formed by

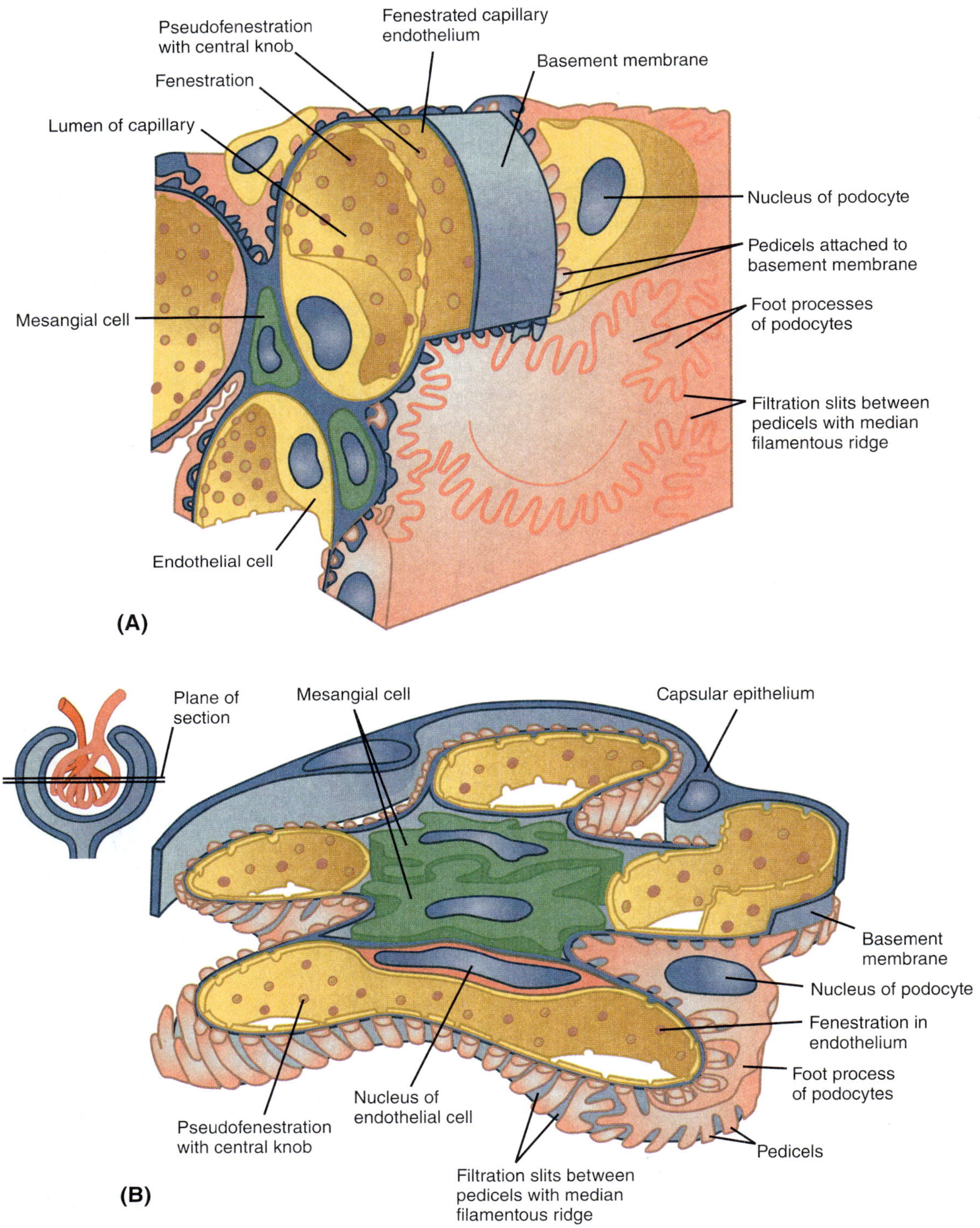

Figure 17-7 A schematic representation of the fine structure of the glomerular filter as visualized by electron microscopy. **(A)** Segment of glomerular capillaries. **(B)** Cross section through the center of the glomerulus, including part of Bowman's capsule.

the endothelium of the glomerular capillaries. The cytoplasm is very thin and is perforated by many small holes termed fenestrations (fenestra = window). This layer is freely permeable to water, many salts, other low molecular-weight molecules, and, in particular, metabolic wastes such as urea and creatinine. The middle layer is the basement membrane, which supports the capillary endothelium. The basement membrane has a negative charge and tends to exclude substances that are anionic while allowing cationic and neutral substances to pass. Filtration by the basement membrane is based primarily on molecular charge. The outer layer of the filtration barrier is composed of the podocytes. Their highly branched cytoplasmic processes are termed foot processes, which are attached to the basement membrane and interdigitate with others from the same cell or adjacent cells. The narrow spaces between adjacent interdigitating pedicels are termed filtration slits. Each slit is covered by a thin membrane termed a slit diaphragm, which is less porous than the other layers of the glomerular filter and is the major barrier to protein loss from the circulation. Damage to the filtration barrier in the glomerulus allows large molecular-weight substances, importantly albumin, to escape into the urine.

Glomerular Function

Filtration

Because the glomerulus is the site where nitrogenous metabolic wastes are filtered from the blood, failure of filtration will result in azotemia, the buildup of nitrogenous wastes in the blood (including urea and related compounds). These waste compounds are broadly toxic and will result in **uremia**, a clinical syndrome which can lead to death from multiorgan failure. For this reason, the **glomerular filtration rate (GFR)** is essential for good health and is carefully regulated. The factors that control GFR are the porosity and the length of the glomerular capillary, the difference in fluid pressure inside the capillary and outside the capillary in Bowman's space, and the oncotic pressure of the plasma in the capillary (note that the oncotic pressure of the filtrate in Bowman's space, which should contain no proteins, is normally zero) (Chapter 2 reviews these concepts). In a healthy person, the length and the porosity of the glomerular capillary is constant but is altered in several diseases. For example, glomeruli may become sclerotic (stiffened) and fail to function, reducing the GFR. In the healthy individual, the renal plasma flow rate (RPF) is carefully regulated because changes affect glomerular capillary pressure and decrease the GFR, and hence the rate of clearance of metabolic toxins decreases. Control of the RPF is complex and occurs at many levels, both external and internal to the kidney. However, within the kidney, changes in the resistance of the afferent glomerular arteriole to flow (afferent arteriolar tone) are most important. Afferent arteriolar tone is "autoregulated" by muscle stretch sensors embedded in the wall of that vessel. Increases in arterial systemic pressure will increase the tone (resistance) of the afferent arteriole regulating pressure within the glomerular capillary (and vice versa), thus keeping RPF and therefore GFR constant. Another important regulating system for GFR is the changes in a group of specialized cells at the macula densa that form the juxtaglomerular apparatus. Cells in the macula densa (located at the thick ascending limb of the loop of Henle) sense increases in the fluid pressure (to be accurate, increased sodium ion influx into the cells) within the tubule associated with an increase in GFR and promote vasoconstriction (increase in tone) of the adjacent afferent arteriolar capillary, reducing the GFR. Additional regulators of GFR are a number of neurohumoral factors that, when released into the

Uremia An excess of urea and other waste products in the blood, resulting from renal failure.

Glomerular filtration rate (GFR) Measure of the volume of body fluid cleared by the kidneys per unit of time.

circulation, control the overall degree of vascular tone, one important example being the renin–angiotensin–aldosterone system (discussed later in this chapter). Neurohumoral regulation is of particular importance in disease states and therapy. Declining GFR occurs in many common chronic conditions of the elderly, including hypertension and diabetes.

Control of Plasma Osmolality

The glomerulus of the kidney is freely permeable to water, sodium, other electrolytes, and many small soluble molecules. In a day, about 200 liters of fluid are filtered by the kidneys. Normal urine output is 1 to 2 liters per day. Clearly most fluid (and sodium) filtered through the glomerulus must be reabsorbed and returned to the circulation in the normal kidney. Reabsorption of water and ions occurs in the tubules and collecting ducts of the nephron. The process requires careful regulation, which is accomplished by two (mostly) independent systems.

Hyponatremia Lower than normal concentration of sodium ions in the plasma and extracellular fluid.

Plasma osmolality is controlled by the sodium ion concentration. **Hyponatremia** (low sodium concentration) results in a hypotonic plasma, the result of which would be cell swelling as osmosis draws water into cells. Consider the potentially catastrophic effects of the brain swelling within the inflexible skull. Hyponatremia occurs when there is an excess of water in relation to sodium, almost always related to impairment of water excretion. Contrawise, hypernatremia results in a hypertonic plasma, resulting in cell shrinkage, also a serious clinical problem. (It should be noted that levels of other solutes and, in particular, potassium [discussed later in this chapter] also must be carefully regulated, but sodium plays the major role in determining plasma osmolality.) The major cause of hypernatremia relates to increased water loss that is not corrected by thirst. An example might be an unconscious person with a severe infection resulting in increased water losses not being properly hydrated. Certain forms of diarrhea related to infection also result in excessive water loss and an increased concentration of sodium in circulation. Plasma sodium concentration, and hence osmolality, is regulated almost completely by control of water uptake (mediated by thirst) and the role of antidiuretic hormone (ADH, also known as vasopressin), released by the posterior pituitary, both controlled by plasma osmolality sensors in the hypothalamus (see Chapter 22). When plasma osmolality increases, thirst increases water intake and ADH acts to reduce water excretion, decreasing plasma osmolality (sodium concentration) by dilution. Lack of secretion of ADH or failure of the kidneys to respond can lead to copious urine production and thirst, a condition termed diabetes insipidus. The effect of ADH on water regulation in the kidney is discussed later in this chapter.

Control of Circulating Volume

Control of circulating volume is mostly independent of osmoregulation and relies on multiple sensors sensitive to tissue perfusion in different regions of the body, including the heart (consider that plasma osmolality is constant throughout the circulatory system, but tissue perfusion [blood flow] may vary locally). Hypoperfusion of the kidney (resulting from low circulatory volume or blood pressure) results in the release of renin from the kidney into the bloodstream from the juxtaglomerular cells in the walls of the afferent glomerular arterioles, activating the renin–angiotensin–aldosterone system (RAAS). Renin is an enzyme that interacts with a blood protein termed angiotensinogen and splits off a short peptide fragment termed angiotensin I. Then, the newly formed

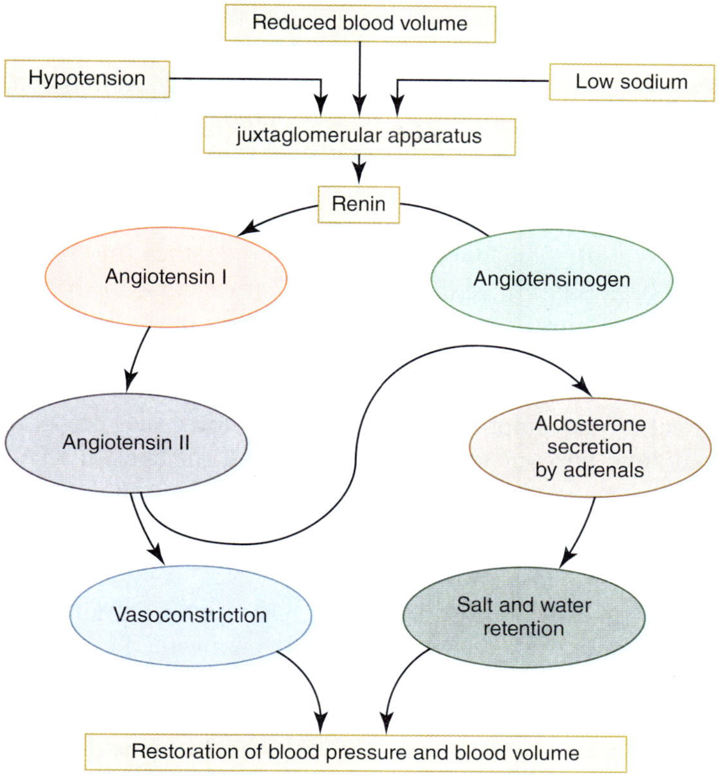

Figure 17-8 The role of the kidneys in the regulation of blood pressure and blood volume.

angiotensin I is almost immediately converted to angiotensin II by an enzyme termed angiotensin converting enzyme (ACE). Angiotensin II is predominantly generated locally in the kidney, although it is also produced by ACE in the pulmonary capillaries.

Angiotensin II is a powerful vasoconstrictor that raises the blood pressure by causing the peripheral arterioles to constrict, enhances sodium absorption by the renal tubules, and also stimulates the adrenal cortex to secrete a steroid hormone, termed aldosterone, which increases reabsorption of sodium by the kidneys and colon. It also increases potassium excretion. As a result, after the blood volume is increased by the greater volume of sodium and water entering the circulation, the blood pressure rises because there is more fluid within the vascular system. Thus, renin regulates blood pressure both by controlling the degree of arteriolar vasoconstriction and by regulating the volume of fluid within the circulation. The system is self-regulating because renin secretion declines as blood pressure, volume, and sodium concentration are restored to normal (**Figure 17-8**).

Structure of Renal Tubules

The renal tubular system and collecting ducts play a critical role in sodium and water homeostasis by their role in reabsorption of these substances.

The renal tubules are long tubes and measure as much as 4 cm in length. The proximal end of the tubule is invaginated by the glomerulus, and its distal end empties into a collecting tubule. The tubule is divided into several parts: the proximal convoluted tubule, the loop of Henle, the distal convoluted tubule, and the collecting tubule (Figure 17-5).

The proximal convoluted tubule is the first part of the tubule that is heavily coiled, its convolutions being located very close to the glomerulus. The loop of Henle is a U-shaped segment composed of descending and ascending limbs joined by a short segment. The descending limb and proximal half of the ascending limb are lined by flat epithelial cells, forming the thin segment of Henle's loop. The distal part of the ascending limb, termed the thick segment of Henle's loop, is lined by tall columnar epithelium similar to that lining the distal tubule. The loop descends from the cortex into the medulla and then bends back sharply, returning to the cortex close to the vascular pole of its own glomerulus (the juxtaglomerular region of the loop of Henle adjacent to the juxtaglomerular apparatus), where it becomes continuous with the distal convoluted tubule. The distal convoluted tubule, much shorter than the proximal tubule, empties into a collecting tubule that passes through the medulla to drain into one of the minor calyces at the apex of a renal pyramid (renal papilla).

Tubular Functions

The renal tubules critically and selectively reabsorb water, minerals, and other substances that are to be conserved and excrete unwanted materials, which are eliminated. Urine is the glomerular filtrate that remains after most of the water and important constituents have been reabsorbed by the renal tubules and other substances excreted by the renal tubules have been added. The functions of the components of the nephron are summarized in **Table 17-2**.

Tubular Sodium Reabsorption

Renal regulation of sodium levels via reabsorption requires the movement of ions from the tubular lumen across the apical membrane (adjacent to the lumen) of the tubular epithelial cell and export of the ions from the basolateral membrane of the cell (adjacent to the renal interstitium) to the interstitium and the capillary network surrounding the tubules. The capillary network

Table 17-2 Functions of the Nephron and the Collecting Duct

Structure	Function
Renal Corpuscle	
Glomerulus	Filters water and dissolved substances from plasma
Glomerular capsule	Receives glomerular filtrate
Renal Tubule	
Proximal convoluted tubule	Reabsorbs 50% of sodium glucose, amino acids, creatinine acids, and ions by active transport; reabsorbs water by osmosis; reabsorbs chloride and other negative ions by electrochemical attraction; actively secretes creatinine and hydrogen ions
Descending limb of nephron loop	Reabsorbs water by osmosis
Ascending limb of nephron loop	Reabsorbs 40% of sodium, potassium, and chloride ions by active transport
Distal convoluted tubule	Reabsorbs 7% of sodium ions by active transport, reabsorbs water by osmosis and secretes hydrogen and potassium ions by electrochemical attraction
Collecting duct	Reabsorbs 3% of sodium and water by osmosis

(vasa recta) is formed from an extension of the efferent glomerular arteriole. Different segments of the tubular network differ in the exact mechanism of sodium ion uptake, but transmembrane carriers and channels are necessary to move the charged ion through the cell's lipid bilayer. The carriers may also co-transport other substances such as glucose and phosphate along with the sodium ions. The basolateral membrane uses a sodium-potassium ATPase pump to move the sodium to the interstitium. The pump maintains a negative charge in the cytoplasm of the tubular cell, allowing sodium co-transporters to function without expenditure of energy (**Figure 17-9**).

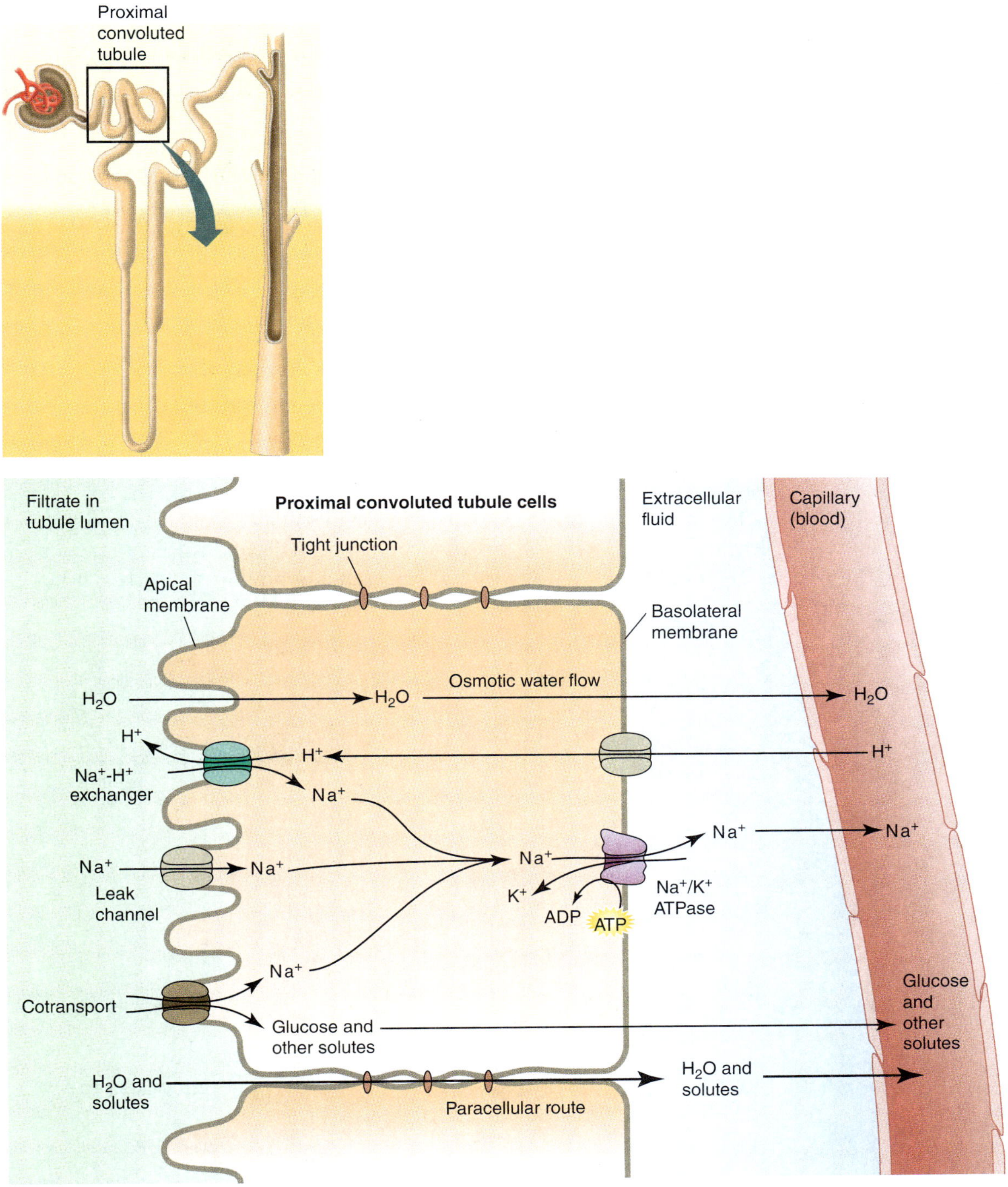

Figure 17-9 Reabsorption of sodium ions via ion exchangers, co-transporters, and sodium potassium pumps in the proximal tubule epithelial cell.

Tubular Water Reabsorption

As noted previously, the glomerulus is freely permeable to water and salts, and hence the glomerular filtrate is isosmotic to plasma. Humans have a highly variable water intake. If water is deprived, a more concentrated hyperosmotic urine must be produced (to conserve water loss) while still excreting waste. After high water consumption, a diluted and hypo-osmotic urine must be produced to remove excess fluid. The secretion of either dilute or concentrated urine is accomplished using a countercurrent amplification mechanism to establish an osmotic gradient combined with the effects of ADH (see the previous discussion) in the collecting ducts. A countercurrent mechanism involves the exchange of a property (heat, a chemical, or, in the renal case, ions and water) between two flowing fluid bodies moving in antiparallel directions. In the kidney this involves filtrate moving in the descending and ascending segments of the loop of Henle. The collecting ducts and tubular capillary network also play an important role. The countercurrent mechanism is most efficient in concentrating the glomerular filtrate in the longer loops that extend from the renal cortex to the medulla (juxtamedullary nephrons). Looking across species, animals that must conserve water and produce concentrated hyperosmotic urine (desert rats, for example) have very long loops compared to animals such as beavers, where a more dilute urine will suffice.

Countercurrent amplification depends on the fact that the descending limb of the loop of Henle is permeable to water but not ions, whereas the ascending limb of the loop is permeable to ions but not water. The only energy expended in concentrating the urine is that used by the ion co-transporter in the ascending limb to reabsorb sodium, pumping it to the interstitium. As sodium flows into the interstitium from the ascending loop, water is osmotically removed from the descending loop, concentrating the filtrate (urine) within. The cycle reoccurs constantly as fresh filtrate enters the descending loop. The net result is the formation of an osmotic gradient in the medulla of the kidney, with osmolality increasing along the length of the loop of Henle and adjacent interstitium (see **Figure 17-10**). As urine leaves the ascending limb in the cortex, it has an

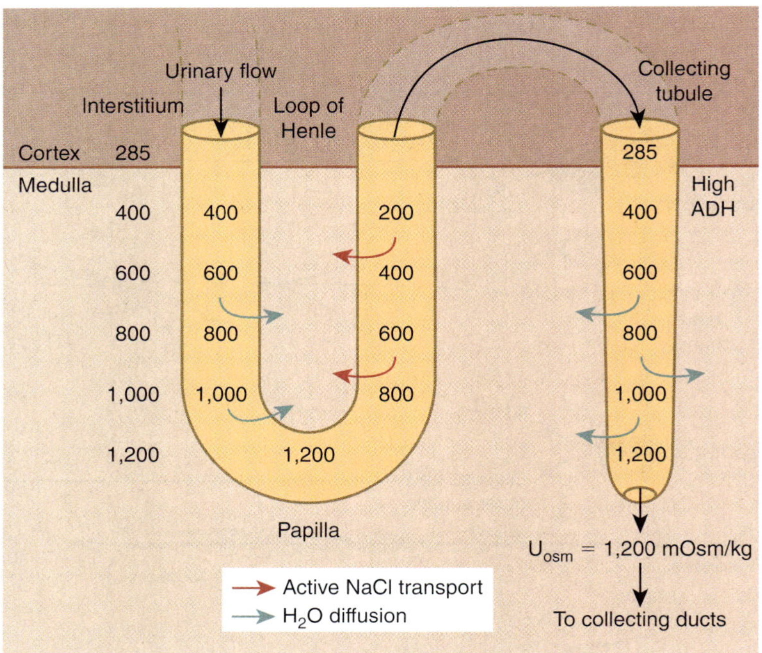

Figure 17-10 Urinary concentration by countercurrent amplification. Numbers represent urinary osmolality (in milliosmoles/kilogram) in the loops of Henle and collecting tubule. Final urine osmolality represents a fourfold concentration of urine.

osmolarity a bit less than plasma (it is not concentrated). It now enters the collecting tubule, descending into the hyperosmotic medullary interstitium. If ADH is present, water channels (aquaporins) open in the collecting tubule, and water is reabsorbed into the hypertonic interstitium. The system can concentrate the urine in the collecting tubule about fourfold versus plasma. In the absence of ADH, the collecting tubule is impermeable to water, and no water reabsorption occurs. Hence, dilute urine is produced. The capillary network (vasa recta) returns the fluid from the interstitium to the circulation.

Diuretics and Renal Function

Diuretics are drugs that increase the excretion of water and sodium and thereby reduce circulating volume. They are often used to treat hypertension and edema caused, for example, by congestive heart failure. The drugs function to reduce sodium reabsorption by inhibiting the movement of the ion across the tubular epithelial cell. There are three major classes of diuretics, which function at different sites in the nephron. Loop diuretics (such as furosemide) block sodium reabsorption in the ascending limb of Henle's loop. Because about 40 percent of sodium is normally reabsorbed at this site, this is the most potent class of diuretics. Thiazide-type diuretics (including hydrochlorothiazide) function in the distal tubule. They are less potent in action than the previous class and are most often used to treat hypertension. Both of these classes result in the loss of potassium and can result in hypokalemia (lower with clinical consequences). The last class of diuretics are potassium-sparing diuretics (such as amiloride and spironolactone), which function in the collecting tubules. A side effect of their action is the inhibition of potassium secretion at a site that is responsible for the greatest loss of potassium in untreated persons. These agents are not as potent as the other classes but are of particular use in patients with diabetes or significant kidney disease. The choice of agent class and dose must be made by the physician based on the particulars of individual patients.

Potassium Homeostasis

The kidney plays an important role in the homeostasis of small molecules other than sodium and water. Defects in sodium concentration include clinical symptoms such as dehydration and cerebral edema. From a clinical point of view, such effects tend to be gradual and can be compensated for. On the other hand, potassium, unlike sodium (the primary extracellular electrolyte), is the major intracellular electrolyte. Defects in potassium concentration are associated with nerve conduction and can result in abnormal cardiac rhythms and muscle function. Hyperkalemia can, if severe, lead to cardiac arrest and death. Hypokalemia, although uncommon, can also lead to EKG changes and cardiac arrhythmias. In addition, hypokalemia inhibits ADH function and can lead to polyuria and increased thirst.

Almost all potassium is intracellular, with only one percent being extracellular. However, an increase of only one percent in the extracellular pool can have drastic consequences. The potassium load of several glasses of orange juice would be sufficient to nearly double normal extracellular potassium if it remained in the extracellular space and could lead to symptoms. Short-term changes in potassium rely on cellular absorption via the sodium–potassium ATPase pump and release of the ion to the extracellular space. Longer term potassium homeostasis is maintained by the kidney. Renal potassium excretion occurs via a subset of cells (principal cells) in the collecting tubules.

Aldosterone release by the adrenal gland (see Chapter 22) increases principal cell secretion. The flow of sodium and water through the collecting tubules is also necessary for potassium secretion. For this reason, diuretics (particularly loop diuretics) increase potassium secretion by increasing sodium in the collecting tubules.

Disturbances of Normal Renal Function

Derangement of any function of the individual nephrons of the kidney results in kidney disease. For a nephron to function normally, there must be free flow of blood through the glomerular capillaries, the glomerular filter must function correctly, the tubules must be able to selectively reabsorb/excrete substances as needed, and the urine formed by the nephron must be able to flow freely from the kidney into the bladder. Therefore, failure of normal renal function, either acute or chronic, may have its roots in pre-renal disease, renal disease, or post-renal disease. An example of pre-renal disease is atherosclerosis of the renal artery, which by compromising blood flow to the kidney can lead to ischemic nephropathy. Post-renal diseases are often obstructive, compromising the ability of urine to flow freely through the bladder and lower urinary tract. Bladder stones, prostatic disease, and cancer may all cause urine to "back up" into the kidney and produce serious damage to the kidney tissue. Several systemic diseases (notably hypertension and diabetes) have both systemic vascular and renal consequences. Many of the diseases of the kidney relate to defects intrinsic to one of the renal compartments mentioned previously, predominantly glomerular or tubular.

Renal Failure (Uremia)

Renal failure is an inability of the kidneys to adequately perform their normal regulatory and excretory functions. Function may decline rapidly, which is termed acute renal injury, or slowly but progressively, which is termed chronic renal injury.

Uremia is the end stage of many different types of kidney disease. Metabolic acidosis occurs because the failing kidneys are unable to efficiently excrete the various acid waste products produced by the body's normal metabolic processes. **ketoacidosis** results from overproduction of the acid ketone bodies, acetoacetic acid, and beta-hydroxybutyric acid, which are derived from the metabolism of fat.

ketoacidosis A buildup of ketone bodies due to increased fat metabolism and decreased carbohydrate metabolism, often resulting in a decrease (acidification) of the plasma or other body fluids.

Chronic Kidney Disease

Definition and Frequency

A normal kidney contains about one million nephrons. In chronic renal failure, renal function declines as the population of functional nephrons decreases, although relatively normal renal function can be maintained until the number of functioning nephrons falls below 20 percent to 30 percent of normal. Unfortunately, all types of chronic renal disease tend to progress because of the way the surviving nephrons respond to the declining renal function. The surviving nephrons are forced to "work harder" to accomplish the functions previously performed by a full complement of nephrons. Each of the remaining nephrons receives a larger volume of blood to process at a higher-than-normal pressure.

Chronic kidney disease (CKD) is defined as an abnormal GFR or the presence of any of a number of other markers of kidney damage (such as albuminuria, the presence of albumin in the urine as a result of a defect in glomerular filtration; electrolyte abnormalities; or abnormal renal pathology) that has persisted for greater than 3 months. Chronic kidney disease may progress through a number of stages with increasing severity, eventually reaching stage 4, where renal function is severely depressed, and stage 5, end-stage renal disease (ESRD), with kidney failure, where treatment such as dialysis or transplantation must be undertaken to prevent uremia and preserve life. About 14 percent of the adult population has CKD, but the prevalence of the condition varies with age, race, and medical status, as does the rate of progression of the condition. For example, ESRD is four times higher in Blacks than Whites. Additionally, compared to Whites, Hispanic and Native Americans are twice a likely to develop ESRD with Asian people having a 1.6 times higher rate. The reason for the difference is partly genetic but probably also related to availability of specialized medical care. About 70 percent of ESRD patients are on dialysis, while the rest have had a renal transplant. Although only a small percentage of CKD patients have ESRD (about 0.4 percent), the economic impact of CKD is high. The mean annual all-cause medical costs for CKD patients are dependent on the stage of disease. Medical costs for patients at either stage 4 or 5 were $46,000 per annum in Medicare patients and $77,000 in non-Medicare patients. Excluding the cost of dialysis, ESRD patients had costs of $87,000 and $122,000 for the two groups. The fact that 40 percent of ESRD patients had type 2 diabetes mellitus and 27 percent had hypertension emphasizes the importance of CKD as a public health concern.

Pathophysiology of CKD

Chronic kidney disease, as noted previously, can result from many disease processes either intrinsic or extrinsic to the kidney (as a result of an extrinsic condition resulting in renal damage). The pathophysiology of CKD often is related to hemodynamic problems. Damage to nephrons leads to reduced renal functional mass. In turn, in an attempt to maintain the GFR, decreased perfusion pressure is sensed by the juxtaglomerular complex, resulting in the release of renin and activation of the RAAS (see the previous discussions). The resulting release of angiotensin II has a number of potentially harmful effects. It is an efficient vasoconstrictor at the level of the efferent glomerular arteriole, increasing intraglomerular filtration pressure, ultimately damaging the glomerular filtration barrier, and causing proteinuria. In addition, angiotensin II results in salt and water retention either at the level of the proximal tubule or via release of aldosterone by the adrenal gland. Activation of the RAAS also leads to non-hemodynamic injury to the kidney, including glomerular fibrosis and inflammation, mediated by the upregulation of several cytokines, including TGF-β. Stimulation by cytokines leads to both endothelial and mesangial hyperplasia and scarring (sclerosis) of glomeruli (**Figure 17-11**).

Hypertensive Nephrosclerosis

Hypertensive **nephrosclerosis** is the result of long-term primary hypertension (essential hypertension; see Chapter 10) and progressive CKD. Arteriolar nephrosclerosis (sometimes termed simply nephrosclerosis) is a complication of severe hypertension altering renal hemodynamics. Because of the extreme elevation of the systemic blood pressure, the small arterioles and arteries throughout the body are called on to carry blood at a much higher pressure

Nephrosclerosis
Thickening and narrowing of the afferent glomerular arterioles.

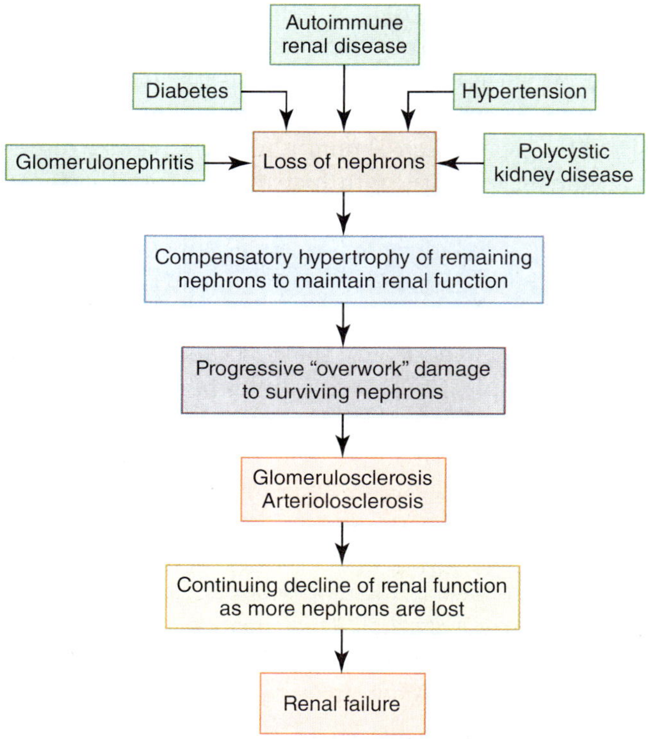

Figure 17-11 Self-perpetuating progression of chronic kidney disease.

than normal. As a result, the blood vessels undergo severe degenerative changes characterized by thickening and narrowing of the lumens, which reduces blood flow through the narrowed arterioles. The name of the disease, which means literally "sclerosis of the arterioles of the nephrons," refers to these characteristic renal vascular changes that result in damage to the nephrons and reduced blood flow to the glomerulus. Glomerular filtration is reduced because the arterioles are greatly narrowed. In addition, the increased glomerular pressure leads to damage to the filtration barrier and the cascade of pathophysiological changes discussed previously. In addition, the renal tubules, which also are supplied by the glomerular arterioles, also undergo degenerative changes. Eventually, the kidneys become shrunken and scarred as a result of reduction of their blood supply, and CKD ensues (**Figure 17-12**). Patients with severe hypertensive nephrosclerosis suffer from ESRD as well as from the systemic effects of severe hypertension.

Diabetic Nephropathy

About half of all patients with ESRD have diabetes, generally type 2 diabetic disease, which is often complicated with hypertension. Once initiated, diabetic CKD cannot be reversed, but the process leading to ESRD can be slowed by control of hypertension and blood sugar levels (strict glycemic control). The beneficial effect of glycemic control suggests that factors other than hypertension are significant in renal disease. This is likely related to modification and damage of the glycocalyx (the carbohydrate-rich layer surrounding the renal cells) resulting from the presence of high circulating sugar levels.

Early changes in diabetic nephropathy (nephros = kidney + path = disease, used when referring to both the characteristic glomerular and the arteriolar lesions) include arteriolar hyalinosis (referring to the deposition of a smooth-appearing, PAS-positive material [PAS being a histologic staining procedure

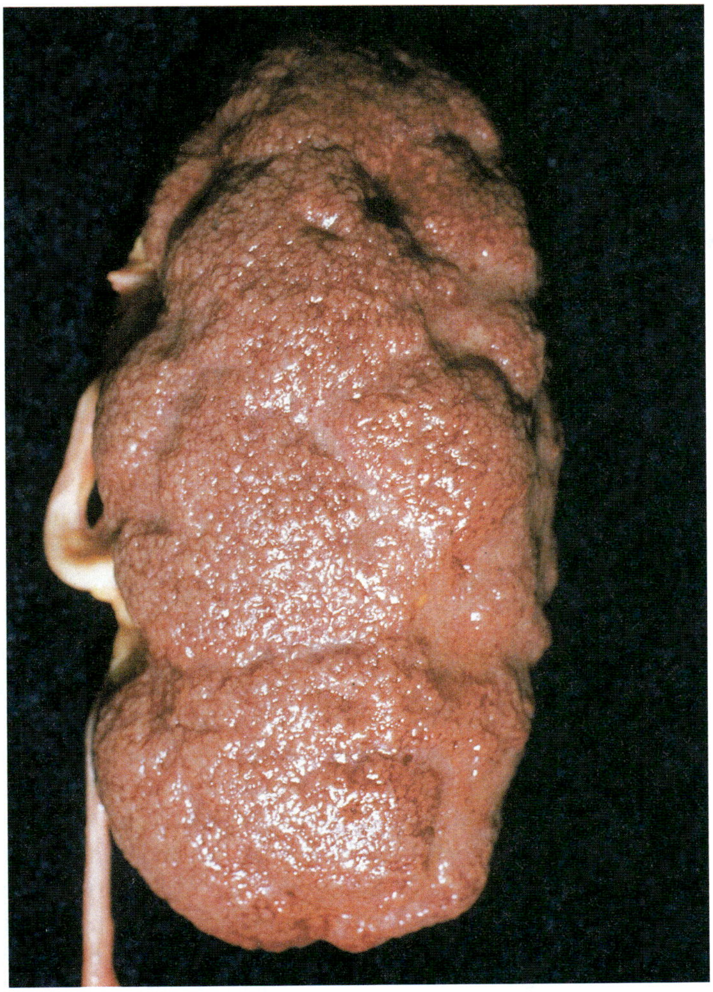

Figure 17-12 Irregular scarring of kidney as a result of nephrosclerosis.
Courtesy of Leonard V. Crowley, MD, Century College.

highlighting carbohydrate-containing components]) in the walls of the afferent and efferent glomerular arterioles, observed by microscopy. Similar material is found deposited in the basement membrane of glomerular capillaries and tubules. Such changes are associated with proteinuria related to damage of the glomerular filtration apparatus. Mesangial expansion occurs with the deposition of such material, which in extreme cases forms nodular structures (Kimmelstiel-Wilson nodules) that are characteristic of severe **diabetic glomerulosclerosis** and occur in about half of the patients (**Figure 17-13**).

Clinically, diabetic nephropathy is characterized by progressive impairment of renal function that eventually will lead to renal failure with increasing proteinuria as protein leaks through the damaged glomeruli and is lost in the urine. No specific treatment can arrest the progression of the disease. A renal transplant may be required if the patient develops renal failure (see Chapter 22).

Diabetic glomerulosclerosis Diffuse and nodular thickening of glomerular basement membranes, a common occurrence in patients with long-standing diabetes mellitus.

End-Stage Renal Disease (ESRD)

Without intervention, CKD will eventually progress to the point where the kidneys are no longer able to perform their regulatory and excretory functions. The patient experiences severe derangements of fluid, electrolyte, and

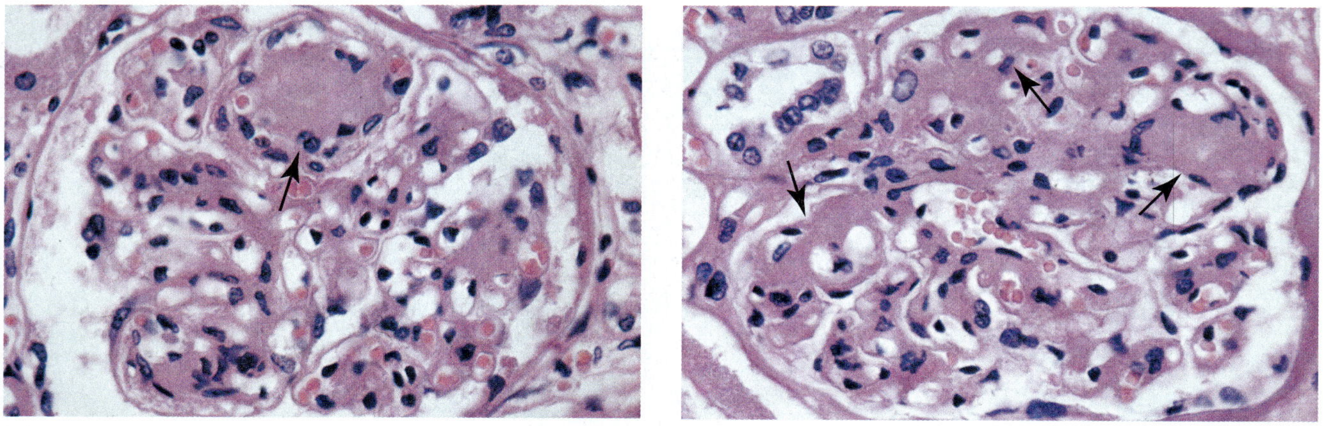

(A) (B)

Figure 17-13 **(A)** Nodular glomerulosclerosis. Nodular areas of glomerular basement membrane thickening (Kimmelstiel-Wilson nodules) (*arrow*) are characteristic of diabetes. **(B)** Diffuse glomerulosclerosis. Diffuse glomerular basement membrane thickening (*arrows*) also occurs in diabetes, but it may occur in other types of glomerular disease as well.
Courtesy of Leonard V. Crowley, MD, Century College.

acid–base balance. Various acids normally excreted by the kidneys are retained, which disturbs the normal pH of body fluids, leading to metabolic acidosis (described in the earlier discussion on water, electrolyte, and acid–base balance). The failing kidneys cannot produce erythropoietin to stimulate bone marrow function, and the patient becomes anemic. As noted previously, renal failure is sometimes termed uremia. This term refers to the characteristic retention of urea in the blood when the kidneys fail. Urea is a normal by-product of protein metabolism and is excreted in the urine. It is not the principal toxic compound but is only one of many toxic substances that accumulates in the blood when the kidneys fail. The amount of urea in the blood, however, correlates with the degree of retention of other waste products and with the clinical manifestations of deteriorating renal function. Therefore, measurement of the concentration of urea in the blood (blood urea nitrogen [BUN] test) provides a rough estimate of the severity of the kidney failure. Another commonly used measure of renal functional impairment is the level of creatinine in the blood.

Symptoms of renal failure are nonspecific. They begin to appear when about 80 percent of renal function has been lost and are quite pronounced by the time when renal function has fallen to 5 percent of normal. Symptoms include weakness, loss of appetite, nausea, and vomiting. Production of red cells by the bone marrow decreases because the failing kidneys cannot produce erythropoietin to stimulate bone marrow function, and the patient becomes moderately anemic. Waste products are not eliminated and increase to toxic levels. Excess salt and water are retained by the failing kidneys, resulting in weight gain. The blood volume increases because of fluid retention, and the blood pressure also tends to rise as the intravascular volume increases. If untreated, the patient in chronic renal failure eventually lapses into coma, may have convulsions, and eventually dies.

Treatment for Renal Failure

The outlook for patients with renal failure and ESRD has improved dramatically in recent years because of three effective methods of treatment: hemodialysis, peritoneal dialysis, and renal transplantation. Hemodialysis and peritoneal dialysis remove waste products from the patient's blood. Both methods are equally effective, and each has advantages and disadvantages. Every year, many new patients with advanced renal disease begin dialysis. Some will continue on dialysis indefinitely. Others will rely on dialysis until a kidney becomes available for transplantation. Renal transplantation, using kidneys from living related donors or recently deceased persons (cadaveric donors), is the most desirable option; however, kidneys for transplantation are in limited supply.

Hemodialysis

Hemodialysis substitutes for the functions of the kidneys. Waste products from the patient's blood diffuse across a semi-permeable membrane into a solution (the dialysate) on the other side of the membrane. The rate of diffusion is determined by several factors: the concentration of the substances on the two sides of the membrane, the rate of blood flow and flow of the dialysate through the dialyzer, and the characteristics of the dialyzer membrane. Waste products, which are present in high concentrations in the patient's blood, diffuse from the blood into the dialysate because of differences in the concentration on the two sides of the membrane. Usually, the patient's blood is dialyzed by an "artificial kidney" machine. This type of hemodialysis is termed extracorporeal hemodialysis (extra = outside + corpus = body) because the blood is transported outside the patient's body for dialysis in the artificial kidney and then returned by means of a system of tubes connected to the patient's circulatory system.

Hemodialysis is usually performed in an outpatient dialysis center three times per week for 3 or 4 hours during each dialysis session, but it can be performed at home by the patient with the assistance of a family member who has been given special training. The patient's blood flows along one side of a synthetic semi-permeable membrane that restricts the passage of blood cells and protein but permits the passage of water and small molecules. The dialysate flows on the other side of the membrane in a direction opposite to the flow of blood. This type of flow pattern, which is termed countercurrent dialysis, promotes more efficient removal of waste products than when dialysate and blood flow in the same direction.

During dialysis, plastic tubes connect the patient's circulation to the dialyzer in the artificial kidney machine. One tube transmits blood to the dialyzer unit, where the blood is cleansed and excess fluid is removed, and the other tube conveys the blood from the dialyzer back to the patient's circulation. Before dialysis begins, the coagulability of the patient's blood is reduced by administration of heparin to prevent the blood from clotting as it flows through the dialyzer.

To perform hemodialysis on a regular basis, one of the patient's arteries and a large vein must be easily accessible so that the tubes that transport blood to and from the dialyzer unit can easily and repeatedly be connected to the patient's blood vessels. Although several methods have been devised to gain access to the patient's circulation, the preferred method consists of surgically interconnecting the radial artery in the wrist and an adjacent vein, forming an artificial communication termed an arteriovenous fistula (**Figure 17-14A**). After the fistula has been created, arterial blood is short-circuited directly into the vein instead of flowing through the peripheral capillaries. The vein, which now receives blood directly under high pressure, becomes much larger and develops a thick wall over a several-month period. When the vein has become suitable for use, dialysis treatments begin. Two needles are inserted through the skin

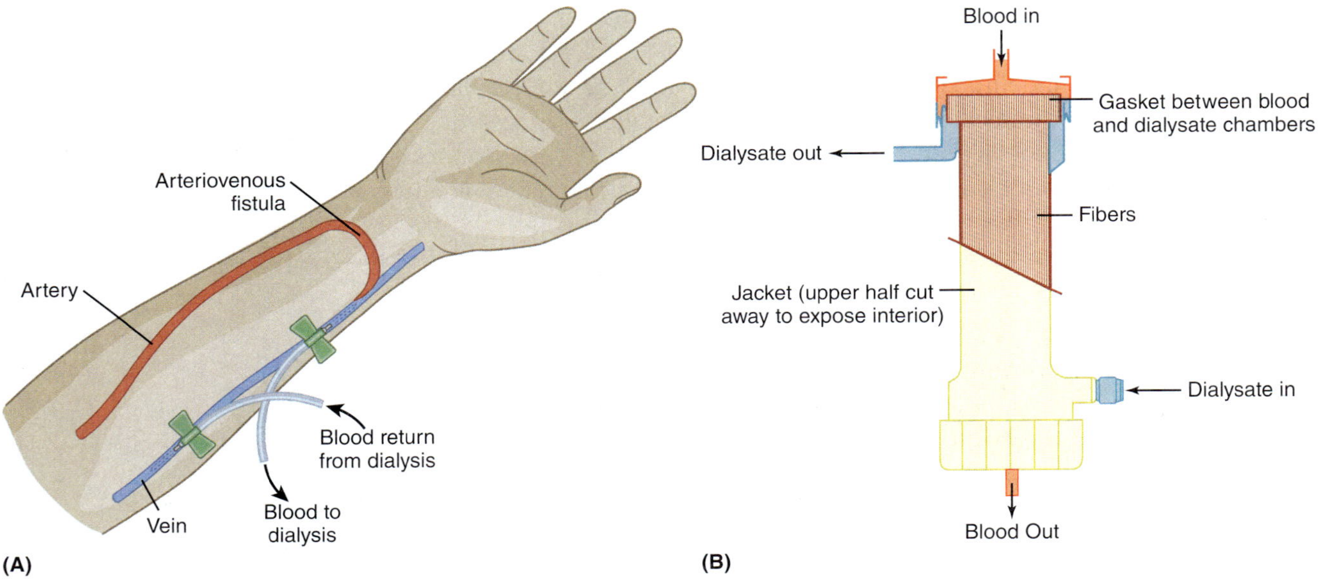

Figure 17-14 **(A)** Arteriovenous fistula created between the radial artery and adjacent vein. **(B)** Hollow fiber dialyzer.

directly into the vein. One needle is attached to the tube that delivers blood to the dialyzer, and the second needle is attached to the tube that returns the blood to the patient. Less commonly, other procedures are used to gain access to the patient's circulation for dialysis.

The essential component of the artificial kidney machine is the dialyzer. Attached to it are the tubes that carry blood to and from the patient and the tubes that carry dialysate to and from the unit. A hollow fiber dialyzer, which is quite compact and efficient and is the most commonly used type, consists of a bundle of hollow synthetic fibers through which the blood passes. The dialysate circulates around the outside of the fibers in the opposite direction (**Figure 17-14B**).

Peritoneal Dialysis

Peritoneal dialysis uses the patient's own peritoneum as the dialyzing membrane. To perform peritoneal dialysis, a large plastic tube must first be inserted into the patient's abdominal (peritoneal) cavity and fixed in position by suturing it to the skin. The dialysis procedure consists of instilling several liters of dialysis fluid through the tube into the peritoneal cavity and allowing the fluid to remain within the peritoneal cavity for a variable time. During this time, waste products diffuse across the peritoneum from the underlying blood vessels into the dialysis fluid that fills the peritoneal cavity. Dialysis fluid is then withdrawn, and fresh fluid is instilled. Peritoneal dialysis can be performed by means of an automated system in which the machine automatically fills and drains the peritoneal cavity at night while the patient is asleep. Another similar method is termed continuous ambulatory peritoneal dialysis. In this procedure, two liters of fluid remain within the peritoneal cavity all the time. The patient replaces the fluid with fresh dialysis fluid four or five times a day. Patients carry out their usual activities when they are not draining and refilling their peritoneal cavities.

Peritoneal dialysis is used less frequently than extracorporeal hemodialysis. Not all patients requiring dialysis are suitable candidates for peritoneal dialysis, but the procedure offers an advantage to patients who wish to continue working full time or part time, as they do not have to spend several daytime hours 3 days each week at a dialysis center, and many patients who choose peritoneal dialysis are quite satisfied with their choice. However, peritoneal dialysis has disadvantages. It is less efficient at removing waste products and carries some risk of peritonitis, which can result if bacteria gain access to the peritoneal cavity around the tube that extends from the skin surface directly into the peritoneal cavity.

Renal Transplantation

When the kidneys fail, a normal compatible kidney sometimes can be transplanted from a close relative, an unrelated volunteer donor, or a recently deceased person (cadaveric donor). Although a renal transplant improves the patient's quality of life and is less costly than dialysis, only 20% of patients with ESRD will receive a transplant because of medical concerns and a limited number of donor kidneys. About one-third of transplants are from living donors, which produce the best outcomes even when such donors are not completely compatible.

In any kidney transplantation, an attempt is made to match the transplanted kidney as closely as possible with the recipient to give the transplant the best chance of survival in the recipient. Unless the transplanted kidney comes from an identical twin, the transplant will invariably contain foreign antigens that the patient lacks. Consequently, the patient's immunologic defenses will respond to the foreign antigens and attempt to destroy (reject) the foreign kidney unless the patient's immune system is suppressed by drugs (see Chapter 5).

The ABO blood group antigens of the proposed donor must be compatible with the blood group antibodies in the blood of the proposed recipient because the ABO blood group antigens are present in body tissues (including the kidney) as well as on red blood cells.

The next group of important antigens are the HLA antigens (discussed in Chapter 5). Unless an identical twin donor is available, the best results are obtained from siblings who have identical HLA antigens. The use of potent immunosuppressive drugs has much improved the overall survival rate of transplanted kidneys even with donors who are not closely matched; however, overall, the closer the match, the better the odds for long-term survival. The overall 1-year survival rate for transplants is as high as 95 percent. A 10-year survival rate of 86 percent is achieved with living donors, 72–76 percent with cadaveric kidney transplants. Some patients, however, reject the transplant despite intensive immunosuppressive therapy. Most rejections occur within the first few months after transplantation. Should this occur, the patient resumes dialysis treatments until another kidney suitable for transplantation becomes available.

Although a well-functioning transplanted kidney permits the patient to lead a relatively normal life, the patient with a renal transplant may have other problems. Immunosuppressive drugs may need to be continued indefinitely to prevent rejection of the foreign kidney, and adverse side effects sometimes result from these drugs. The immunosuppressed patient is also more susceptible to infection because the body's immune defenses have been weakened so the transplant can survive. Occasionally, the disease that destroyed the patient's own kidneys, such as **glomerulonephritis** (see the following discussion), also destroys the function of the transplanted kidney.

Glomerulonephritis An inflammation of the glomeruli caused by either antigen–antibody complexes trapped in the glomeruli or by antiglomerular basement membrane antibodies.

Diseases of the Renal Compartments

Glomerular Disease

Glomerulonephritis

Glomerulonephritis (often referred to as nephritis), an inflammation of the glomeruli often caused by an immune reaction within the glomerulus (including the glomerular capillaries and mesangium), will result in an inflammatory influx of leukocytes and injury to the glomerulus, which, if severe, will result in glomerular necrosis. The signs and symptoms of glomerulonephritis are related to the changes within the glomeruli. When many glomeruli are damaged or destroyed by inflammation, less blood is filtered and less urine is excreted. As urinary output is reduced, waste products are retained and accumulate in the blood. Glomeruli, damaged by inflammatory lysosomal enzymes, are no longer able to function as efficient filters. Protein and red cells leak through the damaged glomerular capillary walls and are excreted in the urine. Frequently, masses of red cells and protein accumulate within the tubules and become molded to the shape of the renal tubules before finally being excreted. These structures, which are termed urinary casts, are an important indication of glomerular injury. Patients with glomerulonephritis are often hypertensive and have some degree of renal failure. Depending on the severity of disease, they may also show proteinuria (but not as severe as that in nephritic syndrome, discussed later in this chapter). In some cases, glomerulonephritis may progress so rapidly that ESRD occurs and dialysis is needed within months to sustain life, a condition termed rapidly progressive glomerulonephritis (RPGN).

The glomerular inflammation can be the result of the formation of antigen–antibody complexes either within the glomerular capillaries or deposited within the glomerulus from the circulation. The interaction of antigen and antibody activates complement and liberates mediators that attract polymorphonuclear leukocytes to the glomerulus. The actual glomerular injury is caused by destructive lysosomal enzymes that are released from the leukocytes that have accumulated within the glomeruli. In some cases (antineutrophil cytoplasmic antibody [ANCA] glomerulonephritis), antibodies bind directly to the surface of the leukocytes and cause them to release the destructive mediators within the glomerulus.

The antigen–antibody reaction within the glomeruli may take place in two ways. Either immune complexes are deposited on the walls of the glomerular capillaries, or an autoantibody can react with the capillary basement membrane. **Figure 17-15** illustrates the histologic appearance of these two types of glomerulonephritis compared with the appearance of a normal glomerulus. In ANCA glomerulonephritis, there is no deposition of antibody within the glomerulus (but rather direct activation of inflammatory cells).

Poststreptococcal Immune-Complex Glomerulonephritis

Immune-complex glomerulonephritis may develop as a complication about 2 weeks after infection by certain beta hemolytic streptococci, the same type of organism that causes the familiar streptococcal sore throat. Fortunately, glomerular inflammation occurs only in a small percentage of patients with streptococcal infections and usually resolves spontaneously. In affected individuals (most often children), the body responds to the streptococcal infection

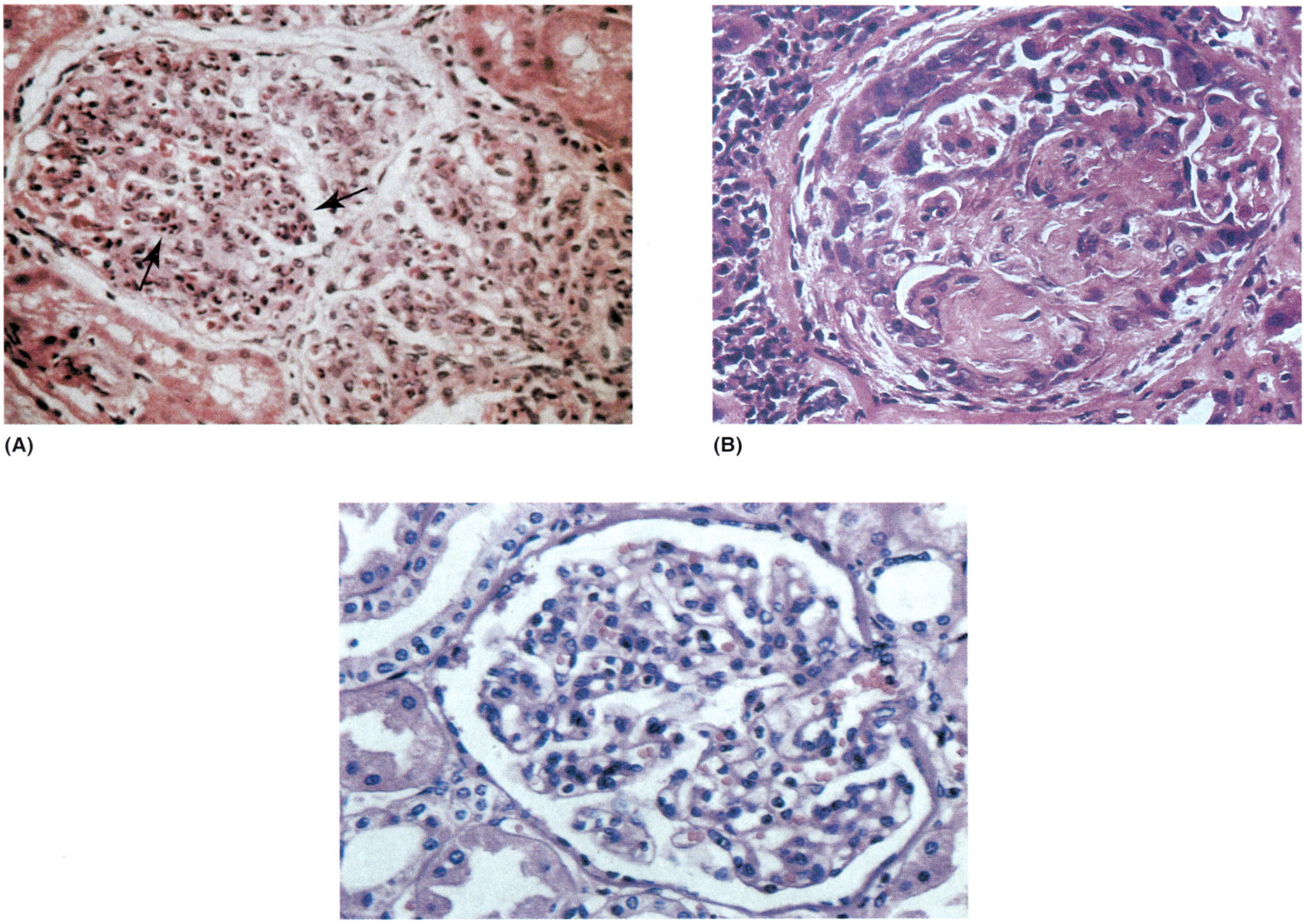

(A) (B) (C)

Figure 17-15 **(A)** Immune-complex glomerulonephritis. Two glomeruli contain large numbers of neutrophils (*arrows*). **(B)** Anti-GBM glomerulonephritis; revealing severe glomerular injury and scarring. **(C)** Normal glomerulus for comparison (original magnification ×400).

Courtesy of Leonard V. Crowley, MD, Century College.

by forming antistreptococcal antibodies that interact with soluble antigens from the streptococci in the bloodstream to form immune complexes. Some of the antigen–antibody complexes are small enough to pass completely through the walls of the glomerular capillaries and be excreted in the urine. Larger complexes, however, pass through the endothelium and basement membranes of the glomerular capillaries but become trapped between the filtration slits of the glomerular epithelial cells in a subepithelial position, where they induce an inflammatory reaction. **Figure 17-16** demonstrates a case of this disease. (The patient recovered slowly, and a biopsy was necessary to confirm the diagnosis.)

Acute glomerulonephritis may at times follow other bacterial or viral infections. **Type I membranoproliferative glomerulonephritis** is a more severe form of the disease associated with infections of the heart, bone, and hepatitis C. In this condition, immune complexes are also found in the mesangium, which results in the influx of inflammatory cells to this location and proliferation of mesangial cells. The basement membrane of the glomerular capillaries becomes markedly thickened (**Figure 17-17**). The mechanism of glomerular injury is similar to that of poststreptococcal glomerulonephritis in that immune complexes play a critical role. Elimination of the infection sometimes

Type I membranoproliferative glomerulonephritis A more severe form of glomerulonephritis associated with infections of the heart, bone, and hepatitis C.

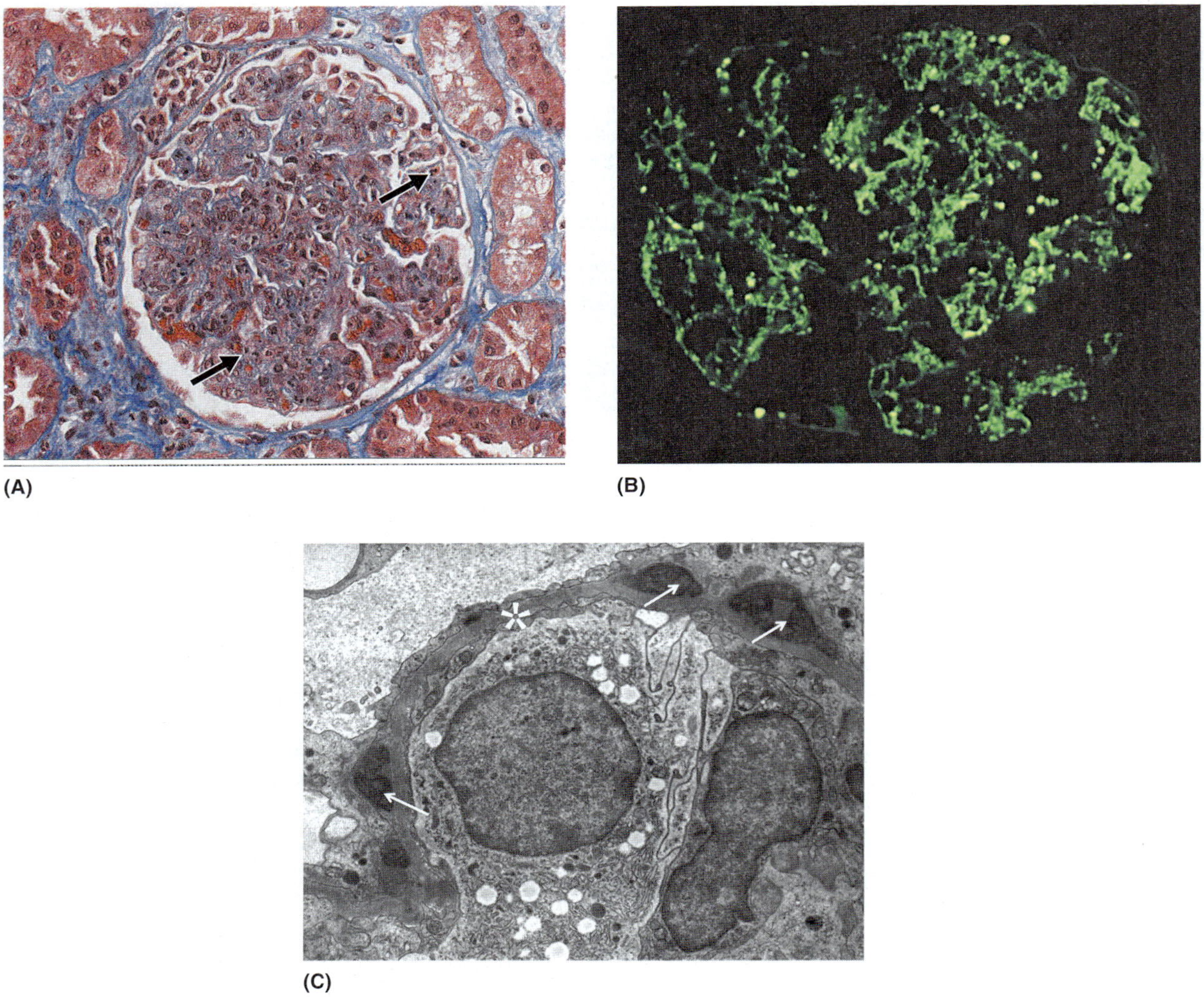

Figure 17-16 **(A)** Glomerulus from a patient with poststreptococcal glomerulonephritis. Several inflammatory cells (neutrophils) are indicated (*arrows*) on the trichrome stain of the biopsy specimen (the blue color highlights connective tissue). Compare with Figure 17-15C. **(B)** Biopsy from the same case stained with a fluorescent antibody that detects human IgG. The "bumpy" green color indicates deposited immune complexes. **(C)** Electron micrograph of biopsy from the case showing immune complexes (*arrows*) trapped beneath the basement membrane (*star*). The lumen of the capillary is filled with inflammatory cells.

results in a cure, whereas in other cases the glomerulonephritis never heals completely. Although poststreptococcal glomerulonephritis is usually acute and self-limited, type I membranoproliferative glomerulonephritis often becomes chronic, progresses slowly, and eventually causes renal failure.

Another relatively common type of immune-complex glomerulonephritis is associated with proliferation of mesangial cells and accumulation of immune complexes containing immunoglobulin A (IgA) within the cells. Because of the type of immunoglobulin associated with the disease, it is often termed IgA nephropathy (or Berger disease). Unfortunately, this type of glomerulonephritis becomes chronic in many patients and is slowly progressive.

Immune-complex glomerulonephritis may also occur in association with autoimmune diseases in which autoantibody-containing immune complexes become trapped in renal glomeruli, as in systemic lupus erythematosus (SLE) (see Chapter 5). Several classes of glomerular disease occur with SLE, and some may be rapidly progressive.

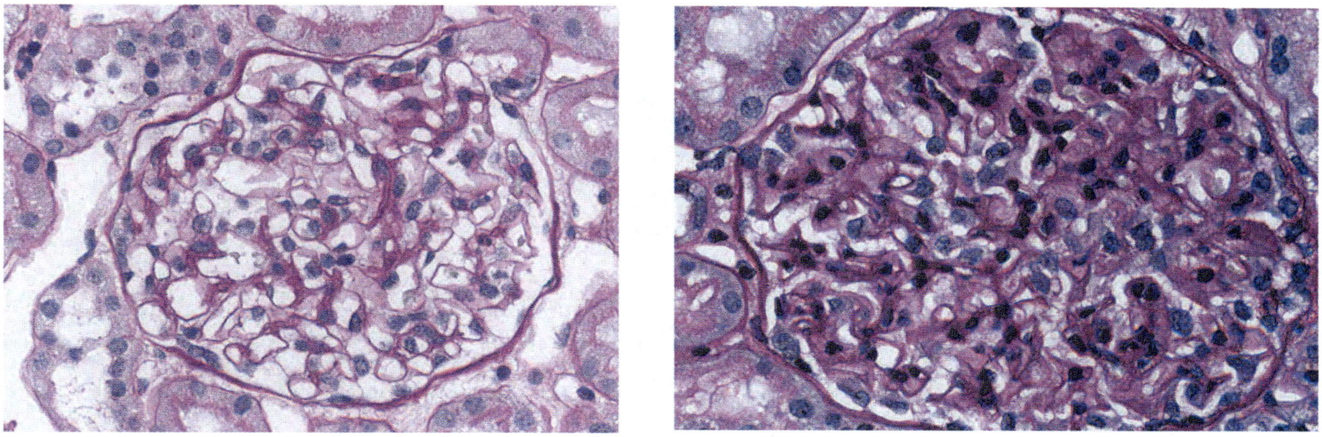

(A) (B)

Figure 17-17 The two glomeruli have been stained with PAS to highlight basement membranes (in fuchsia). **(A)** Normal glomerulus. **(B)** Glomerulus from a patient with membranoproliferative glomerulonephritis. Note the much-thickened basement membranes lining the capillaries.

Courtesy of Drs Singh & Nickeleit, Department of Pathology and Laboratory Medicine, University of North Carolina at Chapel Hill.

Anti-GBM Glomerulonephritis

Glomerulonephritis caused by autoantibodies directed against glomerular basement membranes (anti-glomerular basement membrane [GBM] glomerulonephritis) is a relatively uncommon autoimmune disease. In some patients, the anti-GBM antibodies may also injure the basement membranes of the pulmonary capillaries and may cause intrapulmonary hemorrhage as well as acute glomerulonephritis (Goodpasture syndrome).

Special studies on biopsy tissue can distinguish immune-complex glomerulonephritis from anti-GBM glomerulonephritis. Immune-complex glomerulonephritis is characterized by large, irregular, lumpy deposits composed of antigen, antibody, and complement. These deposits form along the outer surface of the glomerular basement membranes, where the complexes have been trapped between the filtration slits of the glomerular epithelial cells. In contrast, anti-GBM nephritis is characterized by a relatively uniform layer of antibody and complement deposited along the inner surface of the glomerular basement membranes. Anti-GBM disease is severe and rapidly progressive, leading to ESRD if immunosuppressive therapy is ineffective. Patients with anti-GBM disease almost always have **crescentic glomerulonephritis**, in which Bowman's space (surrounding the glomerular capillary tuft) becomes filled with proliferating cells derived from the parietal epithelium of Bowman's capsule, possibly as a result of inflammatory cytokines that leak into the space from the damaged glomerular capillaries (**Figure 17-18**).

Crescentic glomerulonephritis
Form of glomerulonephritis in which Bowman's space (surrounding the glomerular capillary tuft) becomes filled with proliferating cells derived from the parietal epithelium of Bowman's capsule.

ANCA Glomerulonephritis

ANCA-associated glomerulonephritis is the result of autoimmune ANCA antibodies that react with cytoplasmic components of neutrophils. When ANCA antibodies react with their target antigens (which transiently are expressed on the surface of neutrophils), the cells become activated and provoke an inflammatory reaction that destroys the glomerular capillary endothelial cells. ANCA disease is very severe and may progress rapidly, resulting in crescentic glomerulonephritis (Figure 17-18). In the absence of effective immunosuppressive therapy, ESRD will occur in most patients within 5 years.

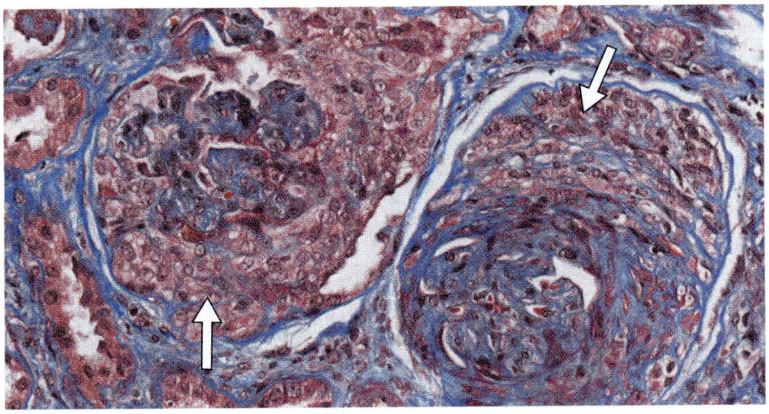

Figure 17-18 Rapidly progressive glomerulonephritis from a patient with ANCA glomerulonephritis. Two glomeruli are trichrome-stained to emphasize connective tissue/scarring (in blue). The glomerulus on the right is necrotic. Both demonstrate crescent formation (*arrows*).

Courtesy of Drs Singh & Nickeleit, Department of Pathology and Laboratory Medicine, University of North Carolina at Chapel Hill.

Many patients with ANCA glomerulonephritis also have small vessel vasculitis (inflammation of capillaries and venules), which results in disease in many additional organ systems.

Nephrotic Syndrome

Glomerular renal disease that is associated with extreme proteinuria (loss of protein into the urine greater than 3 g/24 hr) defines **nephrosis**, also termed **nephrotic syndrome**. Urinary excretion of protein is so great that the body is unable to manufacture protein fast enough to keep up with the losses, resulting in the concentration of protein in the blood plasma decreasing. This, in turn, causes significant edema owing to the low plasma osmotic pressure, which can be widespread and severe (termed **anasarca**) (see Chapter 10). Nephrotic patients also may have hyperlipidemia and secrete lipids in their urine as **fatty casts**, aggregated lipids that maintain the cylindrical shape of the tubule where they were formed.

Nephrosis Renal disease resulting from excessive protein loss in the urine, caused by various types of renal injury. Also referred to as nephrotic syndrome.
Nephrotic syndrome Characterized by severe loss of plasma protein into urine.
Anasarca Widespread edema.
Fatty casts Aggregated lipids that maintain the cylindrical shape of the tubule.
Minimal change nephropathy Common kidney disease of young children that is generally idiopathic.

Nephrotic syndrome may be produced by a number of different types of renal diseases. The basic cause is injury to the glomerular filtration barrier, allowing proteins to leak into the urinary space. Because the albumin molecule is much smaller than the globulin molecule, a disproportionately large amount of albumin is lost in the urine. The osmotic pressure of the plasma falls to such an extent that excessive amounts of fluid leak from the capillaries into the interstitial tissues and body cavities. Patients with the nephrotic syndrome have marked leg edema, and fluid often collects in the abdominal cavity (termed ascites); sometimes fluid also accumulates in the pleural cavities (termed hydrothorax).

When the nephrotic syndrome occurs in children, it is usually caused by extensive loss of the foot processes (termed effacement) of the glomerular epithelial cells (see the previous discussion). Because no abnormality is seen in the glomerulus by light microscopy, this is termed **minimal change nephropathy**. Nephrotic syndrome caused by this type of glomerular abnormality responds to corticosteroid therapy, and most children recover completely.

In contrast to the favorable outcome in children, nephrotic syndrome in adults is usually a manifestation of progressive, more serious renal disease in which there are marked structural changes in the glomeruli. The most

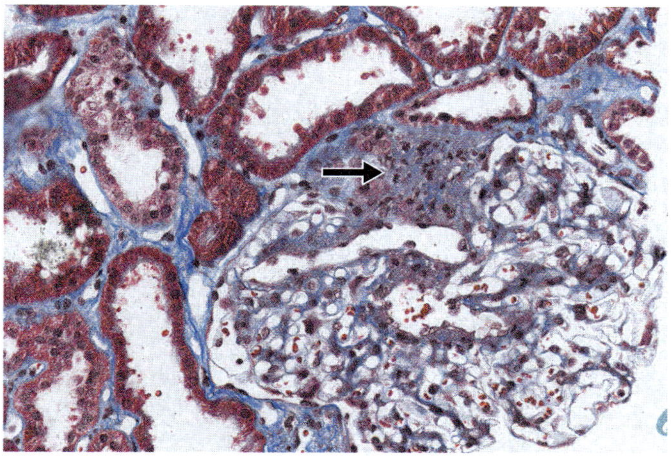

Figure 17-19 Renal biopsy from a patient with focal segmental glomerulosclerosis (FSGS), stained with trichrome stain. The glomerulus (on the edge of the biopsy) shows focal sclerosis (scarring) (*arrow*).

Courtesy of Drs Singh & Nickeleit, Department of Pathology and Laboratory Medicine, University of North Carolina at Chapel Hill.

common nephrotic disease in White and Asiatic adults is **membranous glomerulopathy**. The disease is characterized by markedly thickened capillary basement walls as a result of immune complex formation. In many cases, the immune complexes form within the glomerulus as a result of circulating autoantibodies that react with a component of podocytes. The disease is very variable; sometimes it may go into remission, while at other times it may continue to progress. In adult Blacks, **focal segmental glomerulosclerosis (FSGS)** is most common. The name derives from the fact that only some glomeruli show abnormalities, and often only a portion of a given glomerulus is affected. As previously noted, sclerosis refers to the production of collagen-containing scars within the glomerulus. The disease is not related to immune complex formation but is associated with a variety of etiologic agents, including viruses, familial mutations, drugs, and "overwork," and is seen in people with obesity or occasionally in people with only a single functioning kidney. The disease prognosis depends on the cause and is usually slowly progressive (**Figure 17-19**).

Membranous glomerulopathy A slowly progressive disease of the glomeruli most often found in White and Asian patients between the ages of thirty and fifty.

Focal segmental glomerulosclerosis (FSGS) Scar tissue in the filtering unit of the kidney.

Acute Renal Tubular Injury

Acute tubular injury is the cause of more than half of all intrinsic renal diseases. Renal tubular injury without accompanying glomerular disease may be encountered in two situations: tubular injury as a result of impaired renal blood flow or tubular injury caused by toxic drugs, chemicals, infectious agents, and particularly allergic responses to antibiotics. The blood supply to the renal tubules is derived from the efferent glomerular artery, and minor degrees of tubular injury are seen in many diseases affecting the renal glomeruli. Any condition associated with shock and a marked drop in blood pressure leads to impaired blood flow to the kidneys, which often causes damage and flattening of proximal tubular epithelial cells. Edema in the interstitium of the kidney and debris within the tubular lumens also occur. Many drugs (such as aminoglycoside antibiotics) and chemicals that are ingested or absorbed by the body are excreted by the kidneys. Thus, they may cause direct toxic injury to the tubular epithelium, which may be associated with necrosis of the epithelial cells (**Figure 17-20**).

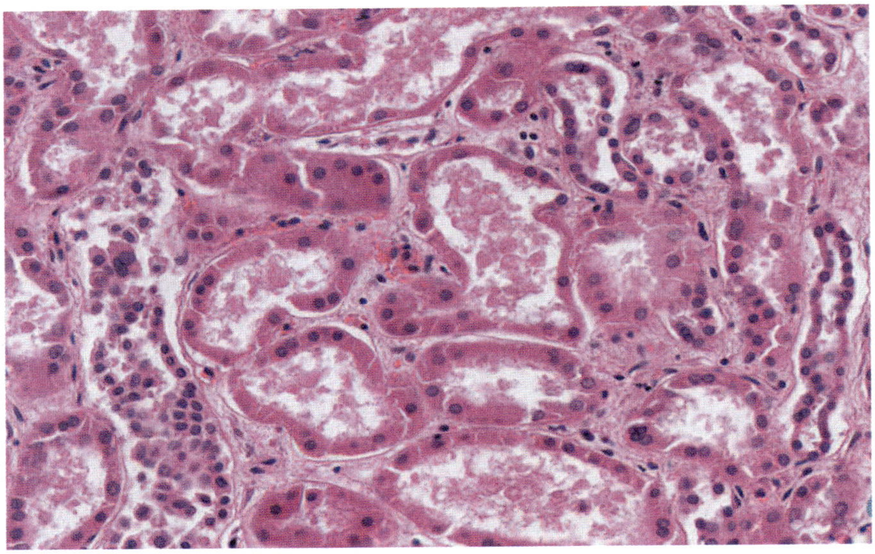

Figure 17-20 Acute tubular injury. Most of the tubules demonstrate flattening of epithelial cells and cellular necrosis shown by loss of nuclei and detachment from basement membranes. The tubules are filled with cellular debris and detached epithelial cells.

Courtesy of Department of Pathology and Laboratory Medicine, University of North Carolina at Chapel Hill.

Acute kidney injury (AKI) Injury to any part of the kidney. May also be defined as prerenal or postrenal.

Acute tubular injury causes severe impairment of renal function characterized by a marked decrease in urine output (oliguria) or complete suppression of urine formation (anuria). This condition is termed **acute kidney injury (AKI)** (or sometimes acute renal failure). The reason urine output is reduced is not well understood. Apparently, marked constriction of renal arterioles reduces blood flow to the kidneys and decreases glomerular filtration. Other factors also may contribute to the reduction of urine output. Many of the tubules are blocked by casts and necrotic debris. The damaged tubular epithelium also has lost its capacity for selective tubular reabsorption, and the glomerular filtrate diffuses back through the damaged tubular epithelium into the adjacent peritubular blood vessels. After a period of several weeks, tubular function is slowly restored by regeneration of the damaged epithelium, but several months may be required before renal function returns to normal completely. During the period of acute renal injury, waste products must be removed from the blood by means of dialysis until tubular function has been restored.

Tubulointerstitial Nephritis

Both tubules and the surrounding renal interstitium may be involved in both acute and chronic disease (tubulointerstitial nephritis). This may be related to an infectious process (pyelonephritis) or to an inflammatory immune process associated with the reaction to a drug, termed hypersensitive acute interstitial nephritis. Several days to weeks after taking the inciting agent, a sudden impairment in renal function may occur. This is most often mild and associated with low-grade fever, rash, and joint pain. Eosinophils, characteristic of an allergic reaction, are often present in the interstitial tissue. A more serious chronic form of the condition is associated with long-term abuse of analgesics, such as aspirin and non-steroidal anti-inflammatory drugs.

Other Renal Diseases

Renal Cysts

Solitary cysts of the kidney are relatively common. They vary in diameter from a few millimeters to about 15 cm. They are most often found in the cortex and may extend outside of the body of the kidney. Simple cysts are generally filled with fluid and are lined by a single layer of cells. They are not associated with impairment of renal function and are of no significance to the patient. Complex renal cysts may infiltrate into the body of the kidney and have a complex internal structure. Complex cysts may be associated with cancer or genetic disease and are of clinical concern.

Genetic Polycystic Kidney Disease

Although several different conditions are associated with the formation of kidney cysts, the most common (affecting as many as 1 in 400 people) and clinically most important of these conditions is autosomal (adult) dominant polycystic kidney disease (ADPKD). Two different genes, designated PKD1 and PKD2 (for **P**olycystic **K**idney **D**isease), located on separate chromosomes, are associated with such disease. About 85 percent of cases result from mutation of PKD1. In most of the others, the mutation involves PKD2, which is associated with later onset and slower progression of the disease. A few unfortunate people have mutations of both PKD1 and PKD2, which cause severe and rapidly progressive disease. The disease is characterized by excessive proliferation of tubular epithelial cells, leading to the formation of cysts that become detached from the tubules. The epithelium lining the cysts secretes fluid that accumulates within the cysts and causes them to enlarge. As the cysts gradually increase in size, they cause progressive enlargement of both kidneys, where they compress and destroy adjacent renal tissue. Eventually, almost no normal kidney tissue remains, and renal failure supervenes (**Figure 17-21**). Sometimes small numbers of cysts also form in the liver, but usually they do not disturb liver function. Some affected people also have small cyst-like outpouchings extending from the cerebral arteries at the base of the brain, which are termed congenital cerebral aneurysms. Because congenital cerebral aneurysms may

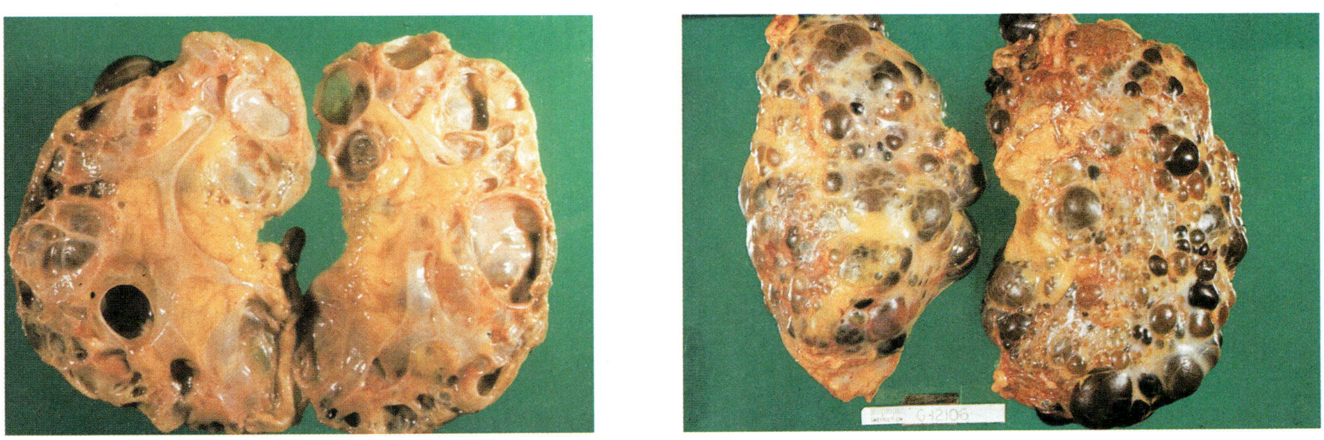

(A) (B)

Figure 17-21 **(A)** Greatly enlarged abnormal kidneys characteristic of congenital polycystic kidney disease. **(B)** Cut surfaces of diseased kidneys, illustrating multiple large cysts. No normal renal tissue remains.

Courtesy of Leonard V. Crowley, MD, Century College.

rupture and cause brain hemorrhage, some physicians have advocated routine magnetic resonance screening of all patients with autosomal dominant polycystic kidney disease. Congenital aneurysms and their complications are described in Chapter 24.

Because renal tissue is destroyed slowly, renal insufficiency does not usually occur until the patient reaches middle age, and some patients do not experience problems until they are in their 40s. Many individuals with congenital polycystic kidney disease are free of symptoms until the disease has markedly progressed, but some experience hypertension, periodic urinary tract infections, or episodes of bloody urine (hematuria) caused by bleeding into one of the enlarging cysts.

Polycystic kidney disease can often be suspected by physical examination, which reveals the greatly enlarged kidneys and can be confirmed by ultrasound or CT examination. There is no specific treatment. When the kidneys fail, dialysis treatments or a kidney transplant may be required. A much less common congenital polycystic disease of the kidney (autosomal recessive polycystic disease) occurs in infants, many of whom die in the neonatal period.

Tumors of the Urinary Tract

Tumors may arise from the epithelium of the renal tubules in the cortex of the kidney, from the transitional epithelium lining the urinary tract, or, rarely, from remnants of embryonic tissue within the kidney.

Renal Cortical Tumors

Benign tumors termed renal cortical adenomas sometimes arise within the kidney. Usually, a benign adenoma is small, well circumscribed, located within the renal cortex, and can be removed by a limited resection. Unfortunately, much more common are malignant tumors, renal cell carcinoma being the most prevalent. Less well-differentiated carcinomas are larger, grow more rapidly, extend into the renal medulla, and exhibit aggressive behavior. Often, the first manifestation of an aggressive carcinoma is blood in the urine (hematuria) as a result of ulceration of the epithelium of the pelvis or calyces caused by the growing tumor. The tumor eventually invades the renal vein.

Transitional Cell Tumors

Almost all tumors arising from the transitional (urothelial) epithelium of the urinary tract are malignant and are termed transitional cell carcinomas. Most arise from bladder epithelium, are of low-grade malignancy, and carry a good prognosis. The tumors are often quite vascular, and they tend to bleed; hematuria may be the first manifestation of the neoplasm. Bladder tumors can be visualized by means of a cystoscope inserted into the bladder through the urethra and often can be resected by means of a similar type of instrument inserted through the urethra. Sometimes it is necessary to resect part of the bladder to remove the tumor completely.

Nephroblastoma (Wilms Tumor)

An unusual, highly malignant tumor composed of primitive cells sometimes arises in the kidney of infants and young children. Histologically, the tumor bears some resemblance to the structure of an embryonic kidney and is termed a nephroblastoma, or Wilms tumor. The neoplasm often metastasizes widely. Treatment is by nephrectomy followed by radiotherapy and chemotherapy.

Diseases of the Urinary Tract (Urological Disease)

Infections of the Urinary Tract

Urinary tract infections are common and may be either acute or chronic. An infection that affects only the bladder is termed **cystitis** (cystis = bladder). If the upper urinary tract is infected, the term is **pyelonephritis** (pyelo = pelvis + nephros = kidney + itis = inflammation). Most infections are caused by gram-negative intestinal bacteria. These organisms often contaminate the perianal and genital areas and gain access to the urinary tract by ascending the urethra.

Cystitis/pyelonephritis Urinary tract infections affecting only the bladder or upper urinary tract.

Free urine flow, large urine volume, and complete emptying of the bladder protect against urinary tract infections because many bacteria that enter the bladder are soon flushed out during urination instead of being retained to multiply in the bladder urine. An acid urine is an additional defense against infection, because most bacteria grow poorly in an acid environment. On the other hand, several conditions predispose to urinary tract infections, including impaired free urine drainage, injury to the mucosa, or introduction of a catheter. Any condition that impairs free drainage of urine increases the likelihood of infection because stagnation of urine favors multiplication of any bacteria that enter the urinary tract. Injury to the mucosa of the urinary tract, as by a kidney stone (calculus) or foreign body, disrupts the protective epithelium, permitting bacteria to invade the deeper tissues and set up an infection. Introduction of a catheter or instrument into the bladder may carry bacteria into the urinary tract and may also injure the bladder mucosa.

Cystitis

Cystitis is more common in women than in men, probably because the short female urethra allows infectious organisms to enter the bladder more easily. Young, sexually active women are especially predisposed because sexual intercourse promotes transfer of bacteria from the distal urethra into the bladder and may cause minor injury to the mucosa at the base of the bladder (trigone). Cystitis is also common in older men who cannot empty their bladders completely because of an enlarged prostate gland (see Chapter 18). The urine remaining in the bladder after voiding favors multiplication of bacteria and may lead to infection.

The manifestations of cystitis result from congestion and inflammation of the bladder (vesical) mucosa. The patient complains of burning pain on urination and a desire to urinate frequently. The urine contains many bacteria and leukocytes. Cystitis is not usually a serious problem and generally responds promptly to antibiotics. Sometimes, however, the infection may spread into the upper urinary tract to affect the renal pelvis and kidney.

Pyelonephritis

Most cases of pyelonephritis are secondary to the spread of infection from the bladder (ascending pyelonephritis), but occasionally the organisms are carried to the kidneys through the bloodstream (hematogenous pyelonephritis). The symptoms of pyelonephritis are those of an acute infection, together with localized pain and tenderness over the affected kidney. Histologically, the infected portion of the kidney is infiltrated by masses of leukocytes and bacteria, and many of the renal tubules in the inflamed area are filled with

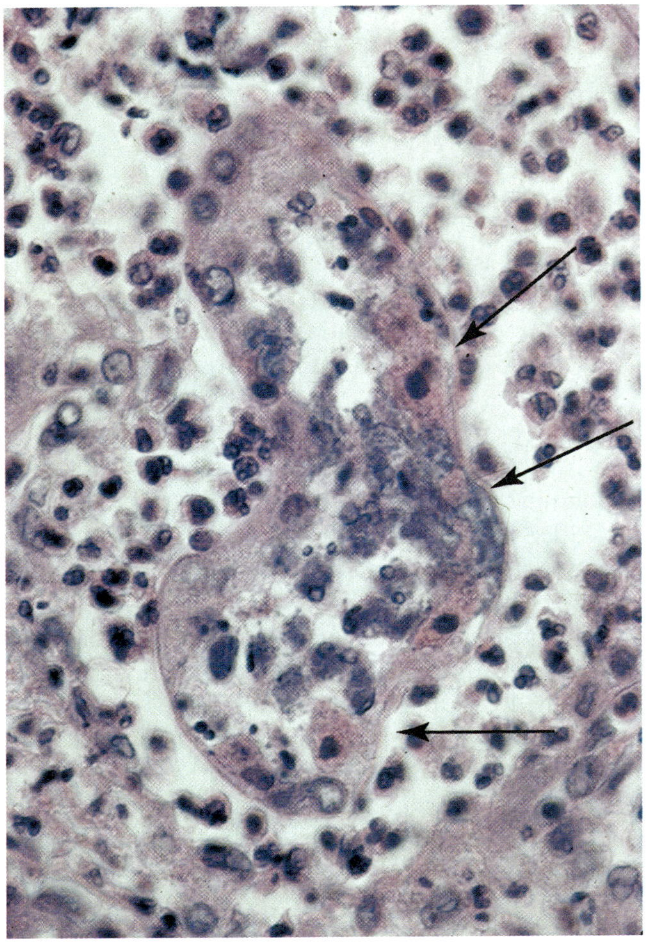

Figure 17-22 Acute pyelonephritis. The tubule in the center of field contains masses of bacteria that extend through wall of tubule (*middle arrow*). Some tubule cells are necrotic (*upper and lower arrows*). Many neutrophils surround the tubule (original magnification ×400).

leukocytes (**Figure 17-22**). Because cystitis and pyelonephritis are frequently associated, the patient also experiences high urinary frequency and pain on urination; the urine contains many bacteria and leukocytes. Treatment involves taking the appropriate antibiotics, together with measures directed at correcting any abnormalities in the lower urinary tract that may impede drainage of urine and predispose to infection.

Most episodes of pyelonephritis respond promptly to treatment. If part of the kidney is severely damaged by the infection, the injured area heals by scarring. The main danger of pyelonephritis lies in the tendency of the disease to become chronic and recurrent. With each subsequent attack, more kidney tissue may be destroyed and healed by scarring. After many episodes of infection, the kidneys may become markedly scarred and shrunken, until the patient eventually exhibits manifestations of renal insufficiency.

Vesicoureteral Reflux and Infection

Normally, effective mechanisms prevent urine from flowing upward from the bladder into the ureters during urination. Sometimes, however, these mechanisms are defective, permitting urine to flow retrograde (reflux) into one or both ureters when the bladder contracts during urination. This condition is termed **vesicoureteral reflux**. It predisposes to urinary tract infection by preventing complete emptying of the bladder. The urine forced into the ureters during voiding flows back into the bladder at the completion of urination, so residual urine remains in the bladder. Bacteria also may be carried into the upper urinary tract by the reflux of urine; this predisposes to pyelonephritis.

Vesicoureteral reflux Retrograde flow of urine from the bladder into the ureter during voiding.

Calculi Stones formed within the body, as in the kidney or gallbladder.

Gout A disorder of nucleoprotein metabolism characterized by elevated uric acid and deposition of uric acid in and around the joints.

Shock wave lithotripsy A method for removing stones from the urinary tract by breaking them into small bits that can be excreted in the urine.

Urolithiasis

Stones may form anywhere in the urinary tract. They are usually termed "**calculi**" (singular, "calculus"), which is a Latin word meaning "little stone" or "pebble." Nephrolithiasis refers to stone formation in the kidney; urolithiasis is a more general term for stone formation at any location in the urinary tract. Most calculi are composed either of uric acid or of a mixture of calcium salts. Three factors predispose to stone formation: increased concentration of salts in the urine, most often due to low fluid intake; infection of the urinary tract; and urinary tract obstruction.

A greatly increased excretion of salts in the urine causes the urine to become supersaturated, and the salts may precipitate to form calculi, especially if the urine is concentrated. For example, in the disease termed **gout** (see Chapter 24), excretion of uric acid is often greatly increased, which may cause uric acid to precipitate from the urine and form uric acid calculi. However, many individuals with urate stones have neither gout nor elevated urate levels. In conditions characterized by hyperfunction of the parathyroid glands, which regulate calcium metabolism (see Chapter 22), or other conditions where excessive calcium is excreted in the urine, subsequent formation of urinary tract calculi composed of calcium salts is common. Infection predisposes to calculi primarily by reducing the solubility of the salts in the urine. Clusters of bacteria also serve as sites where urinary salts may crystallize to form the stone.

Most calculi are small, but occasionally they may gradually increase in size to form large branching structures that adopt the contour of the renal pelvis and calyces where they have formed. This kind of structure is termed a staghorn calculus because it vaguely resembles the antlers of a male deer (**Figure 17-23**). Smaller stones sometimes pass into the ureter. The smooth muscle of the ureter contracts spasmodically to propel the stone along the ureter, causing renal colic—paroxysms of intense flank pain radiating into the groin. Frequently, the rough edges of the stone injure the lining of the ureter, causing red blood cells to appear in the urine. Many stones can be passed through the ureter and excreted in the urine, but some become lodged in the ureter and must be removed. A stone lodged in the distal ureter can usually be removed by inserting a cystoscope into the bladder and then passing a specially designed catheter-like instrument through the cystoscope into the ureter. The instrument is constructed to snare the stone, which is then pulled through the ureter into the bladder and extracted through the cystoscope. A stone lodged in the proximal ureter may be broken into fragments by **shock wave lithotripsy**, a procedure that can break a large stone too big to pass through the ureter into small fragments that can be excreted in the urine instead of requiring a surgical procedure to remove the stone. The usual method for fragmenting a calculus involves positioning the recumbent patient on a specially designed table. Above the table is X-ray equipment capable of visualizing the location of the stone within the kidney. Below the table is a device termed a lithotriptor, which can generate electrically produced shock waves capable of fragmenting the stone. When the exact location of the stone has been determined by X-ray

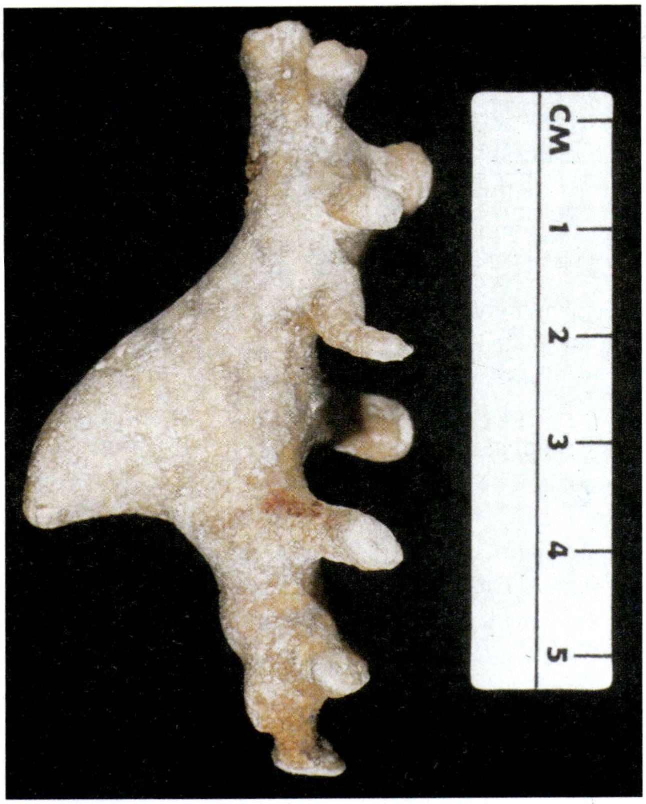

Figure 17-23 Large staghorn calculus of kidney.

Courtesy of Leonard V. Crowley, MD, Century College.

examination, the shock wave–generating equipment is focused very precisely on the kidney stone, and shock waves directed at the stone fragment the stone into fine particles that are excreted in the urine. The success of the technique depends on the size and composition of the stone and, to some degree, the size of the patient. In a large-sized patient, the shock wave may be prevented from impacting on the stone.

Sometimes stones form in the bladder. Usually, this stone formation is secondary to the combined effect of infection and stasis of urine, which decrease the solubility of dissolved salts in the urine. Sometimes bladder calculi can be removed through the bladder by means of a cystoscope. The stones are first broken up by an instrument that is passed through the cystoscope into the bladder and are then flushed out.

Urinary Obstruction

For urine to be excreted normally, the urinary drainage system that transports the urine must permit free flow of urine. Obstruction or marked narrowing of the system at any point (stricture) causes the system proximal to the blockage to dilate progressively because of the pressure of the retained urine. Dilatation of the ureter is termed **hydroureter**. Dilatation of the renal pelvis and calyces is termed **hydronephrosis** (hydro = water + nephros = kidney + osis = condition) (**Figure 17-24**). The distention of the calyces and pelvis in turn causes progressive atrophy of the kidney on the affected side because of the high pressure of the urine within the obstructed drainage system. Eventually, if the obstruction is not relieved, the affected kidney is reduced to a thin shell of atrophic parenchyma covering the overdistended pelvis and calyces.

Hydroureter A dilatation of the ureter secondary to obstruction of the urinary drainage system, often associated with coexisting dilatation of the renal pelvis and calyces (hydronephrosis).

Hydronephrosis A dilatation of the urinary drainage tract proximal to the site of an obstruction.

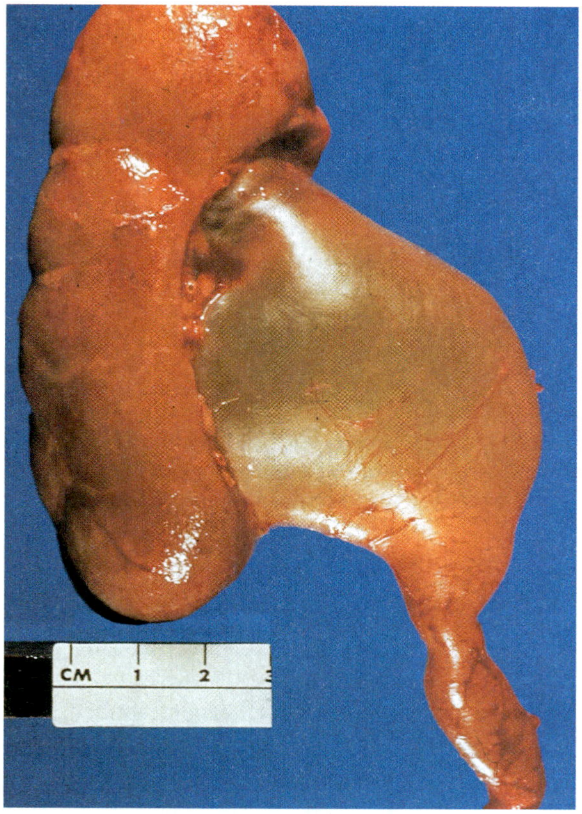

(A)

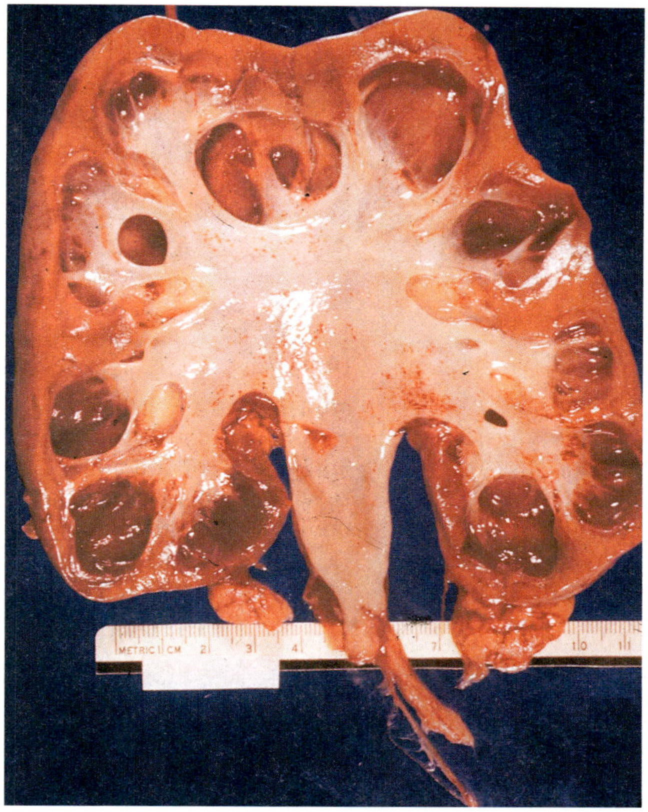

(B)

Figure 17-24 **(A)** Marked hydronephrosis and hydroureter. **(B)** Bisected hydronephrotic kidney, illustrating enlargement of calyces with atrophy of the renal parenchyma caused by the increased pressure exerted by the urine within the distended renal pelvis and calyces.

Which part of the drainage system is affected by the obstruction depends on the location of the block. Obstruction to the outflow of urine from the bladder, as by an enlarged prostate gland or stricture in the urethra, leads to bilateral hydronephrosis and hydroureter, as well as causing overdistention of the bladder (**Figure 17-25A**). Hydronephrosis and hydroureter are unilateral if the obstruction is located low in the ureter, as might be caused by an obstructing calculus impacted in the ureter or an obstructing tumor of the ureter (**Figure 17-25B**). If the obstruction is located at the junction of the renal pelvis and ureter, as might be caused by scarring of the ureter in this area, a unilateral hydronephrosis develops, but the ureter on the affected side is of normal caliber (**Figure 17-25C**).

Diagnosis of urinary tract obstruction is usually made by means of a pyelogram or by a CT scan (procedures described in Chapter 1). These procedures demonstrate the dilatation of the urinary tract. Treatment is directed toward relieving the obstruction by appropriate means before the kidneys are irreparably damaged.

Diagnostic Evaluation of Kidney and Urinary Tract Disease

A variety of methods are used to detect disease of the kidneys and urinary tract, to evaluate the degree to which renal function is disturbed, and to define the type of disease present.

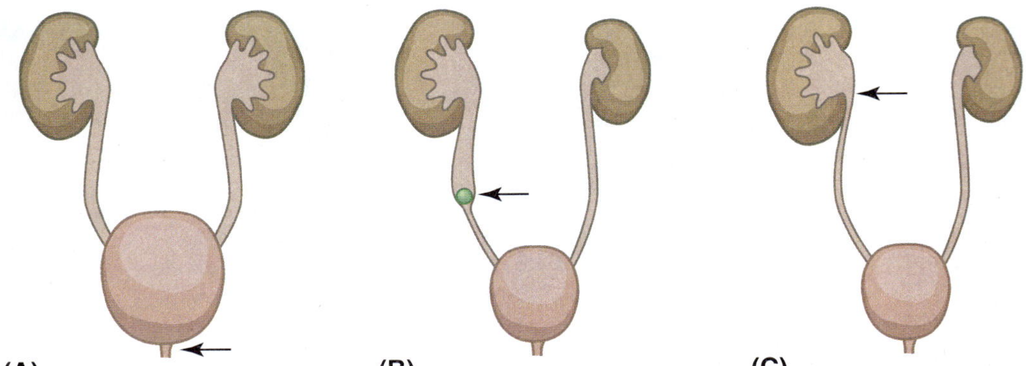

Figure 17-25 Possible locations and results of urinary tract obstruction. The arrows indicate sites of obstruction. **(A)** Bilateral hydronephrosis and hydroureter with distension of the bladder caused by urethral obstruction. **(B)** Unilateral hydroureter and hydronephrosis caused by obstruction of the distal ureter. **(C)** Unilateral hydronephrosis caused by obstruction at the ureteropelvic junction.

Urinalysis

Urinalysis A commonly performed chemical and microscopic analysis of the urine.

Albumin-to-creatinine ratio (ACR) Measurement of urine albumin levels compared to amount of creatinine.

The most widely used diagnostic test is an examination of the urine termed **urinalysis**. The examination is useful for detecting whether urinary tract disease is present and for detecting other systemic diseases that alter renal function. The examination includes determinations of urine pH (acidity) and specific gravity (a measure of urine concentration) and simple tests for glucose and protein. The urinalysis may also include tests for bile pigment, acetone, and other constituents that may appear in the urine in association with various diseases. A sample of the urine is also centrifuged, and the sediment is examined microscopically. If the urinalysis is normal, renal disease is unlikely. Alternatively, the presence of red cells and protein in the urine may indicate damage to the glomerular filter, allowing these substances to leak into the glomerular filtrate, or that bleeding is occurring somewhere in the urinary tract. Renal casts, which are collections of protein and cells molded into the shape of the kidney tubules, are an indication of glomerular or tubular disease. Leukocytes and bacteria in the urinary sediment indicate urinary tract infection.

Additional tests may be performed on the urine as indicated by the patient's clinical condition. If a urinary tract infection is suspected, for example, the urine is cultured for pathogenic bacteria, and antibiotic sensitivity tests are performed if bacteria are present. Measurement of urine albumin levels is an accurate determination of the function of the glomerular filtration barrier. The value is usually expressed as the **albumin-to-creatinine ratio (ACR)** and is often used to monitor kidney damage in type 2 diabetes. Urine levels of the protein beta 2 microglobulin (B2M) increase in the case of renal tubular damage because the renal tubules normally resorb this protein. For this reason, an elevated B2M level suggests a tubular rather than a glomerular defect.

Kidney Function Tests

Impairment of renal function can be recognized by measuring the concentration of various substances in the blood, such as urea (BUN) and serum creatinine, which are waste products excreted by the kidneys. Elevated levels indicate impaired renal function, and the degree of elevation is a measure of the degree of impairment.

The efficiency of the glomerular filtration apparatus can be an early indicator of impaired renal function, even before elevated levels of waste products are present in the blood. The glomerular filtration rate (GFR) is a measure of the volume of body fluid cleared by the kidneys per unit of time. This is generally reported in milliliters/minute. The GFR is usually measured by the ability of the kidney to clear creatinine using the **creatinine clearance test**. This test calculates how much blood plasma must flow through the kidney each minute and be completely cleared of creatinine to provide the quantity of creatinine that appears in the urine within the same period of time. Clearance tests provide a rough estimate of the degree of kidney damage, and periodic clearance tests can be used to follow the progress of renal disease. A gradual fall in the renal clearance of a substance means that renal function is declining. The test requires a cumbersome 12- or 24-hour collection and measurement of urine volume as well as measuring the creatinine level and the serum creatinine level. Often the GFR is calculated based solely on the patient's serum creatinine level, age, gender, and race. The calculated value has some limitations but is easier to obtain and is often used to follow kidney function in chronic renal disease.

Creatinine clearance test A test of renal function that measures the ability of kidneys to remove (clear) creatinine from the blood and excrete it in the urine.

Additional Techniques

Many other specialized procedures can be used to study the kidneys and urinary tract, including various X-ray examinations, ultrasound examinations, and cystoscopy. These examinations are described in Chapter 1. Their specific diagnostic applications also have been considered in conjunction with the various renal and urinary tract diseases for which they provide useful information. X-ray examination of the abdomen, for example, can identify the size and location of the kidneys and can detect radiopaque calculi in the kidneys or urinary tract. CT scans and intravenous pyelograms can detect anatomic abnormalities within the kidneys, such as cysts and tumors, and many abnormalities of the urinary drainage system, such as hydronephrosis (**Figure 17-26**). Renal arteriograms, using techniques similar to those used to study the coronary arteries, can determine the caliber of the renal arteries, can detect segmental areas of

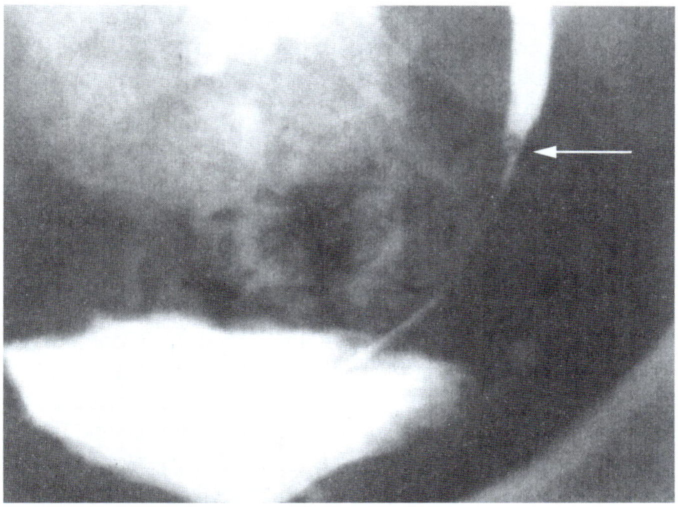

Figure 17-26 Intravenous pyelogram. Contrast material fills the bladder at the bottom of the image and the proximal portion of the right ureter. A stone (*arrow*) is lodged in the ureter, causing dilation of the ureter above the stone and preventing urine from filling the distal portion. The dye in the bladder comes from urine passing through the opposite ureter.

narrowing in the renal arteries, and can identify areas of increased vascularity within the kidney, which often occur when a tumor is present.

Sometimes the clinician cannot make an exact diagnosis concerning the type of renal disease without resorting to biopsy of the kidney. This can be accomplished without undue difficulty or serious risk to the patient by introducing a small biopsy needle through the skin of the flank directly into the substance of the kidney. A small bit of kidney tissue is removed for histologic study. Examination of the biopsy material by the pathologist is often necessary to allow the pathologist to provide an exact diagnosis as to the nature and extent of the renal disease, which serves as a guide to proper treatment. Material for several of the figures in this chapter have been obtained by this technique.

Case 17-1

Antoine is a 3-year-old male child of Black parents. He had just recovered from a mild upper respiratory infection when his parents noticed that his face appeared "swollen." On closer examination, they noted that his legs and scrotum also appeared to be "puffy" (a clinician would say "edematous"). Antoine also seems tired and has little appetite. Concerned, his parents take him to the family pediatrician. The pediatrician confirms marked facial and dependent edema (accumulation of fluid in tissue predominantly below the heart, such as the legs). Careful examination of the patient's fingernails shows a pattern of horizontal lines (Muehrcke lines) in the bed of the nails, which blanch when the nail is pressed. The physician remembers that such lines are sometimes associated with vascular changes that occur when plasma albumin levels are very low, and he orders a urinalysis.

Antoine's urine shows extreme proteinuria. The albumin-to-creatinine ratio is 6 and the urine has a very high specific gravity. These findings would be consistent with loss of protein in the urine because of impaired urinary filtration. The patient's serum albumin is 2.3 g/dl (dl is the abbreviation for deciliter, or 100 ml), which is abnormally low. These findings taken together are consistent with the diagnosis of nephrotic syndrome. Because at least 90 percent of nephrosis in children of Antoine's age is minimal change disease, no invasive investigation of the kidney (such as a renal biopsy) is undertaken. Even if that were done, light microscopy would not be expected to disclose any changes in the glomerulus.

The physician decides to try corticosteroid therapy using prednisone because about 90 percent of children with minimal change disease will respond within 2 weeks. His parents are told to reduce Antoine's salt intake to help reduce his edema.

The Happy Ending

Antoine's proteinuria clears after 10 days of therapy, as does his edema. Drug therapy is continued for four weeks at a reduced dose, and no relapse is noted.

The Not-So-Happy Ending

No change is noted in the degree of nephrosis after 2 weeks of therapy. Antoine complains of increasing abdominal pain, and his blood pressure begins to increase. Therapy with diuretics and antihypertensive medication becomes necessary. His disease is now classified as steroid-resistant nephrotic syndrome (SRNS). Because of his continuing disease, the nephrologist in charge of Antoine's case decides to request a needle biopsy of Antoine's kidney. Light microscopic analysis of the glomerular disease is consistent with focal segmental glomerulosclerosis (FSGS) (see Figure 17-19). This is not surprising, because 70 percent of children with SRNS have FSGS. Aggressive treatment with increased doses of prednisone and immunosuppressive agents was ineffective. Ultimately Antoine developed end-stage renal disease and required a kidney transplant.

Discussion

Minimal change disease is thought to be related to an increased level of a number of cytokines that cause T cells to release an agent that damages the function of the epithelial cell foot processes; however, the exact mechanism is unclear. Although no changes to affected glomeruli are noted by light microscopy, damage to the foot processes (fusion or effacement), as disclosed in EM (electron microscope) studies, is characteristic of the disease (**Case Figure 17-1**). The etiology of the disease remains obscure (although it may occur following an upper respiratory tract infection or allergic reaction). Ninety percent of children with minimal change disease respond to prednisone therapy. Failure of response (SRNS) is an indicator of the likelihood of a different disease process, and, as noted, about 70 percent of children with SRNS have focal segmental glomerulosclerosis. FSGS is significantly increasing in frequency in White and, notably, Black populations, where it is the most common cause of adult nephrosis. FSGS is associated with diverse etiologies and diagnostic subclassifications, including primary (idiopathic) disease or secondary disease-related infection (HIV), drugs, reduced renal mass and hereditary defects in podocyte genes, and (particularly in Blacks) a circulating protein, apolipoprotein L1. The frequency of the variant of the apoL1 gene associated with FSGS susceptibility is more than 10 times higher in Blacks than in Whites and is associated with an increased risk of FSGS and

(A)

(B)

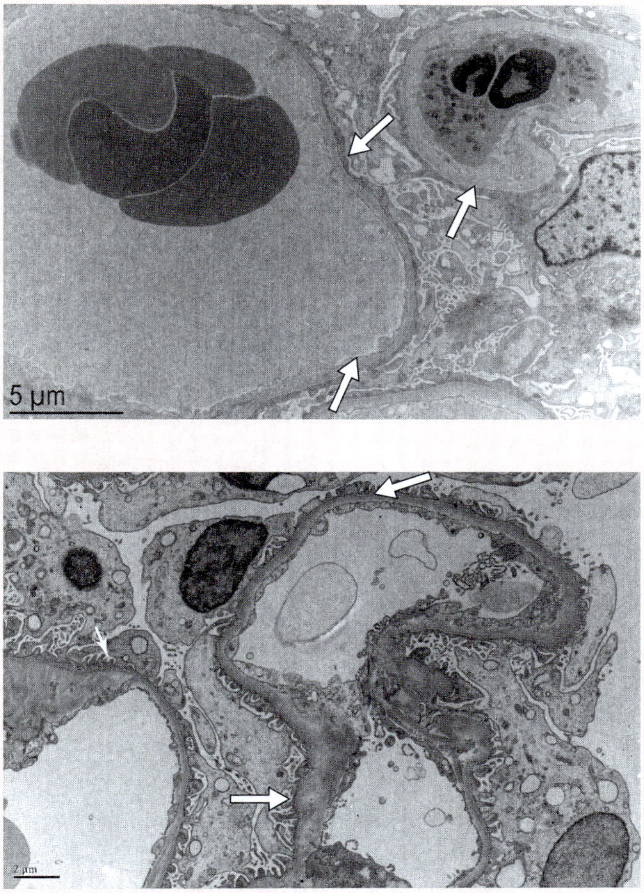

Case Figure 17-1 Electron micrograph images. **(A)** Glomerular capillaries in minimal change disease. Both capillaries show effacement (flattening) of podocytes (*arrows*). One capillary has red cells in the lumen, the other a neutrophil. **(B)** Normal glomerular capillaries demonstrating podocytes (*arrows*).

(continues)

Case 17-1 *(Continued)*

hypertensive end-stage renal disease. The presence of two high-risk alleles of apoL1 is responsible for nearly 20 percent of FSGS. The high-risk alleles of apoL1 are associated with the ability to lyse trypanosomes associated with African sleeping sickness. Individuals with a single high-risk allele are relatively resistant to this parasitic disease, whereas inheritance of two high-risk alleles is associated with a much higher risk of kidney disease. This pattern of heterozygous advantage (versus homozygous disadvantage) is analogous to that seen with sickle cell trait and disease (discussed in Chapter 12). The lack of response by Antoine to steroids and immunosuppressive therapy is consistent with a hereditary condition, but no additional family history or genetic studies are available. However, it is clear that Blacks are at increased risk of FSGS, and hypertensive renal disease is likely to be related in part to hereditary factors.

Etiology and Pathogenesis

Minimal change disease of unknown etiology or steroid-resistant nephrosis associated with focal segmental glomerulosclerosis, possibly of hereditary origin involving apoL1 high-risk alleles or podocyte protein defects.

Questions

1. Clearly distinguish between nephrosis and nephritis. Which is Case 17-1 a good example of and why?
2. Why would immediate renal biopsy of a child with nephrosis be inappropriate? When would this be appropriate?
3. Correlate the laboratory findings in Case 17-1 with the disease process.
4. Correlate the EM findings in Case 17-1 with the disease process.

Questions for Review

1. What are the homeostatic mechanisms by which the kidneys regulate salt and water balance?
2. What role do the renal tubules play in the process?
3. What are metabolic and respiratory alkalosis/acidosis? How do the metabolic and respiratory conditions differ?
4. What are the most common causes of chronic kidney disease?
5. What mechanisms are responsible for loss of kidney function in CKD?
6. What is ESRD?
7. What is the mechanism of glomerular filtration?
8. What is the result of failure of glomerular filtration?
9. What is the difference between glomerulonephritis and pyelonephritis? What is the relationship between glomerulonephritis and beta-streptococcal infection? What factors predispose to urinary tract infection?
10. What is the difference between nephrotic syndrome and nephrosclerosis? Why does edema develop in a patient with nephrosis?
11. What are the common causes of urinary tract obstruction? What are the effects on the kidneys and lower urinary tract?
12. What conditions lead to renal tubular necrosis? What are its clinical manifestations?
13. What is uremia? What are its manifestations? How is it treated? What is the role of urea in producing the clinical manifestations of uremia?
14. What methods does the clinician use to establish a diagnosis of renal disease?

15. What is congenital polycystic kidney disease? What are its clinical manifestations? What is its pattern of inheritance? How is it treated?
16. What is the difference between acute and chronic renal failure?
17. What is the difference between hemodialysis and peritoneal dialysis? How is the patient's circulation connected to the artificial kidney for hemodialysis?
18. Why does a kidney transplant from a donor who is a close relative usually have a greater likelihood of survival than does a cadaver transplant?
19. How does diabetes affect the kidneys? What are the clinical manifestations? How does gout affect the kidneys?

References

Jennette JC, Gasim AMH. Pathology of medical renal disease. In Reisner HM, ed. *Pathology: A Modern Case Study*. 2nd ed. McGraw Hill Lange; 2020:Chapter 13.

Faubel S, Topf J. The Fluid, Electrolyte & Acid-Base Companion. October 26, 2009. http://pbfluids.com/2009/10/the-fluid-electrolyte-and-acid-base-companion-for-free/

- The two texts provide a detailed overview of renal pathology and pathophysiology. The second is a freely available text that is an excellent introduction to renal physiology. Although aimed at medical students and residents, it is so clearly written and well-illustrated that anyone with even an undergraduate biology background will be able to follow it (and it is free).

Chen TK, Knicely DH, Grams ME. Chronic kidney disease diagnosis and management. *JAMA*. 2019;322(13):1294-1304.

Coresh J, et al. Decline in estimated glomerular filtration rate and subsequent risk of end-stage renal disease and mortality. *JAMA*. 2014;311(24):2518-31.

- The two papers concentrate on risk assessment and diagnosis of chronic kidney disease.

National Institute of Diabetes and Digestive and Kidney Diseases. Kidney Disease. https://www.niddk.nih.gov/health-information/kidney-disease

- The portal to a wealth of current information on renal diseases. An excellent first place to go for current information on a wide array of topics.

Rastogi A, et al. Autosomal dominant polycystic kidney disease: Updated perspectives. *Ther Clin Risk Manag*. 2019;15:1041-1052. https://www.ncbi.nlm.nih.gov/pmc/articles/PMC6716585/

- A recent article on the important concepts regarding this disease, including pathogenesis, genetics, associated conditions, complications, clinical manifestations, monitoring disease progression, and treatment.

Zazzeroni L, et al. Comparison of quality of life in patients undergoing hemodialysis and peritoneal dialysis: A systematic review and meta-analysis. *Kidney Blood Press Res*. 2017;42(4):717-727.

- An interesting review of the status of a long-standing controversy over the relative utility of conventional hemodialysis versus peritoneal dialysis, emphasizing quality of life issues. Also provides data on patient survival with two approaches.

Collins BH. Kidney Transplantation. Published 2019. Last updated December 17, 2021. https://emedicine.medscape.com/article/430128-overview

National Kidney Foundation. Organ Donation and Transplantation https://www.kidney.org/transplantation

- The first reference is a recent overview of many aspects regarding renal transplantation. The section on outcomes has some current (and rather surprising) data. The role of comorbidities in graft survival is highlighted. The second is an informative site giving much practical information on both donation and transplantation.

Matas AJ, Vock DM, Ibraham HN. GFR 25 Years Postdonation in Donors with (vs without) a 1st Degree Relative with ESRD. *Am J Transplant*. 2018;18:625-631. https://www.ncbi.nlm.nih.gov/pmc/articles/PMC5820146/

Dormagala P, et al. Successful transplantation of kidneys from deceased donors with terminal acute kidney injury. *Ren Fall*. 2019;41(1):167-174.

- Renal transplantation, although the optimal solution for most patients with ESRD, is associated with several major problems. Donor access is limited, and kidneys from donors with a variety of diseases may (or may not) be as likely to function as well as those from living donors. Are living donors at increased risk of kidney disease? These three papers review important areas of the discussion. The two articles address these issues.

Wrobel G, Kuder T. The role of selected environmental factors and the type of work performed on the development of urolithiasis—a review paper. *Int J Occup Med Environ Health.* 2019;32:761-775.

Hiller SC, Ghanki GR. Frontiers of stone management. *Curr Opin Urol.* 2019. doi:10.1097/MOU.0000000000000698

- Urolithiasis remains an important urological problem. What are some of the environmental factors involved, and what should one do about it?

Silva ACSE, Oliveira EA, Mak RH. Urinary tract infections in pediatrics: An overview (Free access). 2019.

Kumar S, Dave A, Wolf B. Urinary tract infections. *Dis Mon.* 2015;61(2):45-59.

- Clinically oriented detailed reviews of this very common medical condition.

Freedman B, et al. APOL1-Associated Nephropathy: A Key Contributor to Racial Disparity in CKD. *Am J Kidney Dis.* 2018;72 (5 suppl 1):S8-S16 (Free access).

Rosenberg AZ, Kopp JB. Focal Segmental Glomerulosclerosis. *Clin J Am Soc Nephrol.* 2017;12: 502-517 (Free access).

- These two references were useful in the case construction. The first entry highlights an exciting new finding in genetic risk factors for serious renal disease in African Americans that has similarities to sickle cell disease. The second article reviews other inherited diseases associated with FSGS.

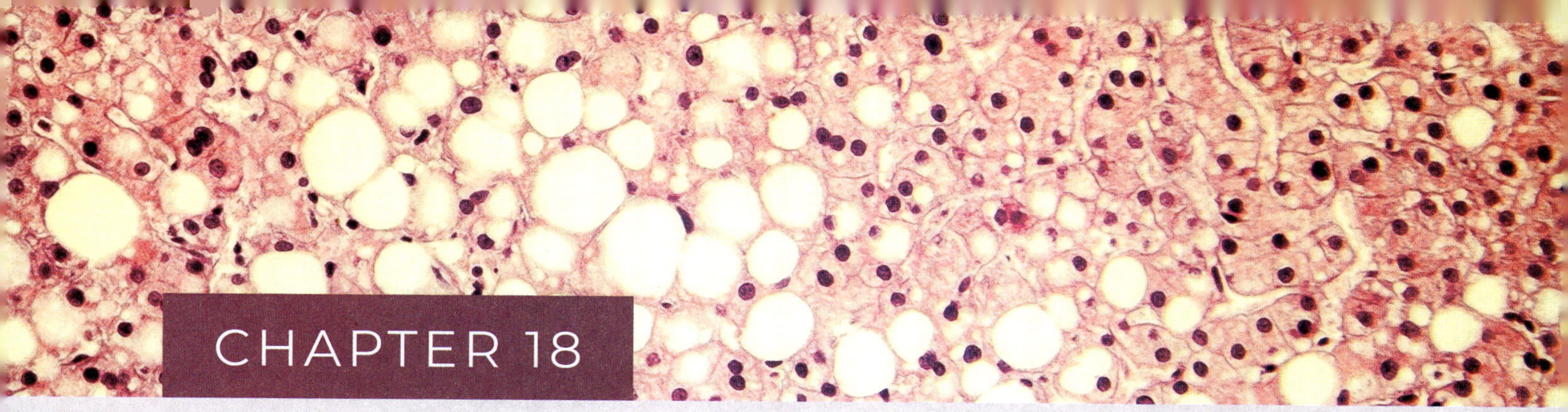

CHAPTER 18

The Female and Male Reproductive Systems

LEARNING OBJECTIVES

1. Describe the common infections of the genital tract and relate them to sexually transmitted infections (STI).
2. Explain the pathogenesis, clinical manifestations, and treatment of toxic shock syndrome.
3. Describe the common diseases of the vulva, cervix, and uterus.
4. List the common causes of irregular uterine bleeding.
5. Describe the clinical manifestations and complications of endometriosis.
6. List the common types of cysts and tumors of the ovary.
7. Name the anatomic structures of the male reproductive system. Describe their functions as they relate to diseases affecting them.
8. Differentiate between benign prostatic hyperplasia and prostatic carcinoma. Describe clinical manifestations and methods of treatment.
9. Discuss symptoms and treatment for erectile dysfunction.

The chapter considers the pathophysiology and pathology of the female and male reproductive systems. Sexually transmitted diseases are of great importance in the pathology of both males and females. As is common in many other organ systems, neoplastic disease and in particular malignancies (cancer) play a major role in female health where cancer of the cervix, uterus, and ovaries are a major cause of disease and death. Likewise, in males, cancer of the prostate and, less commonly, of the testes plays a significant role. An important consideration noted in this chapter is the role of viral infection in promoting cancer, most notably in females, less commonly in males.

Sexually Transmitted Infections (HIV)

Although HIV infection often occurs predominantly as a sexually transmitted infection, HIV may also be transmitted congenitally, parenterally (most commonly via blood-contaminated needles and improperly sterilized instruments), and, in the past, by contaminated blood products.

Rates of infection have declined by about two-thirds since the peak of the infection in the 1980s and continue to decrease. The 13–24 age group has shown a 305 percent decrease in infection rate between 2018 and 2022, most likely related to the use of pre-exposure prophylaxis (PrEP) drugs (Truvada) and increased HIV testing. PrEP is pre-exposure prophylaxis designed to prevent disease in HIV-negative individuals who may be at risk of contracting the disease. PrEP is 99% effective at preventing sexually transmitted HIV as compared to about 70–80% effectiveness of condoms.

For more information regarding HIV and the pathophysiology of **acquired immune deficiency syndrome (AIDS)**, see Chapter 5.

Acquired immune deficiency syndrome (AIDS) An infection caused by the human immunodeficiency virus. The virus attacks and destroys helper T lymphocytes, which compromises cell-mediated immunity, leading to increased susceptibility to infection and some tumors.

Communicable disease A disease transmitted from person to person.

Human papillomavirus (HPV) A virus that stimulates epithelial cell proliferation. Causes warts and genital tract condylomas.

Sexually Transmitted Infections Other Than HIV

Sexually transmitted infections are **communicable diseases** that spread primarily by sexual contact. They can be transmitted by sexual relations between heterosexual or lesbian and gay partners, by genital–genital, genital–oral, and anal contact. The four major sexually transmitted infections are syphilis, gonorrhea, genital herpes infection, and genital chlamydial infections (**Table 18-1**).

Cervical cancer also may be considered a sexually transmitted disease caused by **human papillomavirus (HPV)** infection. In addition, HPV infection transmitted by sexual contact is associated with genital warts; cancer of the vulva, vagina, penis, and anus; and cancers occurring at the back of the throat (oropharyngeal cancer). HPV infection is common (the CDC estimates about 40% of males and females are positive for HPV at some point), and many individuals do not know they are infected. Vaccination against HPV is safe and effective in both males and females, and it is the only method to prevent disease transmitted by oral–genital contact other than the use of dental dams. Men are

Table 18-1 Comparison of Four Major Sexually Transmitted Diseases

	Syphilis	Gonorrhea	Herpes	Chlamydia
Organism	*Treponema pallidum*	Gonococcus (*Neisseria gonorrhoeae*)	Herpes virus	*Chlamydia trachomatis*
Major clinical manifestations	Primary: Chancre Secondary: Systemic infection with skin rash and enlarged lymph nodes Tertiary: Late destructive lesions in internal organs	Urethritis Cervicitis Pharyngitis Infection of rectal mucosa (proctitis)	Superficial vesicles and ulcers on external genitalia and in genital tract Regional lymph nodes often enlarged and tender	Cervicitis Urethritis
Tests used to establish diagnosis	Demonstration of treponemas in chancre Serologic tests	Culture of organisms from sites of infection Nonculture tests also available	Demonstration of intranuclear inclusions in infected cells Virus cultures Serologic tests in some cases	Detection of chlamydial antigens in cervical/urethral secretions Fluorescence microscopy Cultures Nonculture tests also available

	Syphilis	Gonorrhea	Herpes	Chlamydia
Major complications	Damage to cardiovascular system and nervous system in tertiary syphilis may be fatal	Disseminated bloodstream infection Tubal infection with impaired fertility Spread of infection to prostate and epididymides	Spread from infected mother to infant	Tubal infection with impaired fertility Epididymitis
Treatment	Antibiotics	Antibiotics	Antiviral drug shortens infection but not curative	Antibiotics

susceptible to HPV-related oropharyngeal cancer at a relatively early age suggesting the importance of immunization at an early age (10–11 years).

Other common but less serious sexually transmitted diseases are anal and genital warts (**condylomas**; see later in this chapter) caused by HPV as mentioned previously, nonspecific vaginitis caused by pathogenic microorganisms such as *Gardnerella* in conjunction with anaerobic vaginal bacteria, and vaginitis caused by the protozoan parasite *Trichomonas vaginalis* (see Vaginitis in this chapter). Other diseases, including scabies and crabs (body lice), animal parasites, hepatitis B, and some gastrointestinal tract infections, are also sometimes transmitted sexually.

Condyloma A warty, tumor-like overgrowth in the squamous epithelium of the anorectal or genital tract, caused by a virus that is spread by sexual contact.

Treponema pallidum A spirochaete bacterial pathogen that causes syphillis.

Chancre Small ulcer at site of syphilis inoculation.

Syphilis

Syphilis, caused by the spirochete ***Treponema pallidum***, is a very serious sexually transmitted disease because it may cause severe damage in almost any organ of the body. If the disease is not treated, it progresses through three stages: primary, secondary, and tertiary syphilis. Each stage has its own characteristic clinical manifestations (**Figure 18-1**). Although often thought of as an uncommon disease well under control in the population, this is not the case.

During 2023, there were 209,000 new cases of syphilis (all stages), the highest level since 1950. Gay, bisexual, and men who have sex with men (MSM) are experiencing extreme effects of syphilis. They account for 33 percent of all primary and secondary (P&S) syphilis cases in 2023 (58% among the group with known sex partners). However, incidences are increasing among heterosexual men and women in recent years. Congenital syphilis continues to be a concern in the United States. Congenital syphilis occurs when a pregnant person passes syphilis to their baby. Final 2023 data show more than 3900 cases of congenital syphilis.

Primary Syphilis

Contact with an infected partner enables the treponemes to penetrate the mucous membranes of the genital tract, oral cavity, or rectal mucosa, or to be introduced through a break in the skin. The organisms multiply rapidly and spread throughout the body. After an incubation period of up to several weeks, a small ulcer termed a **chancre** develops at the site of contact. It is easily seen if it is on the penis or vulva, but it may be undetected if it is within the vagina, oral cavity, or rectum (Figure 18-1A).

The chancre, which contains large numbers of treponemes and is highly infectious, persists for about 4 to 6 weeks and eventually heals even if the disease

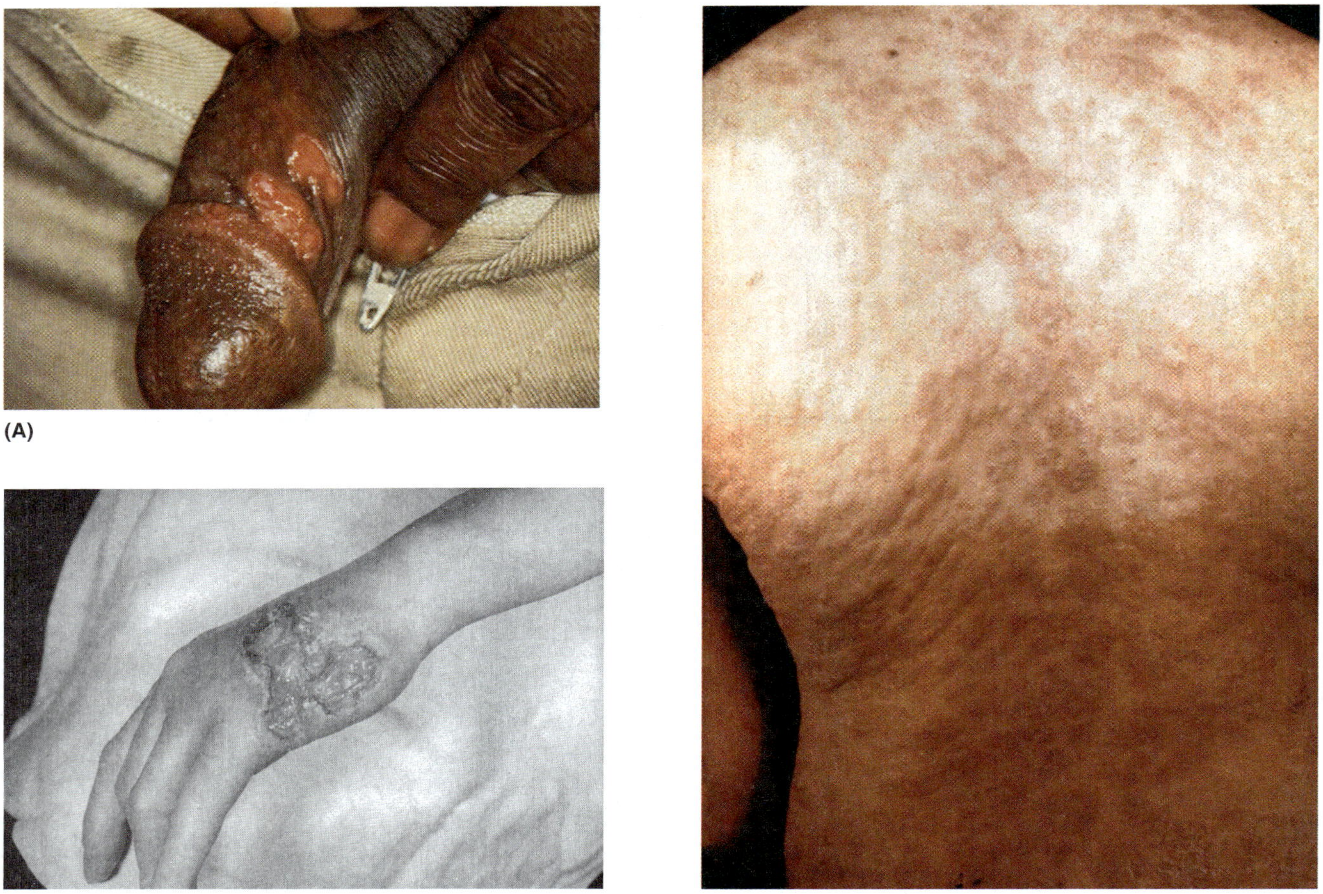

(A) (C) (B)

Figure 18-1 The stages of syphilis. **(A)** The chancre of primary syphilis as it occurs on the penis. The chancre has raised margins and is usually painless. **(B)** A skin rash is characteristic of secondary syphilis. **(C)** The gumma that forms in tertiary syphilis is a granular diffuse lesion compared with the primary chancre.

(A) Courtesy of M. Rein VD/CDC; (B) Courtesy of Dr. Gavin Hart/CDC; (C) Courtesy of Susan Lindsley/CDC.

is untreated. Even though the chancre has healed, however, with progress to secondary syphilis, the treponemes become widely disseminated through the body and continue to multiply.

Secondary Syphilis

The secondary stage of syphilis begins several weeks to months after the chancre has healed. The infected individual develops manifestations of a systemic infection characterized by elevated temperature, enlargement of lymph nodes, a skin rash, and shallow ulcers on the mucous membranes of the oral cavity and genital tract (mucous patches) (Figure 18-1B). This stage of the disease is also extremely infectious because the skin and mucous membrane lesions contain large numbers of treponemes. The secondary stage persists for several weeks and, like the chancre, eventually subsides even if no treatment is administered. Some people experience one or more recurrences of secondary syphilis, but each recurrence subsides spontaneously.

Tertiary Syphilis

After the second stage subsides, the infected individual appears well for a variable period of time, but the organisms are still active and may cause irreparable damage to the cardiovascular and nervous systems and to other organs as well.

Gumma (granulomatous lesions often found in the skin or bones) are characteristic of this stage of the disease (Figure 18-1C). Chronic inflammation and scarring of the aortic valve lead to valve malfunction and heart failure. Often, the aortic wall just above the aortic valve also is damaged by the treponemes. This weakens the aortic wall, causing it to balloon out and eventually rupture. Degeneration of fiber tracts in the spinal cord caused by syphilis impairs sensation and disturbs walking. Damage to the brain and spinal cord by the treponemes (neurosyphilis) causes mental deterioration and eventual paralysis. The late manifestations of the disease, which can appear as long as 20 years after the initial infection, define tertiary syphilis. This stage is not generally communicable because the organisms are relatively few and are confined to the internal organs.

Diagnosis and Treatment

There are several different types of testing protocols, including serologic tests to detect and monitor syphilis progression. Some tests are sensitive as early as 9 days post-potential exposure. Most are reliable at 6 weeks, and testing at 3 months is most reliable. The CDC recently updated the recommended testing protocol for better control and tracking of the infection. Such tests are used both for screening and to also confirm an initial diagnosis.

Syphilis can be treated successfully by penicillin G and, in special circumstances, certain other antibiotics. Treatment stops the progression of the disease and prevents serious late complications.

Congenital Syphilis

A syphilitic mother often transmits the disease to her unborn infant (vertical transmission). The intrauterine infection may cause death of the fetus, or the infant may be born with congenital syphilis. An infected mother should be treated as soon as the maternal infection is identified without regard to the stage of her pregnancy.

Gonorrhea

Gonorrhea, caused by the gonococcus ***Neisseria gonorrhoeae***, is one of the most common communicable diseases. In 2023 there were more than 601,000 cases reported to the CDC, a modest decrease since 2022. This figure is probably an underestimate. The organism primarily infects mucosal surfaces: the linings of the urethra, genital tract, pharynx, and rectum (**Figure 18-2**). Symptoms of infection appear about a week after exposure, and the clinical manifestations differ in the two sexes.

Neisseria gonorrhoeae Bacterium causing gonorrhea.

Gonorrhea in the Female

In the female, the gonococci primarily infect the mucosa of the uterine cervix and the urethra and may also cause inflammation of the fallopian tubes (salpingitis). Therefore, it is a common cause of pelvic inflammatory disease (ascending infection of the female genital tract). The gonococcal infection may also spread into Bartholin glands, which are located adjacent to the vaginal orifice. The cervical infection usually causes profuse vaginal discharge; the urethral involvement is manifested by pain and burning on urination. Some women, however, have few or no symptoms of infection but are nevertheless capable of transmitting the disease to their sexual partners.

The gonococcal infection may also spread upward from the cervix through the uterus into the fallopian tubes, where, as previously noted, it

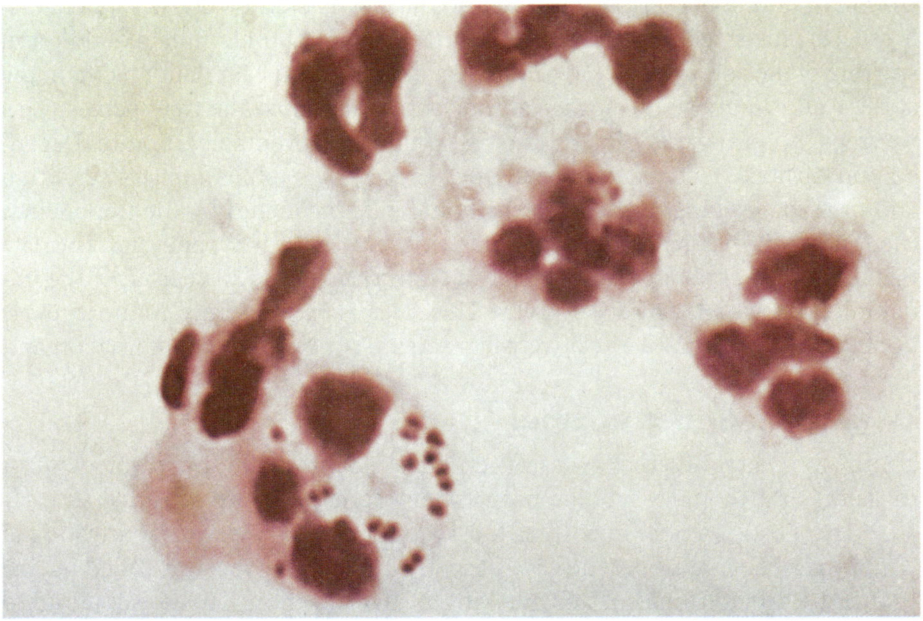

Figure 18-2 Gram stain of pus from the urethra, illustrating many Gram-negative intracellular diplococci characteristic of gonorrhea (original magnification x1,000).
Courtesy of Leonard V. Crowley, MD, Century College.

Salpingitis Inflammation of the fallopian tubes.
Ectopic pregnancy A pregnancy outside the endometrial cavity.
Posterior urethra The section of the male urethra encompassing the membranous urethra and the prostate urethra.

causes an acute **salpingitis** (salpinx = tube). Sometimes, the tubal infection is followed by the formation of an abscess within the fallopian tube or an abscess involving both the tube and the adjacent ovary. Gonococcal salpingitis is manifested by abdominal pain and tenderness together with elevated temperature and leukocytosis. Scarring following the tubal infection may delay transport of the fertilized ovum through the fallopian tube, causing the pregnancy to develop in the tube instead of the uterus, a condition termed an **ectopic pregnancy** (described in Chapter 15). Complete obstruction of both tubes by scar tissue blocks the transport of a fertilized ovum through the tubes and leads to sterility.

Gonorrhea in the Male

In the male, gonococci cause an acute inflammation of the mucosa of the anterior part of the urethra. The infection is usually manifested by a purulent urethral discharge and considerable pain on urination, and if untreated, urethral strictures. Occasionally the infected male may have relatively few symptoms, although he is still capable of infecting others. However, gonorrhea is less likely to be asymptomatic in men than in women.

From the anterior urethra, the infection often spreads by direct extension into the **posterior urethra**, prostate, seminal vesicles, vasa deferentia, and epididymides. An infection in both epididymides and vasa deferentia may lead to sterility because the scarring after the infection may obstruct the duct system and thus block transport of sperm into the seminal fluid.

Extragenital Gonorrhea

Recently, the incidence of gonococcal infection in extragenital sites has increased, particularly in the MSM population. Gonococcal infection of the rectal mucosa causes anorectal pain and tenderness associated with purulent bloody mucoid discharge from the rectum. Rectal infection results from contamination of the rectal mucosa either by infected vaginal secretions or from anal intercourse. Gonococcal infection of the pharynx and tonsils results from oral–genital sex. The infection may be asymptomatic but often causes a sore throat. Neonatal gonorrhea, a result of infection during birth, is most often expressed as conjunctivitis. It is still a major cause of blindness in areas with poor neonatal care, but it is prevented by ocular antibiotic instillation in the United States.

Disseminated Gonococcal Infection

In a small proportion of infected patients, the organism gains access to the bloodstream and spreads throughout the body. This serious complication is characterized by elevated temperature, joint pain, multiple small abscesses in the skin, and sometimes infections of the joints, tendons, heart valves, and covering of the brain (meninges).

Diagnosis and Treatment

Diagnosis of gonorrhea is most commonly established by the use of nucleic acid–based tests on urine or localized swabs. Culturing gonococci from suspected sites of infection—urethra, cervix, rectum, and pharynx—can also be used.

Currently only the antibiotic cephalosporin is used as a first-line treatment. There is increasing concern that strains of gonorrhea are becoming less sensitive to this agent, requiring higher doses for therapy.

Trichomonad Genital Tract Infections

The trichomonads are small motile parasites. One species, *Trichomonas vaginalis*, sometimes causes an acute inflammation of the vagina characterized by itching, burning, and a profuse, frothy vaginal discharge. The infection can be transmitted to the male by sexual intercourse and causes an inflammation of the urethra. In females, *T. vaginalis* infection is a common cause of a common type of vaginitis (see Vaginitis, this chapter). Overall, it is one of the most common sexually transmitted infections (STIs). Infection increases the risk of HIV transmission and is associated with problems in pregnancy, including low birth weight and intrauterine infection (**Figure 18-3**).

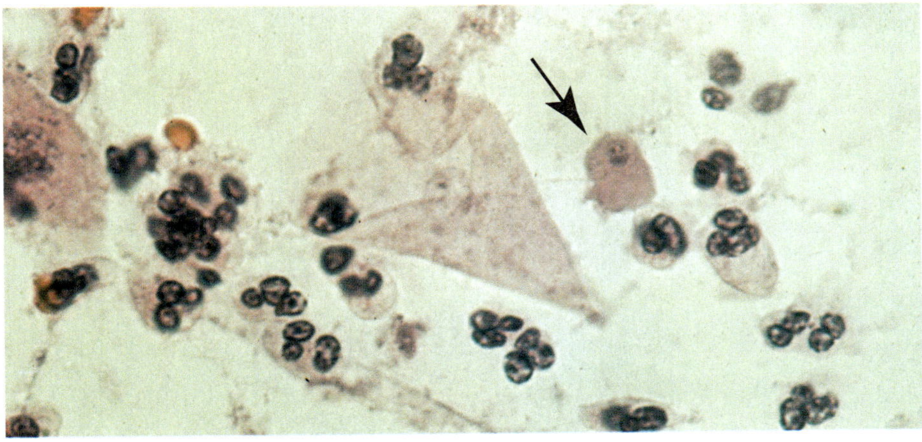

Figure 18-3 Vaginal secretions from women with trichomonad infection, illustrating parasite (*arrow*) and many neutrophils.

Courtesy of Leonard V. Crowley, MD, Century College.

Herpes

The herpes simplex virus is one of several herpes viruses that infect people. There are two forms of the herpes simplex virus, designated types 1 and 2 (HSV-1 and HSV-2). HSV-1 usually infects the oral mucous membrane, where it causes the familiar fever blisters. Most individuals are infected in childhood, and most adults have antibodies to the virus, indicating a previous infection. HSV-2 usually infects the genital tract, and most infections occur after puberty. However, the two types are not restricted in their distribution. Either HSV-1 or HSV-2 may infect either site. Genital herpes is common and an estimated 1 in 6 persons between 14 and 49 years of age are infected with the virus, although many infections are asymptomatic or mild. Serological evidence of infection is common to both forms of the virus. About 12 percent of persons in the United States are HSV-2 positive, but the great majority of them have never been clinically diagnosed.

The clinical course of genital disease caused by either HSV-1 or HSV-2 is indistinguishable, although HSV-2 tends to reoccur more frequently. About 80 percent of genital lesions are associated with HSV-2, although genital HSV-1 infections are becoming more common. The lesions caused by the viral infection usually appear within a week after sexual exposure. They consist of clusters of very small, painful blisters (vesicles) that soon rupture, forming painful shallow ulcers that often coalesce. This may be accompanied by fever, headache, and other systemic symptoms. The lesions contain large quantities of virus and are infectious upon sexual contact. Usually the lymph nodes draining the infected areas are swollen and tender. In men, the vesicles usually appear on the glans or shaft of the penis (**Figure 18-4**). In women, the lesions may be quite extensive (**Figure 18-5**). They may be on the vulva, in the vagina, or on the cervix. Vulvar lesions are quite painful, but those deep in the vagina or on the cervix may cause little discomfort because these regions are relatively insensitive. The ulcers heal slowly in a few weeks. However, the virus persists in the tissues of the infected person and may flare up periodically, causing recurrent infections. Some patients have repeated flare-ups for several years after the initial infection.

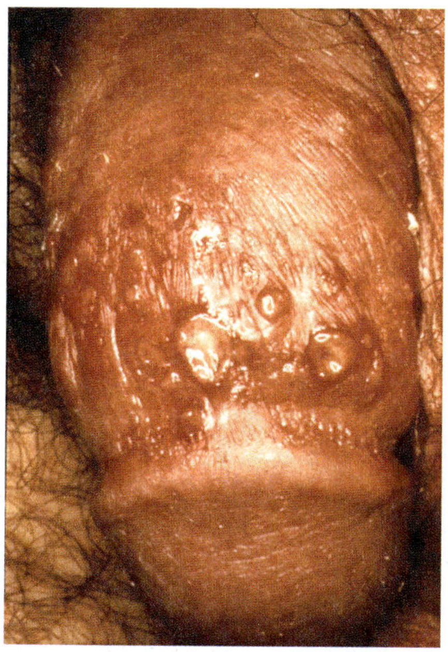

Figure 18-4 Several small superficial herpetic ulcers on the shaft of the penis behind the glans.

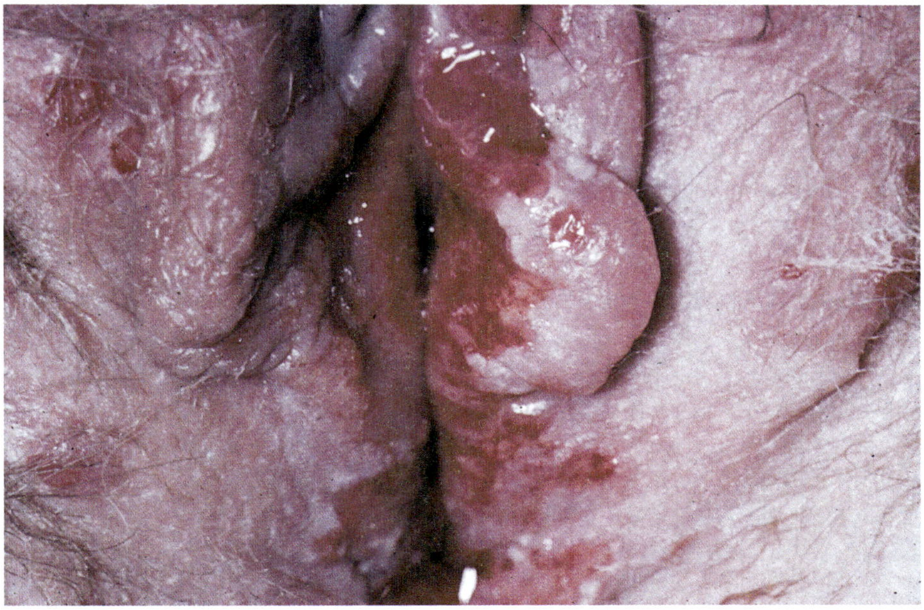

Figure 18-5 Multiple confluent ulcers of the vulva as a result of herpes.
Courtesy of Leonard V. Crowley, MD, Century College.

Active herpetic ulcers shed large amounts of virus, and sexual partners of patients with active lesions are readily infected. Unfortunately, patients without active lesions or symptoms also may excrete small amounts of virus periodically and may infect their sexual partners.

Diagnosis and Treatment

Herpes can usually be suspected from the clinical appearance of the lesions and can be confirmed by smears obtained from the lesions, which reveal the characteristic intranuclear inclusions in infected cells (**Figure 18-6**).

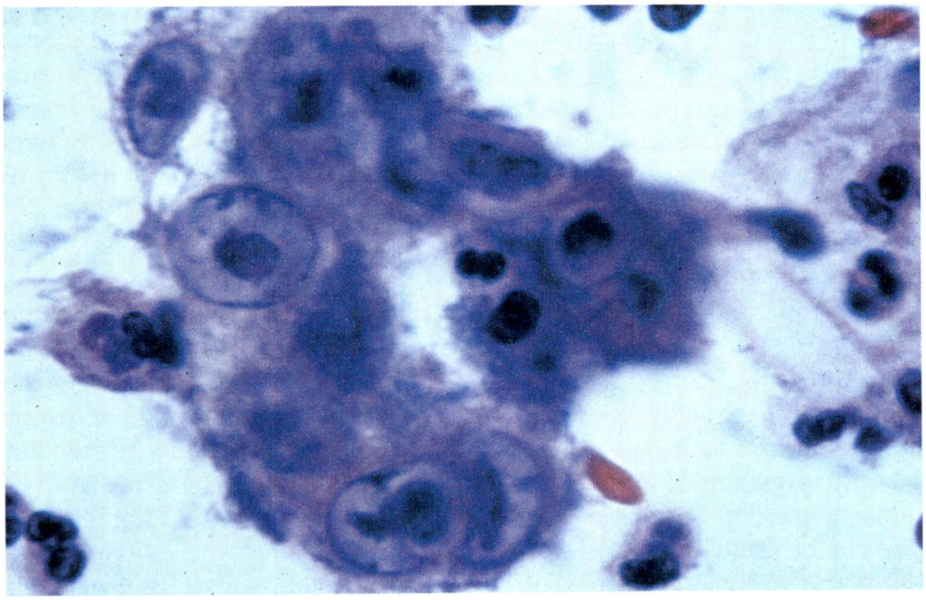

Figure 18-6 Vaginal smear illustrating clusters of herpes-infected epithelial cells containing intranuclear inclusions (original magnification ×1000).
Courtesy of Leonard V. Crowley, MD, Century College.

Antiviral drugs are available that shorten the course and reduce the severity of an acute infection; they do not eradicate the virus but do decrease (but not prevent) transmission. Depending on the severity of the infection, they can be administered intravenously or, more commonly, orally or applied as an ointment to the lesions. Patients with frequent and disabling recurrent infections sometimes benefit from long-term oral treatment, which seems to reduce the frequency and severity of recurrences.

Herpes Infection and Pregnancy

A pregnant person with a genital herpes infection may infect her infant. If the mother has active herpetic lesions in her genital tract, the infant may acquire the virus when passing through the genital tract during delivery. Consequently, a mother with an active infection is usually delivered by cesarean section to prevent infection of the newborn infant. Neonatal herpetic infections may infect the central nervous system and many other visceral organs and, if untreated, have a high risk of mortality.

Genital Chlamydial Infections

The chlamydiae are very small, Gram-negative, nonmotile bacteria once thought to be large viruses. They are deficient in certain enzymes and can live only as parasites inside of the cells of the individual that they infect. They are taken into the cells of the host by phagocytosis, where they divide and form large intracytoplasmic clusters of organisms termed inclusion bodies. These resemble inclusion bodies formed in some viral diseases. Their growth can be inhibited by various antibiotics that inhibit protein synthesis.

Genital tract infection caused by *Chlamydia trachomatis* is now the most commonly reported sexually transmitted disease. In 2023, an estimated 1.6 million new infections with *Chlamydia trachomatis* occurred in the United States among adults aged 15 to 49 years. The global prevalence among people aged 15–49 years was estimated to be 4.0% for women and 2.5% for men in 2020. The incidence is almost three times that of gonorrhea. Part of this increase reflects the availability of new diagnostic tests that enable the healthcare provider to recognize chlamydial infections in patients who have few symptoms, and these cases probably would previously have gone undetected. Many chlamydial infections are asymptomatic, and detection is the result of routine screening. The risk of male–female transmission in unprotected sex is between 10 and 20 percent, and rates of transmission from infected mother to newborn are 50 percent or greater. About 1.4% of newborns develop signs of chlamydial disease.

Chlamydia causes much the same type of inflammation and clinical symptoms as gonorrhea. In women, the initial infection is usually in the uterine cervix and is associated with moderate vaginal discharge. Men often develop acute inflammation of the urethra associated with frequency and burning on urination. Like gonorrhea, the chlamydial infection may spread to the fallopian tubes in women, followed by scarring and impaired fertility, and may cause acute epididymitis in men. As in gonorrhea, many infected individuals may have no symptoms of infection but are still able to infect their sexual partners and may develop complications related to the spread of the infection to other parts of the genital tract.

Another species of chlamydiae causes an uncommon sexually transmissible disease termed lymphogranuloma venereum. This disease is characterized by marked enlargement and inflammation of the lymph nodes in the groin and around the rectum.

Diagnosis and Treatment

Highly sensitive and specific tests are available that can detect chlamydial antigens in cervical secretions and secretions from the male urethra, and the tests can also be performed on urine. Nucleic acid amplification tests, similar to the tests used to identify gonococci, can also be used to diagnose a chlamydial infection by identifying characteristic groups of chlamydial nucleic acids. Currently, azithromycin and doxycycline are preferred for therapy and are 95 percent effective. Both the patient and the partner should be treated.

Condylomas of the Genital Tract and HPV Infection

Condylomas, sometimes termed venereal warts, are benign, warty, tumor-like overgrowths of squamous epithelium caused by human papillomavirus (HPV). Infection with HPV is the most common sexually transmitted disease in the United States, with 30 percent to 40 percent of women between the ages of 20 and 30 being infected. HPV occurs as different strains termed **serotypes**, two of which (6 and 11) are responsible for most cases of condylomas. However, other serotypes (16, 18, and other high-risk types) are major risk factors for **squamous intraepithelial lesions (SILs)** and invasive squamous cell cancers in regions of the female genital tract, including the vulva and cervix (see later in this chapter).

Serotype Immunologically detected pathogen strains.

Squamous intraepithelial lesions (SILs) Precancerous results of infection with some HPV serotypes.

Condylomas vary in size from a few millimeters to more than 1 cm in diameter and frequently occur in multiples. Condylomas develop most often on the vulvar mucosa, on the mucosa of the cervix and vagina (**Figure 18-7**), and around the vaginal opening and anus. Treatment consists of destroying the lesions; this may be accomplished by applying a strong chemical (podophyllin), electrocoagulation, freezing (cryocautery), or surgical excision. Condylomas caused by HPV types 6 and 11 rarely become malignant. However, other condyloma-like skin lesions are associated with high-risk HPV types

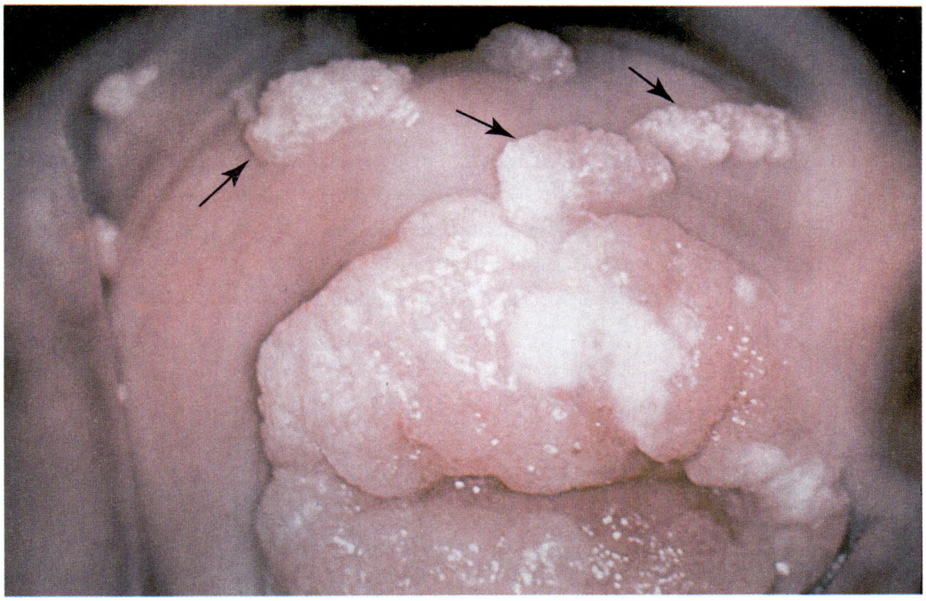

Figure 18-7 Cervical and vaginal mucosa viewed through a vaginal speculum, revealing multiple condylomas (*arrows*) arising from the mucosa.

Courtesy of Leonard V. Crowley, MD, Century College.

and may present a risk for becoming malignant. HPV vaccination in women and men protects against infection with both cancer-causing and condyloma-causing strains of the agent.

HPV Vaccine

The U.S. FDA licensed Gardasil 9 for use in the United States, which protects against 9 strains of the virus. Vaccination at about age 11 to 12 is optimal since most children are unlikely to have been infected with the HPV types included in the vaccines. Even in immunized females, regular gynecologic care and Pap smears are required because other carcinogenic serotypes not covered by the vaccine may still cause papillomas, dysplasia, and cervical cancer. However, the vaccine is nearly 100 percent effective against the serotypes it covers.

Infections of the Female Genital Tract

Infections of the genital tract are common. Frequently involved sites include the vagina, cervix, and fallopian tubes. In addition, certain virus infections of the genital tract cause highly characteristic lesions termed condylomas. Most of the infectious agents of the female genital tract are sexually transmitted.

Vaginitis

Vaginal infections are common. They frequently cause vaginal discharge, together with vulvovaginal itching and irritation. These infections are caused by the fungus *Candida albicans*, (yeast infection), the protozoan parasite *Trichomonas vaginalis*, (see above) or a small gram-negative bacterium termed *Gardnerella (Haemophilus) vaginalis*, in conjunction with various anaerobic vaginal bacteria.

The protozoan parasite *Trichomonas vaginalis* causes the third common type of vaginitis, often termed nonspecific vaginitis, and is usually associated with a profuse, foul-smelling vaginal discharge. So-called nonspecific vaginitis often results from *Gardnerella* infection. Highly specific methods of treatment are available for each type of vaginitis. Unlike *Trichomonas* and *Gardnerella* infections, candidiasis is not sexually transmitted but often occurs with diabetes, antibiotic use, or pregnancy.

Cervicitis

Mild chronic inflammation of endocervical glands is very common in women who have had children. Cervicitis causes few symptoms and is of little clinical significance. More severe cervical inflammation may result from a gonococcal infection or a chlamydial infection. Both infections are sexually transmitted and may be followed by the spread of the infection into the fallopian tubes and adjacent tissues.

Salpingitis and Pelvic Inflammatory Disease

Salpingitis means an inflammation of the fallopian tube (salpinx = tube). The more general term **pelvic inflammatory disease (PID)** refers to any infection that affects the fallopian tubes and adjacent tissues. Sometimes the ovaries are infected along with the fallopian tubes. Most cases are secondary to the spread of a cervical gonorrheal or chlamydial infection through the uterus into the fallopian tubes and surrounding tissues. Less commonly, other pathogenic organisms are involved. An acute pelvic infection causes severe lower abdominal pain and tenderness, together with elevated temperature and leukocytosis.

Pelvic inflammatory disease (PID) A general term for an infection affecting the fallopian tubes and adjacent pelvic organs.

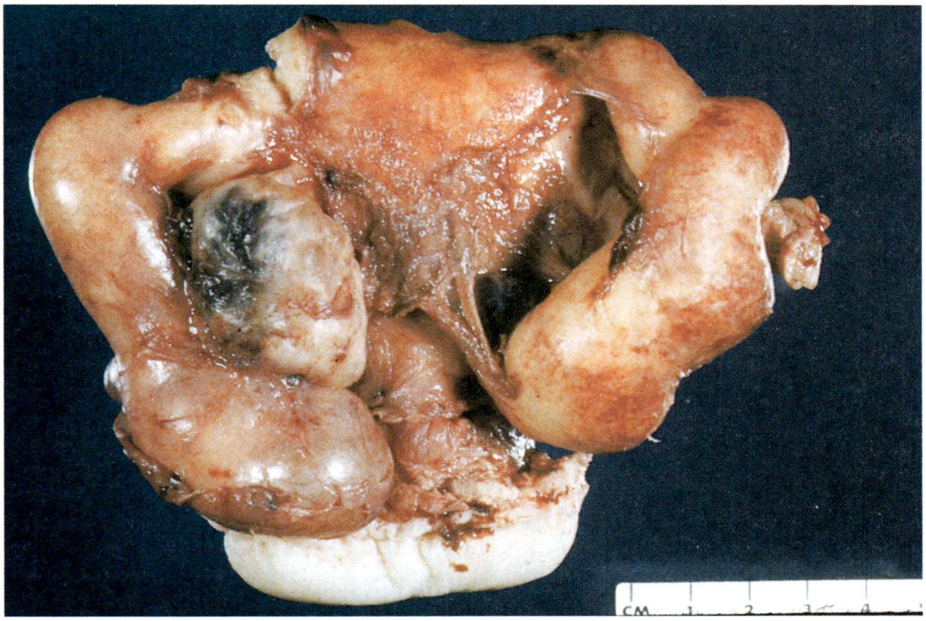

Figure 18-8 Chronic pelvic inflammatory disease. Resected uterus, tubes, and left ovary viewed from behind. Tubes are swollen, and fimbriated ends are occluded. There are numerous adhesions between the tubes and the uterus.

Courtesy of Leonard V. Crowley, MD, Century College.

Both gonorrheal and nongonorrheal salpingitis respond to appropriate antibiotic treatment; healing of the inflammation, however, may be associated with scarring and obstruction of the tubal lumen. Sterility may result if the tubal obstruction is bilateral (**Figure 18-8**). Sometimes, even if the tubes are not completely occluded, the scarring may delay the transport of a fertilized ovum through the tube and lead to an ectopic pregnancy, which is considered in Chapter 15.

Toxic Shock Syndrome

Toxic shock syndrome (TSS) was first recognized 35 years ago in menstruating women who used high-absorbency tampons for prolonged periods of time. The frequency declined as other menstrual products replaced them, although no tampon or menstrual cup is entirely free from risk. Currently, half of the cases of TSS arise from conditions other than menstruation, such as commonly infected wounds. Cases are also associated with non-gynecologic infections involving surgery and burns. A quarter of cases occur in men.

Toxic shock syndrome (TSS) Disease characterized by elevated temperature, vomiting and diarrhea, muscular aches, and a fall in blood pressure.

Superantigens Antigens that cause widespread activation of T cells and release of cytokines.

Clinically, the disease is characterized by elevated temperature, vomiting and diarrhea, muscular aches and pains, a fall in blood pressure (often to shock levels), and various other systemic manifestations. A characteristic feature of the disease is an erythematous (sunburn-like) skin rash that is followed by flaking and peeling of the affected skin (somewhat like the peeling that occurs after a severe sunburn).

The clinical manifestations of toxic shock syndrome are caused by toxins (TSST-1 and infrequently, a number of enterotoxins) produced by *Staphylococcus aureus* or group A *Streptococcus* (*Streptococcus pyogenes*). The toxins act as **superantigens**, causing widespread activation of T cells and the release of cytokines (T cell products) that cause shock and tissue damage. Although TSS is not common (1–3 cases per 10,000), the overall mortality rate is high (over 30 percent). Menstrual-related TSS has a much lower fatality rate of about 2 percent.

Diseases of the Vulva

Vulvar Intraepithelial Neoplasia

Vulvar intraepithelial neoplasia (VIN) Cancer of the vulva.

There are two different forms of **vulvar intraepithelial neoplasia (VIN)**, either of which can progress to invasive squamous cell carcinoma if untreated. The first (classic or usual VIN [UVIN]) comprises about 40 percent of cases and is caused by infection with high-risk HPV serotypes (usually HPV 16, sometimes 18, or others). It has the same risk factors as condylomas and tends to occur in younger women (40 to 50 years of age) with multiple sexual partners and a young age at first intercourse. Whereas condylomas are classified as squamous intraepithelial lesions of low risk, untreated UVIN has about a 6 percent risk of becoming invasive with time (6 years or longer) and may develop into high-risk squamous intraepithelial lesions (HSIL). Lesions may be warty (condyloma-like) or flat (basaloid). See **Figure 18-9**.

The more common form of VIN, termed differentiated VIN (DVIN), occurs in older, usually postmenopausal women in the seventh decade. DVIN is not associated with HPV but tends to occur in the setting of chronic vulvar inflammatory/dermatological conditions. The epithelium of the vulva may exhibit irregular areas of thickening and inflammation that appear as white patches. Histologically, the affected epithelium appears heavily keratinized, and the epithelial cells show variable abnormalities of maturation. Clinically, the condition can present with intense itching and tenderness of the affected areas. The nonspecific descriptive term leukoplakia (leuko = white + plakia = patch) describes this type of lesion. Untreated DVIN has an appreciable frequency of progression to invasive cancer (33 percent). Various types of local treatment are mostly effective. If significant precancerous changes are present in the epithelium, the affected areas need to be surgically removed. As noted, vulvar carcinoma (invasive squamous cell carcinoma) may occur in both pre- and postmenopausal women (**Figure 18-10**).

When occult invasion is unlikely, local excision, laser therapy, or topical drugs may be used for treatment. If invasive disease is suspected, wide local excisions or even resection of the vulva (vulvectomy) along with the inguinal lymph nodes may be undertaken.

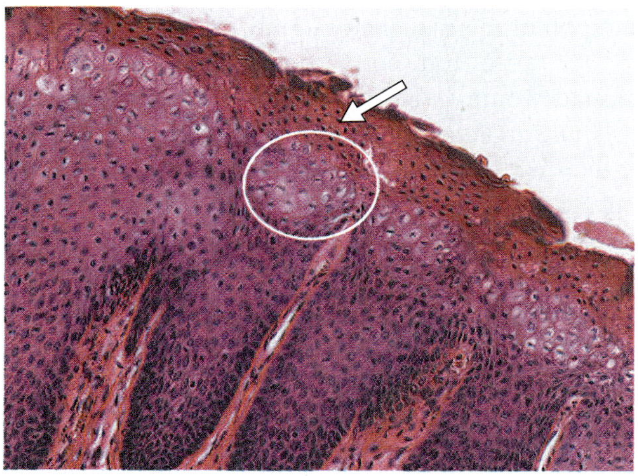

Figure 18-9 UVIN lesion of the vulva (flat, basaloid type). The lesion has a thickened keratinized layer and is hyperkeratotic (*arrow*). Many cells show koilocytosis; they have enlarged and irregular nuclei surrounded by a perinuclear halo (*circled area*). This is indicative of infection with HPV.

Courtesy of Department of Pathology and Laboratory Medicine, University of North Carolina at Chapel Hill.

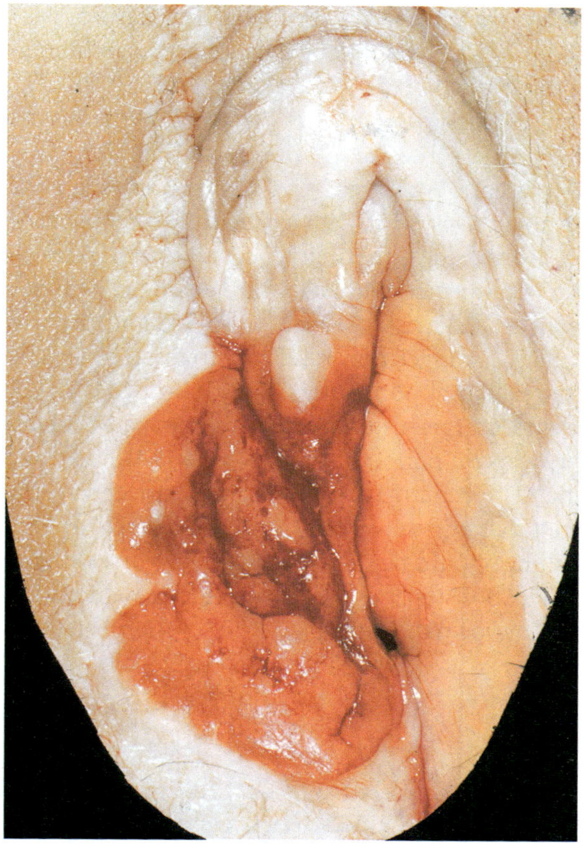

Figure 18-10 A large carcinoma of the vulva. The white appearance of the skin adjacent to the carcinoma is caused by preexisting vulvar dystrophy.
Courtesy of Leonard V. Crowley, MD, Century College.

Conditions of the Cervix

Cervical Polyps

Occasionally, benign polyps arise from the cervix. Usually, they are small and do not cause symptoms, but some may be quite large. Sometimes the tip of the polyp becomes eroded and causes bleeding. Treatment consists of surgically removing the polyp.

Cervical Intraepithelial Lesions (CIN)

In the past, cervical cancer was the number one cause of cancer-related death in American women. Although worldwide it remains the fourth most common cancer in women and is the most common cancer among women in 25 countries, mortality has fallen drastically in the United States (13,000 new cases and 4,000 deaths in 2025) as a result of cytological screening of cervical cells (Pap smear and related techniques). Cervical cancer is the ultimate result of untreated, high-risk squamous intraepithelial lesions (HSIL) of the cervix. As is the case with UVIN, cervical intraepithelial neoplasia (CIN) is related to infection with HPV and bears the same risk factors. Low-risk squamous intraepithelial lesions (LSIL) are classified as CIN I or mild dysplasia and are related to infection with low-risk HPV serotypes (6 and 11), which may be expressed as genital warts on the cervix. Such lesions rarely progress and may disappear spontaneously. Low-risk HPV does not become integrated into host cell DNA but remains as an episome. Virus accumulates in the infected cell, eventually killing it. High-risk squamous intraepithelial lesions are classified as CIN II moderate dysplasia or CIN III severe dysplasia or carcinoma *in situ* and are associated with infection by high-risk HPV serotypes (16, 18, and many others). They do not regress spontaneously. Such HPV serotypes integrate into the host cell DNA and synthesize viral proteins that allow for tumor progression into invasive disease. Although rates of infection with HPV are substantial (20 percent of women ages 18 to 59 were found to be infected with high-risk serotypes in the last decade), the incidence of cancer is far lower. The small proportion of women infected with a cancer-causing HPV type who are unable to eliminate the virus are at risk of severe dysplasia and cervical carcinoma.

Dysplastic changes range from mild disturbances of epithelial maturation (CIN I) to severe cellular abnormalities (CIN II and CIN III). Severe dysplasia does not regress and progresses to in situ carcinoma and eventually to invasive carcinoma after a variable period of time (**Figure 18-11**).

Currently the ACS recommends that cervical cancer screening should begin at age 25 and continue every five years until age 65. If HPV testing is unavailable, a Pap test alone should be done every three years. Recently an "in-home" cervical cancer detection test has been introduced, which does not require a healthcare worker or vaginal dilation.

Diagnosis and Treatment of Cervical Dysplasia

The cellular abnormalities indicative of CIN (dysplasia and carcinoma *in situ*) develop first in the cells at the junction between the squamous epithelium covering the exterior of the cervix and the columnar epithelium lining the cervical canal. This region is termed the squamocolumnar junction, or **female transition zone**, and is usually located at the external opening (external os) of the cervix. During a Pap smear, cells are collected both from the area of the transition zone and from the endocervical canal because adenocarcinoma of the endocervical canal can result from HSIL occurring in that area.

Female Transition zone
The junction of the ectocervix (the part of the cervix that protrudes into the vagina) and the endocervical canal (the inner part of the cervix)

An abnormal Pap smear requires further evaluation using HPV testing if not already performed. In cervical dysplasia and carcinoma, characteristic abnormalities in the cervical epithelium and underlying blood vessels can be identified that define the location and extent of the abnormal epithelium. After initial diagnosis, multiple biopsy specimens are taken from the abnormal-appearing areas and material from the endocervical canal. CIN II and CIN III lesions (HSIL) are

(A)
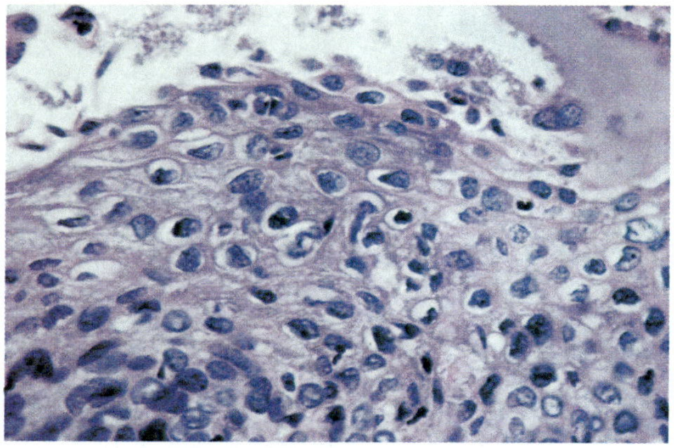
(B)
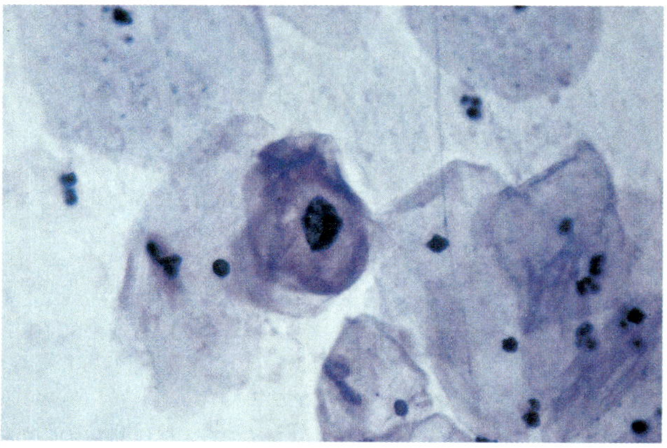

Figure 18-11 **(A)** Cervical epithelial dysplasia (CIN III carcinoma in situ) caused by papilloma virus. **(B)** Dysplastic epithelial cell identified in Papanicolaou smear (original magnification ×400).

usually treated by destruction of the abnormal epithelium by freezing (cryocautery), laser light, or surgical excision. HSIL lesions can be cured by proper treatment and carry an excellent prognosis. These lesions may remain localized within the epithelium of the cervix for as long as 10 years before eventually becoming invasive. Once invasion occurs, however, the neoplasm becomes much harder to treat, with less satisfactory results. The tumor may extend through the cervix into the adjacent tissues and may infiltrate the rectum and bladder. The ureters, which lie on each side of the cervix, may also be invaded and obstructed by the neoplasm. Metastatic spread to regional lymph nodes and distant sites also occurs. Invasive carcinoma is treated either by radiation or by resection of the uterus, fallopian tubes, ovaries, and adjacent tissues (radical hysterectomy).

Other Sites of HPV Infection

As previously noted, in addition to HPV-caused cervical cancer, HPV has also been identified in association with carcinoma of the vulva, penis, rectum, oral cavity, and oropharynx, where it may have been transmitted from a cervical infection.

Conditions of the Uterus

Benign Proliferative Changes in the Uterus

An excess of estrogen unrelated to the usual menstrual cycle may result from a variety of causes, including anovulatory cycles, estrogenic drug therapy, obesity, and polycystic ovary syndrome, and will result in persistent proliferative uterine changes. With continuing stimulation, increased glandular hyperplasia occurs, a condition termed **nonatypical endometrial hyperplasia**, which is characterized by unevenly distributed areas of increasing gland density throughout the uterus (**Figure 18-12**). These glands are often dilated and show a

Nonatypical endometrial hyperplasia Uterine condition characterized by unevenly distributed areas of increasing gland density in the uterus.

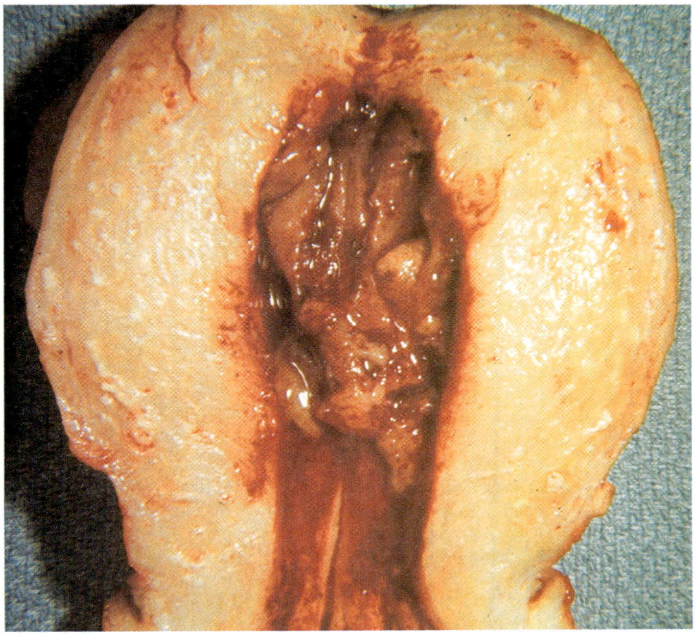

Figure 18-12 Nonatypical endometrial hyperplasia (benign endometrial hyperplasia). The uterus opened to reveal polypoid masses of hyperplastic endometrium filling the endometrial cavity.

Courtesy of Leonard V. Crowley, MD, Century College.

Proliferative phase Growth of endometrial cells lining the uterus.

Endometrial intraepithelial neoplasia (EIN) Result of long-term nonatypical endometrial hyperplasia; a precursor lesion to cancer.

Leiomyomas Benign, smooth muscle tumors in the uterus.

tubular ciliated structure similar to the **proliferative phase** of the menstrual cycle. Although by itself a benign condition, long-term nonatypical endometrial hyperplasia may develop areas of atypical hyperplasia (**endometrial intraepithelial neoplasia (EIN)**), a precursor lesion to cancer. Continued presence of estrogens will result in irregular uterine bleeding, and a sudden lack of estrogen can result in extremely heavy menses.

Benign polyps in the endometrium are also common. An endometrial polyp may cause uterine bleeding if the tip becomes inflamed or ulcerated.

Uterine Leiomyomas

Benign, smooth muscle tumors termed **leiomyomas** (myomas or fibroids) arise in the wall of the uterus (**Figure 18-13**). They are frequently encountered and are estimated to occur in approximately 30 percent of women over 30 years

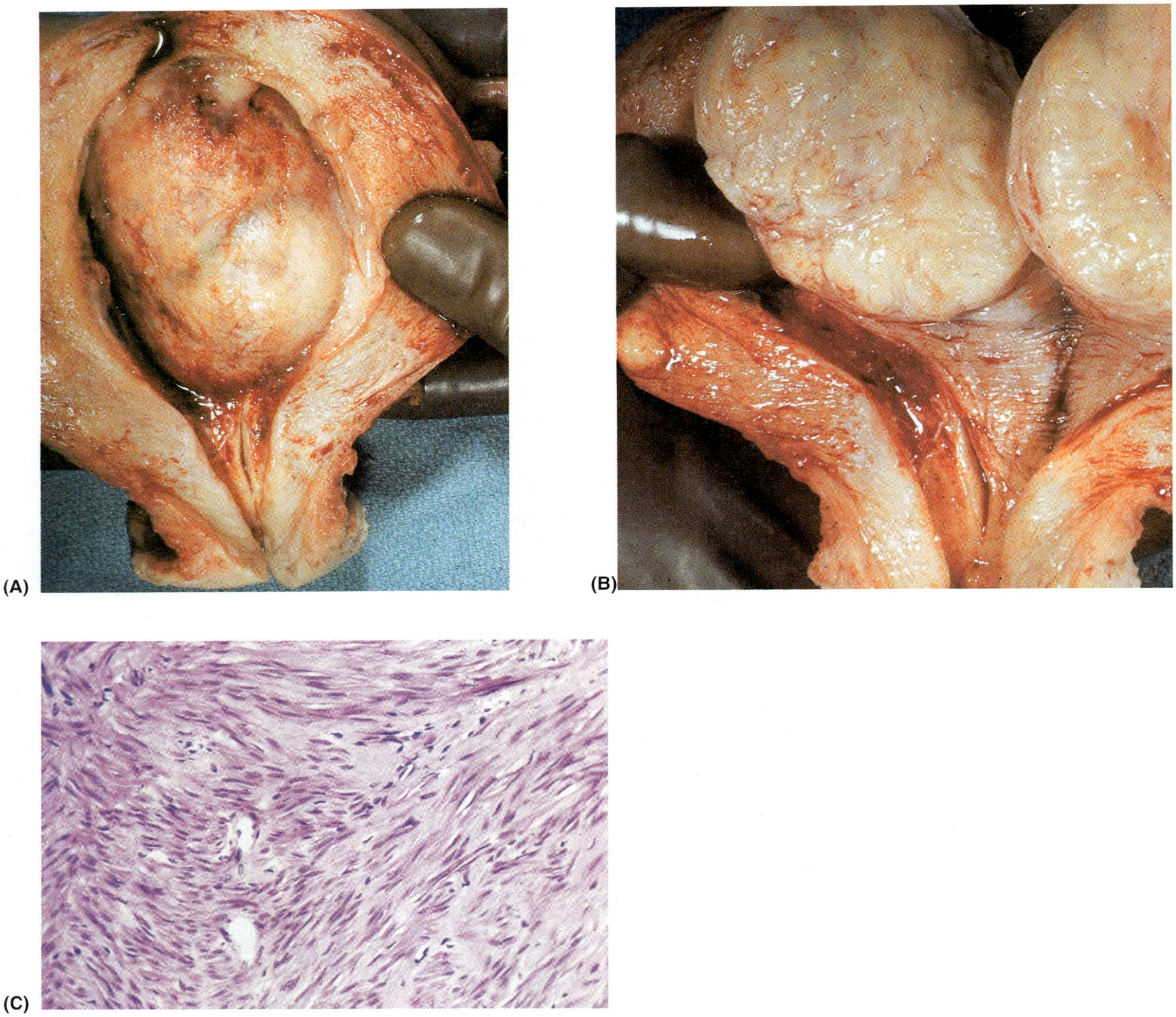

Figure 18-13 Uterine myoma. **(A)** A uterus opened to reveal a large spherical myoma protruding into the endometrial cavity. **(B)** A cross section of myoma illustrating a well-circumscribed tumor without evidence of necrosis, features suggesting a benign neoplasm. **(C)** Histologic appearance, revealing interlacing bundles of mature smooth muscle cells that resemble the normal muscle cells from which the tumor arose (original magnification ×100).

Courtesy of Leonard V. Crowley, MD, Century College.

of age. Occasionally, leiomyomas may be responsible for excessive or irregular uterine bleeding or may produce symptoms related to pressure on the adjacent bladder or rectum. When symptomatic, myomectomy (removal of the leiomyoma) or hysterectomy (removal of the uterus) may be required.

Neoplastic Proliferative Changes in the Uterus

Endometrial intraepithelial neoplasia (EIN) is the precursor lesion to endometrial adenocarcinoma. Uterine (endometrial) cancer is the most common gynecologic cancer. Uterine cancer has two major types. Type I carcinoma is endometroid; that is, it resembles the proliferative glands seen in nonatypical endometrial hyperplasia in its earliest stages (grade 1 lesions). Increasingly advanced stage (grades 2 and 3) is poorly differentiated, with loss of glandlike structures showing increasing degrees of cellular atypia, including increased and abnormal mitosis (**Figure 18-14**). Type I carcinoma has its origin in continued unopposed estrogen stimulation of the uterus. It comprises about 80 percent of cases and tends to occur either in older premenopausal women or at the time of menopause. The disease usually has a favorable course and is detected at a low grade while confined to the uterus. Type II endometrial carcinoma occurs in older women and has a much more serious course with a poor prognosis because the cancer is invasive and often discovered at a late stage. The most common form of type II carcinoma (serous adenocarcinoma) may spread through the fallopian tubes and invade the peritoneal surface. It is not related to estrogen-induced hyperplasia. Endometrial cancer is not reliably detected by routine cervical cancer screening but is suspected when abnormal uterine bleeding occurs in older (peri- or postmenopausal) women. Transvaginal ultrasound is helpful in diagnosis. Type I carcinoma confined to the endometrium may be treated by hysterectomy (sometimes accompanied by radiation). Type II carcinoma is often accompanied by metastases to the lung and lymph nodes associated with the aorta.

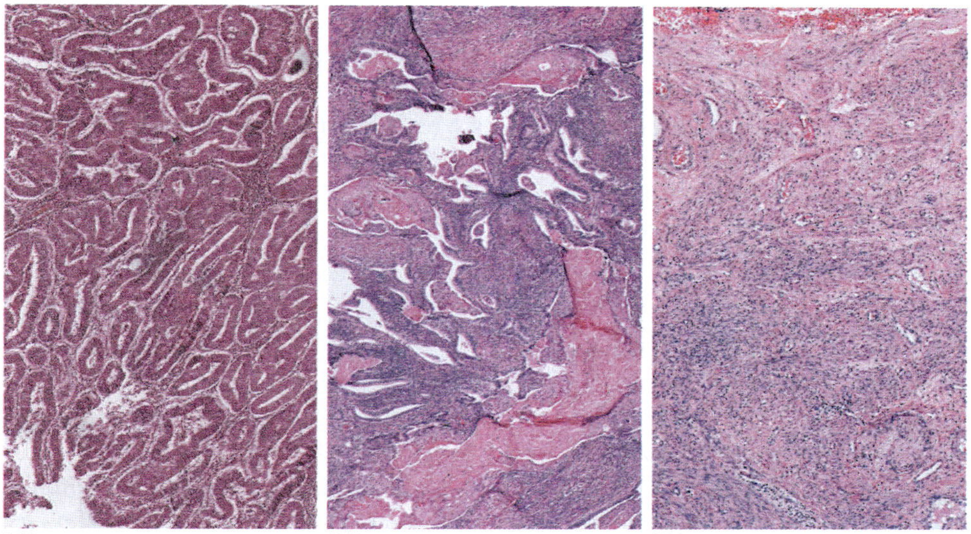

(A) (B) (C)

Figure 18-14 Uterine adenocarcinoma demonstrating increasingly advanced grades. **(A)** Grade 1. **(B)** Grade 2. **(C)** Grade 3.

Courtesy of Department of Pathology and Laboratory Medicine, University of North Carolina at Chapel Hill.

Irregular Uterine Bleeding

Excessive or irregular uterine bleeding is a common gynecologic problem. Most cases in younger women result from a disturbance of the coordinated activity of estrogen and progesterone on the endometrium in the normal cyclic. This is usually termed dysfunctional uterine bleeding. In older women, bleeding can be the result of many causes, including neoplastic disease.

Dysfunctional (Abnormal) Uterine Bleeding

Dysfunctional uterine bleeding (also referred to as abnormal uterine bleeding) arises from the disruption of the network of endocrine glands that control uterine function, rather than any abnormality of the uterus itself. Most cases of dysfunctional uterine bleeding occur because the follicle fails to mature to the point of ovulation and, consequently, no corpus luteum forms. As a result, the endometrium is subjected to continuous estrogen stimulation and responds by shedding irregularly instead of all at once as in a normal period. This condition is also termed anovulatory bleeding (ana = without + ovulation). It tends to occur at both extremes of reproductive life: when normal menstrual cycles are being established at puberty and near menopause when ovarian function is declining. Less commonly, irregular bleeding is the result of continuous secretion of progesterone from a corpus luteum that fails to involute. This prolongs the secretory phase of the endometrium, which sometimes sheds irregularly.

Dysfunctional uterine bleeding is treated by administering hormones to restore the proliferative–secretory sequence in the endometrium that is characteristic of a normal menstrual cycle. In one common treatment, the patient is given a synthetic steroid hormone having progesterone activity. The hormone induces secretory changes in the endometrium and stops the bleeding. The hormone treatment is then stopped, and the endometrium sheds as in a normal period. Frequently, the next cycle becomes normal and usually no further treatment is required. Multiple recurrent episodes of dysfunctional bleeding that lead to anemia resulting from excessive blood loss may require more aggressive treatment such as uterine ablation, destruction of the endometrium by a variety of physical methods, including heat, cold, or microwave radiation. Because the technique has serious consequences (including likely loss or compromise of fertility), medical treatment is preferred when feasible.

Uterine bleeding resulting from causes intrinsic to the uterus is not considered dysfunctional. This includes benign endometrial hyperplasia, endometrial and cervical polyps, uterine leiomyomas, EIN, and uterine carcinoma. For this reason, abnormal uterine bleeding (particularly in peri- and postmenopausal women) must be clinically evaluated with dispatch.

Diagnosis and Treatment

Irregular bleeding is always a cause for concern when it occurs in an older woman nearing the end of her reproductive years or after menopause because it may be the result of an endometrial carcinoma. Bleeding in older women is usually treated with **dilatation and curettage (D&C)**. In some cases endometrial sampling may be done in the medical office by aspiration sampling of more limited areas of the uterus. The tissue removed is examined microscopically by the pathologist. If the endometrial tissue is not malignant, no further treatment is needed. If endometrial carcinoma is detected on histologic examination, further treatment is required, usually consisting of hysterectomy, sometimes preceded by a course of radiation therapy.

Dilatation and curettage (D&C) Procedure involving scraping the lining of the uterus; used to treat irregular bleeding.

Endometriosis

Endometriosis refers to the presence of uterine endometrium in any location outside the endometrial cavity (**Figure 18-15**). Ectopic deposits (ecto = outside) of endometrium occasionally may be encountered most commonly in the ovary (**Figure 18-16**), in the wall of the uterus, or elsewhere in the pelvis. Sometimes endometrial tissue is found in the appendix or in the rectum. Endometriosis is a common problem, occurring in about 10 percent of women, and results in pelvic pain, irregular menses, or **dysmenorrhea**. Endometriosis results in infertility in as many as 30 percent of the patients. Often, the condition appears to occur in families, and a woman is more likely to develop endometriosis if her mother had it. Ectopic endometrial deposits respond to normal hormonal stimuli and therefore undergo cyclic menstrual desquamation and regeneration. Because the misplaced endometrial tissue is outside of the endometrial cavity, the "menses" tissue is not discharged through the vagina. Old blood and desquamated material are retained in the ectopic sites, leading to considerable scarring and causing crampy pain during menstrual periods. With time, ectopic foci become inflamed and fibrotic. Obstruction of the fallopian tubes by scarring may cause sterility. Infertility is a common complaint along with pain.

Endometriosis Presence of endometrial tissue in abnormal locations, such as in the ovary or pelvis.

Dysmenorrhea Painful menstruation.

The reason endometrial deposits occur in unusual locations is unknown, although many hypotheses have been proposed. Some cases seem to be caused by reflux of bits of shed endometrium along with menstrual blood through the fallopian tubes into the peritoneal cavity during menstruation (retrograde menstruation), which then implant and grow in the pelvis. This does not provide a complete explanation, as endometriosis is occasionally found in the lungs and lymph nodes, suggesting transport through the blood or lymph.

Diagnosis of endometriosis is usually established by visualizing the ectopic deposits within the pelvis. Treatment consists of removing or destroying the deposits surgically or impeding the progression of endometriosis by

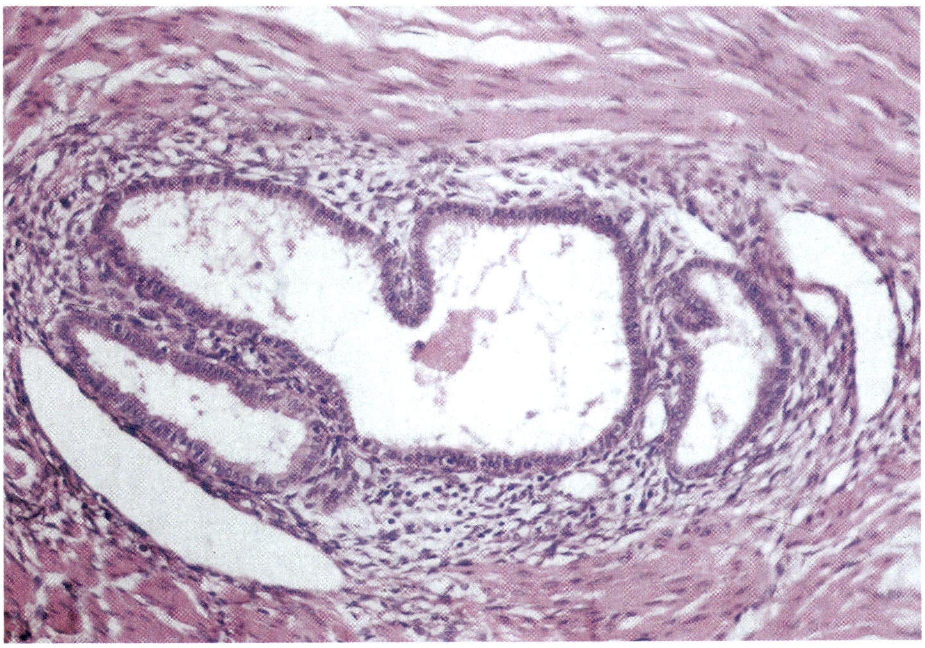

Figure 18-15 A photomicrograph of endometriosis in the uterine wall. Normal endometrial glands and stroma are surrounded by uterine muscle (original magnification ×100).

Courtesy of Leonard V. Crowley, MD, Century College.

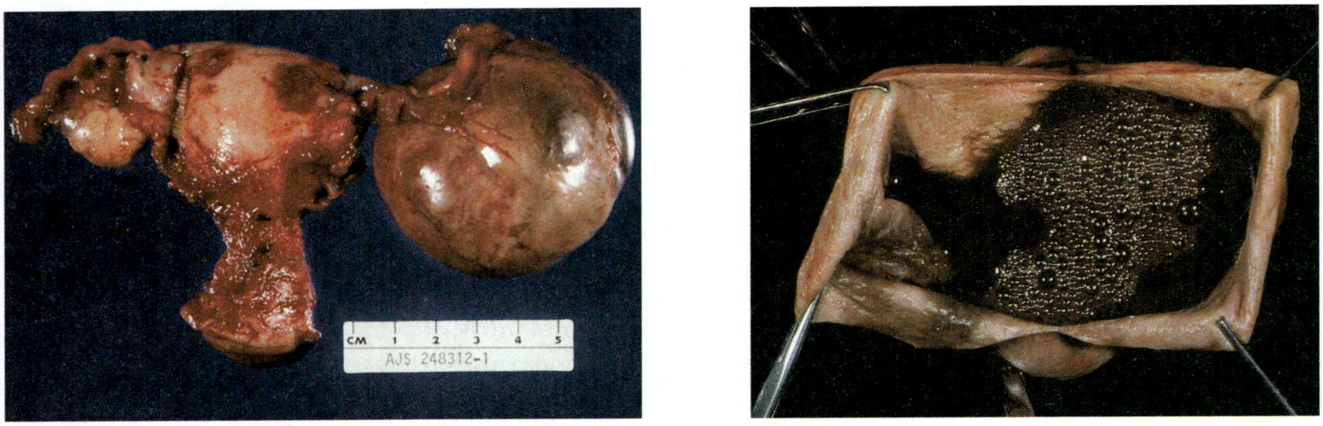

(A) (B)

Figure 18-16 **(A)** Endometriosis of the ovary. An accumulation of blood and debris within the ovarian endometriosis has led to formation of an endometrium-lined cyst filled with old blood and desquamated endometrial tissue within the right ovary (*right*). **(B)** Endometrial cyst opened, revealing contents consisting of old blood and debris derived from the endometrium lining the cyst.

administering drugs or hormones. Hormone treatments commonly used include synthetic hormones having progesterone activity that completely suppress the menstrual cycles or birth control pills that suppress ovulation, which affects the endometrium so that it becomes thin and atrophic. The subsequent menstrual periods are very light. Another treatment is to administer drugs that suppress the output of gonadotropins from the pituitary gland. This, in turn, leads to a decline in ovarian function, similar to that occurring in menopause. The deposits of endometrium, deprived of cyclic estrogen-progesterone stimulation, undergo regression.

Dysmenorrhea

Dysmenorrhea means painful menstruation. There are two types: primary dysmenorrhea, in which the pelvic organs are normal, and secondary dysmenorrhea, which results from various diseases of the pelvic organs, such as endometriosis.

Primary dysmenorrhea is the more common type. The pain is crampy, begins just prior to menstruation, and lasts for one or two days after onset of the menstrual flow. Usually, menstrual periods are painless for the first year or two after onset of menses during adolescence because early menstrual cycles are usually anovulatory, and primary dysmenorrhea does not occur unless ovulation occurs. Dysmenorrhea does not usually become a problem until regular ovulatory menstrual cycles are established.

Prostaglandin A series of derivatives of arachidonic acid that have widespread physiologic effects.

Crampy menstrual pain is caused by a class of compounds termed **prostaglandins**. Prostaglandins synthesized within the endometrium under the influence of progesterone are released when the endometrium breaks down during menstruation. When they diffuse into the myometrium, they cause the spasmodic myometrial contractions that are responsible for the crampy menstrual pain. Dysmenorrhea does not occur if cycles are anovulatory because no corpus luteum forms and no progesterone is produced to stimulate prostaglandin synthesis.

Treatment consists of aspirin or another anti-inflammatory drug such as ibuprofen, which is administered before the onset of menses. These drugs suppress the synthesis of prostaglandins within the endometrium. Primary dysmenorrhea can also be treated very effectively with oral contraceptive pills, which prevent dysmenorrhea by suppressing ovulation.

Cysts and Tumors of the Ovary

Nonneoplastic Lesions

The ovary gives rise to a wide variety of cysts and tumors, and only the more common ones are considered here. Benign ovarian cysts may arise from invaginated surface epithelium (serous cysts) from ovarian follicles or from corpora lutea (**Figure 18-17**) that have failed to regress normally and instead become converted into fluid-filled cysts. Follicle cysts and corpus luteum cysts are often termed functional cysts because they represent a derangement of the normal maturation and involution of a follicle or corpus luteum. Functional cysts do not usually become very large, and most regress spontaneously. Endometrial deposits in the ovary resulting from endometriosis may form cysts lined by endometrium and filled with old blood and debris. These are termed **endometrial cysts**.

Endometrial cyst An ovarian cyst lined by endometrium and filled with old blood and debris. A manifestation of endometriosis.

Polycystic Ovary Syndrome

Polycystic ovary syndrome (PCOS), also termed Stein-Leventhal syndrome, is a common endocrine disorder affecting 10 percent of women in the United States and is a common cause of infertility. It is often diagnosed in the second to third decade because PCOS is a very common cause of anovulatory infertility. The disease is also associated with obesity, insulin resistance (pre-diabetes), hirsutism (excess body hair), and other virilizing signs such as

Polycystic ovary syndrome (PCOS) Common endocrine disorder and common cause of anovulatory infertility; associated with obesity, diabetes, and hirsutism.

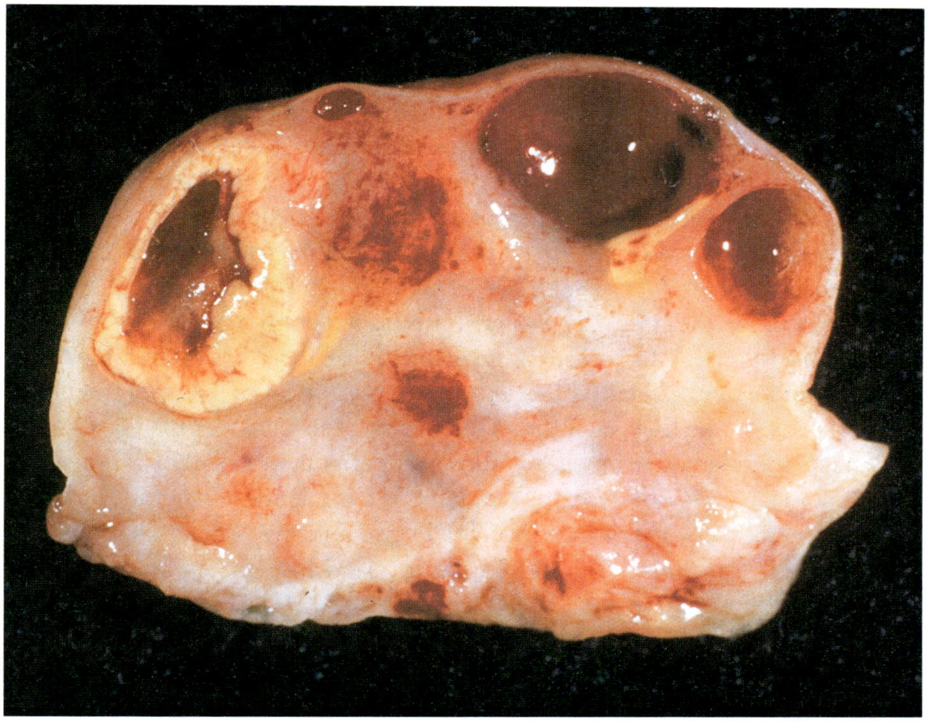

Figure 18-17 Section of normal ovary. There are two follicles beneath the capsule (*right side*) and a corpus luteum (*left side*).

Courtesy of Leonard V. Crowley, MD, Century College.

acne. Ovaries are enlarged and contain multiple cysts related to high levels of circulating gonadotrophins. The disease is associated with hyperandrogenism (excess production of male hormones), most likely in the ovary. Some of these androgens are converted to estrogens in the ovary, resulting in excess estrogen production. PCOS occurs with hyperinsulinemia and resistance of target tissue to insulin (insulin resistance), the cause of which is uncertain. The defect in insulin function appears to contribute to the hormonal imbalance that occurs.

Ovarian Neoplasms

Serous tumor Ovarian tumor resembling cells in the fallopian tube.

Mucinous tumor Ovarian tumor made of cells resembling the mucus-secreting epithelium of the endocervix.

Endometrioid tumor Tumor epithelium resembles endometrium.

Clear cell carcinoma Glycogen-rich tumors similar to endometroid carcinoma.

Transitional cell tumor/ Brenner tumor Benign tumor containing nests of urothelial-like cells.

Ovarian tumors are the second most common gynecologic cancer, and they account for the second greatest number of deaths. Because they are difficult to detect, most patients present with disseminated disease. Only 15 percent of cases are diagnosed with stage I disease. Ovarian cancer is predominantly a disease of older women and is most often diagnosed around age 60, with an increasing frequency of occurrence through the eighth decade. Ninety percent of ovarian cancers are high-grade **serous tumors** believed to arise in the fallopian tubes. Although rare, the disease can occur in the very young. The disease has a strong genetic component, with about 10 percent of cases being familial. In these cases, the disease appears a decade earlier. Mutations in a number of genes are associated with common types of ovarian cancer, notably BRCA1 and BRCA2. Individuals harboring these mutations have risks as high as 45 percent and 20 percent for the respective gene. Because of the difficulty in early diagnosis, patients may elect to undergo oophorectomy and salpingectomy (removal of the ovaries and fallopian tubes).

Ovarian neoplasms may arise in one or both ovaries. They may be either benign or malignant, cystic or solid, and derive from several cell types, including the surface epithelium, germ cells, or stromal cells. Of these, epithelial tumors are the most common. The epithelial cells on the surface of the ovary and the epithelium of the tumor cells may resemble the cells found in other parts of the genital tract. If the tumor epithelium resembles the cells lining the fallopian tube, the tumor is classified as a serous tumor, the most common type. Many of these tumors may, in fact, derive from cells of the fallopian tube. If the tumor epithelium resembles the mucus-secreting epithelium of the endocervix, it is termed a **mucinous tumor**; if the tumor epithelium resembles endometrium, it is termed an **endometrioid tumor**. In many of these serous tumors, the neoplastic epithelium may extend onto the external surface of the tumor (**Figure 18-18**). When this occurs, small pieces of the projecting tumor may break off and implant elsewhere in the pelvis, peritoneal cavity, and omentum, where they continue to grow. Tumors manifesting this behavior may be difficult to remove completely. A mucinous tumor is designated as either a mucinous cystadenoma, which is benign, or a mucinous cystadenocarcinoma. Mucinous tumors generally consist of multiple small cysts and may be very large in size (**Figure 18-19**). Any tumor demonstrating invasion into the ovarian stroma is suggestive of malignancy.

Most of the ovarian tumors with endometrium-like epithelium are malignant and are termed endometrioid carcinomas. Less common are **clear cell carcinoma**, glycogen-rich tumors similar to the endometrioid carcinoma (and may be associated with endometriosis) and **transitional cell (Brenner) tumors**, which are benign tumors containing nests of urothelial-like cells (those lining the bladder) surrounded by a fibrous stroma. Malignancy

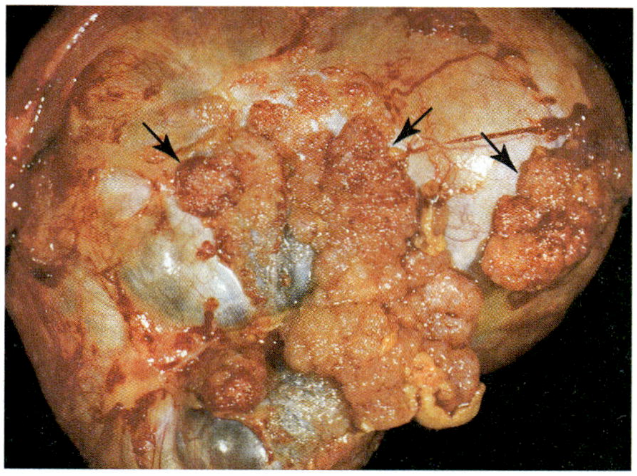

(A)

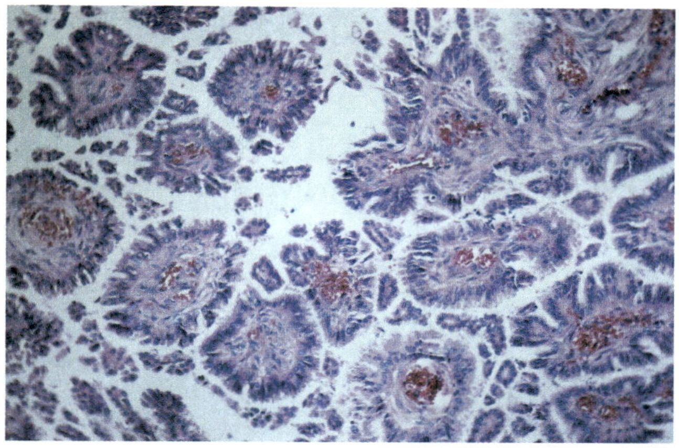

(B)

Figure 18-18 **(A)** A resected serous tumor of the ovary measuring 10 cm in diameter. Several masses of tumor (*arrows*) project from the surface. **(B)** Histologic appearance of the tumor, which forms papillary processes covered by well-differentiated epithelial cells (original magnification ×100).

is most common in the high-grade serous category (70 percent), followed by endometroid and clear cell carcinomas (10 percent).

About 25 percent of ovarian tumors derive from germ cells and, in adults, almost all are benign (although in children they are most often malignant). Ovarian tumors are very similar to testicular germ cell tumors, as both derive from germ cells. The most common of these, **mature teratomas** (also termed mature cystic teratoma, **dermoid cysts**), arise from unfertilized ova that have

Mature teratomas/ dermoid cyst A common type of benign cystic teratoma that commonly arises in the ovary.

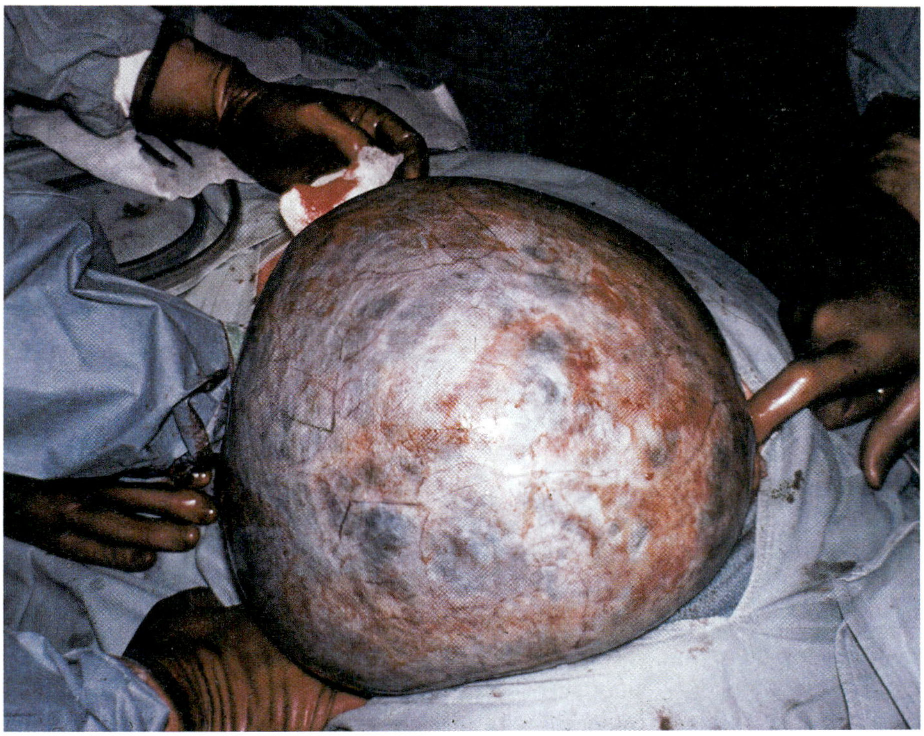

Figure 18-19 A large benign cystic ovarian tumor removed from a pregnant woman. The tumor weighed 35 lbs.

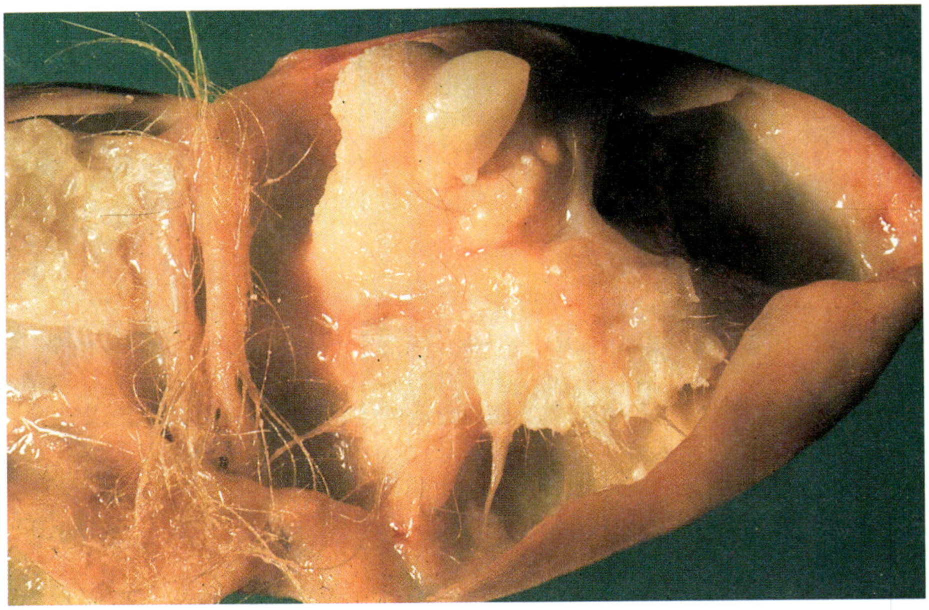

Figure 18-20 Opened dermoid cyst of ovary (benign cystic teratoma) with contents removed. The cyst contains a well-formed jawbone with two teeth (*center*). Note the hair arising from the skin that lines the cyst.

Courtesy of Leonard V. Crowley, MD, Century College.

undergone neoplastic change. The haploid cells develop by parthenogenesis to yield 46,XX cells. The teratomas often contain skin, hair, teeth, bone, parts of the gastrointestinal tract, thyroid, and other tissues growing in a jumbled fashion (**Figure 18-20**). In contrast with the frequency of benign ovarian teratomas, malignant teratomas of the ovary are quite rare.

The last group of ovarian tumors derive either from the fibrous connective tissue of the ovary (**fibromas**) and are almost always benign or from the developing sex cords and may produce female or, rarely, male sex hormones. One type arises from the estrogen-producing cells lining the follicles (granulosa cells) and the closely associated cells adjacent to the follicle cells (theca cells). These cells produce estrogen, and so does a tumor arising from these cells, termed a **granulosa cell tumor** or a **thecoma**. The former may be fibroma-like and benign; the latter are of low-grade malignant potential. The tumors may induce endometrial hyperplasia caused by excessive endometrial stimulation from the estrogen produced by the tumor. A granulosa cell tumor in a postmenopausal woman may induce irregular uterine bleeding. A few rare types of ovarian tumor (Sertoli-Leydig cell tumors) produce male sex hormones instead of estrogen and may induce masculinization.

Fibroma Benign tumor arising from the fibrous connective tissue of the ovary.

Granulosa cell tumor/thecoma An ovarian tumor arising from the estrogen-producing granulose cell of an ovarian follicle.

Hypospadias A congenital abnormality of penile development.

Diseases of the Male Reproductive System

Diseases of the male reproductive system include infectious diseases such as gonorrhea, chlamydia, and herpes simplex virus (discussed in Sexually Transmitted Infections previously in this chapter), scrotal pathologies such as hydroceles, benign prostatic hyperplasia, and carcinoma of various sites, including the penis and testes. Developmental abnormalities can result in **hypospadias**, cryptorchidism, and neonatal testicular torsion (Chapter 16). Functional abnormalities can include erectile or ejaculatory dysfunction.

Nongonococcal Urethritis

In addition to the STIs covered at the beginning of the chapter, a variety of pathogens of the urinary tract, such as *E. coli*, are associated with urethritis and prostatitis. These can be difficult to distinguish in the presence of concurrent cystitis (bladder inflammation). Urinary tract infections in men can be the result of benign prostatic hyperplasia causing bladder outlet obstruction.

Prostatitis

Acute prostatitis may result from either an infectious or noninfectious process. Acute bacterial prostatitis may follow a gonococcal infection of the posterior urethra or be associated with concurrent infectious cystitis or urethritis. Chronic prostatitis is often an inflammatory process and may present with few symptoms or be associated with dysuria and pain in the perineal or suprapubic area. In some cases, no causative organism can be identified (nonbacterial prostatitis).

Benign Prostatic Hyperplasia

Moderate enlargement of the prostate gland is relatively common in older men, affecting 50 percent to 60 percent of males in their sixties and 80 percent to 90 percent of men over the age of 70. The condition usually involves the inner group of glands surrounding the urethra (**Figure 18-21**) termed the transition zone. Hyperplasia results from stimulation of the gland by a potent male sex hormone termed dihydrotestosterone (DHT). The enzyme 5-alpha reductase converts testosterone to DHT in the stromal cells of the prostate. Prostatic enlargement may obstruct the bladder outlet, leading to incomplete emptying of the bladder. Symptoms of bladder outlet obstruction can include increased urinary frequency, urinary urgency, or even complete urinary tract obstruction resulting in urinary retention. Urinary retention and stagnation of urine in the bladder caused by benign prostatic hyperplasia can lead to other pathologies, such as cystitis, pyelonephritis, hydronephrosis, and/or bladder stone formation.

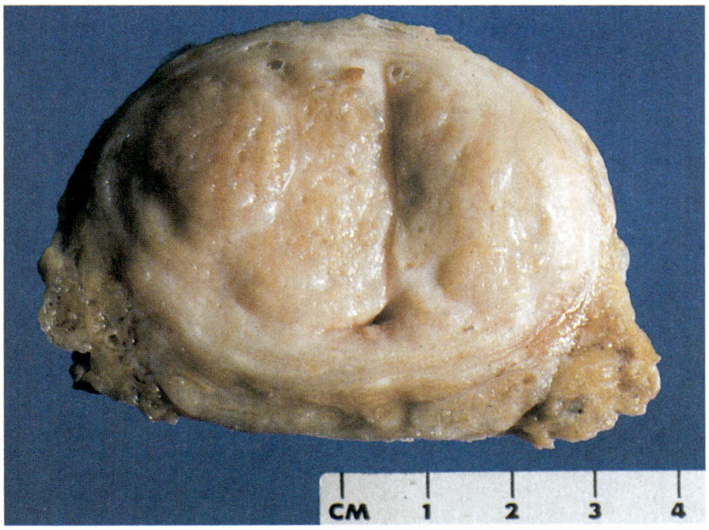

Figure 18-21 Cross section of prostate, showing nodules of hyperplastic tissue compressing urethra.

Courtesy of Leonard V. Crowley, MD, Century College.

Treatment for benign prostatic hyperplasia offers many options depending upon factors such as the size of the gland, the severity of symptoms, the patient's comorbidities, and, of course, the patient's preference. Treatment options include oral medications to relax the smooth muscle in the prostate by blocking prostatic alpha-adrenergic receptors, resulting in more effective bladder emptying. Tadalafil, a phosphodiesterase type 5 inhibitor, is useful in improving bladder emptying and also indicated for erectile dysfunction. There are drugs that shrink the prostate size by blocking prostatic 5-alpha reductase–mediated conversion of testosterone to DHT. These drugs are proven to be effective in alleviating symptoms of benign prostate hyperplasia; a synergistic effect can be achieved when used in combination with tadalafil. Side effects from alpha-adrenergic receptor blockers might include dizziness, low blood pressure, changes in ejaculatory function, and potentially serious problems during cataract surgery. Side effects from 5-alpha reductase inhibitors can be fatigue and decreased libido.

Several procedures exist to address benign prostatic hyperplasia causing bladder outlet obstruction. These procedures aim to remove or remodel the hyperplastic tissue causing the obstruction. The classic procedure utilized is termed a transurethral resection of the prostate (TURP). This very effective treatment remains the "gold standard" compared to all other treatments. A scope is inserted through the penis into the urethra. At the site of the prostatic urethra, a hook-like instrument connected to electrocautery removes the obstructing tissues. This procedure enlarges the prostatic urethral lumen as well as the bladder neck, so the patient can void (urinate) more easily. A pathologist examines the resected tissue histologically to establish the diagnosis of benign prostatic hyperplasia and exclude prostatic carcinoma as a cause of the obstruction (**Figure 18-22** and **Figure 18-23**). The lining of the urethra covering the enlarged prostate is removed along with the obstructing part of the gland, but the epithelial lining soon regenerates, and the continuity of the urethral

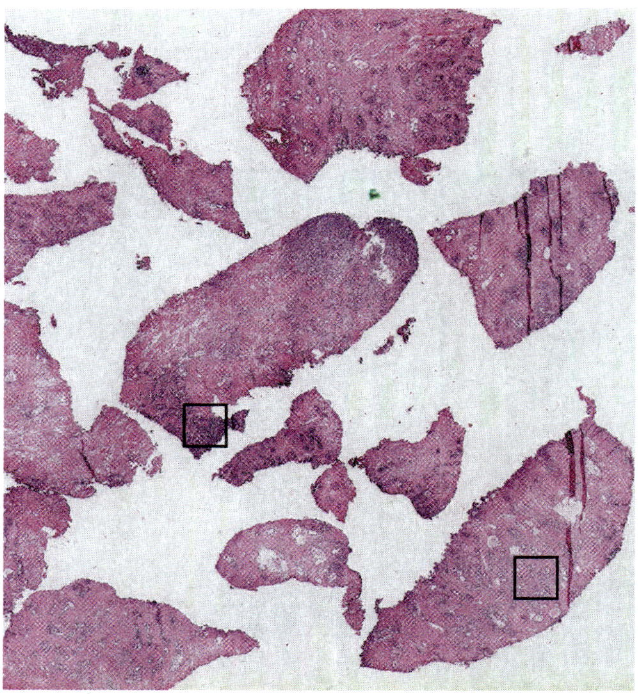

Figure 18-22 Microscopic appearance of tissue removed by transurethral resection (TURP). Boxed areas are shown at higher power in Figure 18-23.

Courtesy of Department of Pathology and Laboratory Medicine, University of North Carolina at Chapel Hill.

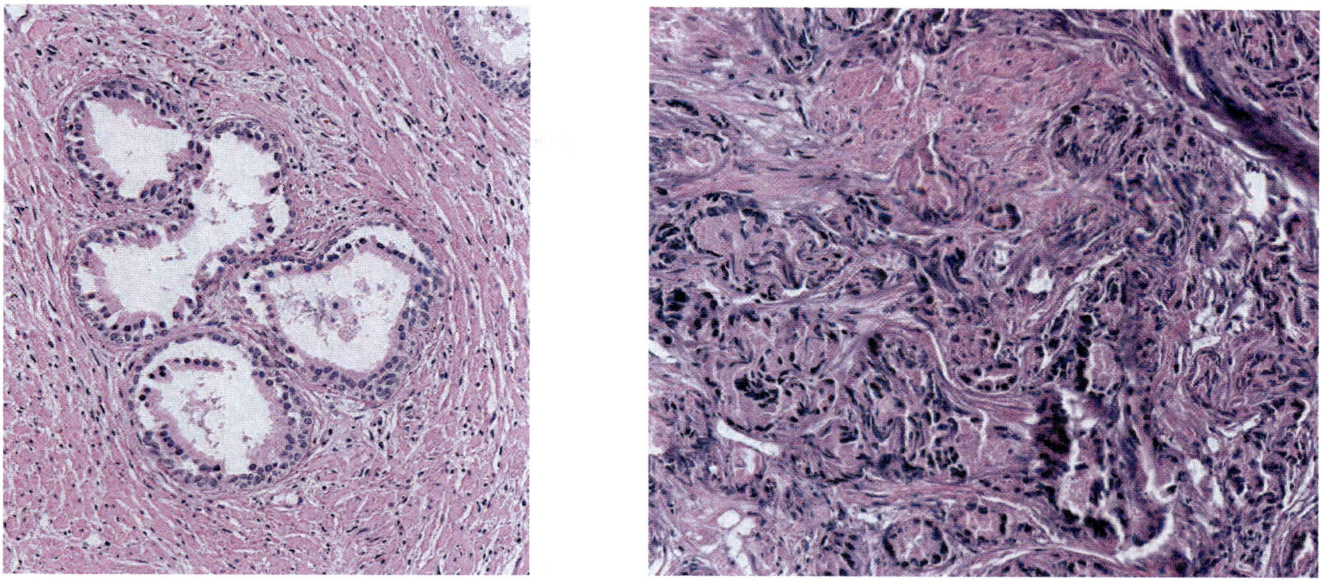

(A) (B)

Figure 18-23 **(A)** An area from TURP specimens shown in Figure 18-22 showing benign prostatic hypertrophy. **(B)** An area from TURP specimens in Figure 18-22 showing prostatic adenocarcinoma.

Courtesy of Department of Pathology and Laboratory Medicine, University of North Carolina at Chapel Hill.

lining restored. Other surgical modalities to remove or remodel excess prostate tissue include a variety of laser technologies, photovaporization, microwave, steam convection, or even the placement of surgical implants. More recently, a system is available to mechanically pull the prostate away from the urethra using small implants in a minimally invasive procedure (Urolift system). Other techniques are available as well. Each modality has patient-specific pros and cons, including invasiveness and durability of results.

Adenocarcinoma of the Prostate

Adenocarcinoma of the prostate is the most common cancer in men, primarily affecting older men, with an average of 68 years at the time of diagnosis. In contrast to benign prostatic hyperplasia, which involves the inner group of glands, the tumor usually originates in the outer group of prostatic glands (**peripheral zone**). The use of **prostatic-specific antigen (PSA)** as a screening test to detect prostate carcinoma allows diagnosis roughly 10 years earlier than was previously possible. Elevated levels of PSA, secreted by prostatic epithelial cells, appear in the blood of many patients with prostate inflammation, benign hypertrophy, and prostate cancer. Hence, the test is not specific for prostate adenocarcinoma. An elevated PSA, or an abnormal digital rectal examination (no longer strongly recommended for screening) in which an area of irregularity or nodularity on the posterior surface of the prostate is detected through the rectum by the examiner's finger, can be further evaluated by several diagnostic tools and tests. MRI (Chapter 1) of the prostate can be an effective tool at identifying high-risk prostate cancers. However, diagnosis of prostate adenocarcinoma requires a biopsy. During a transrectal ultrasound (TRUS)–guided needle biopsy of the prostate, a needle is inserted into a suspected abnormal area in the prostate. Multiple sites within the prostate are sampled to increase the chances of detection. The accuracy of these biopsies can be improved with the fusion of an MRI image denoting an area of concern, which can then be targeted by the ultrasound operator. Increasingly, transperineal biopsies taken through

Peripheral zone Part of the prostate that surrounds the other zones.

Prostatic-specific antigen (PSA) An antigen produced by prostatic epithelial cells that is often found in higher-than-normal concentrations in the blood of patients with prostatic cancer and other diseases of the prostate.

the skin between the anus and scrotum are being used. The procedure reduces the risk of infection versus a transrectal approach, In the absence of early detection, the first manifestations of prostate adenocarcinoma may appear when the growing tumor partially obstructs the bladder neck, causing symptoms similar to those of patients with benign prostatic hyperplasia. The tumor may eventually infiltrate the tissues surrounding the prostate and metastasize to the bones of the spine and pelvis. Diagnostic screening of asymptomatic individuals by the use of prostatic-specific antigen testing has led to an increase in the diagnosis of prostate cancer. Somewhat controversially, statistical studies questioned the utility of such screening programs because most studies report no significant reduction in prostate cancer–specific deaths resulting from screening. One study demonstrated that the screening of about 1000 men between the ages of 55 and 69 would prevent a single prostate cancer death over a span of 11 years. These results suggest that prostate cancer is relatively benign in many men and that men with prostate cancer are far more likely to die of other causes. Screening may lead to overdiagnosis, which can result in complications such as increased anxiety, infection, and bleeding associated with biopsy procedures. Currently the American Cancer Society suggests starting screening at age 50 for individuals with a 10-year expected life expectancy and at 45 years for high-risk individuals, men who have a first-degree relative (father or brother) diagnosed with prostate cancer at an early age (younger than age 65), and at age 40 for men at even higher risk (those with more than one first-degree relative who had prostate cancer at an early age). Current studies indicate that specialized types of MRI could be an effective screening technique for the diagnosis of possible cancer. However, questions of cost and availability are of concern. Clearly better, more predictive screening for prostate cancer is necessary, in particular to detect those cases most likely to progress to life-threatening disease.

Treatment depends on the degree of differentiation of the tumor, the age of the patient, and most importantly, whether the tumor has spread beyond the prostate gland. A well-differentiated (low-grade) localized tumor may progress slowly and may not produce symptoms for as long as 10 years. Many patients in whom prostatic carcinoma is diagnosed fall into this group and may elect active surveillance, being followed by their physician without any treatment unless the tumor appears to be progressing. Tracking for progress could include monitoring PSA, MRI imaging, and repeating biopsies as indicated. In contrast, a less well-differentiated tumor in a younger man may require more aggressive treatment. A small, localized prostatic carcinoma can be treated by radical prostatectomy, removing the entire prostate and surrounding tissues (**Figure 18-24**). Although this operation may eradicate the tumor, it may also disrupt the nerve supply to the penis, which can lead to erectile dysfunction (impotence). Another potential complication is injury to the rhabdosphincter, which can result in urinary incontinence. Primary radiation therapy offers a different option. Radiation therapy can be delivered by several modalities, including external beam therapy and localized implantation of radioactive seeds, termed brachytherapy. As with all disease processes, many factors must be considered when selecting treatment for patients with prostate cancer. These include the patient's age and comorbidities and the grade and stage of their disease, as well as their preferences. A patient's access to health care in general and the availability of specific treatments to that patient will affect treatment decisions and outcomes as well.

When a prostatic carcinoma spreads to where it is found beyond the prostate, it is often possible to induce regression of the tumor by altering the level of male sex hormones in the body. Most prostatic carcinomas are initially dependent on the male sex hormone testosterone for their continued growth. Therefore, many

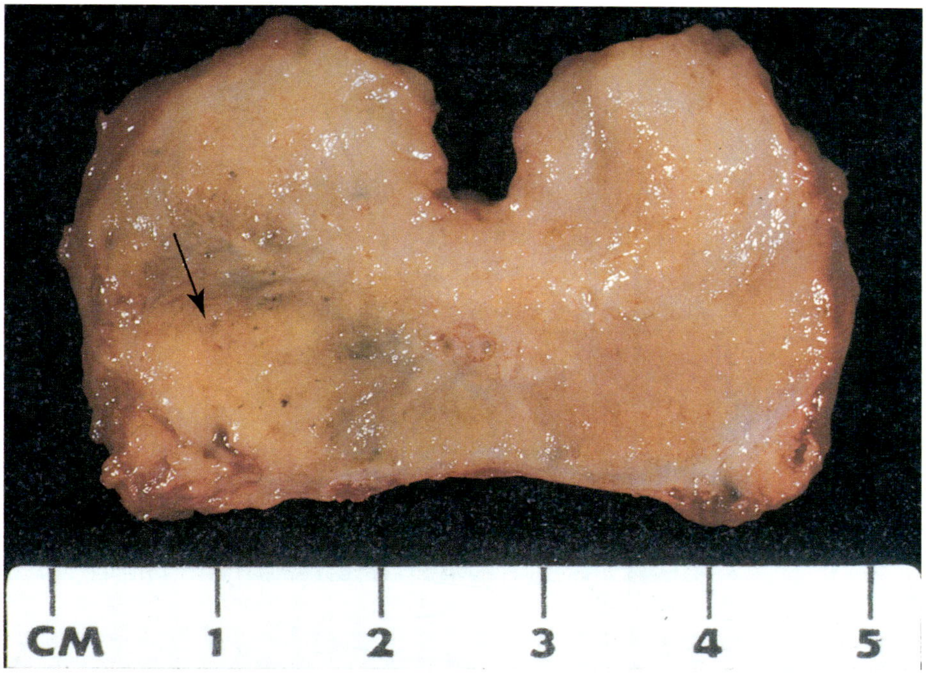

Figure 18-24 A cross section of a resected prostate illustrating a small carcinoma arising from outer prostate glands (*arrow*).

Courtesy of Leonard V. Crowley, MD, Century College.

advanced prostatic tumors can be treated effectively by surgical removal of the testes, eliminating the source of the male sex hormone. Alternatively, drugs that suppress output of pituitary gonadotropic hormone (GnRH, Chapter 22) would result in inhibition of testicular testosterone secretion. Castration, surgical or hormone-induced, or hormone treatment usually causes a temporary regression of the tumor. Widespread metastatic spread to lymph nodes, bones, liver, and lungs is often accompanied by hormone-independent tumor growth, and traditional chemotherapy and local radiation can be used palliatively.

Testicular Torsion

If the fibrous tissue derived from the gubernaculum that attaches the testis to the scrotum is a relatively long and narrow band rather than a short broad attachment, the testis may undergo a rotary twist on its axis, which also twists the spermatic cord and interrupts the blood supply to the testis (**Figure 18-25A**). The thin-walled veins in the cord are compressed first, which impedes the return of venous blood from the testis, but flow through the arteries continues for a time, leading to marked engorgement of the testis with blood, which is soon followed by complete hemorrhagic necrosis of the testis, termed a hemorrhagic infarction (**Figure 18-25B**). The condition may occur in the neonatal period (either in the fetus or soon after birth), where it is not associated with an anatomic defect. Adult testicular torsion is most common in adolescents but may occur at any age. A testicular torsion is characterized by an acute onset of severe testicular pain associated with swelling of the involved testis and is an acute surgical emergency. If the torsion can be untwisted and the testis is properly anchored in the scrotum within a few hours after the onset of the torsion, the testis probably can be salvaged. The longer the delay, the less likely the testis will survive. Adult testicular torsion is associated with **bell-clapper defect**, an anatomic abnormality responsible for increased testicular mobility.

Bell-clapper defect
Anatomic abnormality responsible for increased testicular mobility.

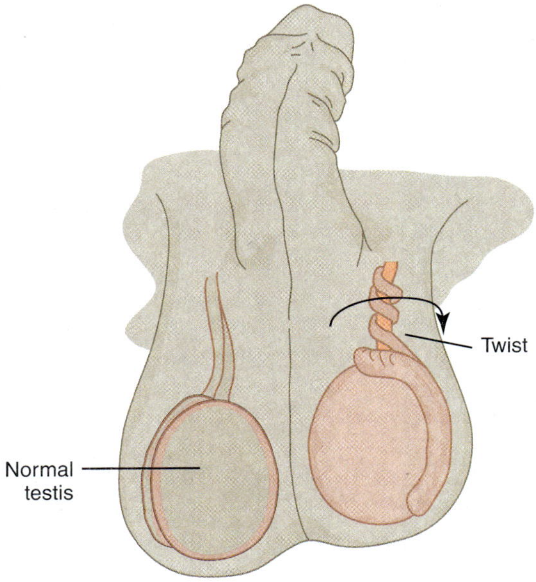

(A)

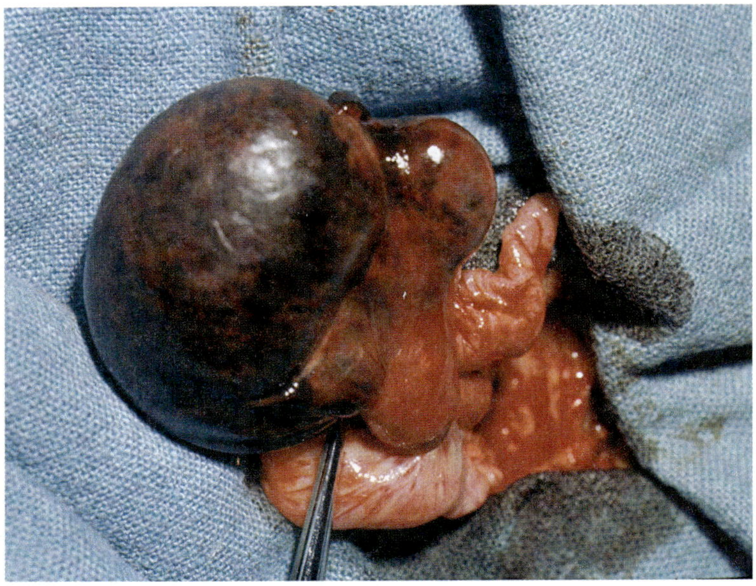

(B)

Figure 18-25 Cause and effect of testicular torsion. **(A)** Rotary twist of the testis also twists the spermatic cord, interrupting blood supply to the testis. Normally, the epididymis is located along the posterior surface of the testis, but the torsion has rotated the testis and also rotated the epididymis anteriorly. **(B)** Hemorrhagic infarction of the testis caused by torsion.

Scrotal Abnormalities

Hydrocele

Normally the sac-like tunica vaginalis contains only a very small amount of fluid (**Figure 18-26A**), but when a much larger amount of fluid accumulates in the sac, a **hydrocele** (*hydro* = water + *cele* = swelling) results (**Figure 18-26B**). The condition may be congenital or result from trauma, infection, or other causes. Although this usually does not require therapy, the scrotal swelling may be uncomfortable. Long-standing hydrocele can cause testicular atrophy and may require surgical excision of the sac.

Hydrocele An accumulation of excess fluid within the tunica vaginalis of the testis.

Varicocele Varicose veins that develop within the spermatic cord veins.

Varicocele

The term "**varicocele**" (*varix* = dilated vein + *cele* = swelling) refers to varicose veins that develop within the spermatic cord veins that drain blood from the testis, caused by failure of the vein valves to function properly and allowing

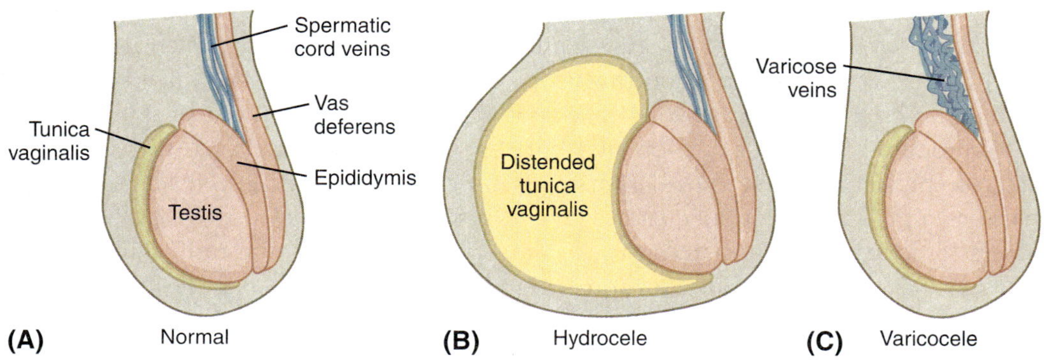

Figure 18-26 **(A)** Normal tunica vaginalis containing a small amount of fluid. **(B)** Hydrocele. **(C)** Varicocele.

for backflow, pooling of blood, and venous dilation (**Figure 18-26C**). When the scrotum is examined while the patient is standing, the scrotal varicose veins located above the testis are sometimes described as "feeling like a bag full of worms." When the patient lies down, blood drains easily from the veins and the varicocele can no longer be felt. Generally, a varicocele does not cause symptoms. However, varicoceles may occasionally reduce fertility by impairing spermatogenesis, possibly as a result of the higher scrotal temperature caused by warm venous blood pooling in the varicose scrotal veins.

Carcinoma of the Testis

Testicular tumors are uncommon; they most frequently develop between the ages of 30 and 40. Both benign and malignant testicular tumors are rare in prepubertal males. Most tumors arise from the germinal epithelium of the testicular tubules and are malignant.

The type with the most favorable prognosis is termed a **seminoma**. (This is an exception to standard terminology, as the term refers to a malignant neoplasm that resembles spermatogonia rather than to a benign tumor.) The tumor, which is detectable as a growing scrotal mass, is highly sensitive to radiation therapy; a greater than 90 percent cure rate is possible using orchiectomy and radiation and, in the case of large tumors, chemotherapy.

A second class of testicular tumors encompasses several histologically distinct varieties and are known collectively as nonseminomatous germ cell tumors. Within this category, tumors derived from undifferentiated embryonal cells are termed **embryonal carcinomas**. More differentiated embryonal cells give rise to **teratocarcinomas**, also termed **malignant teratomas**, composed of many different types of malignant tissues, some of which demonstrate the characteristics of a variety of somatic or extraembryonic cells of the developing embryo. Some other testicular tumors resemble placental trophoblastic tissue. An example is **choriocarcinoma**, which is the same kind of tumor that arises from trophoblastic tissue in the uterus (described in Chapter 15).

The neoplastic cells of many testicular tumors produce **human chorionic gonadotropin (hCG)**, which is the same hormone made by the placenta in pregnancy. Consequently, a pregnancy test given to a man with testicular cancer may be positive. Some testicular tumors also produce **alpha-fetoprotein (AFP)**, which is a protein produced by the fetus early in prenatal development but not normally found in adults. If a testicular carcinoma produces these substances, the concentrations may fall after successful treatment of the tumor and rise again if the tumor recurs. Consequently, the healthcare provider can monitor the response to treatment by serial determinations of hCG and AFP (described in Chapter 6). Nonseminomatous tumors are not as sensitive to radiation and often require the use of chemotherapy.

Carcinoma of the Penis

Carcinoma of the penis is uncommon and is almost never encountered in a circumcised male. It is hypothesized that chronic inflammation due to poor hygiene underneath preputial skin can be a progenitor of penile carcinoma. However, other factors also may account for the low incidence of carcinoma in circumcised males. Carcinogenic strains of HPV, the same virus that appears related to cervical dysplasia and carcinoma in women, play a major role in causing penile cancer. Treatment usually consists of partial or complete resection of the penis.

Seminoma One type of malignant tumor of the testis.

Embryonal carcinoma A malignant testicular tumor in which the malignant cells have features resembling rapidly growing trophoblastic tissue.

Teratocarcinomas/ malignant teratomas A malignant testicular tumor composed of many different types of malignant tissues.

Choriocarcinoma A malignant proliferation of trophoblastic tissue.

Human chorionic gonadotropin (hCG) A hormone made by the placenta in pregnancy that has actions similar to pituitary gonadotropins. The same hormone is made by neoplastic cells in some types of malignant testicular tumors.

Alpha-fetoprotein (AFP) Protein produced by the fetal liver early in gestation. Sometimes produced by tumor cells. Level is elevated in amniotic fluid when the fetus has a neural tube defect.

Erectile Dysfunction

Physiology of Penile Erection

The penis consists primarily of three cavernous bodies, which are cylinders of extremely vascular erectile tissue: two laterally placed corpora cavernosa and the midline corpus spongiosum that surrounds the penile urethra. Each cylinder, surrounded by a thick fibrous tissue capsule, is composed of a spongy meshwork of endothelium-lined blood sinuses supported by trabeculae (partitions) composed of connective tissue and smooth muscle. The blood sinuses of the erectile tissue are supplied by arteries and drained by veins. Normally, the arteries are constricted, and very little blood flows into the cavernous bodies, and the vascular sinuses are collapsed. During sexual excitement, parasympathetic nerve impulses arising from the sacral part of the spinal cord release the neurotransmitter nitric oxide, which causes relaxation of the smooth muscle in the walls of the penile arteries and in the trabeculae between the sinuses. Nitric oxide functions by stimulating the enzyme guanylate cyclase, resulting in an increase in cyclic guanine monophosphate (cGMP), which plays an important role in arterial vasodilation. As a result, the penile arteries dilate, and the sinuses in the cavernous bodies expand. Blood enters under arterial pressure into the blood sinuses within the cavernous bodies. The greatly increased arterial blood flow and rising pressure within the blood sinuses compress the draining veins, which retard the outflow of blood from the penis and contribute to the engorgement of the blood sinuses. The penis rapidly becomes rigid and erect (**Figure 18-27**). Detumescence (loss of erection) occurs by activation of adrenergic nerves producing vasoconstriction of penile vessels. Additionally,

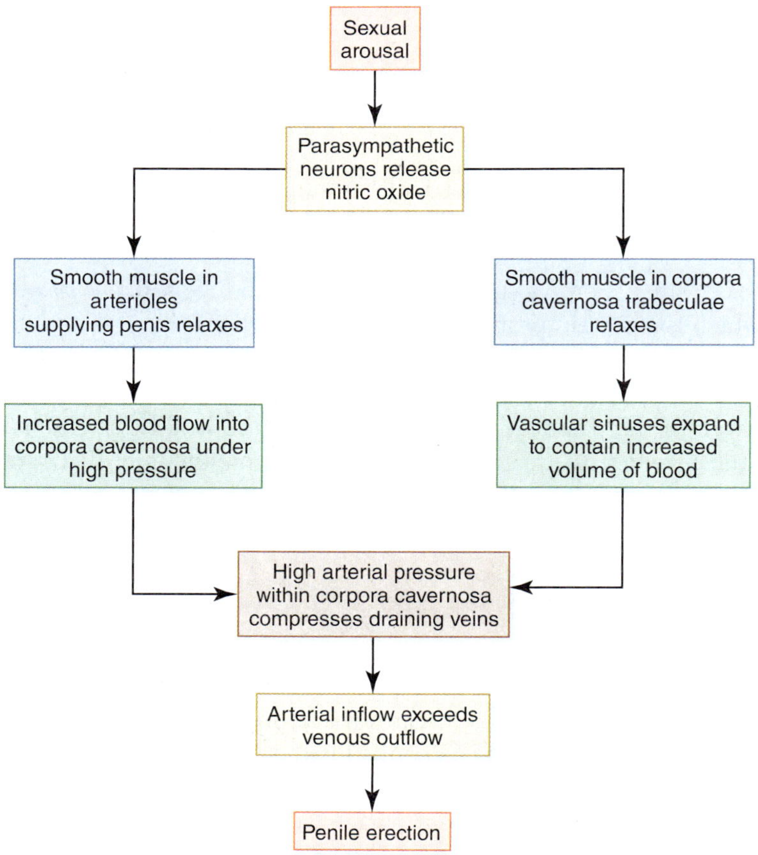

Figure 18-27 Physiology of penile erection.

phosphodiesterases hydrolyze the cGMP to an inactive form and play a role in detumescence.

Erectile dysfunction is an inability to achieve and maintain a penile erection of sufficient rigidity to penetrate the vagina and maintain the erection during sexual intercourse. This is a relatively common problem that increases in frequency with advancing age. Penile erection is a complex process. First, sexual desire is required to initiate the physiologic events that increase blood flow to the penis. Second, the arteries supplying the cavernous bodies must dilate enough to deliver a large volume of blood to the penis. Third, the pressure of the blood within the cavernous bodies must be sufficiently high to compress the draining veins. Blood must flow into the penis faster than it drains out, or an erection cannot be maintained.

Causes of Erectile Dysfunction

To achieve and sustain a penile erection, the sensory, motor, and autonomic nerve supply to the penis must be intact, and the blood vessels supplying the penis must be able to deliver an adequate volume of blood to the penis. Various factors may disturb these physiologic processes, including a low testosterone level, which inhibits sexual desire and arousal; damage to the nerves supplying the penis resulting from radical prostate surgery or neurologic diseases; impaired blood supply to the penis resulting from arteriosclerosis of the blood vessels that deliver blood to the penis; the effect of drugs used to treat hypertension that target the autonomic nervous system, including the branches supplying the penis; and stress, emotional factors, or chronic illnesses, which may impair the person's quality of life and also adversely affect sexual performance.

Treatment

Both medical and surgical procedures can be used to treat erectile dysfunction, depending on the etiology and the patient's preference. One well-known treatment involves drugs that inhibit phosphodiesterase and consequently promote increased blood flow to the penis. Several phosphodiesterase-inhibiting drugs are available (sildenafil, vardenafil, tadalafil), which differ primarily in their duration of action. They are relatively safe drugs when used properly. However, serious complications may arise with improper use or when used by people with other underlying health concerns. The best known of these drugs is sildenafil, better known by its trade name Viagra.

Case 18-1

Fifteen-year-old Janice was becoming increasingly depressed by the constant teasing of her female friends. Breast development started normally at age 11, followed by menarche (first menstrual period) at age 12. Now, 3 years later, Janice had experienced only three additional menstrual periods. This concerned her because her friends were all "regular" with their menstrual cycles. She had annoying outbreaks of acne, and her skin was very oily. When she was 13, her mother took her to their family physician, concerned about irregular periods. At that time, the physician explained that menstrual cycles often take a long time to regulate. He also explained that acne and some facial hair were not unusual during early adolescence and tended to decrease with time.

Currently, Janice's major complaint was how hairy she had become. She had noticeable coarse dark hair above her upper lip, on her chin, and around

(continues)

Case 18-1 *(Continued)*

her nipples. She would not wear a two-piece bathing suit at the beach because she had a streak of dark hair running from her pubis up the center of her abdomen. Her thighs and lower back also grew dark hair. Her friends who had seen her undressed said she had hair "like a boy," and the teasing increased. She also began to put on weight. Janice visited her physician again. The physician carefully examined Janice and confirmed that she had an unusual amount of hair that was distributed in a male pattern (hirsutism). Janice had persistent oligomenorrhea (few menstrual periods) and had remained amenorrheic for over 3 months. The physician was also concerned about Janice's weight gain and referred her to a gynecologist who specialized in endocrine and developmental problems.

The gynecologist confirmed a diagnosis of hirsutism. This finding, along with acne, prolonged amenorrhea, and increasing weight gain, suggested that Janice was suffering from an excess of androgens (male hormones), which could be responsible for her symptoms. A very common endocrine disorder, polycystic ovary syndrome (PCOS), occurs in up to 10 percent of females and is associated with hyperandrogenism. PCOS is often diagnosed during adolescence. The gynecologist ordered a series of additional tests for Janice to rule out other possible causes of hyperandrogenism. These included determination of blood testosterone levels (and a number of other endocrine hormone level determinations), ovarian ultrasound, insulin levels, and glucose tolerance testing. Test results disclosed abnormally high androgen levels without an indication of adrenal or thyroid dysfunction. Janice had high levels of circulating insulin and an abnormal glucose tolerance test, suggesting the early onset of insulin resistance. Abdominal ultrasound suggested increased ovarian volume (but this is a common finding in adolescents). Janice underwent transvaginal ultrasound and was found to have an excess of cystic areas on her ovaries, consistent with PCOS. Janet's gynecologist diagnosed PCOS based on the findings of hyperandrogenism and ovulatory dysfunction (in the absence of other factors), polycystic ovaries, and the suggestion of early onset type 2 diabetes with obesity.

Janice was treated with combination birth control pills (containing both estrogen and progesterone) and an androgen-blocking agent (spironolactone). This regularized her menses and reduced the hirsutism. She was counseled regarding a healthy lifestyle, including exercise and weight control. The drug metformin was also prescribed because of increasing concern about her diabetes.

Discussion

One might imagine that PCOS would be relatively easy to diagnose in an adolescent considering the distinctive signs and symptoms. This is incorrect. Normal body hair distribution varies greatly from person to person, dependent upon both degree of sexual development and, in particular, ethnic origin. For example, what might be considered an abnormal amount of hair in a person of Chinese (Han) origin might be quite normal in a White or Black female. The semiquantitative Ferriman-Gallwey score can be used in the clinical assessment of hair, but half of women with isolated hirsutism are found not to have excess androgens. For this reason, only moderate to extreme excess of hair (particularly in a male growth pattern) is suggestive of PCOS.

Laboratory testing for levels of circulating androgens (testosterone) is difficult to perform and interpret. There is no universally accepted "normal" level, particularly in developing female adolescents. Another complicating factor is that much of the testosterone in circulation is bound to steroid hormone-binding globulin and thus is not hormonally active. Hence, determination of androgen level must be done by a reliable laboratory that has established accurate and appropriate normal controls for both sexes at different ages. In the absence of other symptoms, a single high androgen level should be interpreted with caution. In addition, abnormally high androgen levels in a female can be caused by ovarian and adrenal tumors and adrenal hyperplasia.

Primary ovarian failure (not related to excess androgen levels) can result from a variety of other hormonal abnormalities. Determining whether the ovaries show a polycystic morphology is most commonly accomplished using transvaginal ultrasound, but there is no widely accepted definition for an "abnormal" polycystic ovarian morphology in adolescents. A large number of adolescent females without hyperandrogenism show evidence of such an ovarian morphology. It is accepted that there is a high level of insulin resistance and obesity associated with PCOS in adolescents. Hence, the diagnosis of PCOS requires multifactorial evaluation coupled with clinical expertise to avoid errors in diagnosis.

The etiology of PCOS remains uncertain. Clearly, abnormally high androgen levels, produced in the ovary and adrenals, are central in pathogenesis. There is a clear genetic component to PCOS and suggestions of association with a variety of genes in the population. The relation of high insulin level, insulin resistance, and obesity to hyperandrogenism remains speculative but clearly contributes to the hormonal abnormality. To date, the exact cause-effect relationship between PCOS and the associated metabolic disturbances is undefined.

Questions

1. How might a clinician distinguish hyperandrogenism resulting from PCOS from that resulting from other causes (such as a tumor)?
2. What are the differences in distribution of body hair in a normal male and female?

Case 18-2

The patient is an 18-year-old male who visits his physician at the urging of his girlfriend. She has noted bilateral enlargement of his breasts and is concerned that he might have breast cancer. The physician confirms nontender gynecomastia (breast enlargement in a male). The patient states that he has had mild dyspnea (shortness of breath) for about a month. On questioning, he notes that he has had a painless mass in the right testis in the last several months. His history is also pertinent; he had cryptorchidism that was surgically repaired at 24 months. He does not know which testis was cryptorchid. The physician confirms a painless hard right testicular mass by palpation with otherwise normal male genitalia showing obvious distortion visible through the scrotum. Questionable supraclavicular lymphadenopathy (enlargement of the lymph nodes above the clavicle) is also noted. The physician orders laboratory tests for hCG (chorionic gonadotrophin) and AFP (alpha fetoprotein), both of which are positive. The physician refers the patient to a urologist who performs a testicular ultrasound and notes that a "fluffy" density has replaced much of the right testis. The left testis appears normal. A chest X-ray shows multiple lesions consistent with metastatic disease. The patient undergoes orchiectomy of the right testis. Histopathological examination of the testis discloses a nonseminomatous germ cell tumor (NSGCT) described as a teratocarcinoma (malignant teratoma). The patient has high-stage disease with pulmonary metastases. After undergoing several cycles of chemotherapy using platinum-based agents, he has been disease-free for 3 years.

Discussion

About 50 percent of all germ cell tumors of the testes are NSGCTs, and about two-thirds of these are teratocarcinomas. The tumors are believed to derive from embryonal carcinoma cells that have differentiated into a mixture of

(continues)

Case 18-2 *(Continued)*

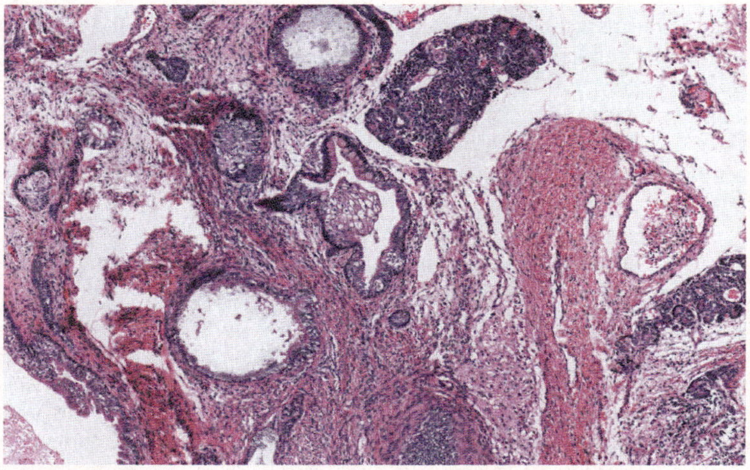

Case Figure 18-1 Nonseminomatous germ cell tumor (NSGCT) of teratocarcinoma type. The tumor shows a mixture of mature-appearing tissue elements.

Courtesy of Department of Pathology and Laboratory Medicine, University of North Carolina at Chapel Hill.

mature-looking tissues normally found in a variety of organs (**Case Figure 18-1**). These tumors are often "mixed" and also contain embryonal cells that are not differentiated and maintain malignant potential.

It is of interest that the mature-appearing cells (as shown in Case Figure 18-1) may survive chemotherapy, whereas the malignant embryonal component forming metastases is eliminated. In fact, there is an excellent potential for a cure even in advanced-stage disease. The presence of gynecomastia can be physiological and is a common transient finding in pubertal boys. However, the occurrence of gynecomastia should prompt examination for testicular tumors. Between 5 percent and 10 percent of testicular germ cell tumor patients will show gynecomastia. Over 70 percent of NSGCTs secrete hCG or AFP. The hCG molecule shares components with a number of other human hormones. hCG tends to increase the level of the female hormone estrogen more than that of testosterone, and the increased ratio of the former to the latter results in gynecomastia.

Etiology and Pathogenesis

Nonseminomatous germ cell tumor (NSGCT) of the subclass containing mixed differentiated tissue components (malignant teratoma) with metastatic disease to lymph nodes and lungs. Gynecomastia is related to the production of hCG by the tumor.

Questions

1. Considering that testicular cancer is uncommon and quite curable, propose a simple screening protocol for early detection of this disease.
2. Propose a likely mechanism for the secretion of hCG by embryonal tumors.
3. Assume you are a male of 40 years of age with no prior family history of prostatic cancer. Your doctor suggests screening for this disease. (A) What tests is your doctor likely to perform? (B) Your test results are of "borderline significance" for the presence of prostatic cancer. What tests is your physician likely to suggest? (C) Would you agree to the testing procedure? Support the logic of your answer.

Questions For Review

1. What are the possible results of HPV infection?
2. A patient consults her healthcare provider because of irregular uterine bleeding. What are some of the diseases of the genital tract that can cause this bleeding?
3. What is endometriosis? What symptoms does it produce? What are some complications that may be associated with endometriosis?
4. What is the difference between *in situ* and invasive cervical carcinoma? How is the Pap smear used in the diagnosis of carcinoma?
5. What is a dermoid cyst?
6. What is toxic shock? What role do staphylococci play?
7. What is benign prostatic hyperplasia? What are its clinical manifestations? How is it treated?
8. How does administration of female sex hormones affect prostatic carcinoma? What is the effect of castration on prostatic carcinoma?
9. A young man has a positive pregnancy test. Under what circumstances could this occur?
10. What factors predispose to the development of carcinoma of the penis? How may the disease be prevented?
11. What is cryptorchidism? What are the clinical manifestations? How is the condition treated? Why should it be treated?
12. What is a testicular torsion? What are its manifestations and complications? How is the condition treated?
13. A young man has an undescended testis within the abdomen. How does this affect testicular function? What complications may result from this condition?
14. Which sexually transmitted infections (STIs) can be difficult to diagnose in females?
15. What is the natural course of events if syphilis is untreated?
16. What is the connection between STIs and infertility?

References

Pommerville JC. *Fundamentals of Microbiology*. 11th ed. Jones & Bartlett Learning; 2018.

Shors T. *Understanding Viruses*. 3rd ed. Jones & Bartlett Learning; 2017.

- Those interested in the study of infectious disease should start by consulting texts in the area of microbiology and virology. Although somewhat advanced, both of these texts are easy to read and up-to-date.

Centers for Disease Control and Prevention. Sexually Transmitted Infections (STIs). www.cdc.gov/std

- A first place to look for accurate and up-to-the-minute information on any aspect of infectious disease is the United States Centers for Disease Control and Prevention. This is a gateway to current information on essentially all aspects of sexually transmitted diseases.

Centers for Disease Control. HIV. www.cdc.gov/hiv

HIVinfo. National Institutes of Health. https://hivinfo.nih.gov/

- These sites provide accurate information on all aspects of HIV. HIVinfo has highly detailed technical information on current therapeutic guidelines as well as an excellent glossary and series of illustrations. Both sites are highly recommended.

Old Blind Dogs. Pills of white mercury. On *Tall Tails*. Lochshore; 1994. https://www.youtube.com/watch?v=6iiJMgUlIR8

- One doesn't usually think of syphilis as a topic for singing. This is a rather chilling song performed by a Scottish folk group that describes the effects of the disease and its treatment (likely the highly toxic mercuric chloride) prior to antibiotics.

Papp JR, Park IU, Fakile Y, Pereira L, Pillay A, Bolan GA. CDC laboratory recommendations for syphilis testing, United States, 2024. *MMWR Recomm Rep.* 2024;73(1):1-32. DOI:10.15585/mmwr.rr7301a1

- This report provides new CDC recommendations for tests that can support a diagnosis of syphilis, including serologic testing and methods for the identification of the causative agent *Treponema pallidum*.

Centers for Disease Control and Prevention. About Congenital Syphilis. https://www.cdc.gov/syphilis/about/about-congenital-syphilis.html

Gilroy, SA. HIV Infection and AIDS Treatment & Management. Updated January 2, 2025. https://emedicine.medscape.com/article/211316-treatment

- Consult this site for a summary of current practice in HIV disease treatment and management. Also an excellent source on opportunistic infections associated with HIV and their therapy.

Faria NR, et al. The early spread and epidemic ignition of HIV-1 in human populations. *Science.* 2014;346(6205):56-61.

Oster AM, et al. Identifying clusters of recent and rapid HIV transmission through analysis of molecular surveillance data. *J Aquir Immune Defic Syndr.* 2018;79(5):543–550. https://www.ncbi.nlm.nih.gov/pmc/articles/PMC6231979/

- The original scientific literature on HIV is endless. These two references review areas of research that have been of recent interest. The first article, although very technical in its details, presents a fascinating picture of how the AIDS epidemic developed and spread based on modern genetic technology and is now a "classic." The second article discusses an interesting example of epidemiological cluster analysis to highlight areas of unusually rapid HIV transmission. The methods are highly technical, but the introduction and discussion are interesting.

Brondani MA, Siqueira AB, Alves CMC. Exploring lay public and dental professional knowledge around HPV transmission via oral sex and oral cancer development. *BMC Public Health.* 2019;19(1):1529. https://www.ncbi.nlm.nih.gov/pmc/articles/PMC6858745/

- There is a surprising amount of ignorance about HPV and cancer and, in particular, the risk of HPV transmission via oral sex. This is a timely review of current literature.

Gray-Swain MR, Peipert JF. Pelvic inflammatory disease in adolescents. *Curr Opin Obstet Gynecol.* 2006;18(5):503.

Rolle CJ, et al. Unilateral twin ectopic pregnancy in a patient with a history of multiple sexually transmitted infections. *Infect Dis Obstet Gynecol.* 2006;2006:10306.

Marion LL, Meeks GR. Ectopic pregnancy: History, incidence, epidemiology, and risk factors. *Clin Obstet Gynecol.* 2012;55(2):376-386.

- The case presented in this chapter is based on information contained in the following three references. The third has a very interesting historical introduction.

Boston Women's Health Book Collective. *Our Bodies, Ourselves*. Atria Books; 2011.

Corinna H. S.E.X. 2nd ed. The All-You-Need-To-Know Sexuality Guide to Get You Through Your Teens and Twenties. Da Capo Lifelong Books; 2016.

Planned Parenthood. http://www.plannedparenthood.org/

- The book referenced in the first entry covers a wide range of subjects dealing with sexual anatomy, physiology, and pathology in a clear and concise manner, although some consider it dated. The second suggested book is a more up-to-date guide, which some find a bit explicit. The third entry has extensive information on birth control, emergency contraception, and STDs.

Banet N, Scanga L, Lininger RA. "The female reproductive tract." In Reisner H, ed. *Pathology: A Modern Case Study.* 2nd ed. McGraw Hill Lange; 2020.

Shors T. *Understanding Viruses*. 3rd ed. Jones & Bartlett Learning; 2017.

Tan HH, Chan R. Genital warts. In Zenilman JM, Shamanesh M, eds. *Sexually Transmitted Infections: Diagnosis, Management, and Treatment*. Jones & Bartlett Learning; 2012.

- The three recommended texts contain useful additional background information relating to diseases discussed in this chapter. The first entry has many additional short cases and illustrations of gynecological pathology. It provides a brief overview aimed at undergraduate medical students. Several chapters on HPV in the second reference provide additional information on the role of HPV in human cancer. The third entry is specifically cited for the chapter on genital warts, but other chapters have useful background on many sexually transmitted diseases.

Rivlin K, Isley MM. Patient-centered contraceptive counseling and prescribing. *Clin Obstet Gynecol.* 2018;61(1):27-39.

Lee JK, Schwarz EB. The safety of available and emerging options for emergency contraception. *Expert Opin Drug Saf.* 2017;16(10):1163-1171.

ACOG Practice Bulletin No. 206: Use of hormonal contraception in women with coexisting medical conditions. *Obstet Gynecol.* 2019;133(2):e128-e150.

- The first two references provide useful short reviews of current practice and options in birth control. The failure rates provided in the first publication are higher than many shown in other sources but represent "real-world" findings. The last reference (at least the first ten or so pages) provide information that all women should consider before making a choice as to birth control methods. In addition, the website https://www.acog.org has a list of other definitive but very technical guidelines published by the American College of Obstetricians and Gynecologists.

National Cancer Institute. Human Papillomavirus (HPV) Vaccines. https://www.cancer.gov/about-cancer/causes-prevention/risk/infectious-agents/hpv-vaccine-fact-sheet

- The site provides information on the utility, efficacy, and safety of HPV immunization.

Office on Women's Health. Endometriosis. U.S. Department of Health and Human Services. https://www.womenshealth.gov/a-z-topics/endometriosis

Lagana AS, et al. The pathogenesis of endometriosis: Molecular and cell biology insights. *Int J Mol Sci*. 2019;20(22):5615. https://www.ncbi.nlm.nih.gov/pmc/articles/PMC6888544/

- The first site provides an excellent overview and extensive links to additional resources. The second reference is a thorough review of the scientific literature aimed at the etiology and pathogenesis of the disease.

PDQ Adult Treatment Editorial Board. Endometrial Cancer Treatment: Health Professional Version. Published February 12, 2025. https://www.ncbi.nlm.nih.gov/books/NBK65829/

PDQ Adult Treatment Editorial Board. Ovarian Epithelial, Fallopian Tube, and Primary Peritoneal Cancer Treatment: Health Professional Version. Published February 12, 2025. https://www.ncbi.nlm.nih.gov/books/NBK66007/

- The PDQ Professional series of online ebooks are much more than therapeutic summaries but present an up-to-the-minute overview of the diseases. The second volume covers an interesting topic in gynecologic cancer (fallopian tube disease) about which there is much current interest in relation to ovarian disease.

Loeffler AG, Hart MN. *Introduction to Human Disease*. 7th ed. Jones & Bartlett Learning; 2020.

- Those interested in the detailed study of male reproductive disease should consult a work on human pathology aimed at the undergraduate medical curriculum. However, a good place to start at a less advanced level is by reading Chapter 16 in this book.

Tests to Diagnose and Stage Prostate Cancer. American Cancer Society. https://www.cancer.org/cancer/prostate-cancer/detection-diagnosis-staging/how-diagnosed.html

Descotes J-L. Diagnosis of prostate cancer. *Asian J. Urol*. 2019;6(2):129. https://www.ncbi.nlm.nih.gov/pmc/articles/PMC6488713/

Fenton JJ, Weyrich MS, Durbin S, Liu Y, Bang H, Melnikow J. Prostate-Specific Antigen-Based Screening for Prostate Cancer: A Systematic Evidence Review for the U.S. Preventive Services Task Force. Agency for Healthcare Research and Quality (US); May 2018. https://www.ncbi.nlm.nih.gov/pubmed/30085502

- One of the more controversial areas in urology is the appropriate role of prostate cancer screening. This is combined with the advent of new screening mechanisms such as fusion MRI and cell-free DNA-based detection. The first two references review both the more standard and new approaches to detection. The last is an extensive review of the much-quoted U.S. Preventive Task Force analysis. It is rich in detail and statistical data.

Hennigan ST, et al. Low abundance of circulating tumor DNA in localized prostate cancer. *JCO Precis Oncol*. 2019. doi:10.1200/PO.19.00176. https://www.ncbi.nlm.nih.gov/pmc/articles/PMC6746181/

- There is great interest in molecular aspects of prostate cancer and, in particular, the use of such methods in diagnosis. This reference shows one very popular approach in the use of circulating DNA derived from the tumor.

Elzinga-Tinke JE, et al. Etiology and early pathogenesis of malignant testicular germ cell tumors: Toward possibilities for preinvasive diagnosis. *Asian J Androl*. 2015;17(3):381-393. https://www.ncbi.nlm.nih.gov/pmc/articles/PMC4430936/

Can Testicular Cancer Be Found Early? American Cancer Society. https://www.cancer.org/cancer/testicular-cancer/detection-diagnosis-staging/detection.html

- The review covers multiple aspects of testicular cancer, including the various types and the molecular biology. The American Cancer Society site has a discussion of self-screening.

Bing Z, Bai S. Gynecomastia: An uncommon but important clinical manifestation for testicular tumors. *Open J Pathol*. 2012;2(1):6-13.

- This reading reviews gynecomastia in relation to testicular tumors and was useful in constructing the second case for this chapter.

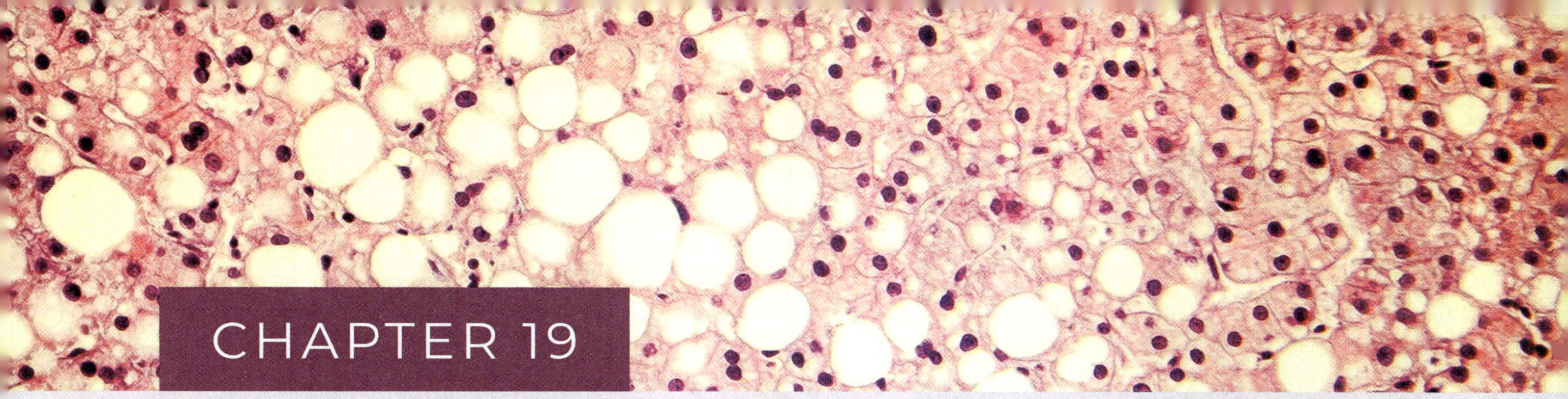

CHAPTER 19

The Liver and the Biliary System

LEARNING OBJECTIVES

1. Describe the normal structure and function of the liver and explain how they relate to major liver diseases.
2. List the major causes of liver injury and describe their effects on hepatic function.
3. Compare the three major types of viral hepatitis in terms of their pathogenesis, incubation period, incidence of complications, and frequency of carriers. Explain the diagnostic tests used to identify each type of viral infection and describe their methods of prevention.
4. Explain the adverse effects of excess alcohol intake on liver structure and function.
5. Explain how gallstones are formed and describe their causes and effects.
6. Compare the three major causes of jaundice.
7. Outline the pathogenesis of liver disease from normal function to end-stage cirrhosis.

Structure and Function of the Liver

The liver, the largest organ in the body, has a roughly triangular shape and is located beneath the diaphragm in the upper abdomen (**Figure 19-1**). Its many functions include the following:

- Storage of glycogen, iron, copper, triglycerides, and lipid-soluble vitamins such as B_{12}.
- Synthesis of certain serum proteins, including albumin, proteins important in coagulation and inflammation, and binding or carrier proteins for many substances.
- Metabolism of glucose and free fatty acids.
- Catabolism of both endogenous substances, such as hormones, and exogenous toxic agents. The liver also removes ammonia derived from amino acid breakdown.
- Production and excretion of bile.

The liver possesses a double blood supply. About 70 percent of the blood flowing through the liver is provided by the portal vein, which drains the spleen

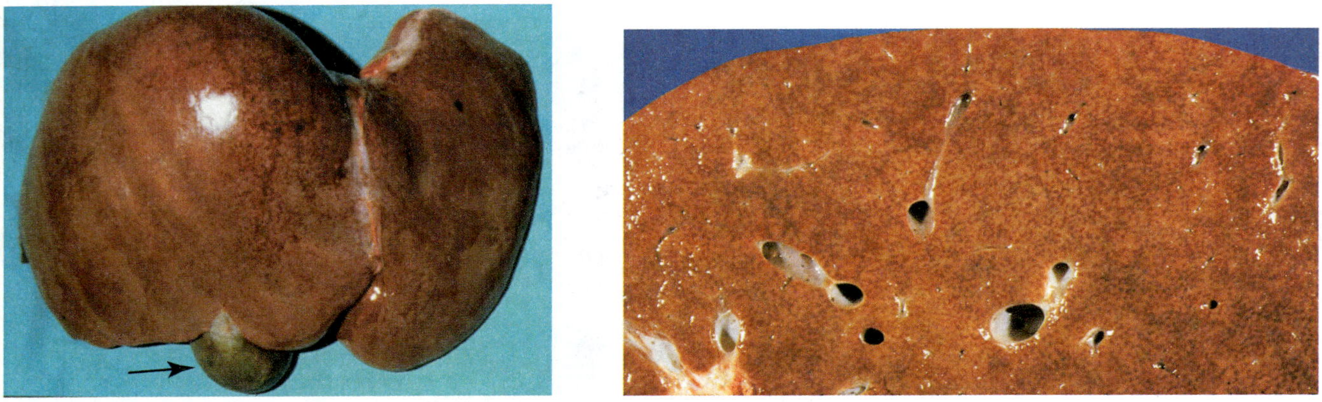

(A) (B)

Figure 19-1 **(A)** A normal liver viewed from above to show its superior and anterior surfaces. The gallbladder is located on the undersurface of the liver, and the fundus of the gallbladder projects slightly beyond the anterior edge of the liver (*arrow*). **(B)** Section of liver illustrating the uniform appearance of the hepatic parenchyma and the large blood vessels (branches of the portal vein) transporting blood into the liver from the gastrointestinal tract.

Courtesy of Leonard V. Crowley, MD, Century College.

and gastrointestinal tract. Portal blood, while rich in nutrients absorbed from the intestines, is low in oxygen content. The rest of the blood supply, which comes from the hepatic artery, has a high oxygen content but is low in nutrients. Blood flowing from the hepatic artery and the portal vein mixes as the blood flows through the liver and is eventually drained into the right and left hepatic veins, which flow into the inferior vena cava.

Liver cells exhibit an easily recognized histological arrangement. They form long, wide plates interconnected at angles to form a lattice. The hepatic **sinusoids** occupy the spaces between the plates (**Figure 19-2A**). Branches of the hepatic artery, portal vein, **bile** ducts, and lymphatic vessels travel together within the liver and are termed the **portal tracts**, also referred to as **triads** (**Figure 19-2B**). The terminal branches of both the hepatic artery and the portal vein discharge their blood into the hepatic sinusoids (**Figure 19-2C**). In histologic sections, the liver plates appear as cords surrounded on each side by sinusoids that converge toward the central veins. The portal tracts appear at the periphery. This anatomic configuration, which is termed a **liver lobule**, is illustrated diagrammatically in **Figure 19-3A**.

Sinusoid Small, irregularly shaped blood vessel, which in the livers is found between the sheets of hepatocytes.

Bile A secretion of the liver containing bile salts, cholesterol, and other substances.

Portal tract/triad Branches of the hepatic artery, portal vein, and bile duct are located at the periphery of liver lobule.

Liver lobule A histologic subdivision of the liver in which columns of liver cells converge toward a central vein and portal tracts are located at the periphery.

Bile canaliculi Small terminal bile channels located between liver cords.

Blood flow in the liver runs from portal tracts through the sinusoids into central veins (**Figure 19-3B**). Consequently, the liver cells nearest the portal tracts receive the most oxygen and nutrients, with those nearest the central veins much less well supplied. Because of their relatively poor nutritional state and lower degree of oxygenation, the liver cells nearest the central veins are more vulnerable to injury from toxic agents or circulatory disturbances, as might occur in shock and heart failure, than are the cells nearer the portal tracts. For this reason, centrilobular necrosis is a common result of such liver injury.

The small terminal bile channels, termed **bile canaliculi** (singular canaliculus), are located between adjacent liver cords and drain into the bile ducts traveling in the portal tracts. The direction of the bile flow is opposite that of the blood flow in the sinusoids (Figure 19-3B). The bile ducts gradually converge to form larger ducts, which finally unite as the large right and left hepatic ducts. The two hepatic ducts join to form the common hepatic duct. The gallbladder joins the common hepatic duct by means of the cystic duct to form the common bile duct that enters the duodenum (**Figure 19-4**).

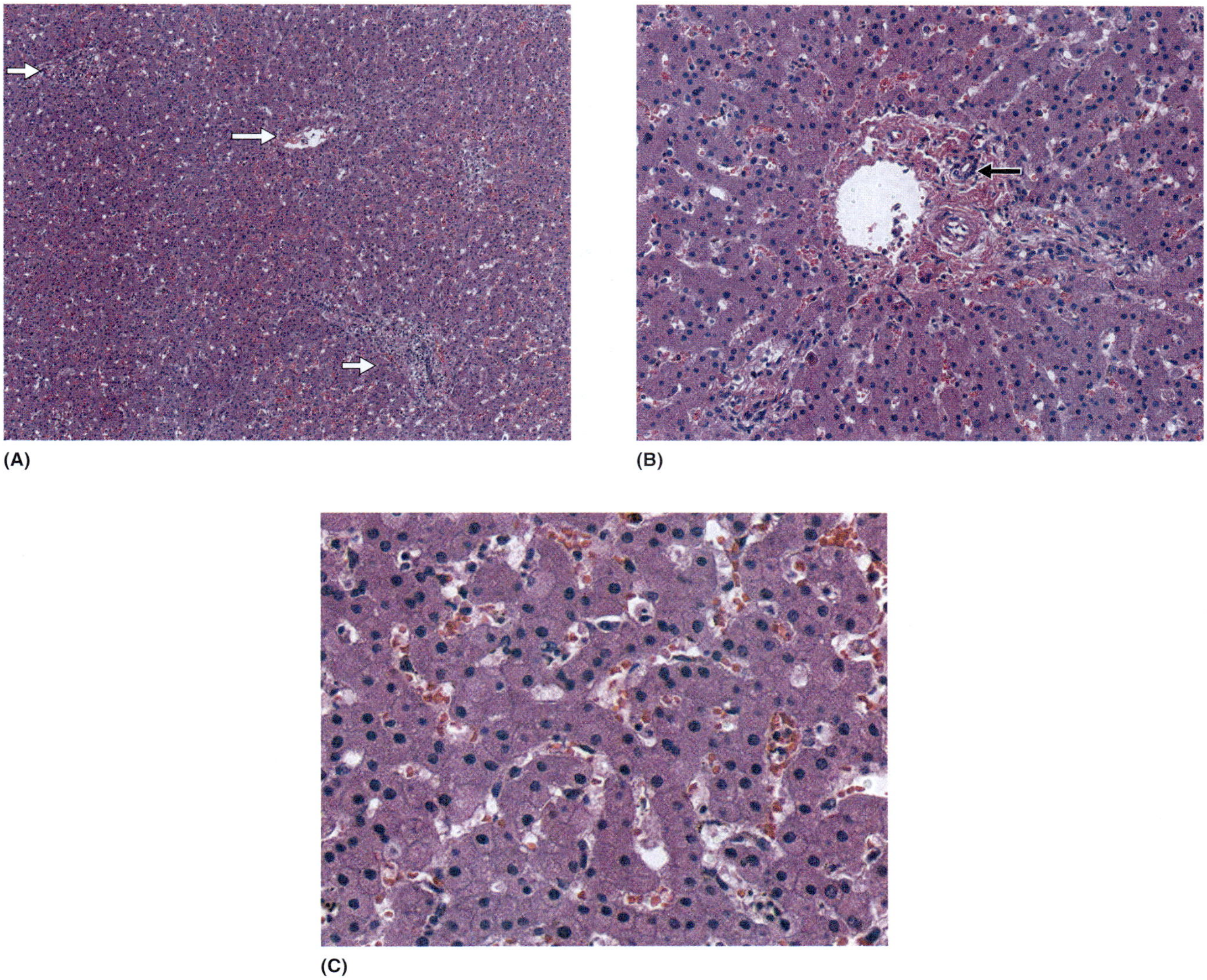

Figure 19-2 Photomicrographs showing the cellular structure of a normal liver. **(A)** Low-magnification photomicrograph illustrating plates of liver cells, which appear as cords in histologic sections, and sinusoids between cords, which drain into central veins (*arrows*). Short arrows indicate portal triads. **(B)** Higher magnification illustrating portal tract. A branch of the hepatic artery is below the bile duct (*arrow*), and a branch of the portal vein is left and below the bile duct. **(C)** High magnification of liver cell cords and hepatic sinusoids. Sinusoids show some residual blood cells.

Causes and Effects of Liver Injury

The liver is vulnerable to injury by many agents, including viral infection, consumption of alcohol, and many toxic agents and drugs. Histologically, injury to liver cells can activate either necrosis (unprogrammed cell death) or apoptosis (programmed cell death); cause the accumulation of fat within the liver cell cytoplasm, often the initial sign of liver injury; or a combination of these events. Some injurious agents primarily cause cell death, whereas others chiefly induce fatty changes in liver cells.

Many times, the exact cause and extent of liver disease is difficult to determine. In such cases, a biopsy of the liver can be performed by inserting a needle through the skin directly into the liver and extracting a small bit of liver tissue, which can be examined microscopically by the pathologist for better understanding of the nature and severity of the liver disease.

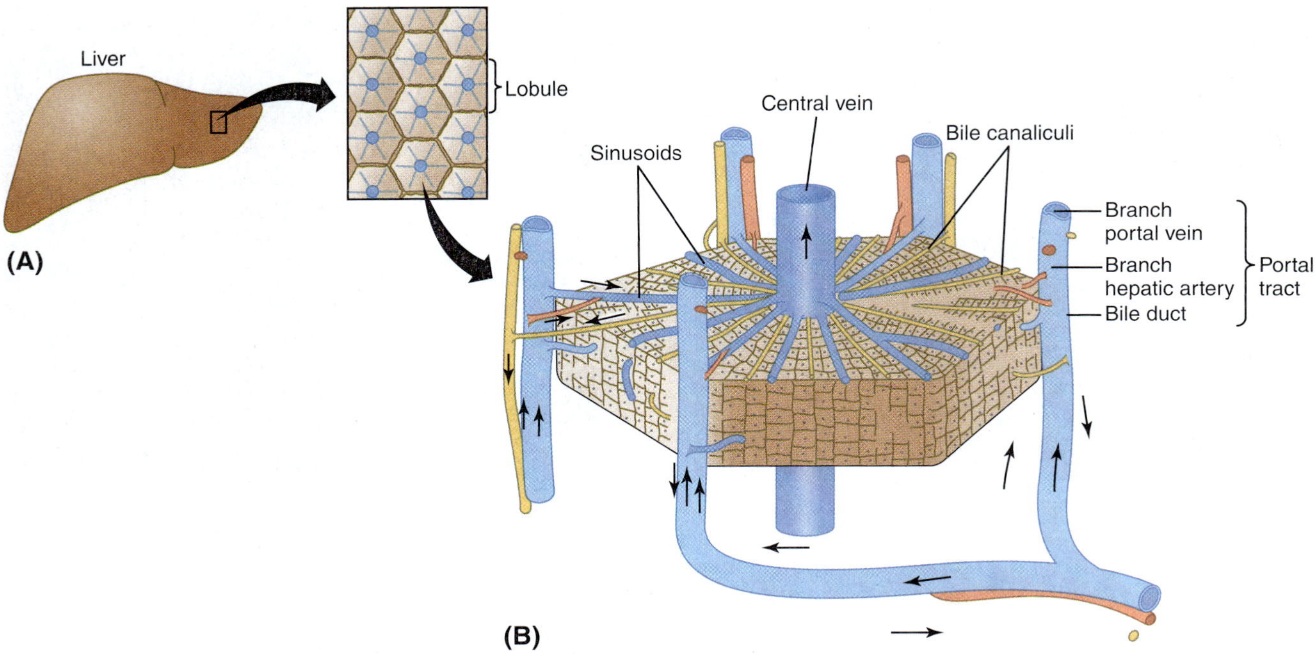

Figure 19-3 **(A)** Concept of liver lobule, consisting of cords of cells radiating toward central vein with portal tracts at the periphery. Lobules are outlined in the diagram. **(B)** Blood flow in sinusoids toward the central vein; flow of bile toward portal tract.

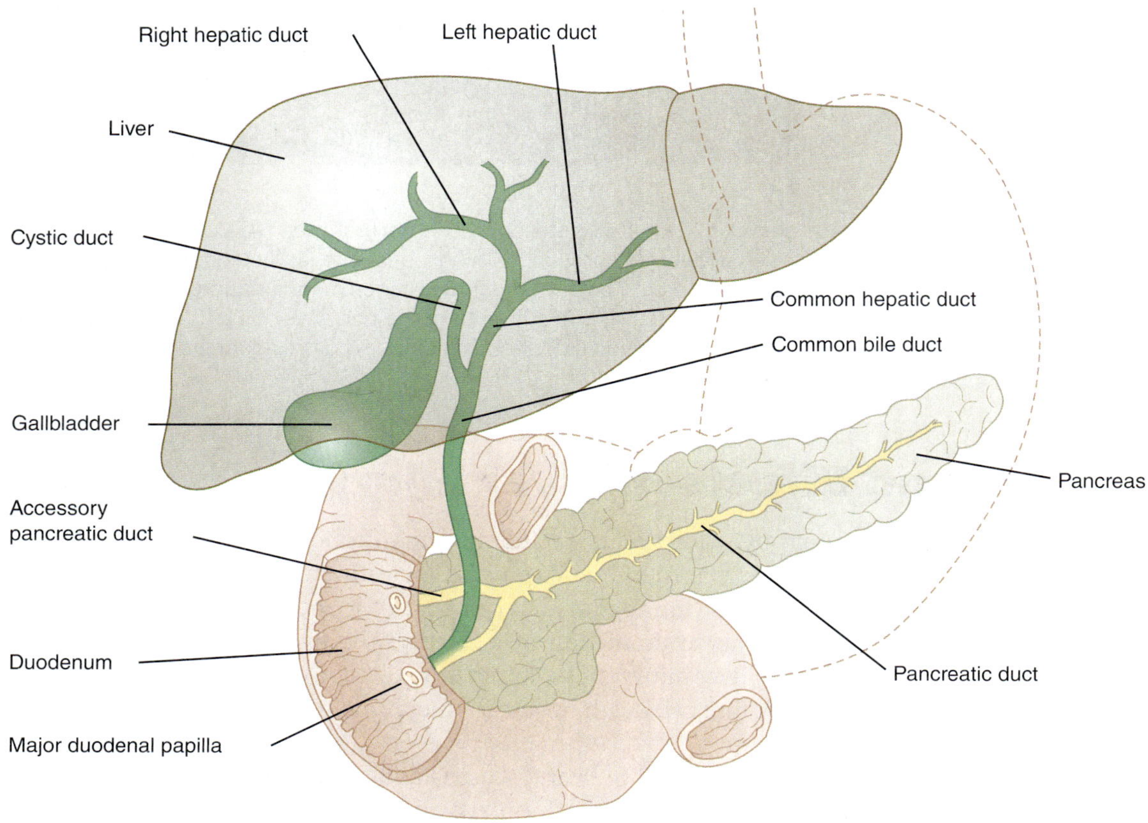

Figure 19-4 Anatomy of the biliary duct system. The right and left hepatic ducts form the common hepatic duct, which is joined by the cystic duct to form the common bile duct, which opens into the duodenum along with the pancreatic duct through a common channel.

The effect of hepatic injury depends on the extent of damage induced by the injurious agent. If liver injury is mild, the liver cells will regenerate and recover, restoring liver function to normal. Fortunately, this is the usual outcome. If the injury is extremely severe, destroying large amounts of liver tissue, not enough liver tissue may remain to sustain life. If the patient does survive, healing of the severe injury may be associated with severe scarring, and liver function may never return to normal. Multiple episodes of relatively mild liver injury may have a cumulative effect, leading to scarring (fibrosis) and permanent impairment of liver function. Chronic liver cell injury from any cause may in turn be followed by diffuse scarring throughout the liver, which is termed **cirrhosis of the liver** (**Figure 19-5**). Cirrhosis can be considered end-stage liver disease. Long-standing cirrhosis may be associated with the development of liver cancer.

Clinically, the most common types of liver disease characterized by injury to liver cells include viral **hepatitis** and injury-associated alcohol toxicity (**alcoholic liver disease**). **Nonalcoholic fatty liver disease (NAFLD)** (now sometimes termed metabolic dysfunction–associated steatotic liver disease—MASLD), is associated with obesity and impaired glucose metabolism with insulin resistance, termed **metabolic syndrome**. Metabolic syndrome ranks as the most common cause of chronic liver disease as a result of increasing levels of obesity in the Western population. Although it is normal

Cirrhosis of the liver A disease characterized by diffused intrahepatic scarring and circulatory disturbance within the liver.

Hepatitis Inflammation of the liver.

Alcoholic liver disease Long-term injury to the liver resulting from frequent and heavy alcohol consumption.

Nonalcoholic fatty liver disease (NAFLD) Fatty liver without significant inflammation or scarring within the liver, which usually occurs in insulin-resistant obese people with lipid abnormalities.

Metabolic syndrome A syndrome characterized by obesity and insulin resistance often associated with nonalcoholic fatty liver disease.

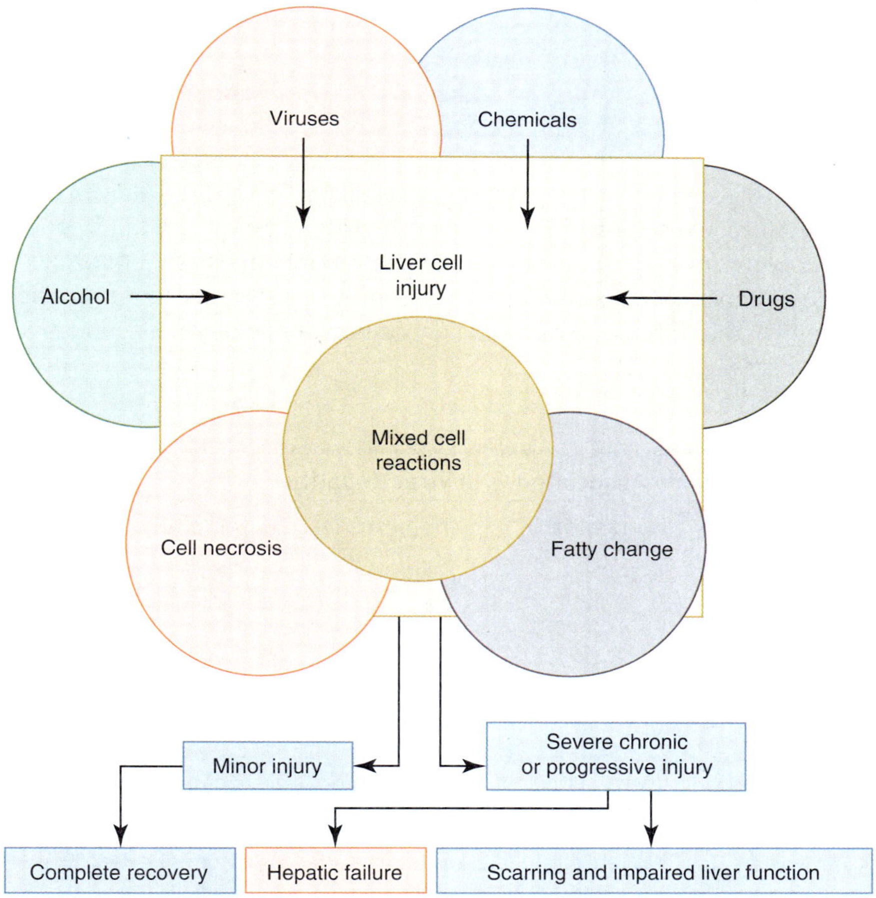

Figure 19-5 Summary of causes and effects of liver injury. Many agents can cause injury to liver cells, manifested as fatty change, cell death, or a combination of both. Mild injury is followed by complete recovery. Severe, chronic, or progressive injury may lead to hepatic failure or diffuse scarring with impaired hepatic function.

Steatosis Abnormal storage of fat in the liver. Can result from alcoholic damage or some other cause.

Councilman/apoptotic bodies Cell shrinkage/apoptotic cell death in inflammation of the liver.

Jaundice Yellow discoloration of skin and the white part of the eyes (sclera) resulting from an accumulation of bilirubin in the body.

for less than 5–10 percent of the liver weight to consist of fat, larger amounts are termed **steatosis** (fatty liver). This, when severe, is associated with liver damage (steatohepatitis).

Viral Hepatitis

The term viral hepatitis applies to several clinically similar infections that result in inflammation and necrosis of the liver. Hepatitis A, B, and C (HAV, HBV, and HCV, respectively) account for almost all cases of viral hepatitis in the United States and Europe. Two additional types of viral hepatitis have also been identified: hepatitis D, or delta hepatitis, which occurs in people already infected with the hepatitis B virus; and hepatitis E, which is infrequently encountered in North America. HBV and HCV can lead to chronic infection associated with cirrhosis and liver cancer. It is estimated that about 300 million people have these chronic infections, resulting in 60 percent of cirrhosis and up to 80 percent of primary liver cancer cases. Hence, viral hepatitis is a significant public health concern worldwide. The overall properties of the agents causing viral hepatitis are summarized in **Table 19-1**.

Clinical Manifestations and Course

All of the hepatitis viruses produce similar histologic changes in the liver, characterized by diffuse inflammation throughout the liver lobules associated with liver cell swelling and necrosis of scattered individual liver cells or cells in small groups. Apoptotic cell death characterized by cell shrinkage and dark red color (termed **Councilman** bodies, also termed **apoptotic bodies**) is also seen (**Figure 19-6A**). When the acute disease is severe (most commonly in HBV infection), confluent areas of the liver may undergo necrosis resulting in destruction of essentially all hepatocytes and collapse of the liver (**Figure 19-6B**). The clinical manifestations of acute viral hepatitis are variable and correlate with the degree of liver cell injury and associated inflammation. Some affected individuals experience loss of appetite, feel ill or malaise, become **jaundiced** (yellowing of the skin as a result of the deposition of bile products), and exhibit abnormal laboratory tests.

Table 19-1 Comparison of Viruses Most Commonly Associated with Viral Hepatitis

Virus	Hepatitis A	Hepatitis B	Hepatitis C	Hepatitis D	Hepatitis E
Type	RNA	DNA	RNA	RNA	RNA
Route of transmission	Fecal–oral	Parenteral, perinatal, sexual contact	Parenteral	Parenteral	Fecal–oral, rarely foodborne (from pork)
Chronic liver disease	Never	10%	~80%	5%	Never
Diagnosis	IgM	HBsAg or antibody to HBcAg	Molecular test for HCV RNA	IgM, IgG, or viral-specific antigens	IgM, IgG, or viral-specific antigens
Highest prevalence	Rural areas with poor sanitation and hygiene	Asia	Western nations, United States	Requires HBV for infection	Zoonotic reservoir, India
Fatality	<1%	<1%	20% 10 years post-infection	20%	Unusual but highest in pregnant women

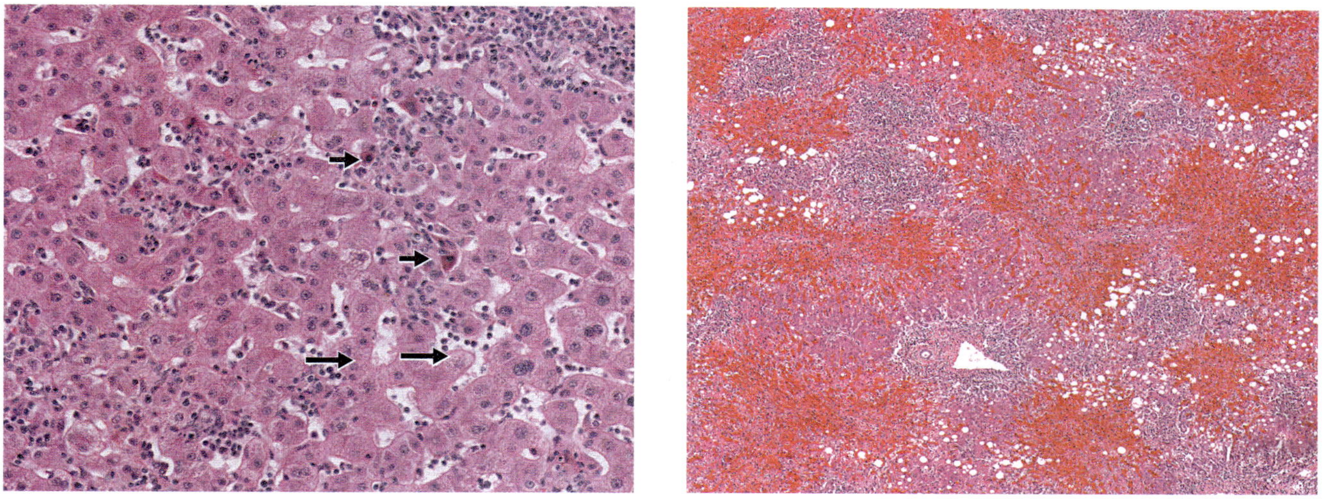

(A) (B)

Figure 19-6 **(A)** Acute viral hepatitis. Cords of liver cells have lost their orderly arrangement and appear disrupted by swelling of liver cells (*arrows*), necrosis of individual cells, and scattered aggregates of inflammatory cells throughout the liver lobules. Apoptotic bodies are visible as condensed intensely red cells (*short arrows*). **(B)** Confluent hepatic necrosis showing geographic areas of hemorrhage and necrosis throughout the liver.

As a result of hepatic viral infection, some individuals become ill with abnormal laboratory tests but never develop jaundice. This condition is termed **anicteric hepatitis** (ana = without + icterus = jaundice). Still others have few symptoms and do not seek medical attention, but laboratory tests reveal liver injury. Their infection, which could easily escape detection, is sometimes termed **subclinical hepatitis**. Despite the absence of symptoms, these individuals can transmit the infection to others.

Anicteric hepatitis Symptoms of hepatitis without the appearance of jaundice.

Subclinical hepatitis Liver inflammation resulting in few symptoms.

A number of blood tests contribute to the diagnosis of liver injury and hepatitis. Alanine aminotransferase (ALT) and aspartate aminotransferase (AST) are enzymes released from injured liver cells into the blood, often before jaundice occurs. The amount of AST and ALT released into the blood and the ratio of increase between them indicate the severity of injury and hint at the cause. Alkaline phosphatase (ALP) is an enzyme that increases with injury to the bile ducts. Increased levels in the blood suggest biliary disease (but are not specific for such).

The outcome of viral hepatitis depends primarily on which virus caused the infection. Many cases of hepatitis caused by the hepatitis A infection can be quite mild, and patients recover completely without complications. An unfavorable outcome occurs in only a very small percentage of cases. In contrast, people infected with hepatitis B virus or hepatitis C virus may become chronic carriers of the virus and develop chronic progressive hepatitis that eventually leads to cirrhosis and liver failure.

Hepatitis A

The hepatitis A virus is an RNA-containing virus measuring 27 nm. Hepatitis A has a relatively short incubation period that varies from 2 to 6 weeks. The virus is excreted in oropharyngeal secretions and in the feces during the late incubation period and for about 2 weeks after the onset of symptoms. Transmission is by direct person-to-person contact or by fecal contamination of food or water. Food- or waterborne infections may occur in epidemics or during natural disasters where the water supply has become compromised. The infection is self-limited, and there are no chronic carriers of the virus.

Antibodies to the hepatitis A virus appear in the blood after recovery, providing immunity against the hepatitis A virus but not against the other hepatitis viruses. Hepatitis A is a common infection in the United States, and almost half the adult population has antibodies against the virus. A highly effective inactivated hepatitis A vaccine has been available since 1995 and is recommended to immunize people with a relatively high risk of becoming infected, such as healthcare workers who have frequent contact with infected patients or people traveling in foreign countries where there is a high incidence of hepatitis A in the population. Although not universally required, the CDC recommends immunization of all children ages 12–23 months, often given in combination with vaccination for hepatitis B. Increased levels of immunization correlate with a marked decrease in hepatitis A in the United States. If an unvaccinated individual is exposed to hepatitis A, hepatitis immune globulin–containing antibodies to HAV can prevent infection if given within 2 weeks of exposure. During 2022 a total of 2300 hepatitis A cases were reported to the CDC by 50 states. This is likely to be an underestimate but a marked decrease from historic levels, a result of immunization. In the United States, contamination of food products and transmission by restaurant staff contribute to the transmission of the virus. An increase in the disease among the homeless and IV drug abusers can occur. This argues strongly for more aggressive use of vaccination.

Hepatitis B

The hepatits B virus is a DNA-containing virus measuring 42 nm, somewhat larger than the hepatitis A virus, with an inner core and an outer surface envelope. The core contains a partially double-stranded circular DNA and an enzyme, DNA polymerase, enclosed within a protein shell. The inner protein shell forms the **hepatitis B core antigen (HBcAg)**. The same gene that codes for the core antigen also produces a somewhat larger protein that forms the **hepatitis B e-antigen (HBeAg)**. Continued presence of HBeAg in the blood of an infected person is a marker for continued viral replication and indicates continued infectivity and likely chronic infection. The outer surface envelope is composed of lipid and glycoproteins, the latter of which constitutes the **hepatitis B surface antigen (HBsAg)**. Infected hepatocytes secrete large amounts of this antigen into the blood. The viral core and surface envelope together form the complete virus particle, which is often termed the Dane particle after the pathologist who first described it.

Hepatitis B core antigen (HBcAg) The antigen contained in the core of the hepatitis B virus.

Hepatitis B e-antigen (HBeAg) Antigen associated with active hepatitis B virus proliferation.

Hepatitis B surface antigen (HBsAg) The coating of the hepatitis B virus that is also found in great excess in the blood of infected patients.

Hepatocellular carcinoma (HCC) Most common liver cancer.

The clinical features of HBV infection are indistinguishable from those of HAV, although HBV has a longer incubation period, which varies from 2 weeks to 6 months. Also, unlike hepatitis A, HBV disease can progress in several patterns. Initial HBV infection may be asymptomatic in 50 percent of cases or can produce an acute hepatitis that may end in viral clearance and recovery or may (uncommon) result in fulminant hepatitis with liver necrosis. Acute hepatitis, if not cleared by the immune system, can lead to a chronic disease state that may, in turn, progress to cirrhosis. Some chronic carriers may be asymptomatic but nevertheless infectious. Also, HBV-induced chronic liver disease is associated with the development of liver cancer, or **hepatocellular carcinoma (HCC)**.

The host immune response to HBV is the major factor in the course of disease. The virus does not directly cause hepatocyte injury. In chronic disease, the host T cells' response to virally infected cells continually damages host

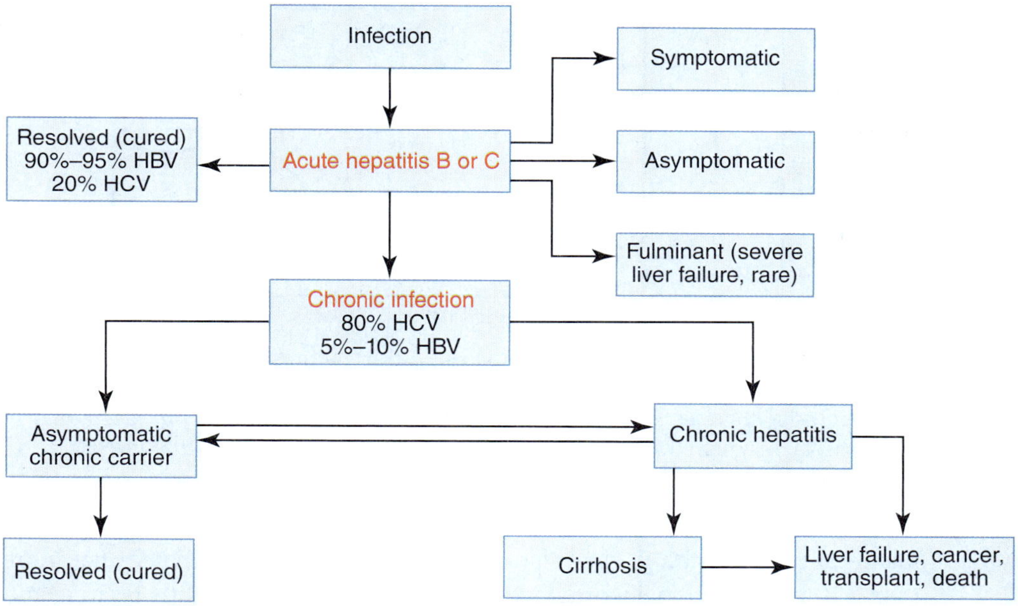

Figure 19-7 Natural history of hepatitis B and C infections.

liver cells while not eliminating the virus, resulting in scarring and cirrhosis (**Figure 19-7**).

When an individual becomes infected, the virus invades the liver and multiplies within the hepatic cells. The core of the virus is produced in the cell nucleus, and the surface antigen is produced in the cytoplasm. For some unexplained reason, much more surface antigen is produced within the infected cells than is necessary to coat the virus particles, and, as noted, the large excess is released into the bloodstream, where it can be detected by laboratory tests. Such blood is termed surface-antigen (HBsAg) positive. Although the laboratory tests detect only the surface antigen, HBsAg-positive blood is infectious because it also contains complete virus particles.

Serological testing of blood is critical in the diagnosis of HBV infection and in charting the progress of the disease. In the course of an infection, HBsAg appears during the incubation period and can be detected during the first few weeks. It is a marker for the infectious state of the patient. Normally, it does not persist in the blood for more than 2 or 3 weeks and disappears during convalescence. Antibody to the surface antigen (anti-HBs) then begins to appear and provides lifelong immunity to future infections. Antibody to the viral core (anti-HBc) appears early in the course of infection and does not provide future immunity. Antibody to HBe generally indicates clearance of the virus and recovery. However, some patients with these antibodies have persistent chronic infection (**Figure 19-8**). Many people possess antibodies against the virus resulting from deliberate immunization or as a result of prior infection. Unlike infection, immunization results only in antibodies to HBsAg (not HBc or HBe) because the vaccine contains a recombinant form of pure HBsAg.

Most infected individuals eliminate the virus from the bloodstream within a few weeks and recover completely, but as many as 90 percent of infants, 50 percent of children, and 5–10 percent of adults become chronic carriers of the virus. Some of the carriers develop chronic hepatitis, which results in progressive liver damage. About 0.5 percent of the U.S. population are asymptomatic chronic carriers of the virus, although the rate may be as high as 20 percent in some areas of the world. In these areas, the high rate is a result of

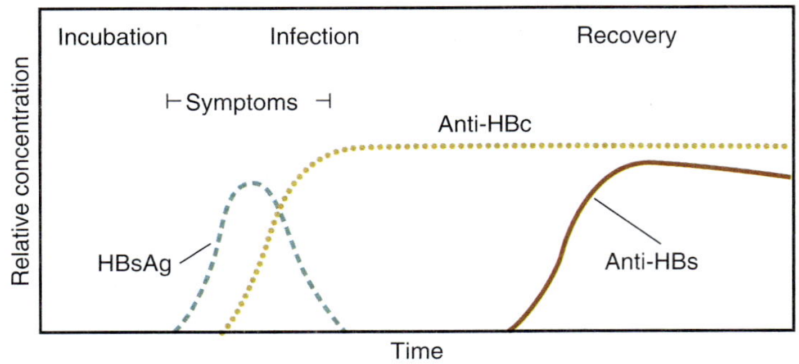

Figure 19-8 Acute HBV infection and recovery, illustrating serial changes of major antigens and antibodies used to aid in the diagnosis of HBV infection and monitor its course. Serial changes in HBeAg and anti-HBe are not shown. HBeAg rises along with HBsAg during active infection, and anti-HBe appears along with anti-HBc during recovery.

maternal transmission to the infant at birth. Overall, it is estimated that more than 350 million people worldwide are infected with the hepatitis B virus, and about 800,000 people die each year of complications of the disease. Although the availability of childhood immunization to HBV has drastically cut the number of cases seen in the United States, in 2022, a total of 2100 cases of acute hepatitis B were reported to the CDC (with an estimated total of 14,000 cases), for an overall incidence rate of 0.7 cases per 100,000 people. After adjusting for under-ascertainment and under-reporting, an estimated 17,000 chronic hepatitis B cases occurred in 2020. An estimated 900,000 people live with chronic HBV infection in the United States, two-thirds of whom may be unaware of their infection.

The highest levels of hepatitis B virus are found in the blood, with lower levels being present in semen and saliva. The virus is not excreted in stool, tears, sweat, or urine. Consequently, transmission does not occur by means of contaminated food or water. HBV infections result only from mucosal or parenteral contact with the blood or body fluids of HBsAg-positive individuals. In the United States, the most common route of transmission is by sexual contact. Infection via blood transfusion and other therapeutic infusions of blood products no longer occurs as a result of careful donor blood–screening procedures. However, healthcare workers are still at risk from accidental contact with contaminated material or surfaces, as are people who share needles. High-risk sexual behavior and intravenous drug use account for 80 percent of all new cases of hepatitis B in the United States. Over 20 percent of people who inject recreational drugs have chronic hepatitis B infection. Needle sharing increases the risk of transmission. In areas of the world with high levels of chronic infection, perinatal infection is the most common mechanism for transmission. Over 90 percent of infants born to mothers who are HBsAg- and HBeAg-positive become infected, and almost all of these infections will be chronic, with 25 percent dying prematurely of liver failure. Immediate treatment of these children at birth with vaccine and antibody-containing hepatitis B immune globulin reduces the risk to under 5 percent. Pretreatment of the mother with antiviral agents or immune globulin may further reduce the risk.

As noted previously, hepatitis B immune globulin provides good protection if administered promptly after exposure to the virus. Several oral antiviral drugs are available that can suppress viral multiplication and slow disease progression in people with chronic disease. These drugs are used in combination with a type of interferon that helps the immune system clear the virus. However, rigorous adherence to childhood vaccination protocols provides the best way of reducing the public health burden of the disease.

Hepatitis C

The hepatitis C virus is an 80 nm RNA virus transmitted by infected blood and body fluids, as is HBV. There are seven major genotypes (genetic variants) and multiple subtypes, which differ in their response to treatment. Types 1, 2, and 3 are the most common in the United States, with type 1 being responsible for about 75 percent of cases, the most resistant to treatment, and associated with more severe liver disease and a higher risk of chronicity. In many ways, HCV infection is an even more serious problem than HBV infection. HCV is a major cause of chronic liver disease in the United States, accounting for about 10 percent of reported cases. Seventy-five percent of HCV-infected individuals are unable to eliminate the virus and become chronic carriers; of these, between 10 and 20 percent will develop cirrhosis with a potential result of liver failure and a 1 to 5 percent annual risk of developing liver cancer. In 2023, 101,500 persons were newly diagnosed with chronic hepatitis C, of which two-thirds were males. The highest number of cases occurred in the 30–39 years of age group for a case rate of 72.1 cases per 100,000. There were 11,200 deaths, with the highest numbers found in American Indian populations. A 2024 survey by the CDC indicates good progress toward reduction in disease-related deaths, but there continues to be an increase in new hepatitis C infections.

Hepatitis C is transmitted by blood from an HCV-infected person. Currently, the sharing of equipment used to inject drugs is the most common route. For persons engaging in long-term monogamous sexual relationships, the risk of sexual transmission is low. When the number of sexual partners increases, the risk increases as well. Mother-to-child transmission can also spread the disease. Prior to 1992, infected blood transfusions were a major source.

There are no agents like immune globulin that can protect an uninfected person who has been exposed to the virus, e.g., from an accidental needle stick when drawing blood from an infected person. HCV uses an RNA-dependent RNA polymerase during replication, which is prone to making errors. This results in a high rate of natural mutation. One of the envelope proteins of the virus, E2, is particularly prone to mutating, most likely because of selective pressure from antibodies developed by the infected host to the virus. The virus changes rapidly enough that the immune system cannot effectively eliminate it. Thus, no immunizing agent is available that can establish an active immunity against the virus. Diagnosis usually starts with an antibody-based test followed by a molecular-based test for hepatitis C RNA. The CDC encourages screening as one-third of hepatitis C patients are unaware they are infected.

HCV-infected persons may experience symptoms of hepatitis, as previously described, but most infected individuals have few symptoms of infection and those that occur are often not related to the liver. For example, joint and muscle aches, itching, and paresthesias, unusual sensations such as "pins and needles" relating to peripheral nerve damage, are common. Infected people develop antibodies against HCV, usually within 2 months of infection, that remain during the chronic phase of the disease. Viral RNA, a measure of virus particles in the circulation, is an indication of continuing infection, and the amount of viral RNA can be measured in the blood of infected people to monitor the course of the disease. In addition to liver disease, individuals with chronic HCV infection suffer from a wide variety of extrahepatic diseases, many of which are believed to be autoimmune in nature and possibly related to the chronic but ineffective immune response to the virus.

In the past, many HCV infections followed transfusion of HCV-infected blood or blood products. Modern ultrasensitive molecular testing techniques reduce the risk to about 1 in 100,000 units. However, many of those currently suffering chronic disease were infected prior to this testing. Currently, most new HCV infections are acquired from infected blood or body fluids in much the same ways that HBV is acquired.

Because of the potential late complications of HCV infection, all HCV-positive individuals are considered for therapy to reduce viral load and to eliminate the virus. Therapy uses any of several oral antiviral drugs (termed DAA or direct acting antivirals), the choice depending on the presence or absence of cirrhosis and, importantly, the genotype of the viral infection. Therapy significantly reduces the risk of progression of disease and of death. Current therapy can result in a sustained virologic response—lack of detectable virus for 3 months after therapy—and can be considered as a cure in greater than 90 percent of those treated. Treatment requires 8 to 12 weeks of continued dosing with antiviral medications at a potential cost of over $50,000. Cost is much reduced ($3000–$5000) for those covered by insurance (such as Medicare).

Hepatitis D (Delta Hepatitis)

This type of hepatitis is caused by a small defective RNA virus that can only infect people who are already infected with the hepatitis B virus, either chronic carriers of HBV or those with an acute HBV infection (termed superinfection). The delta virus is always associated with an HBV infection because the virus is unable to produce its own outer viral coat and can reproduce itself only by coating itself with HBsAg produced by HBV, thereby forming complete but hybrid virus particles composed of a delta virus core and an HBsAg outer layer. Delta virus superinfection increases the probability that HBV will become chronic and worsen the severity of existing chronic HBV disease. Delta hepatitis is uncommon in the United States, and most cases are found among intravenous drug abusers. The disease is more common in regions where rates of HBV infection remain high.

Hepatitis E

Hepatitis E is caused by an RNA virus most commonly transmitted by the fecal–oral route. Foodborne disease also occurs from a serotype of virus associated with an animal reservoir, most often porcine. As is the case with hepatitis A virus, outbreaks have been traced to contaminated water supplies. Only a few cases have been reported in North America, and most of the infected individuals acquired the disease while traveling outside the United States. A diagnostic test has been developed to detect anti-HEV antibodies as an indication of HEV infection. Although the disease is often acute and self-limited, it is a particular danger to pregnant women, particularly in the second and third trimester where it can result in fulminant liver failure and maternal death in up to 30 percent of cases. A vaccine has been developed but is not licensed for use in the United States.

Other Hepatitis Viruses

Yellow fever virus causes severe hepatitis and remains a serious risk in tropical areas. A vaccine is available for travelers visiting areas where the disease is endemic. Other viruses may, at times, cause mild hepatitis. These include the **Epstein-Barr (EB) virus**, which causes infectious mononucleosis (Chapter 11), and another somewhat similar virus termed **cytomegalovirus** (CMV), which may also cause an infection resembling infectious mononucleosis.

Epstein-Barr (EB) virus A virus that causes infectious mononucleosis.

Cytomegalovirus One of the herpes viruses that causes an infectious mononucleosis-like syndrome in adults; may cause congenital malformation in fetuses (Chapter 16).

Fatty Liver

The liver performs many important functions related to the metabolism of food, including an important role in fat metabolism, so conditions that disturb liver functions can lead to accumulation of fat in liver cells. Fatty liver is a particular type of liver injury (**Figure 19-9**) associated with a number of injurious agents capable of increasing the synthesis or decreasing oxidation of free fatty acids by the liver or impairing the release of lipids bound to carrier proteins. All of these derangements can result in fat accumulation in the organ, leading to an accumulation of fat globules within the liver cell cytoplasm, termed steatosis (**Figure 19-10**). Diffuse fatty change within the liver can be demonstrated by ultrasound examination, by computed tomography (CT) scans, or by magnetic resonance imaging (MRI). A liver biopsy can determine if liver cell damage can be associated with the fatty change. In the United States, the most common causes of fatty liver are excessive alcohol ingestion, alcoholic liver disease or alcoholic steatosis, type II diabetes, and nonalcoholic liver disease or nonalcoholic steatosis. Nonalcoholic liver disease is rapidly increasing in frequency in association with the increase of metabolic syndrome and type 2 diabetes (Chapter 20). Many volatile solvents, drugs, and chemicals, and some poisons can also cause fat accumulation in liver cells.

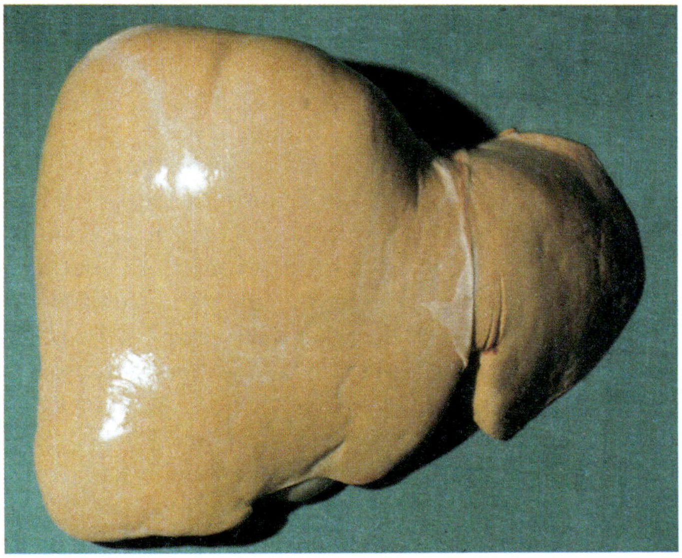

(A)

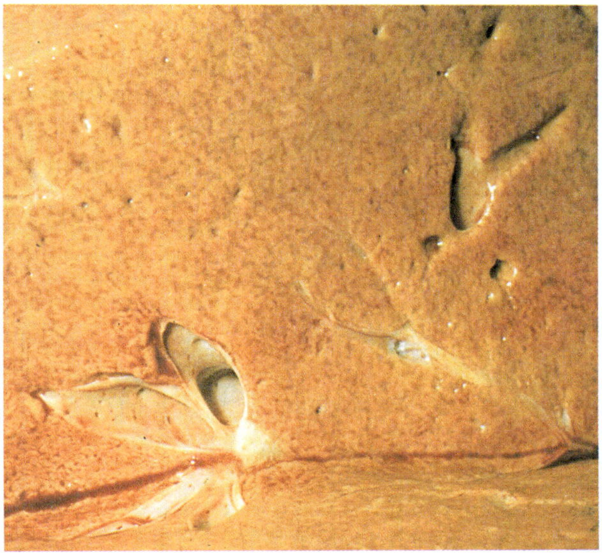

(B)

Figure 19-9 Fatty liver. **(A)** The liver appears yellow because of a large amount of fat within liver cells, but otherwise appears normal. **(B)** A section of liver that appears normal except for the yellow color caused by the fat.

Courtesy of Leonard V. Crowley, MD, Century College.

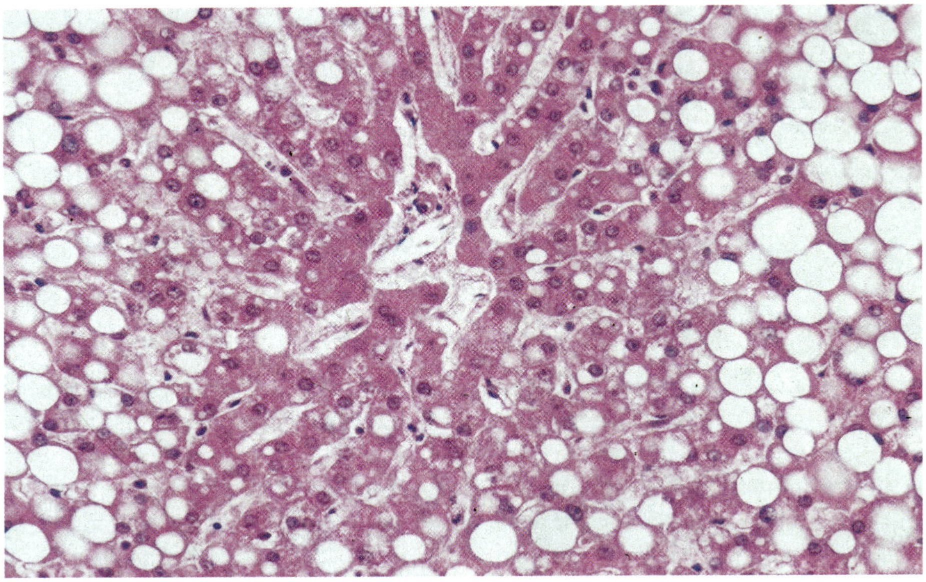

Figure 19-10 Photomicrograph of fatty liver. Liver cord cells (*center*) appear relatively normal. Other cells contain large fat globules that appear as clear spherical vacuoles within the liver cells. Processing the tissue for microscopy dissolves the fat.

Courtesy of Leonard V. Crowley, MD, Century College.

Alcoholic Liver Disease

Alcoholic liver disease refers to a group of structural and functional changes in the liver resulting from excessive alcohol consumption. The severity of the liver injury and its rate of progression are determined not only by how much alcohol is consumed but also by the length of time the person drank excessively. It is convenient to subdivide alcoholic liver disease into three stages of progressively increasing severity: (1) alcoholic fatty liver, (2) alcoholic hepatitis, and (3) alcoholic cirrhosis.

Alcoholic fatty liver is the mildest form of alcoholic liver disease. If the person stops consuming alcohol, the liver function gradually returns to normal, and the fat globules in the liver cells disappear when the liver cells oxidize the accumulated fat.

Alcoholic hepatitis is the next stage in progressive liver injury. In this case, the term hepatitis refers to the inflammatory cell infiltration secondary to liver cell necrosis and does not imply an infection, as in viral hepatitis. Heavy alcohol intake not only promotes fatty change in liver cells but also causes other degenerative changes as well and may actually induce liver cell necrosis. A characteristic feature of severe alcoholic liver injury is the accumulation of irregularly shaped, pink deposits within the cytoplasm of the liver cells. These structures, which are termed **Mallory bodies**, Mallory-Denk bodies, or alcoholic hyaline, indicate that the cell has been irreparably damaged. The bodies consist of cytokeratin filaments. Neutrophilic leukocytes also accumulate in response to the liver cell necrosis. In this situation, which is the second stage in the progression of alcoholic liver disease termed alcoholic hepatitis, the pathology includes progressive fibrous scarring throughout the liver. Alcoholic hepatitis is characterized not only by fatty change but also by liver cell degeneration with Mallory bodies and leukocyte infiltration (**Figure 19-11**).

Mallory body An irregular, red-staining structure in the cytoplasm of injured liver cells, usually resulting from alcohol-induced liver injury.

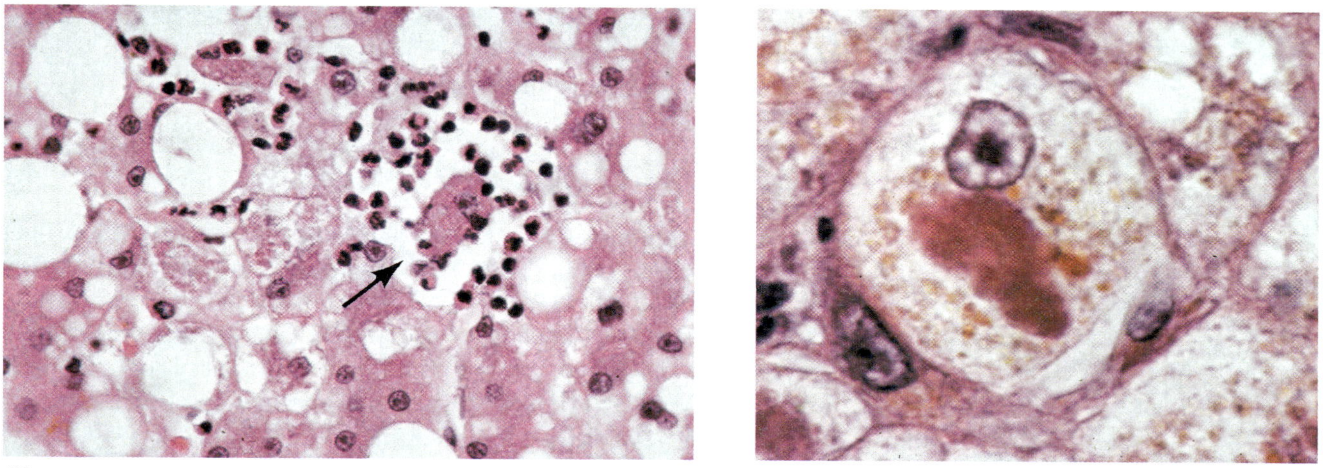

(A) (B)

Figure 19-11 A photomicrograph illustrating hepatic cellular structure in alcoholic hepatitis. **(A)** Many cells contain fat vacuoles. Others are swollen and contain Mallory bodies. One necrotic cell (*arrow*) is surrounded by a cluster of neutrophils. **(B)** A high-magnification photomicrograph of a Mallory body in a swollen liver cell.

Courtesy of Leonard V. Crowley, MD, Century College.

Alcoholic cirrhosis, the third and most advanced stage of alcoholic liver injury, is characterized by diffuse scarring throughout the liver, which disturbs liver function and impedes blood flow through the liver. In the United States, a large number of cases of cirrhosis are related to heavy alcohol ingestion and follow repeated episodes of alcoholic hepatitis. Although there is considerable individual variation in susceptibility to alcoholic liver injury, in general, a person must drink more than 1 pint of whiskey daily, or its equivalent in other alcoholic beverages, for 10 to 15 years to develop alcoholic cirrhosis. Occasionally, the disease develops more rapidly, and it may be seen in teenagers and young adults.

Nonalcoholic Liver Disease

Obese individuals and many people with type 2 diabetes also accumulate excess fat in the liver unrelated to excess alcohol consumption, a condition of increasing importance referred to as nonalcoholic fatty liver disease (NAFLD) or metabolic dysfunction–associated liver disease (MASLD). Usually, the affected individuals have a higher-than-normal blood glucose or type 2 diabetes related to obesity, which causes the body cells to become less responsive to insulin, a key finding in metabolic syndrome. The fatty change in the liver cells is termed nonalcoholic fatty liver to distinguish it from the fatty liver of alcoholic patients. Heavy fat infiltration may impair liver function and cause mild liver injury. However, the liver cell damage usually is reversible. Unfortunately, prolonged and severe fatty infiltration can cause significant liver cell damage associated with inflammation and scarring similar to the liver cell damage encountered in alcoholic patients, termed nonalcoholic steatohepatitis (NASH), which can progress to cirrhosis and eventually to liver failure and hepatocellular carcinoma in a manner similar to the condition that occurs in alcoholic liver disease. Unfortunately, NAFLD and its complications are becoming more frequent in the United States due to the increasing frequency of obesity and diabetes in the population. NASH is now the leading cause of chronic liver disease in the United States. Weight loss, exercise, and diabetic control are effective in controlling NAFLD. Recently, GLP-1 receptor agonists such as semaglutide and liraglutide have been shown to be effective in treating NAFLD, in part by promoting weight loss and controlling type 2 diabetes.

Cirrhosis of the Liver

Cirrhosis of the liver, regardless of cause, refers to obliteration of the normal architecture of the liver and replacement of the parenchyma by regenerating nodules of hepatocytes surrounded by bands of collagen and fibrosis (**Figure 19-12**). Any substance capable of injuring the liver may cause cirrhosis under certain conditions. The most common cause of cirrhosis is chronic hepatitis caused by HBV or HCV infections, alcoholic liver disease resulting from repeated episodes of alcoholic hepatitis and, increasingly, NAFLD.

Less common causes of cirrhosis include use of recreational drugs, some prescribed pharmaceuticals, and chemicals that damage liver cells; genetic diseases that directly or indirectly lead to liver damage, such as hemochromatosis (Chapter 12); $alpha_1$ antitrypsin deficiency, which also causes some types of pulmonary emphysema (Chapter 13); or long-standing bile duct obstruction, which causes a special type of cirrhosis termed **biliary cirrhosis**.

Biliary cirrhosis Diffuse liver cell damage and scarring with the distortion of liver cell structure and function (cirrhosis) caused by obstruction of bile ducts.

Portal hypertension Characterized by increased resistance to blood outflow and impaired liver function.

In cirrhosis, the liver is converted into a mass of scar tissue containing nodules of degenerating and regenerating liver cells, proliferating bile ducts, and inflammatory cells (**Figure 19-13**). The normal architectural pattern of the liver is completely disorganized, and the intrahepatic branches of the hepatic artery and portal vein are surrounded by scar tissue and ultimately isolated from the vascular outflow tract (central vein). This results in **portal hypertension** characterized by increased resistance to blood outflow and impaired liver function, followed by hepatic encephalopathy as a possible sequela.

Impaired Liver Function

As a result of liver cell damage, scarring, and impairment of blood supply to the liver caused by scarring, the number of functioning liver cells is greatly reduced and function impaired. Eventually, a patient with cirrhosis may die of

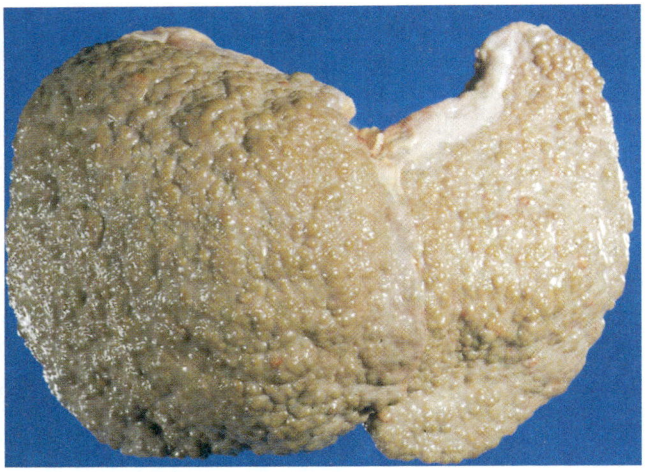

(A)

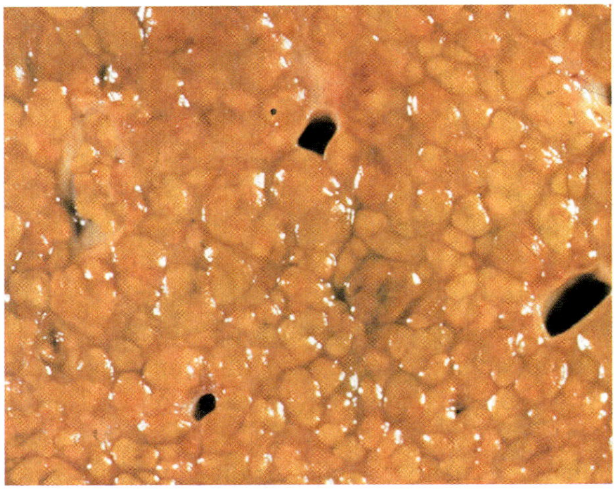

(B)

Figure 19-12 Advanced hepatic cirrhosis illustrating elevated nodules of liver tissue surrounded by depressed areas of scar tissue. **(A)** Exterior of liver. **(B)** A closer view of the liver in cross section.

Courtesy of Leonard V. Crowley, MD, Century College.

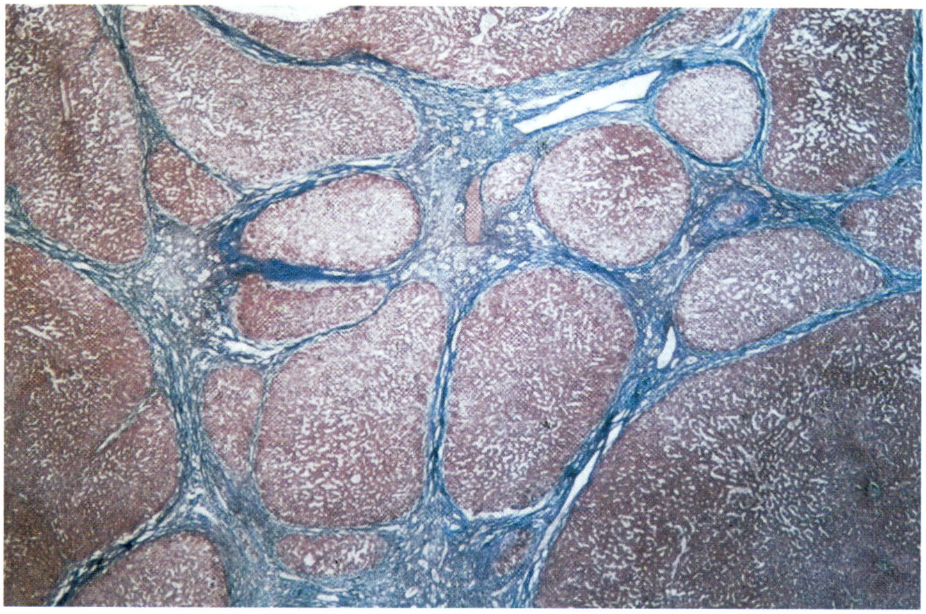

Figure 19-13 A low-magnification photomicrograph of cirrhotic liver illustrating nodules of liver cells circumscribed by dense scar tissue (blue-green stain). The normal architectural pattern is lost. The number of functioning liver cells is reduced and replaced by scar tissue, and the scar tissue disrupts blood flow through the liver. Compare with Figure 19-2.

Courtesy of Leonard V. Crowley, MD, Century College.

liver failure. Clinical manifestations commonly found in men with advanced cirrhosis are testicular atrophy, loss of sex drive, and breast hypertrophy. These manifestations result from impaired liver function and appear to be the result of an excess of estrogen. Normally, men produce not only the male sex hormone (testosterone) but also small amounts of estrogen. The estrogen is usually inactivated by the liver and exerts little effect. The cirrhotic liver, however, is unable to accomplish this function efficiently; consequently, estrogen accumulates and produces these associated clinical manifestations.

Albumin, which is produced by the liver, is reduced in cirrhosis. This can result in **ascites** because albumin is crucial to maintaining the normal colloid osmotic pressure of the blood, which is the force that tends to hold fluid in the capillaries (Chapter 12). Because most proteins important in blood coagulation are produced in the liver, individuals with impaired liver function may be susceptible to hemorrhage.

Ascites The buildup of fluid in the abdomen, causing a swollen belly, most often occurring because of cirrhosis, a liver disease.

Reye's syndrome Acute illness following mild viral infection in infants, children, and teens, characterized by brain swelling associated with aspirin consumption.

In addition to liver impairment from alcohol ingestion, other diseases can result in liver impairment. An example is **Reye's syndrome** (rhymes with "eye"), now an extremely uncommon acute illness that develops most frequently in infants, children, and teens after a mild viral infection and is characterized by both marked swelling of the brain with neurologic dysfunction and accumulation of fat within the cytoplasm of liver cells associated with impaired liver function.

Current evidence suggests that Reye's syndrome is related in some way to acetylsalicylic acid (aspirin) given to treat the fever and discomfort associated with the viral infection and likely also with otherwise undiagnosed inborn errors of metabolism. The recommended use of acetaminophen to treat symptoms of viral infections in infants and children has led to a much-diminished frequency of the condition, with two cases or less being reported per year in the United States. However, it should be noted that an acetaminophen overdose can be associated with severe acute liver disease, which may require transplantation (see **Case 19-1**).

Portal Hypertension

Normally, the portal vein blood passes through sinusoids into the hepatic veins and then into the inferior vena cava. In cirrhosis, venous return through the portal system and liver sinusoids to the central veins is impaired because of scar tissue leading to portal hypertension. The high pressure affects the portal capillaries, contributing to excessive leakage of fluid. Eventually, the abdomen becomes distended by ascites, fluids that accumulate within the abdominal cavity (**Figure 19-14**).

Because of the obstruction of portal venous return, a collateral circulation develops in response to increased portal pressure in an attempt to bypass the intrahepatic obstruction and deliver portal blood directly into the systemic

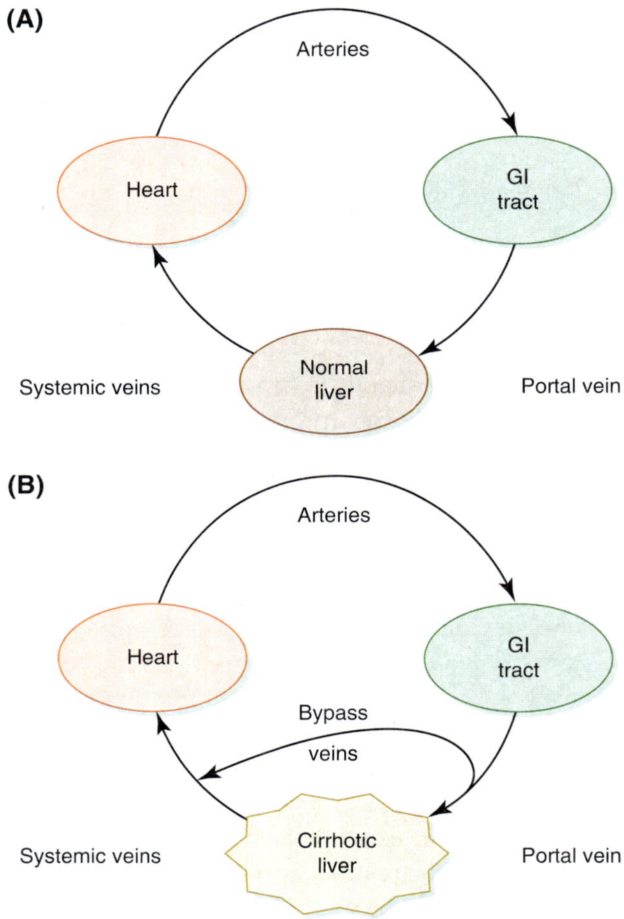

Figure 19-14 A comparison of normal blood flow pathways with those in cirrhosis. **(A)** Normal flow pattern. The heart pumps blood through the aorta to the gastrointestinal tract, from which blood collects in the portal vein and flows through hepatic sinusoids into hepatic veins, then into the vena cava, and finally, back to the heart to be repumped. **(B)** The flow pattern in cirrhosis. Blood pumped to the gastrointestinal tract is collected in the portal vein; however, flow through hepatic sinusoids is interrupted by intrahepatic scarring, and portal vein pressure rises. Bypass channels shunt blood into the superior or inferior vena cava to return blood to the heart. Bypass veins cannot handle increased blood flow under increased pressure and become dilated.

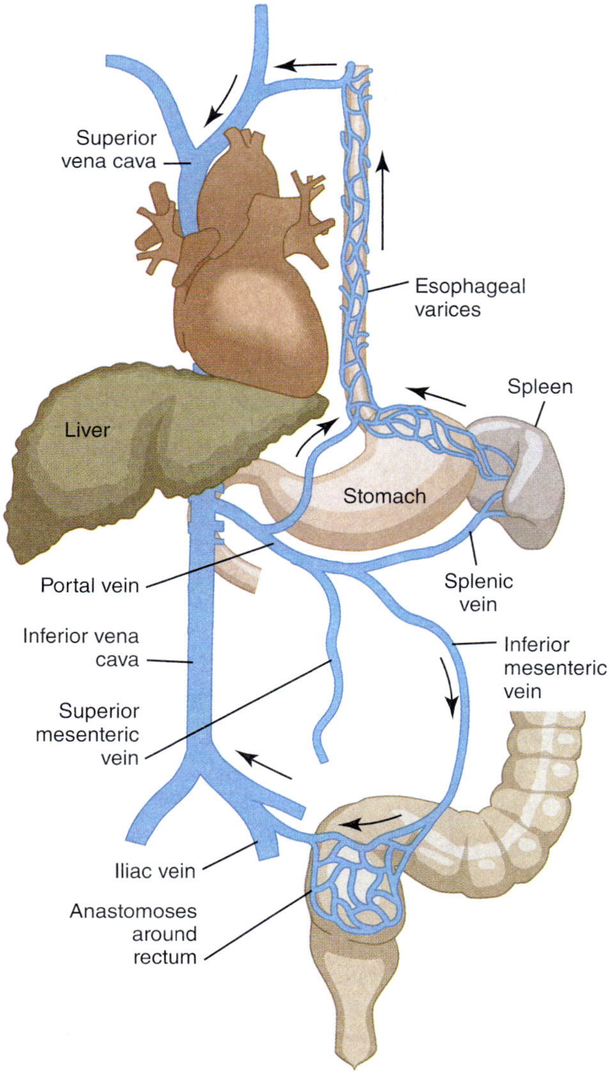

Figure 19-15 Formation of collateral venous channels that return blood to the systemic circulation when portal the blood flow is impeded by cirrhosis. The arrows indicate direction of blood flow.

circulation. Anastomoses develop where tributaries of portal and systemic veins are closely associated, and they shunt blood from the veins of the portal system, where the pressure is high, into the veins of the systemic circulation, where the pressure is much lower. The communications that are most important clinically are the anastomoses developing between veins around the stomach and spleen, which drain into the portal vein, and the esophageal veins that eventually drain into the superior vena cava by way of the intercostal veins and azygos veins (**Figure 19-15**). The esophageal veins are not equipped to handle the increased blood flow and high pressure. In 90 percent of patients with cirrhosis, these veins become dilated and form varicose veins (**esophageal varices**). Esophageal varices are thin-walled vessels covered by a thin layer of esophageal epithelium (**Figure 19-16**) and frequently rupture, leading to profuse and often fatal hemorrhage.

Although this chapter has focused on causes of portal hypertension related to the sinusoid (intrahepatic causes), occlusive disease of the portal vein can result in **presinusoidal portal hypertension**, and thrombosis of the hepatic vein (**Budd-Chiari syndrome**) can lead to **postsinusoidal portal hypertension**.

Esophageal varices Thin-walled vessels that can rupture.

Presinusoidal portal hypertension Portal hypertension resulting from occlusions in the portal vein.

Budd-Chiari syndrome Thrombosis of the hepatic vein.

Postsinusoidal portal hypertension Hypertension resulting from thrombosis of the hepatic vein.

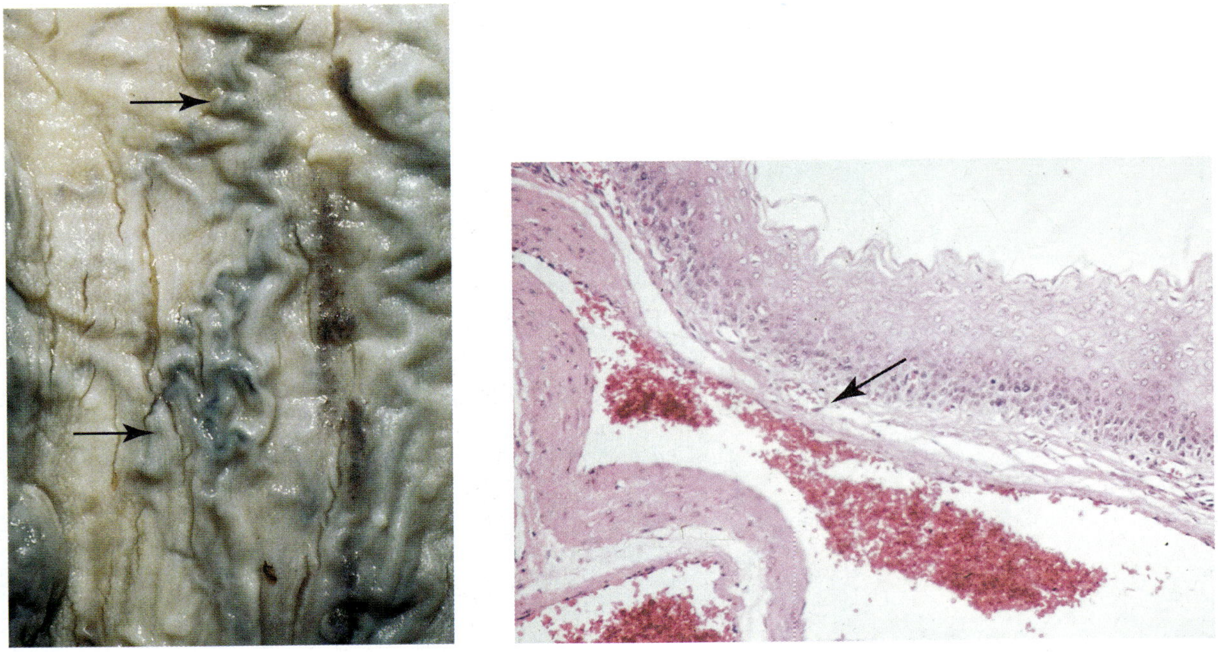

(A) (B)

Figure 19-16 **(A)** Mucosal surface of esophagus illustrating varices, wh ch appear as tortuous elevations of the mucosa (*arrows*). **(B)** A photomicrograph of a varix. The very thin wall (*arrow*) is covered only by a thin layer of esophageal squamous epithelium and is very susceptible to rupture.

Courtesy of Leonard V. Crowley, MD, Century College.

Hepatic Encephalopathy

The cirrhotic liver is not able to detoxify or excrete toxic substances that accumulate in the bloodstream. Hepatic encephalopathy (encephalon = brain + pathy = disease) is a deterioration of brain function characterized by impaired consciousness, confusion, disorientation, and eventually coma. Not all of the toxic products have been identified, but many of them are products of protein digestion, especially ammonia, which comes from deamination of amino acids and other products derived from bacterial decomposition of material in the colon. In a person with advanced liver disease, any event that further compromises liver function may precipitate hepatic encephalopathy. This includes such events as an episode of binge drinking in a person with alcoholic liver disease; a hemorrhage into the gastrointestinal tract, which drops blood pressure and reduces hepatic blood flow; or a systemic infection with a fever that reduces hepatic blood flow and increases liver cell metabolism.

Procedures to Treat Manifestations of Cirrhosis

If a patient has developed esophageal varices and is acutely bleeding, a variety of endoscopic treatment procedures are available at the level of the esophagus. The varices may be endoscopically ligated (EVL procedure), or an attempt may be made to obliterate them by injecting them with a sclerosing solution. The solution, which is irritating, causes an inflammation in and around the dilated veins, which is followed by scarring and eventual obliteration of the varices. Multiple injections over a period of several months are usually required. The vasoconstrictive somatostatin-like drug octreotide is often combined with

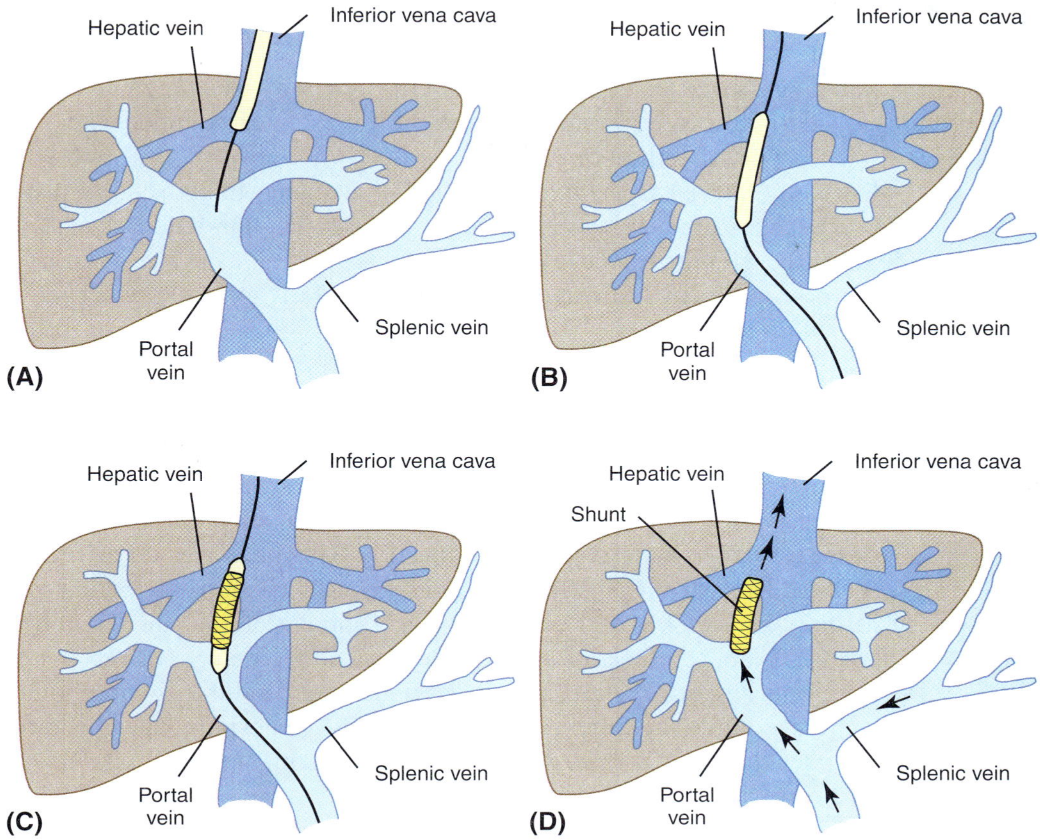

Figure 19-17 The TIPS procedure. **(A)** Intrahepatic communication (tract) established between the hepatic and portal veins. **(B)** Angioplasty balloon dilates tract. **(C)** Expandable metal stent inserted into the tract and dilated by angioplasty balloon. **(D)** Completed shunt between the hepatic vein and portal vein lowers portal vein pressure. Esophageal varices become smaller as portal vein pressure falls.

endoscopic esophageal therapy, but control is often temporary at best. To achieve a more permanent solution, endoscopic or surgical procedures are available that attempt to shunt the portal to the venous systemic circulation, thereby bypassing the liver and reducing portal pressure. A nonsurgical portal–systemic communication can be accomplished by means of a procedure termed a **transjugular intrahepatic portosystemic shunt** (the TIPS procedure). Under X-ray guidance, a stent is placed via the jugular and inferior vena cava within the liver to join portal and systemic circulation. The stent placement creates a shunt that artificially connects one of the hepatic veins (which drain blood from the liver into the inferior vena cava) with a large intrahepatic branch of the portal vein, thus bypassing the hepatic sinusoids (**Figure 19-17**). As a result, the high pressure in the portal vein falls toward normal. The dilated esophageal veins decrease in size, and the risk of hemorrhage from varices is greatly reduced. The shunt also may improve the patient's ascites because the lower portal pressure resulting from the shunt lowers the venous pressure in the capillaries draining into the portal system, and less fluid is forced from the capillaries to accumulate in the abdominal cavity.

Transjugular intrahepatic portosystemic shunt A nonsurgical method used to lower portal vein pressure in a person with cirrhosis by connecting an intrahepatic branch of the portal vein to a hepatic vein branch.

Liver Transplantation

In cases of continued cirrhosis-related disease, liver transplantation is now considered the treatment of choice. Formerly, this was most commonly associated with chronic hepatitis C infection, but that is currently declining as a result of effective anti-viral therapy. (In fact, some HCV-positive organs may be used in transplants.) Cirrhosis related to nonalcoholic liver disease is likely to become the leading indicator for transplantation in the next few years. Acute liver failure related to toxic agents (acetaminophen overdose being a common example) is also an important indication.

Currently, liver transplantation is second in frequency to kidney transplantation. The most common source of organs is deceased donors, and lack of such is a major constraint to increased use of the procedure. The 5-year survival rate for post-transplant patients is 75 percent, and early graft failure occurs in 10 percent of cases.

Bile: Formation and Excretion

Bile is an aqueous solution excreted by the liver that contains various dissolved substances, including **conjugated bilirubin**, **bile salts**, **lecithin**, **cholesterol**, water, minerals, and other materials that have been detoxified by liver cells and excreted. Cholesterol is a lipid with a complex ring structure that is classified as a sterol. Bile salts, the major constituent of bile, are derivatives of cholesterol and certain amino acids. They function as detergents because of their molecular structure, which contains both a lipid-soluble, hydrophobic, and a water-soluble, hydrophilic part. Lecithin is a phosphorous-containing lipid, a phospholipid, that has detergent properties similar to bile salts. Bile is secreted continually and is concentrated and stored in the gallbladder. During digestion, the gallbladder contracts, squirting bile into the duodenum. Bile does not contain digestive enzymes but functions as a biologic detergent. Bile salts emulsify fat into small globules, increasing the surface area so that the fat can be acted on more readily by pancreatic enzymes. Digestion of fat is much less efficient in the absence of bile.

The excretion of bile, containing a product of the breakdown of the pigment in red blood cells, is an important function of the liver. Red cells normally survive for about 4 months. The worn-out erythrocytes are broken down by mononuclear phagocytes, predominantly in the spleen, liver, and bone marrow. The iron derived from the hemoglobin is conserved by the body and reused to synthesize new hemoglobin. The iron-free heme pigment forms **bilirubin**. Because the breakdown of red cells proceeds in mononuclear phagocytes in several locations, small quantities of bile pigment are continually present in the blood, complexed to albumin. When the blood passes through the liver, the bilirubin is removed from the albumin and taken up by the hepatocytes. Excretion is accomplished by combining bilirubin with glucuronic acid. This process, termed conjugation, requires certain specific enzymes (uridine diphosphate-glucuronyl transferase, UGT). Most of the bilirubin is conjugated with glucuronic acid and excreted as bilirubin glucuronide. The conjugated bilirubin is much more water soluble and less toxic than the unconjugated material. **Gilbert syndrome** is a very common inherited condition, occurring in 5 to 10 percent of the population, related to a mild lack of sufficient levels of synthesis of UGT. The condition is most often not associated with disease. However, a complete lack or extreme deficiency of UGT (**Crigler-Najjar syndrome**) causes severe disease in early childhood related to the effects of unconjugated bilirubin on the brain (kernicterus). After the bile pigment is excreted into the small bile channels between the liver cell cords, it is collected into large ducts at the periphery of the lobules, which eventually unite to form the major bile ducts. Figure 19-4 summarizes the basic anatomy of the biliary duct system.

Conjugated bilirubin A more soluble form of bilirubin produced by the addition of two molecules of glucuronic acid to the bilirubin molecule.

Bile salts Derivatives of bile acids present in bile that act as emulsifiers to promote fat digestion and absorption.

Lecithin A phosphorus-containing lipid (phospholipid) having detergent properties similar to bile salts.

Cholesterol A complex lipid (sterol) containing several hydrocarbon ring structures.

Bilirubin One of the bile pigments derived from the breakdown of hemoglobin.

Gilbert syndrome Common inherited condition related to a mild lack of uridine diphosphate-glucuronyltransferase (UGT).

Crigler-Najjar syndrome Lack of UGT, which causes a severe disease of early childhood.

Jaundice

Jaundice, a yellow discoloration of the skin and the sclerae resulting from accumulation of bilirubin in the tissues and body fluids, can have several causes. Jaundice is generally classified on the basis of the disturbance responsible for the retention of bile pigment, either hemolytic, hepatocellular, or obstructive. Proper classification can be achieved on the basis of certain laboratory tests in conjunction with clinical features. Physiological neonatal jaundice occurs transiently in up to 70 percent of newborns and is related to a low level of liver UGT in combination with normally increased red cell destruction. In severe cases or in premature infants, phototherapy by exposure of the neonate to selected wavelengths of visible light converts unconjugated bilirubin to several water-soluble forms.

Hemolytic Jaundice

Under conditions associated with the accelerated breakdown of red cells, excessive bile pigment is delivered to the liver beyond the liver's ability to conjugate and excrete the pigment. Therefore, unconjugated bile pigment accumulates in the blood. Hemolytic jaundice is sometimes seen in adults with hemolytic anemia and in the case of certain congenital disorders of red blood cells, such as sickle cell disease, but it is encountered most frequently in newborn infants with hemolytic disease as a result of blood group incompatibility between mother and infant (Chapter 15).

Hepatocellular Jaundice

If the liver is severely damaged, as in hepatitis or cirrhosis, or conjugation of bilirubin is impaired, jaundice may occur. The condition may be related to a number of genetic conditions that interfere with the mechanism of bilirubin conjugation or that prevent transport of conjugated bilirubin into the bile canaliculi, which lead to the bile ducts. Moreover, the excretion of conjugated bilirubin may be hampered because of injury to liver cells and disruption of the canaliculi that lie between liver cell cords. As a result, conjugated bilirubin leaks back into the blood through the ruptured intrahepatic bile channels. **Cholestasis** refers to decreased bile flow and bile stasis in the liver, which may result from intrahepatic or extrahepatic obstruction of bile flow. This leads to local damage to hepatocytes and ultimately to cirrhosis. As serum bile acids increase, intense itching may result.

Cholestasis Decreased bile flow and bile stasis.

Obstructive jaundice Symptom from a blocked common bile duct.

Obstructive Jaundice

In **obstructive jaundice**, the extraction and conjugation of bilirubin by liver cells are not impaired, but jaundice develops because the bile duct is obstructed, preventing delivery of bile into the duodenum. Often, the obstruction is caused by an impacted stone in the common duct. Carcinoma of the head of the pancreas is another common cause of common bile duct obstruction. The common duct passes very close to the head of the pancreas as it enters the duodenum (**Figure 19-18**). Therefore, a pancreatic tumor frequently compresses and invades the common duct. As previously described, long-standing common bile duct obstruction leads to obstructive biliary cirrhosis.

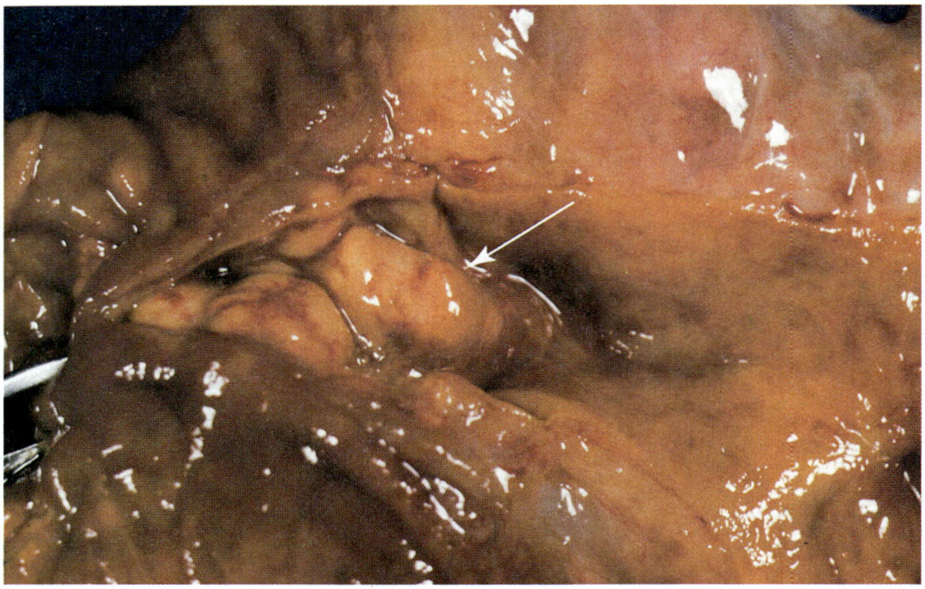

Figure 19-18 Carcinoma arising from the common bile duct (*arrow*) blocking outflow of bile into the duodenum. The common bile duct has been opened and is distended, a result of the increased pressure of the bile within the common duct caused by the duct obstruction.

Courtesy of Leonard V. Crowley, MD, Century College.

Biliary Cirrhosis

In some types of cirrhosis, the initial pathology of the liver damage is the epithelium of the bile ducts rather than the functional cells (hepatocytes) of the liver lobules. This type of cirrhosis is termed biliary cirrhosis to distinguish it from the more common type of cirrhosis in which hepatocyte injury is the primary event. The cirrhotic component of the disease is a late complication representing secondary damage to hepatocytes. There are two main types of biliary cirrhosis. The first, which is termed primary biliary cirrhosis, is an autoimmune disease that targets the small intrahepatic bile ducts. The second, termed secondary biliary cirrhosis or obstructive biliary cirrhosis, results from long-standing obstruction of the large extrahepatic bile ducts.

Primary Biliary Cirrhosis

Primary biliary cirrhosis (now often termed primary biliary cholangitis), a progressive, chronic disease found almost exclusively in women, is characterized by inflammation and destruction of the small intrahepatic bile ducts. Bile excretion is disrupted and followed by scarring, which begins in the portal tracts and eventually spreads into the liver lobules. The disease appears to be caused by autoantibodies that are directed against bile duct epithelial cells. Antinuclear autoantibodies and antimitochondrial antibodies can usually be demonstrated in the blood of affected patients.

Because excretion of bile is impeded, products accumulate in the blood that are normally excreted in the bile, including bile pigment (bilirubin), bile salts, and cholesterol. Accumulation of bile pigment in the blood results in jaundice and pruritus (itching). As a result of the high blood cholesterol, masses of cholesterol accumulate in the skin and form small yellow skin nodules termed xanthomas. Unfortunately, there is no effective treatment for this condition, which progresses slowly over many years and eventually leads to liver failure. Ultimately, a liver transplant may be required.

Secondary (Obstructive) Biliary Cirrhosis

This condition is caused by long-standing blockage of the large extrahepatic bile ducts associated with obstructive jaundice. The bile duct obstruction leads to stasis of bile within the ducts. The pressure within the ducts rises, and the larger ducts become dilated. The elevated intraductal pressure is transmitted back into the smaller intrahepatic bile ducts and from there into the small bile channels (bile canaliculi) that carry bile from the liver lobules into the bile ducts within the portal tracts at the periphery of the lobules. The elevated intraductal pressure and bile stasis damage the intrahepatic bile ducts, which is followed by portal tract inflammation and scarring.

The clinical manifestations of the extrahepatic bile duct obstruction are much the same as those caused by primary biliary cirrhosis. Treatment consists of various surgical procedures to unblock the obstructed bile duct. If this is not possible, some type of surgical procedure is used to bypass the obstruction and reestablish bile flow into the duodenum.

Cholelithiasis (Gallstones)

Factors Affecting the Solubility of Cholesterol in Bile

Because cholesterol is a lipid, it is not soluble in an aqueous solution such as bile but is brought into solution by bile salts and lecithin, which aggregate in clusters termed **micelles**. In a micelle, the lipid-soluble (hydrophobic) parts of the bile salt molecules are oriented toward the center of the cluster, and the opposite water-soluble (hydrophilic) ends face outward. Cholesterol becomes soluble by dissolving in the hydrophobic center of the micelles, and the cholesterol-containing micelles dissolve in the bile because the peripheral hydrophilic parts of the bile salt molecules are water soluble. Lecithin participates in the formation of the micelles by fitting between the molecules of the bile salts (**Figure 19-19**).

Approximately seven molecules of bile salts interspersed between lecithin molecules in a micelle are required to dissolve one molecule of cholesterol. Consequently, the solubility of cholesterol in bile depends not only on its cholesterol content but also on its content of bile salts and lecithin, because these substances are needed to hold the cholesterol in solution. Cholesterol remains soluble provided its concentration is not excessive in relation to the amounts of available bile salts and lecithin.

Micelle Spherical structure formed by the aggregation of surfactant molecules. In aqueous solution the hydrophobic regions face inward and the hydrophilic areas interact with the aqueous solution.

Cholelithiasis Formation of gallstones.

Formation of Gallstones

Whenever bile contains a relative excess amount of cholesterol, it becomes supersaturated with cholesterol, and under proper conditions the cholesterol may precipitate to form the beginnings of gallstones. The formation of stones within the gallbladder is termed **cholelithiasis** (chole = bile + lith = stone) (**Figure 19-20**). This situation may arise because of an increased excretion of cholesterol in the bile, a reduced excretion of bile salts and lecithin, or a combination of both factors. As long as the bile remains supersaturated, cholesterol

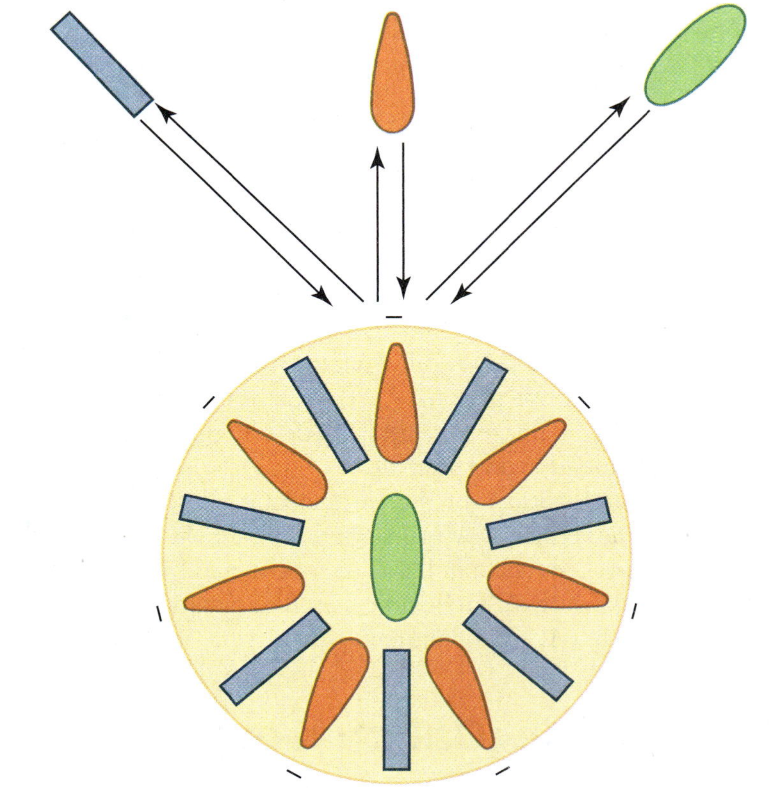

Figure 19-19 The manner in which cholesterol dissolves in micelles composed of bile salts and lecithin. If the bile salt concentration is insufficient relative to that of cholesterol, cholesterol will precipitate and form gallstones.

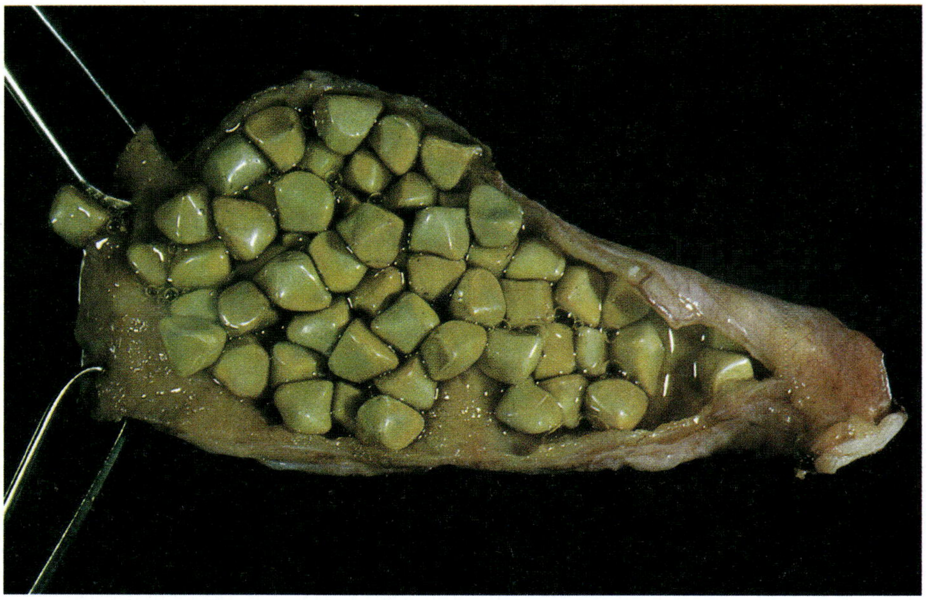

Figure 19-20 Opened gallbladder filled with gallstones composed of cholesterol.
Courtesy of Leonard V. Crowley, MD, Century College.

crystals continue to accumulate around those that have already precipitated, and the gallstones slowly increase in size. Eventually, the gallbladder may become filled with gallstones, the end stage of a process that began several years earlier. This process often leads to **cholecystitis**, inflammation of the gallbladder.

Some people are known to have an increased risk of forming gallstones. The incidence of gallstones is higher in women than in men, higher in obese women, and higher in multipara than in childless women. Certain contraceptive pills containing drospirenone may result in a slightly increased (but possibly not clinically significant) risk of gallstones compared to women not using oral contraception. Higher estrogen levels are also likely to account for the increased risk. Obesity predisposes to gallstones because extremely overweight individuals often have a higher blood cholesterol and excrete more cholesterol in their bile than do people of normal weight. Less commonly, gallstones form as a result of infection of the gallbladder. Infection predisposes to "brown pigment" gallstones by deconjugating bilirubin and thereby reducing its solubility.

Cholecystitis Inflammation of the gallbladder.

Biliary colic Abdominal pain that results when a gallstone enters the biliary duct system.

Acute calculous cholecystitis Mucosal injury from concentrated bile within the gallbladder.

Chronic cholecystitis Ongoing irritation of the gallbladder by repeated bouts of acute disease.

Complications of Gallstones

Gallstones that remain in the gallbladder rarely cause symptoms. Unfortunately, gallstones are sometimes extruded into the cystic duct or common bile duct when the gallbladder contracts after a fatty meal, and they may become impacted within the biliary ducts. This event causes severe abdominal pain termed **biliary colic**. The pain results from spasm of the smooth muscle in the ducts combined with forceful contractions of the gallbladder that attempt to propel the stone through the ducts. Sometimes a stone can be passed through the ducts into the duodenum, but often it becomes impacted. If the stone lodges in the cystic duct, bile can neither enter nor leave the gallbladder, but the flow of bile from the liver into the duodenum is not disturbed. However, if the stone blocks the common duct, bile can no longer be excreted into the duodenum, and it accumulates in the bloodstream. This condition is termed obstructive jaundice. Such blockage is also a common cause of acute pancreatitis, a serious and painful inflammatory condition of that organ (discussed in Chapter 20). Blockage of the cystic duct by a stone can lead to bacterial infection, distension of the gallbladder, compromise of blood flow, and, ultimately, inflammation, ischemia, and necrosis of the mucosa. In addition, concentrated bile within the gallbladder may lead to mucosal injury. The result is **acute calculous cholecystitis** (**Figure 19-21**). If there is no underlying gallbladder infection, the bile trapped within the gallbladder by the impacted stone is gradually absorbed into the bloodstream, and eventually the contents of the gallbladder consist only of mucus that has been secreted by the epithelial cells lining the gallbladder. **Chronic cholecystitis** is generally associated with gallstones but is also likely to involve chronic ongoing irritation of the gallbladder by repeated bouts of acute disease. Uncomplicated cholecystitis related to gallstones may be treated with antibiotics and analgesics. Recurrent or severe, intractable disease is treated by laparoscopic surgical removal of the diseased gallbladder (cholecystectomy). In some cases, an acute bout of obstructive jaundice may be treated by endoscopic removal of the stone blocking the duct. Adenocarcinoma of the gallbladder is associated with cholelithiasis and is an incidental finding in about 2 percent of surgically removed organs.

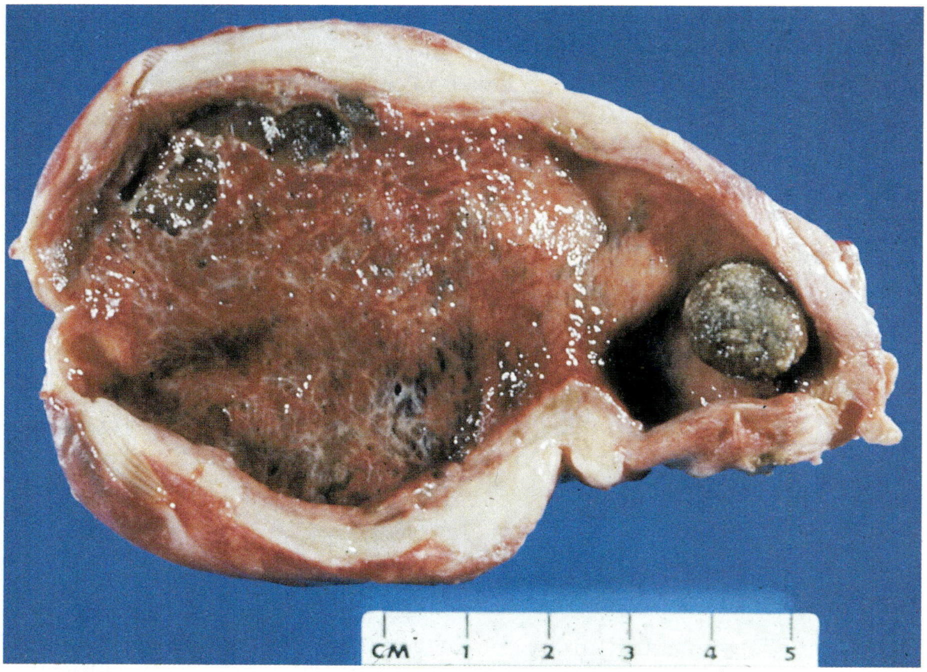

Figure 19-21 An inflamed, thick-walled gallbladder with a stone impacted in the neck of the gallbladder.
Courtesy of Leonard V. Crowley, MD, Century College.

Tumors of the Liver

The most common primary malignant tumor of the liver, hepatocellular carcinoma (HCC), may be the most common human cancer when viewed worldwide. Almost 90 percent of HCC cases occur in countries with high levels of HBV and HBC carriers. As noted, HCC is associated with cirrhosis in such patients (**Figure 19-22**). Once rare in industrialized countries, liver cancer has the most rapidly increasing incidence of any cancer in the United States. Most of the increase is due to preventable risk factors, such as obesity and the risk

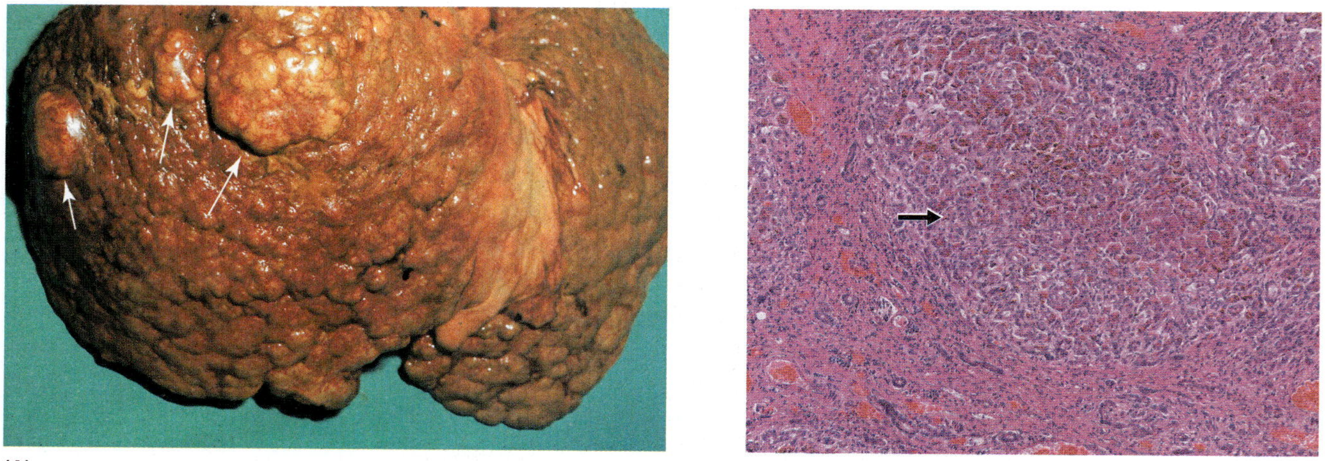

(A) (B)

Figure 19-22 **(A)** Cirrhosis of the liver complicated by hepatocellular carcinoma (*arrows*). **(B)** Hepatocellular carcinoma in a cirrhotic liver (*arrow*) (microscopic view).
(A) Courtesy of Leonard V. Crowley, MD, Century College; **(B)** Courtesy of Department of Pathology and Laboratory Medicine, University of North Carclina at Chapel Hill.

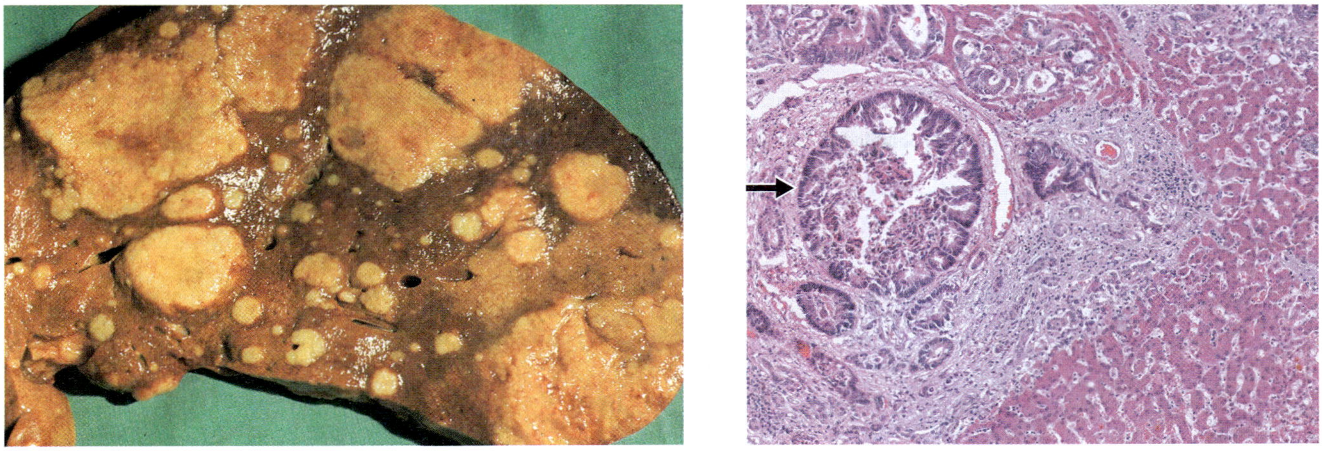

(A) (B)

Figure 19-23 **(A)** A cross section of the liver containing multiple nodules of metastatic carcinoma. **(B)** Nodules of metastatic adenocarcinoma in the liver (*arrow*). The likely source was colonic adenocarcinoma (microscopic view).

(A) Courtesy of Leonard V. Crowley, MD, Century College; **(B)** Courtesy of Department of Pathology and Laboratory Medicine, University of North Carolina at Chapel Hill.

of type 2 diabetes and metabolic syndrome, excess alcohol consumption, and chronic hepatitis B and C infections.

HCC occurs in some areas of the world as a result of contamination of groundnut meal, corn, and sorghum by a fungus that produces a potent carcinogen, aflatoxin B. Warm, moist areas such as Southeast Asia and Sub-Saharan Africa are at particular risk. This carcinogen produces a specific mutation in the TP53 gene, which is associated with HCC that occurs in these areas. Aflatoxin contamination may occur in agricultural products in parts of the United States. For example, fungal-contaminated corn in bovine feeds results in aflatoxin levels in milk. Mandatory monitoring of milk and other products is carried out to reduce risk.

The liver is a common site of metastatic carcinoma (**Figure 19-23**). Carcinoma arising in the gastrointestinal tract may spread to the portal venous blood. Tumors from the breast, lung, and other sites also often spread to the liver. The tumor cells are carried in the blood delivered to the liver by the hepatic artery. Various diagnostic procedures can be used to identify tumors in the liver.

Case 19-1

John is a 16-year-old high school student who is interested in trying out for the school wrestling team. One week before tryouts, he badly sprains his back playing touch football. He is in considerable pain and is concerned that he will not be able to make the team. He visits his physician, who confirms that the injury is not serious, although it is quite painful. To relieve John's discomfort, the physician prescribes a mild opiate anti-inflammatory medication (Endocet [oxycodone and acetaminophen] 7.5/500, 24 pills). John is instructed to take two pills three times a day for pain relief. Concerned about his ability to compete for the team, John takes the pills four times a day until he runs out. In addition, he self-medicates with extra strength acetaminophen (Tylenol™), taking three pills every 4 hours in combination with the Endocet™. On the weekend prior to his injury, John attended a party and overindulged in drinks containing alcohol. Four days after seeing his physician, John becomes

(continues)

Case 19-1 *(Continued)*

severely nauseated, sweaty, and "flulike." John's mother notes that he seems sluggish and confused and brings her son to the local emergency room.

In the emergency room, the physician carefully reviews John's history of medication. John's liver is noted to be tender and mildly enlarged on physical examination. The physician is concerned about possible drug toxicity. John has consumed 4 grams of acetaminophen (from the Endocet™) and 6 grams of acetaminophen by self-medication per day. Thus, John has consumed 10 grams of acetaminophen per day for 3 days. The maximum recommended dose of acetaminophen is 3 grams per day for an adult. Concerned about hepatic toxicity, the physician orders liver function tests that indicate acute liver failure. A serum acetaminophen assay discloses a potentially toxic amount of the drug. John is treated on an emergency basis with oral N-acetylcysteine and medication to control nausea. He recovers with normalization of liver function tests over the period of several weeks. He does not make the wrestling team.

Discussion

Acetaminophen (better known by its trade name Tylenol™) has gained popularity as an over-the-counter pain medication and aspirin replacement over the last several decades, in part because of the association of Reye's syndrome with aspirin in children and the reduced level of gastric side effects. Although acetaminophen is generally a safe medication, with a toxic dose (generally considered to be above 8 grams per 8 hours or less) far above the recommended maximum therapeutic dose of 3 grams per day, it is often abused. This is related to a lack of knowledge about potential toxicity and the widespread availability of the drug, which is often combined with other medications and hence is not obvious to the user. It may surprise individuals to learn that acetaminophen is responsible for over half of all cases of drug-induced liver injury, almost 80,000 ER visits, and more than 30,000 hospitalizations per year in the United States. Acetaminophen overdose was responsible for more than 3500 deaths per year—half accidental, half suicidal—and is the most common cause of acute liver failure requiring transplantation.

Ninety-five percent of ingested acetaminophen is detoxified and chemically modified in the liver and ultimately excreted in the urine. About 5 percent of acetaminophen is modified by the cytochrome P-450 enzymes to a toxic intermediate termed NAPQI. NAPQI binds to mitochondrial proteins and leads to the formation of reactive oxygen species, which result in hepatocyte death and, if levels are high enough, acute hepatic necrosis. Two factors influence the degree of toxicity. Cytochrome P-450 enzymes are increased by alcohol consumption, leading to the formation of more of the toxic metabolite NAPQI. Liver cells have a detoxifying chemical termed GSH (reduced glutathione), which binds to NAPQI and renders it harmless. However, large amounts of NAPQI can deplete available glutathione. The drug used to treat John (N-acetylcysteine) replenishes stores of GSH, reducing the toxic effects of NAQPI.

Etiology and Pathogenesis

Drug-induced acute liver injury resulting from acetaminophen overdose.

Questions

1. What metabolic factors influence the toxicity of ingested acetaminophen?
2. What over-the-counter drugs are likely to contain "hidden" acetaminophen? It would be instructive to read the contents of the drugs found in your own medicine cabinet.
3. Given the potential toxicity of acetaminophen, what additional controls on its sales (if any) might be reasonable to control accidental overdosing?

Questions For Review

1. What are some of the principal functions of the liver? How does the blood supply to the liver differ from that to other organs? Why does severe liver disease cause disturbances in blood clotting?
2. What is the difference between hemoglobin and bilirubin? How does conjugated bilirubin differ from unconjugated bilirubin? What is the difference between bilirubin and bile? What role does bile play in digestion?
3. What are the possible causes and effects of liver injury (see Figure 19-5)? What is the usual outcome of a liver injury?
4. What is viral hepatitis? What are its major symptoms? How is hepatitis transmitted?
5. What is the difference between hepatitis A and hepatitis B? What is anicteric hepatitis? What is subclinical hepatitis?
6. What effect does alcohol have on the liver? What types of liver disease are associated with excessive alcohol ingestion?
7. What is cirrhosis? What liver diseases may lead to cirrhosis? Why does portal hypertension develop in patients with cirrhosis? Why does ascites develop in patients with cirrhosis? Why do esophageal varices develop?
8. What is jaundice? How is jaundice classified? Under what circumstances do gallstones cause jaundice?
9. What factors predispose to the development of gallstones?
10. What is the difference between viral hepatitis and alcoholic hepatitis?

References

Greene KG. "Pathology of the liver, gall bladder and extrahepatic biliary tract." In: Reisner H, ed. ed. *Pathology: A Modern Case Study.* 2nd ed. McGraw Hill Lange; 2020.

Loeffler AG, Hart MN. *Introduction to Human Disease*. 7th ed. Jones & Bartlett Learning; 2020.

- Those interested in the detailed study of liver disease should consult a work on human pathology aimed at the undergraduate medical curriculum as their first reference. However, a good place to start at a less advanced level is by reading Chapter 14 of the second reference.

Centers for Disease Control and Prevention. Viral Hepatitis. 7https://www.cdc.gov/hepatitis/index .html

- The CDC has an extensive online compilation of information about all forms of viral hepatitis.

Shors T. *Understanding Viruses*. 3rd ed. Jones & Bartlett Learning; 2017.

- A thorough discussion of infectious viral hepatitis with an emphasis on molecular aspects of the infectious agents is presented.

National Institute of Diabetes and Digestive and Kidney Diseases. Cirrhosis. https://www.niddk .nih.gov/health-information/liver-disease/cirrhosis

American Liver Foundation. Cirrhosis of the Liver. https://liverfoundation.org/for-patients/about -the-liver/diseases-of-the-liver/cirrhosis/

- Both resources present current detailed information on cirrhosis. The American Liver Foundation website has an extensive library of information on all liver diseases.

Rabaan AA, et al. Overview of hepatitis C infection, molecular biology, and new treatment. *J Infect Public Health*. 2020. doi:10.1016/j.jiph.2019.11.015

- An up-to-date overview of one of the great success stories in the treatment of chronic liver disease, which has had a major impact on public health and led to discussion of the very high cost of therapy.

Centers for Disease Control and Prevention. Liver Cancer. https://www.cdc.gov/cancer/liver/index .htm

Craig AJ, et al. Tumor evolution in hepatocellular carcinoma. *Nat Rev Gastroenterol Hepatol*. 2019. doi:10.1038/s41575-019-0229-4

- A good general source of information with recent epidemiological and survival data, along with a review stressing the molecular biology of hepatocellular carcinoma.

Heuman DM. Gallstones (Cholelithiasis). Medscape. Updated April 1, 2019. https://emedicine.medscape.com/article/175667-overview

- Current information on the pathophysiology, etiology, and medical aspects of gallstones (cholelithiasis).

National Institute of Diabetes and Digestive and Kidney Diseases. Nonalcoholic Fatty Liver Disease (NAFLD) & NASH. https://www.niddk.nih.gov/health-information/liver-disease/nafld-nash

Ganguli S, Deleeuw P, Satapathy SK. A review of current and upcoming treatment modalities in non-alcoholic fatty liver disease and non-alcoholic steatohepatitis. *Hepat Med.* 2019;11:159-178. https://www.ncbi.nlm.nih.gov/pmc/articles/PMC6863115/

- A brief overview of the condition and a review of potential therapies, including life-style modification and pharmacological approaches not discussed in the text.

McGill MR, Jaeschke H. Metabolism and disposition of acetaminophen: Recent advances in relation to hepatotoxicity and diagnosis. *Pharm Res.* 2013;30(9):2174-2187.

- Additional information on the mechanism of acetaminophen toxicity with an emphasis on pharmacology. Used in case construction.

Toshikuni N, Tsutsumi M, Arisawa T. Clinical differences between alcoholic liver disease and nonalcoholic fatty liver disease. *World J Gastroenterol.* 2014;20(26):8393-8406. doi:10.3748/wjg.v20.i26.8393. PMID: 25024597; PMCID: PMC4093692

- This article provides a nice explanation of the differences and similarities between alcoholic liver disease and nonalcoholic liver disease, which would include metabolic syndrome.

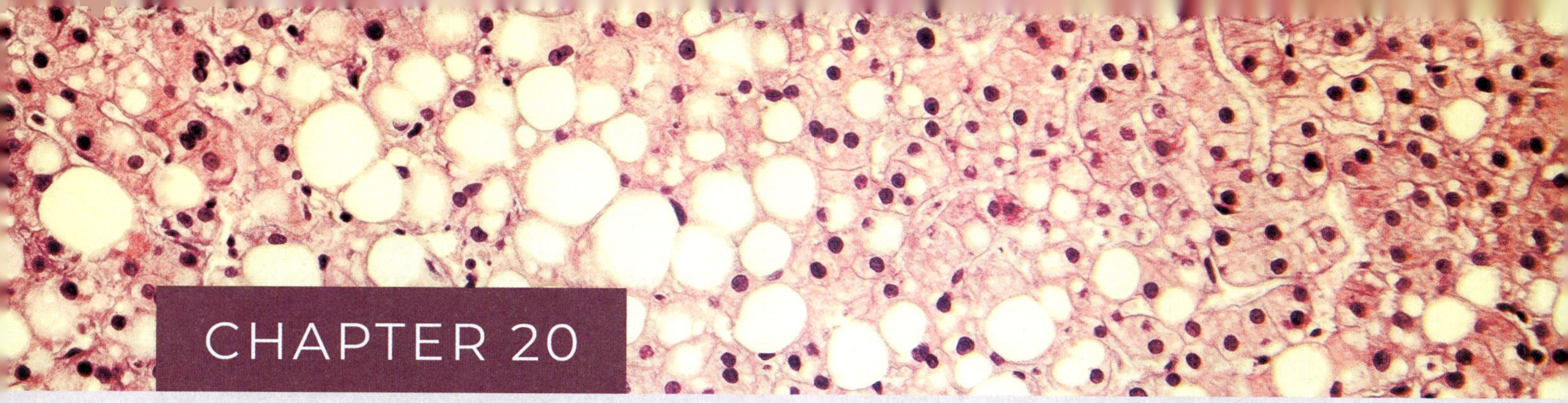

CHAPTER 20

The Pancreas and Diabetes Mellitus

LEARNING OBJECTIVES

1. Describe the pathogenesis and treatment of acute and chronic pancreatitis.
2. Describe the pathogenesis, manifestations, complications, and prognosis of pancreatic cystic fibrosis.
3. Understand the current treatment/management of pancreatic cancer.
4. Differentiate between the two principal types of diabetes mellitus with respect to pathogenesis, incidence, manifestations, complications, and treatment.
5. Compare and contrast diabetes with metabolic syndrome.

Structure and Function of the Pancreas

The pancreas is actually two glands in one: a digestive exocrine gland and an endocrine gland. The exocrine tissue of the pancreas, which is concerned solely with digestion, secretes an alkaline pancreatic juice rich in digestive enzymes into the duodenum through the pancreatic duct. The powerful digestive enzymes break down proteins (trypsin and chymotrypsin), carbohydrates (amylase), and fats (lipase). The protein-digesting (proteolytic) enzymes are secreted in an inactive form and are activated after they are discharged into the duodenum. Exocrine pancreatic tissue makes up more than 80 percent of the pancreas and consists of enzyme-secreting **acini** arranged around ductules that ultimately drain into the pancreatic duct. The endocrine tissue of the pancreas consists of multiple small clusters of cells scattered throughout the gland called the pancreatic islets, or **islets of Langerhans**, which discharge their secretions directly into the bloodstream. Each islet is composed of several different types of cells, including alpha cells, beta cells, and delta cells. Alpha cells secrete a hormone called glucagon. The more numerous beta cells secrete insulin in response to a rise in blood glucose after eating, which restores blood glucose to normal. Both glucagon and insulin regulate the level of glucose in

Acini/acinar Acini are small grape-like clusters of glands composed of a cavity surrounded by secretory cells. "Acinar" means having the properties of acini.

Islets of Langerhans Cluster of endocrine cells in the pancreas.

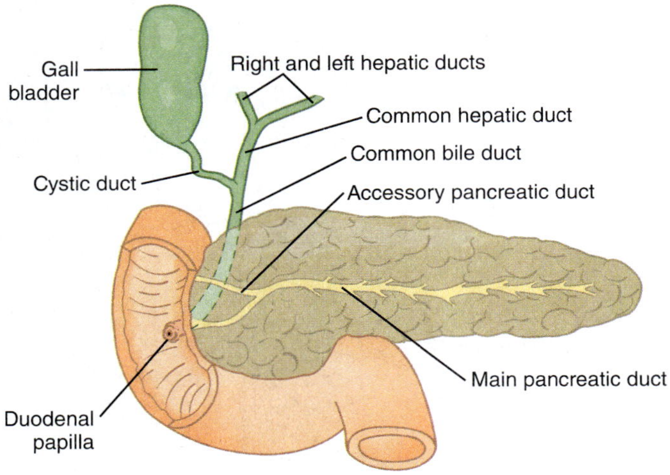

(A)

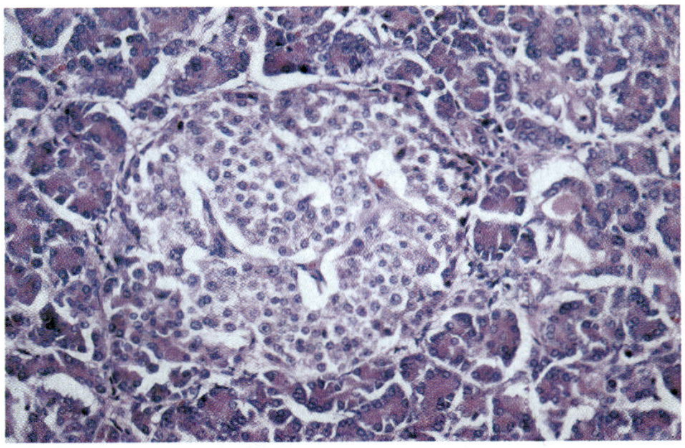

(B)

Figure 20-1 **(A)** Duct system of pancreas. The main pancreatic duct usually joins the common bile duct to form a common channel (ampulla of Vater) that enters the duodenum by a single opening at the apex of a nipple-like projection called the duodenal papilla. A much smaller accessory pancreatic duct is frequently present and opens into the duodenum by a separate opening proximal to the duodenal papilla. **(B)** A photomicrograph of a pancreatic islet surrounded by exocrine pancreatic tissue.

(B) Courtesy of Leonard V. Crowley, MD, Century College.

the blood but have opposing effects. Glucagon raises blood glucose; insulin lowers it. Delta cells produce a hormone called **somatostatin**, which inhibits secretion of both glucagon and insulin. Diffuse islets of Langerhans occur in the head of the pancreas as cords between pancreatic **acinar cells**. The diffuse islets contain predominantly beta cells and cells that secrete human pancreatic polypeptide (HPP), which helps regulate both pancreatic and gastrointestinal function and may also play a role in regulating food intake. **Figure 20-1** shows the anatomy and cellular structure of the pancreas.

Somatostatin Hormone produced by the delta cells of the pancreas.

Acinar cells The main functional units of the exocrine pancreas, responsible for producing, storing, and secreting crucial digestive enzymes.

Pancreatitis

Pancreatitis refers to the inflammation of the pancreas occurring for any reason, presenting as either acute or chronic pancreatitis.

Acute Pancreatitis

Acute pancreatitis is caused by the presence of pancreatic juice from the ducts into the substance of the pancreas, leading to the destruction of pancreatic acinar and islet tissue by activated pancreatic enzymes, accompanied by acute inflammation of the affected pancreatic tissue. Some of the enzymes leak from the damaged tissue into the bloodstream, where elevated levels of amylase and lipase can be detected by laboratory tests. The clinical manifestations of acute pancreatitis depend on how much pancreatic tissue has been damaged. Mild episodes are accompanied by abdominal pain with elevated pancreatic enzymes; however, the pain subsides, and the patient recovers. Patients with severe acute pancreatitis have marked abdominal pain and tenderness and are seriously ill. The activated pancreatic enzymes not only destroy much of the pancreas but also damage pancreatic blood vessels, which leads to marked hemorrhage in the damaged tissues. This condition is often referred to as

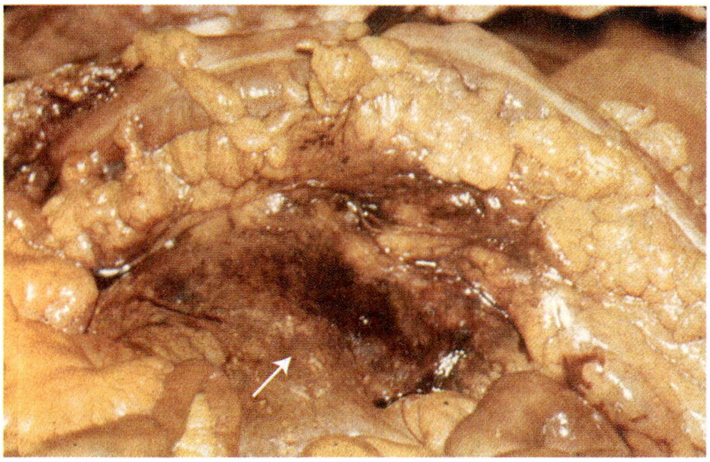

(A)

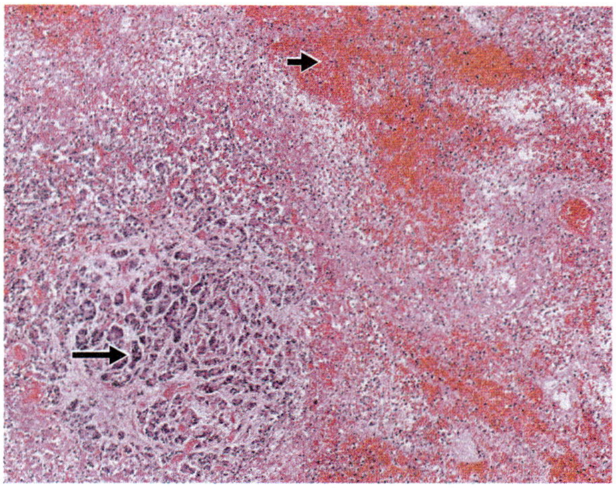

(B)

Figure 20-2 **(A)** Acute pancreatitis. The transverse colon (*upper part of photograph*) has been elevated to reveal the pancreas (*arrow*), which is inflamed and contains large areas of hemorrhage. **(B)** Photomicrograph of acute hemorrhagic pancreatitis. Damaged exocrine gland of pancreas (*arrow*). An area of hemorrhage is visible on the right of the image (*short arrow*).

(A) Courtesy of Leonard V. Crowley, MD, Century College; (B) Courtesy of Department of Pathology and Laboratory Medicine, University of North Carolina at Chapel Hill.

acute hemorrhagic pancreatitis, and it may be associated with multiple organ systemic disease, shock, and death (**Figure 20-2**).

The pathogenesis of acute pancreatitis usually involves active secretion of pancreatic juice while the pancreatic duct is obstructed at its entrance into the duodenum. The buildup of obstructed secretions greatly increases the pressure within the duct system, causing the ducts to rupture and the pancreatic juice to escape. Autoactivation of the digestive enzymes occurs within the pancreas and surrounding tissue, leading to digestion of the affected areas. Two factors predisposing to acute pancreatitis are disease of the gallbladder and excessive alcohol consumption.

Pancreatitis often develops in patients with gallstones because in most individuals, the common bile duct and common pancreatic duct enter the duodenum through a common channel (the **ampulla of Vater**). If a stone becomes impacted in the ampulla, it can obstruct the pancreatic duct and precipitate pancreatitis.

People who drink excessive amounts of alcohol also are prone to pancreatitis. Alcohol is a potent stimulus of pancreatic secretions, and it may induce edema and spasm of the pancreatic sphincter in the ampulla of Vater. Pancreatitis develops because alcohol-induced hypersecretion of digestive enzymes combined with sphincter spasm leads to high intraductal pressure, followed by duct necrosis, and escape of pancreatic juice. In addition, acute pancreatitis may be associated with certain therapeutic drugs, viruses, and trauma related to endoscopic or surgical procedures. A number of cases have no known cause (are idiopathic); other cases relate to inherited defects in the precursor protein for trypsin (trypsinogen) and in otherwise undiagnosed forms of cystic fibrosis. Such inherited lesions often result in chronic disease.

For acute and severe acute pancreatitis, pain management medicine, fluid resuscitation, and enteral nutrition supplements are necessary. Antibiotics may be prescribed to prevent infectious complications. Additionally, ERCP (endoscopic retrograde cholangiopancreatography) might be performed to find and treat the problems of the bile and pancreatic ducts.

Acute hemorrhagic pancreatitis Severe pancreatic inflammation with necrosis of pancreatic ducts and release of pancreatic enzymes that damage the pancreas and blood vessels.

Ampulla of Vater The area in the duodenum where the pancreatic duct and common bile duct come together, also known as the hepatopancreatic ampulla or hepatopancreatic duct.

Chronic Pancreatitis

Chronic pancreatitis often results from repeated episodes of mild acute pancreatitis associated with chronic alcoholism or other forms of recurrent pancreatic injury. Each bout of pancreatitis destroys some pancreatic tissue, but the inflammation subsides, and the damaged pancreatic tissue is replaced by scar tissue. Eventually, as progressively more pancreatic tissue is destroyed, the affected person has difficulty digesting and absorbing nutrients because there is not enough surviving pancreatic tissue to produce adequate digestive enzymes. The associated destruction of pancreatic islets may also lead to diabetes. Chronic pancreatitis is often accompanied by debilitating pain. Death may occur with recurrent acute attacks.

For chronic pancreatitis, the treatment is to help the patient relieve pain and manage complications. If the conditions don't improve, removal of the whole pancreas (total pancreatectomy) followed by islet auto-transplantation might be needed. These islets will make hormones and release them into the bloodstream.

Cystic Fibrosis of the Pancreas

The rate of those affected with cystic fibrosis varies by ancestry. For those of Northern European descent, the rate is 1 in 3,500, and for Black people, the rate is 1 in 15,000. However, for unknown reasons, the prevalence is much lower in Asia (1:30,000). Cystic fibrosis is a multisystem disease related to the production of abnormally viscous epithelial cell secretions (mucus). The abnormality results from a mutation of the CFTR gene, which stands for cystic fibrosis transmembrane conductance regulator, a rather formidable term meaning that the gene regulates the movement of chloride in most epithelial cells by means of ion channels located on the cell membranes. The CFTR gene, localized to the long arm of chromosome 7, currently has a total of 2,114 mutations identified, including 709 CF-causing mutations. The most common mutation in the CFTR gene is a deletion of three bases, which removes a single amino acid, phenylalanine, from the CFTR protein at position 508 (termed ΔF508).

The mutation blocks maturation of the protein, which is not transported to the cell surface and is degraded. In some individuals, the disease is relatively mild; others experience severe symptoms and morbidity. Most people with cystic fibrosis live into their fourth decade before needing a lung transplant. Modern therapy has much improved the quality of life for cystic fibrosis patients as well as the median age of survival. It is predicted that the median age of survival of CF patients who were born between 2020 and 2024 is 65 years.

As a result of the gene mutation, there is decreased secretion of chloride and increased reabsorption of sodium from epithelial cells in many organ systems. The defect in ion transport leads to increased cellular uptake of water from the lumen of organs and hence increased viscosity of the mucus secreted by the epithelial cells of the pancreas, bile ducts, mucosa of the respiratory tract, and other mucus-secreting cells throughout the body. As a result, the mucus becomes abnormally thick and tends to form dense plugs that obstruct the pancreatic ducts, bronchi and bronchioles, and bile ducts.

Although lung disease characterized by chronic viscid mucus–obstructed bronchioles and bronchi leading to repeated bouts of infection is the major cause of illness and death in cystic fibrosis patients, about 85 percent of patients

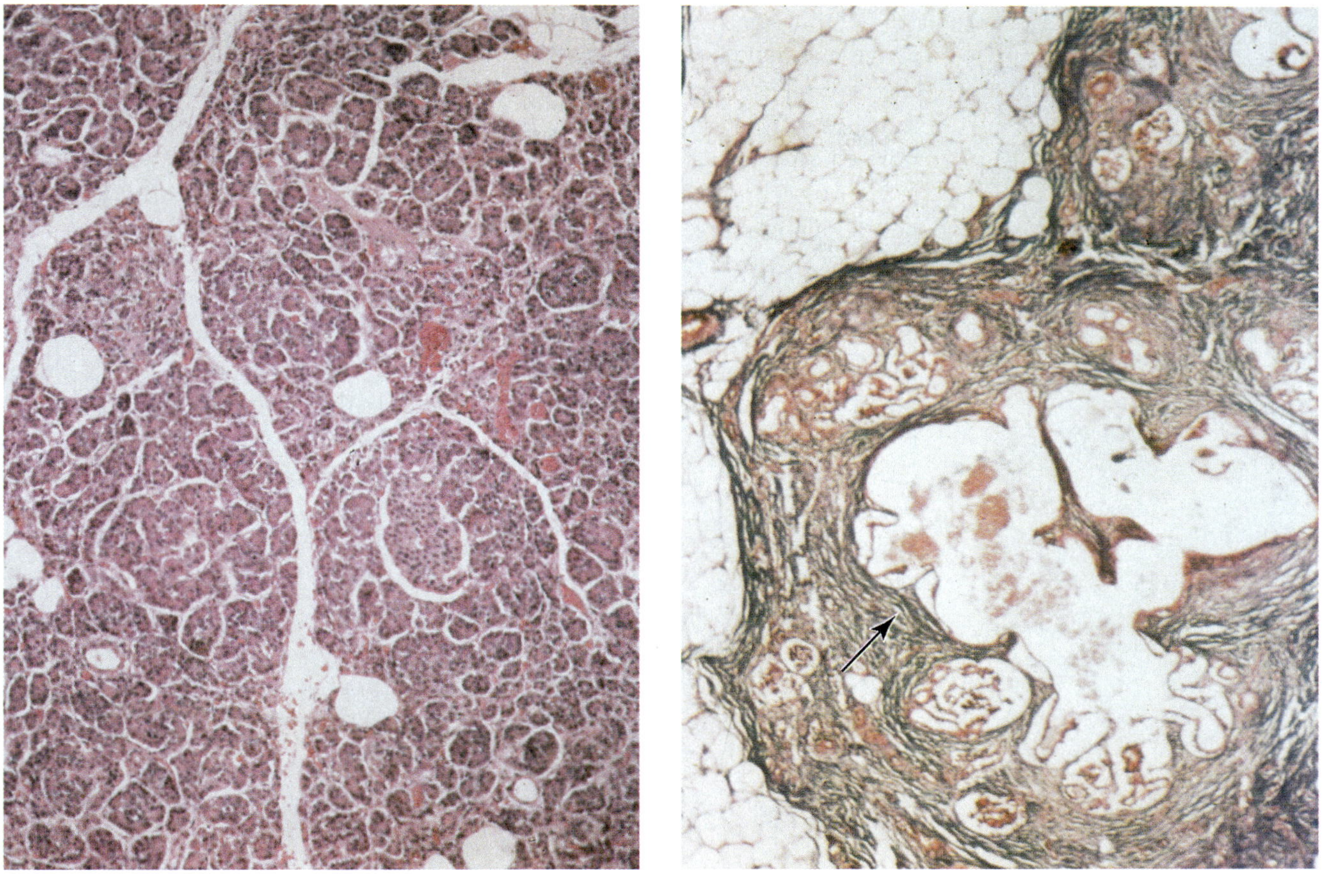

(A) (B)

Figure 20-3 Low magnification photomicrographs comparing a normal pancreas **(A)** with the pancreas of a patient with cystic fibrosis **(B)**. The duct in the center of the field (*arrow*) exhibits dilation. Most of the pancreatic glandular tissue has undergone atrophy and has been replaced by fibrous tissue.

have chronic pancreatitis as well. Mucous plugs in the small pancreatic ducts block the secretion of pancreatic juice, which accumulates under increased pressure within the obstructed ducts. Eventually, the ducts become cystically dilated. The pancreatic secretory cells, unable to discharge their secretions into the duodenum, undergo atrophy and are replaced by fibrous tissue, but the pancreatic islets are unaffected because they discharge their hormones directly into the bloodstream. Eventually, the pancreas becomes converted into a mass of cystically dilated ducts surrounded by dense fibrous tissue (**Figure 20-3**). For this reason, many cystic fibrosis patients need to take capsules containing pancreatic enzymes to digest and absorb food properly because their own pancreas has been destroyed by the disease. The name of the disease derives from these characteristic structural abnormalities.

The function of sweat glands is also abnormal in cystic fibrosis. The sweat glands are unable to reabsorb sodium and chloride, so the sweat of affected individuals contains an excessively high salt concentration. This biochemical abnormality has served as the basis of a diagnostic test for cystic fibrosis called a **sweat test**. A small quantity of sweat is collected, and the sodium and chloride concentrations are determined. The salt concentration of the sweat is low in normal persons and high in persons with cystic fibrosis. In addition, molecular analysis of the gene can allow characterization of the specific mutation responsible.

Sweat test Diagnostic test for cystic fibrosis.

The discovery of the CFTR gene and its defective counterpart stimulated active research efforts that recently have led to the development of drugs that improve CFTR protein function, as demonstrated by more efficient chloride transport across the cell membrane, which leads to improved pulmonary function. CFTR modulators (potentiators) target the defective protein produced by certain susceptible mutations and serve to potentiate the CFTR chloride channel, allowing more chloride flow with water following the chloride, so consequently, the mucus produced is less thick and sticky. Other modulators are termed "correctors," which help the defective protein produced by the ΔF508 mutation form the right three-dimensional shape to allow it to move to the cell surface and be retained. A combination of both types of modulators (for example, in Trikafta) is effective in treating not only the common ΔF508 mutation but also another 170 additional CF-causing mutations. Such drugs have much improved the life quality of CF patients and increased the lifespan of patients born after 2019 by over 20 years, with some individuals living into their 80s. However, the cost of such drug therapy is high and may exceed $300,000 per year. Prophylactic use of antibiotics remains critical to impede the occurrence of bacterial lung disease related to the viscid mucus–obstructed bronchioles and bronchi in the lung.

More traditional therapies for CF are aimed at preventing infections, thinning mucus, and clearing the airways. CF patients may consider a lung transplant.

Role of Insulin in Metabolism

The insulin made by the pancreas has a number of critical roles in controlling energy metabolism. Insulin is responsible for stimulating the movement of glucose transport proteins to the cell surface, resulting in insulin entering the cell and being available for cellular metabolism. With glucose entering into cells, blood glucose levels will be lowered. In addition, insulin stimulates the conversion of hepatic glucose into glycogen (a storage molecule that is a polymer of glucose) while suppressing the conversion of glycogen into glucose. Insulin also plays an important role in stimulating liver lipid synthesis. This enables the liver to "store" excess calories in a more efficient and osmotically inactive form that ultimately is deposited as visceral fat contained in adipocytes. Insulin also promotes entry of amino acids into the cells and stimulates protein synthesis. Insulin stimulates endothelial cells to produce nitric oxide (NO), a potent vasodilator increasing blood flow to skeletal muscle. The main stimulus for insulin release is elevation of the level of glucose in the blood, as occurs after a meal. In **diabetes mellitus**, glucose is absorbed normally. However, because of a lack of insulin or insulin insensitivity, which occurs in the various forms of diabetes mellitus, glucose is not used to produce energy and is not stored as glycogen as in a healthy person. Consequently, glucose accumulates in the bloodstream, resulting in hyperglycemia. The excessive glucose "spills over" in the urine and is excreted. Because insulin must be excreted in aqueous solution in the urine, the body loses excessive amounts of water and electrolytes along with the glucose. This may lead to a disturbance in the water balance and the acid–base balance. (Water and electrolyte balance is discussed in Chapter 17.) Protein synthesis is also compromised, and body protein is broken down into amino acids. The liver converts these amino acids into glucose, augmenting the hyperglycemia and leading to additional losses of glucose, water, and electrolytes in the urine.

Diabetes mellitus
A metabolic disease characterized by hyperglycemia and caused by insufficient insulin secretion or inefficient utilization of insulin.

Diabetes Mellitus

Diabetes mellitus is a very common and important metabolic disease that results either because of a deficit in the secretion of insulin by the pancreatic islets or because the targets of insulin action become resistant to its effects. The major symptom is a high level of glucose in the blood (**hyperglycemia**). A normal fasting blood glucose concentration is considered to be 70–100 mg per 100 mL of plasma (abbreviated 70–100 mg/dL). A diagnosis of diabetes requires a fasting glucose of 126 mg/dL or higher, or over 200 mg/dL in two random tests with symptoms, or a glucose concentration over 200 mg/dL determined by an oral glucose tolerance test (75 g of oral glucose 2 hours prior to testing of plasma glucose levels). Fasting blood glucose levels between 110 and 125 mg/dL are considered to be impaired and indicative of a "prediabetic" condition. Another test, called a **glycated hemoglobin test** (also called the **hemoglobin A1c test**), is based on the observation that hemoglobin in the blood is non-enzymatically glycated to a degree based on the level of plasma glucose. Fasting plasma glucose or postglucose tolerance testing levels are both "snapshots" of glucose metabolism at the time of the test. The A1c test represents the "historical" average levels of plasma glucose during the life of the red cell (100 to 120 days). An A1c level of 6.5 percent or greater is diagnostic of diabetes; levels between 5.7 percent and 6.4 percent indicate a prediabetic state.

Hyperglycemia Blood glucose levels higher than the normal range.

Glycated hemoglobin test/hemoglobin A1c test A test that measures the amount of glucose permanently attached to hemoglobin, which is higher than normal in many people with diabetes.

Type 1 diabetes mellitus (T1DM) Diabetes resulting from a deficit in insulin production.

Type 2 diabetes mellitus (T2DM) Diabetes resulting from the resistance of target tissue to the effect of insulin with a compensatory oversecretion by the pancreas.

Latent autoimmune diabetes of adults (LADA) Subtype of type 1 diabetes first appearing in adults.

The hyperglycemia of diabetes affects carbohydrate, fat, and protein metabolism. These derangements may result in acute and life-threatening disease and serious and chronic disturbances of multiple organ systems, notably the cardiovascular system, kidney, retina, and nervous system, leading to significant excess mortality and morbidity. The risk factors for diabetes include being age 45 or older, having a sibling with type 2 diabetes, being physically active less than 3 times a week, having non-alcoholic fatty liver disease (NAFLD) (see Chapter 19), having a history of gestational diabetes (diabetes during pregnancy; see Chapter 15), or having given birth to a baby who weighed over 9 pounds. There is an increase in risk in some ethnic groups, which may be related to lifestyle and other social determinants of health.

More than 11 percent of the U.S. population has diabetes, rising to 29 percent in the population over age 65. In 2022 the disease was the eighth most common cause of death in the United States. The death rate from cardiovascular disease is about seven times as high in diabetics. Diabetic kidney disease is the most common cause of kidney failure. In 2023 the overall annual cost of diabetes in the United States was over 412 billion dollars.

Diabetes is divided into two major groups, depending on whether the diabetes results from an autoimmune disease, leading to the destruction of beta cells in the pancreas and hence a deficit in insulin production (**type 1 diabetes mellitus [T1DM]**), or from the resistance of target tissue to the effect of insulin and a compensatory oversecretion of insulin by the pancreas (**type 2 diabetes mellitus [T2DM]**). T2DM (formerly noninsulin-dependent diabetes mellitus) is the more common form, often associated with the previously mentioned risk factors, often occurring in adults as part of the metabolic syndrome. T2DM also affects children and teens. T1DM accounts for fewer than 10 percent of cases and usually occurs in a population less than 20 years of age. A subtype of T1DM, termed **latent autoimmune diabetes of adults (LADA)**, occurs in older individuals and may be misdiagnosed as T2DM. Because LADA also relates to autoimmune damage to beta cells, the terms "juvenile" and "adult-onset diabetes" are somewhat inaccurate and no longer used. **Table 20-1** compares the

Table 20-1 Comparison of Two Major Types of Diabetes Mellitus

	Type 1	Type 2
Usual age of onset	Child to young adult	Middle age or later
Body build	Normal	Overweight
Plasma insulin	Absent or low	Normal or high
Complications	Ketoacidosis	Hyperosmolar coma
Response to insulin	Normal	Reduced
Response to oral antidiabetic drugs	Unresponsive	Responsive

Gestational diabetes Elevated blood glucose caused by insulin resistance resulting from elevated hormones related to pregnancy. Blood glucose returns to normal postpartum, but the woman has an increased risk of diabetes later in life.

Ketone bodies Three related compounds (acetone, acetoacetic acid, and beta-hydroxybutyric acid) are produced during the metabolism of fats. These molecules are small and water-soluble.

major features of the two types of diabetes. Diabetes may also occur in association with pregnancy (**gestational diabetes** (Chapter 15)) or in association with mutations in single genes (monogenic diabetes). Certain drugs and viral infections may lead to islet destruction independent of autoimmune reactivity.

Type 1 Diabetes Mellitus

Type 1 diabetes is an autoimmune disease in which cytotoxic CD8− T lymphocytes attack and destroy the pancreatic islets. The production of autoantibodies to beta cell products and components, including insulin, accompanies beta cell destruction. Such antibodies may be found before there is any evidence of clinical disease. The rate at which islets are destroyed by the immune system and the rate at which insulin secretion declines vary among affected individuals, but the disease usually has a long onset, with severe disease being present after about 80 percent of beta cells are destroyed. In some cases, the onset may be so slow as to not be noted until adulthood (LADA). However, the peak incidence of T1DM occurs primarily in children and young adults, most often around puberty. There is a clear hereditary predisposition to type 1 diabetes. People who inherit certain HLA-D types are at increased risk of acquiring this type of diabetes as well as other autoimmune diseases of the endocrine system. (HLA types and predisposition to disease are considered in the discussion on immunology in Chapter 5.) Other nongenetic factors are also important in the causation of T1DM. More than 80 percent of patients do not have an affected relative, and fewer than half of identical twins both develop the disease. Seasonal variation in frequency and changes in the frequency of T1DM with time in a population suggest that environmental agents (and in particular, infectious disease) may have a role in T1DM etiology. An infection with the Coxsackie B virus has been noted to precede some cases of the disease.

The pathogenesis of T1DM is clearly related and proportional to the lack of insulin and consequent metabolic changes associated with it. Uncontrolled hepatic glucose output and lack of storage into muscle and fat tissue lead to high blood sugar (hyperglycemia). The osmotic effect (hyperosmolarity) leads to excessive urination (polyuria) with dehydration, increased thirst (polydipsia), and loss of minerals. People with type 1 diabetes, lacking insulin, are unable to use carbohydrates because insulin is required to promote entry of glucose into the cells where the glucose can be metabolized to yield energy. Metabolism falls into a starvation-like state. When glucose is not used as a fuel source, adipose stores are used as an energy source. Oxidation of fat produces **ketone bodies**, which are released from the liver into the blood. Production of ketone bodies occurs in everyone when the blood glucose levels are lower and

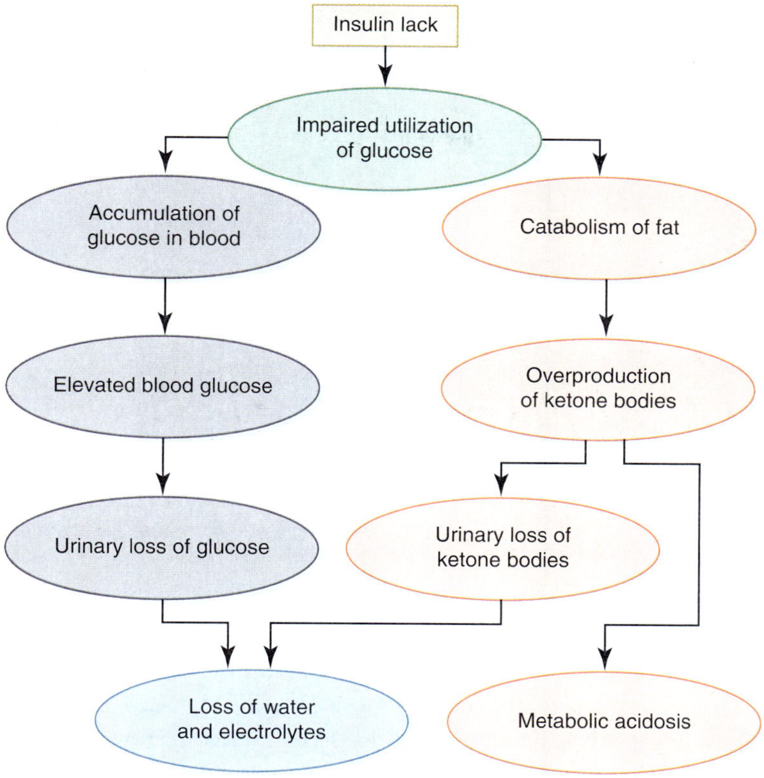

Figure 20-4 Major metabolic derangements in type 1 diabetes mellitus.

stops when there is sufficient glucose available for cellular metabolism. Without sufficient insulin to promote cellular absorption of glucose, fat oxidation is the major source of fuel production, resulting in excess production of ketone bodies, leading to metabolic acidosis (**diabetic ketoacidosis**). Together the acidosis, dehydration, and loss of ions can lead to coma and ultimately death if left untreated by provision of exogenous insulin.

All these effects can be reversed by supplying insulin, which promotes normal utilization of glucose and storage of glycogen. The disturbances of fat and protein metabolism also are reversed by the action of insulin. **Figure 20-4** summarizes the major metabolic disturbances in type 1 diabetes.

Diabetic ketoacidosis A disturbance of the body's acid–base balance (acidosis) caused by an inability to utilize glucose, which requires the body to use fat as an energy source. Fat metabolism generates excessive amounts of ketone bodies, which disrupts the normal alkalinity of body fluids.

Type 2 Diabetes Mellitus

Type 2 diabetes, by far the more common type, is a complex metabolic defect associated with risk factors mentioned previously. While type 2 diabetes often occurs in those middle-aged or older, it has become more prevalent in teens and even children. The pancreatic islets secrete insulin normally, followed by increasing amounts of insulin, but target tissues are relatively insensitive to the action of insulin and are unable to respond appropriately (termed **insulin resistance**). Eventually insulin output becomes unable to meet demand, and hyperglycemia ensues. Unlike the case in T1DM, there is no autoimmune destruction of islet cells, although with increasing age, fibrosis and deposition of amyloid (abnormally precipitated protein composed of a beta cell–secreted protein termed amylin) can occur in the islets (**Figure 20-5**). There is increasing evidence that there are reduced numbers of islets/beta cells associated with T2DM, which is related to increased beta cell death. The cause of the loss and its relation to the etiology of T2DM remain unclear.

Insulin resistance Condition when target tissues are relatively insensitive to the action of insulin.

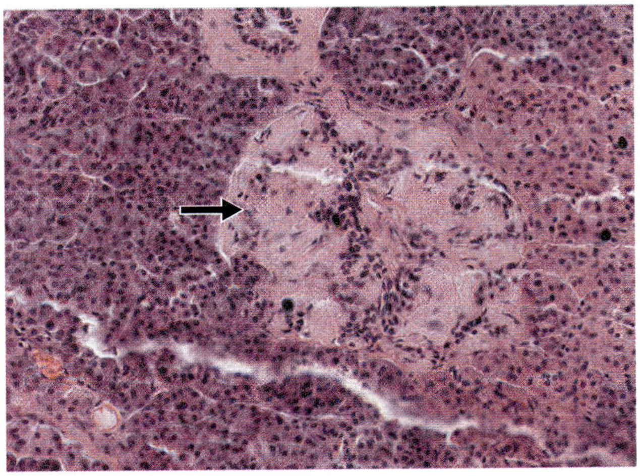

Figure 20-5 Amyloid deposition in pancreatic islet in long-standing T2DM. An islet where most cells have been replaced by amyloid (*arrow*) is visible as amorphous pink material.

Courtesy of Department of Pathology and Laboratory Medicine, University of North Carolina at Chapel Hill.

The reason for the impaired response to insulin is not completely understood, but it is central to the pathogenesis of T2DM. T2DM in some cases can be alleviated with weight loss and lifestyle changes. However, congenital genetic diseases that prevent normal deposition of visceral fat (lipodystrophies) are often associated with severe insulin resistance. Hence, an optimal amount of visceral fat is necessary to buffer excess calories and prevent insulin resistance. The root cause of insulin resistance remains speculative. Excess adipose tissue associated with T2DM may contain inflammatory cells that secrete a number of cytokines, which can lead to insulin resistance in experimental animal models. However, the evidence supporting this in T2DM is limited.

Early symptoms of type 2 diabetes may be mild, with the disease disclosed only on routine testing. The early symptoms are similar to that of type 1 diabetes, with polyuria, polydipsia, increased hunger, and sometimes unexplained weight loss. Itchiness and fatigue may also occur. Ketoacidosis does not usually occur as a complication of type 2 diabetes, but affected individuals may develop another complication called **hyperosmolar coma**, which results from the marked hyperglycemia. Of critical concern are the chronic effects of the disease, which are expressed in essentially every organ, and most notably, in the cardiovascular and renal systems. Many of the chronic effects of T2DM relate to dyslipidemia (increased triglycerides and reduced high-density lipoprotein cholesterol). Dyslipidemia is expressed in essentially every organ system in the body as a chronic disease state. The risk of atherosclerotic vascular disease with an increased incidence of hypertension, heart attack, and strokes; nonalcoholic fatty liver disease, which may progress to steatohepatitis; endocrine disease; renal disease; retinal disease; and an increased risk of cancer are all associated with the chronic dyslipidemia of T2DM.

Hyperosmolar coma Coma resulting from neurologic dysfunction caused by hyperosmolarity of body fluids as a consequence of severe hyperglycemia.

Type 2 diabetes is in part a hereditary disease in which genetic factors play an even greater role than in type 1 diabetes. The risk of diabetes occurring in both of a pair of monozygotic (identical) twins is nearly 100 percent. A study comparing the Pima Indians of Arizona with the Pima Indians of Mexico, who are essentially genetically identical, reinforced the idea that a modern sedentary lifestyle increases the risk of developing diabetes. Although genetics is clearly important in this population, environmental and nutritional factors also play a major role.

More than two hundred genetic loci are associated with increased risk for type 2 diabetes, but these loci contribute only about 10 percent of the overall disease risk attributable to genetic background. However, variants (polymorphisms) of one gene (TCF7L2) are involved in about 20 percent of all cases of type 2 diabetes, and people homozygous for the high-risk allele of the gene have about a twofold increased risk of disease. The gene appears to be involved in beta cell function rather than insulin resistance. The biological function of many of these genes in increasing the risk of disease remains unknown. Obesity (central obesity, the accumulation of visceral fat), a clear risk factor for T2DM, also has a strong genetic as well as an environmental component. About 40 to 70 percent of the risk for central obesity relates to multiple genetic factors. Hence, it is not surprising that genes that contribute to the risk of central obesity also may increase the risk of T2DM. The best characterized of these is a set of genes on chromosome 16 located near the FTO (fat mass and obesity–associated) gene. Genetic variants of the FTO gene have a marked effect on the risk of adult obesity. The effects are likely to be mediated through a second gene, Irx3, whose level of expression is controlled by FTO. Irx3 is expressed in an area of the brain (the hypothalamus) critical in energy regulation. Additional information is available in the discussion of obesity in Chapter 21.

An uncommon autosomal dominant genetic form of diabetes representing 1 to 2 percent of cases of adult diabetes is maturity onset diabetes of the young (MODY). The name is a misnomer because the disease is not related to T2DM (generally associated with adult onset) but rather relates to mutations in a number of genes associated with impaired insulin secretion/beta cell function occurring at an early age. At least a dozen genes have been associated with MODY. The most common form of MODY (MODY1) results from mutations in the HNF1A gene, which leads to progressive beta cell failure and a reduction in important steps in glucose transport and metabolism. The disease is progressive with age and associated with diabetic complications. The second most common form (MODY2) is associated with mutations in the glucokinase gene (GCK). These mutations interfere with the formation of glucose-6 phosphate, which ultimately stimulates the "glucose sensor" on the beta cell, but the beta cells cannot respond appropriately to the degree of glycemia. This disease is mild and does not progress with age.

Prediabetes

Many people who eventually develop diabetes present with blood glucose that is higher than normal but not high enough to establish a diagnosis of diabetes (the cut-off is arbitrary). This condition is closely associated with visceral obesity and, in particular, with deposition of adipose tissue in the abdominal region (as opposed to the hips and buttocks) and is associated with metabolic syndrome. This borderline abnormality in blood glucose level is termed **prediabetes**, indicating that increased beta cell insulin production can no longer completely keep pace with the increasing resistance of insulin targets to the effect of the hormone. Currently, there are several working definitions of the criteria for a diagnosis of prediabetes, making it difficult to estimate the public health burden of this condition. Reducing the demands on the pancreas may be accomplished by weight loss and moderate exercise (which reduce the insulin resistance of body cells so less insulin is required) and by healthy eating habits, emphasizing fruits, vegetables, and whole grains (called the "Mediterranean-style diet"). Certain medications (such as metformin, which inhibits the

Prediabetes Higher than normal blood glucose but not high enough to establish diagnosis of diabetes.

production of glucose by the liver) may also be required. All these measures help preserve beta cell function and promote more efficient utilization of glucose so that blood glucose does not rise as high after eating.

Gestational Diabetes

The high levels of placental hormones in pregnancy (see Chapter 15) cause the pregnant woman to develop insulin resistance, but most women can compensate by secreting more insulin, and the blood glucose does not rise excessively. Women who are unable to secrete enough additional insulin develop pregnancy-related diabetes caused by their insulin resistance. Gestational diabetes is distinct from preexisting T2DM or LADA. Gestational diabetes is not uncommon, affecting nearly 10 percent of pregnancies. The condition is treated in a manner similar to prediabetes, with some physicians preferring supplementary insulin rather than metformin because hyperglycemia is harmful to the developing fetus. Although blood glucose returns to normal after delivery, a woman who has demonstrated significant insulin resistance/gestational diabetes during pregnancy is at risk of developing T2DM in later years.

Diabetes and Metabolic Syndrome

Metabolic syndrome is defined as abnormal fasting plasma glucose caused by insulin resistance, mild hypertension, and dyslipidemia (elevated plasma triglycerides and low plasma high-density lipoprotein [HDL] cholesterol). The syndrome occurs with abdominal obesity and a sedentary lifestyle. Metabolic syndrome may progress to diabetes-associated complications as well as to cardiovascular disease and its complications. Metabolic syndrome is an independent risk factor for many poor health outcomes. Its individual components should be treated with medication and behavioral changes to reduce cardiovascular risk and prevent diabetes and its complications.

Monitoring Control of Diabetes

The current goal of treatment is to achieve control of blood glucose (glycemic control) that is as close as possible to normal, as close control of hyperglycemia reduces the long-term complications caused by diabetes. It is clear that such stringent management of hyperglycemia is associated with lower risk, increased life expectancy, and reduced vascular complications. As noted previously, two methods are used to assess the degree of glycemic control (i.e., the level of blood glucose). Self-monitoring of blood glucose by the patient (SMBG) can be accomplished with several different methods. If the patient recognizes the signs of low blood glucose (which can result in confusion and fainting), it can be rectified in a timely manner. Insulin dosage (when used) needs to be carefully tailored to help achieve as near to normal blood glucose levels as possible.

Tests for the level of glycated hemoglobin (also called hemoglobin A1c and often abbreviated as HbA1c) as an index of long-term control of hyperglycemia are generally done twice a year, or more frequently when therapy is changed. These tests are useful predictors of diabetic complications. Urine tests may be used in special circumstances to check for ketone bodies as an indication of diabetic ketoacidosis. The goal of frequent in-home blood glucose testing (or continuous glucose monitoring) is to monitor and control insulin dosage to achieve an optimal level of blood glucose with minimal variation in the face of varying nutrition and stress.

Treatment of Diabetes

Type 1 diabetics require insulin at doses adjusted to control the level of blood glucose as close to normal as possible to reduce late complications. Most type 1 diabetics require several insulin injections spaced throughout the day to maintain blood glucose within reasonably normal limits. A variety of insulins are used that provide prolonged effects with relatively slow onset (basal insulins) or that act rapidly with shorter periods of action (bolus insulins). The exact dosing regimen optimal for a T1DM patient must be determined individually. Frequent measurements of blood glucose permit better regulation of insulin dosage and improve control of diabetes.

An insulin pump is a small, battery-operated device that can be attached to the patient's belt. A short length of tubing extends from the pump to a fine (27 gauge) needle inserted into the subcutaneous tissue of the abdominal wall and secured with tape. The pump is programmed to deliver a small, constant infusion of insulin, supplemented by larger doses just before meals, simulating the release of insulin by the pancreas. Despite the convenience, use of an insulin pump requires very close medical supervision because complications can arise from pump malfunction or infections at the site of needle placement. Great progress has been made on achieving the goal of combining these pumps with continuous blood glucose monitoring.

Type 2 diabetic patients can often be managed by diet and weight reduction alone. If they do not respond adequately, oral and now parenteral hypoglycemic drugs are added. Metformin, a biguanidine class drug, is the recommended preferred initial cost-effective agent. The drug's principal mode of action is inhibiting gluconeogenesis, the production of glucose by the liver from non-carbohydrates. The drug also appears to increase the body's sensitivity to insulin. If sufficient control cannot be achieved, either an additional oral agent or insulin is added. There are many additional oral pharmacologic agents other than metformin available, each with potential advantages and disadvantages. Recently the use of incretins or incretin analogues has seen increasing use in diabetes therapy but also in weight control, a use that has received much public attention. Incretins are gut hormones that, in response to food, promote insulin production by the pancreas. Glucagon-like peptide-1 (GLP-1) and glucose-dependent insulinotropic polypeptide (GIP) are incretins that have been used as therapeutic targets in the treatment of type-2 diabetes. Perhaps best known are the GLP-1 receptor agonists (GLP-1RA), which mimic how GLP-1 functions. Semaglutide (Ozempic) and liraglutide (Victoza) are examples currently seeing much use not only to improve glycemic control in patients but also to promote weight loss and reduce cardiovascular risk, benefits that are valuable in dealing with the effects of metabolic syndrome. The choice is determined by the patient in consultation with the physician and is based on effectiveness, potential side effects, effects on weight, the likelihood of causing **hypoglycemia**, and cost. Many of these agents are extremely expensive, requiring parenteral dosing, and the choice of a second agent is often very limited.

Hypoglycemia Lower than normal concentration of glucose in the blood.

Complications of Diabetes

Complications of diabetes include increased susceptibility to infection, apparently related to the high levels of blood glucose, or development of diabetic coma as a result either of ketoacidosis or of the greatly increased osmolarity of body fluids resulting from hyperglycemia. Diabetics have a greater incidence of renal disease, arteriosclerosis and its associated vascular complications such as strokes and heart attacks, and gangrene of the legs and feet as a result of poor circulation. The vascular problems probably result both from abnormalities in fat metabolism associated with diabetes and from the elevated blood lipids frequently found in diabetics. Patients with diabetes are also subject to other late complications, which increase in frequency with the duration of the disease. The small blood vessels supplying the retina of the eye often undergo degenerative changes, which may eventually lead to blindness in some patients. The glomerular arterioles and capillaries within the kidneys also undergo degenerative changes, which impair renal function and may result in renal failure (discussed in Chapter 17). The peripheral nerves may undergo degenerative changes, called peripheral neuritis, which causes pain and disturbed sensations in the extremities. In addition, host responses to infection by bacteria and fungi are also impaired. How high glucose leads to organ damage is not completely understood, but the organ damage is related either directly or indirectly to hyperglycemia. One concept proposes that hyperglycemia causes the proteins in the retina, peripheral nerves, and capillary basement membranes to undergo the same type of glycation as hemoglobin. These glycated proteins undergo further interactions with other cell components, leading eventually to the blood vessel and organ damage characteristic of long-standing, poorly controlled diabetes.

Other Causes of Hyperglycemia

Other conditions may lead to hyperglycemia, but they are much less common than true diabetes mellitus. These conditions include chronic pancreatic disease, in which the hyperglycemia results from damage or destruction of pancreatic islets; endocrine diseases associated with overproduction of pituitary or adrenal hormones, which also raise blood glucose; ingestion of certain drugs, such as diuretics or antihypertensive drugs, that impair glucose metabolism as a side effect; and a few rare hereditary diseases in which carbohydrate metabolism is disturbed.

Hypoglycemia

The normal pancreas continually monitors the blood glucose and automatically adjusts its output of insulin to maintain the blood glucose level within the normal range. The type 1 diabetic patient, however, must adjust the dose of insulin to match the amount of carbohydrate to be metabolized. If there is insufficient insulin, the blood glucose is too high. If there is too much insulin, the blood glucose is too low, a condition called hypoglycemia (hypo = under). Two conditions predispose to hypoglycemia in a diabetic patient taking insulin. The first is a reduced intake of food, such as skipping a meal; blood glucose falls because carbohydrate intake is insufficient in relation to the amount of insulin injected. The second condition is increased activity, such as vigorous exercise, which lowers blood glucose by increasing glucose utilization. As a result, there is a relative excess of insulin. Too much insulin causes a precipitous drop in the level of glucose in the blood and initiates a chain of events called an **insulin reaction**, also called **insulin shock**. The adrenal medulla responds to the hypoglycemia by discharging epinephrine (adrenaline), which tends to raise blood glucose by converting liver glycogen into glucose. Epinephrine exerts widespread systemic effects as well: rapid heart rate, rise in blood pressure, constriction of cutaneous blood vessels causing the skin to appear pale, stimulation of sweat glands causing a cold sweat, and stimulation of the nervous system leading to increased excitability, anxiousness, hyperactive reflexes, and tremors.

Insulin reaction/insulin shock Condition in which there is too much insulin in the blood.

Table 20-2 Differentiation of Insulin Shock from Ketoacidosis and Hyperosmolar Coma

Diagnostic Feature	Insulin Shock	Ketoacidosis	Hyperosmolar Coma
Food intake	May be insufficient	Normal or excessive	Normal or excessive
Insulin	Excessive	Insufficient	Normal or increased
Onset of symptoms	Rapid	Gradual (several days)	Gradual (several days)
Skin	Cold sweat, pale	Dry and flushed	Dry and flushed
Respirations	Normal or shallow	Slow and deep	Usually normal
Reflexes	Hyperactive	Depressed	Normal
Heart rate	Rapid	Rapid	Usually normal
Blood pressure	Normal or slightly elevated	Low	Usually normal
Glucose in urine	Absent	Large amount	Large amount
Blood glucose	Very low	High	Extremely high
Blood bicarbonate and pH	Normal	Low	Normal
Acetone in blood and urine	Absent	Present	Absent

Neurologic manifestations appear if the blood glucose continues to fall, because the nervous system requires glucose to carry out its metabolic processes and begins to malfunction when deprived of its energy source. The individual becomes confused, loses consciousness, may also have convulsions, and could lapse into a deep coma. Prolonged severe hypoglycemia may cause permanent brain damage.

If the patient is still conscious and able to swallow, the insulin reaction can be stopped by ingesting a quick-acting carbohydrate, such as a piece of candy or a glucose tablet. The diabetic patient should always have a quick-acting carbohydrate available for such emergencies. If the patient is unconscious, an injection of glucagon can be given; this raises blood glucose by mobilizing glucose from liver glycogen. A concentrated glucose solution may also be given intravenously.

Insulin shock must be distinguished from diabetic ketoacidosis or hyperosmolar nonketotic coma, two other conditions to which the diabetic patient is predisposed (**Table 20-2**). Determination of blood sugar level (low in insulin shock) is a first step.

Tumors of the Pancreas

Carcinoma of the pancreas is relatively common (67,000 new cases and 52,000 deaths per year) and develops most often in the head of the pancreas. In this location, the neoplasm blocks the common bile duct, resulting in obstructive jaundice. Carcinoma elsewhere in the pancreas is usually far advanced when first detected and produces no specific symptoms. Little progress has been made in the treatment of exocrine tumors of the pancreas, and 5-year survival rates for these tumors are much lower than for other cancers. Endocrine pancreatic tumors have a better prognosis. Sometimes, benign or malignant tumors arise from the islet cells and produce symptoms as a result of overproduction of hormones. Beta cells give rise to insulin-secreting tumors (insulinomas) that cause episodes of severe hypoglycemia similar to those experienced by a diabetic who receives too much insulin. It is often difficult to predict if endocrine tumors of the pancreas will behave in a malignant fashion. Other cells of the islets of Langerhans may also form tumors that cause paraneoplastic disease—that is, disease not directly related to local tumor growth but rather to materials synthesized by the tumor and released into the body. The nature of the disease will depend on the particular type of cell from which the tumor arose. For example, alpha cells may form glucagonomas associated with anemia, mild diabetes, skin disease, and sometimes psychiatric disturbances.

As noted previously, the treatment of pancreatic cancer (particularly of the exocrine pancreas) can be challenging since patients with pancreatic cancer are often diagnosed at advanced stages when treatment options are very limited. For cancer that has not spread into the major blood vessels near the tumor, surgical removal, such as the Whipple procedure (developed by Dr. Allen Oldfather Whipple in the 1930s), total pancreatectomy, or distal pancreatectomy is occasionally an effective approach, but only a small number of patients are eligible for surgery.

When cancer cells have spread and cannot be removed surgically, chemotherapy and radiotherapy are often used to control the growth of the tumor and keep it from further spreading. A recently approved drug combination (Nalirifox) for metastatic disease has been shown to marginally prolong overall survival to eleven months.

In some cases, palliative surgery, such as biliary bypasses, endoscopic stent placement, and gastric bypasses is utilized to relieve the symptoms and improve the quality of patients' lives.

Prevention and early detection become crucial given the poor prognosis for advanced disease. The glycan carbohydrate antigen 19-9 (CA 19-9), identified in the 1980s, remains the commonly used clinical marker of limited utility to aid pancreatic cancer diagnosis. In families with known risk, genetic testing may be helpful. Certain predisposing factors should be recognized and avoided. These include smoking, obesity, chronic pancreatitis, and diabetes.

Case 20-1

Case 1: Jane is a 12-year-old female who has begun to have a variety of problems at school. She has been losing weight and is concerned because she has not yet achieved menarche, unlike many of her friends. Her schoolwork has begun to suffer. She is fatigued and has trouble concentrating; she has difficulty participating in athletics, and her vision is occasionally blurred. She is embarrassed because her teacher has noticed that she frequently must ask to go to the restroom and is constantly drinking. While trying to exercise in the gym, she faints and is taken to the hospital by ambulance. Her temperature is normal. Respirations are rapid and deep. Blood pressure is normal. She is comatose but responds to painful stimuli. Her skin is warm and dry. The remainder of the physical signs are normal. The patient's urine contained large amounts of glucose. There was a strongly positive reaction for acetone and other ketone bodies. Blood glucose was 565 mg/dL (normal range 60–100 mg/dL). Other laboratory studies revealed a low blood pH and reduced plasma bicarbonate of 8 mEq/L (normal range 24–28 mEq/L). The patient was considered to have severe diabetic acidosis, probably precipitated by stress during exercise. After intensive treatment with intravenous fluids and insulin, her condition gradually improved. The following day she was conscious and oriented and was able to take fluids orally. She continued to improve and was eventually discharged from the hospital. Testing revealed a moderately elevated level of hemoglobin A1c. She was diagnosed with type 1 diabetes mellitus and instructed in the details of a diabetic diet and taught to do frequent self-monitoring for blood glucose levels. She required a minimum of two injections of insulin with occasional supplementation with a rapid-acting inhaled insulin prior to strenuous exercise. She is now doing well in school and is monitored regularly by a physician specializing in diabetes in the young.

Case 2: John is an obese, 68-year-old man who was diagnosed several years ago as being prediabetic on the basis of a borderline abnormal glucose tolerance test and minimally elevated hemoglobin A1c. He was also found to be moderately hypertensive at that time, but John has not seen a physician since, nor has he modified his sedentary lifestyle. He has experienced increased urinary output and thirst for the last 2 weeks. He attends the North Carolina State Fair on an extremely warm and humid day and consumes large quantities of sugar-containing soft drinks, cotton candy, and fried chocolate candy bars. He becomes progressively more confused and collapses in a coma. He is brought to the hospital by the local emergency rescue squad with a suspicion of heat exhaustion, but his temperature is only slightly elevated. On admission, he is comatose and dehydrated. His respiratory rate is not increased. Blood pressure is normal. The urine contains a large amount of glucose but no ketone bodies. Blood pH and bicarbonate are normal. Blood glucose is 1750 mg/dL (normal range 60–100 mg/dL), and the osmolarity of the plasma is 396 mOsm/liter (normal range 280–295 mOsm/liter). A diagnosis of hyperosmolar nonketotic coma is made. He is treated with large volumes of hypotonic (0.45 percent) saline solution and with insulin. His condition gradually improves over the next several days. His blood glucose falls toward normal and eventually reaches 150 mg/dL on the fourth day. Plasma osmolarity also returns to normal as the elevated blood glucose declines. He is diagnosed as having type 2 diabetes mellitus and is instructed to lose weight and begin a moderate exercise program. He is placed on an oral hypoglycemic agent (metformin) but also requires supplemental insulin to control his blood glucose level. He does forswear high-sugar snacks in future visits to the fair.

Discussion

The purpose of these cases is to illustrate some of the typical symptoms of type 1 and type 2 diabetes mellitus and acute medical problems associated with each. It is not uncommon for emergency medical responders to be required to diagnose and begin therapy for ketoacidosis, hyperosmolar coma, and insulin shock (the latter not illustrated in the cases). Table 20-2 summarizes the differential signs of each. Type 1 and type 2 diabetes mellitus are both characterized by hyperglycemia, but the etiologies and presentations of the diseases are quite different. Although acute complications of both diseases may differ, the chronic multisystem effects of poorly controlled disease are similar.

Etiology and Pathogenesis

Case 1 is undiagnosed type 1 diabetes mellitus associated with autoimmune destruction of the pancreatic islets and consequent lack of sufficient insulin production. A common acute presentation (diabetic ketoacidosis) relates to the production of acidic metabolic products of excessive lipid metabolism, which exceeds the buffering capacity of the plasma. Case 2 demonstrates the progression of prediabetes into symptomatic type 2 diabetes in an individual suffering from uncontrolled metabolic syndrome. In this case, increasing insulin resistance related to obesity and lifestyle progress to the point at which extreme hyperglycemia related to the sudden intake of massive amounts of sugar occurs.

(continues)

Case 20-1 *(Continued)*

Questions

1. Type 1 diabetes mellitus (unlike type 2 diabetes mellitus) is often discovered when a person suffers from the sudden occurrence of ketoacidosis. Why do the two diseases differ in this respect?
2. Type 1 and type 2 diabetes mellitus both result in hyperglycemia, but the etiologies are distinct. What are the likely etiologies for the two conditions?
3. How are the symptoms and clinical signs of both forms of diabetes related to the pathophysiology of the diseases?
4. The second case description states the patient has metabolic syndrome. What is this syndrome, and how does the description of the patient support this? What is the relationship of metabolic syndrome to type 2 diabetes mellitus?

Questions For Review

1. What is the difference between acute and chronic pancreatitis?
2. What are the major metabolic disturbances in type 1 diabetes? How does insulin correct these disturbances?
3. What are the major complications of diabetes?
4. Which type of diabetes can be treated by diet alone?
5. What is meant by the following terms: sweat test, hyperglycemic coma, and insulin resistance?
6. What is cystic fibrosis of the pancreas? What are its clinical manifestations? What is its pattern of inheritance?
7. What is hypoglycemia? What are its clinical manifestations? How is it treated?
8. What are the major differences between diabetic ketoacidosis and insulin shock?
9. What is gestational diabetes? Why does it occur?
10. Compare and contrast diabetes mellitus and metabolic syndrome.

References

MedlinePlus. Pancreatitis. National Library of Medicine. https://medlineplus.gov/pancreatitis.html

Tang JCF. Acute Pancreatitis. Medscape. https://emedicine.medscape.com/article/181364-overview

Huffman JL. Chronic Pancreatitis. Medscape. https://emedicine.medscape.com/article/181554-overviewcape

- The first entry presents a useful overview. The last two entries are recent reviews of the etiology and pathogenesis and clinical aspects of the most significant forms of pancreatitis.

Cystic Fibrosis Foundation. Managing CF. https://www.cff.org/Life-With-CF/Treatments-and-Therapies/

Cuyx S, De Boeck K. Treating the underlying cystic fibrosis transmembrane conductance regulator defect. *Semin Respir Crit Care Med*. 2019;40(6):762-774.

- These two references review current approaches to the treatment of cystic fibrosis using both pharmacology and molecular biology.

Varkki SD, et al. *CFTR* mutations and phenotypic correlations in people with cystic fibrosis: A retrospective study from a single centre in south India. *Lancet Reg Health Southeast Asia*. 2024; 27:100434.

American Diabetes Association. Important Updates to the Standards of Medical Care in Diabetes–2022 Incorporate New Evidence. https://www.diabetes.org/

- This paper reviewed how several environmental factors trigger islet autoimmunity and promote progression into type 1 diabetes.

Rewers M, Lundvigsson J. Environmental risk factors for type 1 diabetes. *Lancet*. 2016;387(10035): 2340-2348. https://www.ncbi.nlm.nih.gov/pmc/articles/PMC5571740/

- The American Diabetes Association has an excellent website. Of particular value is their newly released standards of care (also available as an app) which are essential reading for anyone with diabetes. The second reference, although a bit dated, is an interesting review of the controversies surrounding environment and type I diabetes.

Schulz LO, Chaudhari LS. High-risk populations: The Pimas of Arizona and Mexico. *Curr Obes Rep*. 2015;4(1):92-98. doi:10.1007/s13679-014-0132-9. PMID: 25954599; PMCID: PMC4418458.

- A study comparing the Pima Indians of Arizona with the Pima Indians of Mexico, who are essentially genetically identical, reinforced the idea that a modern sedentary lifestyle increases the risk of developing diabetes.

Moodley N, et al. Historical perspectives in clinical pathology: A history of glucose measurement. *J Clin Pathol*. 2015;68(4):258-264.

- Glucose testing is the key to diabetes diagnosis and therapy. This is a fascinating review of methods for glucose testing in body fluids from ancient Egypt to the present.

National Heart, Lung, and Blood Institute (NIH). What is Metabolic Syndrome? https://www.nhlbi.nih.gov/health-topics/metabolic-syndrome

Banerjee S, et al. Type II diabetes mellitus and obesity: Common links, existing therapeutics and future developments. *J Biosci*. 2019;44(6):150.

Saklayen MG. The global epidemic of the metabolic syndrome. *Curr Hypertens Rep*. 2018:20(2):12. https://www.ncbi.nlm.nih.gov/pmc/articles/PMC5866840/

- The three references have the common theme of how environmental factors, nutrition, and exercise (or lack thereof) are involved in the etiology of metabolic syndrome and type II diabetes.

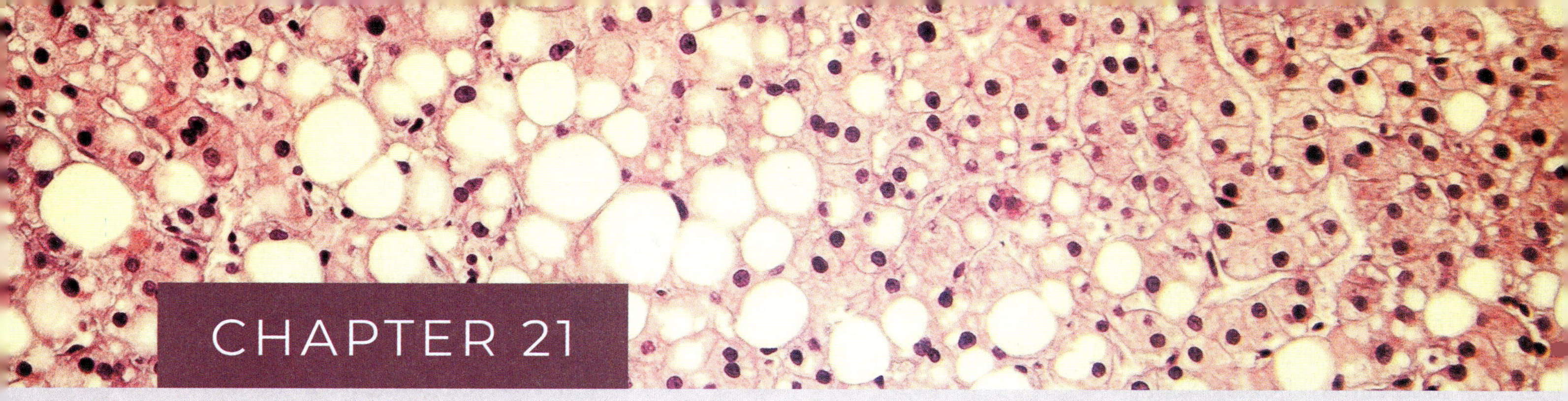

CHAPTER 21

The Gastrointestinal Tract

LEARNING OBJECTIVES

1. Explain the pathogenesis of dental caries and periodontal disease and describe prevention and treatment.
2. Name and describe the three most common lesions of the esophagus that lead to esophageal obstruction.
3. Describe the common types of gastritis and their clinical manifestations.
4. Explain the pathogenesis of peptic ulcers. Describe the three major complications of peptic ulcers. Describe the three major types of peptic ulcer and their treatment. Name the methods of treatment.
5. Differentiate between appendicitis and Meckel diverticulitis in terms of pathogenesis, clinical manifestations, and treatment.
6. Describe the common types of chronic and acute enteritis, their clinical manifestations, and the treatment/management.
7. Describe the pathogenesis of diverticulitis and explain the role of diet in the development of lesion.
8. Name the causes, clinical manifestations, and complications of intestinal obstruction, carcinoma of the colon, and diverticulosis of the colon. Explain their treatment.
9. Understand the major eating disturbances and their effects.

Structure and Functions

The gastrointestinal tract, which functions in the digestion and absorption of food, reabsorption of water, and elimination of wastes, comprises the oral cavity and related parts of the face, the esophagus, the stomach, the small and large intestines, the rectum, and the anus.

Abnormalities of the Oral Cavity

Dental Caries and its Complications

The oral cavity contains a diverse collection of both aerobic and anaerobic bacteria. Masses of these bacteria intermixed with bacterial products and proteins from saliva form a biofilm termed **dental plaque**, which adheres to the teeth and predisposes to tooth decay.

Caries, the term for tooth decay, is a Latin word meaning dry rot. The condition is a decalcification of the tooth structure caused by mouth bacteria acting on bits of retained food material, including sugar and highly refined, starchy

Dental plaque Masses of bacteria, bacterial products, and salivary proteins adherent to teeth, which predispose to tooth decay.

Dentine Bony structure of the tooth.
Dental cavity A loss of tooth structure caused by the combined action of mouth bacteria and organic acids derived from bacterial fermentation of retained food particles.
Xerostomia Dry mouth, which is lacking in saliva.
Caries Tooth decay.
Pulpitis Inflammation of the dental pulp.
Periapical abscess Infection of the tooth root.
Root canal treatment Replacement of tooth root canal with a filling material.
Gingivitis Gum inflammation.
Periodontal disease Pockets of infection between teeth and gum.
Stomatitis Inflammation of the oral cavity.

foods. Bacterial fermentation liberates organic acids that erode the covering enamel, exposing the underlying **dentine**, which is then attacked by the acids and invaded by mouth bacteria. The loss of tooth structure that results from the combined acid and bacterial action is termed a **dental cavity**. The affected area appears discolored and is quite soft when probed with a dental instrument. Dental X-rays reveal the cavity as an area of decreased density in the affected tooth. Saliva buffers the bacterially produced acid. For this reason, people who lack saliva (have **xerostomia**, a dry mouth) have a high incidence of **caries**.

If the cavity is not treated and continues to enlarge, the decay eventually reaches the dental pulp. The bacteria invade the pulp and incite an inflammation (**pulpitis**) that causes the throbbing pain, characteristic of a toothache. Unchecked, the infection may spread to the apex of the tooth root, which is embedded in the jawbone, and from there spread to the bone surrounding the dental root. The result may be an abscess surrounding the apex of the tooth, which is termed a **periapical abscess** (peri = around).

The incidence of tooth decay can be reduced by proper mouth hygiene, including frequent brushing of the teeth and use of dental floss to remove food particles that promote bacterial growth. Fluoride added to water supplies (a public health action becoming increasingly contentious) and toothpaste helps to prevent cavities by promoting formation of a more acid-resistant tooth structure that retards decay; however, excess use of fluoride from dental products can lead to tooth discoloration. Dental cavities are treated by removing the decayed area and packing the defect with some type of dental filling material. After infection of the pulp and dental root has occurred, more extensive treatment and possibly the use of antibiotics are required. The root of the tooth tends to be resistant to antibiotics, and the pulp of the tooth, along with the nerve, may need to be removed and the area sealed. This procedure is referred to as a root canal or **root canal treatment**. Sometimes the tooth cannot be salvaged and must be extracted.

Masses of bacteria and debris accumulating around the base of the teeth may incite inflammation. Initially, inflammation affects only the gums surrounding the roots of the teeth; such inflammation is termed **gingivitis** (gingiva = gum). Later, the inflammation extends between the teeth and the adjacent gums, leading to the formation of small pockets of infection between the teeth and gums. This condition is termed **periodontal disease** (peri = around + dens = tooth). If pus is discharged from the margins of the infected gums, the descriptive term pyorrhea (pyo = pus + rhea = flow) is often used. The infection may spread into the sockets that anchor the teeth in the jawbone, causing the teeth to loosen and eventually fall out. Various methods of treatment to the gums and teeth may control or arrest the condition, an important contributor to tooth loss. Chronic periodontal disease is associated with a number of systemic conditions, including heart disease and preterm or low-birth-weight pregnancies; however, this remains an area of controversy.

Inflammation of the Oral Cavity

An inflammation of the oral cavity, termed **stomatitis** (stoma = mouth), may be caused by a number of irritants and infectious agents. Common irritants are alcohol, tobacco, and hot or spicy foods. Infectious agents include herpes virus, human papilloma virus (HPV), and several other viruses; the fungus *Candida albicans*, particularly in immunosuppressed individuals and diabetics; and a combination of two bacteria (*Fusobacterium* and spirochetes) that cause acute necrotizing gingivitis (termed trench mouth or Vincent angina when it affects the tonsils and pharynx).

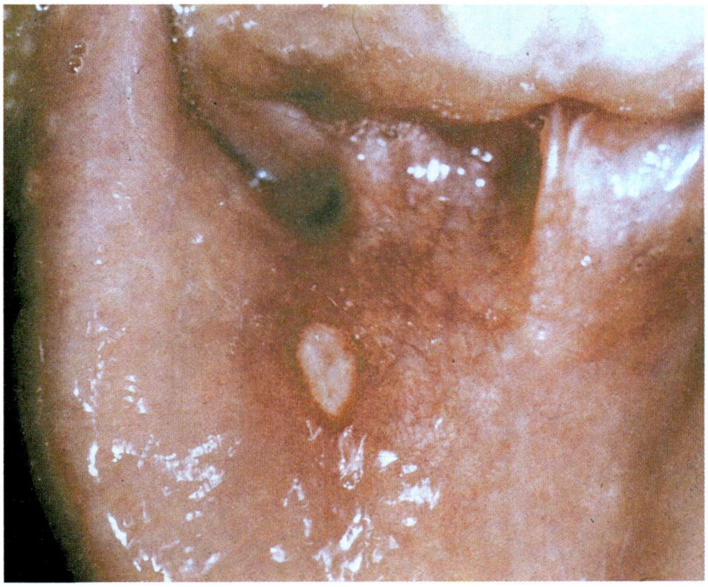

Figure 21-1 Superficial shallow ulcer of oral mucosa caused by a canker sore.
Courtesy of Leonard V. Crowley, MD, Century College.

Canker (aphthous ulcers) is another relatively common inflammatory disease involving the oral cavity. A **canker sore** appears as a small, painful, superficial ulcer of the oral mucosa surrounded by a narrow zone of inflammation that appears as a red border surrounding the ulcer (**Figure 21-1**). The cause of the sores is unknown, but an immune reaction to oral bacteria has been suggested as a cause.

Canker sore Small, painful ulcer developed in the oral cavity.

Leukoplakia A white patch of hyperplastic and usually atypical squamous epithelium on the oral mucosa or genital tract mucosa.

Erythroplakia Depressed red lesions on the oral mucosa.

Tumors of the Oral Cavity

Leukoplakia, the presence of white lesions on the mucosa of the oral cavity, is common, and about 20 percent demonstrate cellular dysplasia, a precursor to oral cancer. **Erythroplakia**, depressed red lesions on the oral mucosa, are of more concern and are frequently associated with dysplasia and even carcinoma in situ. Dentists are careful to search for and evaluate such lesions, often by biopsy. Carcinoma of the oral cavity, which may arise from the squamous epithelium of the lips, cheeks, tongue, palate, or back of the throat, is relatively common, with about 60,000 cases per year in the United States (**Figure 21-2**). Squamous cell carcinoma of the oral cavity is similar to that seen at other sites and frequently metastasizes. The nasal cavities and sinuses also may develop squamous cell carcinomas that may be associated with industrial exposure to nickel and other agents and also are associated with HPV infection.

Both benign and malignant tumors of the salivary glands occur (most frequently in the parotid gland). The most common benign tumor (pleomorphic adenoma) is slow growing and painless, consisting of a mixture of epithelial and duct-like cells, but it can be difficult to completely remove. Malignant salivary gland tumors consist of a number of different carcinomas that require surgery and sometimes radiation therapy.

Tumors of the Oropharyngeal Cavity

Cancers of the oropharyngeal cavity are responsible for about 13,000 deaths per year in the United States. In the past these were diagnosed in the elderly and were strongly associated with tobacco and alcohol use. Such cancers are

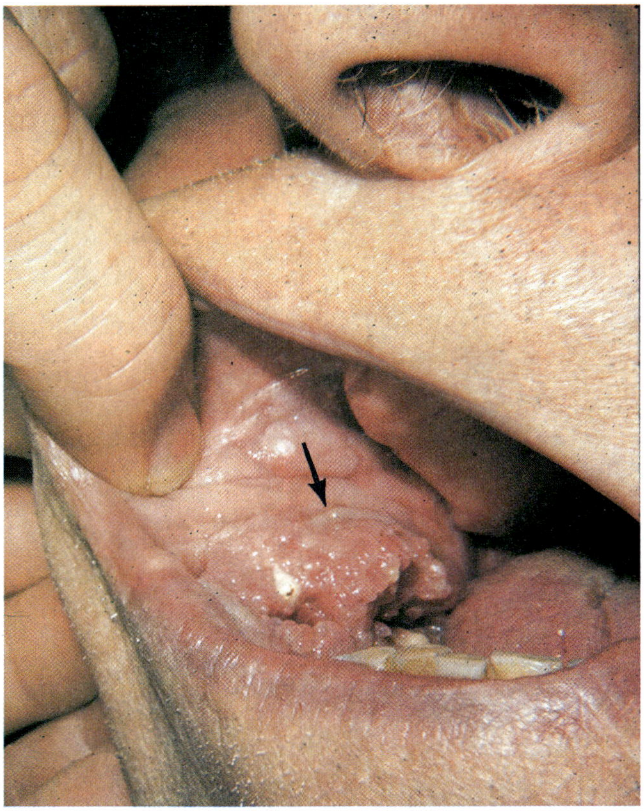

Figure 21-2 Squamous cell carcinoma of oral mucosa (*arrow*), which appears as an irregular overgrowth of tissue arising from the mucosa of the cheek.
Courtesy of Leonard V. Crowley, MD, Century College.

decreasing in frequency with a decrease in tobacco use. Oropharyngeal cancers are also termed throat cancer: This cancer forms in tissues of the oropharynx (the middle part of the throat, behind the mouth). Most oropharyngeal cancer (70 percent) is caused by HPV. Oropharyngeal cancer is different than oral cavity cancer, which forms in the mouth; both are types of head and neck cancer.

The HPV vaccine is estimated to prevent up to 90 percent of cancers caused by HPV infection and genital warts. HPV vaccination is recommended by the Centers for Disease Control and Prevention (CDC)'s Advisory Committee on Immunization Practices to prevent new HPV infections and HPV-associated cancers and other diseases. HPV vaccination offers the most protection when given to girls and boys at ages 9–12.

HPV-associated cancers have a better response to chemotherapy and radiation and hence have a better prognosis than non-HPV disease in the more elderly population.

Diseases of the Esophagus

The esophagus is a muscular tube extending from the pharynx to the stomach with sphincters at both upper and lower ends. The upper sphincter relaxes to allow passage of swallowed food, which is propelled down the esophagus by rhythmic peristaltic contractions. The lower esophageal sphincter (termed the **gastroesophageal sphincter** or the **cardiac sphincter**) relaxes when the food reaches the lower end of the esophagus and allows the food to pass into the stomach. Problems with the esophagus include malfunction of the lower sphincter, tears in the lining, obstruction, inflammation, and neoplasia.

Gastroesophageal/ cardiac sphincter Lower esophageal sphincter.

Symptoms of esophageal disease include difficulty swallowing (**dysphagia**) together with variable degrees of substernal discomfort or pain (often termed "heartburn"). Complete obstruction of the esophagus leads to an inability to swallow, which is often associated with regurgitation of food into the trachea, causing episodes of choking and coughing. Irregularities in the esophageal mucosa (esophageal webs and rings) may occur as congenital lesions or as the result of disease. **Diverticula** in the esophagus may occur as a result of motor disturbances. Elderly patients may acquire a **Zenker diverticulum**, which is an outpouching in the upper portion of the esophagus that traps food and causes regurgitation.

Cardiac Sphincter Dysfunction

The two major disturbances of cardiac sphincter function are failure of the cardiac sphincter to open properly, which is termed **achalasia** (formerly cardiospasm), and inability of the sphincter to remain closed properly, which is termed an incompetent cardiac sphincter and leads to **reflux esophagitis**.

Achalasia

Sometimes the cardiac sphincter fails to open properly, caused by a malfunction of the nerve plexuses in the esophagus that control its functions. As a result, food cannot pass normally into the stomach, and the smooth muscle in the wall of the esophagus must contract more vigorously to force the food past the constricted sphincter. Eventually, the esophageal muscle undergoes marked hypertrophy, and the esophagus becomes dilated proximal to the constricted sphincter because of food retention. This results in dysphagia and sometimes in food regurgitation. A number of drugs are useful in helping to relax the muscle, including endoscopic injection of botulinum toxin, which blocks the transmission of nerve impulses from the nerve plexuses to the muscle fibers for several months. More permanent therapy consists of periodic stretching of the sphincter or by surgically cutting the muscle fibers in the constricted area.

Incompetent Cardiac Sphincter and Its Complications

In this relatively common condition, acid gastric juice leaks back into the esophagus through the improperly closed, incompetent lower esophageal sphincter. The squamous epithelial lining of the esophagus, which was not "designed" to tolerate high-acid secretions, becomes irritated and inflamed, leading to reflux esophagitis. The condition is most commonly found in people after the age of 40 and is associated with obesity, smoking, and alcohol consumption. In some patients, the squamous mucosal lining may actually become ulcerated and scarred. Sometimes the squamous lining responds to the acidity by undergoing a change (metaplasia) into a more acid-resistant columnar gastric type of mucosa. This condition is termed **Barrett esophagus**, after the person who first described it. Unfortunately, the metaplastic columnar epithelium is frequently abnormal and poses an increased risk of developing adenocarcinoma (**Figure 21-3**). Patients with a significant degree of Barrett esophagus require periodic endoscopic monitoring and biopsy to detect early cancer. The condition may be treated endoscopically by using radiofrequency-induced heating or related therapies to ablate affected areas or, in some cases, endoscopic surgery. The treatment of reflux esophagitis to prevent progression to Barrett esophagus consists of avoiding lying down soon after eating because the recumbent position promotes reflux, sleeping with the head of the bed elevated to minimize

Dysphagia Difficulty swallowing.

Diverticula/diverticulum An outpouching from an organ, as from the mucosa of the colon, that projects through the muscular wall.

Zenker diverticulum Outpouching in the upper portion of the esophagus.

Achalasia Inability of a gastrointestinal sphincter to relax. Formerly known as cardiospasm.

Reflux esophagitis Inflammation of the lining of the esophagus caused by reflux of acidic gastric secretions through an incompetent lower gastroesophageal sphincter.

Barrett esophagus Squamous lining changes to a more acid-resistant columnar mucosa.

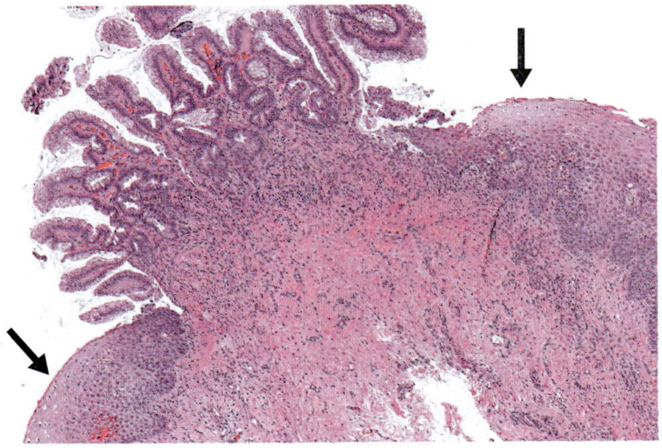

Figure 21-3 Barrett esophagus. A biopsy specimen from a patient with Barrett esophagus. The two arrows indicate areas of normal squamous mucosa. The area between them demonstrates mucosal metaplasia where the squamous epithelium has been replaced by columnar epithelium.

Courtesy of Department of Pathology and Laboratory Medicine, University of North Carolina at Chapel Hill.

reflux, and avoiding alcoholic beverages because alcohol not only stimulates gastric acid secretion but also tends to relax the lower esophageal sphincter, facilitating reflux. Drugs such as proton pump inhibitors and H2 receptor antagonists that reduce secretion of gastric acid and antacids that neutralize gastric acid are helpful.

Gastric Mucosal Tears

Retching and vomiting may cause linear tears in the mucosa of the gastroesophageal junction where the esophagus passes through the diaphragm or in the lining of the distal esophagus, and these tears can bleed profusely (Mallory-Weiss syndrome) (**Figure 21-4**). The repetitive, intermittent, vigorous contractions of the abdominal muscles associated with vomiting raise intragastric pressure while lowering the intrathoracic pressure and lead to distension and extremely forceful ejection of stomach contents through the esophagus. The additional stresses resulting from vigorous contractions of the muscular walls of the stomach and esophagus associated with vomiting probably place additional stress on the mucosa, which also plays a role in causing the laceration. This vomiting-related complication is not uncommon and is responsible for up to 10 percent of cases of bloody vomiting (**hematemesis**). It often follows the retching and vomiting related to excess alcohol intake, but it may follow vomiting from any cause, including self-induced vomiting to control weight. Far more serious, although very uncommon, is Boerhaave syndrome, in which the esophagus ruptures (rather than tears) after severe and forceful vomiting. The syndrome is associated with high mortality.

Hematemesis Bloody vomit, an indication of bleeding in upper GI, a medical emergency.

Esophageal Obstruction

Carcinoma of the Esophagus

Carcinoma may arise anywhere in the esophagus, either from the squamous epithelium (squamous cell carcinoma) or from the columnar epithelium associated with Barrett esophagus (adenocarcinoma). Worldwide, squamous cell carcinoma is more common and is related to alcohol intake, smoking, the consumption of near-boiling beverages (often tea), HPV infection, and a variety of

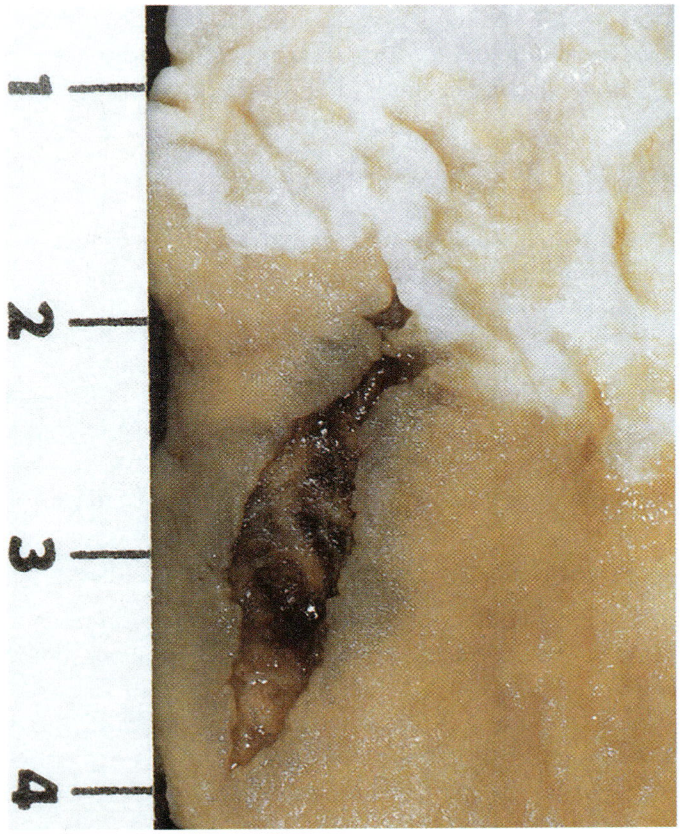

Figure 21-4 Gastric mucosal tear caused by retching and vomiting. The opaque mucosa in the upper part of the photograph is the normal stratified squamous of the esophagus. The 2 cm-long tear extends distally from the gastroesophageal junction and caused a fatal gastric hemorrhage.

Courtesy of Leonard V. Crowley, MD, Century College.

environmental agents. Adenocarcinoma is more frequent in the United States, possibly due to the increased prevalence of Barrett esophagus associated with changes in dietary habits. In either case, the tumor gradually narrows the lumen of the esophagus, frequently infiltrates the surrounding tissues, and may invade the trachea. Necrosis of the tumor extending between the esophagus and trachea may lead to the formation of an abnormal communication between these two structures termed a **tracheoesophageal fistula** (fistula = tube). The tumor is often discovered at an advanced stage, requiring esophagectomy, chemotherapy, and radiation.

Tracheoesophageal fistula Abnormal connection between the esophagus and trachea.

Food Impaction

Obstruction of the esophagus may be caused by the impact of poorly chewed meat in the distal part of the esophagus. This is sometimes encountered in people who are unable to chew their food properly because they have poor teeth or improperly fitting dentures or who have poor eating habits.

Stricture

A stricture is a narrowing caused by scar tissue. Reflux esophagitis with ulceration and scarring is the most common cause of stricture. Esophageal scarring also may result from accidentally or deliberately swallowing a corrosive chemical that causes necrosis and inflammation. Severe scarring eventually follows.

A common cause of esophageal stricture in children is accidental swallowing of commercial lye solutions (used for cleaning clogged drains). The ingestion of other household cleaning agents and disc batteries is also a frequent cause.

Diseases of the Stomach

Gastritis Inflammation of the stomach.

Cyclooxygenase Enzyme needed for synthesis of prostaglandins.

Diseases of the stomach include acute and chronic **gastritis**, peptic ulcer, carcinoma of the stomach, and gastroenteritis.

Gastritis

Inflammation of the stomach is termed gastritis, and the inflammation may be either acute or chronic. Many patients with gastritis have few symptoms, but some experience abdominal discomfort and nausea. However, acute gastritis may be severe enough to result in a life-threatening hemorrhage.

Acute Gastritis

In most cases, acute gastritis is a self-limited inflammation of short duration. However, at times, the acute inflammation may be quite severe and may be complicated by ulceration of the mucosa with bleeding from the ulcerated areas. Patients with acute gastritis associated with mucosal ulceration often have more pronounced symptoms, and the ulcerated areas may bleed profusely, a condition termed acute hemorrhagic gastritis.

There are many causes of acute gastritis, but the most common is related to the use of nonsteroidal anti-inflammatory drugs (NSAIDs) such as aspirin, ibuprofen, and naproxen. These drugs are widely used to treat symptoms of arthritis and related musculoskeletal pain problems. The drugs act by inhibiting an enzyme termed **cyclooxygenase**, which is required for the synthesis of prostaglandins (potent mediators discussed in Chapter 4). Prostaglandins are produced by many different cells and have many different functions. Those produced by gastric epithelial cells help protect the stomach from the damaging effects of gastric acid by promoting the secretion not only of sodium bicarbonate to counteract the acid but also of mucin to coat and protect the stomach lining. Consequently, NSAIDs cause the mucosa to become more vulnerable to injury from acidic gastric juice, which may lead to acute inflammation of the mucosa and in some cases even be followed by mucosal ulceration with bleeding.

There are two forms of cyclooxygenase. One form (COX-1) is constitutive (is always active) and promotes the synthesis of the prostaglandins that protect gastric mucosa. The other form (COX-2) is involved in the synthesis of the prostaglandins that function as mediators of inflammation and the symptoms associated with infections. COX-2 is not always active but is induced by these inflammatory conditions. NSAIDs such as aspirin, which are available "over the counter," inhibit both forms of the enzyme, suppressing the symptoms of inflammation (fever, aches, and pains) but also placing the gastric mucosa at risk. Some NSAIDs are more selective for COX-2, thereby reducing the risk of damaging gastric mucosa. NSAIDs also pose a low risk of causing heart attacks and strokes compared to COX-2 inhibitors. Currently only one selective COX-2 inhibitor is available in the United States (celecoxib). The drug carries a warning of increased cardiovascular risk and still may be associated with gastrointestinal risk. Hence, many physicians favor limiting the use of COX-2 selective inhibitors unless their benefits outweigh the possible cardiovascular risks.

Excess ingestion of alcoholic beverages is another common cause of acute gastritis because alcohol is a gastric irritant and also stimulates gastric acid secretion. In addition, any type of stress (such as burns, surgery, or serious systemic infections) may compromise the circulation to the stomach and contribute to the formation of acute gastritis, erosion of the stomach wall, and, if severe, stress ulcers.

Chronic Gastritis and Its Complications: The Role of Helicobacter pylori

Many cases of chronic gastritis are related to growth (colonization) of a small, curved, gram-negative organism termed *Helicobacter pylori* on the surface of the gastric mucosa. This unique organism grows in the layer of mucus covering the epithelial cells lining the stomach, where it can be identified by special bacterial stains, by culture, or by other specialized tests. The organism produces an enzyme termed "urease," which decomposes urea, a normal by-product of protein metabolism that is present in small amounts in blood and body fluids. Decomposition of urea yields ammonia, a substance that neutralizes the gastric acid and allows the organism to flourish in an acid environment that would destroy other bacteria. Helicobacters also produce enzymes that can break down the layer of protective mucus that covers the epithelial surface. Presumably, chronic gastritis is caused by the ammonia and other products produced by the organism that damage the gastric mucosa of susceptible individuals.

Colonization of the gastric mucosa by *H. pylori* is very common, and not all people who harbor the organism have chronic gastritis. About 30 percent of people younger than 30 years of age are colonized by *H. pylori*. By age 50, the proportion increases to about 50 percent and may be as high as 65 percent in people older than age 65. The spread of the organisms appears to be by mouth-to-mouth contact and also by the fecal-oral route; the organism has been cultured from both dental plaque material and from fecal material.

There are also some uncommon but important long-term harmful effects of Helicobacter infection. Chronic gastritis caused by this organism slightly increases the risk of two different gastric tumors: gastric carcinoma and malignant lymphoma arising from lymphocytes in the gastric mucosa (termed mucosa-associated lymphoid tissue, MALT). The gastric carcinoma risk occurs because gastritis often leads to atrophy of the gastric mucosa (atrophic gastritis) and causes the gastric epithelium to change into an abnormal intestinal-type epithelium (a process termed intestinal metaplasia). It is these cellular changes in the gastric mucosa that predispose to gastric carcinoma. Patients with severe atrophic gastritis associated with *H. pylori* may have up to a 90-fold increased cancer risk. The lymphoma risk probably results because gastritis overstimulates the mucosa-associated lymphoid tissue, which may lead to unregulated growth of lymphocytes that eventually progresses to gastric lymphoma.

Peptic Ulcer

Peptic ulcer is a chronic ulcer that usually involves the distal stomach or proximal duodenum (**Figure 21-5**). The ulcer results from digestion of the mucosa by acid gastric juice. People who secrete large volumes of acidic gastric juice and who are infected with *H. pylori* are prone to ulcers. The bacterium is present in nearly all patients with duodenal ulcer disease but is not, in itself, sufficient to cause the disease; many people harboring the agent do not develop ulcers.

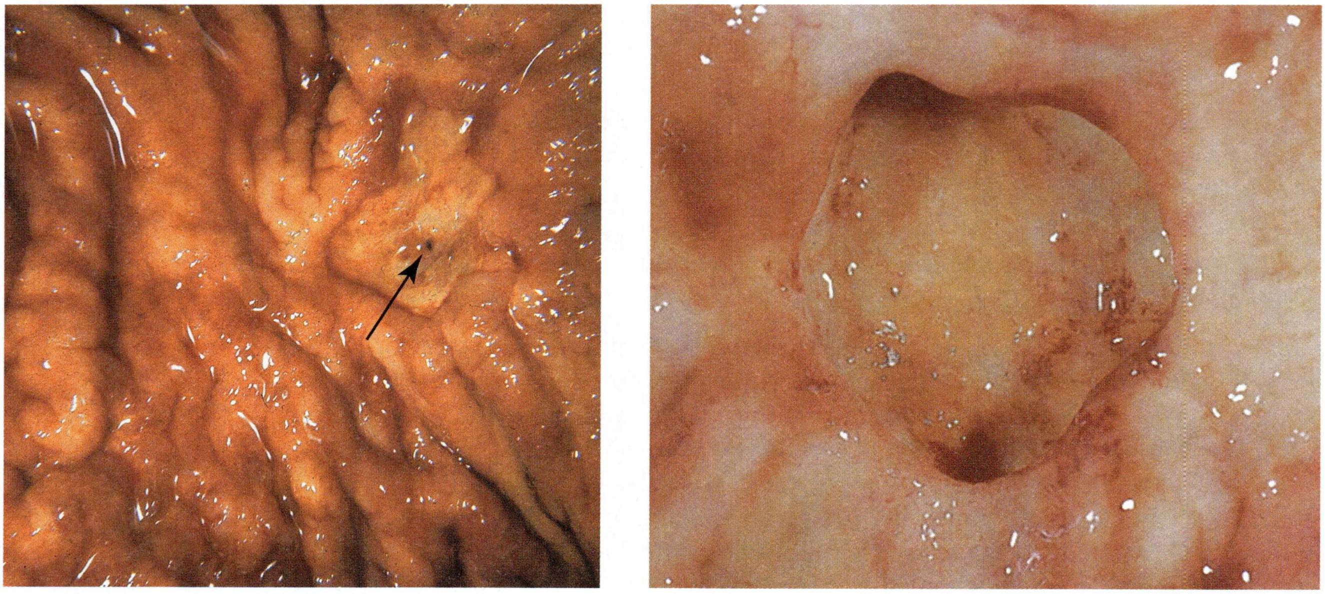

(A) (B)

Figure 21-5 Peptic ulcers. **(A)** Gastric ulcer, which eroded a blood vessel in the base of the ulcer (*arrow*) and bled profusely. **(B)** Large chronic duodenal ulcer.

Courtesy of Leonard V. Crowley, MD, Century College.

Only about 75 percent of patients with gastric ulcers have *H. pylori* infection, and cases in noninfected patients are likely related to other causes.

The initial event is probably a small, superficial erosion of the gastric or duodenal mucosa. Gastric acid and pepsin begin to digest the deeper tissues, which have been denuded from protective epithelium. The hypersecretion of acid (in part related to inflammation caused by *H. pylori* infection) appears important in this process. *H. pylori* are not generally found in the duodenum (but rather the gastric mucosa), so an indirect role for the organism in stimulating acid secretion seems likely. Attempts at healing in the presence of continuing digestion eventually lead to considerable scarring at the base of the ulcer. Clinically, ulcers produce pain that is usually relieved by ingestion of food or antacids that neutralize the gastric acid.

Peptic ulcer complications include hemorrhage, perforation, and obstruction. An ulcer may erode into a large blood vessel, causing severe hemorrhage, or erode completely through the wall of the stomach or duodenum, causing a perforation through which gastric and duodenal contents leak into the peritoneal cavity, resulting in a generalized inflammation of the peritoneum (peritonitis). Sometimes the scarring that follows healing of a gastric ulcer may be so severe as to cause obstruction of the outlet of the stomach, termed the pylorus, preventing the stomach from emptying properly.

Triple therapy Treatment of ulcer with proton pump inhibitors combined with two antibiotics.

Peptic ulcer is generally treated by antacids, which neutralize the excess gastric acid, or by drugs that block the secretion of acid by the gastric epithelial cells (histamine receptor blockers and proton pump inhibitors). Antibiotics are used to eliminate *H. pylori*. **Triple therapy**, using a proton pump inhibitor combined with two antibiotics (often clarithromycin and amoxicillin, sometimes combined with metronidazole), is successful in up to 90 percent of cases and is often undertaken in the absence of laboratory-confirmed bacterial infection. Sometimes quadruple therapy is used when triple therapy has failed. In such cases, bismuth subsalicylate (Pepto-Bismol) may be added along with other antibiotics.

Carcinoma of the Stomach

At one time, carcinoma of the stomach was the most common malignant tumor, but the incidence has been markedly decreasing. This is likely related to the decreased consumption of smoked and cured meat products with the advent of refrigerators for the preservation of fresh foods. The initial symptom may be only vague, upper abdominal discomfort. Sometimes the first manifestation is an iron deficiency anemia, the result of chronic blood loss from the ulcerated surface of the tumor. Gastric carcinoma is often treated by resection of a large part of the stomach together with the surrounding tissues and draining lymph nodes (**Figure 21-6**). This is often combined with adjuvant therapy using both radiation and chemotherapeutic drugs. Unfortunately, gastric carcinoma is often far advanced and has metastasized by the time it causes symptoms; consequently, long-term survival of patients with stomach carcinoma is relatively poor. Some cases of gastric carcinoma may be restricted to mucosa or submucosa (termed early gastric cancer). Such very early-stage cancer is sometimes treated using an endoscopic procedure to remove localized lesions. Sometimes gastric carcinoma may produce

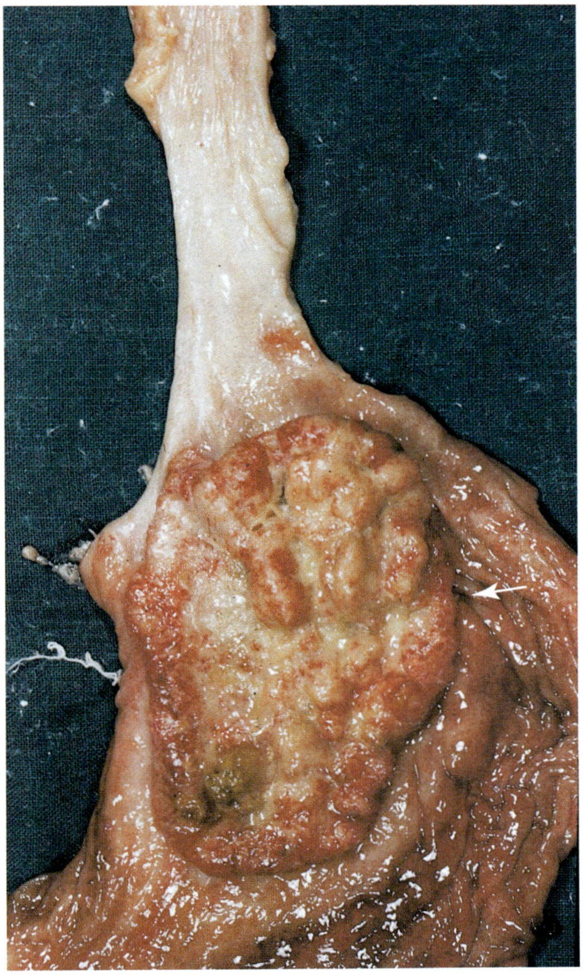

(A)

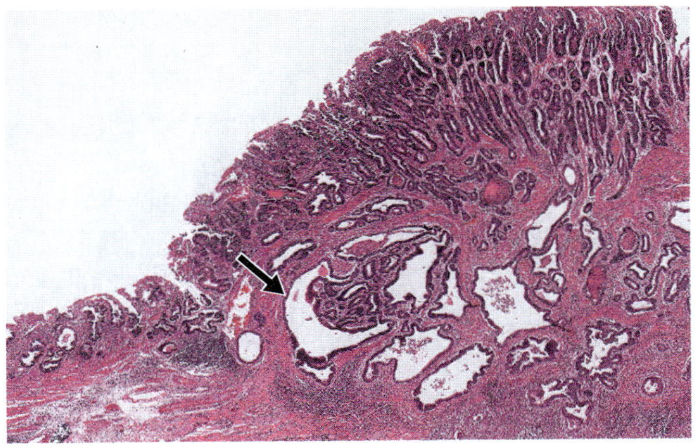

(B)

Figure 21-6 Carcinoma of the stomach. **(A)** The stomach has been opened, revealing a large, ulcerated neoplasm arising from the gastric mucosa (*arrow*) and extending upward to the gastroesophageal junction. The esophagus is seen in the upper part of the photograph. **(B)** Photomicrograph of carcinoma of the stomach in the setting of chronic gastritis. Glands (adenocarcinoma) invading the body of the stomach are highlighted (*arrow*).

(A) Courtesy of Leonard V. Crowley, MD, Century College; **(B)** Courtesy of Department of Pathology and Laboratory Medicine, University of North Carolina at Chapel Hill.

symptoms similar to those of a benign peptic ulcer. The distinction usually can be made by endoscopic techniques (gastroscopy) and, if necessary, via examination of biopsy material.

Diseases of the Small Intestine

Enteritis Inflammation of the intestinal tract.
Rotavirus An RNA virus that is transmitted primarily through the oral-fecal route and causes severe gastroenteritis in children.
Norovirus An extremely infectious RNA virus easily spread from person to person and by contaminated food or water.

Diseases of the intestine can be divided into those that predominantly affect the small bowel or the large (colon), although there is some overlap. Acute viral and bacterial **enteritis** predominantly affect the small intestine (and in some cases the stomach, so the term gastroenteritis is sometimes used).

Acute Viral Gastroenteritis

Viral gastroenteritis is commonly caused by either **rotavirus** or **norovirus**, both having RNA genomes. The condition is characterized by an abrupt onset of nausea, vomiting, abdominal cramps, and profuse diarrhea, which may affect only a few people or may occur as an epidemic affecting large numbers of people. Usually, the illness subsides spontaneously within a few days, and no specific treatment is required. Severely affected people may require intravenous fluids to replace depleted body fluids and electrolytes resulting from diarrhea.

Rotavirus primarily affects infants and young children, most commonly in the winter and spring. It is spread via an oral–fecal route and can contaminate food and surfaces. Outbreaks occur in the daycare setting and occasionally as widespread epidemics related to contaminated food or water. An effective oral vaccine is now available.

Norovirus is extremely contagious and is now the leading cause of illness from contaminated food in the United States. Contaminated leaf greens, fresh fruits, and shellfish are the most common sources. The illness is also spread from person to person, stool and vomitus being viral sources. Outbreaks tend to occur in closed places such as daycare centers and nursing homes and on cruise ships. Unlike the case with rotavirus, no vaccine is available, and proper sanitary techniques (including frequent hand washing and washing contaminated clothing) are critical for prevention. The virus can remain infective in feces for up to two weeks after symptoms subside. Norovirus is resistant to some disinfecting agents, so the use of agents registered to be effective against the virus (such as 5.3 percent chlorine bleach) is important. There are many strains of norovirus, and recurrent infection is possible.

Acute Bacterial Gastroenteritis

Pathology from acute bacterial infections usually occurs by infection of known pathogens or the toxins they produce (see Chapter 7). These infections are predominantly diseases of the small intestine. They are generally of short duration and may subside without specific treatment or may respond to appropriate antibiotics or other agents. Clinical manifestations include nausea, vomiting, abdominal discomfort, and passage of many loose stools. In severe infections, the bowel mucosa may be ulcerated, and the diarrheal stools may be bloody. Bacterial diarrhea (commonly caused by *Escherichia coli* and *Vibrio* species) is a major cause of death in young children, accounting for more than three-quarters of the deaths of children in developing countries in Africa and Asia.

Cholera, caused by ingestion of the bacteria *Vibrio cholerae* from contaminated water, remains a common and in some regions endemic cause of severe and potentially fatal diarrhea. An outbreak of cholera in Yemen associated with the ongoing civil war is reported to be the largest in recorded history, with more than 1.2 million cases through 2018 and over 2500 deaths, the majority in children. By comparison, there are usually fewer than 20 cholera cases per year in the United States, and these are usually imported by travelers. The bacteria do not invade the mucosa of the small bowel but rather multiply in the mucous layer, where they secrete a cholera toxin that causes the intestinal cells to secrete large amounts of water and sodium ions into the intestinal lumen, which results in profound diarrhea and salt loss leading to dehydration, shock, and death if untreated. Replacement of lost fluids and salt with oral rehydration fluids consisting of water, salt, and glucose is a simple and highly effective therapy. Antibiotics shorten the course of the disease.

Disturbances of Bowel Function: Food Intolerance

Some patients manifest crampy abdominal pain, abdominal distention, flatulence (excessive gas in the intestinal tract), and frequent loose stools as a result of food intolerance. The two most common types are lactose intolerance and gluten intolerance.

Lactose Intolerance

Lactose is a disaccharide found in milk and dairy products. During digestion, lactose must be split into its two monosaccharides, glucose and galactose, before it can be absorbed. This process is catalyzed by an enzyme termed lactase, which is present on the mucosal surface of the epithelial cells in the small intestine. The enzyme is abundant in infants and young children. In many populations, however, the concentration of lactase gradually declines to very low levels during adolescence and early adult life. However, some populations tend to have persistent levels of lactase into adulthood. The enzyme is deficient in about 20 percent of adult Whites, 70 percent of American Blacks, 90 percent of American Indians, and almost all Asians. A complete deficiency of lactase is a rare autosomal recessive trait found in some Finnish families. It has serious consequences because neonates cannot digest milk.

People with lactase deficiency are unable to digest lactose. Consequently, lactose cannot be absorbed and remains within the intestinal lumen, where it raises the osmotic pressure of the intestinal contents. Because of the high intraluminal osmotic pressure, fluid is retained within the intestinal tract instead of being absorbed normally, leading to abdominal discomfort, cramps, and diarrhea. Some of the unabsorbed lactose is fermented by bacteria in the colon, yielding lactic acid and other organic acids that further raise the intraluminal osmotic pressure and contribute to the person's discomfort. The symptoms are related to ingestion of lactose containing dairy products and abate promptly when intake of dairy products is reduced or discontinued. Lactase-containing supplements are available and are effective for some individuals.

Gluten Intolerance

Gluten is composed of several macropolymers of proteins found in wheat, rye, oats, and barley. The gluten in wheat flour is responsible for imparting the elasticity to bread dough necessary during rising. Some people have a hereditary predisposition to become sensitive to one of the proteins in gluten termed **gliadin**. During digestion gluten is broken into its component proteins, including gliadin, which is not completely digested. Within the layers of the wall of

Gliadin A protein component of gluten causing an adverse immune response that damages the small intestine.

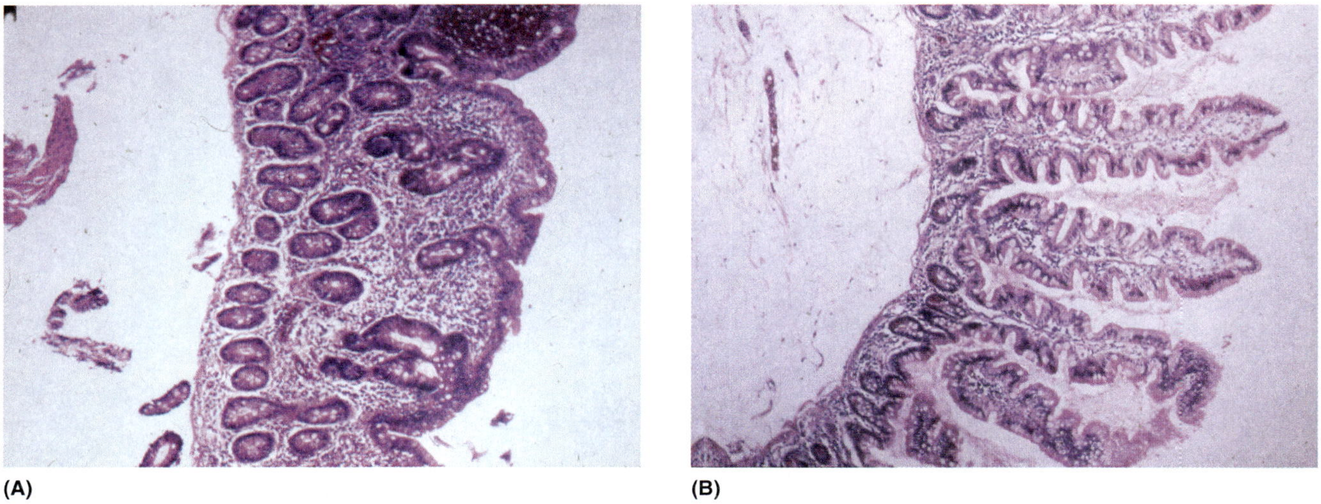

Figure 21-7 Low-magnification. Photomicrographs comparing appearance of a trophic intestinal villi caused by gluten sensitivity **(A)** with normal-appearing villi after excluding gluten from the diet for several months **(B)**.

Tissue transglutaminase Human enzyme target of antibodies detected in gluten sensitivity.

Gluten-sensitive enteropathy (GSE) Damage to intestinal villi in gluten-sensitive people caused by ingestion of gluten-containing food; characterized by passage of large, bulky stools containing a large amount of poorly absorbed fat.

the small intestine, a naturally occurring enzyme, **tissue transglutaminase** (tTG), acts by deamidating glutamic acid residues in the gliadin, making it highly immunogenic in genetically susceptible individuals. Levels of tTG become elevated as a result of inflammation and also act as an autoantigen in susceptible people. These individuals form antigliadin antibodies and activated gliadin-sensitized T cells and anti-tTG antibodies. The autoimmune response leads to atrophy of the intestinal villi in the duodenum and proximal jejunum (**Figure 21-7**). As a result, digestion and absorption of fats and other nutrients are impaired. Several different names have been applied to this condition. The most descriptive term is **gluten-sensitive enteropathy (GSE)**, but the condition (particularly in severe forms) is also known as celiac disease or celiac sprue. Clinically, the condition is characterized by the passage of frequent, large, bulky stools containing much unabsorbed fat and is associated with weight loss and vitamin deficiencies as a result of the impaired intestinal absorption. Extraintestinal symptoms, including anemia and osteoporosis, may also occur, presumably related to malabsorption. GSE has a major genetic component because essentially all patients have two specific separate genes in different parts of the HLA complex. In addition, infection with adenovirus type 12 may be a factor, because the virus has a protein similar in structure to alpha-gliadin.

A simple serological test for the presence of antibodies (generally of the IgA class) to the human enzyme tissue transglutaminase or tests for the presence of antibodies reactive with the endomysium (muscle fiber sheath rich in tissue transglutaminase) have greatly simplified the diagnosis of GSE and reduced the need for biopsy of the small intestinal mucosa to reveal atrophy of the intestinal villi. When indicated, the specimen for biopsy is obtained by a flexible biopsy device with a small capsule on the end that is swallowed by the patient. The device is positioned in the upper jejunum and is manipulated so that a small bit of intestinal mucosa enters the capsule. Then the capsule is closed, cutting off and retaining a piece of mucosa. Adopting a gluten-free diet promptly cures the condition, and the intestinal villi return to normal in 3 or 4 months. The current wide variety of gluten-free products makes maintenance of such a diet easier. Some potential sources of hidden gluten, such as soy sauce and teriyaki sauce, should also be recognized and avoided. For patients suffering from anemia or nutritional deficiencies, supplements of vitamins, folic acid, and iron are recommended. In severe cases when small intestines are severely damaged or with refractory celiac diseases (persistent or recurrent symptoms despite the treatment/management), steroids may be prescribed to control inflammation. Although the topic is controversial, there is evidence that GSE has been underdiagnosed in the past and has resulted in increased morbidity in the undiagnosed population. Even individuals who test negative in the described clinical assay may appear to be gluten-sensitive and suffer from GSE. Additional discussion is presented in the case for this chapter.

Irritable Bowel Syndrome

Some patients exhibit episodes of cramps, abdominal discomfort, loud gurgling bowel sounds (**borborygmi**), and disturbed bowel function. Frequent loose stools sometimes alternate with periods of constipation, and excessive amounts of mucus are secreted by the colonic mucosal glands. These manifestations are frequently quite distressing to the affected individual, but no structural or biochemical abnormalities can be identified to account for the functional disturbances. This condition is often termed **irritable bowel syndrome (IBS)**. Other terms for this very common condition are spastic **colitis** and mucous colitis. Diarrhea-predominant IBS (IBS-D) and constipation-predominant IBS (IBS-C), along with a mixed form, are recognized subtypes.

The diagnosis of IBS is one of the exclusions, as there is no recognized specific test. The healthcare provider must rule out infections as a result of pathogenic bacteria and intestinal parasites, food intolerance, and various types of chronic enteritis such as **Crohn's disease** and chronic ulcerative colitis (see Chronic Enteritis).

The goal of the treatment of IBS is to alleviate symptoms and enhance the well-being of the patients. This can be achieved by dietary changes and medications (such as smooth muscle relaxants, antidiarrheal medications, and laxatives, to name a few). Antidepressants and psychotherapy might also be helpful. It has been shown that stress plays an important role in the frequency and severity of symptoms in IBS patients.

Borborygmi Loud bowel sounds.

Irritable bowel syndrome (IBS) A condition characterized by frequent loose stools and excessive amounts of mucus. This umbrella term includes Crohn's disease and ulcerative colitis.

Colitis Inflammation restricted to colon.

Crohn's disease A type of chronic enteritis with the potential to impact any areas of the digestive tract. Most frequently involving the end of the small intestine and the beginning of the large intestine, inflammation often spreads to the deeper layer of the bowel.

Inflammatory Diseases of the Bowel

The intestine may be the site of both acute and chronic inflammation. The term *enteritis* (enteron = bowel) is used to describe inflammation of any part of the intestinal tract. The term *colitis* denotes inflammation restricted to the colon, and the general term *bowel inflammation* refers to any part of the intestinal tract, either the small intestine, the colon, or both.

Appendicitis

Appendicitis is the most common inflammatory lesion of the bowel. In many animals, the portion of the bowel represented in humans by the appendix is a large, wide-caliber intestinal segment, similar in appearance to the remainder of the colon. In humans, this segment of bowel is reduced in both size and caliber to the extent that it approaches being a vestigial structure.

The high incidence of acute appendicitis is due primarily to the narrow caliber of the appendix, the base of which often becomes plugged by firm bits of fecal material or, in some cases, plant seeds or parasitic worms. Because of the obstruction, the secretions normally produced by the epithelial cells lining the appendix drain poorly from the area distal to the blockage. The accumulated

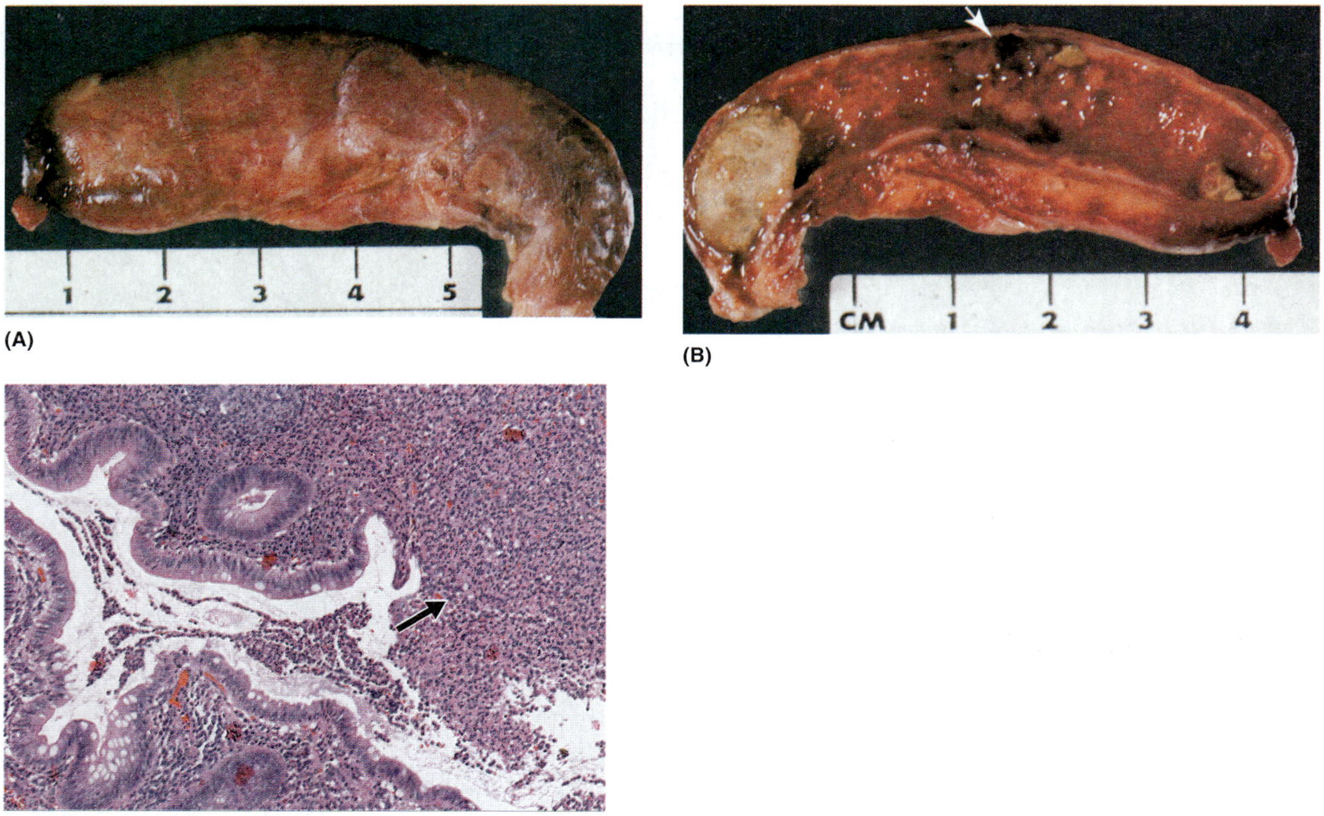

(A)

(B)

(C)

Figure 21-8 Acute appendicitis. **(A)** The exterior of the appendix is swollen, congested, and covered with inflammatory exudate. **(B)** Appendix bisected to reveal interior. Pus within the lumen has been removed. The mucosa is congested and ulcerated (*arrow*). The base of the appendix (*left side*) is plugged by a firm mass of fecal material. **(C)** Photomicrograph of removed appendix. The lumen is filled with inflammatory cells (pus). The wall of the intestine has been destroyed and replaced by an area of inflammatory cells (*arrows*).

(A, B) Courtesy of Leonard V. Crowley, MD, Century College; **(C)** Courtesy of Department of Pathology and Laboratory Medicine, University of North Carolina at Chapel Hill.

secretions create pressure within the appendiceal lumen. This compresses the blood vessels in the mucosa, impairing its viability (**Figure 21-8**). Bacteria normally present in the appendix and colon invade the devitalized wall, causing an acute inflammation.

Clinically, appendicitis is characterized by generalized abdominal pain that soon becomes localized to the right lower part (quadrant) of the abdomen. Examination of the abdomen reveals localized tenderness over the appendix when pressure is applied to the abdomen by the fingers of the examiner. Often, the patient also experiences pain when the pressure is released suddenly (rebound tenderness). In addition, there is usually reflex contraction of the abdominal muscles (abdominal rigidity) in response to the underlying inflammation. Laboratory tests reveal that the number of polymorphonuclear leukocytes in the blood also is increased. Currently, CT examination of the abdominal area and, in some cases (particularly in children), ultrasound are highly accurate in establishing a diagnosis, and laparoscopy is rarely needed.

Patients with suspected appendicitis are treated with antibiotics, which are followed by surgery if the condition does not resolve. However, a significant number of such patients may require surgery because of treatment failure or recurrence. Severe inflammation may lead to rupture of the appendix and peritonitis. For this reason, it is essential to identify appendicitis and, if necessary, remove the appendix.

Chronic Enteritis

Chronic enteritis refers to long-lasting inflammation of the small intestine. It may also include gastroenteritis (stomach inflammation) or enterocolitis (inflammation of the large intestine). It's usually caused by a viral, bacterial, or parasitic infection. Sometimes it's caused by radiation, drugs, or disease. Chronic enteritis is less common and more difficult to treat.

Treatment of Chronic Enteritis

Treatment of inflammatory bowel disease involves symptomatic and supportive measures, including antibiotics, corticosteroids to control disease symptoms during flare-ups, and immunosuppressive drugs, particularly biological inhibitors (monoclonal antibodies) directed to components of the immune system, including TNF (tumor necrosis factor) inhibitors. Eventually, surgical resection of severely diseased bowel segments may be required in many patients. People with severe and extensive chronic ulcerative colitis may require total removal of the entire colon and rectum, both to control the disease and to eliminate the risk of colon carcinoma, which is prone to occur in patients with long-standing chronic disease. Some people taking broad-spectrum antibiotics develop mild diarrhea. Others, unfortunately, develop severe bloody diarrhea with abdominal pain, fever, and other systemic manifestations, which may be life-threatening, that are associated with exudative inflammatory plaques on the colonic mucosa (termed pseudomembranes). The multiple ulcerations of the colonic mucosa are covered by masses of fibrin and inflammatory cells. The most common causative agent is the anaerobic spore-forming intestinal bacterium *Clostridium difficile*.

Broad-spectrum antibiotics cause colitis by changing the intestinal bacterial flora. Most of the normal flora is destroyed, allowing the overgrowth of the more resistant *C. difficile* organism, which produces two toxins that cause intestinal inflammation and necrosis.

The diagnosis of antibiotic-associated colitis is most commonly established by detection of the bacterial toxin in the stool. Treatment consists of stopping the inciting antibiotic and giving antibiotics, such as metronidazole or vancomycin, that inhibit growth of the organism. Treatment should not include drugs that reduce the diarrhea by inhibiting intestinal motility. These drugs prolong the illness by allowing the injurious clostridial toxins to remain in the intestine instead of being eliminated rapidly in the diarrheal stools. The disease may reoccur and in some cases be life-threatening due in part to increased bacterial resistance to antibiotics. In these cases, "fecal transplants" from healthy donors have proved successful as a therapeutic measure for restoring the normal intestinal flora.

Crohn's Disease and Ulcerative Colitis

Crohn's disease can affect the entire gastrointestinal tract (most commonly the terminal ileum and sometimes the right colon), whereas ulcerative colitis (UC) tends to affect the rectum and progresses proximally up the colon. Often, the two diseases are grouped together under the general term chronic inflammatory bowel disease (IBD). Both diseases tend to be chronic, with periodic flare-ups manifested by cramp-like abdominal pain and diarrhea, followed by periods when the disease is inactive. During an active phase, the affected individuals may also have systemic manifestations, including joint inflammation, eye inflammation, and various types of skin nodules and skin infections. Although the diseases have similarities, there are also significant differences between them.

These two diseases appear to have both genetic and environmental components (see Chapter 5). Recent studies have provided further insight into their pathogenesis. Although multiple genes have been associated with susceptibility to each disease, the significance of this remains unclear. It is most likely that multiple factors, both environmental (and in particular gut microflora) and genetic, work together to trigger the inflammatory response that leads to these diseases, including an impaired immune response, defective barrier epithelium leading to penetration by intestinal bacteria, and the presence of activated T lymphocytes. However, it is uncertain whether the inflammatory reaction that damages the bowel is directed against intestinal bacteria that get into the intestinal wall periodically because epithelial barrier function is defective, or whether it is in part an autoimmune response directed against the patient's own cells because they contain some of the same antigenic determinants (cross-reacting antigens) as those possessed by the intestinal bacteria to which the immune system has responded.

Crohn's Disease

Crohn's disease is chronic inflammation and ulceration of the bowel mucosa with marked thickening and scarring of the entire bowel wall (**Figure 21-9**). The inflammation often affects scattered areas of the small bowel (skip lesions), leaving normal intervening segments of bowel between the areas of severe disease. Occasionally, affected individuals have such severe thickening and scarring of an involved segment of bowel that the lumen becomes greatly narrowed or even completely blocked, which impedes passage of bowel contents. Crohn's disease was originally termed regional ileitis because the inflammatory process is often localized to the distal ileum, but other parts of the small intestine may be involved, and the disease may involve the colon as well.

Multiple disposing factors can contribute to the development of Crohn's disease. These include damaged intestinal mucus membrane, dysregulation of innate and adaptive immune responses in the GI tract, and an imbalance between the organisms in the gut microflora (dysbiosis). There is a suspicion

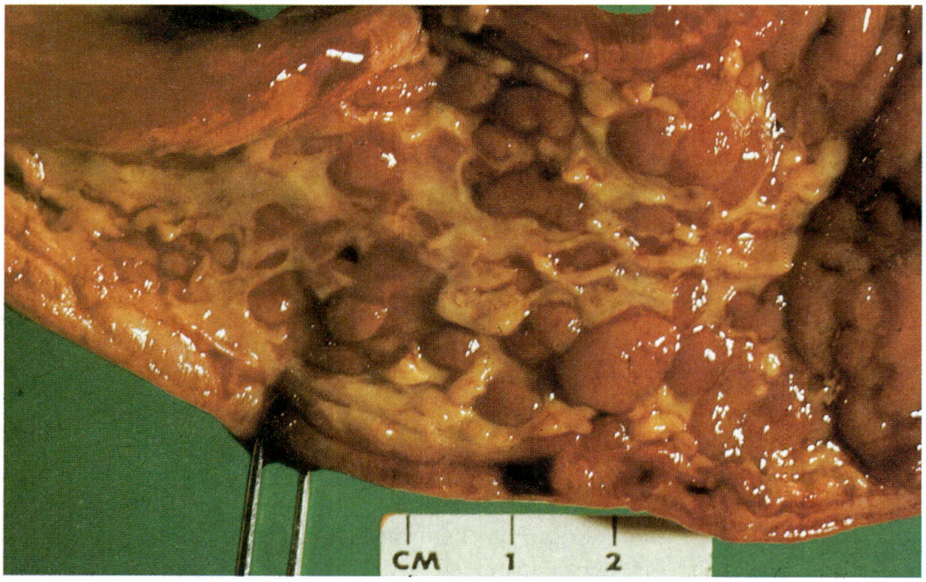

Figure 21-9 Crohn's disease (regional enteritis). Mucosa is ulcerated and covered by inflammatory exudate.

Courtesy of Leonard V. Crowley, MD, Century College.

that certain bacteria in the gut microbiome are associated with Crohn's, but it is unknown if they are causative and provoke an immune-mediated inflammatory disease or are "bystanders." Diagnosis of Crohn's disease can be challenging. It requires a comprehensive assessment of the patient's clinical history, review of physical exam results, and checking for the presence of biomarkers from blood and fecal samples.

There is no cure for Crohn's disease. Treatment involves the use of a variety of anti-inflammatory drugs and agents that modulate the immune response. The goal of the treatment is to promote mucosal healing, keep patients in remission, and increase the quality of life.

Chronic Ulcerative Colitis

In contrast to Crohn's disease, chronic ulcerative colitis targets the colon, not the small intestine. The inflammation is limited to the mucosa, and the bowel wall is not thickened as in Crohn's disease. Frequently, the disease begins in the rectal mucosa but may spread progressively until eventually the entire colon is involved. In severe cases, the ulcerated mucosa may bleed profusely, leading to bloody diarrhea, and at times the inflammatory process becomes so extensive that it leads to a perforation of the colon with escape of bowel contents into the peritoneal cavity. Affected people with long-standing disease also may develop carcinoma arising in the diseased regions of the colon or rectum.

As is the case with Crohn's disease, the cause is unknown and likely to result from the interaction among genetic, immune, and environmental triggers. Like Crohn's disease, the diagnosis of ulcerative colitis involves assessments from different perspectives. These include blood tests for anemia and raised inflammatory markers, endoscopy, fecal calprotectin tests that measure inflammation in the GI tract, radiographic studies including CT and MRI, and biopsies. 5-aminosalicylic acid (5-ASA, an anti-inflammatory aspirin-like agent) is usually the first line of treatment for moderate to mild forms of UC. It can be administrated rectally, or orally. 5-ASA is often used in combination with steroids for better outcomes. A number of immunomodulators and biologic agents are used to reduce inflammation. The treatment of ulcerative colitis is aimed at relieving symptoms and healing disease at the mucosal level, restoring the quality of life for the patient.

Structural Diseases of the Bowel

Intestinal Obstruction

If the normal passage of intestinal contents through the bowel is blocked, the patient is said to have an intestinal obstruction. The site of the blockage may be either the small intestine (high intestinal obstruction) or the colon (low intestinal obstruction). Bowel obstruction is always serious. The severity of the symptoms depends on the location of the obstruction, its completeness, and whether there is interference with the blood supply to the blocked segment of bowel.

Obstruction of the small intestine causes severe, crampy pain as a result of vigorous peristalsis, reflecting the attempt of the intestine to force bowel contents past the site of obstruction. This is associated with vomiting of copious amounts of gastric and upper intestinal secretions, resulting in loss of large quantities of water and electrolytes. As a consequence, the patient becomes dehydrated and develops pronounced fluid and electrolyte disturbances.

Symptoms are much less acute when the distal colon is obstructed. There may be mild, crampy abdominal pain and moderate distention of the abdomen.

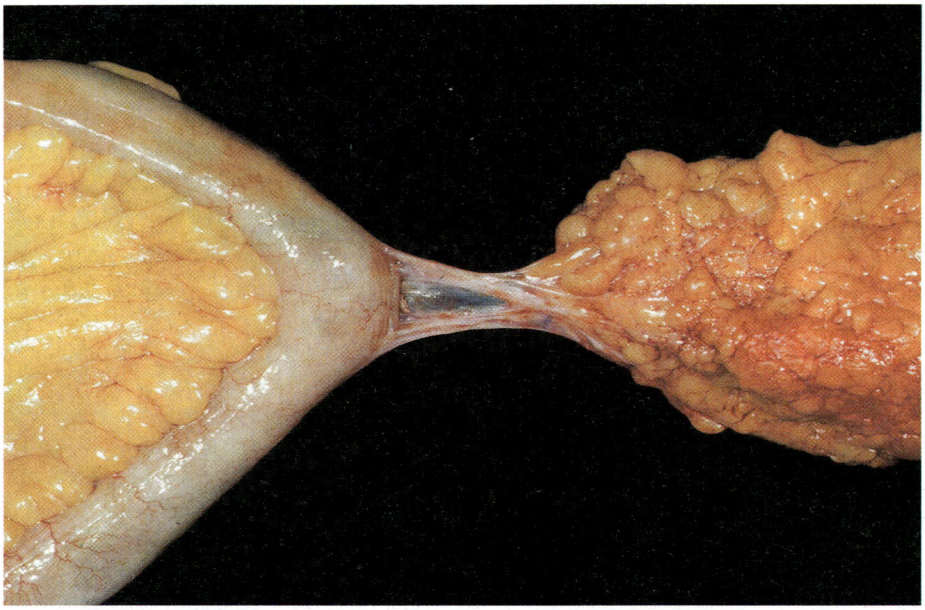

Figure 21-10 Fibrous adhesion between loop of small intestine (*left side*) and omentum.

Courtesy of Leonard V. Crowley, MD, Century College.

However, vomiting with associated loss of fluid and electrolytes is not as serious a problem as in high intestinal obstruction. Disturbances of fluid and electrolytes do not develop as rapidly.

The common causes of intestinal obstruction are intestinal **adhesion**, **hernia**, tumor, **volvulus**, **intussusception**, or neoplastic disease (most commonly carcinoma).

Adhesion Band of fibrous tissue that form subsequent to the inflammatory response, which may include scar tissue formation binding adjacent tissues together.

Hernia A protrusion of a loop of bowel through a narrow opening, usually in the abdominal wall.

Volvulus Rotary twisting of the bowel.

Intussusception Telescoping of a bowel segment into an adjacent segment.

Adhesions

Adhesive bands of connective tissue (adhesions) may form within the abdominal cavity after surgery (**Figure 21-10**). Sometimes a loop of bowel becomes kinked, compressed, or twisted by an adhesive band, causing obstruction proximal to the site of the adhesion. This often results from surgical procedures involving the bowel.

Hernia

A hernia is a protrusion of a loop of bowel through a small opening, usually in the abdominal wall. The herniated loop pushes the peritoneum ahead of it, forming the hernia sac. Inguinal hernia is quite common in men. A loop of small bowel protrudes through a weak area in the inguinal ring and may descend downward into the scrotum. Umbilical and femoral hernias occur in both sexes. In an umbilical hernia, the loop of bowel protrudes into the umbilicus through a defect in the abdominal wall (**Figure 21-11**). In a femoral hernia, a loop of intestine extends under the inguinal ligament along the course of the femoral vessels into the groin. If a herniated loop of bowel can be pushed back into the abdominal cavity, the hernia is said to be reducible. Occasionally, a herniated loop becomes stuck and cannot be reduced. This is termed an incarcerated hernia. Sometimes the loop of bowel is tightly constricted by the margins of the defect, and the blood supply to the herniated bowel is obstructed, causing necrosis of the protruding segment of bowel. This is termed a strangulated hernia and requires prompt surgical intervention.

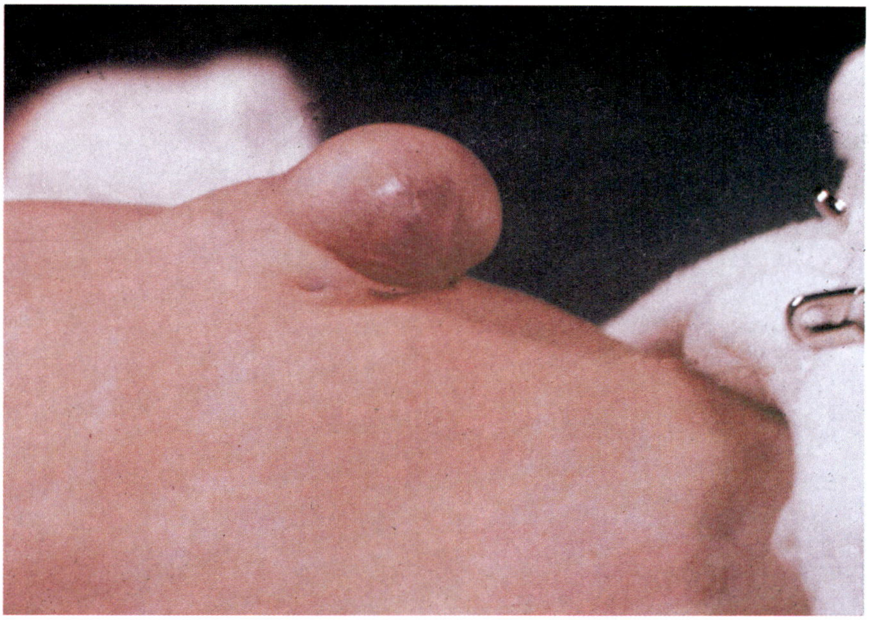

Figure 21-11 A large umbilical hernia in an infant.
Courtesy of Leonard V. Crowley, MD, Century College.

Volvulus and Intussusception

A volvulus is a rotary twisting of the bowel on the fold of peritoneum (the mesentery) that suspends the bowel from the posterior wall of the abdomen. The blood supply to the twisted segment also is impaired because the blood vessels supplying the bowel travel in the mesentery, and they are compressed when the bowel and mesentery become twisted. The sigmoid colon is the usual site for such a condition (**Figure 21-12**).

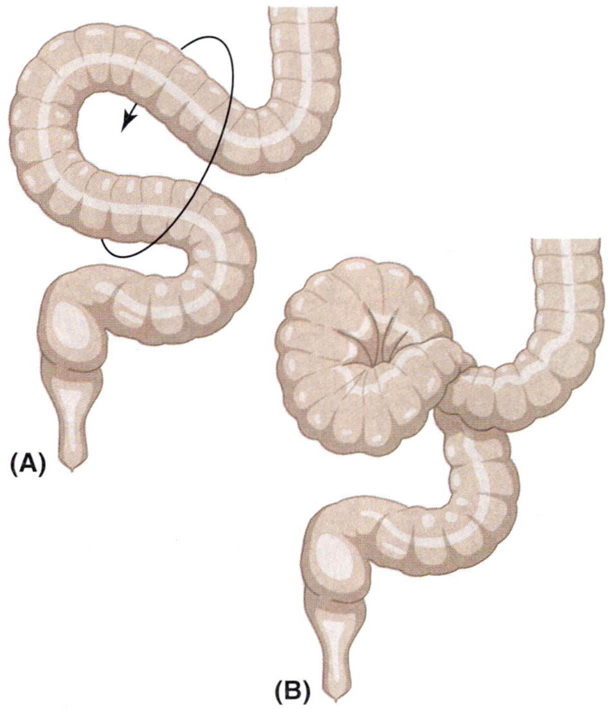

Figure 21-12 Pathogenesis of volvulus. **(A)** Rotary twist of sigmoid colon on its mesentery. **(B)** Obstruction of the colon and interruption of its blood supply caused by volvulus.

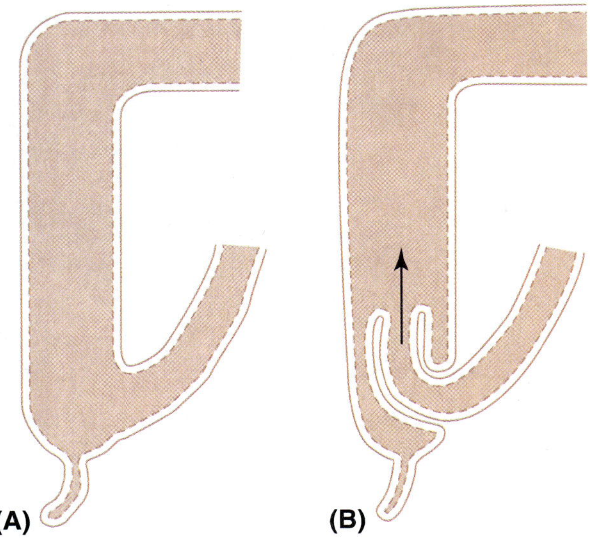

Figure 21-13 Pathogenesis of ileocecal intussusception. **(A)** Normal anatomic relationships. **(B)** Vigorous peristalsis carries the ileum into the cecum. The dashed lines indicate mucosa.

An intussusception is a telescoping of one segment of bowel into an adjacent segment. This is a common cause of intestinal obstruction in children and usually results from vigorous peristalsis that telescopes the terminal ileum into the proximal colon through the ileocecal valve (**Figure 21-13** and **Figure 21-14**). In adults, the condition is usually secondary to a tumor of the bowel that is supported by a narrow stalk. A tumor of this type is often termed a pedunculated tumor, the name being derived from the stalk (pedicle) that supports it (pediculus = little foot). As the tumor is propelled by a peristaltic wave, the base of the tumor exerts traction on the bowel wall at its site of attachment, causing the proximal segment to telescope into the distal bowel (**Figure 21-15** and **Figure 21-16**). In children, the cause is most often unknown but may be related to an intestinal infection or, rarely, to a rotavirus vaccine immunization that causes enlargement of gut lymph, which becomes

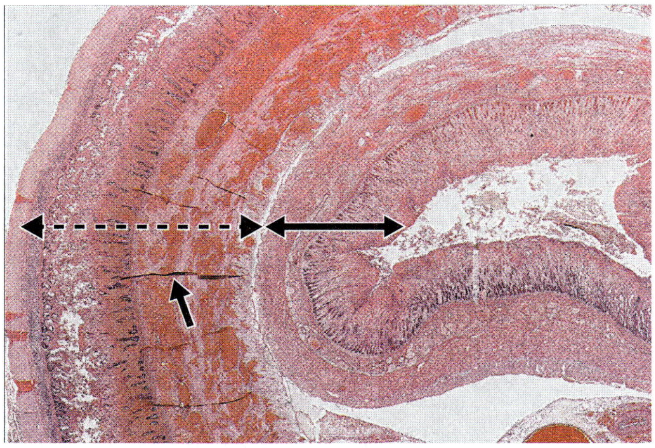

Figure 21-14 Photomicrograph of an ileocecal intussusception. The solid line indicates invaginated ileum, and the dashed line indicates multiple layers of cecum that are necrotic as a result of compromise of blood supply. An artifactual fold in the tissue (*arrow*) occurred during processing.

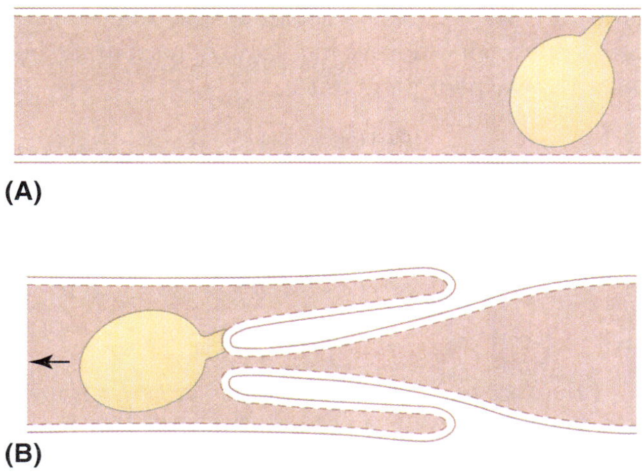

Figure 21-15 Pathogenesis of intussusception caused by tumor. **(A)** Pedunculated tumor protrudes into the lumen of the bowel. **(B)** Peristalsis propels the tumor and produces traction on its base, causing the proximal segment of the bowel to be telescoped into the distal segment. The dashed lines indicate mucosa.

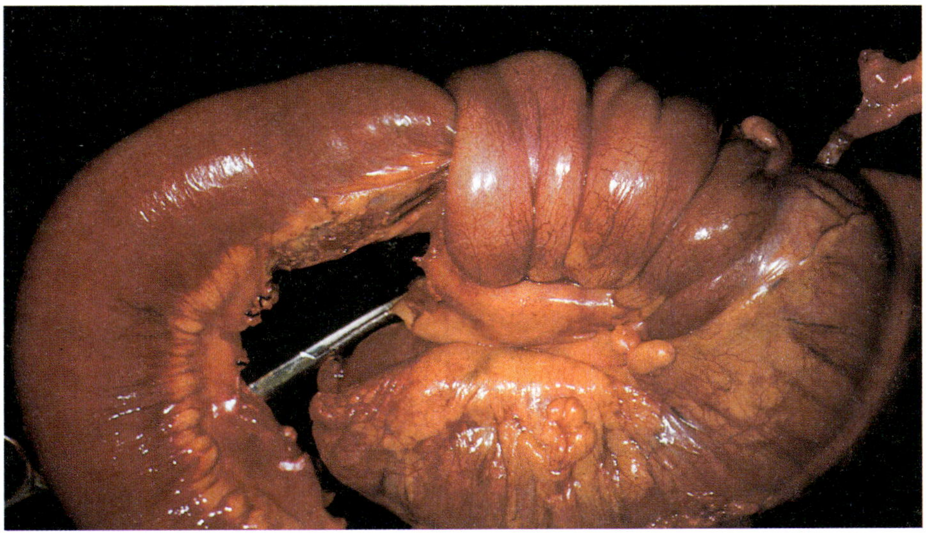

Figure 21-16 Intussusception of the colon as a result of a colon tumor. The midportion of the colon is swollen because of telescoping of the proximal segment (*left side*) into the distal segment (*right side*).

Courtesy of Leonard V. Crowley, MD, Century College.

"caught" in peristalsis and leads to the formation of the intussusception. In children, the use of either an air or barium enema may lead to the unfolding and release of the intussusception. If not relieved, the intussusception can result in bowel infarction (necrosis as a result of compromised blood supply) (**Figure 21-17**).

Mesenteric Thrombosis

The blood supply to the gastrointestinal tract is derived from several large arteries arising from the aorta. The blood supply to most of the bowel is provided by the superior mesenteric artery. This vessel supplies blood to the entire small intestine and the proximal half of the colon. The arteries supplying the gastrointestinal tract may develop arteriosclerotic changes and become occluded by thrombosis in the same way as many other arteries. Thrombosis of the superior mesenteric artery leads to an extensive infarction of most of the bowel, a medical emergency with a very poor prognosis.

Diseases of the Colon and Anus

Diverticulosis A condition characterized by outpouchings of the colonic mucosa through weak areas in the muscular wall.
Diverticulitis An inflammation of a diverticulum.
Hemorrhoids Dilated veins around the anus and the rectum.

Diseases of the colon and anus include **diverticulosis**, **diverticulitis**, tumors both benign and malignant, and **hemorrhoids**.

Diverticulosis and Diverticulitis

Outpouchings of the mucosa of the colon often project through weak areas in the muscular wall of the large intestine. These outpouchings are termed diverticula (singular, diverticulum), and the condition is termed diverticulosis (**Figure 21-17** and **Figure 21-18**). This is an acquired condition, in contrast to Meckel diverticulum, which is a congenital abnormality (Chapter 16). Diverticula, which usually occur in the distal colon, are encountered with increasing frequency in older patients. Highly refined, low-residue diets predispose to diverticula because stools are small and hard, requiring high intraluminal pressure generated by peristalsis to propel them through the colon. This high intracolonic pressure forces the mucosa through weak areas in the muscular wall. In contrast, people who subsist on high-residue diets have large, bulky stools that can be propelled through the colon easily at low intraluminal pressures, and diverticula occur infrequently among them.

Most diverticula are asymptomatic, but occasionally problems arise. Bits of fecal material may become trapped within these pouches and incite an inflammatory reaction termed diverticulitis. The inflammation may be followed by considerable scarring. Occasionally, perforation of a diverticulum

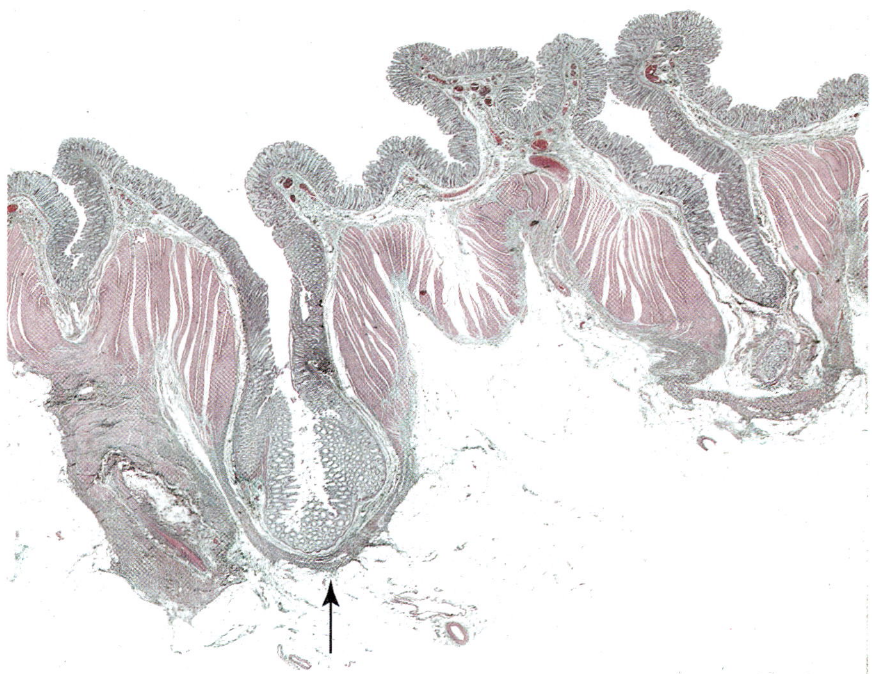

Figure 21-17 A low-magnification photomicrograph of a colon illustrating diverticula. The mucosa of the colon (*upper part*) protrudes through the muscular wall (*arrow*) into the serosa of the colon.

Courtesy of Leonard V. Crowley, MD, Century College.

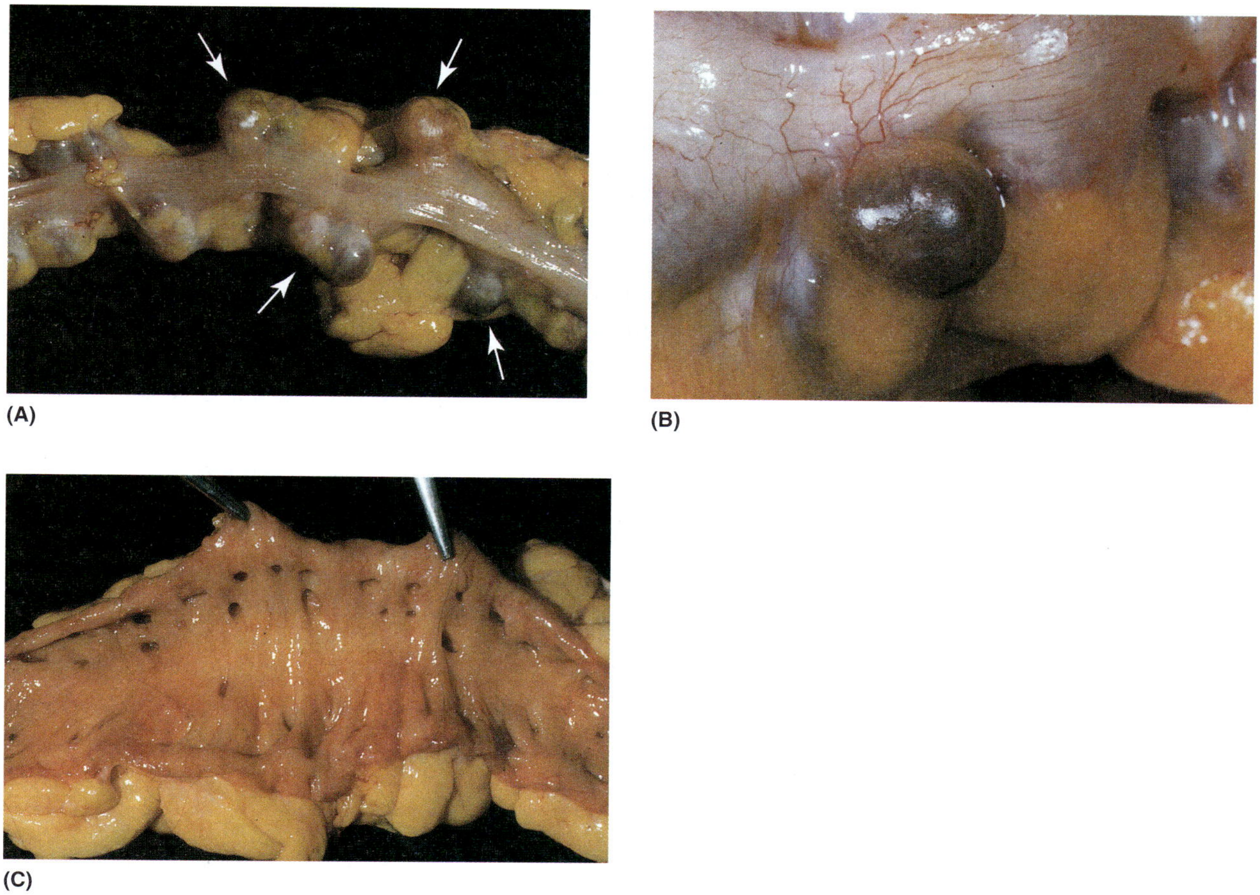

Figure 21-18 Diverticulosis of the colon. **(A)** Exterior of colon illustrating several diverticula projecting through wall of colon (*arrows*). **(B)** A closer view of the diverticulum. **(C)** Interior of colon, illustrating openings of multiple diverticula. Several of the openings are well demonstrated in the mucosa just below the clamps.

Courtesy of Leonard V. Crowley, MD, Century College.

may occur, leading to an abscess in the pelvis. Sometimes blood vessels in the mucosa of the diverticulum become ulcerated by abrasion from the fecal material, resulting in bleeding. Diverticula attended by such complications as infections, perforation, or bleeding may require surgical resection of the affected segment of bowel.

Tumors of the Bowel

Tumors of the small intestine are uncommon. Unfortunately, this is not the case for tumors of the colon and rectum. Ten percent of all new cases of cancer, as well as 9 percent of all cancer deaths, occur as a result of disease in the colon and rectum. It is estimated that 154,000 new cases and 53,000 deaths occur yearly as a result of colorectal cancers. Advanced age contributes to the risk of colorectal cancer (CRC) development. Incidence rates increase by 80–100 percent for each five-year period until age 50, with a reduced increase of 20–30 percent in older groups. Due to colonoscopy screening, the incidence of age-related colorectal cancer has dropped among older adults. However, the rate is increasing in younger age groups. The percentage of cases occurring in individuals younger than 55 years increased from 11 percent in 1995 to 20 percent in 2019. Currently, about 13 percent of all cases of CRC are under the age of 50. When the cancer is detected and confined to the colon, there is a 90 percent 5-year survival rate. When the cancer metastasized to distant locations, the 5-year survival rate is 13 percent. Not only can colonoscopy detect early colon and rectal cancer, but it can also prevent cancer from occurring by detecting precancerous lesions termed adenomas (polyps) and removing them before they have a chance to become cancer (adenocarcinoma). Colonoscopy involves inserting a flexible, tubelike device through the anus into the rectum and colon. The procedure is done under mild sedation and is not painful. The most unpleasant part of the procedure is the bowel cleaning required prior to the test, which involves inducing diarrhea using large volumes of oral fluid or other agents to flush the bowel. The colonoscope enables visualization of the bowel and allows removal of a stalked (pedunculated) polyp by cutting the narrow stalk. Flat lesions can be cauterized when they cannot be removed. Colorectal cancer often develops over many years, evolving slowly from the first precancerous lesion to invasive carcinoma. For this reason, colonoscopy need not be undertaken frequently. In the absence of risk factors, screening every 10 years starting at age 45 and continuing through age 75 is recommended. Cancer and precancerous lesions are often associated with some degree of bleeding into the stool (although this is often low in amount and not evident visually). As an alternative, highly sensitive fecal blood testing can be undertaken yearly, or relatively new tests that detect DNA changes associated with colon cancer in cells shed in the feces can be undertaken every 3 years. Positive results with other testing would require further investigation by colonoscopy.

Familial adenomatous polyposis (FAP) A genetic disease characterized by many polyps in the colorectal region.

As is the case with every cancer, colon cancer begins with a mutation in the DNA of a cell/cells, in this case in the colon/rectum. The first gene to be lost is usually APC, so named because it is associated with a genetic disease termed adenomatous polyposis coli or **familial adenomatous polyposis (FAP)**. People who inherit a germline mutation in the APC gene develop FAP, a disease characterized by the presence of hundreds of polyps (adenomas) in the colorectal region (**Figure 21-19**). By the age of 40, colorectal cancer is inevitable in FAP patients unless the colon is totally removed. However, the great majority (over 99 percent) of individuals who develop colorectal cancer do not have germline (inherited) mutations in the APC gene. Rather, the extraordinary number of dividing cells in the colorectal region develop spontaneous mutations in the APC gene as the person ages. Because APC is a tumor

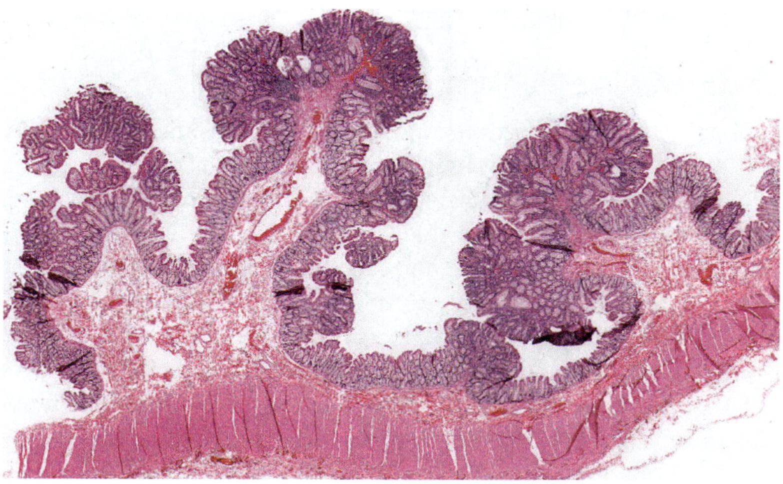

Figure 21-19 Photomicrograph of a segment of colon removed from a patient with FAP demonstrating multiple polyps.

Courtesy of Department of Pathology and Laboratory Medicine, University of North Carolina at Chapel Hill.

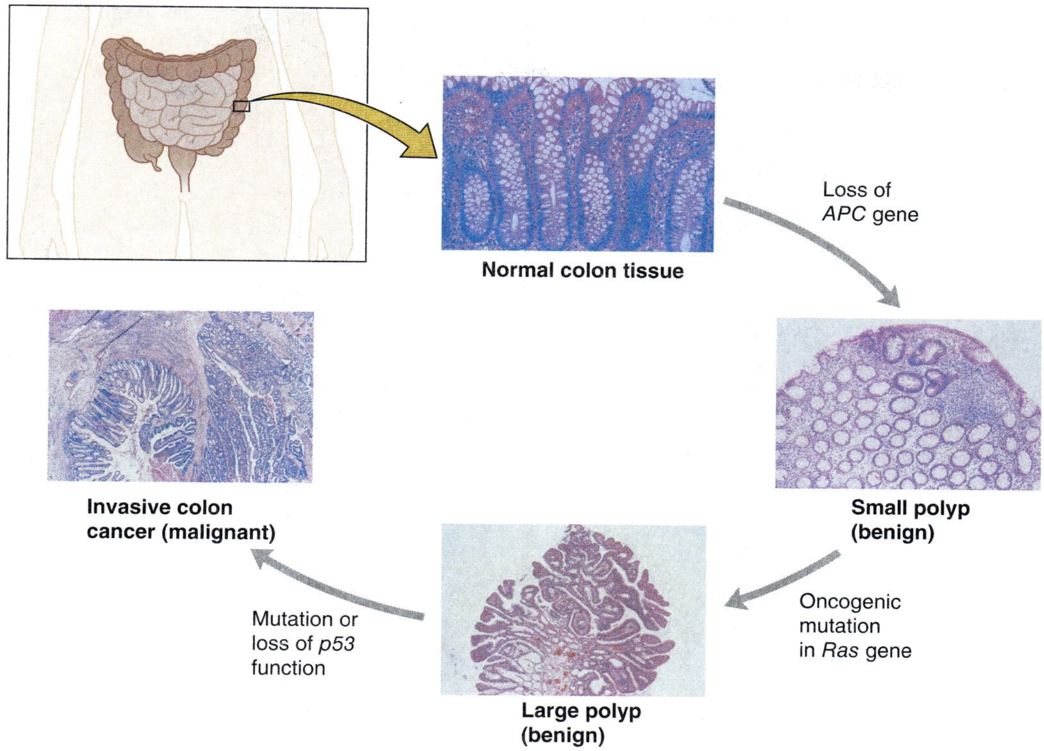

Figure 21-20 Stages in the progression of invasive colon cancer. Malignant colon cancer is defined by its ability to invade distant anatomic sites.

suppressor gene, it must function normally to control cell growth. Cells begin the pathway to colorectal cancer when both copies of APC are non-functional in the same cell. People with sporadic colorectal cancer need "two hits" to begin the process. Hence, sporadic (non-inherited) colorectal cancer is not inevitable and predominantly occurs in aging people. Cells that have lost APC have a growth advantage over their normal counterparts. Because they grow rapidly, they are more likely to accumulate many additional mutations that further dysregulate their growth. Ultimately loss of the TP53 gene, which is important in maintaining DNA integrity, is associated with transformation of the benign adenoma into a malignant adenocarcinoma capable of metastasis to distant sites. This prolonged and stepwise process of carcinogenesis is illustrated in **Figure 21-20**.

Carcinoma of the colon may arise anywhere in the large intestine or rectum. Carcinoma arising in the cecum and right half of the colon generally does not cause obstruction of the bowel because the caliber of this portion of the colon is large, and the bowel contents are relatively soft. However, the tumor often becomes ulcerated and bleeds, leading to chronic iron deficiency anemia. The patient with a carcinoma of the right half of the colon may consult a physician because of weakness and fatigue caused by the anemia, without experiencing any symptoms referable to the intestinal tract, or the lesion may have been detected by screening the stool for occult (not obvious) blood as noted previously. Carcinoma of the distal portion of the colon, which has a much smaller caliber than the proximal colon, often causes partial obstruction of the bowel and leads to symptoms of lower intestinal obstruction (**Figure 21-21** and **Figure 21-22**). Polyps are most often symptom-free until they advance into cancer, but occasionally the tip of the polyp may

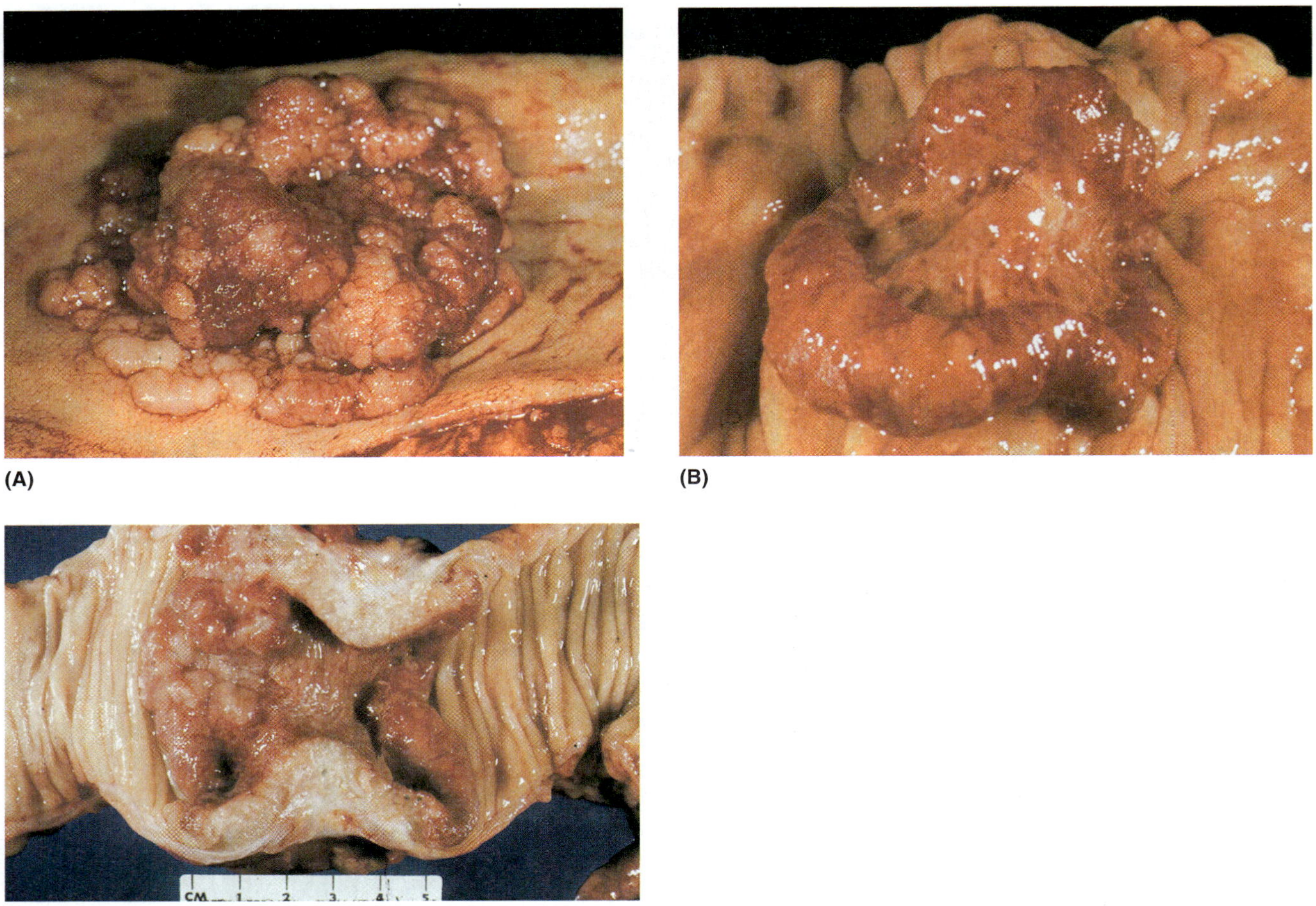

(A) (B) (C)

Figure 21-21 Stages in the progressive growth of a colon carcinoma. **(A)** Broad-based overgrowth of neoplastic epithelium. No ulceration or invasion of the bowel wall. **(B)** Central necrosis within more advanced carcinoma. The tumor invades the bowel wall. **(C)** Ulcerated far-advanced colon carcinoma completely encircles the bowel, reducing the caliber of the lumen, and extends completely through the bowel wall.

Courtesy of Leonard V. Crowley, MD, Century College.

become eroded and cause bleeding. Because removal of a polyp prevents it from becoming cancerous, survey of the bowel by colonoscopy may well prevent cancer.

Hemorrhoids

Hemorrhoids are varicosities, structural dilations of the veins of the venous plexus that drain the rectum and anus (**Figure 21-23**). Constipation and increased straining during bowel movements predispose to their development, as does pregnancy (presumably because of increased abdominal pressure). Internal hemorrhoids, which involve the veins of the lower rectum, may become eroded and bleed, may become thrombosed, or may prolapse through the anus. External hemorrhoids involve the veins of the anal canal and perianal skin. They sometimes become thrombosed, which causes considerable anorectal discomfort.

Symptoms of hemorrhoids can often be relieved by a high-fiber diet rich in fruits and vegetables, which promotes large, bulky stools that can be passed without excessive straining. Stool softeners and local application of rectal ointments may also provide temporary relief. Hemorrhoids can be removed surgically if they do not respond to more conservative therapy.

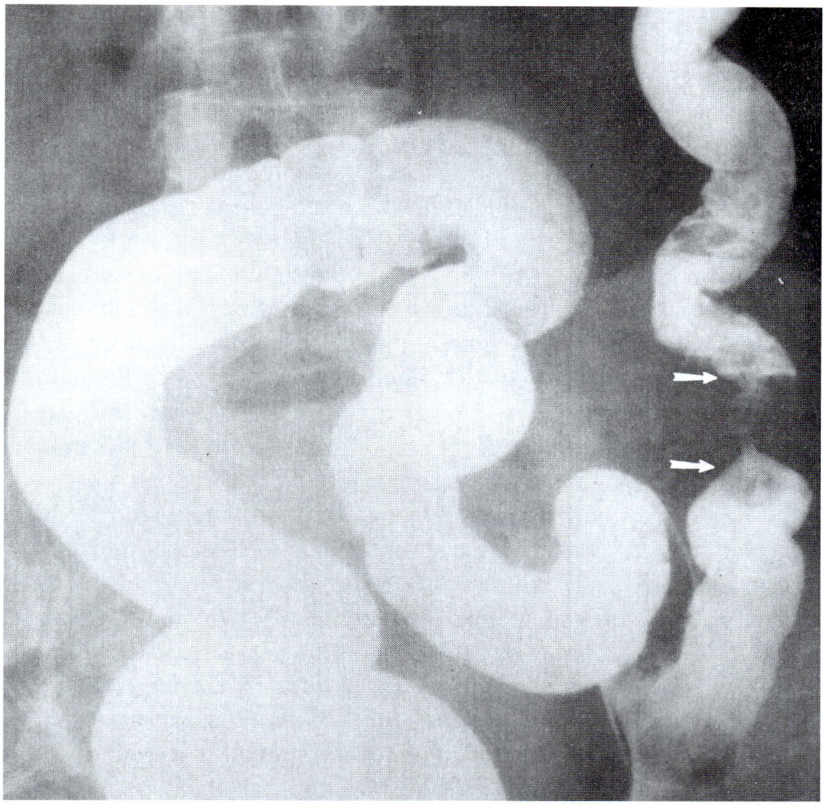

Figure 21-22 Colon carcinoma demonstrated by barium enema. The tumor narrows the lumen of the colon, which appears as a filling defect in the column of barium (*arrows*).

Courtesy of Leonard V. Crowley, MD, Century College.

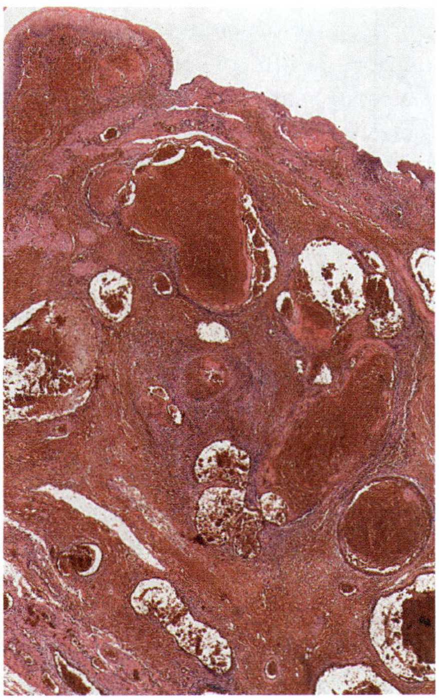

Figure 21-23 Photomicrograph of excised protuberant external hemorrhoids. External perianal epithelium is on top. There are many examples of thrombosed and blood-engorged vessels with abundant inflammatory cells throughout the tissue.

Courtesy of Department of Pathology and Laboratory Medicine, University of North Carolina at Chapel Hill.

Diagnostic Evaluation of Gastrointestinal Disease

Although the gastrointestinal tract cannot be examined as easily as many other parts of the body, it is possible to visualize the interior of the esophagus, the stomach, the duodenum, and the entire colon by endoscopic procedures using specially designed instruments inserted into the gastrointestinal tract either through the oral cavity or the anus. Recent development of "pill cameras," which transmit an image of the region of the gut they pass through, has made it easier to examine regions of the small intestine formerly difficult or impossible to image visually. (Endoscopy is described in Chapter 1.). Endoscopic procedures are generally employed if the patient experiences symptoms suggesting disease of the esophagus, stomach, or colon. Abnormal areas in the mucosa can be visualized, biopsied, and examined histologically.

Areas that cannot be visualized directly can be studied by radiologic examination. Examination of the upper gastrointestinal tract is accomplished by having the patient ingest a radiopaque material (contrast medium), allowing the clinician to visualize the transport of the material through the intestinal tract by X-ray studies. This technique also allows the clinician to visualize the contours of the gastrointestinal mucosa and thereby to identify the location and extent of disease affecting the bowel mucosa, such as ulcer, stricture, tumor, or an area of chronic inflammation. The colon can be studied in a similar manner by instilling radiopaque material into the bowel through the anus to outline the contours of the large intestine. This type of study is termed a barium enema (see Figure 21-22).

Eating Disorders

Eating disorders are conditions in which food intake is inappropriate and harmful because it leads to serious health consequences. Excessive food intake leading to obesity, which has many harmful effects on health, is the most prevalent disorder. However, abnormal eating habits associated with anorexia nervosa, bulimia nervosa, and binge eating disorders also pose serious health problems for those affected.

Obesity

Causes of Obesity

Obesity is a very complex disorder that involves genetic, environmental, and lifestyle-dependent variables. Lifestyle choices such as lack of exercise and an unhealthy diet contribute to the problem. Such a diet often includes too many highly processed foods and excess consumption of sugar, notably sugar-sweetened beverages, and too little consumption of fiber, fruits, and vegetables. There has been recent concern about excess consumption of "ultra-processed food." The definition of such is often unclear but includes foods that are industrially processed and contain excess sugar, preservatives, and food coloring. Behavioral factors include not enough sleep and too much "screen time," the latter because such serves as an alternative to exercise. Stress tends to increase appetite and leads to craving high-sugar, -fat, and -salt snacks. A number of medications are associated with weight gain, including but not limited to antipsychotics, antidepressants, and steroids. Medical conditions associated with weight gain include metabolic syndrome (and associated type 2 diabetes), polycystic ovary syndrome, and a number of endocrine conditions. Defined genetic conditions, single-gene disorders, that directly cause obesity are rare, but nutritional behaviors such as hunger and satiety control are associated with multiple less well-defined genes.

Fat is the storage form of energy. Any caloric intake that exceeds requirements is stored as adipose tissue, and weight is gained. Each excess pound of body weight represents the storage of approximately 3500 calories. Weight is lost if caloric intake is reduced below the amount required for total daily energy expenditure (TDEE). About 60 percent of TDEE is related to basal metabolic rate (the energy expenditure at rest, including the energy necessary for processes vital for life). Smaller proportions of the TDEE are used to digest food, to store resultant calories, and to regulate thermogenesis in response to the environment. The major adjustable component of TDEE is activity thermogenesis, which is the result of physical movement and deliberate exercise, thus emphasizing the importance of exercise on weight management. Many genetic, environmental, and hormonal factors play a role in regulating body weight by affecting appetite and satiety, thereby controlling food intake, and by influencing the metabolic pathways that convert food into energy or into adipose tissue. As noted previously, obesity may be caused by a rare genetic defect, endocrine gland malfunction, hypothyroidism, or adrenal cortical hyperfunction, but these are uncommon situations. Most obese individuals have no detectable genetic, endocrine, or metabolic disturbances. In the majority of cases, obesity is the result of overeating and could be "cured" by reducing food intake—easy in theory, but often difficult in practice because of behavioral issues not easily amenable to control, although recent pharmacologic advances in weight control drugs are extremely successful in helping to reduce food intake.

Using body mass index (BMI) (weight in kilograms divided by height in meters squared), overweight is defined as a BMI of 25 to 25.9 and obesity as a BMI of 30 or greater in individuals 20 years or older. Alarmingly, obesity rates have at least doubled between 1990 and 2021. Current data indicate that 72 percent of adult Americans are overweight or obese. Forty percent of people in this overweight group are classified as obese, which is defined as 20 percent or more over ideal body weight. Rates of childhood obesity increased with age, from 13 percent in ages between 2 and 5 to 22 percent in adolescents aged 12–19. About 10 percent of women and 6 percent of men are more than 100 pounds over their ideal body weight, a condition termed morbid obesity.

Health Consequences of Obesity

Overweight people have a higher incidence of diabetes, hypertension, cardiovascular disease, and several other diseases compared with people with normal weight. Therefore, being significantly overweight is undesirable, and extreme obesity is a major health hazard. Obese people have a mortality rate at least 20 percent higher than that of normal individuals. Excess fat is harmful to the cardiovascular system, and because blood volume and cardiac output must increase in the obese, there is a tendency to high blood pressure, and elevated blood lipids can predispose to arteriosclerosis. The high incidence of diabetes in obese people is the result of an impaired ability to utilize insulin efficiently (described in Chapter 20). Musculoskeletal disabilities such as osteoarthritis are frequent because the excess weight places undue stress on the bones, joints, and ligaments. Finally, an obese individual is at a serious disadvantage if surgery is required. The operative procedure carries a higher risk, and postoperative complications are more frequent. Any surgical procedure is technically much more difficult in an obese person, and wound healing is delayed. The adipose tissue, which has a relatively poor blood supply, heals poorly and is also quite vulnerable to infection, resulting in an increased incidence of postoperative wound infections.

Treatment of Obesity

The treatment of obesity by dieting leads to surprisingly poor results, likely because satiety and appetite are controlled by a complex interaction between behavior (and the environment interacting with such) and genetics. Hence, simply saying "eat less, exercise more," although correct, rarely leads to maintained weight loss. Although the area is extremely controversial, no one diet has proven more effective in the long term. Low-carbohydrate diets and so-called ketogenic diets have gained in popularity, but they have no clear advantages in promoting cardiovascular health and may be associated with additional health risks.

Because of the limited success of treating obesity by diet, various other measures have been proposed. Recent advances in the use of GLP-1RA drugs have proven remarkably successful in promoting weight loss (see also chapter 20). Such drugs mimic the function of natural gut hormones (such as GLP-1) and have several effects. The drugs suppress appetite and improve satiety possibly by acting directly on the brain to reduce hunger signals. They slow digestion by reducing the rate of gastric emptying, leading to feelings of fullness. They increase the release of other gut hormones, which leads to reduced food intake, and, as noted in Chapter 20, they improve insulin sensitivity. Although initially designed for control of type 2 diabetes, there is an increasing number of GLP-1RAs aimed at weight loss. The drugs appear to require prolonged use by injection (from daily to weekly) and are associated with a number of side effects. Rarely such side effects may be severe, such as pancreatitis and thyroid cancer. Other drugs that suppress appetite have been used, but many of these drugs have undesirable side effects and have had very limited success. As a last resort, massive obesity is sometimes treated by various surgical operations (bariatric surgery). The current surgical procedures produce weight loss primarily by restricting the capacity of the stomach without resorting to drastic restriction of nutrient absorption in the small intestine. They can be performed using standard surgical incisions or by laparoscopy using small abdominal incisions and are often grouped together under the general term stomach stapling operations. The best known and most widely used of these procedures is termed the Roux-en-Y gastric bypass, named after the man who devised it (Roux) and the Y-shaped connection made between the small bowel loops in the procedure (**Figure 21-24**). Unfortunately, gastric bypass procedures may lead to late complications in many patients: anemia caused by poor absorption of iron and vitamin B_{12} and weakening of bones (osteoporosis) as a result of inadequate calcium intake and absorption. On the other hand, **adjustable gastric banding**, a solely restrictive surgery, is safer and has lower short-term complications.

Adjustable gastric banding A method for treating obesity by applying an adjustable gastric band to the stomach to reduce its capacity, thereby promoting weight loss.

Anorexia Nervosa and Bulimia Nervosa

These two conditions are characterized by profound eating disturbances. Although they are separate disorders, there is considerable overlap between the two conditions. Both of these conditions can lead to extreme malnutrition caused by inadequate nutrients, along with associated vitamin and mineral deficiencies. These conditions can lead to serious health consequences, which can be fatal if not adequately treated.

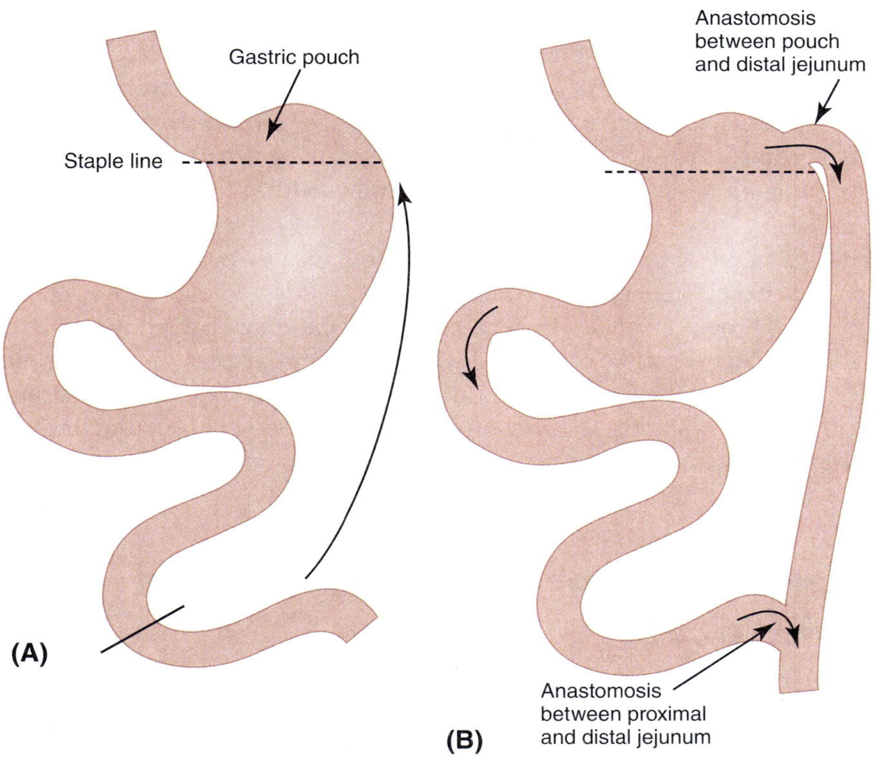

Figure 21-24 Gastric bypass. **(A)** The upper dashed line indicates the location of gastric staples placed to create a gastric pouch. The lower solid line indicates the site where the jejunum is divided. The arrow indicates how the distal segment of the jejunum is moved for anastomosis with the gastric pouch. **(B)** Completed bypass illustrating proximal and distal anastomoses. The arrows indicate the direction of movement of the gastrointestinal contents. An alternative termed gastric banding is no longer frequently used.

Anorexia Nervosa

In this condition, affected individuals have a false perception of being too fat when they are actually much too thin, and they continue to lose weight by restricting food intake, exercising excessively, or using drugs such as laxatives or self-induced vomiting. The condition occurs much more frequently in women than in men and is more prevalent in Western countries, where a slim body is considered ideal and excessive weight is thought to be undesirable. Fashion models, ballet dancers, athletes, and other groups for whom a slender body is required are disproportionately represented.

Excessive weight loss disrupts many of the body's physiologic processes. Menstrual periods cease, thyroid function declines, fluid and electrolyte disturbances develop, and bones become fragile from loss of calcium (osteoporosis). Extreme emaciation is a life-threatening condition that may lead to death if not treated.

Severe anorexia nervosa is difficult to treat, as both medical and psychological problems associated with the condition must be addressed.

Bulimia Nervosa

This condition is another method of weight control that is characterized by repeated episodes of binge eating (rapidly eating an excessively large amount of food) followed by purging (self-induced vomiting) to counteract the effects of the bingeing, along with guilt and remorse at the inability to control the binge-purge behavior. Purging may be supplemented by taking laxatives to decrease food absorption by promoting rapid passage of digested food through the small intestine. The condition occurs most often in young women. Their body weight may fluctuate in relation to their binge-purge behavior, but they do not become emaciated. Their friends and relatives usually are not aware of their problem because they look normal and carefully conceal their binge-purge behavior.

Bulimia nervosa carries with it some serious health problems. Repeated self-induced vomiting leads to dental problems due to the corrosive effect of gastric acid on tooth enamel. The repeated loss of excess gastric juice may lead to metabolic alkalosis and electrolyte disturbances (see Chapter 17). One of the most serious effects of self-induced vomiting is a tear in the mucosa of the stomach near the gastroesophageal junction, which can bleed profusely and may be fatal. Treatment involves the same medical and psychological approaches used to deal with anorexia nervosa.

Chronic Malnutrition: Its Causes and Effects

Causes of Malnutrition

Malnutrition results when the intake of nutrients is insufficient to supply the body's needs either because there is insufficient food available or the food is not being used efficiently. In developing countries, inadequate food to supply the population may result from crop failure, a natural disaster such as a flood or a drought, poor food distribution, an unstable government, or other causes that have an impact on food production or delivery. Often, infants and children are disproportionately affected because they have a greater need for nutrients to sustain their rapid growth rate during infancy and childhood. Such deficiency may be related to overall lack of nutrition (termed **marasmus** when severe) or more specifically to a lack of protein but high in carbohydrates (kwashiorkor). In 2023 in the United States, 17.9 percent of households with children were considered to be food insecure.

Marasmus Global deficiency of caloric intake in infants and children.

Cases of chronic malnutrition may also be caused by diseases that impair food intake, digestion, or absorption or by conditions that increase nutrient and protein requirements, such as an acute illness, a severe burn, or a major surgical procedure. Other people at risk are those living in poverty, the elderly, people who consume alcohol in excess, drug abusers, or those with advanced cancer or eating disorders. Treatment consists of supplying adequate nutrients together with vitamins and minerals before the malnutrition-induced organ damage has progressed to such a degree that a response to treatment is unlikely to be successful.

Global deficiency of caloric intake in infants and children, marasmus, is not uncommon, particularly in children who have been weaned. The child will suffer from growth failure and wasting. Immunosuppression occurs, accompanied by repeated infections. There is general wasting and loss of subcutaneous fat. Kwashiorkor occurs when a diet is sufficient in calories but not in protein, most often in children whose diet consists nearly exclusively of carbohydrates. Severe edema and skin abnormalities occur. The hair takes on a red color. Intestinal changes may interfere with nutrient absorption even when nutrition becomes improved, and diarrhea is likely. However, caloric intake is sufficient, so subcutaneous fat is normal. Under any circumstances, extreme emaciation is a life-threatening condition, and loss of over 30 percent of body weight may be fatal.

Case 21-1

Maddy is a 19-year-old first-year student in a local community college. She has been in good health until recently except for an occasional sinus infection treated by her local family physician. Her medical history is notable only for an appendectomy at the age of 9 years. Recently she noted an increase in weakness and fatigue during midterm week. Her friends began to tease her because she had a "noisy tummy" (borborygmus) and tended to pass gas (be flatulent). She noted an increased incidence of diarrhea followed by periods of constipation. Her digestive disturbances were accompanied by moderate abdominal pain, which was relieved by passing gas.

Several of her friends suggested that she might consider "going gluten-free," stating that such a diet made them "feel better and think more clearly." Maddy began by restricting her intake of pizza to a gluten-free brand and, feeling better, found it easy to switch to a gluten-free or low-gluten diet because the cafeteria in her college provided these products. She also reduced her intake of milk and dairy products, which also seemed to relieve her symptoms. On a weekend trip she consumed a large amount of double cheese pizza. The restaurant did not have a gluten-free product. The next morning, she noted a severe recurrence of abdominal discomfort and did poorly on a series of school examinations. Her friends suggested that she had "gluten sensitivity." Maddy developed an annoying itchy rash on her back and buttocks and decided to consult her physician about the possibility she might have some type of gluten sensitivity or celiac disease; her friends told her this was very common.

Maddy's physical examination noted the following. She had a mild papulovesicular ("bumps and small blisters") rash that appeared to be receding. Maddy noted she had switched to a new shower gel recently and had gone back to her prior product. Maddy had a slightly protuberant abdomen and increased bowel sounds that the physician attributed to intestinal gas. No weight loss was noted. Her blood count was normal, but she did have borderline anemia. On reviewing Maddy's history of abdominal discomfort associated with her consumption of pizza, the physician suggested a possibility of lactose intolerance producing excessive intestinal gas and suggested Maddy keep a food diary to correlate symptoms with food consumption. Maddy was quite upset at the results of the examination, as she (and her friends) believed it was likely she had gluten sensitivity. Her physician suggested two additional blood-based tests useful in diagnosing celiac disease (gluten-sensitive enteropathy). One test looked for autoantibodies to a protein associated with celiac disease. The second test assayed for the presence of certain genetic markers on cells (major histocompatibility markers) that occurred in most individuals who have the disease. Maddy was negative in both tests. She continued to maintain that a gluten-free diet made her feel much better and joined a support group for non-celiac gluten sensitivity.

Discussion (Pathophysiology)

Celiac disease (gluten-sensitive enteropathy) is a complex autoimmune disease associated with the production of an immune response to peptides derived from gluten, a high-molecular-weight seed storage protein found in grass-related grains such as wheat, rye, and barley. The protein is responsible for the ability of bread dough to become elastic, retain gas produced by leavening agents such as yeast, and rise prior to baking. The use of gluten is widespread in many food products. In celiac disease, the immune system recognizes a soluble component of gluten (gliadin), which has many glutamine amino acid residues clustered at one end of the molecule. Gliadin-derived peptides are transported to the gut, where an enzyme (tissue transglutaminase, or tTG) deamidates (removes the side-chain amino group of) certain glutamine residues in the gliadin peptide. In individuals with particular HLA (major histocompatibility) types, the tTG-altered peptides

(continues)

Case 21-1 *(Continued)*

are recognized by CD4+ helper T cells and result in cellular immunity directed toward the altered peptides in the small intestine. This results in the activation of inflammatory pathways leading to immune-mediated damage to the absorptive surface of the small intestine and a variety of malabsorptive and digestive symptoms. A second major component of celiac disease is autoimmune production of antibodies to tTG. Although the exact mechanism remains unclear, gliadin-derived peptides in combination with tTG induce the formation of antibodies to both gliadin and tTG. These antibodies are likely to contribute to the intestinal damage, but antibodies to tTG (and in particular IgA antibodies) are most likely to be responsible for the non-gut-related autoimmune disease seen in celiac disease (as tTG is found in many sites in the body). Hence, celiac disease is associated with a confusing array of symptoms, some of which (diarrhea, malabsorption of fats, flatulence, weight loss, anemia, and osteoporosis) are clearly associated with damage to the absorptive capacity of the intestine. Other symptoms (neurologic, hormonal disturbances, and skin disorders such as dermatitis herpetiformis consistent with Maddy's rash) may be related (at least in part) to a systemic autoimmune response. (It should be noted that this list of symptoms is by no means exhaustive.)

Discussion (Diagnosis)

Until the early 2000s, celiac disease was considered uncommon, with a frequency of about 1 in 6000 people. Diagnosis was costly and invasive, requiring intestinal biopsy and tissue evaluation by a pathologist. However, the development of several relatively easy serological tests that measure antibodies to TG2 defined an increased incidence of the disease to perhaps as high as 1 percent as measured by positivity in these assays. Many "new" cases are diagnosed in women and adults who have symptoms that may be less severe and "nonspecific." The number of seropositive individuals who have celiac disease as defined by intestinal biopsy is also unclear, and the area remains extremely controversial.

What about Maddy? Celiac disease has a very strong genetic component. Well over 90 percent of patients with celiac disease have particular pairs of HLA markers. Tests for these markers are very sensitive (but not very specific) and are excellent for excluding this disease. On this basis alone, Maddy is very unlikely to have celiac disease. The utility of serological testing depends strongly on test specifics. Assuming the best technique was used, sensitivity and specificity are over 90 percent, again arguing that Maddy was unlikely to have celiac disease. However, does this mean Maddy was not sensitive to gluten consumption? In one study, 60 percent of patients with symptoms similar to Maddy's could not be classified as having celiac disease. Maddy's symptoms could have been related to lactose intolerance or irritable bowel disease. Both were hinted at in the case presentation. Maddy's rash could have been related to a shower gel. Because of this uncertainty, which is often a problem with diseases that are solely self-reported, a condition termed non-celiac gluten sensitivity has been defined (predominantly based on the lack of objective symptoms and laboratory tests). Perhaps this is what Maddy had, perhaps stress contributed to irritable bowel disease, or perhaps she was lactose intolerant.

Etiology and Pathogenesis

Undefined, fits the diagnostic category non-celiac gluten sensitivity.

Questions

1. Case 21-1 notes that HLA testing is very useful in diagnosing potential cases of celiac disease. If someone has the appropriate HLA markers, does this mean the person has the disease?

2. Why was HLA typing unlikely to have been offered to Maddy as an initial test?
3. Case 21-1 suggests Maddy might have been lactose intolerant. What characteristics of Maddy's background (deliberately excluded in Case 21-1) might have made this more likely?
4. How could lactose intolerance have been confirmed?
5. Maddy was scrupulous in avoiding gluten-based products, excelled in college, and had much reduced intestinal symptoms. Does this mean she had celiac disease or non-celiac gluten sensitivity?

Questions for Review

1. What factors affect the development of dental caries? What complications may result from dental caries? What are the causes and possible effects of periodontal disease?
2. What are some of the major causes of esophageal obstruction? What symptoms does esophageal obstruction produce?
3. What is a peptic ulcer? In what parts of the gastrointestinal tract are peptic ulcers encountered? What factors contribute to the development of peptic ulcers? What are the complications of a peptic ulcer?
4. What is the difference between Crohn's disease and chronic ulcerative colitis? Diverticulosis and diverticulitis?
5. What is a Meckel diverticulum? Where is it located? What clinical manifestations can it produce?
6. What is intestinal obstruction? What symptoms does it produce? What are some of the common causes of intestinal obstruction?
7. What is the pathogenesis of acute appendicitis?
8. What symptoms and physical findings are likely to be encountered in a patient with a carcinoma of the colon? Why?
9. What is an intussusception? How is it caused? What is the difference between volvulus and intussusception?

References

Loeffler AG, Hart MN. "Gastrointestinal tract." In: *Introduction to Human Disease*. 7th ed. Jones & Bartlett Learning; 2020.

- The chapter presents an overview and some additional details on gastrointestinal disease. Any of a number of pathology texts used in undergraduate medical education will provide additional details.

NIH, National Cancer Institute. HPV and Cancer. https://www.cancer.gov/about-cancer/causes-prevention/risk/infectious-agents/hpv-and-cancer

- Provides the content on the HPV vaccine's ability to prevent cancer.

American Cancer Society. What is Colorectal Cancer? https://www.cancer.org/cancer/colon-rectal-cancer/about/what-is-colorectal-cancer.html

National Cancer Institute. Genetics of Colorectal Cancer (PDQ). https://www.cancer.gov/types/colorectal/hp/colorectal-genetics-pdq

Menter DG, et al. Back to the colorectal cancer consensus molecular subtype future. *Curr Gastroenterol Rep*. 2019;21(2):5. https://www.ncbi.nlm.nih.gov/pmc/articles/PMC6622456/

- The first site has a good overview of colorectal cancer; the second summarizes the genetics of the disease. The third reference is a somewhat technical review of the modern state of knowledge of the mutations involved in colorectal cancer and the definition of "molecular subtypes" in an analogous approach to that used with great success in breast cancer.

National Institute of Diabetes and Digestive and Kidney Diseases, NIH. Treatment for Peptic Ulcers (Stomach or Duodenal Ulcers). https://www.niddk.nih.gov/health-information/digestive-diseases/peptic-ulcers-stomach-ulcers/treatment

The Helicobacter Foundation. www.helico.com

- The first entry is a general overview of peptic ulcer disease and is strong on therapy. The second entry is for Dr. Barry Marshall's website; he established the relationship of *H. pylori* to gastrointestinal disease. It has an up-to-date reference list and excellent quick reviews as well as being enjoyable.

American Society for Metabolic and Bariatric Surgery. Bariatric Surgery Procedures. Updated May 2021. http://asmbs.org/patients/bariatric-surgery-procedures

Mayo Clinic. Obesity. http://www.mayoclinic.org/diseases-conditions/obesity/basics/definition/con-20014834

Centers for Disease Control and Prevention. Obesity. https://www.cdc.gov/obesity/

- These three references describe the magnitude of the "obesity epidemic" and the applications and limitations of various surgical procedures used to treat morbid obesity.

National Lipid Association. https://www.lipid.org/

Kirkpatrick CF, et al. Review of current evidence and clinical recommendations on the effects of low-carbohydrate and very-low-carbohydrate (including ketogenic) diets for the management of body weight and other cardiometabolic risk factors. A scientific statement from the National Lipid Association. *J Clin Lipidol*. 2019;13(5):689-711. https://www.lipid.org/nla/review-current-evidence-and-clinical-recommendations-effects-low-carbohydrate-and-very-low

- The National Lipid Association is a treasure trove of information on nutrition and diet of great value to anyone interested in the area. The second reference is a Scientific Statement from the NLA and its investigation of popular weight reduction diets. This should be read by anyone considering keto, paleo, and any of a number of current diet fads.

Centers for Disease Control and Prevention. Norovirus. http://www.cdc.gov/norovirus/

Centers for Disease Control and Prevention. Rotavirus. http://www.cdc.gov/rotavirus/

- These two CDC web pages will tell you everything you need to know about the two viral forms of gastroenteritis. They contain useful and detailed lists of publications, most of which are available online.

Wang Y, et al. Research progress in fecal microbiota transplantation as treatment for irritable bowel syndrome. *Gastroenterol Res Pract*. 2019;2019:9759138. doi:10.1155/2019/9759138

Liwinski T, Elinav E. Harnessing the microbiota for therapeutic purposes. *Am J Transplant*. 2020;20(6):1482-1488. doi:10.1111/ajt.15753

- In addition to the treatment of clostridial pseudomembranous colitis, fecal transplantation is being investigated for a wide variety of (sometimes seemingly unlikely) conditions. The first paper reviews one of the more popular areas of investigation, and the second is an excellent recent overview of the role of changing the gut microbiota as a therapeutic intervention.

Peters Y, et al. Barrett oesophagus. *Nat Rev Dis Primers*. 2019;5(1):35.

- An overview of the epidemiology, pathogenesis, diagnosis, and treatment of Barrett's and gastroesophageal reflux syndrome.

Huang L, et al. Comparison of antibiotic therapy and appendectomy for acute uncomplicated appendicitis in children: A meta-analysis. *JAMA Pediatr*. 2017;171(5):426-429. https://www.ncbi.nlm.nih.gov/pmc/articles/PMC5470362/

Wonski S, Ranzenberger LR, Carter KR. Appendix Imaging. StatPearls. Last updated April 1, 2023. https://www.ncbi.nlm.nih.gov/books/NBK549903/

- The treatment and diagnosis of appendicitis is a far from settled medical issue. The current views on such issues are reviewed in these two references.

Aziz I, Branchi F, Sanders DS. The rise and fall of gluten! *Proc Nutr Soc*. 2015;74(3):221-226.

Husby S, Murray JA. Diagnosing coeliac disease and the potential for serological markers. *Nat Rev Gastroenterol Hepatol*. 2014;11(11):655-663.

Meresse B, Malamut G, Cerf-Bensussan N. Celiac disease: An immunological jigsaw. *Immunity*. 2012;36:907-919.

- These three references were the most valuable for use in constructing the case. The first is an amusing overview that touches on the controversial aspects of celiac disease diagnosis. The second presents a more in-depth analysis of diagnostic technology, and the third details the immunopathology of the disease.

U.S. Department of Agriculture, Economic Research Service. Food Security in the U.S. – Key Statistics & Graphs. https://www.ers.usda.gov/topics/food-nutrition-assistance/food-security-in-the-us/key-statistics-graphics

- This USDA source provides information on food security used in the chapter.

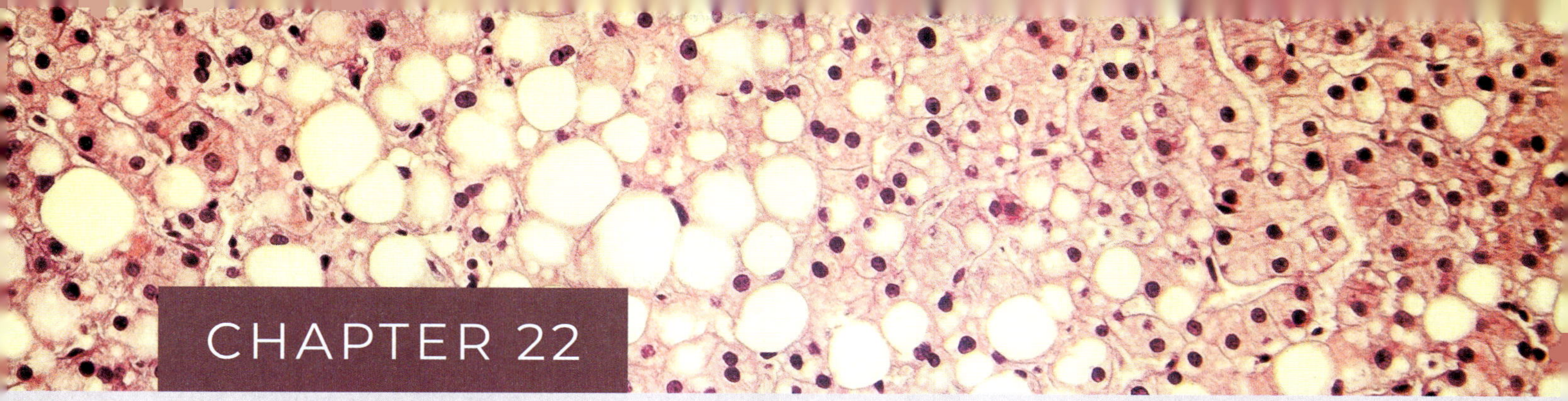

CHAPTER 22

The Endocrine Glands

LEARNING OBJECTIVES

1. Explain the normal physiologic functions of the pituitary hormones. Name the common pituitary hormonal disturbances and describe the methods of treating each disturbance.
2. Describe the major endocrine disturbances caused by thyroid dysfunction, their clinical manifestations, and explain the methods of treatment.
3. Compare and contrast toxic and non-toxic goiter. Identify major factors that predispose to the development of non-toxic goiter.
4. Explain the normal physiologic functions of the endocrines secreted by adrenal cortex and medulla. Name the related hormonal disturbances and describe methods of treatment.
5. Define the causes and effects of parathyroid dysfunction and describe the methods of treatment.
6. Understand the concept of ectopic hormone production by nonendocrine tumors.
7. Explain how stress affects the endocrine system.

Endocrine Functions and Dysfunctions

Cell signaling or communication occurs through different mechanisms in the human body. Secreted cellular products may act on the same cells that release them, a process known as autocrine activity; on the vicinity of the cells, termed paracrine activity; or at distant sites, known as endocrine activity. Endocrine glands secrete their products directly into the bloodstream and exert a regulatory effect on various metabolic functions distant from the gland. The major endocrine glands are the pituitary, thyroid, and parathyroid glands, along with the adrenal cortex and medulla. Other organs such as the pancreatic islets (Chapter 20) and the ovaries and testes also secrete endocrine hormones (Chapter 18). In addition, many other groups of specialized cells also secrete hormones. Renin and erythropoietin are secreted by the kidneys; the hormones gastrin, secretin, and cholecystokinin are produced by the mucosa of the gastrointestinal tract. Of increasing interest are the incretins, gut peptide hormones that sense food intake and stimulate insulin release after eating. By convention, these hormones are considered along with the organs with which they are associated and are not generally regarded as part of the endocrine system (**Figure 22-1**).

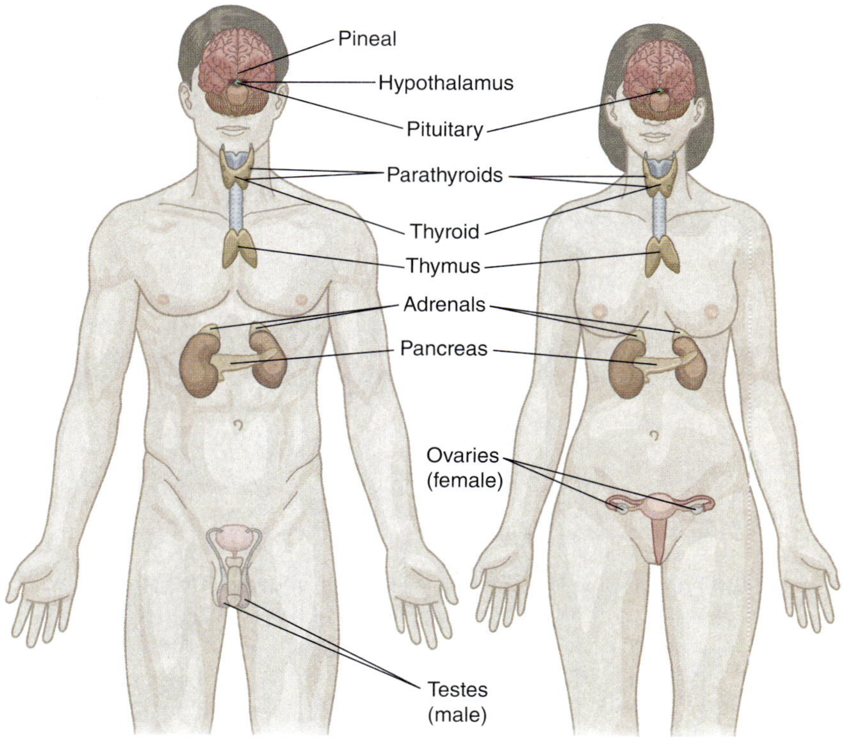

Figure 22-1 Endocrine organs and tissues.

Feedback mechanisms Biological control using levels of output, such as hormones, to control further production of substances.

Thyroid-stimulating hormone (TSH) Hormone secreted by the anterior lobe of the pituitary that regulates thyroid function.

The amount of hormone synthesized and released into the circulation by an endocrine gland may be regulated directly by the level of hormone circulating in the blood or indirectly by the level of a substance under hormonal control, such as the concentration of glucose or sodium in the blood. Mechanisms of this type are termed **feedback mechanisms**. In a negative feedback mechanism or feedback inhibition mechanism, usually an increase in the level of hormone or hormone-regulated substance suppresses further hormone output. These mechanisms modulate the output of the pituitary hormones and the hormones they regulate. Trophic hormones secreted by the pituitary control the level of secretion of hormones by other endocrine glands, which they target. For example, the pituitary will secrete additional **thyroid-stimulating hormone (TSH)** in response to low circulating levels of thyroid hormones. Conversely, high levels of thyroid hormone suppress the production of TSH by the pituitary. A disorder in an endocrine gland may consist of either hypersecretion or hyposecretion of the hormone(s), manifested as abnormal activity of the organ controlled by the gland. This may result from intrinsic abnormalities of the endocrine gland itself (the thyroid in the example) or from a deficit or excess secretion of tropic hormones by the pituitary (**Figure 22-2**).

The clinical effects of a disturbance of endocrine gland function are determined by the degree of dysfunction of the gland and by the age and sex of the affected individual. Symptoms of dysfunction range from barely detectable variations from normal to extreme hypofunction or hyperfunction. The age of the person when the endocrine disturbance becomes manifest contributes to a pronounced effect on the clinical features. Some endocrine glands, such as the thyroid gland, affect growth and development as well as metabolic processes. Therefore, disturbed function in a child will produce a somewhat different clinical picture from a similar disturbance in an adult. The sex of the individual also influences the effect of disturbed endocrine function because many hormones

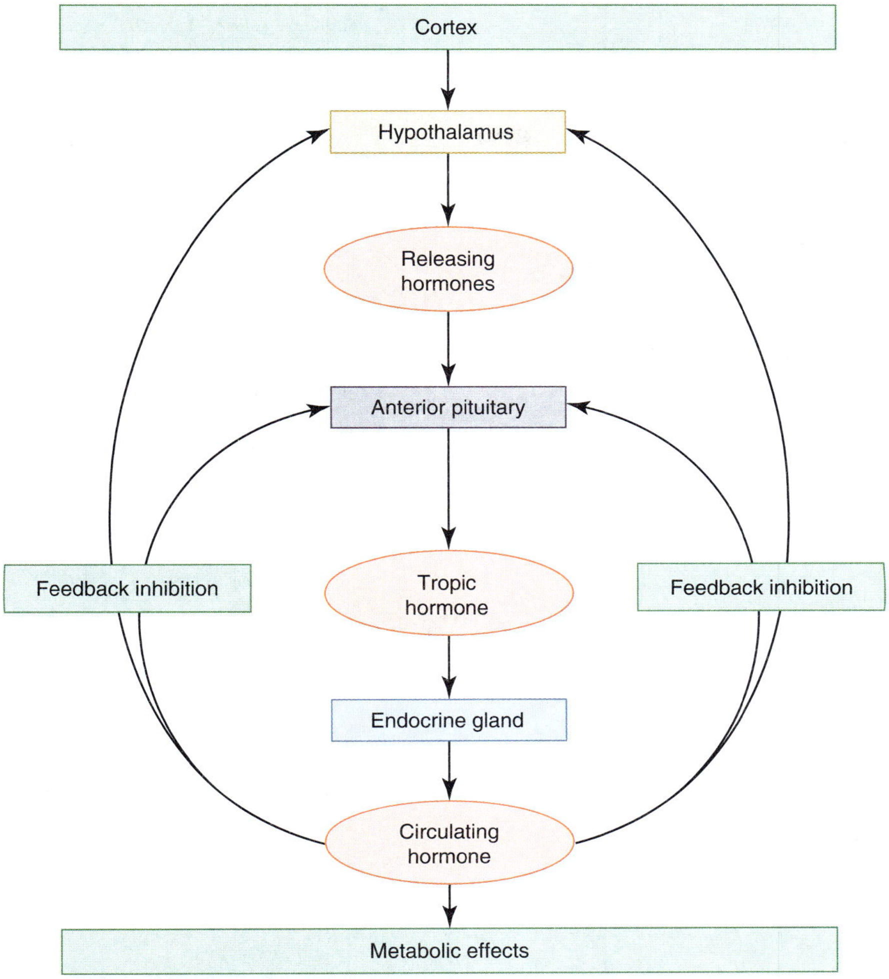

Figure 22-2 Normal mechanisms controlling elaboration of tropic hormones by the pituitary gland.

are concerned with the development and maintenance of sexual function and secondary sexual characteristics. Some endocrine disturbances cause alterations in sexual development in children, whereas the effects are much less pronounced in adults. Overproduction of an inappropriate sex hormone in some endocrine diseases causes masculinization, or virilization, of the female or feminization of the male; conversely, overproduction of a sex hormone appropriate to the sex of the individual has little clinical effect.

The Pituitary Gland

The pituitary gland is a small, pea-shaped gland suspended by a narrow stalk from the hypothalamus at the base of the brain. The gland, composed of an anterior lobe and a posterior lobe, is located in a small depression within the sphenoid bone, termed the pituitary fossa or sella turcica (named because of a supposed resemblance to a Turkish saddle), just behind the optic chiasm. Many mammals possess an intermediate lobe located between the anterior and posterior lobes that produces **melanin-stimulating hormone (MSH)**. However, in humans, the intermediate lobe consists only of a series of small cystic cavities whose function is unclear and is no longer discernable as a distinct structure (**Figure 22-3**).

Melanin-stimulating hormone (MSH) One of the hormones produced by the pituitary. Causes darkening of the skin.

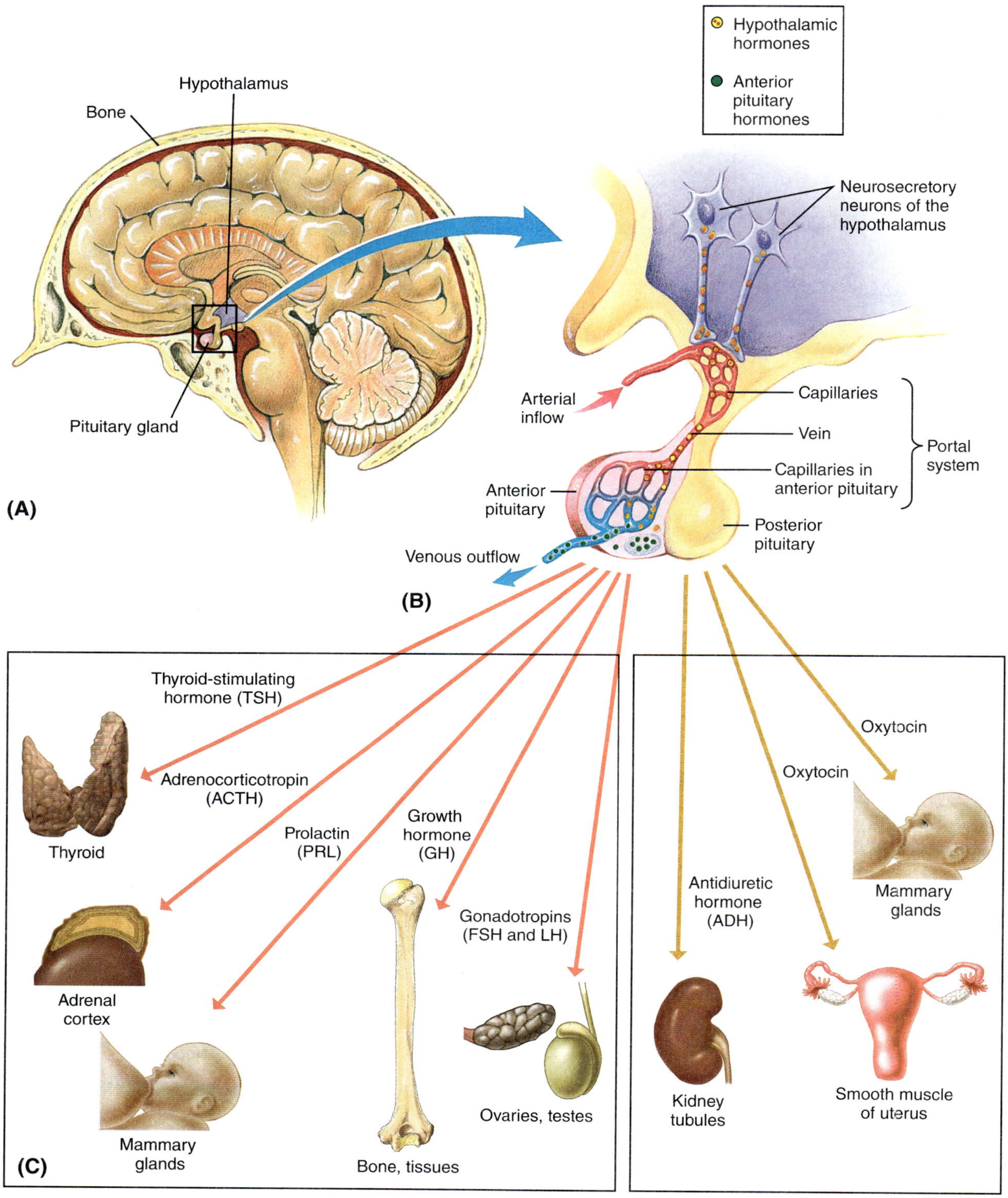

Figure 22-3 The pituitary gland. **(A)** Cross section of the brain showing the location of the pituitary and hypothalamus. **(B)** The structure of the pituitary gland. **(C)** Releasing and inhibiting hormone travel via the hypothalamus to the anterior pituitary where they affect tropic hormone secretion as indicated.

The anterior lobe (also known as the adenohypophysis) is composed of cords of epithelial cells containing hormones that are synthesized and stored within the lobe. Anterior lobe cells have been classified on the basis of the staining reaction of their cytoplasmic granules using routine staining methods. Three cell types were recognized: eosinophilic, which contain bright-red-staining cytoplasmic granules; basophilic, which have abundant purple-staining granules in their cytoplasm; and **chromophobe cells**, which contain sparse, poorly stained granules. Currently, five different cell types are defined based on the specific hormone each produces as detected using immunological staining procedures. For example, those cells secreting thyroid-stimulating hormone are termed thyrotrophs; the most common cell type is somatotrophs, which secrete **growth hormone (GH), or somatotropin**.

The anterior lobe is connected to the hypothalamus by a special system of blood vessels termed a portal system, which begins as capillaries in the hypothalamus and extends down the pituitary stalk to terminate as capillaries around the cells of the anterior lobe. Release of the hormones stored within the anterior lobe is regulated by the hormonal substances termed **releasing hormones**, which are synthesized in the hypothalamus and carried to the anterior lobe through the portal system.

Usually, a hypothalamic releasing hormone stimulates a single cell type within the anterior pituitary, resulting in the release of a pituitary hormone that activates or inhibits functions at the target. For example, corticotropin-releasing hormone (CRH) stimulates the release of **adrenocorticotropic hormone (ACTH)** from corticotroph cells in the pituitary. In turn, ACTH stimulates the adrenal cortex. Some releasing hormones stimulate several cell types in the pituitary. Thyrotropin-releasing hormone (TRH) stimulates both thyrotroph and lactotroph cells in the pituitary, resulting in the release of hormones stimulating both the thyroid gland and breast. Some hypothalamic hormones inhibit rather than stimulate specific pituitary cells, and the hormone response of the target gland reflects the net effect of the interaction between releasing and inhibiting hormones (**Table 22-1**).

The posterior lobe (also known as neurohypophysis) consists of a meshwork of nerve fibers intermixed with modified neuroglial cells and is connected to the hypothalamus by bundles of nerve fibers extending through the pituitary stalk rather than by the portal circulation. The hormones in the posterior lobe are synthesized within the hypothalamus and are then transmitted down the nerve axons in the pituitary stalk to the posterior lobe, where they are stored.

Chromophobe cells Anterior lobe pituitary epithelial cells containing sparse, poorly stained granules.

Growth hormone (GH), or somatotropin An anterior lobe pituitary hormone that stimulates the growth of bone and other body tissues.

Releasing hormones Hormones synthesized in the hypothalamus, which act to stimulate release of specific hormones from the anterior pituitary.

Adrenocorticotropic hormone (ACTH) A hormone secreted by the anterior lobe of the pituitary that stimulates the adrenal cortex to manufacture and secrete adrenal cortical hormones.

Table 22-1 Hypothalamic Hormones and Their Targets

Hypothalamic Hormone	Response of Pituitary and Target Gland
Thyrotropin-releasing hormone (TRH)	Stimulates release of thyroid-stimulating hormone (TSH), which in turn stimulates production and release of thyroid hormone Stimulates prolactin production and release
Corticotropin-releasing hormone (CRH)	Stimulates release of adrenocorticotropic hormone (ACTH), which in turn stimulates production and release of adrenal cortical hormones
Gonadotropin-releasing hormone (GnRH)	Stimulates follicle-stimulating hormone (FSH) and luteinizing hormone (LH), which in turn affect gonadal function
Growth hormone–releasing hormone (GHRH)	Stimulates synthesis of growth hormone, which in turn promotes production of growth factors that promote general tissue growth
Prolactin inhibitory hormone (Dopamine)	Inhibits prolactin release from pituitary gland Inhibits FSH and LH
Somatostatin	Inhibits secretion and release of growth hormone, which in turn inhibits growth factors that promote general tissue growth Inhibits TSH

They are then released from the posterior lobe in response to nerve impulses transmitted from the hypothalamus down the pituitary stalk.

The hypothalamus, which controls the release of hormones from both the anterior and posterior pituitary lobes, is in turn under the control of higher cortical centers. Consequently, pituitary secretion is to some extent influenced by emotional stimuli such as anxiety, rage, and fear and is also influenced by sensory impulses that enter the nervous system and are in turn relayed to the hypothalamus.

Pituitary Hormones

The pituitary gland secretes a total of eight separate hormones, which have multiple functions. Six are produced by the anterior lobe: growth hormone (GH), **prolactin**, thyroid-stimulating hormone (TSH), adrenocorticotropic hormone (ACTH), **follicle-stimulating hormone (FSH)**, and **luteinizing hormone (LH)**. Two, **antidiuretic hormone (ADH)** and **oxytocin**, are produced by the posterior lobe. Melanocyte-stimulating hormone (MSH) is sometimes considered a ninth hormone secreted by the pituitary gland. The four anterior lobe hormones that regulate other endocrine glands are termed tropic hormones (Figure 22-3C).

Prolactin Hormone produced by the anterior lobe of the pituitary gland that stimulates milk secretion.

Follicle-stimulating hormone (FSH) One of the gonadotropic hormones secreted by the anterior lobe of the pituitary; it stimulates the growth of ovarian follicles in females and sperm production in males.

Luteinizing hormone (LH) One of the gonadotropic hormones secreted by the anterior lobe of the pituitary; it triggers ovulation in females, and production of testosterone in males.

Antidiuretic hormone (ADH) Posterior lobe pituitary hormone that regulates urine concentration by altering the permeability of the renal collecting tubules.

Oxytocin A hormone that is stored and released in the posterior lobe of the pituitary gland that causes uterine contractions during labor and ejection of milk from the breast lobules into the larger ducts.

Glucocorticoid An adrenal cortical hormone that regulates carbohydrate metabolism.

Anterior Lobe Hormones

Growth hormone (GH), also termed somatotropin, has multiple actions, all concerned with general tissue growth. GH also indirectly exerts its growth-promoting effects on tissues by stimulating the liver to produce a peptide termed insulin-like growth factor 1, or somatomedin (soma = body + medin = mediator of growth). The growth factor enters the circulation and travels throughout the body where it promotes growth of the skeletal system and internal organs. Prolactin stimulates the secretion of milk by the breast, which has been previously stimulated by estrogen and progesterone. Levels are normally low in males. TSH, also termed thyrotropin, stimulates the thyroid gland to secrete thyroid hormone. ACTH, also termed corticotropin, stimulates the adrenal cortex to manufacture and secrete adrenocortical hormones. ACTH exerts its main effect on the adrenal hormones that control carbohydrate metabolism, **glucocorticoids**, and it is produced from a large precursor molecule that gives rise not only to ACTH but also to MSH as a by-product. MSH causes darkening of the skin by stimulating melanocytes, but normally not enough is produced to have any significant effect when the output of ACTH is normal. However, darkening of skin may be a result of excess ACTH synthesis. FSH and LH are gonadotropic hormones. They regulate the growth and development of the gonads (ovaries and testes) and control the output of sex hormones, which are responsible for the development of male and female secondary sex characteristics.

Posterior Lobe Hormones

ADH, also referred to as vasopressin, causes the cells of the renal collecting tubules to become more permeable to water so that more water is reabsorbed and concentrated urine is excreted. Secretion of ADH is regulated by receptors in the hypothalamus, which respond to variations in the osmolarity of the extracellular fluid. If the osmolarity rises, the hypothalamic neurons send impulses to the posterior lobe to stimulate the release of ADH. Water is retained instead of being excreted, which dilutes the extracellular fluid and lowers its osmolarity. Conversely, if the extracellular fluids become too diluted, the hypothalamus directs the pituitary to decrease its output of ADH. More water is excreted in the urine, which causes the osmolarity of the body fluids to rise.

Oxytocin stimulates the contraction of the pregnant uterus and causes the release of milk from the lactating breast. It also promotes maternal bonding with the neonate. Oxytocin also contributes to aspects of the human sexual response. When an infant nurses, oxytocin is secreted in response to stimulation of the nipples during nursing. The sensory nerve impulses are transmitted to the hypothalamus, and the hypothalamic neurons in turn send impulses to the posterior lobe, which causes the release of oxytocin.

Physiologic Control of Pituitary Hormone Secretion

The level of each of the various trophic hormones produced by the pituitary is regulated by the level of circulating hormone produced by the target gland (Figure 22-2). Cells in the hypothalamus measure the level of the various chemicals and hormones in the blood. They respond by adjusting, releasing, and inhibiting hormones that control the release of pituitary hormones into the circulation. Several hormones produced by the hypothalamus and pituitary gland are released in pulses rather than as a continuous output. Many hormone levels also may vary over a 24-hour period with a circadian rhythm. This is most notable for ACTH; the highest levels occur in the early morning, followed by a gradual fall throughout the day. When the concentration of the hormone falls below a threshold level, releasing hormones increase and travel by the hypophyseal portal system to the pituitary gland, causing the release of the tropic hormone. This, in turn, affects the target organ. The level of the hormone produced by the target organ rises until it reaches the upper range of normal. At this point, the high level of circulating hormone "shuts off" further excretion of tropic hormones. This mechanism maintains a relatively steady hormone output from the target organ and prevents wide fluctuations in hormonal levels that might disrupt the smooth functioning of the body's hormonally regulated organ systems. It should be noted that the set point at which a hormone produced by a target gland turns off tropic hormone secretion varies considerably from individual to individual.

Prolactin secretion is regulated by a somewhat different mechanism than the other pituitary hormones. With other hormones, the main effect of hypothalamic releasing hormones is to stimulate secretion. For prolactin, however, the principal control is by an inhibitory substance, the neurotransmitter **dopamine**. Secretion of prolactin would continue unabated if it were not continuously suppressed. Release of prolactin is affected by stimuli from the nipples during nursing. The stimuli are relayed to the hypothalamus, which responds by releasing less dopamine, and prolactin secretion increases.

Dopamine Chemical mediator released by some neurons of the central nervous system. Dopamine also serves as a neurotransmitter in the nervous system.

Effects of Abnormalities in the Secretion of Tropic Hormones

Abnormalities in the secretion of tropic hormones may involve either a single or multiple hormones and may be manifested as either a hypofunction or an overproduction of pituitary hormone.

Pituitary Hypofunction

Panhypopituitarism Failure of secretion of all anterior lobe pituitary hormones.

Pituitary dwarfism Stunted growth caused by a deficiency of growth hormone in a child.

Diabetes insipidus A condition resulting from a deficiency of antidiuretic hormone, characterized by the excretion of a large volume of very diluted urine.

Pituitary hypofunction can occur when the anterior lobe of the pituitary gland is destroyed by a tumor, neurological injury, or cranial radiation therapy or undergoes necrosis owing to a disturbance of its blood supply, as sometimes occurs in the postpartum period, termed Sheehan syndrome. Rare congenital defects in the development of the pituitary can also occur and result in pituitary hypofunction. In a condition termed **panhypopituitarism** (pan = multiple + hypo = decrease), the anterior lobe fails to secrete the normal level of any hormones. The functions of the thyroid gland, adrenal glands, and gonads are impaired because tropic hormone stimulation is lost. Pituitary hypofunction can lead to **pituitary dwarfism** or **diabetes insipidus**, resulting from a lack of growth hormone or ADH, respectively.

Pituitary dwarfism, an isolated deficiency of growth hormone in a child, is characterized by delayed growth and development. In some cases, a mutation in the growth hormone gene is responsible, but in most cases, the cause is unknown. Normal growth and development can be restored by administering growth hormone. Diabetes insipidus is a disease usually caused by failure of the posterior lobe of the pituitary gland to secrete ADH due to injury, tumor, or some other pathologic process involving the posterior lobe. Because of the lack of ADH, the affected person is unable to reabsorb water from the renal collecting tubules and excretes a large volume of extremely diluted urine. Large amounts of water must be consumed to compensate for the excessive water loss and to prevent dehydration. In some cases of diabetes insipidus, however, the problem is not with inadequate output of ADH but with an inability of the kidneys to respond to the hormone. This condition is termed "nephrogenic diabetes insipidus" to set it apart from the disease caused by posterior lobe malfunction. Treatment differs depending on the cause of the diabetes insipidus. If the posterior lobe is at fault, treatment consists of supplying ADH. If it is a kidney problem, drugs are given to make the kidney more responsive to ADH.

Pituitary Tumors

Many conditions affecting the pituitary gland result from pituitary tumors involving the anterior lobe of the gland, many of which are considered functional since they produce hormones. Tumors that do not produce hormones are designated nonfunctional tumors. Although no hormones are produced, a nonfunctional tumor may cause problems resulting from the mass effect of the enlarging tumor. Because the location of the pituitary is close to the optic chiasm, optic nerves, and other vital structures at the base of the brain, an enlarging tumor may erode the pituitary fossa, encroach on the optic chiasm, and disrupt the hormone-producing functions of adjacent normal anterior lobe cells that are compressed by the expanding tumor. As well as disrupting pituitary function, nonfunctional tumors may result in visual disturbances, headaches, and other neurological abnormalities.

Clinical manifestations of a functional tumor are determined by what hormone it makes, how much hormone it produces, the size of the tumor, and the age of the individual. The two most common functional pituitary tumors produce growth hormone and prolactin. Generally, each type of tumor produces a characteristic clinical syndrome. The great majority of pituitary tumors are adenomas; that is, they are benign glandular tumors that do not metastasize but may be associated with significant disease (**Figure 22-4**).

Treatment of a pituitary tumor is determined by the type of tumor, the hormones it produces, and the size of the tumor. A small prolactin-secreting

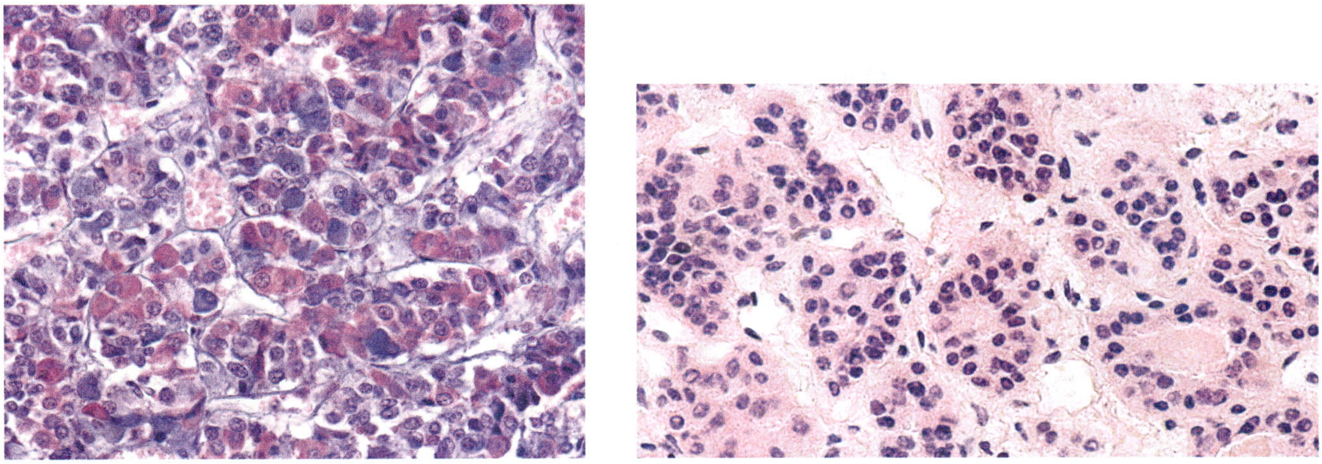

Figure 22-4 Histology of a normal pituitary gland and a pituitary gland with an adenoma. **(A)** Normal pituitary tissue showing characteristic multiple cell types. **(B)** Uniform cell population of the pituitary adenoma.

adenoma may respond well to drugs that shrink the tumor. A tumor secreting growth hormone can be suppressed by drugs. In many cases, however, the treatment of a pituitary tumor is surgical removal, occasionally followed by radiation treatment in selected patients.

Because a pituitary tumor is so difficult to approach through the cranial cavity, it is usually resected through the nasal cavity and sphenoid sinus, a procedure termed a transsphenoidal resection (**Figure 22-5**). The transsphenoidal method for resecting all types of pituitary tumors involves entering the nasal cavity either directly or through an incision under the upper lip and removing part of the nasal septum. Then the sphenoid sinus is entered, and the anterior part of the pituitary fossa, the sella turcica, is opened to expose the pituitary tumor, which is resected. Finally, the nasal incision is repaired.

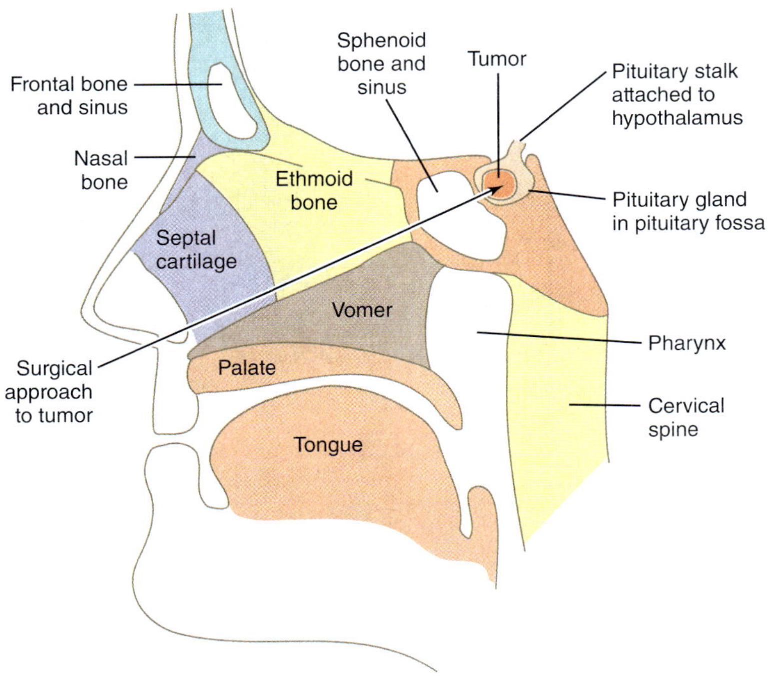

Figure 22-5 Transsphenoidal resection of a pituitary tumor.

Overproduction of Growth Hormone

Overproduction of growth hormone might be the result of a functional adenoma in children and adolescents, whose epiphyses have not yet fused, causing excessive growth in the length of bones. The person becomes exceptionally tall. This condition is termed **pituitary gigantism**. Some coarsening of the facial features usually occurs in response to the effect of growth hormone on the structure of the facial bones.

Pituitary gigantism A condition resulting from excessive secretion of growth hormone in the child.

Acromegaly A condition resulting from excessive secretion of growth hormone in the adult.

Galactorrhea Secretion of milk by breast not associated with pregnancy or normal lactation.

Amenorrhea Absence of menses.

In adults, excessive growth hormone causes **acromegaly**. Because the epiphyses have fused, there can be no growth in height, but the growth hormone produces thickening and coarsening of bones and generalized enlargement of the viscera. Affected individuals have coarse facial features, large prominent jaws, and large spade-like hands, but they are no taller than normal (**Figure 22-6**). The term acromegaly (acron = extremity + megas = large) describes one prominent feature of the disease. Growth hormone excess is almost always associated with pituitary adenomas. In addition to the hormonal effects, manifestations related to the size and location of the tumor may also occur. As noted previously, surgery is curative.

Overproduction of Prolactin

In a nonpregnant woman, excess secretion of prolactin (hyperprolactinemia) may cause spontaneous secretion of milk from the breasts, **galactorrhea**, and cessation of menstrual periods, **amenorrhea**. Galactorrhea results from the effect of the hormone on breast tissue. Amenorrhea occurs because high levels of prolactin also inhibit secretion of pituitary gonadotropins FSH and LH, which in turn leads to cessation of ovulation and menstrual cycles. This is

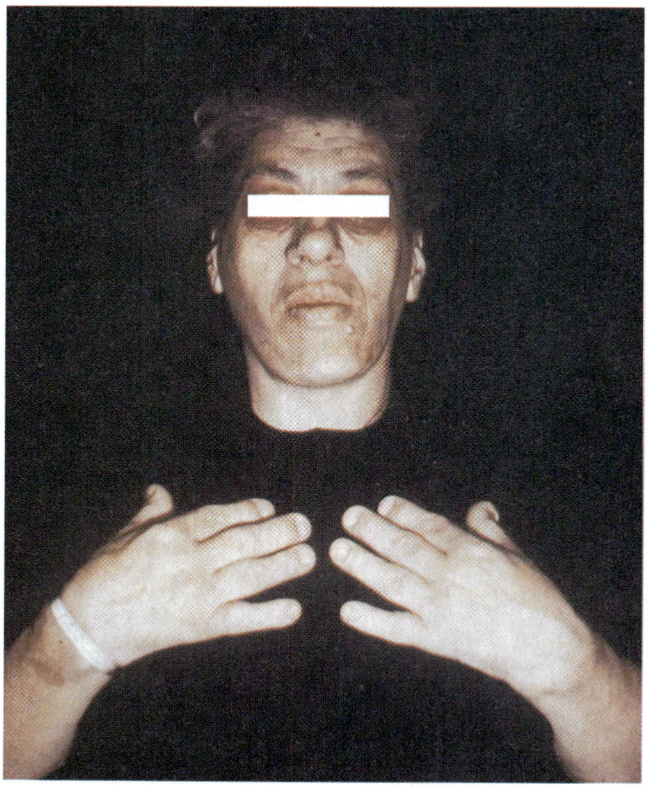

Figure 22-6 The appearance of an individual with advanced acromegaly.

Courtesy of Leonard V. Crowley, MD, Century College.

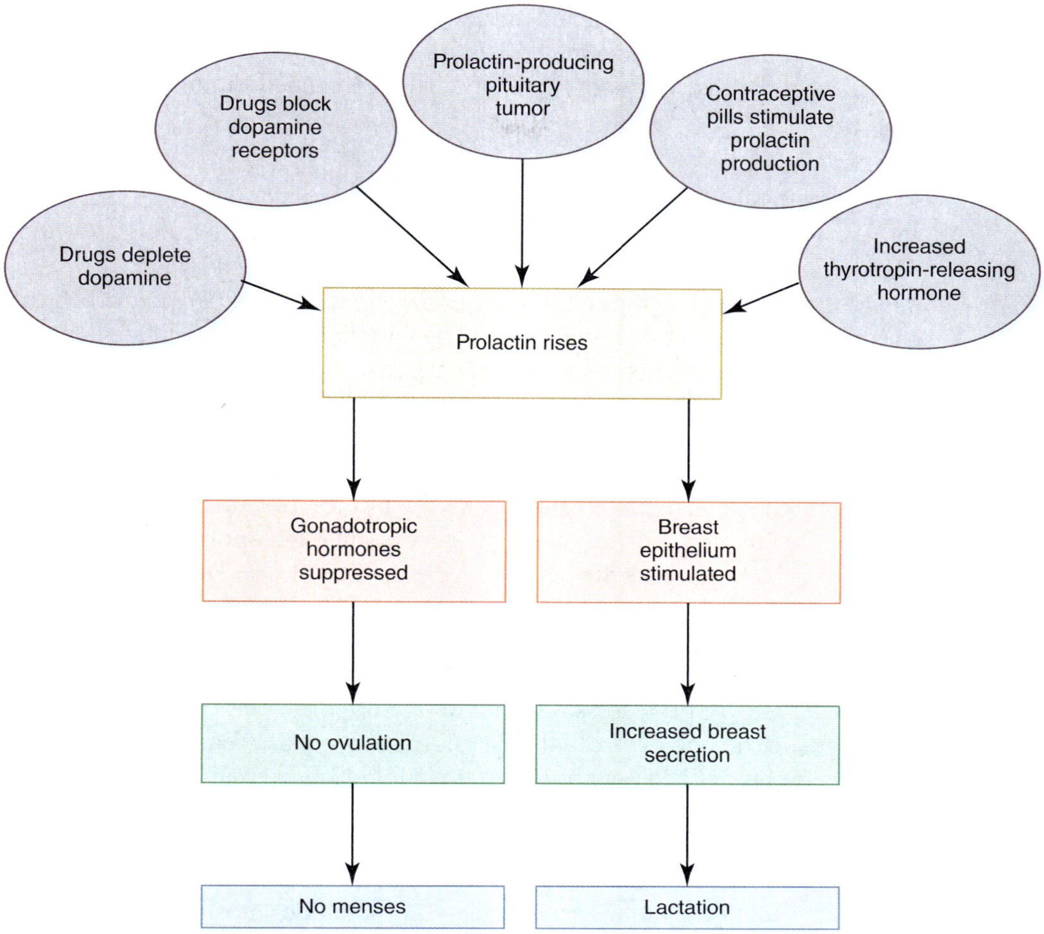

Figure 22-7 Factors regulating prolactin secretion and pathogenesis of amenorrhea–galactorrhea syndrome.

sometimes termed the amenorrhea–galactorrhea syndrome. In males, overproduction of prolactin by a functional tumor is associated with infertility, hypogonadism, reduced sexual function, and occasionally gynecomastia, breast tissue enlargement. However, headaches, visual disturbances, and neurological defects most often bring attention to such tumors in males before hormonal changes manifest.

The various causes of the amenorrhea–galactorrhea syndrome are summarized in **Figure 22-7**. A prolactin-secreting pituitary adenoma is the most likely possibility. Sometimes the tumor is quite small (termed a microadenoma) and causes few symptoms other than those related to the increased prolactin production. Larger tumors may cause enlargement of the pituitary fossa and visual disturbances like those caused by adenomas that secrete growth hormone. A prolactin-secreting pituitary adenoma can be removed surgically, but a small adenoma can often be inhibited by a **dopamine agonist** drug (agon = competitor), which is a drug that functions like dopamine, such as bromocriptine or a similar drug that attaches to dopamine receptors on the prolactin-secreting anterior lobe cells. The attachment suppresses the output of prolactin, which in turn suppresses the growth and secretion of the prolactin-secreting adenoma.

Dopamine agonist A drug such as bromocriptine that binds to the dopamine receptors on the anterior pituitary cell and mimics the function of dopamine, producing effects such as inhibition of prolactin secretion.

There are other causes of hyperprolactinemia. Some drugs and medications may at times raise prolactin levels, resulting in amenorrhea and galactorrhea. These include estrogens, antihypertensive drugs, and drugs used to treat mental or emotional problems. Antihypertensive drugs, phenothiazine drugs (used to treat mental illness), and antidepressant drugs raise prolactin levels by depleting dopamine or blocking dopamine receptors in the hypothalamus. Prolactin levels also rise in hypothyroidism, which is related indirectly to reduced thyroid hormone secretion.

The Thyroid Gland

The thyroid gland, consisting of two lateral lobes connected by a narrow isthmus (**Figure 22-8A**), is located in the neck overlying the upper part of the trachea and is regulated by pituitary TSH. The parathyroid glands (most often four in number) are located on its posterior surface.

Histologically, the thyroid gland is composed of multiple minute spherical vesicles (acini, singular acinus) designated as thyroid follicles. Each follicle consists of a central mass of eosinophilic protein material termed "**colloid**", containing the protein **thyroglobulin**, which is the precursor of thyroid hormones. The colloid is surrounded by a layer of cuboidal epithelial cells termed follicular cells (**Figure 22-8B**). Under the influence of TSH, the follicular cells synthesize two hormones—triiodothyronine (T_3) and tetraiodothyronine, or thyroxine (T_4), which require iodination of the thyroglobulin protein. Newly synthesized T_3 and T_4 are attached to the thyroglobulin protein. Thyroglobulin is cleaved by proteases, releasing T_3 and T_4 into the circulation, where they regulate the body's metabolic processes and are also required for the normal development of the nervous system. Thyroid hormone is a general term referring to the two metabolic hormones, T_3 and T_4; the numbers indicate the number of iodine atoms attached to the molecules (**Figure 22-9**). More than 80 percent of T_3 (the more active hormone) is derived in circulation from secreted T_4. Both hormones can circulate in the blood, mostly in bound form (they usually bind to thyroid-binding globulin) or less than 1 percent in a free state. They are biologically active only when circulating in free form.

Specialized parafollicular cells located between the thyroid follicles elaborate a third hormone termed **calcitonin**. This hormone tends to lower blood calcium but plays a relatively minor role in regulating the level of calcium in the blood and may also have a role in bone formation.

Colloid Homogenous substances with particles dispersed throughout the substance and include gels, sols an emulsions. Colloidal osmotic pressure contributes to water balance throughout the body.

Thyroglobulin A protein within the colloid of the thyroid follicles, which is a precursor of thyroid hormone.

Calcitonin A hormone that lowers blood calcium, produced by the interfollicular cells of the thyroid gland.

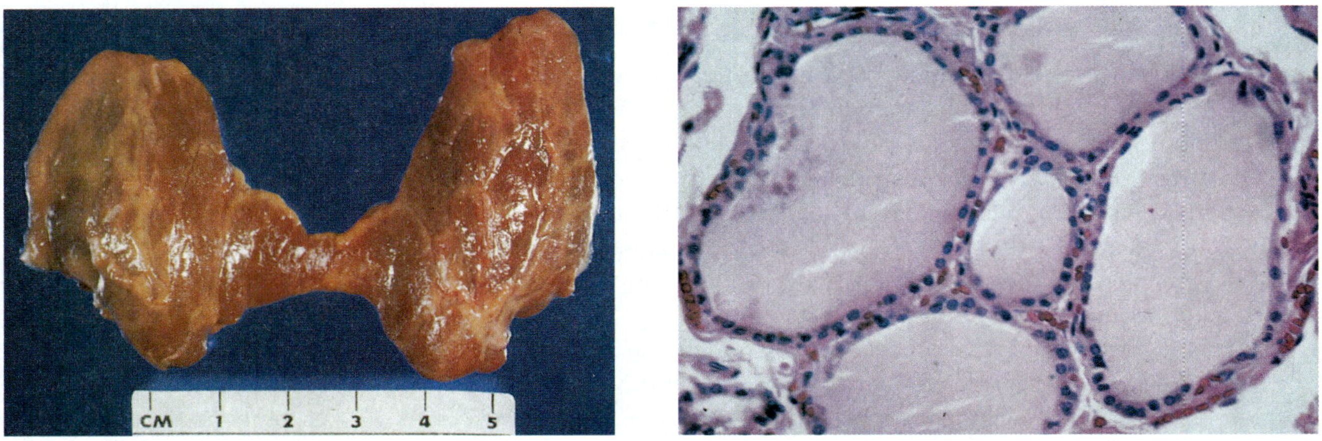

(A) (B)

Figure 22-8 **(A)** Normal thyroid gland, illustrating two lateral lobes connected by a narrow isthmus. **(B)** High-magnification photograph of normal thyroid follicles, illustrating central masses of colloid surrounded by follicular epithelial cells (original magnification ×400).

Courtesy of Leonard V. Crowley, MD, Century College.

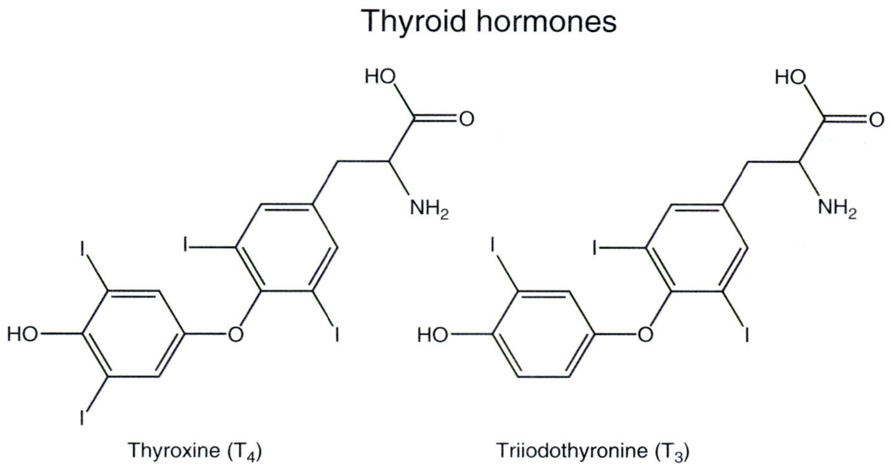

Figure 22-9 Structural formula of thyroid hormones: thyroxin (T_4) and Triiodothyronine (T_3).

Actions of Thyroid Hormone

Thyroid hormone controls the rate of metabolic processes and is required for normal growth and development. Too much thyroid hormone leads to a condition termed hyperthyroidism, characterized by an acceleration of all bodily metabolic functions. Conversely, a decrease in the level of thyroid hormone, termed hypothyroidism, slows metabolic processes.

Clinically, some of the most pronounced effects of excess thyroid hormone are manifested in the cardiovascular and neuromuscular systems. The heart rate is accelerated. Reflexes are hyperactive, and frequently a fine tremor of the muscles is apparent. The hormone also has conspicuous effects on emotional and intellectual functions. Individuals with excess thyroid hormone are hyperactive, emotionally labile, and often quite irritable. They may have difficulty concentrating because mental processes are accelerated excessively.

The effects of thyroid hypofunction are the reverse of those in hyperthyroidism. The hypothyroid individual is slow and lethargic. Bodily metabolic functions are subnormal. Reflexes and speech are slow and sluggish. **Table 22-2** summarizes the major clinical effects resulting from abnormal levels of thyroid hormone.

Table 22-2 Comparison of Major Effects of Hyperthyroidism and Hypothyroidism

	Hyperthyroidism	Hypothyroidism
Cardiovascular effects	Rapid pulse, increased cardiac output	Slow pulse, reduced cardiac output
Metabolic effects	Increased metabolism, skin hot and flushed, weight loss	Decreased metabolism, cold skin, weight gain
Neuromuscular effects	Tremor, hyperactive reflexes	Weakness, lassitude, sluggish reflexes
Mental, emotional effects	Restlessness, irritability, emotional lability	Mental processes sluggish and retarded, personality placid and phlegmatic
Gastrointestinal effects	Diarrhea	Constipation
General somatic effects	Warm, moist skin	Cold, dry skin

Goiter

Goiter Any enlargement of the thyroid gland.

An enlargement of the thyroid gland is termed a **goiter** (from the Latin *guttur*, throat). A nontoxic goiter does not secrete excess thyroid hormone. The gland may be uniformly enlarged, a diffuse goiter. Most commonly, multiple nodules of proliferating thyroid tissue can be visualized, termed a nodular goiter. Occasionally, patients with nontoxic multinodular goiters may develop nodules that secrete hormones, resulting in hyperthyroidism. Such goiters are termed toxic.

Both nodular and diffuse nontoxic goiters can result in inadequate secretion of thyroid hormone. The enlargement of the gland results from stimulation of the gland by TSH. The increased TSH release occurs due to the low thyroid hormone output resulting from low iron intake (**Figure 22-10**). As a result, the gland enlarges to produce more hormones. However, many nontoxic goiters do not result in hormonal irregularities but rather come to medical attention for cosmetic reasons.

Three major factors predispose one to the development of a nontoxic goiter: iodine deficiency, deficiency of enzymes required for the synthesis of thyroid hormone or ingestion of substances that interfere with the function of these enzymes, or increased hormone requirements due to the individual's developmental stage.

Iodine Deficiency

If iodine is deficient in the diet, the production of thyroid hormone will be inadequate for the needs of the individual. The enlargement of the gland is a result of an attempt to make more hormone in response to TSH stimulation.

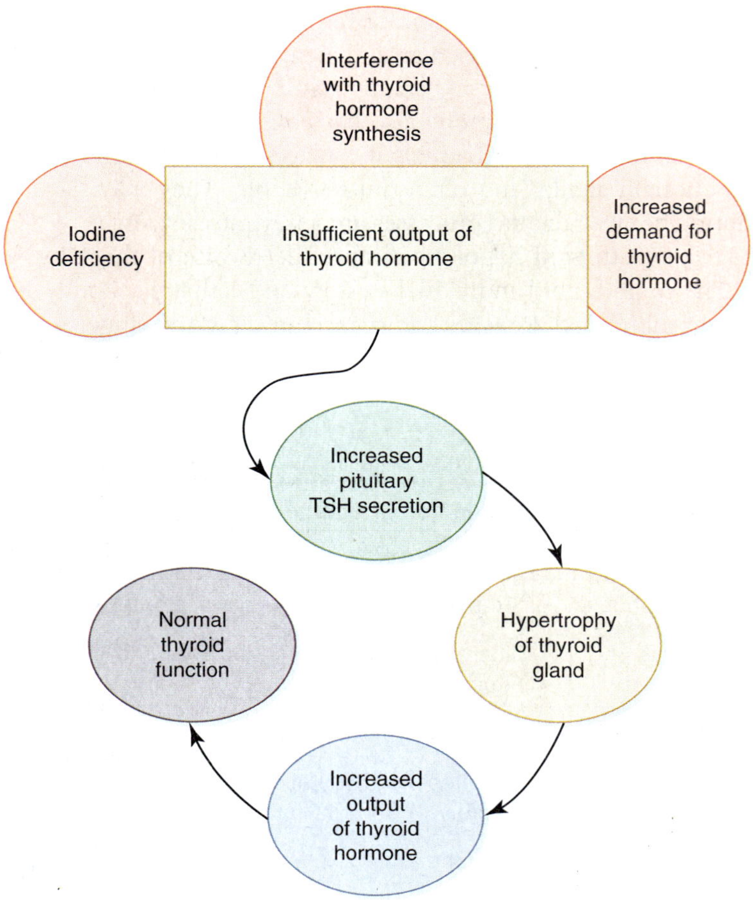

Figure 22-10 The pathogenesis of nontoxic goiter.

Now iodine deficiency is rarely a cause of goiter in the United States because table salt, bread, and many other foods fortified with iodine are available. However, it continues to be a problem in some countries where food sources are naturally low in iodine and salt is not routinely fortified.

Enzyme Deficiency or Impaired Enzyme Function

Goiter more commonly results from a mild deficiency in a glandular enzyme that is required for hormone synthesis; the enzyme-deficient gland is unable to produce sufficient hormone without enlarging. Less commonly, the enzymes are present in normal amounts, but their functions are impaired by ingestion of drugs or other substances that interfere with the action of the enzymes. Even some "natural" foods, such as cabbage and turnips, contain small amounts of substances that interfere with thyroid-hormone synthesis, but these foods are not usually eaten in quantities sufficient to cause difficulty.

Increased Hormone Requirements

Normally, the need for thyroid hormone increases in puberty, during pregnancy, and under conditions of stress. In some individuals, the thyroid gland may be able to produce adequate hormone under normal circumstances but may be unable to increase its output in response to increased requirements without enlarging.

Whenever hormone output is inadequate, no matter what the cause, more TSH is released to step up hormone production. Because hormone requirements often fluctuate, a gland may undergo successive alternating periods of enlargement and reduction in size. At first, the gland enlarges uniformly in response to TSH stimulation, returning to its original size when increased hormone output is no longer required. Eventually, however, the gland may respond in an irregular manner to TSH stimulation. If this occurs, the enlargement of the gland is not uniform, and a nodular goiter results (**Figure 22-11**).

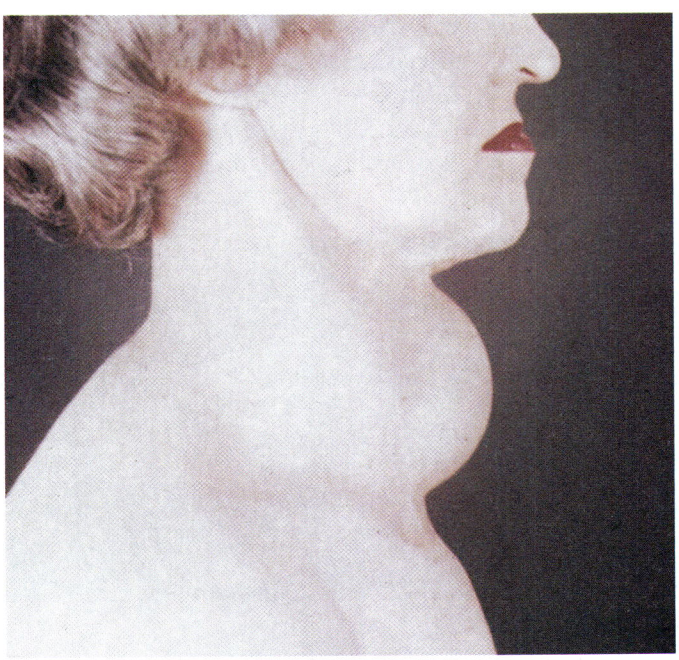

Figure 22-11 Large nodular goiter.

Courtesy of Leonard V. Crowley, MD, Century College.

Treatment of Nontoxic Goiter

Because a nontoxic goiter results from excessive stimulation of the thyroid gland by TSH, it is usually treated by administration of thyroid hormone, which suppresses TSH output by the negative feedback mechanism. Treatment usually causes the enlarged gland to shrink because it is no longer being stimulated by TSH. A large nodular goiter may have to be removed surgically if it compresses the trachea, interferes with respiration, or obstructs the neck veins returning blood to the heart.

Hyperthyroidism

Many different conditions can cause an excess secretion of thyroid hormone. Sometimes a nodular goiter or a solitary thyroid adenoma may produce excess hormone and cause hyperthyroidism. A few other uncommon conditions may also increase hormone output. However, hyperthyroidism usually is caused by an autoimmune disease in which various autoantibodies target thyroid cells. This condition is usually termed either **Graves' disease**, after the Irish physician who described the condition, or **exophthalmic goiter**, after a common eye manifestation of the disease, Graves' ophthalmopathy. The most significant of the antithyroid autoantibodies in this disease is the one that mimics the function of TSH and binds to TSH receptors on thyroid cells, driving the thyroid to secrete excess hormone. This excess and inappropriate hormone secretion remains unresponsive to the inhibitory feedback control mechanisms. The autoantibody continues to mimic thyroid hormone by binding to the receptor, enabling the thyroid gland to produce hormones. In most patients, the thyroid gland is diffusely enlarged, but the degree of enlargement is not always marked (**Figure 22-12**).

Graves' disease An autoimmune thyroid disease in which autoantibodies resembling thyroid-stimulating hormone stimulate an excessive output of thyroid hormone, causing hyperthyroidism.

Exophthalmic goiter A manifestation of Graves' disease, named for the protrusion of the eyes seen in many patients with this disease. It is also referred to as thyroid eye disease.

The eye changes that occur in many subjects with Graves' disease are also caused by the autoimmune disease. Activated T lymphocytes infiltrate the fat, connective tissue, and muscles that move the eyes, extraocular muscles, located in the orbital cavities behind the eyes. The T lymphocytes cause inflammation and swelling of the tissues, which pushes the eyes forward. The eye protrusion may interfere with the ability of the eyelids to close the eyes and/or with the function of the extraocular muscles. In severe cases, the eyes may be pushed so far forward that the optic nerves are stretched to the point of injury. Fortunately, although some degree of eye protrusion is present in many affected individuals, extreme eye protrusion and its complications are uncommon.

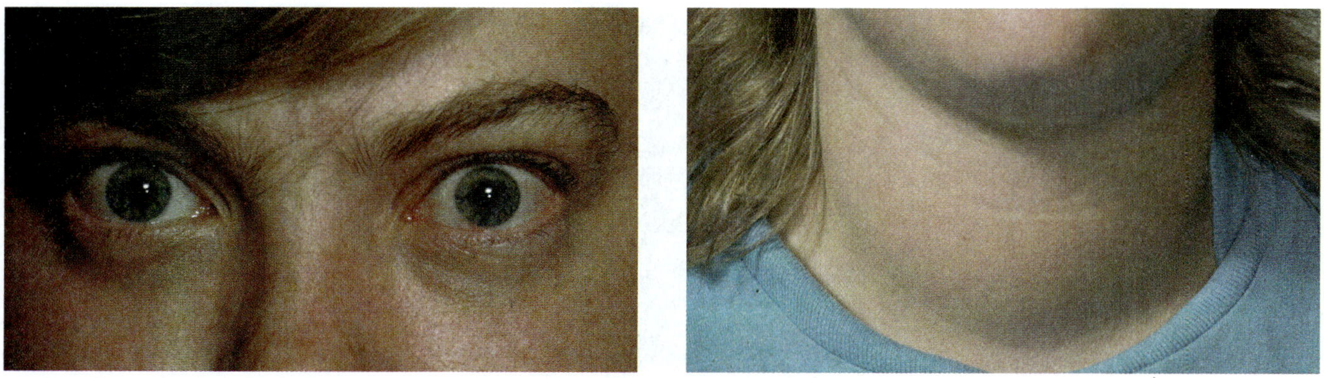

(A) (B)

Figure 22-12 Graves' disease. **(A)** Exophthalmos is characterized by a wide-eyed staring gaze. **(B)** Diffuse swelling of the neck due to goiter.

Courtesy of Dr. Don Schalch, Division of Endocrinology, University of Wisconsin School of Medicine and Public Health.

At present, no method is available to block the stimulation of the thyroid gland by the autoantibodies causing the unregulated hypersecretion of thyroid hormone. It is possible, however, to control the hyperthyroidism. Three different methods of treatment can be used. Antithyroid drugs can be administered to block the synthesis of hormone by the hyperactive gland. A large portion of the gland can be removed surgically, reducing the source of the hormone. A dose of radioactive iodine can be administered to be taken up by the thyroid gland. The irradiation destroys part of the gland and reduces its hormone output.

Successful treatment of hyperthyroidism may stop further protrusion of the eyes, but sometimes the protrusion progresses even though the hyperthyroidism has been controlled.

Hypothyroidism

Hypothyroidism in the Adult

Hypothyroidism in the adult is sometimes termed **myxedema** (**Figure 22-13**) and is manifested by a general slowing of the body's metabolic processes. Frequently, there are localized accumulations of mucinous material in the skin, from which the disease received its name (myx = mucin + edema = swelling). Hypothyroid individuals have low levels of circulating thyroid hormone and high levels of TSH that reflect stimulation of the gland in an unsuccessful attempt to increase hormone output. The condition is treated by supplying the deficient hormone, which results in clinical improvement, return of thyroid hormone level to normal, and a fall in TSH.

Myxedema Hypothyroidism in the adult.

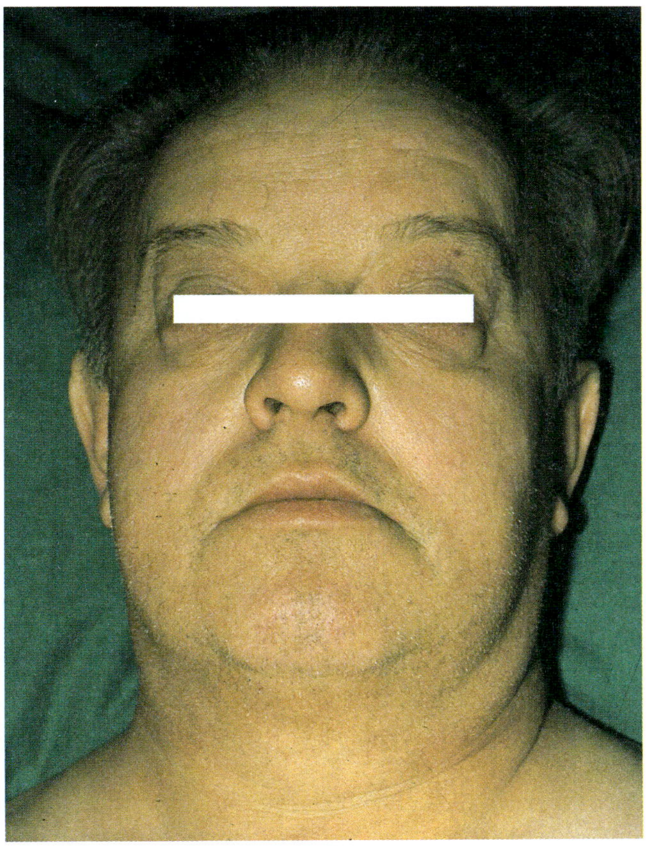

Figure 22-13 The appearance of a patient with myxedema.

Courtesy of Leonard V. Crowley, MD, Century College.

Neonatal Hypothyroidism

Hypothyroidism in the newborn infant is termed congenital hypothyroidism. This condition may be caused by failure of the thyroid gland to develop or may result from a genetically determined deficiency of enzymes necessary for thyroid hormone synthesis. In the latter condition, the gland undergoes hyperplasia caused by excessive TSH stimulation but is unable to produce adequate hormone because of the enzyme deficiency.

Usually, the affected infant appears normal at birth because the placenta supplied the fetus with significant amounts of thyroid hormone. However, as the level of passively transferred maternal thyroid hormone gradually falls, clinical manifestations of hypothyroidism appear within the first few months after birth. Thyroid hormone not only regulates metabolic processes but is also required for normal growth. The hormone is essential for the normal development of the nervous system, which continues for several months after birth. If neonatal hypothyroidism is recognized and treated promptly, the affected infant will usually grow and develop normally. If the condition remains undetected, the unfortunate infant will remain permanently stunted in growth and mentally disabled. Historically, this condition was termed **cretinism** and was associated with endemic congenital iodine deficiency. In the United States and Europe, defects in thyroid development or in hormone production are usually responsible. Areas with low levels of iodine in the soil (or lacking iodized food products) continue to experience environmental hypothyroidism in young children. Hypothyroidism and cretinism in children resulting from nutritional lack of iodine remain an important source of childhood neurological disease in some areas of the world. Screening tests for neonatal hypothyroidism are performed routinely on newborn infants to identify neonatal congenital hypothyroidism by detecting the low levels of thyroid hormone and elevated levels of TSH.

Cretinism Hypothyroidism in the infant.

Hashimoto thyroiditis An autoimmune disease in which an autoantibody is directed against thyroid epithelial cells, causing progressive destruction of the thyroid gland, leading to chronic hypothyroidism.

Chronic Thyroiditis: Hashimoto Thyroiditis

Thyroiditis, or inflammation of the thyroid gland, may result from a bacterial or viral infection and can compromise thyroid function. The inflammation can be acute or chronic, depending on its clinical manifestations and the type of inflammatory cells involved. However, not all forms of thyroiditis are infectious. **Hashimoto thyroiditis**, a chronic thyroiditis, is an autoimmune disease in which antithyroid autoantibodies and activated T lymphocytes target thyroid antigens and destroy the thyroid gland. This is the most common cause of hypothyroidism in adults, and it occurs predominantly in middle-aged women. One of the autoantibodies formed in this disease targets and destroys the TSH receptors on the thyroid cells, preventing TSH from binding and stimulating the thyroid gland. Consequently, the output of thyroid hormone falls as TSH receptor damage progresses. The normal feedback control system that regulates hormone output (Figure 22-2) responds to the low hormone level, and TSH rises as thyroid hormone falls. The behavior of the autoantibody in Hashimoto thyroiditis is quite different from that of the autoantibody in hyperthyroidism (Graves' disease). In the first case, the antibody destroys the receptors, causing hypothyroidism; in the second case, the autoantibody stimulates the receptors, causing hyperthyroidism.

The thyroid gland of a person with Hashimoto thyroiditis is usually enlarged due to the diffused infiltration of activated T lymphocytes and plasma cells that are destroying the thyroid tissue (**Figure 22-14**). No specific treatment is available to arrest the relentless progression of the disease. Hypothyroidism can be

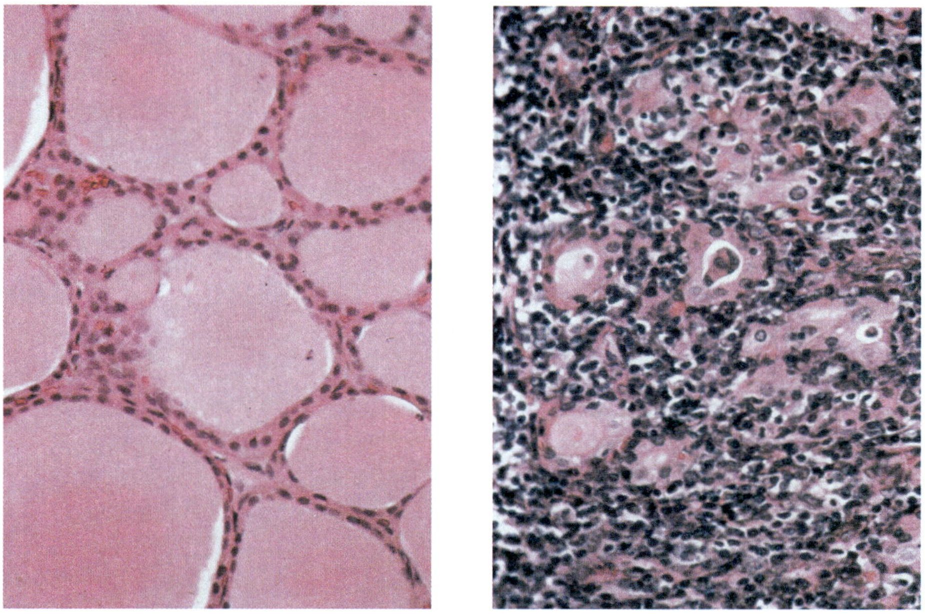

(A) (B)

Figure 22-14 Low-magnification photomicrographs comparing the cellular structure of a normal thyroid gland **(A)** with that in chronic thyroiditis **(B)**. The gland is heavily infiltrated by lymphocytes. Follicles are small and lack colloid (original magnification ×100).

Courtesy of Leonard V. Crowley, MD, Century College.

treated by the administration of thyroid hormone. Both the level of thyroid hormone in the blood and the level of TSH are considered to determine how much thyroid hormone to give the patient.

Tumors of the Thyroid

The thyroid gives rise to benign adenomas and several different types of carcinomas. Thyroid follicular adenomas contain completely encapsulated nodules composed of cells that differ in pattern from the thyroid gland outside the nodule (**Figure 22-15**). Thyroid nodules are very common (over 50 percent of

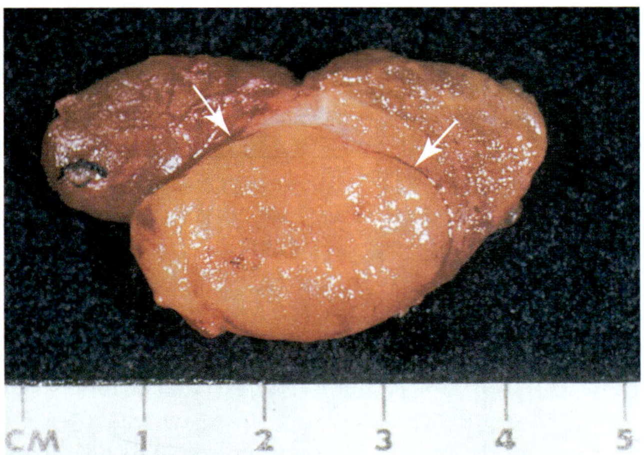

Figure 22-15 A benign, well-circumscribed adenoma of the thyroid gland (*arrows*). The surrounding thyroid tissue appears normal.

Courtesy of Leonard V. Crowley, MD, Century College.

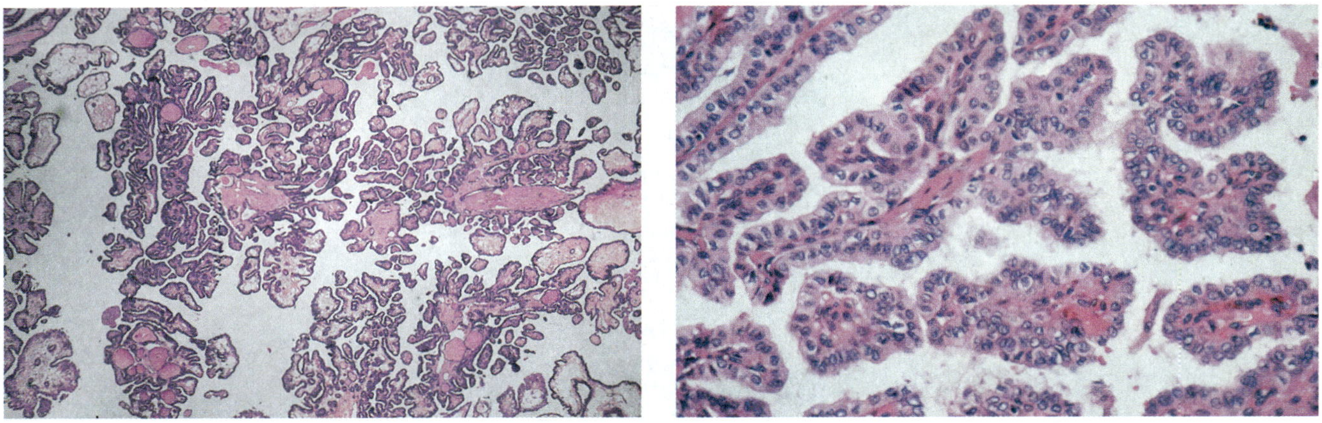

(A) (B)

Figure 22-16 Well-differentiated papillary carcinoma of the thyroid. **(A)** A low-magnification view illustrating the papillary structure (original magnification x 40). **(B)** Higher magnification of papillary process covered by well-different ated neoplastic thyroid epithelium (original magnification × 160).

Courtesy of Leonard V. Crowley, MD, Century College.

the population have them present at autopsy). Although most such nodules are benign, up to 20 percent may be malignant. Three distinct types of follicular cell–derived thyroid carcinoma are recognized: follicular, papillary, and anaplastic.

The most common type, illustrated in **Figure 22-16**, is termed a papillary carcinoma, because the tumor is composed of well-differentiated papillary processes covered by well-differentiated thyroid epithelial cells. It is strongly associated with radiation exposure in children (such as from the Chernobyl disaster or from therapeutic procedures). It has an excellent prognosis in the young, but it may present as an aggressive disease in older males. A less common type of tumor is termed a follicular carcinoma, because the tumor cells form colloid-filled follicles, which resemble normal thyroid tissue. They occur in an older population and, unlike papillary carcinomas, may be associated with metastatic disease. Treatment of both types is by surgical resection of the thyroid gland (thyroidectomy). Partial resection may be undertaken in the case of papillary cancer; however, total resection followed by treatment with radioactive iodine is used in treating follicular cancer.

Undifferentiated (anaplastic) carcinoma is uncommon and develops in older people. The disease is composed of rapidly growing bizarre tumor cells and has poor prognosis. Treatment is by means of surgical resection combined with radiation and chemotherapy.

Medullary carcinoma is an uncommon tumor derived from the calcitonin-secreting parafollicular cells of the thyroid with a characteristic histologic pattern in which small cells are embedded in a hyalinized (glasslike) framework containing collagen and a calcitonin precursor (**Figure 22-17**). Measurement of calcitonin levels in the blood has been used as a diagnostic test for this type of thyroid cancer because the tumor cells often secrete calcitonin. Although the effect of calcitonin is to lower blood calcium, the excess hormone secretion has no significant effect on blood calcium because the effect of the calcitonin is counteracted by an increased secretion of parathyroid hormone, preventing blood calcium from falling. (The physiologic effects of parathyroid hormone are considered in conjunction with diseases of the parathyroid glands.) Thyroid tumors may not produce symptoms initially but as they enlarge, they may cause neck swelling, swallowing

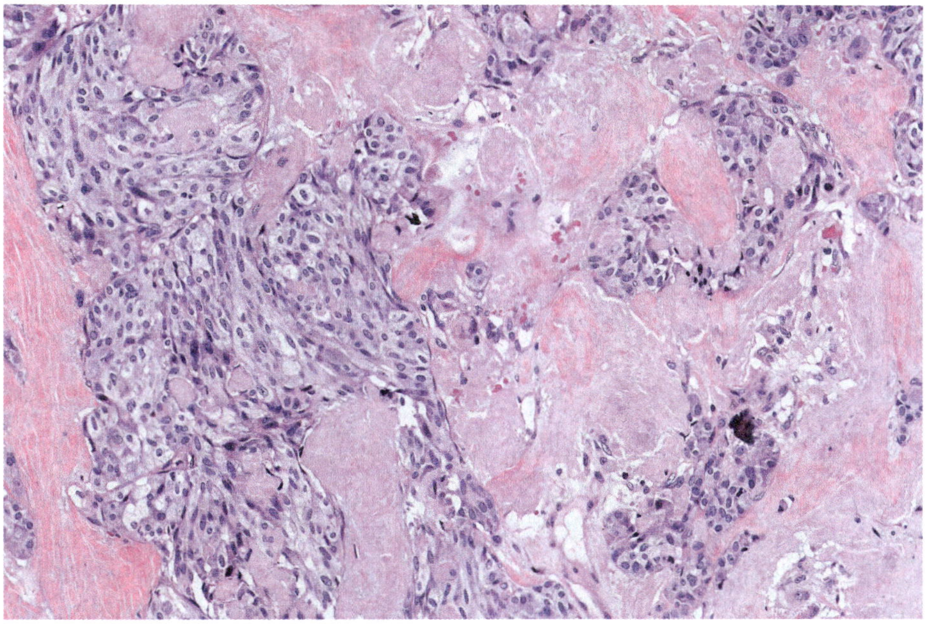

Figure 22-17 Medullary thyroid carcinoma. Small, polygonal tumor cells are embedded in a hyalinized collagenous acellular framework.

difficulties, and changes in the voice. An increase in the frequency of such "incidental" thyroid tumors is related to their finding in CT and MRI studies for other reasons.

The Parathyroid Glands and Calcium Metabolism

The parathyroid glands are located on the posterior surface of the lateral lobes of the thyroid gland and produce a hormone that regulates the level of calcium in the blood. Although the most common number of glands is 4, this may vary from 1 to more than 10. Usually, the blood calcium is in equilibrium with the calcium salts present in bone. Half the blood calcium is present as calcium ions (Ca^{2+}) and is the active form. The other half is bound to blood proteins and is biologically inactive. An adequate concentration of ionized calcium is required for normal cardiac and skeletal muscle contraction, for transmission of nerve impulses, and for coagulation of the blood. A subnormal level of ionized calcium causes increased excitability of nerve and muscle cells, leading to spasms of skeletal muscles, which is termed **tetany**. Conversely, a high level of ionized calcium diminishes neuromuscular excitability and leads to generalized muscular weakness.

Tetany Spasm of skeletal muscles caused by a subnormal level of ionized calcium in the blood or certain bacterial toxins.

The parathyroid hormone regulates the level of calcium by regulating the release of calcium from bone, the absorption of calcium from the intestine, and the rate of excretion of calcium by the kidneys. The secretion of parathyroid hormone (PTH) is regulated by the level of ionized calcium in the blood rather than by a tropic hormone elaborated by the pituitary gland. If the level of ionized calcium in the blood decreases, the parathyroids secrete more hormone. If the ionized calcium level rises, parathyroid hormone secretion declines. Any abnormality in the secretion of parathyroid hormone changes the concentration of ionized calcium in the blood and will eventually alter the amount of calcium deposited in bone. The PTH also indirectly leads to the activation of vitamin D, increasing intestinal absorption of calcium and the release of calcium from bones. High levels of active vitamin D suppress the secretion of PTH.

Hyperparathyroidism

Primary hyperparathyroidism is a relatively common problem and is usually the result of a hormone-secreting parathyroid adenoma. In response to increased output of hormone, the blood calcium rises (hypercalcemia), and excessive calcium is withdrawn from bone. The bones become excessively fragile and are easily broken.

Excessive amounts of calcium are excreted in the urine (hypercalciuria), sometimes leading to the formation of calcium stones within the urinary tract. Occasionally, calcium precipitates out of the blood and becomes deposited in the kidneys, lungs, and other tissues, producing tissue injury and functional impairment. Treatment consists of surgical removal of the tumor. Secondary hyperparathyroidism occurs with chronic renal disease rather than an abnormality of the parathyroids. Secondary hyperparathyroidism is the result of hypocalcemia related to chronic renal failure leading to decreased vitamin D activation.

Hypoparathyroidism

Hypoparathyroidism usually results from accidental removal of all parathyroid glands during an operation for a diffuse toxic goiter or a nodular goiter in which most of the thyroid gland is removed. Blood calcium falls precipitously, which leads to increased neuromuscular excitability and tetany. Treatment consists of raising the level of blood calcium by the administration of a high-calcium diet and supplementary vitamin D, which promotes absorption of calcium from the intestinal tract. Congenital and autoimmune-mediated forms of hypoparathyroidism also occur. Patients with congenital DiGeorge syndrome, associated with T cell immunodeficiency and craniofacial defects, also have neonatal hypoparathyroidism in about half of the cases.

The Adrenal Glands

The adrenals are paired glands located above the kidneys. Each adrenal consists of two separate endocrine glands: an inner adrenal medulla surrounded by an outer adrenal cortex. The adrenal cortex may be further divided into three zones: the zona glomerulosa, just under the capsule; the zona fasciculata; and the zona reticularis, adjacent to the medulla. The adrenal cortex and medulla secrete different hormones (**Figure 22-18**).

The Adrenal Cortex

Mineralocorticoid
Adrenal cortical hormone that regulates salt and water metabolism.

The adrenal cortex secretes three major classes of steroid hormones: glucocorticoids, **mineralocorticoids**, and sex hormones. Different zones of the adrenal cortex differ in their synthetic profile. The zona glomerulosa is responsible for mineralocorticoids; the zona fasciculata produces most of the glucocorticoids and some sex hormones; the zona reticularis produces most of the sex hormones (and some glucocorticoids).

Glucocorticoids raise the blood glucose by decreasing glucose utilization in many tissues, except the brain, and promote fat breakdown with utilization

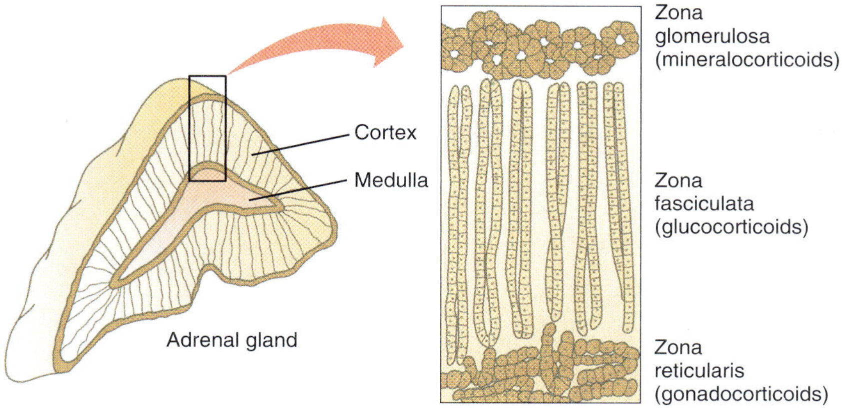

Figure 22-18 The adrenal gland.

of fatty acids rather than glucose as an energy source. They inhibit protein synthesis and promote breakdown of body proteins, some of which are converted into glucose by the liver. The net effect is to deplete tissue proteins and raise blood glucose. The adverse effect of glucocorticoids on wound healing and tissue repair is a result in part of their protein-depleting effects. Also, they act at multiple sites to suppress the inflammatory reaction. The use of adrenal corticosteroids to treat various types of inflammatory disease, such as the synthetic **cortisol**-like drug prednisone, is related to the anti-inflammatory property of the glucocorticoids.

Cortisol The major glucocorticoid.

Aldosterone A steroid hormone produced by the adrenal cortex that regulates the rate of sodium absorption from the renal tubules.

Glucocorticoids are secreted in response to stimulation by ACTH, and their output is controlled by the same type of negative feedback mechanism that regulates secretion of thyroid hormone. The major glucocorticoid is cortisol.

Mineralocorticoids regulate electrolyte and water balance by promoting absorption of sodium and water and excretion of potassium by the renal tubules. The major mineralocorticoid is **aldosterone**, whose secretion is regulated by more than one mechanism. Although ACTH increases aldosterone secretion to some extent, the most potent stimulus for aldosterone secretion is the renin–angiotensin system (Chapter 17), which responds to a reduction in renal blood flow or blood pressure. The kidneys respond to the reduced blood flow and pressure as if the blood volume is low; aldosterone secretion is then called for to promote retention of sodium and water, thus increasing blood volume.

Sex Hormones

The adrenal cortex also produces weak androgenic, testosterone-like steroid hormones in response to ACTH stimulation, which are further metabolized into testosterone and into estrogens by both males and females. In men, the estrogens have little effect because of the much greater testicular production of testosterone. In women, the testosterone is responsible for sex drive and is important in maintaining bone and muscle health and fertility. Its physiological role in women is overshadowed by estrogen produced by the ovaries. The additional estrogens made from adrenal androgenic hormones do not add much to the large amount already made by the ovaries. However, in estrogen-deficient postmenopausal women, the estrogens produced from adrenal androgens may be very significant (Chapter 18). In some diseases, the output of adrenal androgens is greatly increased, which may exert undesirable masculinizing effects.

Disturbances of Adrenal Cortical Function

Abnormal adrenal cortical function causes abnormalities in the metabolism of carbohydrates and protein as a result of abnormal glucocorticoid secretion, as well as disturbances of salt and water metabolism caused by disturbed mineralocorticoid secretion.

Addison's Disease

Addison's disease
A disease caused by chronic adrenal cortical hypofunction.

Adrenal cortical hypofunction, termed **Addison's disease**, results from atrophy or destruction of both adrenal glands, leading to a deficiency of all of the steroid hormones produced by these glands. In most cases, the disease results from an autoimmune disorder in which destructive autoantibodies directed against adrenal cortical cells and invading cytotoxic lymphocytes destroy the cortex. Less commonly, the adrenal destruction is caused by tuberculosis, histoplasmosis, or metastatic carcinoma involving both adrenal glands.

As a result of a glucocorticoid deficiency, the blood glucose level is subnormal and may decline during fasting to such a low level that symptoms develop. The body's ability to regulate the content of sodium, potassium, and water in body fluids is disturbed as a result of the mineralocorticoid deficiency. Blood volume and blood pressure fall, as does the concentration of sodium in the blood, and blood potassium rises. The blood volume may become so reduced that the circulation can no longer be maintained efficiently.

People with Addison's disease also frequently exhibit increased pigmentation of the skin, which is caused by increased secretion of ACTH, along with MSH, produced from the same precursor molecule that gives rise to ACTH. The MSH simulates the melanin-producing cells in the skin and is responsible for the increased skin pigmentation characteristic of Addison's disease. Fatigue and muscle weakness are common (**Figure 22-19**).

ACTH output is regulated by a negative feedback mechanism. In Addison's disease, secretion of cortisol is greatly diminished, which causes ACTH to rise in response to decreased cortisol levels. Treatment of Addison's disease consists of administering the deficient corticosteroids.

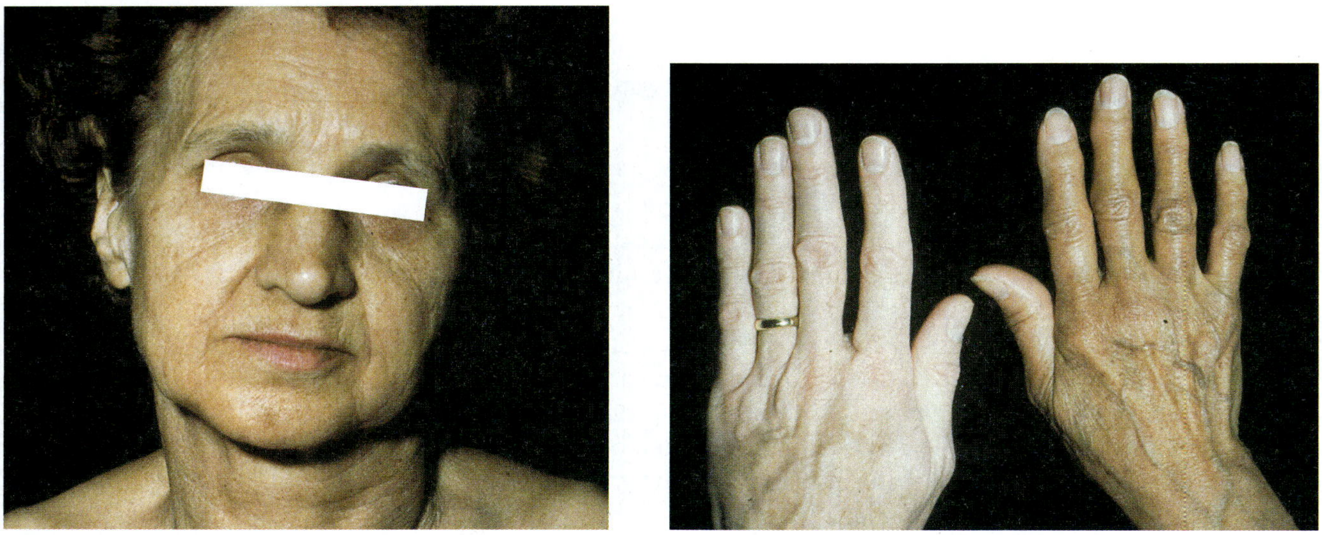

(A) (B)

Figure 22-19 Patient with Addison's disease. **(A)** Appearance of face illustrating increased skin pigmentation. **(B)** Appearance of hand (*right side*) compared with the hand of a normal person.

Cushing's Disease and Cushing's Syndrome

Adrenal cortical hyperfunction causes a characteristic clinical syndrome that results from excess production of adrenal corticosteroids. The glucocorticoid excess causes disturbances of carbohydrate, protein, and fat metabolism. The blood glucose rises. Protein synthesis is impaired, and body proteins are broken down, which leads to loss of muscle fibers and muscle weakness. Bones become weaker and more susceptible to fracture, or osteoporosis, as the protein breakdown leads to loss of the connective tissue framework of the bones. The amount and distribution of body fat are altered. Fat tends to accumulate on the trunk, and the extremities appear thin and wasted because of muscle atrophy.

The skin becomes thin and bruises easily. Stretch marks (striae) often appear in the skin as fat deposits accumulate in the subcutaneous tissues of the trunk. The face appears full and rounded, which is sometimes termed a "moon face." Salt and water are retained because of the increased output of mineralocorticoids, leading to an increase in blood volume and a rise in blood pressure. Excess adrenal androgens may lead to increased growth of facial and body hair in women.

Corticosteroid excess can result from different causes. Exogenous Cushing's syndrome results from excessive use of drugs such as prednisone often prescribed for inflammatory diseases. Endogenous causes of Cushing's syndrome include pituitary tumors (most often adenomas) secreting excessive ACTH. This is somewhat confusingly known as **Cushing's disease**. Other causes are adrenal gland tumors, which can be either adenomas or carcinoma, and lastly, uncommonly, some tumors in other organs (lungs and pancreas are common sources).

Cushing's disease Caused by an ACTH-producing tumor of the pituitary gland that stimulates the adrenal glands to enlarge.

The treatment of this condition depends on the cause. If it is Cushing's disease caused by a pituitary microadenoma, the usual method of treatment is transsphenoidal resection of the tumor. Cushing's syndrome caused by an adrenal cortical tumor is treated by resection of the adrenal tumor. Successful treatment is followed by regression of the clinical manifestations of the disease (**Figure 22-20**).

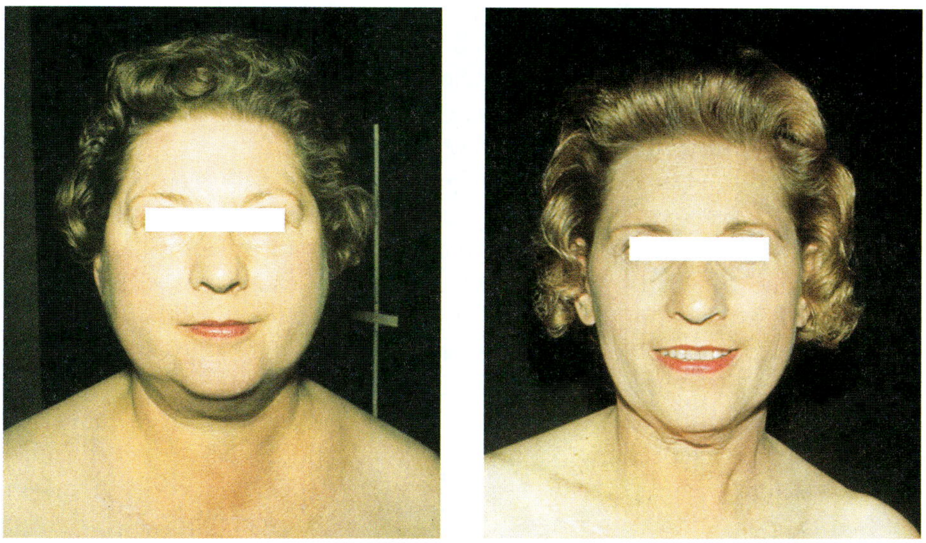

(A) (B)

Figure 22-20 Cushing's disease before and after treatment. **(A)** Full, rounded face ("moon face") prior to treatment. **(B)** Normal facial appearance after treatment.

Courtesy of Leonard V. Crowley, MD, Century College.

Overproduction of Aldosterone

Aldosterone promotes absorption of salt and water by the kidneys in exchange for potassium, which is excreted; its secretion is regulated primarily by the renin–angiotensin–aldosterone mechanism (Chapter 17). However, sometimes the adrenal cortex gives rise to an aldosterone-secreting adenoma termed an aldosteronoma. This condition is termed Conn's syndrome. The excess aldosterone produced by the tumor promotes excessive absorption of sodium and excessive excretion of potassium by the kidneys. Because water is absorbed along with the sodium, the blood volume increases along with the sodium concentration, and the blood pressure also rises along with the blood volume. The excessive hormone-induced excretion of potassium lowers blood potassium, which impairs neuromuscular function and leads to muscle weakness. The high aldosterone output exerts a negative feedback effect on renin production by the kidneys, and plasma renin falls.

Although an aldosterone-secreting adenoma is not a common cause of hypertension, it may be suspected by the physician when the hypertension is associated with an elevated plasma sodium and a low plasma potassium. This can be confirmed by additional laboratory studies that reveal an elevated plasma aldosterone and low renin. Treatment consists of identification of the adrenal tumor, often accomplished by CT or MRI examinations, followed by removal of the tumor. Many cases of hyperaldosteronism are sporadic and idiopathic.

Overproduction of Adrenal Sex Hormones: Congenital Adrenal Hyperplasia

Adrenal gland dysfunction associated with abnormal production of sex hormone is uncommon. This may result from congenital hyperplasia of the adrenal glands or, very rarely, from an adrenal sex hormone–producing tumor.

Congenital adrenal hyperplasia is the result of a congenital deficiency of certain enzymes required for the synthesis of various steroid hormones. In the normal biosynthesis of hormones by the adrenal cortex, cholesterol is initially converted into an intermediate compound (pregnenolone), which is a precursor of the other steroids produced in the adrenal cortex (**Figure 22-21**). The chief metabolic pathways are concerned with the conversion of the intermediate compound into aldosterone, the major mineralocorticoid (pathway 1), and into the glucocorticoid cortisol (pathway 2). A third minor metabolic pathway leads to the production of adrenal androgens (pathway 3).

Biosynthesis of hormones in the major pathways (1 and 2) requires a series of additions of hydroxyl groups to the steroid molecules, catalyzed by enzymes termed hydroxylases. If certain hydroxylases are absent or deficient, synthesis of aldosterone and cortisol will be impaired. This leads to increased ACTH secretion since the pituitary responds to low steroid levels in the blood as a signal to produce more ACTH. ACTH stimulation produces hyperplasia of the adrenal glands and increased synthesis of precursor compounds, a condition termed congenital adrenal hyperplasia (CAH). However, because an enzymatic block affects the major pathways of steroid production, biosynthesis is shifted in the direction of androgenic steroids (pathway 3). Consequently, the major steroid output from the adrenals consists of androgenic compounds.

The clinical disorder produced by these enzymatic defects in CAH is often termed the adrenogenital syndrome. This syndrome has several clinical varieties depending on which of the hydroxylases is deficient and the extent of the deficiency. All have the common feature of causing premature sexual

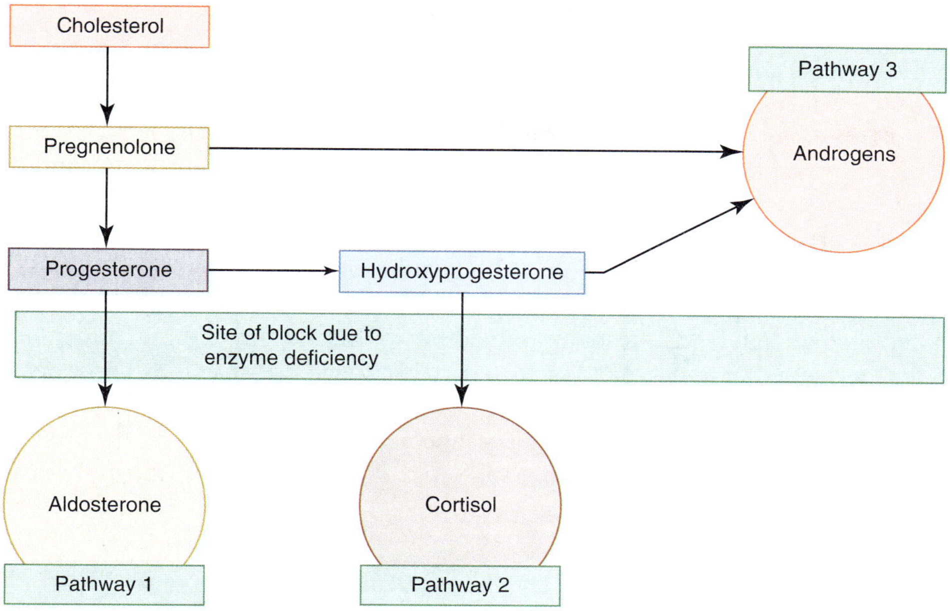

Figure 22-21 Biosynthesis of adrenal cortical hormones and the site of enzymatic block leading to overproduction of adrenal androgens.

development, known as precocious puberty. In the female, sexual development is masculine because of the effect of the androgens. The age at which the hormonal effects become manifest depends on the degree of the enzyme deficiency. Congenital virilization, which may be noted at birth (**Figure 22-22**), is the most common cause of ambiguous genitalia in neonatal females. If the deficiency is less severe, symptoms may not appear until the child is older. In males, sexual organs are normal, but there may be precocious sexual development. Some forms of CAH are also associated with hypoaldosteronism and severe loss of sodium and potassium; the associated dehydration and hypotension are potentially fatal soon after birth.

Adrenal tumors that elaborate sex hormones are extremely rare and may secrete either androgen or estrogen (or sometimes both).

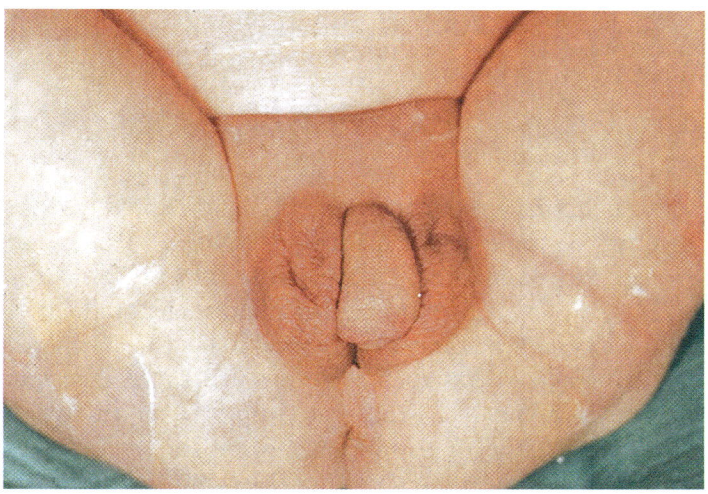

Figure 22-22 Masculinization of external genitalia of infant girl. The enlarged clitoris resembles a penis. Vulvar labia are wrinkled and resemble a scrotum.

Courtesy of Leonard V. Crowley, MD, Century College.

Norepinephrine Is both a neurotransmitter in the autonomic nervous system and a hormone secreted by the adrenal medulla.

Epinephrine Is both a neurotransmitter in the autonomic nervous system and a hormone secreted by the adrenal medulla.

Catecholamines A class of molecules that act as neurotransmitters and hormones in various body regions. These chemical messengers include dopamine, norepinephrine (noradrenaline), and epinephrine (adrenaline), which are derived from the amino acid tyrosine.

Pheochromocytoma Catecholamine-secreting tumor of the adrenal medulla.

The Adrenal Medulla

The adrenal medulla produces two similar hormones termed **norepinephrine** (also termed noradrenaline) and **epinephrine** (also termed adrenaline), which belong to a class of compounds termed **catecholamines**. The hormone-producing cells of the medulla are arranged in small groups surrounded by a rich network of capillaries. The cell cytoplasm is filled with fine granules that become dark brown when treated with chromium salts, and the cells are termed chromaffin cells because of this staining affinity.

The catecholamines produced by the chromaffin cells are stored within the cells and are released in response to nerve impulses transmitted to the medulla by the sympathetic nervous system. Any emotional stress such as anger, fear, or anxiety activates the sympathetic nervous system and causes the adrenal medulla to release its hormones. The liberated catecholamines cause a rapid heart rate, a rise in blood pressure, and other effects that prepare the individual to cope with the stress of an emergency.

Tumors of the Adrenal Medulla

Rarely, a benign tumor termed a **pheochromocytoma** arises from the chromaffin cells of the medulla. A pheochromocytoma often secretes large amounts of catecholamines and produces severe effects on the heart and vascular system. The tumor may discharge catecholamines intermittently and induce periodic episodes of high blood pressure and increased heart rate. At times, the blood pressure may rise so severely that a cerebral blood vessel ruptures, causing a cerebral hemorrhage. In other cases, the increased output of catecholamines by the tumor is continuous and causes a sustained high blood pressure. Treatment consists of surgical removal of the tumor. Pheochromocytomas may also occur outside the adrenal gland. In such cases they are termed paragangliomas.

Multiple Endocrine Neoplasia Syndrome (MEN)

Most pheochromocytomas occur sporadically. However, in some cases pheochromocytomas and other tumors of endocrine glands are associated with autosomal dominant inherited diseases associated with mutations of two genes, MEN 1 and MEN 2. MEN type 1 is associated with pituitary and parathyroid adenomas and islet cell tumors of the pancreas. Almost all patients with MEN type 2 suffer from medullary thyroid cancer and about half from pheochromocytoma.

Hormone Production By Nonendocrine Tumors

Sometimes nonendocrine tumors secrete hormones that produce the same clinical manifestations as those of tumors arising from endocrine glands. These hormones are termed ectopic hormones because they are formed outside the endocrine glands, which are the normal sites of hormone production. An ectopic hormone is a molecule that is either identical to the true hormone produced by the endocrine gland or has such a close resemblance that it mimics the action of the true hormone. Many different ectopic hormones have been identified, including ACTH, TSH, gonadotropins, ADH, parathyroid hormone, and insulin. Most hormone-producing nonendocrine tumors are malignant and are associated with carcinomas of the lung, pancreas, or kidneys, or with malignant connective-tissue tumors. These effects are often referred to as paraneoplastic syndrome.

Endocrine Function of the Pancreatic Islets

In addition to manufacturing digestive enzymes, the pancreas functions as an endocrine gland. Scattered throughout the pancreas are more than a million small clusters of cells termed the "pancreatic islets" or "islets of Langerhans," which produce three different hormones: insulin, glucagon, and somatostatin. Diseases of the islets are considered in conjunction with diseases of the pancreas (Chapter 20).

The Gonads

The gonads have two functions: the production of germ cells, either eggs or sperm, and the production of sex hormones responsible for the development of secondary sexual characteristics. This function is controlled by the gonadotropic hormones of the pituitary gland.

Occasionally, sex hormone–secreting tumors develop in the ovary or testis. They may secrete sex hormones appropriate to the sex of the individual or, paradoxically, sex hormones characteristic of the opposite sex. No endocrine symptoms result from a tumor that produces the "proper" sex hormone; however, elaboration of the inappropriate sex hormone by the tumor causes masculinization in the female or feminization in the male. Sex hormone–secreting tumors of the gonads are usually benign, and the disorder can be cured by surgical excision.

Stress and the Endocrine System

The maintenance of **homeostasis** by the body's internal organ systems is the result of regulatory mechanisms that attempt to maintain the steady state under which the body functions most effectively. In a general sense, stress can be defined as any event that disturbs this stable internal environment. The event may be physical trauma, such as an injury or surgical operation; prolonged exposure to cold, vigorous exercise, or pain; or a strong emotional stimulus, such as anxiety or fear. Any of these events result in a response that helps the body maintain homeostasis. There are two distinct but overlapping responses to stress, and their activation depends on both the intensity and the duration of the stress. The acute, short-term response is mediated by the sympathetic nervous system and the adrenal medulla, and the chronic, longer-term response includes the participation of several endocrine glands, with the adrenal cortex playing the major role. Both the acute and the chronic responses are initiated in the hypothalamus, which regulates both the autonomic nervous system and many endocrine glands. During this process, the hypothalamus also receives input from higher cortical centers (the cerebral cortex).

Homeostasis A dynamic process where the body maintains stable internal conditions while reacting to changes in both the internal and external environments.

The acute stress response is the well-known fear–fight–flight reaction triggered by the sympathetic nervous system. Norepinephrine released from sympathetic nerve endings, supplemented by norepinephrine and epinephrine released from the adrenal medulla in response to sympathetic nerve impulses, prepares the body to deal with acute situations. Blood glucose rises as liver glycogen is broken down into glucose and released into the bloodstream. Peripheral vessels constrict, diverting more blood to the brain, heart, and skeletal muscles. The blood pressure rises, and the heart beats more forcefully. All of these systemic effects are of short duration and gradually subside when the stressful event is no longer present.

In contrast, long-term stress of any type, either physical or emotional, initiates a slower but more complex chain of events. Hypothalamic-releasing hormones, acting through the pituitary gland, cause the adrenal cortex to increase its output of cortical hormones; they also increase the output of growth hormone and thyroid hormone while suppressing the output of gonadotropic hormones. Excess cortisol production has pronounced effects on glucose, protein, and fat metabolism, as described earlier in connection with Cushing's disease. Cortisol excess also dampens the inflammatory response and reduces the responsiveness of the immune system. In addition, cortisol excess tends to raise blood pressure by making the peripheral arterioles more responsive to the vasoconstrictor effect of norepinephrine released from sympathetic nerve endings. Increased aldosterone output promotes retention of salt and water, which also tends to raise blood pressure by increasing intravascular fluid volume.

The stress-related fall in gonadotropin output impairs gonadal function, which has widespread physiologic effects, and in women may lead to stress-related cessation of menstrual periods. Stress-related amenorrhea has well-defined adverse effects on the skeletal system (Chapter 24).

The increased output of thyroid hormone speeds up metabolic processes to allow the body to deal more effectively with the stress, as does increased output of growth hormone, which also stimulates the body's metabolic processes.

Unfortunately, chronic stress takes its toll on the body and, over the long term, may predispose to illness. Excessive demands are placed on the cardiovascular system, which may contribute to heart disease, and the chronic corticosteroid excess places undue demand on the vascular system, as well as on other organ systems. Perhaps even more important, the chronic corticosteroid excess may increase our susceptibility to many types of illnesses by reducing our ability to generate an effective inflammatory reaction and by reducing the responsiveness of our immune system.

Stress initiates many physiologic responses that are designed to help protect us from harm, but chronic, unrelieved stress can cause us harm, and stress-relieving activities can help protect us from its long-term injurious effects.

Case 22-1

Irene is the second child of the Mikros family. She is currently 5.5 years old and is the product of an uneventful pregnancy. Her brother Georgio, who is 9 years old, has no outstanding health problems, although his pediatrician is a bit concerned about his weight gain. His height is appropriate for his age, but he is in the 85th percentile for weight.

The Mikros family always wanted a female child, and Irene's mother Eleni made an effort to record Irene's development by measuring her height twice a year on a standard growth chart for girls. **Case Figure 22-1** is an example of such a chart and has patient height data from age 2 to the present. Although Irene was a healthy and well-behaved child for the first 4 years of her life, her mother has become concerned. Irene was always small in stature, being in the 25th percentile for her age and sex through the fourth year. Irene's pediatrician was reassuring, noting that the child's weight was appropriate for her height and that she was meeting (and in some cases exceeding) her developmental milestones. Eleni has now noted that in Irene's fifth year there has been a marked drop in her rank in height to the fifth percentile. Eleni and her husband are considerably taller than average, so they do not understand Irene's slow gain in stature.

In addition, Irene's parents have noticed that she has begun to have what they call "sinking spells" in the late afternoon when she returns from day

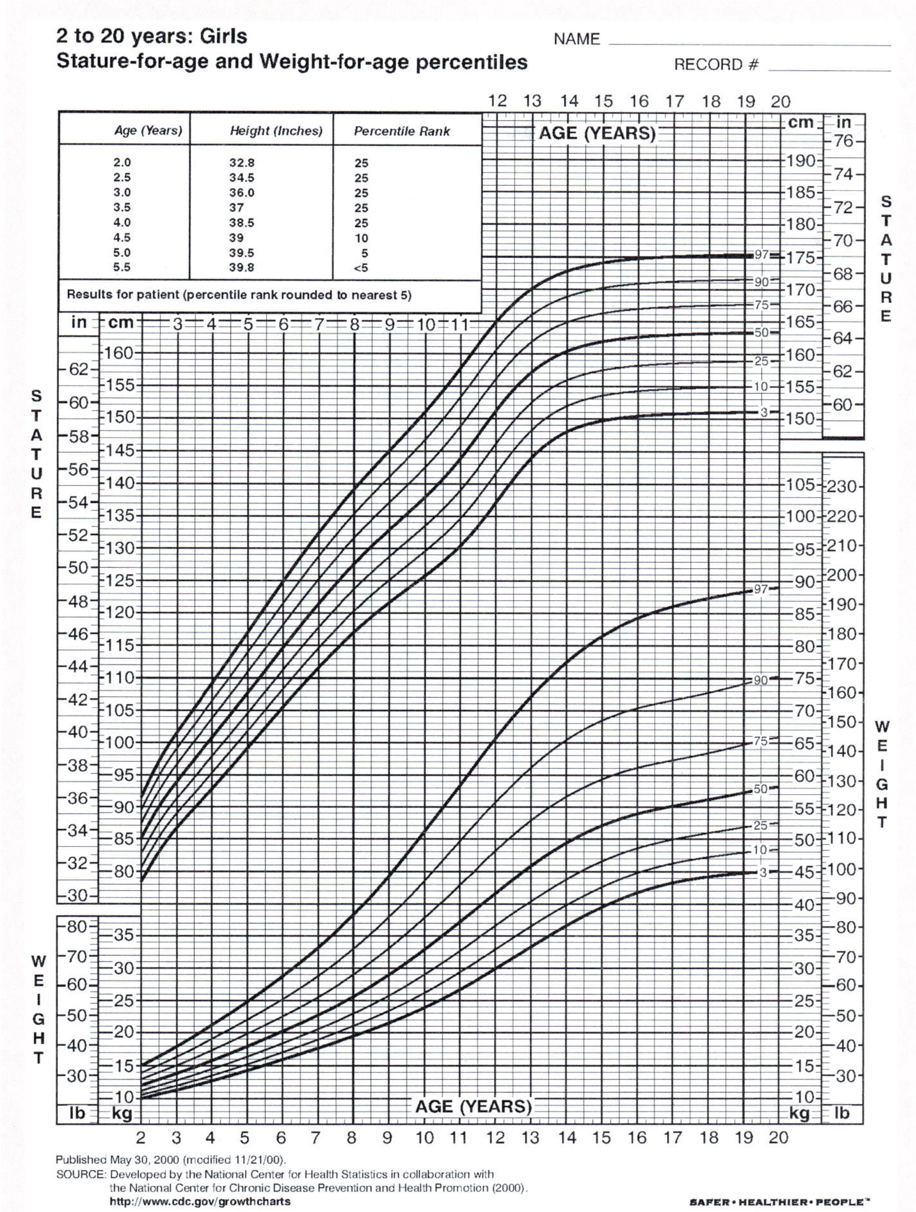

Age (Years)	Height (Inches)	Percentile Rank
2.0	32.8	25
2.5	34.5	25
3.0	36.0	25
3.5	37	25
4.0	38.5	25
4.5	39	10
5.0	39.5	5
5.5	39.8	<5

Case Figure 22-1 Standard growth chart for girls age 2 to 20 years. Data for Irene Mikros is included for years 2 to 5.5.

Growth chart is published by the CDC and is available at http://www.cdc.gov/growthcharts

care. Although her food intake is normal at day care, she becomes "fussy" and complains of being dizzy. Providing Irene with a predinner snack of fruit and crackers appears to perk her up, so her mother suspects she may have mild hypoglycemia.

Irene recently caught a gastrointestinal virus at day care and refused all food for 24 hours. By morning she was sweating, confused, and lethargic. At the pediatrician's urging, her parents took her to the local pediatric emergency room. On examination, Irene is found to be markedly hypoglycemic and suffering from mild ketonuria (Chapter 20). She is treated with an intravenous glucose infusion and is asymptomatic within several hours.

Marked metabolic derangement after a 24-hour fast is unusual in a healthy child. Hence, Irene's pediatrician suspects that the child may be suffering from an endocrine disorder that is affecting her growth and refers the Mikros family

(continues)

Case 22-1 *(Continued)*

to a pediatric endocrinologist who is expert in auxology, the study of growth and development in children.

Irene's past medical history is significant with a continued but stable history of small stature with recent marked slowing of her rate of growth, termed height velocity. At birth she was not noted to be small for her gestational age. Her mother's pregnancy was uneventful, and there is no family history of endocrine or genetic diseases. Irene's parents are of above average height and reached puberty at average ages. Irene is noted to be well dressed and comes from a family that does not have financial problems. Although clearly small for her age, she is well proportioned, has no obvious signs of developmental disease, and has normal facies (facial appearance that, when abnormal, can provide clues to possible congenital disease). Irene shows normal to accelerated developmental signs.

The pediatric endocrinologist orders a karyotype analysis and a battery of tests for the level of pituitary and other hormones. This includes measurement of the level of growth hormone IGF-1, insulin-like growth factor 1, thyrotropin, and ACTH. The pediatrician also orders an MRI study of the brain with emphasis on the region of the sella. Although the results indicate a low level of growth hormone and markedly reduced levels of IGF-1, no other hormonal abnormalities are noted. Irene's karyotype reveals a normal female chromosomal complement. Her brain MRI discloses no abnormalities. The pediatric endocrinologist diagnoses isolated growth hormone deficiency of potentially genetic origin, most likely autosomal recessive in nature, and offers the Mikros family the opportunity for extensive molecular testing and further genetic counseling, an offer that is deferred.

Irene is started on subcutaneous recombinant growth hormone treatment. She is taught to dose herself three times weekly using an automated injector "pen." After 4 weeks of therapy, her IGF-1 level is near normal, and she achieves a normal height velocity. Ongoing monitoring every 6 months to continue to measure her continuing growth and development is recommended. With continued treatment, it is hoped she will have a normal puberty and attain an adult height consistent with that predicted from the height of her parents (the midparental height, which can be easily calculated based on parental heights and the child's sex).

Discussion

The factors that control the rate of growth in developing children and eventual adult height are exceedingly complex and depend on both environmental factors and multiple genetic determinants. Clearly, expected adult height (target height) is highly dependent on parental height and can be calculated. Thus, a child of two short parents might be expected to fall below the average age for height but ultimately reach their target height predicted by that of the parents. When evidence appears that the target height will be reached and that bone growth is normal, such a short child is defined as having familial short stature (FSS). These cases generally need no therapy, although in severe cases of FSS, growth hormone therapy may be undertaken. A variant of FSS is constitutional delay of growth and puberty (CDGP). In CDGP, bone development is delayed compared to chronological age, but the growth rate is appropriate if compared to bone age rather than chronological age. These individuals are often "late bloomers" with delayed puberty, but they eventually reach their target height. These patients are not considered pathological, and other organic defects affecting growth would not be expected. However, a variety of chronic disease states can cause a pathological failure of bone growth. The list is long and includes infectious diseases such as recurrent ear infections and diseases associated with immunodeficiency. Chronic inflammatory diseases, such as Crohn's disease with gastrointestinal symptoms, juvenile idiopathic arthritis, and severe asthma, are all associated with growth delay and failure. Prolonged use of glucocorticoids (perhaps as part of asthma therapy) is also associated with growth defects.

Having ruled these out (as was the case with the Mikros family), endocrine disease (either congenital or acquired) must be considered as well as other nonendocrine genetic diseases associated with growth failure. For example, Turner syndrome is characterized by an XO karyotype and has symptoms of recognizable abnormalities such as disproportionate growth, skeletal and cardiovascular abnormalities, and marked short stature (see Chapter 3). Turner syndrome is not rare (about 1 in 2000 female births) and varies in severity of symptoms. For this reason, the establishment of a normal female karyotype in Irene was a reasonable diagnostic approach. Many other nonendocrine syndromes are associated with short stature, one example being achondroplasia, the failure of bone ossification associated with short-limb dwarfism. These syndromes are almost always recognizable in a thorough physical examination, and Irene had no evidence of such.

The low growth hormone (GH) level in Irene in the presence of normal levels of other pituitary hormones suggests an isolated defect in growth hormone synthesis or release. This is an important finding, as about 25 percent of GH deficiency is associated with an organic (nongenetic) etiology. The two most common of these are tumors of the central nervous system (notably craniopharyngioma, a tumor derived from the sellar region that may damage or destroy the pituitary). Developmental defects of the pituitary (some of which are of known genetic origin) can result in a missing, malformed, or hypoplastic pituitary that does not synthesize a normal array of hormones. An isolated defect in GH would not be expected from this, and the normal brain imaging study in Irene rules out a tumor or maldevelopment of the pituitary.

Unfortunately, GH is difficult to measure in the laboratory. The hormone is released in pulses, generally during the evening, and blood levels vary markedly with time. Because growth hormone stimulates the release of IGF-1 (which mediates most or all of the biological effects of GH), IGF-1 is commonly used as a surrogate marker for GH because it is easier to assay and its level correlates with the average level of GH secreted. Hypoglycemia in newborns is associated with GH deficiency in about 20 percent of severe cases. Hypoglycemic events also may occur in fasting children with low GH levels. The mechanism is complex but may be related to low liver glycogen and decreased glucose production related to low IGF-1 levels.

The frequency of mutations in the GH gene is poorly defined, but it is certain that a percentage of cases of isolated GH deficiency (i.e., in the absence of other pituitary hormonal defects) are related to mutations in GH (and in about 10 percent of cases to a mutation in the hypothalamic receptor that binds the growth hormone–releasing hormone). Irene has no evidence of any other disease process, suggesting that she does, in fact, have a defect in the GH gene, which is presumed to be recessive, as neither parent is affected. Type IA growth hormone mutations result in the total absence of GH synthesis and in severe growth retardation by the age of 6 months. Type IB disease is associated with low but detectable levels of GH and a milder form of growth retardation that may become obvious with time. The relatively sudden slowing of Irene's rate of growth at age 4 is suggestive of type IB GH deficiency disease, but further molecular analysis would be required for confirmation. The successful use of recombinant growth hormone in Irene's case does confirm the relationship between her low GH (and IGF-1) and her slow rate of growth.

Questions (and Some Things to Try)

1. Although not specifically stated, the Mikros family is of Greek origin. Why might ethnic background have been important in this case? The physician neglected to ask an important question in obtaining family history. Do you know what that question is and why it is important?
2. The pattern of Irene's increase in stature is sometimes termed "line crossing" and is considered to be a very important observation in the

(continues)

Case 22-1 *(Continued)*

investigation of a child's development. Why is this term used, and why is it important? (Hint: plot Irene's data on the appropriate growth chart.)

3. Many families keep data on children's height over time. If your data is available, plot your height on a growth chart and observe the pattern of development. (The reference by Rogol and Hayden explains how to calculate target height, and calculators to establish midparental height are available on the internet.) Calculate your target height (midparental height) and observe whether it works in your case.
4. Human growth hormone was originally prepared from cadaveric pituitary glands. This material was used from the late 1950s until the mid-1980s, when it was suddenly withdrawn from the market until recombinant growth hormone became available in 2005. What prompted the withdrawal? What are the risks of using human material in therapeutic agents?
5. Human growth hormone is a carefully regulated substance because of widespread off-label use and misuse. Currently, how is growth hormone being used by adults in settings other than to treat growth deficiency? Do you believe this is inappropriate or not, and why?

Questions For Review

1. What are the major hormones produced by the pituitary gland? What factors regulate secretion of pituitary hormones?
2. What is the effect of overproduction of growth hormone?
3. What factors regulate the rate of production of thyroid hormone? What are the major effects of an abnormal output of thyroid hormone? What is the difference between cretinism and myxedema?
4. Why does the thyroid gland become enlarged as a result of iodine deficiency?
5. What is the difference between Cushing's disease and Cushing's syndrome?
6. What are the main classes of hormones elaborated by the adrenal cortex? What diseases result from adrenal cortical dysfunction?
7. What factors regulate the output of parathyroid hormone? What are the possible effects of parathyroid dysfunction?
8. What factors regulate the release of prolactin? What are the clinical effects of hyperprolactinemia? What are the causes of hyperprolactinemia?
9. What is Addison's disease? What is the cause of the skin pigmentation?

References

Hammett-Stabler CA, Maygarden SJ, Cotten SW. Pathology of the endocrine system. In: Reisner HM, ed. *Pathology: A Modern Case Study*. 2nd ed. McGraw Hill Lange; 2020.

Cotten SW, Hamett-Stabler CA. Clinical practice: Laboratory medicine and patient care. In: Reisner HM, ed. *Pathology: A Modern Case Study*. 2nd ed. McGraw Hill Lange; 2020.

Endocrine Diseases. National Institute of Diabetes and Digestive and Kidney Diseases (NIDDK). https://www.niddk.nih.gov/health-information/endocrine-diseases

- Endocrinology is an exceedingly complex area that is heavily dependent on clinical laboratory medicine for diagnosis. These two chapters are aimed at undergraduate medical students and provide a brief and targeted presentation toward understanding clinical case presentations. The first chapter includes brief reviews of the physiology of endocrine hormones. The second chapter provides a good overview of how laboratory medicine affects patient care. This is particularly pertinent in the evaluation of endocrine disease. The NIDDK website provides useful introductory information on common endocrine diseases as well as recent advances and news in the field.

Inaba H, et al. Comprehensive research on thyroid diseases associated with autoimmunity. *Endocr J*. 2019;66(10):843-852.

Roman BR, et al. The thyroid cancer epidemic, 2017 perspective. *Curr Opin Endocrinol Diabetes Obes*. 2017;24(5):322-336.

Yamamoto H, et al. Association between the detection rate of thyroid cancer and the external radiation dose-rate after the nuclear power plant accidents in Fukushima, Japan. *Medicine (Baltimore)*. 2019;98(37):e17165.

Kamiya K, et al. Long-term effects of radiation exposure on health. *Lancet*. 2015;386(9992): 469-478.

- The first entry presents a recent overview of autoimmune disease in the thyroid and is of relevance to other endocrine organs. The second and third entries are concerned with changes in the epidemiology of thyroid cancer and the relation of such to potential environmental agents (such as radiation) and overdiagnosis. The fourth entry provides an excellent overview of the biological effects of radiation. Although not specific to endocrine disease, it is a first-rate primer on the subject.

Hannah-Shmouni F, Stratakis CA. An update on the genetics of benign pituitary adenomas in children and adolescents. *Curr Opin Endocr Metab Res*. 2018;1:19-24.

- This article reviews our current understanding of the molecular pathogenesis of pituitary adenomas with emphasis on children.

Colao A, et al. Acromegaly. *Nature Rev Dis Primers*. 2019;5(1):20.

- The case in this chapter delves into the complexities of growth hormone deficiency. This is an overview of diseases associated with growth hormone excess. Although Nature Reviews Disease Primers are not open access, they are an excellent resource for up-to-date reviews on diseases of interest.

Yaribeygi H, et al. The impact of stress on body function: A review. *EXCLI J*. 2017;16:1057-1072.

- The role of stress in endocrine disease is sometimes underemphasized. This is a review of the mechanisms by which stress can affect homeostatic mechanisms and produce disease.

Ergun-Longmire B, Wajnrajch M. Growth and Growth Disorders. Last updated March 4, 2025. http://www.ncbi.nlm.nih.gov/books/NBK279142/

Rogol AD, Hayden GF. Etiologies and early diagnosis of short stature and growth failure in children and adolescents. *J Pediatr.* 2014;164(5 Suppl):S1-S14.

Kotch JB. *Maternal and Child Health*. 3rd ed. Jones & Bartlett Learning; 2013.

- The first two articles were the major resources used in the case construction and presented an overview of short stature and growth hormone deficiency. The first entry is notable as an example of a series of freely available review texts produced by Endotext (www.endotext.org) in the field of endocrinology. Many additional texts on related topics are available. The third entry is a classic text that goes into detail on developmental stages in children and their evaluation.

Suggested Readings

Chaker L, Razvi S, Bensenor IM, et al. Hypothyroidism. *Nat Rev Dis Primers*. 2022;8(1):30.

- This article reviews our current understanding of the epidemiology, pathophysiology, diagnosis, and treatment/management and prevention of different types of hypothyroidism, including primary, central, and peripheral, based on the pathology.

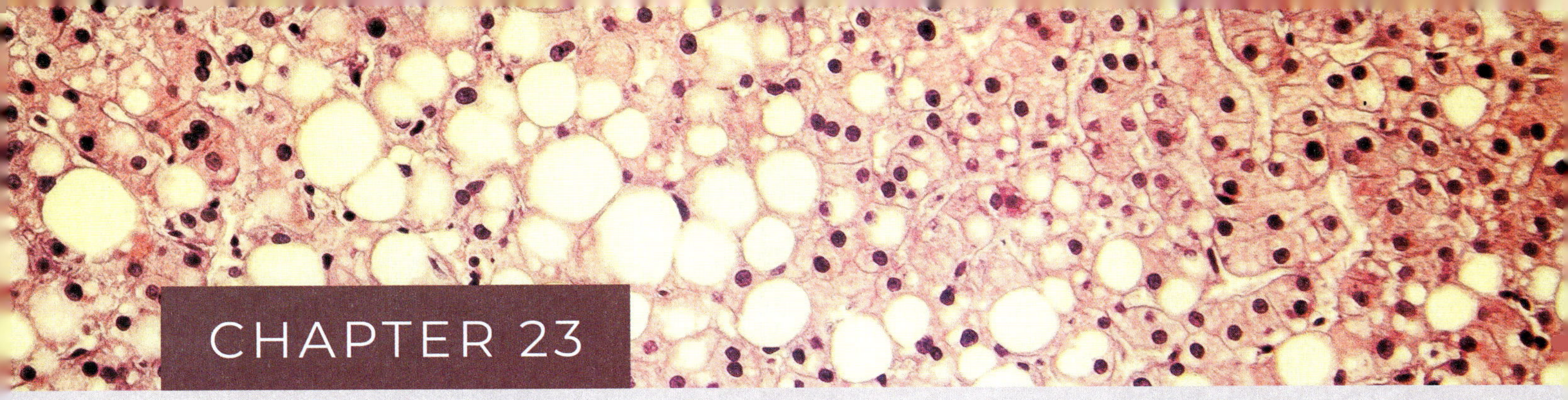

CHAPTER 23

The Nervous System

LEARNING OBJECTIVES

1. Describe the normal structure and basic functions of the brain, meninges, and cerebrospinal fluid.
2. Define muscle tone and voluntary motor activity, and relate these concepts to the two forms of muscle paralysis.
3. Describe the pathogenesis and manifestations of rabies.
4. Name the causes, manifestations, and treatment of transient ischemic attacks.
5. Differentiate the principal types of stroke in regard to pathogenesis, prognosis, and treatment.
6. Describe the pathogenesis, manifestations, and treatment of congenital cerebral aneurysms.
7. Name the types of tumors that affect the central nervous system, and explain their origin, pathogenesis, clinical manifestations, and treatment.
8. Explain the pathogenesis, major clinical manifestations, and general principles of treatment of Parkinson's disease, meningitis, multiple sclerosis, and Guillain-Barré syndrome.

Structure and Function

The central nervous system (CNS) consists of the brain, the **brain stem**, the **cerebellum**, and the spinal cord, all surrounded by several membranes termed **meninges**. The membranes include the **dura**, a firm, fibrous outer membrane; the **pia**, a thin inner membrane that adheres to the surface of the brain and spinal cord; and the **arachnoid**, the middle membrane, interposed between the pia and dura. The term mater is often included in the names of these membranes: dura mater, pia mater, and arachnoid mater. The space between the arachnoid and the underlying pia is termed the **subarachnoid space**, which contains cerebrospinal fluid (CSF) together with fine strands of arachnoid connective tissue that extend through the space and attach to the tips of the gyri (convolutions on the surface of the cerebral hemispheres separated by the sulci, the intervening spaces).

The brain contains four interconnected cavities termed **brain ventricles**. Arterial blood is supplied to the brain by large blood vessels entering the base of the skull that join to form a circle of vessels (the circle of Willis) at the base of the brain. Branches from the circle extend outward to supply all parts of the brain. Venous blood is returned from the brain into large venous sinuses in the dura, which eventually drain into the jugular veins (**Figure 23-1**).

Brain stem The brain stem is the elongated central portion of the brain connecting the cerebral hemispheres with the spinal cord. It controls the flow of messages to the rest of the body and is critical for autonomic functions such as breathing.

Cerebellum Part of the brain regulating muscle tone, coordination, posture, and balance.

Meninges The membranes covering the brain and spinal cord.

Dura (mater) The outer covering of the brain and spinal cord.

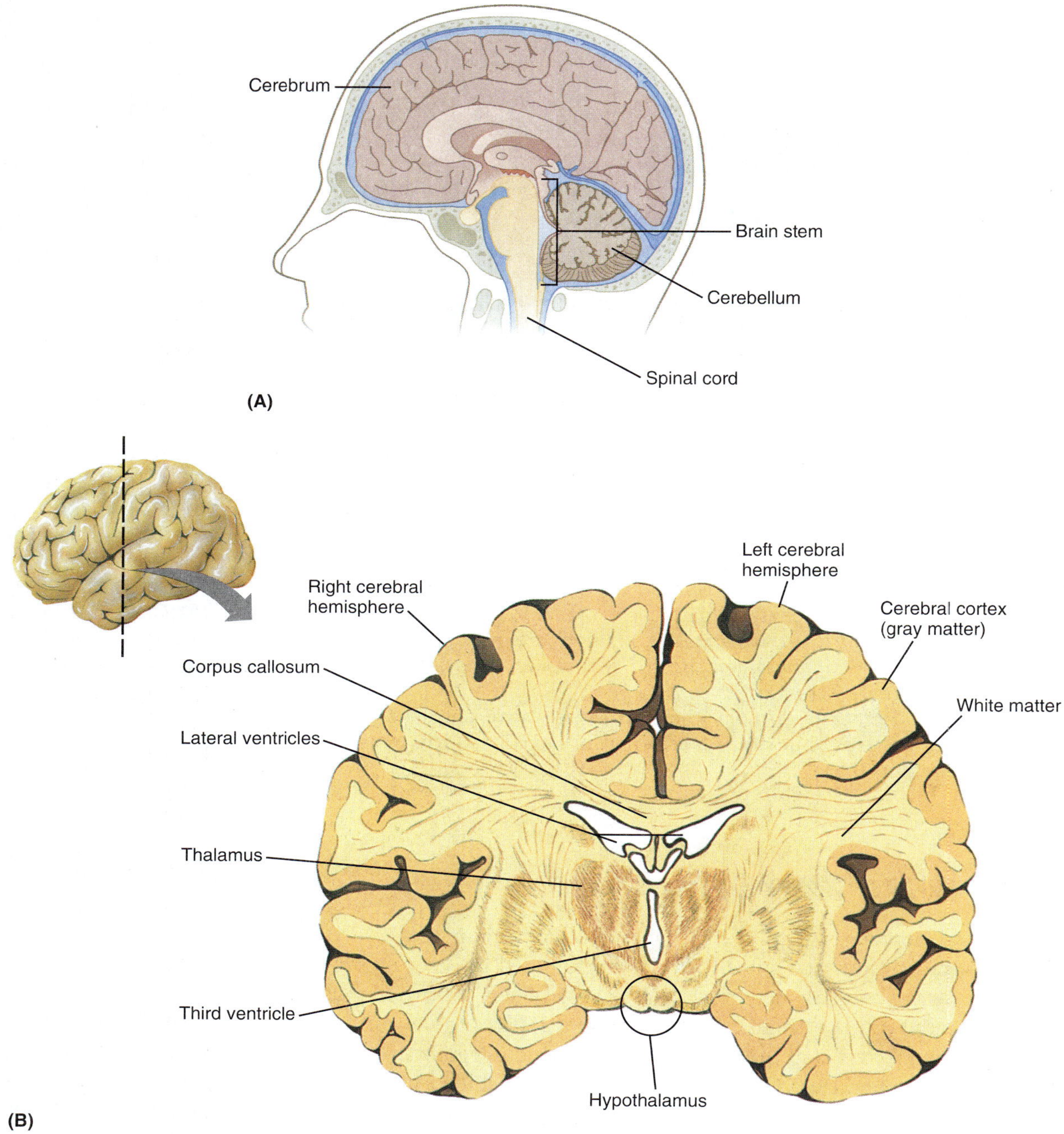

Figure 23-1 **(A)** Parts of the central nervous system. **(B)** Structures of the brain. A cross section through the brain showing gray and **white matter** of the cortex, ventricles, and deeper structures.

Pia (mater) The innermost of the three membranes covering the brain and spinal cord.

Arachnoid (mater) The middle of the three meninges that cover the brain.

The brain and spinal cord, surrounded by cerebrospinal fluid (CSF), are encased within protective bony structures: the cranium and the vertebral column. This bony case protects the soft and rather fragile nervous tissue; the cerebrospinal fluid acts as a hydrostatic cushion to insulate the brain from shocks and blows. Because the brain and surrounding cerebrospinal fluid form a closed system within the skull, changes in the volume of either brain tissue or CSF are poorly tolerated, particularly if they occur rapidly. Increases in the volume of either will cause injury to the substance of the brain, leading to death if not relieved (**Figure 23-2**).

The neural tissue of the brain and spinal cord is composed of nerve cells termed **neurons** with supporting and protective cells termed **neuroglia**.

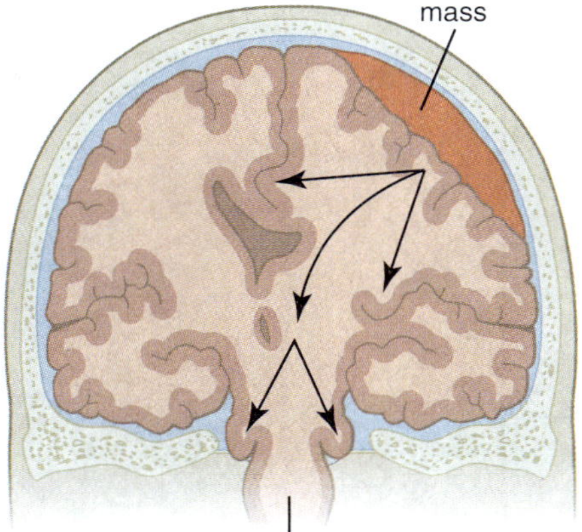

Figure 23-2 Forces resulting from increased intracranial pressure pushing the brain into the foramen magnum (the hole in the base of the skull through which the spinal cord passes). This results in injury to vital brain structures, including the brain stem and, ultimately, leads to death.

Taken together, the neurons and neuroglial cells form the **neuropil**, the substance of the CNS. Grossly, the neuropil is divided into the **gray matter** and white matter. The gray matter contains the neuronal cell bodies and supportive glial cells, which support the neurons and play a role in the response of the CNS to injury. The **microglia**, which are macrophage-like mononuclear phagocytes often localized at the site of CNS injury. The white matter of the CNS consists predominantly of the portions of the neurons that conduct impulses away from the neuronal cell body, termed axons. Many nerve axons are covered by a fatty insulating material, the myelin sheath, produced and maintained by specialized glial cells, the oligodendrocytes, also found in the white matter along with other macroglial cells. When a myelinated nerve fiber leaves the central nervous system and becomes part of the peripheral nervous system (PNS), it will be covered with myelin produced by **Schwann cells**.

Each individual neuron consists of a central body and one or more long processes extending from the cell body to transmit the impulses. Standard scientific convention defines a process that transmits impulses toward the cell body, a **dendrite**, and one conducting impulses away from the cell body, an **axon**. The term "nerve fiber" may also be used when describing nerve cell processes because it can be applied to any nerve process without regard to its direction of impulse transmission.

Neurons are frequently arranged in arrays. Although the neurons interconnect with other neurons to transmit impulses, they are not in direct contact with one another. Instead, they are separated by minute gaps termed **synapses**. The transmission of a nerve impulse across a synapse uses a chemical neurotransmitter that is released from the end of an axon and activates receptors on the dendrite or cell body of the adjacent neuron. Some of the more important neurotransmitters are acetylcholine (ACh), norepinephrine (NE), and dopamine, which is closely related to norepinephrine. A nerve that transmits impulses into the nervous system is termed a sensory nerve or afferent nerve (ad = to + ferre = carry). A motor nerve, or efferent nerve (e = away), conducts impulses from the brain or spinal cord to muscles.

The nervous system may be regarded as a motherboard receiving sensory impulses and relaying this information to the brain and spinal cord centers

Subarachnoid space The space between the arachnoid and the pia, containing large blood vessels supplying the brain.

Brain ventricle A small hollow cavity in the brain.

White matter Area of the CNS that contains a lot of nerve axons, many of which are myelinated, giving those areas a white appearance.

Neuron A nerve cell, including the nerve cell body and its processes.

Neuroglia Supporting cells of the nervous system that do not conduct electrical impulses.

Neuropil The densely packed interworven areas of the central nervous system containing nerve and glial cells that form the gray matter.

Gray matter Part of the brain containing the neuronal cell bodies and many of the supportive glial cells.

Microglia Macrophage-like cells that regulate brain development, maintenance of neuronal networks, and injury repair.

Schwann cells Cells making myelin for nerve fibers in the peripheral nervous system.

Dendrite Nerve process conducting impulses toward the nerve cell body.

Axon Portion of the neuron that conducts impulses away from the neuronal cell body.

Synapse Gap between connecting neurons.

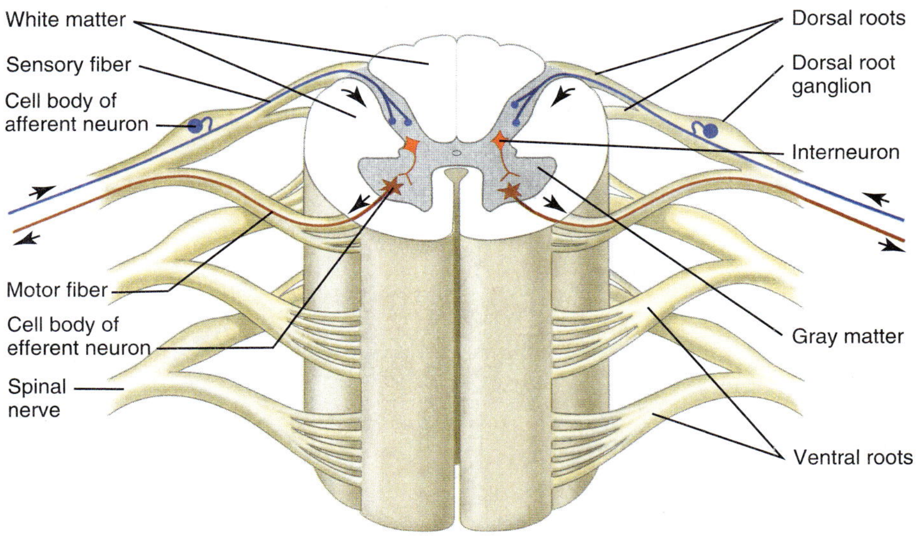

Figure 23-3 Spinal nerves are attached to the spinal cord by two roots, the dorsal and ventral roots. The dorsal root carries sensory information into the spinal cord. The ventral root carries information out of the spinal cord. Spinal nerves often contain both sensory and motor fibers. Dorsal root ganglia contain the cell bodies of multiple sensory neurons.

Cerebral cortex Receives sensory input and initiates voluntary motor activity.

Muscle tone The slight contractility (tension) present in resting muscles.

concerned with perception of sensation and with motor activity. The **cerebral cortex** receives sensory input either directly or relayed from other structures and initiates motor activity. The midbrain contains important information-processing areas and information-relaying areas such as the thalamus and the basal ganglia (basal nuclei).

The brain stem is the elongated central portion of the brain connecting the cerebral hemispheres with the spinal cord. It controls the flow of messages to the rest of the body and is critical for autonomic functions, such as breathing. It contains neurons that are involved in multiple functions not under direct cortical control; it also carries the bundles of nerve fibers that pass to higher and lower levels within the central nervous system. The cerebellum is the part of the brain regulating **muscle tone**, coordination, posture, and balance (Figure 23-1).

The spinal cord is the continuation of the brain stem. Its central gray matter receives sensory input from spinal nerves entering the cord, and motor neurons exit from the cord to innervate muscles. Spinal sensory and motor neurons are involved in many reflex functions not under cortical control, but spinal motor neurons are also activated by motor impulses originating from cortical neurons. The spinal motor neurons in turn discharge impulses to the skeletal muscles that they supply, causing them to contract (**Figure 23-3**).

The fiber tracts conveying sensory impulses to the cortex and those conveying motor impulses from the cortex cross within the brain stem to the opposite side as they transmit impulses to their destination. Consequently, the right hemisphere registers sensation from the left half of the body and innervates the muscles on the left side. Conversely, the left hemisphere receives sensation from the right side of the body and activates muscles on the right side.

Interaction of Nervous System with Muscles

A skeletal muscle contracts in response to impulses discharged from lower motor neurons, motor neurons in the spinal cord, or from corresponding neurons of the cranial nerves in the brain stem. Voluntary motor activity, controlled by nerve impulses originating in motor neurons in the cerebral cortex (sometimes termed upper motor neurons), is managed by two separate motor systems: the pyramidal system, which controls voluntary motor functions, and the extrapyramidal system, which regulates muscle groups concerned primarily with balance, posture, and coordination.

The pyramidal system and the extrapyramidal system function together as a single system under cortical control to produce the smooth integrated functions of muscle groups involved in voluntary motor activity. Malfunction of the extrapyramidal system leads to loss of coordinated motor functions. The muscles do not function smoothly, and the malfunction also gives rise to abnormal uncontrollable muscular movements (ataxia).

Muscle tone refers to the firmness of a muscle and its resistance to stretching. A muscle lacking tone is limp and offers no resistance when stretched. Conversely, a muscle with excess tone is firm, resists stretching, and is said to be **spastic**. Muscle tone results from the reflex contraction of muscle in response to stretching. Specialized receptors located in the muscle are activated, and afferent impulses are conveyed to the lower motor neuron, causing reflex discharge of motor impulses that stimulate the muscle to contract and resist the stretching force. Muscle tone is also influenced by impulses discharged from higher centers in the nervous system, which adjust the responsiveness of the stretch receptors when stimulated.

Spastic Describes muscle with excess tone that resists stretching.

Hydrocephalus Dilatation of the cerebral ventricular system caused by pressure arising from accumulation of cerebrospinal fluid within the ventricles.

Muscle Paralysis

A muscle that is no longer subject to voluntary control is said to be paralyzed. There are two different types of paralysis: flaccid paralysis, caused by disease of the lower motor neurons or their fibers; and spastic paralysis, which results from disease affecting the cortical motor neurons or their fibers. Spastic paralysis occurs more frequently than flaccid paralysis because cortical neurons are more often damaged by disease than spinal motor neurons.

Flaccid Paralysis

If the lower motor neuron in the spinal cord is destroyed by a disease, such as poliomyelitis (polio), or if the peripheral nerve supplying the muscle (which contains the nerve fibers of the spinal neurons) is interrupted, the reflex arc responsible for muscle tone is interrupted or abolished because the muscle is deprived of its innervation. The muscle becomes limp and undergoes severe atrophy.

Spastic Paralysis

If cortical motor neurons or their fibers that travel in the motor pathways are interrupted, as in a stroke, voluntary control of the muscles supplied by the affected neurons is lost because the pyramidal tract pathway is interrupted. However, because the reflex arc that maintains muscle tone is not disturbed and the muscle retains its innervation, significant atrophy of the muscle does not occur. Generally, muscle tone is increased because extrapyramidal motor impulses descending from the cortex tend to inhibit muscle tone, and this inhibitory effect is lost after an upper motor neuron injury.

Acquired Hydrocephalus

Blockage of CSF flow after the ventricular system is termed "communicating **hydrocephalus**." In these cases, all the ventricles dilate; this is generally an acquired condition.

Meningitis Inflammation of the meninges.

Concussion A temporary loss of consciousness caused by a head injury, often without any memory of the events that occurred shortly before or after the head injury.

Contusion Injury resulting from severe blunt force.

Acquired hydrocephalus is most commonly caused by obstruction of the circulation of the cerebrospinal fluid in the fourth ventricle by fibrous adhesions, which sometimes form after a bacterial infection of the meninges (**meningitis**) and block the outflow of fluid from the fourth ventricle, or by blockage of the ventricular system secondary to a brain tumor. Acquired hydrocephalus develops after the skull bones fuse, so the skull cannot enlarge as in the congenital form of hydrocephalus. (See also Chapter 16 for additional discussion of congenital hydrocephalus.)

Treatment of Hydrocephalus

Hydrocephalus can often be treated successfully by a shunting procedure in which a plastic tube inserted into one of the dilated ventricles can reroute the fluid into another part of the body where it can be absorbed. The fluid can be shunted into either the right atrium via the jugular vein (ventriculoatrial shunt) or into the peritoneal cavity (ventriculoperitoneal shunt). Whatever type of shunt is used, a one-way valve is incorporated in the tube to prevent any reflux of blood or peritoneal fluid into the ventricles.

Cerebral Injury

The brain is well protected from moderate trauma but may be injured by a blow to the head that jars the brain within its protective cranial cavity. The mildest form of head injury is termed a **concussion**, which may be caused by any force injury that causes a temporary loss of consciousness, as might occur in contact sports such as football or boxing. A concussion usually is characterized by temporary loss of consciousness without any memory of the events that occurred shortly before and after the head injury (amnesia). The concussion may be associated with a headache, temporary disorientation, and confusion but does not result in any neuropathology detected grossly. However, repeated head injuries related to football, boxing, or other contact sports may lead to permanently impaired cerebral function associated with axonal damage. Such repeated trauma to the brain can result in chronic traumatic encephalopathy (CTE), which may become evident only long after the episodes that produced the trauma. CTE is likely to be associated with an increase in neurodegenerative disease later in life. This has been well documented in boxers who develop dementia pugilistica, but is likely to also occur in individuals who engage in other contact sports such as football or in veterans of military service exposed to repeated blast exposure. Documentation about CTE is leading to concern about contact sport exposure (and in particular football) in youth and the potential for cognitive deficits later in life. Likewise, branches of the military are studying the effects of assignments where service members are exposed to repeated forms of head trauma such as explosions and bouncing around in small high speed boats.

More severe force injuries are termed **contusions**, and they can result in detectable (and sometimes permanent) damage to brain tissue and are the equivalent to bruising in other tissues. If sufficiently severe, a blow may injure the brain and fracture the skull (**Figure 23-4**). Force injury to the brain may be manifested by loss of consciousness and various neurologic disturbances depending on the severity and nature of the insult. The injured brain becomes swollen and often shows evidence of pinpoint hemorrhages caused by disruption of small intracerebral blood vessels, resulting in increased intracranial pressure that may be life-threatening. Usually the brain injury is located

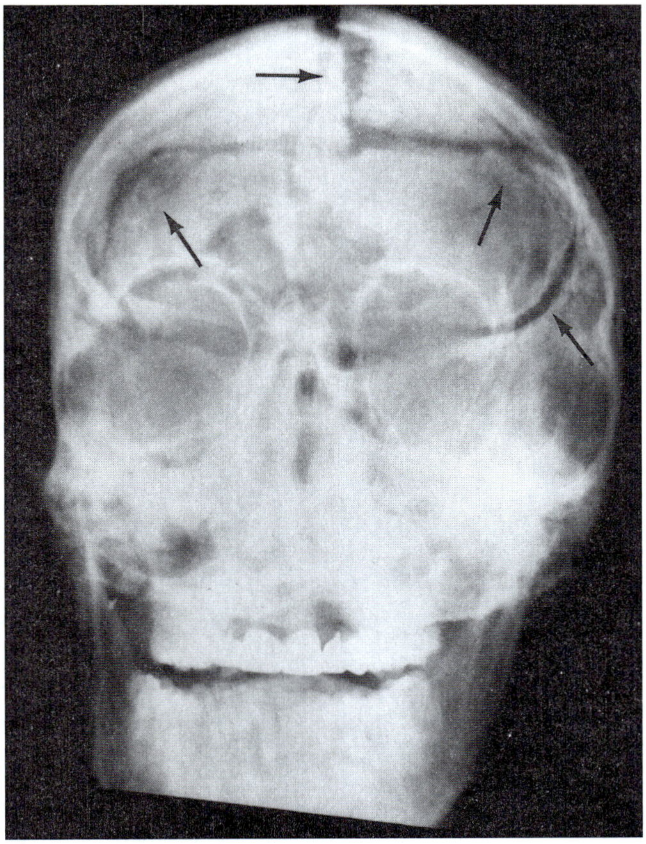

Figure 23-4 Skull X-ray illustrating a large skull fracture (*arrows*) associated with extensive injury to the underlying brain.
Courtesy of Leonard V. Crowley, MD, Century College.

immediately adjacent to the site of the blow (a coup injury), but sometimes the brain injury is caused by violent contact of the displaced brain against the cranial cavity on the side opposite the injury. For example, the force of a blow to the back of the head may displace the brain forward, injuring the front of the brain where it strikes against the front of the bony cranial cavity (a contrecoup injury) (**Figure 23-5**).

Sometimes, a head injury tears blood vessels located between the cranial bones and the dura, or under the dura. The escaping blood may accumulate in any of several locations, depending on which vessels have been damaged: epidural hemorrhage (between the outer layer of dura and the cranial bones), subdural hemorrhage (between the dura and the arachnoid), or subarachnoid hemorrhage (between the arachnoid and the pia) (**Figure 23-6**).

Epidural hematomas are most often associated with skull fractures that damage the middle meningeal arteries that lie in grooves in the bone of the skull. If torn, blood from the meningeal artery rapidly fills the epidural space and continues to expand. The hematoma, if not removed, will compress the brain within the unyielding skull, leading to irreversible brain damage and death within a day or two. Subdural hematomas tend to enlarge more slowly because the source of bleeding is from veins. The condition may become chronic with healing within the hematoma followed by occasional rebleeding. The hematoma may ultimately be resorbed and heal, calcify, or continue to expand. Although serious symptoms may be delayed by even months from the occurrence of the injury, seizures, weakness, and lethal brain damage may ultimately occur. In a subarachnoid hemorrhage, the blood often mixes with the

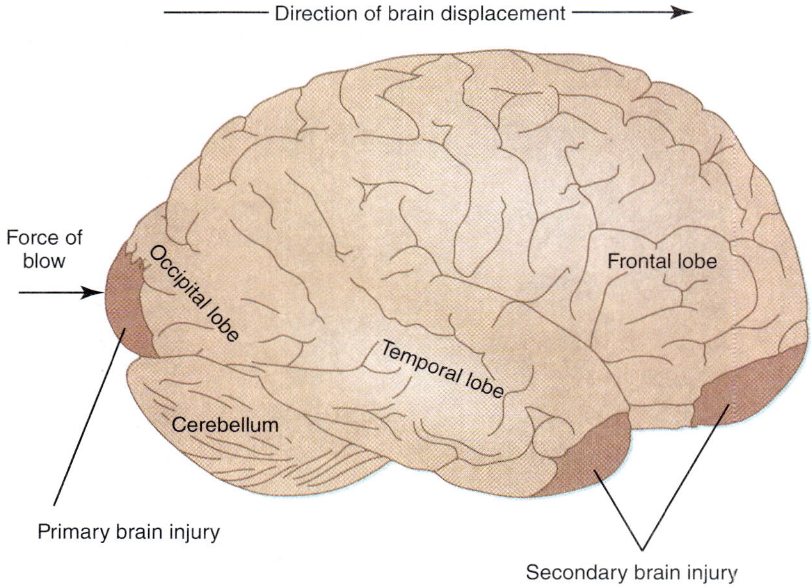

Figure 23-5 Mechanism of injury to frontal and temporal lobes of brain caused by a blow to the back of the head.

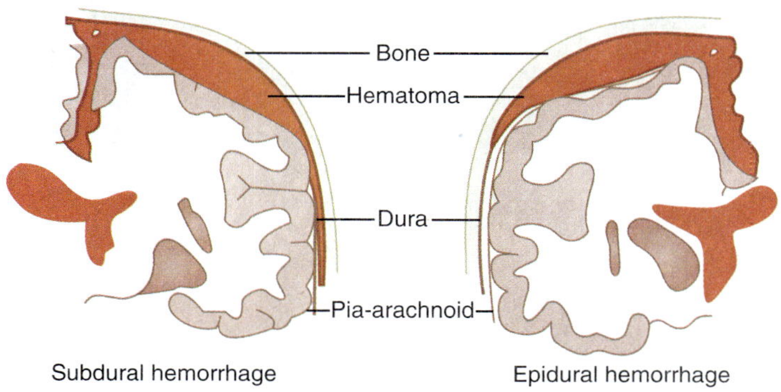

Figure 23-6 Comparative locations of epidural and subdural hemorrhages.

Aneurysm A dilatation of a structure, such as the aorta, a cerebral artery, or a part of the ventricular wall.

Stroke/cerebrovascular accident (CVA) An injury to the brain resulting in a disturbance of cerebral blood flow caused by a cerebral thrombosis, cerebral embolism, or cerebral hemorrhage.

Cerebral embolus A stroke caused by blockage of a cerebral artery by a blood clot that had formed elsewhere, a fat globule, or air bubble, which was transported in the bloodstream to the brain.

Cerebral thrombosis A stroke caused by thrombosis of an arteriosclerotic cerebral artery.

cerebrospinal fluid and spreads diffusely through the subarachnoid space. Subarachnoid hemorrhages may occur as a result of trauma but often are a result of rupture of congenital **aneurysms** (berry aneurysms), outpouchings that occur in the base of the brain in the vasculature of the Circle of Willis.

Stroke

A **stroke**, also termed a **cerebrovascular accident (CVA)**, designates any injury to brain tissue resulting from disturbance of blood supply to the brain and encompasses three conditions: cerebral thrombosis, cerebral embolism, and cerebral hemorrhage. Cerebral thrombosis, as indicated by the name, results from thrombosis of a cerebral artery narrowed by arteriosclerosis and is the cause of most strokes. Strokes are the fifth leading cause of death in the United States.

A **cerebral embolus**, which occurs less frequently than a **cerebral thrombosis**, is caused by blockage of a cerebral artery by a fragment of a blood clot, fat globule, or air bubble. Three cardiac conditions predispose to cerebral emboli: (1) a mural thrombus that forms on the wall of the left ventricle adjacent to a healing myocardial infarct, (2) a thrombus that forms on the rough surface of a diseased mitral or aortic valve, and (3) a small thrombus in a left atrium demonstrating fibrillation. A **cerebral hemorrhage**, the most serious type of stroke, is caused by a rupture of a cerebral artery, most often in a person with hypertension. Blood under high pressure escapes from the ruptured vessel and causes marked damage to the brain.

Cerebral hemorrhage A stroke caused by rupture of a cerebral artery, usually in a person with hypertension that allows blood to escape under high pressure into the brain.

Cerebral infarct Brain tissue that became necrotic after a stroke.

Cerebral Thrombi

When a cerebral artery is blocked by either a thrombus or an embolus, the brain tissue in the distribution of the blocked vessel becomes necrotic and degenerates, resulting in a **cerebral infarct** (**Figure 23-7** and **Figure 23-8**). The myelin

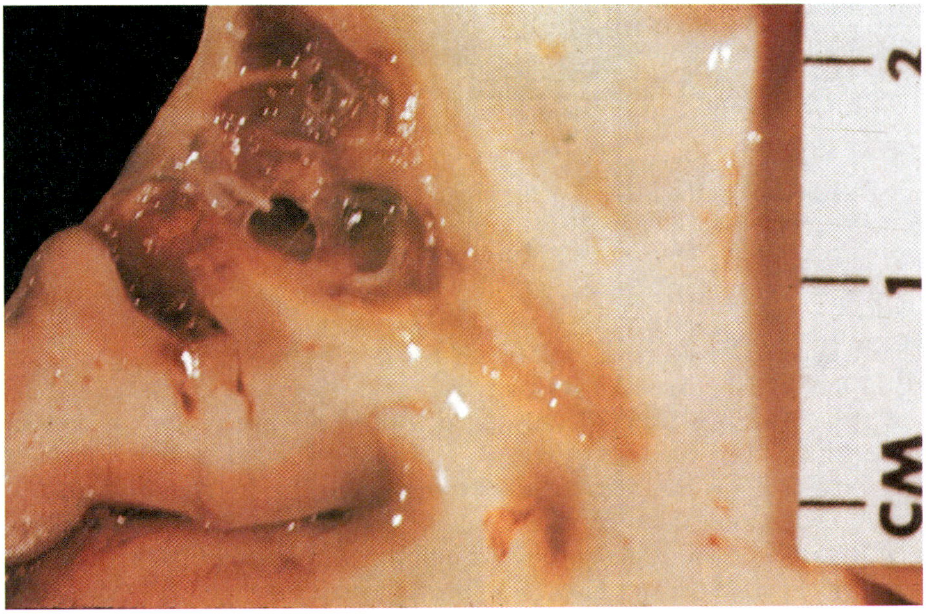

Figure 23-7 A small, older infarct of the cerebral cortex that is undergoing a cystic breakdown (encephalomalacia).

Courtesy of Leonard V. Crowley, MD, Century College.

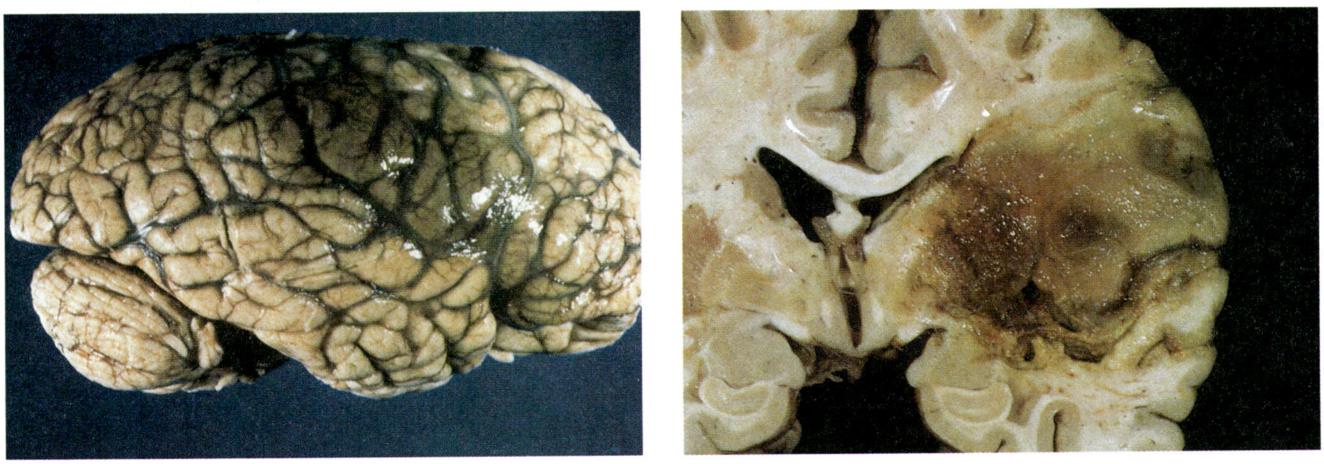

(A) (B)

Figure 23-8 A large recent infarct of the right cerebral hemisphere caused by a thrombosis of middle cerebral artery. **(A)** External surface of a brain illustrating the swollen, dark, infarcted area in the right hemisphere. **(B)** Coronal section through hemispheres at level of basal ganglia. A cerebral tissue is necrotic and discolored and involves a large part of the hemisphere.

Courtesy of Leonard V. Crowley, MD, Century College.

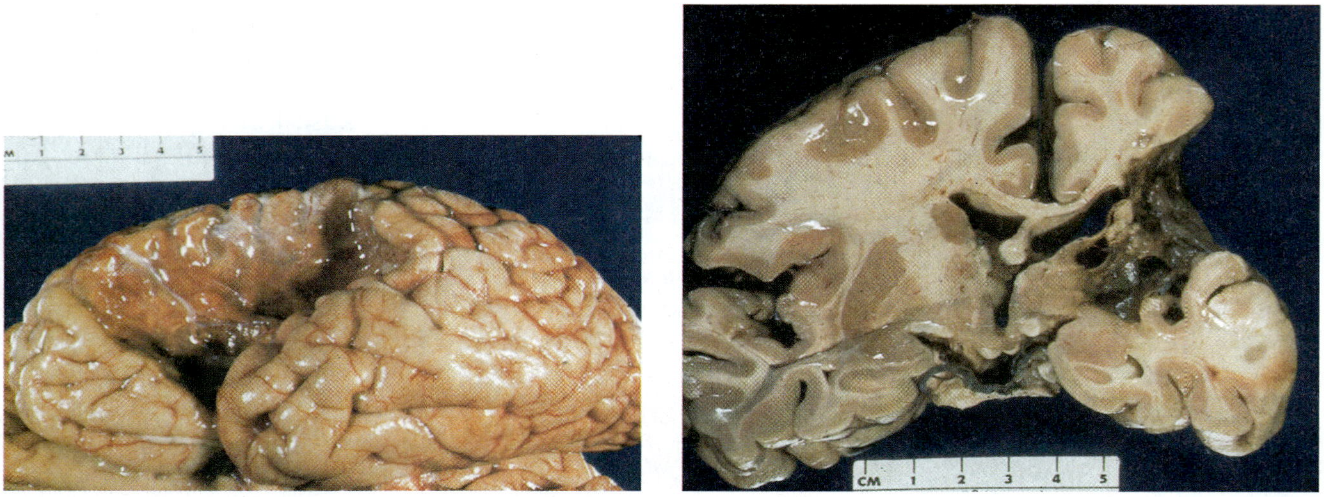

(A) (B)

Figure 23-9 A large old infarct in the left hemisphere sustained several years previously, which caused paralysis of the right side of the body and loss of speech. **(A)** External surface of the brain, illustrating the large defect in the hemisphere at the site of the old infarct. **(B)** Coronal section through the hemisphere revealing complete loss of cerebral tissue at the site of the old infarct, leaving only a few strands of glial tissue.

Courtesy of Leonard V. Crowley, MD, Century College.

Encephalomalacia
Cystic lesion of degenerated brain tissue as a result of obstruction of cerebral blood supply. Same as cerebral infarct.

sheath material breaks down, and the debris resulting from the necrosis of brain tissue is eventually cleaned up by phagocytes, leaving a cystic cavity. Because the end stage of a brain infarct is cystic, in contrast to the appearance of infarcts in other tissues, the term **encephalomalacia** (encephalon = brain + malacia = softening) is sometimes used to describe this kind of lesion (**Figure 23-9**).

Although most thrombotic cerebral infarcts are not associated with bleeding, a small amount of blood can leak into the degenerated brain tissue from adjacent damaged cerebral blood vessels, as illustrated in Figure 23-8. Bleeding is more common in embolic infarcts because the "plugged" vessel tends to leak beyond the point of blockage. This type of infarct is sometimes termed a hemorrhagic infarct, but the term should not be confused with a cerebral hemorrhage, which is a large hemorrhage within the brain resulting from a ruptured cerebral artery, a very different and much more serious condition.

Some patients who have had a cerebral thrombosis may benefit from the same type of thrombolytic drugs used to dissolve blood clots in coronary arteries (see Chapter 10). Unfortunately, flow through a blocked cerebral artery must be restored almost immediately or permanent brain damage occurs; also, sometimes the thrombolytic drug treatment may be complicated by hemorrhage within the damaged brain tissue.

Stroke Caused by Arteriosclerosis of Extracranial Arteries

A stroke also may be caused by arteriosclerosis (specifically atherosclerosis) of one of the major arteries arising from the aorta to supply the brain. A commonly affected site is at the origin of the internal carotid artery in the neck, where atheromatous plaques may narrow the lumen and reduce cerebral blood flow. The plaques may become ulcerated, with thrombi forming on the roughened surfaces. Bits of atherosclerotic debris or thrombus material may break loose from the plaque and be carried into the intracerebral circulation, where they may block small cerebral arteries and cause embolic strokes. A 50 percent reduction in the lumen of the artery corresponds to a 75 percent reduction in

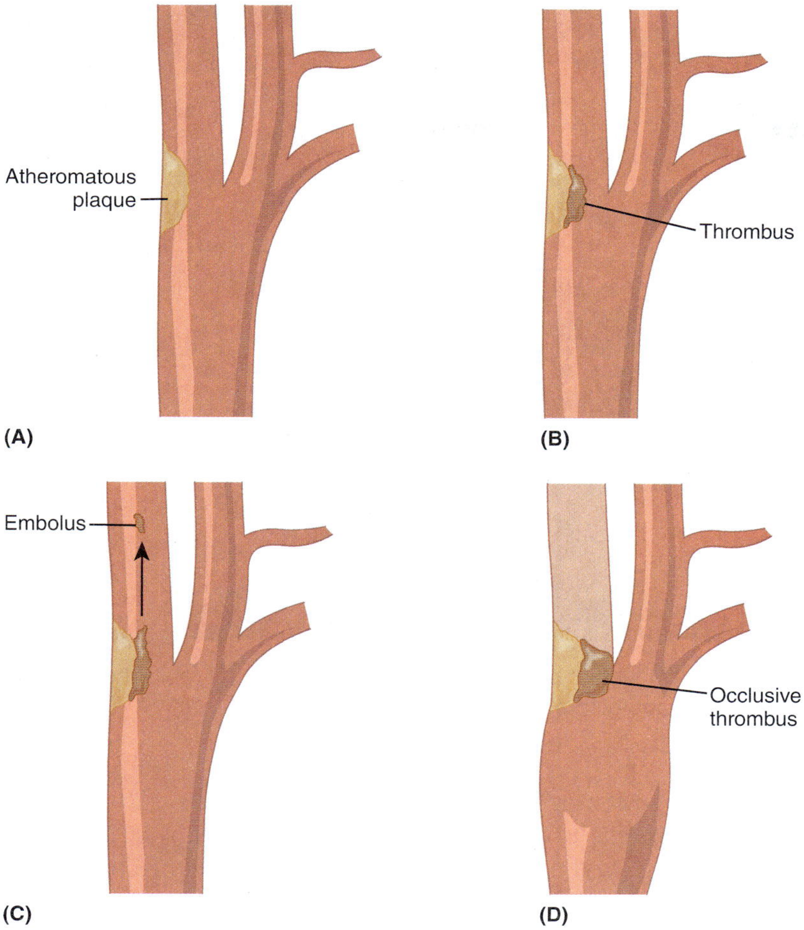

Figure 23-10 Effects of atherosclerosis of the carotid artery in the neck. **(A)** Atherosclerotic plaque narrows the lumen, and the surface frequently becomes ulcerated. **(B)** Formation of thrombus on ulcerated surface of plaque, further narrowing vessel. **(C)** Thrombus material dislodged from plaque to form emboli, which is carried to the brain. **(D)** Complete occlusion of artery by thrombus.

the cross-section area of the lumen and is associated with a large reduction in flow rate through the artery. Rarely, the internal carotid artery may become completely blocked by a thrombus that has formed on the roughened surface of the artery, leading to a large cerebral infarction. **Figure 23-10** illustrates the possible effects of atherosclerosis of the internal carotid artery in the neck. Ultrasound analysis of blood flow in the carotid artery (duplex carotid ultrasound) is used to diagnose the degree of blockage of the carotid. Atherosclerotic plaques that occlude the carotid artery and impede cerebral blood flow can be removed surgically using a procedure termed a carotid endarterectomy (endo = within + artery + tome = incision). Other less invasive methods include the same type of balloon angioplasty and stent insertion procedures that are used to treat coronary artery plaques (discussed in Chapter 10).

Cerebral Hemorrhage

A cerebral hemorrhage is a much more serious type of stroke, most often found in people who have high blood pressure. Blood from the ruptured vessel escapes into the brain under high pressure and causes extensive damage to brain tissue. A large cerebral hemorrhage is frequently fatal (**Figure 23-11**).

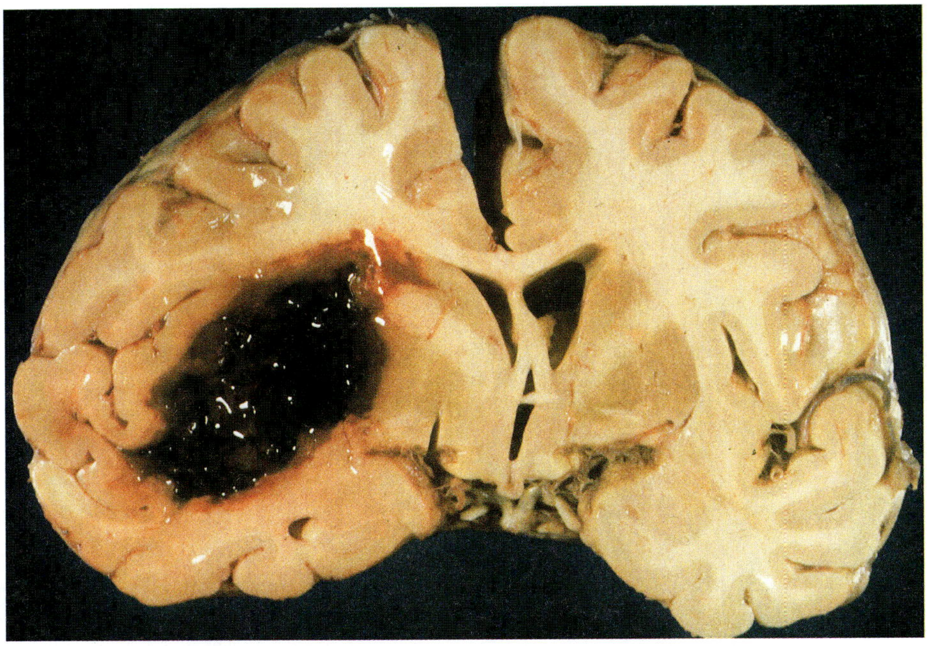

Figure 23-11 Coronal section of brain illustrating a large cerebral hemorrhage that has compressed and displaced the cerebral ventricles.

Courtesy of Leonard V. Crowley, MD, Century College.

It is possible to distinguish a cerebral infarct (caused by a thrombosis) from a cerebral hemorrhage using either computed tomography (CT) or magnetic resonance imaging (MRI) scans. In a CT image, a cerebral hemorrhage appears as a dense area within the brain because blood is denser than normal brain tissue (**Figure 23-12**). However, an infarct may be somewhat less dense and difficult

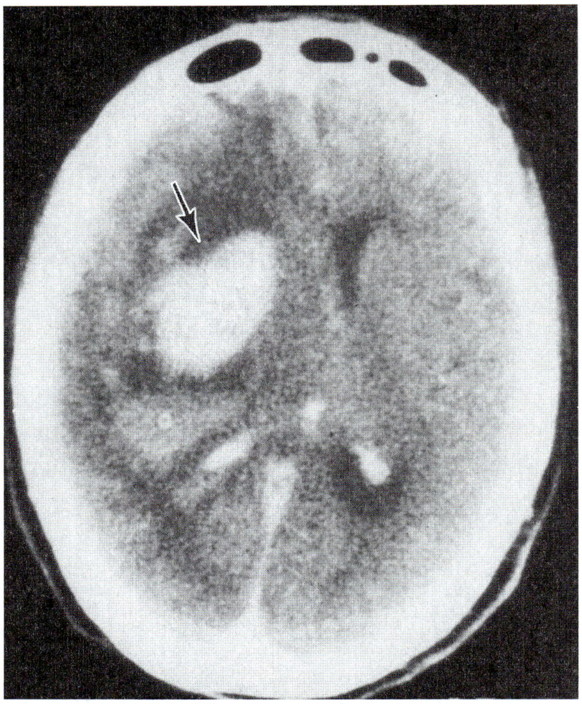

Figure 23-12 A CT scan of a patient with cerebral hemorrhage (*arrow*), which appears white because blood is denser than brain tissue.

Courtesy of Leonard V. Crowley, MD, Century College.

to detect. MRI scans have particular utility in the early diagnosis of cerebral infarcts and are much more sensitive than CT scans.

Manifestations of Stroke

The clinical effects of a stroke depend on the location of the brain damage and the amount of brain tissue injured. Small infarcts may cause little functional disturbance and are usually followed by prompt recovery with little or no residual disability. Unfortunately, many strokes resulting from occlusions of the middle cerebral artery or one of its major branches or from a hemorrhage in a part of the brain supplied by the artery cause major damage, including partial paralysis by disrupting the nerve fibers that carry impulses to the spinal motor neurons and motor neurons of the cranial nerves (lower motor neurons). Nerve fibers carrying sensory impulses to the cortex are often damaged as well, leading to various sensory disturbances.

Sensory and motor fiber tracts cross in the brain stem as they ascend or descend. Consequently, a stroke involving one cerebral hemisphere often leads to weakness or paralysis on the opposite side, termed **hemiplegia** (hemi = half + plege = stroke) or hemiparesis (paresis = weakness), with some sensory impairment on the same side as the affected hemisphere as well. Visual changes are more complex since peripheral visual pathways do not cross to the opposite hemisphere. Speech also may be affected, and the affected individual may or may not lose consciousness.

Hemiplegia Paralysis of one side of the body.

Transient ischemic attack (TIA) Temporary cerebral dysfunction as a result of transient obstruction of a cerebral vessel by a bit of atheromatous debris or blood clot, usually embolized from an arteriosclerotic plaque in the carotid artery.

Rehabilitation of the Stroke Patient

Many patients who suffer a major stroke are partially paralyzed and may have speech impairment as well. Rehabilitation, which needs to start as soon as possible, helps the patient achieve several goals: regain the ability to walk, relearn self-care activities, prevent stiffness and limitation of motion in the joints of the paralyzed limbs, and make an emotional adjustment to the disability. These goals are achieved primarily by a program of exercises and relearning. If speech is impaired, speech therapy is also necessary. Many patients can learn to walk again, although in some cases a leg brace and cane may be required. It is difficult to regain useful function in a paralyzed upper limb.

Other Types of Neurologic Dysfunction

Transient Ischemic Attack

Transient ischemic attack (TIA) refers to brief episodes of neurologic dysfunction, such as temporary paralysis of an arm or leg, loss of speech, or disturbances of vision. The episodes, which tend to occur in older people, often last only a few minutes to a few hours and clear completely. They are usually caused by bits of thrombus or arteriosclerotic debris that break loose from an ulcerated plaque and obstruct a small cerebral artery. The episodes are brief because the obstructing debris or small clot becomes fragmented and dissolved, and the circulation through the blocked vessel is restored before permanent damage to brain tissue occurs.

About one-third of patients with transient ischemic attacks suffer a major stroke within 5 years (most often within a month of the initial event), but the majority experience no further complications. Treatment consists either of surgical resection of the ulcerated plaque, if possible, or stenting along with administration of drugs such as antiplatelet agents that decrease the likelihood that thrombi will form on the ulcerated plaques, thereby reducing the risk of embolization.

Multi-Infarct Vascular Dementia

Vascular dementia/ multi-infarct dementia Compromise of cerebral function caused by blockage of small cerebral blood vessels.

Not all cerebral infarcts result in paralysis. In people with vascular disease caused by hypertension, diabetes, or abnormal blood lipids, the smaller cerebral blood vessels are affected as well as the large cerebral arteries. Those affected may have repeated small strokes caused by blockage of smaller cerebral blood vessels that damage brain tissue but may not affect motor neurons or lead to muscle paralysis. Each additional small stroke further compromises cerebral function. Eventually the cumulative brain damage causes dementia. The condition is termed "**vascular dementia**," also termed "**multi-infarct dementia**," and is the most common cause of dementia after Alzheimer's disease. Diagnosis of vascular dementia is made by CT or MRI studies which can reveal the marked brain damage caused by multiple small strokes. Progression of vascular dementia can be slowed or even prevented by treating the conditions that predispose to cerebrovascular disease.

In addition to multi-infarct dementia, dementia can result from additional diseases that damage small vessels of the brain. Disease of the white matter (Binswanger's disease) results from degenerative changes in small arteries and larger vessels. The deposition of an abnormal insoluble protein (amyloid) in cerebral vessels leads to cerebral amyloid angiopathy. The affected vessels are prone to repeated cerebral hemorrhages that can result in dementia. Such diseases may be mistaken for Alzheimer's disease.

Cerebral Aneurysm

Occasionally, an aneurysm occurs in the large cerebral arteries at the base of the brain. The most common type, a congenital cerebral aneurysm, results from a congenital defect in the elastic and muscular tissue of the vessel wall, usually at the point where the artery branches. Because of the congenital weakness, the lining of the arterial wall (intima) eventually protrudes through the defect at the point of branching, leading to the formation of a saclike outpouching, commonly in the vessels of the Circle of Willis (**Figure 23-13**).

Although the weakness of the vessel wall is congenital, the actual aneurysm does not develop until young adulthood or middle age. People with congenital polycystic kidney disease (see Chapter 17) are prone to develop aneurysms of this type. Congenital aneurysms are hazardous because they may rupture, producing severe and often fatal hemorrhage within the cranial cavity (**Figure 23-14**). Individuals with high blood pressure are especially prone to this complication. The initial symptoms of a ruptured aneurysm (a subarachnoid hemorrhage) are a severe headache and a stiff neck. The headache results from the increased intracranial pressure caused by the sudden escape of blood into the subarachnoid space. The stiff neck occurs because the escaping blood irritates the meninges, setting off reflex contraction of the neck muscles. The location of the aneurysm can be determined by a cerebral angiogram. Radiopaque material (contrast medium) is injected into the arteries supplying the brain and fills the aneurysm sac, defining both its size and position (**Figure 23-15**).

Treatment usually consists of occluding (closing off) the aneurysm by applying a small metal clip to the narrow neck of the sac at its attachment to the arterial wall. Another approach involves filling the aneurysm sac with coils of

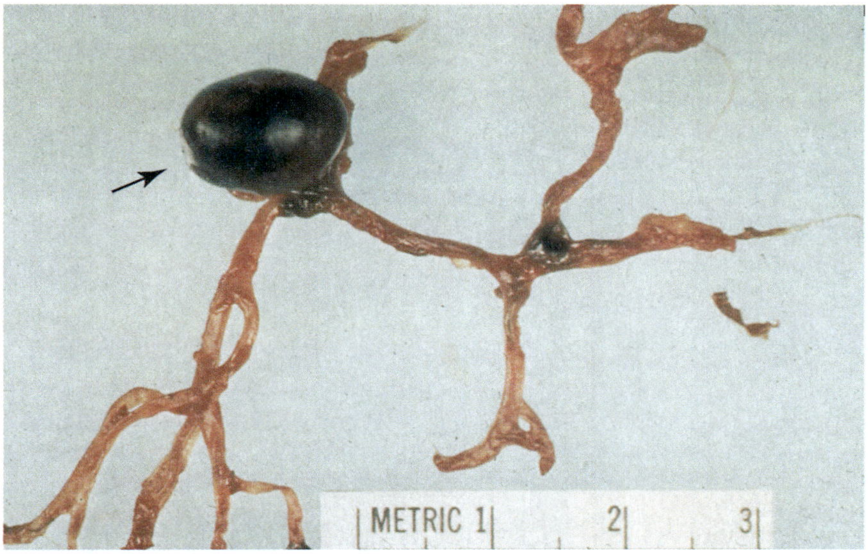

Figure 23-13 Dissection of vessels from the brain of a person with large congenital cerebral aneurysm.

Courtesy of Leonard V. Crowley, MD, Century College.

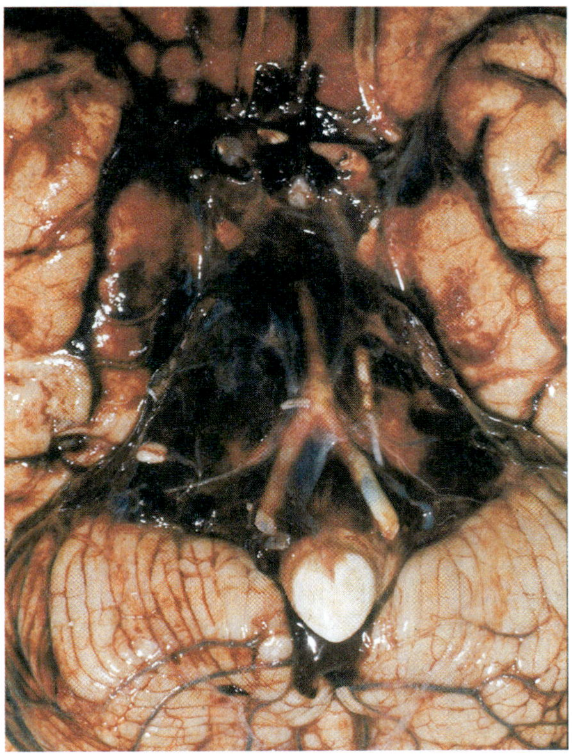

Figure 23-14 Undersurface of a brain, illustrating subarachnoid hemorrhage secondary to ruptured cerebral aneurysm.

Courtesy of Leonard V. Crowley, MD, Century College.

material to stop blood from filling the aneurysm. To perform the coiling procedure, a catheter is inserted into the femoral artery, advanced through the aorta into the carotid artery, and then advanced to the base of the aneurysm. Then, multiple coils of material are passed through the catheter into the aneurysm to completely fill the aneurysm sac.

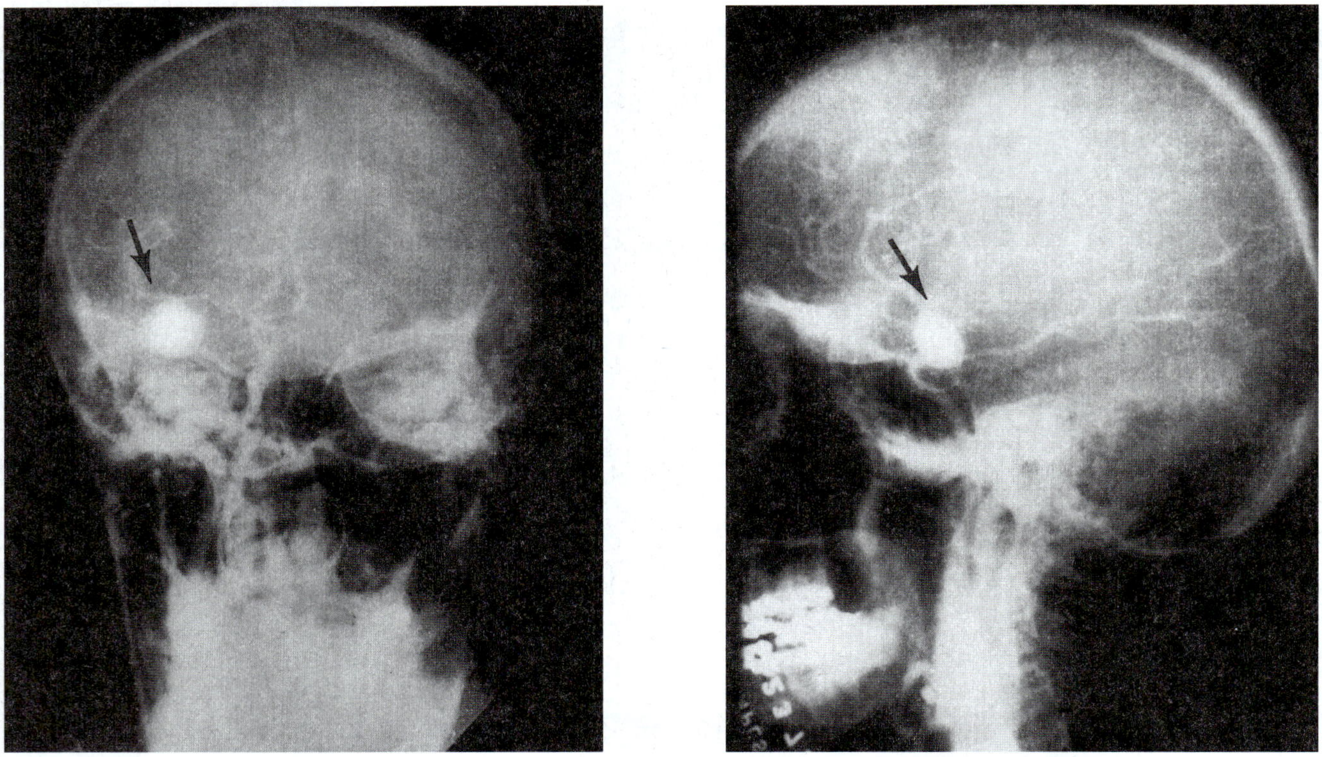

(A) (B)

Figure 23-15 A cerebral aneurysm (*arrow*) demonstrated by an angiogram. **(A)** Front view. **(B)** Side view.

Infections of the Nervous System

Encephalitis An inflammation of the brain.
Meningocele A protrusion of meninges through a defect in the spinal vertebral arches.
Myelitis An inflammation of the spinal cord.

Many different organisms can infect the nervous system, including bacteria, viruses, and fungi. An infection that predominantly affects the meninges surrounding the brain and spinal cord is termed meningitis. An infection of the brain tissue is termed an **encephalitis**. If both the brain and meninges are affected, the term **Meningocele** is often used. An infection of the spinal cord is termed a **myelitis**.

The manifestations of an infection of the central nervous system are those of any systemic infection: elevated temperature and other nonspecific symptoms. In addition, there are manifestations of meningeal irritation, consisting of a headache and a stiff neck. Involvement of brain tissue is associated with alteration of consciousness and neurologic symptoms resulting from dysfunction of localized areas within the brain.

Diagnosis of a central nervous system infection is established by examination of the cerebral spinal fluid, which contains a large number of leukocytes and an elevated protein concentration if infection is present. In bacterial infections, the leukocytes are primarily neutrophils, whereas lymphocytes predominate in viral infections. In bacterial and fungal infections, the organism responsible for the infection can often be identified in stained smears prepared from the spinal fluid and by culture of the cerebral spinal fluid.

Meningitis Caused by Bacteria and Fungi

Two organisms are responsible for most cases of bacterial meningitis: the meningococcus (*Neisseria meningitides*) and the pneumococcus (*Streptococcus pneumoniae*). Until recently, a third organism, *Haemophilus influenzae*, was a common cause of meningitis in children (see the case in this chapter). Infants and children are now routinely immunized against this organism, so Haemophilus influenzae meningitis, as well as other infections caused by this organism, occur much less frequently than in the past.

The use of a vaccine that prevents many (but not all) strains of meningococcus has reduced the incidence of this disease in many parts of the world. Because meningococcal infections occur primarily in young adults and often become epidemic where people live in close quarters, such as college dormitories and army camps, mandatory vaccination for these individuals is becoming frequent. If an individual does develop meningococcal meningitis, people who have had close contact with the infected individual are treated with prophylactic antibiotics. In contrast, pneumococcal meningitis occurs sporadically in older adults and in children. Currently *S. pneumoniae* is the most common cause of bacterial meningitis in children under 5 years of age. The disease is generally not transmitted from person to person, as is meningococcal meningitis. Consequently, people who have had contact with an individual who develops pneumococcal meningitis do not require antibiotic prophylaxis, and communitywide immunizations are not required. However, immunization for children under 2 years of age and some individuals with medical conditions is recommended. Other bacteria may occasionally cause meningitis, especially in neonates, where *Escherichia coli* is a common causative agent, or in people whose immunologic defenses have been weakened by disease or immunosuppressive therapy or under conditions in which bacteria are introduced directly into the nervous system.

Bacterial meningitis is often preceded by a mild upper-respiratory infection, during which small numbers of bacteria gain access to the bloodstream. They are carried to the meninges, where they localize and initiate an acute infection (**Figure 23-16**). Occasionally, the pathogens may spread directly to the meninges from a sinus or middle-ear infection or may be introduced into the nervous system directly from a serious head injury such as a gunshot wound or severe skull fracture.

Meningitis caused by the tubercle bacillus or pathogenic fungi is uncommon and tends to be chronic rather than acute. Both tuberculous meningitis and fungal meningitis result from the spread of organisms from a primary infection in the lung (see Chapter 13). Many cases of fungal meningitis develop in immunocompromised individuals. The most common type of fungal meningitis is caused by *Cryptococcus neoformans* (see Chapter 7). Disease may also occur in immunocompetent individuals after exposure to excreta from birds, which are a major host for the fungus. Several other fungal pathogens, including *Coccidioides immitis* (found predominantly in the San Joaquin Valley of California and other locations in the Southwest), and *Histoplasma capsulatum* (found in areas surrounding the Mississippi basin) may occasionally result in pulmonary disease that spreads to the brain. Bacterial and fungal infections are treated with appropriate antibacterial or antifungal drugs.

Viral Infections

Many viruses can infect the nervous system, including rabies, measles, and mumps viruses, various intestinal and respiratory viruses (enteroviruses), the herpes simplex virus, cytomegalovirus, poliomyelitis virus, and an important group of viruses termed arboviruses, which are zoonotic diseases spread from a viral animal host to humans by insects.

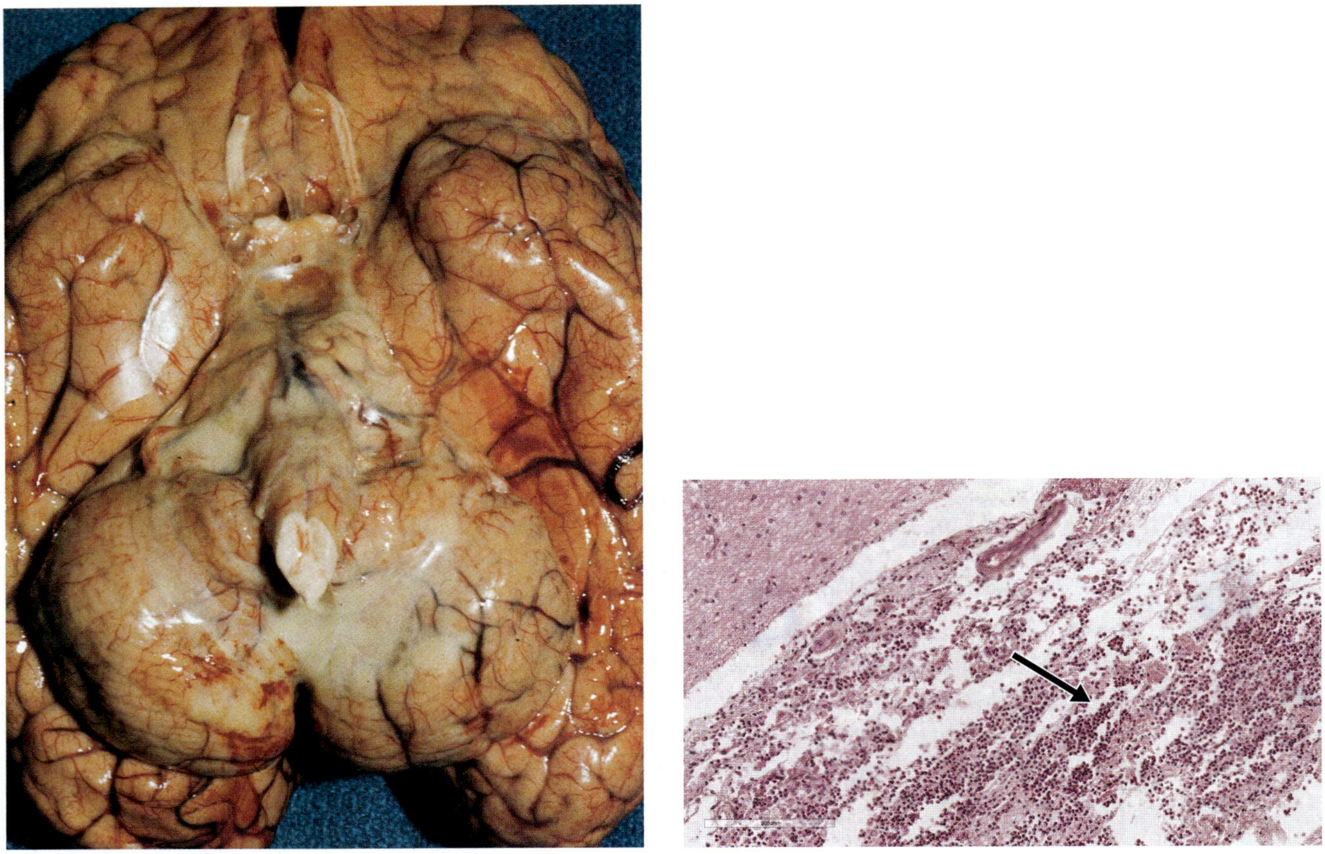

(A) (B)

Figure 23-16 **(A)** Bacterial meningitis, illustrating purulent exudate in the meninges. Exudate is most noticeable over the pons (*middle*) and cerebellum. **(B)** Microscopic view of bacterial meningitis showing purulent exudate containing neutrophils (*arrow*) in the arachnoid space.

(A) Courtesy of Leonard V. Crowley, MD, Century College; **(B)** Courtesy of Department of Pathology and Laboratory Medicine, University of North Carolina at Chapel Hill.

Manifestations of Nervous System Virus Infection

A viral infection may affect either the meninges (meningitis) or the brain tissue (encephalitis). A viral infection restricted to the meninges is often termed "aseptic meningitis" to distinguish it from "suppurative" (pus-producing) meningitis caused by pathogenic bacteria. The affected individual has an elevated temperature, headache, and a stiff neck but does not usually appear seriously ill and recovers completely. Viral encephalitis is a much more serious infection. Affected patients are often very sick and exhibit various neurologic disturbances, such as confusion, disorientation, coma, cranial nerve dysfunction, weakness, and paralysis. Some cases, such as rabies, are fatal (although there are an extremely small number of survivors [less than 0.1 percent]), and some cases have a high degree of morbidity and mortality (such as Eastern equine encephalitis). Patients who recover may be left with some permanent neurologic disability. Unfortunately, there is no specific treatment for most cases of viral encephalitis. However, some antiviral drugs may be effective in herpes simplex encephalitis if administered early in the course of the disease (antiviral drugs are considered in Chapter 7).

Rabies

Rabies encephalitis is essentially an invariably fatal disease caused by an RNA virus transmitted from infected animals to humans via virally contaminated saliva introduced in bites or other forms of contact. The CDC collects and analyzes data on rabies cases in animals and people from state health departments. The latest report, Rabies Surveillance in the United States, indicates that wild animals account for more than 90 percent of reported cases, with bats (35 percent), raccoons (29 percent), skunks (17 percent), and foxes (8 percent) most often exposing Americans to rabies. From 2015 to 2024, 17 cases of human rabies were documented, two of which were contracted outside of the United States. Although fatal rabies is rare in the United States, it is endemic in many parts of the world, with nearly 60,000 annual deaths.

The rabies virus is carried from the site of infection via peripheral nerves upward through the spinal cord and brain, resulting in destruction of the brain stem and generalized encephalopathy. The virus may take from 10 days to several months to reach the brain, so symptoms may occur remotely in time from the initial infection. Rapid postexposure vaccination and treatment with hyperimmune antirabies globulin (from immune donors) are absolutely critical for survival, because death is inevitable once symptoms occur. Individuals who have occupational exposure to potentially rabid animals, such as veterinarians, are preimmunized to the agent.

Arbovirus Infections

Arbovirus is responsible for many cases of meningitis and encephalitis. The viruses infect birds and animals as well as humans and are transmitted by mosquitoes. The term **arbovirus** is a contraction of the words **arthropod-borne virus**. Several different types of arboviral encephalitis are recognized, and they are named for the location where they were first characterized. In the United States, Western equine encephalitis occurs primarily in the West, and Eastern equine encephalitis in the eastern part of the county. As the names imply, the viruses also cause encephalitis in horses (equus = horse). Two other types of encephalitis, St. Louis encephalitis and La Crosse encephalitis, are not limited to the area implied by their names but are quite widely distributed. Eastern equine encephalitis is the most serious of the arboviruses with potential to cause neurological disease. The risk of death can be as high as 30 percent of the cases. From 2003 to 2024, a total of 215 cases have been reported. In 2024 the CDC reported 19 cases. As expected, most cases occur in the summer months. Encephalitis caused by various other arboviruses occurs in other countries, but until recently "foreign" arbovirus infections were uncommon in the United States and Canada. This situation changed with the arrival of the **West Nile virus** in the United States in 1999; the first case was identified in a person living in the New York City area.

Arthropod-borne virus/arbovirus Viruses that are transmitted to humans primarily through the bites of infected mosquitoes, ticks, sand flies, or midges.

West Nile virus An arbovirus that infects birds, animals, and humans.

West Nile Virus Infections

Since the first U.S. case was identified in 1999, the virus has spread rapidly through the United States, as well as into Canada and Mexico, and has caused the largest outbreak of arbovirus infections ever recorded in the Western Hemisphere. The West Nile virus infects many species of wild birds, horses, and other animals, as well as humans, and can be transmitted by many species of mosquitoes. The virus has also been transmitted by transfusion of blood from blood donors infected with the virus and by organ transplants. These routes of transmission are no longer possible because all blood collected for transfusion and all organ transplants are screened to exclude West Nile virus infections today. The virus also can be transmitted across the placenta from a pregnant, virus-infected person to their infant or via breast milk. For 2023, 2,628 cases were reported with 194 deaths. Currently, about 1300 cases and 100 deaths are reported per year (predominantly in the elderly). Since most cases are mild (only about one in five show symptoms, which are generally mild), this is certain to be an underestimation. Infected individuals develop a fever and neurologic manifestations that can vary from mild aseptic meningitis to severe and fatal encephalitis (in less than 1 percent or fewer cases). However, simple precautions, such as the use of insect repellents and protective clothing, are effective barriers to mosquitoes.

Zika Virus Infections

Zika virus is an arbovirus spread by the *Aedes* mosquito or via sex with an infected person. Although the great majority of adults either do not know they are infected or have only mild symptoms, the risk is to the fetus of infected women. By 2018, over 4800 pregnancies occurred in women with Zika infections. About 14 percent of babies resulting from such pregnancies showed signs of congenital Zika syndrome (see Chapter 16). Local transmission was reported in the United States (in Florida and Texas) in 2017; however, aggressive mosquito control appears to have alleviated insect-borne transmission in the continental United States. Although as of early 2020 there is no risk of Zika infection in the United States and no known international outbreaks, pregnant women are advised to check with the CDC prior to international travel to areas where Zika has formerly been reported, including tropical Africa, South America, Southeast Asia, and the Pacific Islands (see also Chapter 16 for additional details).

Poliomyelitis

Poliomyelitis was formerly an important and serious disease that caused much disability and many deaths. The virus enters the body through the gastrointestinal tract, localizing in the gray matter of the spinal cord and sometimes also in the cell bodies of cranial nerves in the brain stem. Destruction of motor neurons leads to paralysis of the muscles supplied by the affected neurons. The name of the disease refers to the affinity of the virus for the gray matter of the spinal cord (polios = gray). Although polio is currently found in Afghanistan and Pakistan, efforts are being made to eliminate it totally. Rarely, the virus in a weakened live oral polio vaccine mutates and may spread from person to person (VDPV [vaccine-derived poliovirus]). Current immunization vaccines (including those that have been used in the United States for many years) prevent this, but VDPV disease still occurs occasionally in Africa.

The Post-Polio Syndrome

Between 25 and 40 percent of individuals who survived paralytic poliomyelitis begin to experience slowly progressive muscular atrophy, weakness, and muscle fatigue, beginning many years after the original episode of acute poliomyelitis from which they had recovered. This late-onset muscle weakness and muscle atrophy have been termed the post-polio syndrome. The weakness usually involves muscles or muscle groups that had been affected during the original bout of poliomyelitis and from which the individual had made a partial or apparent complete recovery. The exact cause of post-polio syndrome is unknown. One likely explanation is that overuse of the reinnervated muscles, which compensated for the initial effects of the disease for many years, eventually caused the overworked neurons to fail, leading to weakness and atrophy of the involved muscles as they gradually lost their nerve supply. Unfortunately, no specific treatment can restore function to the muscles that have become weak and atrophic. A program of mild exercise that does not overstress the muscles may be helpful, and measures to improve pulmonary function may be required if respiratory muscles are affected.

Neurologic Manifestations of Human Immunodeficiency Virus Infections

The nervous system is often involved in people infected with the human immunodeficiency virus (HIV). A generalized discussion of HIV and subsequent AIDS is included in Chapter 5. Neurologic manifestations fall into three large categories: direct infections by virus, indirect infections by opportunistic pathogens, or HIV-related tumors of the nervous system (discussed later in this chapter).

HIV-infected monocytes can transport the virus into the brain, where it can injure the nervous system. In some patients, the infection may be manifested as acute viral meningitis occurring soon after the initial infection with the HIV virus. In others, the infection causes a more chronic progressive degeneration of the brain with symptoms similar to those of Alzheimer's disease (HIV-related dementia or HIV encephalopathy [encephalon = brain + pathy = disease]). ART therapy, particularly if started early, can prevent the most severe symptoms of AIDS-associated neurological disease, but slowly progressive chronic neurological symptoms may still occur, albeit in a mild form. Possibly this is related to chronic infection of the brain glial cells by the HIV virus. The immunosuppressive effect of the HIV virus is associated with infection by many of the opportunistic viruses, bacteria, fungi, and parasites, which can cause a primary infection of the nervous system. Some of the more common opportunistic infections are those caused by the herpes virus, cytomegalovirus (**Figure 23-17**), the fungus *Cryptococcus neoformans* (see Chapter 7), and the protozoan parasite *Toxoplasma gondii* (see Chapter 8).

Manifestations of Prion Infection

A **prion** (a contracted form of proteinaceous infectious particles) is an abnormal form of specific proteins. The infectious agent is unusually resistant to inactivation by heat or many disinfectants or ultraviolet light, but it can be destroyed by autoclaving or by household bleach. The normal form of the protein (the "good prion," designated PrP^{C}) is found in the cell membranes of neurons and in some other tissues. The abnormal form of the protein (the "bad prion," designated PrP^{Sc}) is identical except for the way the protein is

Prion A protein infectious particle responsible for Creutzfeldt-Jakob disease and some other degenerative diseases of the nervous system, such as Kuru.

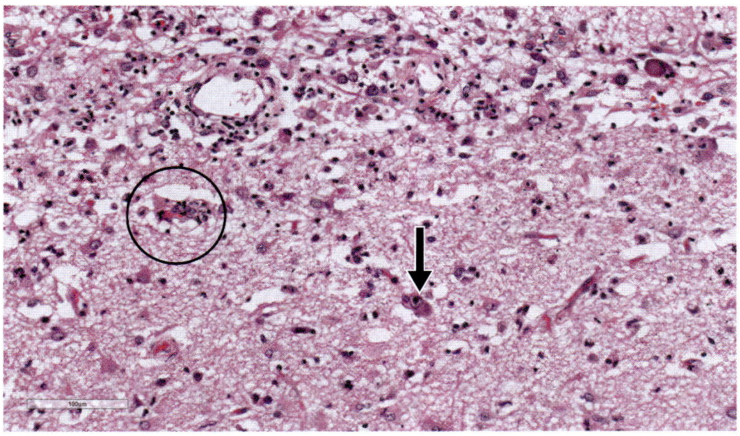

Figure 23-17 Cytomegalovirus encephalitis in an AIDS patient. A neural cell demonstrates the characteristic "owl eye" nuclear viral infection of the CMV virus (*arrow*). A multinucleated giant cell characteristic of HIV virus encephalitis is also present (*circle*).

Courtesy of Department of Pathology and Laboratory Medicine, University of North Carolina at Chapel Hill.

folded, which causes the protein to have a different configuration (conformation) when viewed in three dimensions. The abnormal prion is able to function as an infectious agent because of its ability to convert normal prions into abnormal forms (i.e., it acts like a catalyst). As progressively more prion proteins are converted into abnormal forms, a self-perpetuating chain reaction occurs as the newly formed abnormal prions convert more normal prions. As the abnormal prion proteins continue to accumulate, they disrupt the functions of the brain cells, which leads to the characteristic clinical and histologic manifestations of Creutzfeldt-Jakob (CJD) disease and several other uncommon conditions.

Creutzfeldt-Jakob Disease

Sporadic Creutzfeldt-Jakob disease accounts for about 75 percent of CJD cases. The disease occurs in older adults by an unknown mechanism as the PRNP gene (which produces the PrP protein) shows no mutations. However, certain inherited variants (polymorphisms) of PRNP found in the population are associated with susceptibility to sporadic CJD. Sporadic CJD is found worldwide and is uncommon (about one case per million). Some cases of CJD have resulted from the medical use of materials such as pituitary growth hormone or dura mater used in surgical grafting procedures that have been derived from CJD patients. Careful monitoring and the use of recombinant growth hormone has eliminated this risk. Kuru, the first human prion disease to be characterized, was transmitted by ritual cannibalism practiced by the Fore people of New Guinea and is now extinct.

Inherited (familial) CJD is associated with mutations in PRNP located on the short arm of chromosome 20 and is responsible for 15 to 20 percent of cases. Although we are not certain of the function of the protein coded by the normal gene (it may play a role in neuronal development and synapse formation), we know that certain mutations of the gene are associated with a high probability of forming the abnormal prion protein that is responsible for Creutzfeldt-Jakob disease. Certain mutations in this protein are responsible for other rare prion-related diseases (such as fatal familial insomnia and Gerstmann-Sträussler-Scheinker disease).

Clinically, Creutzfeldt-Jakob disease is characterized by rapidly progressive mental deterioration (dementia) associated with neurologic disturbances in individuals with an average age of 65. The disease is usually fatal within 6 months after the onset of symptoms. Histologically, the brains of affected individuals contain a large number of vacuoles within the neurons, which causes the affected brain tissue to have a spongy appearance; hence, the disease is referred to as a spongiform encephalopathy. The affected neurons degenerate, and **astrocytes** proliferate in response to the neuron loss; however, there is no inflammatory reaction (**Figure 23-18**). Unfortunately, no treatment is available for this devastating disease.

Astrocytes Participate in numerous physiological processes, such as regulation of axonal growth support, blood–brain barrier formation, and immune responses, as well as participating in higher cognitive functions, including memory.

Mad Cow Disease

A somewhat similar prion disease occurs in animals and can be transmitted between animals of the same or, in some cases, different species by feeding animal tissues from infected animals to healthy animals. One such disease occurs in cattle and sheep. Bovine spongiform encephalopathy, or mad cow disease, is associated with a form of Creutzfeldt-Jakob disease (variant Creutzfeldt-Jakob disease, vCJD) found in humans that is characterized by an earlier onset of

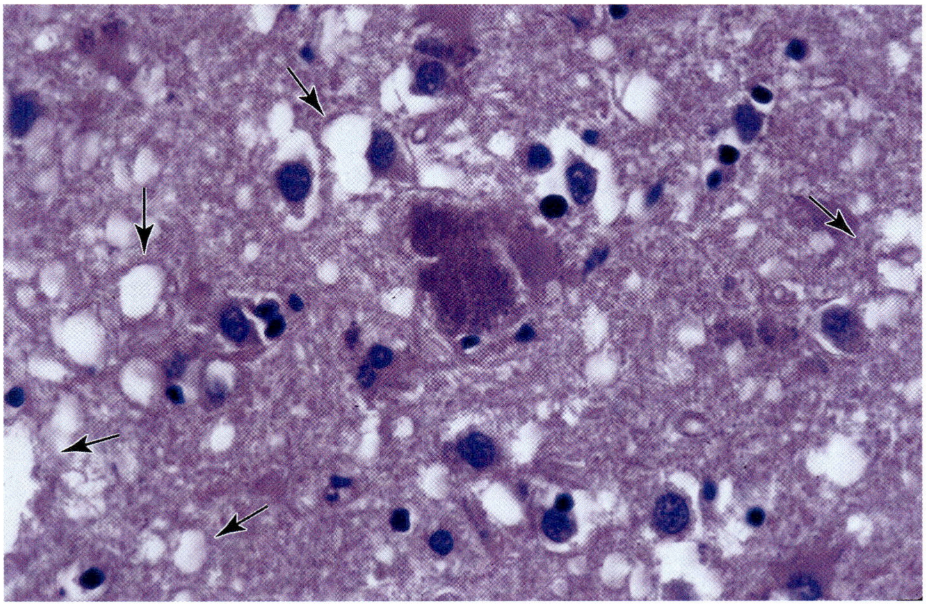

Figure 23-18 A photomicrograph of cerebral tissue from a patient with Creutzfeldt-Jakob disease illustrating multiple small vacuoles throughout the cortex (*arrows*) with loss of neurons and proliferations of astrocytes but no inflammatory reaction. The clump of eosinophilic material in the center of the photograph is an aggregate of abnormal prion protein (original magnification: ×400).

illness (average age about 25), a longer course, and a different clinical course (behavioral and sensory changes) from that of sporadic CJD.

In 1985, several dairy cows in the United Kingdom were diagnosed with bovine spongiform encephalopathy because of the bizarre behavior of the infected animals. During subsequent years, the number of infected cows increased to more than 170,000. This epidemic was traced to cattle feed that had been mixed with protein-rich tissues obtained from sheep that had been infected with another prion disease, scrapie (as well as tissue from discarded sick cattle). After this incident, the feeding practice was discontinued, and the frequency of the cattle disease declined. Use of animal tissues in animal feed is banned in both Britain and the United States today.

The disease in cattle was followed several years later by cases of vCJD. This variant disease was contracted from eating meat from infected cows, and many people were concerned that more cases would be found because there was a lag time between the consumption of infected beef and the onset of clinical manifestations. Such an increase in new cases has not materialized. A total of about 225 cases of vCJD were reported as of 2011, most of which were in the United Kingdom. Four cases have been reported in the United States. Two of the cases were associated with ingestion of infected beef in England; the other two cases were possibly related to the ingestion of infected beef from Saudi Arabia. There is some concern about possible transmission of a prion-based disease to humans from the ingestion of squirrels and from deer infected with prion-based cervid wasting disease occurring in free ranging deer, elk, and moose now found in at least 36 states, Canada, and Scandinavia. The disease has also occurred in farmed cervid herds. The concern over the possibility of transmission to humans is theoretical, but no such cases have been found to date.

Other Diseases of the Nervous System

Alzheimer's Disease

Alzheimer's disease is a chronic progressive disease that primarily affects people older than 65 years, with a frequency increasing with advancing age. Approximately 1.5 percent of people under age 65 have the disease (early onset Alzheimer's disease), increasing to 35 percent in people older than age 85. Overall, about 11 percent of people over 65 have the disease. Alzheimer's disease is characterized by progressive failure of recent memory, followed by difficulties in thinking, reasoning, and judgment; it is often associated with emotional disturbances such as depression, anxiety, and irritability. Alzheimer's disease is the most common cause of dementia in elderly people. An Alzheimer's disease diagnosis is preceded by about 6 years of declining cerebral function (mild cognitive impairment). The course of the disease differs among individuals but usually is fatal in 6 to 8 years, although some of those affected survive more than 20 years. Currently, about 6.7 million people suffer from Alzheimer's disease in the United States. Women have about a twofold increased risk of the disease versus men. Most Alzheimer's cases are sporadic, but 5 to 10 percent of cases are associated with inherited autosomal dominant disease and are often early in onset.

The brains of affected patients exhibit progressive loss of neurons with atrophy of the cerebral cortex and compensatory ventricular enlargement (hydrocephalus ex vacuo). Two characteristic histologic changes characterize the disease: neurofibrillary tangles and neuritic (senile or Aβ amyloid) plaques. Neurofibrillary tangles result from degenerative changes affecting the thin, delicate, wirelike neurofilaments located within the cytoplasm of the neurons. They become converted into thick, tangled, insoluble masses encircling the nuclei of nerve cells and are demonstrated by special stains containing silver compounds (**Figure 23-19A**). Neurofibrillary tangles are mostly composed of a protein termed tau, which in Alzheimer's disease is hyperphosphorylated (i.e., has an excessive number of phosphorus groups added to it after it is synthesized). Tau is associated with the pathogenesis of Alzheimer's disease but is also found in other degenerative neurological diseases (termed tauopathies).

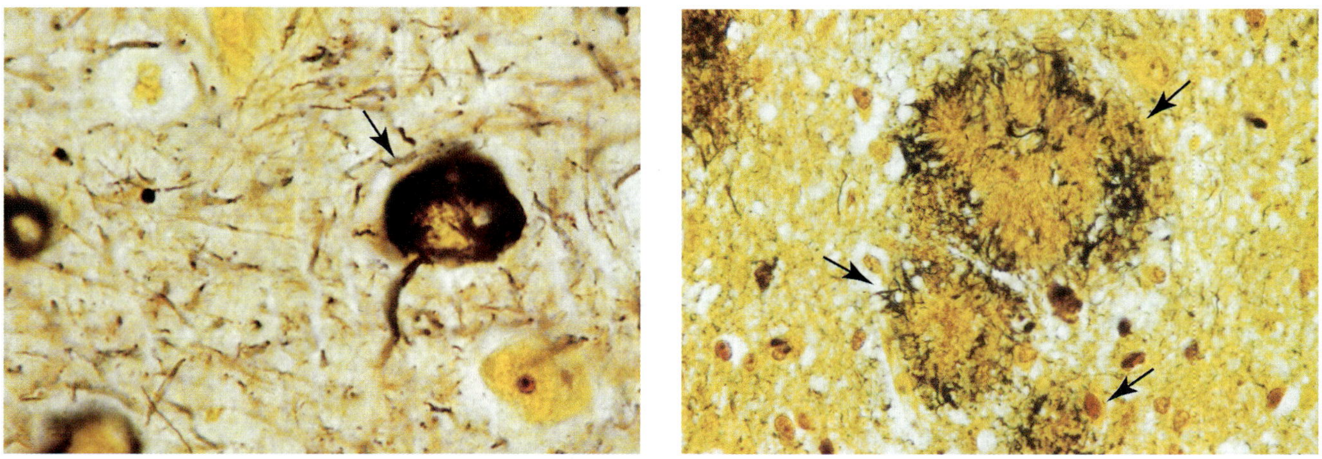

(A) (B)

Figure 23-19 Alzheimer's disease. **(A)** Thickened neurofilaments encircle and obscure the nucleus of nerve cells (*arrow*), forming a neurofibrillary tangle (silver stain, original magnification x400). **(B)** Three neuritic plaques (*arrows*) composed of broken masses of thickened neurofilaments (silver stain, original magnification ×100).

Neuritic plaques are masses of broken, thickened nerve filaments that stain intensely with silver-containing stains and that surround a core of acellular protein material, termed amyloid protein, with distinct staining properties (**Figure 23-19B**). In general, there is a correlation between the degree of intellectual deterioration and the severity of the histopathologic changes. The brains of patients with advanced Alzheimer's disease contain large numbers of neuritic plaques and neurofibrillary tangles, whereas those with mild disease have less striking changes.

The Aβ amyloid protein found in neuritic plaque is produced from a membrane protein of unknown function termed APP. APP is cleaved from cells by specific proteases following two different pathways, one of which results in the formation of Aβ amyloid (the amyloidogenic pathway). The other pathway produces a soluble protein that is not associated with disease (the nonamyloidogenic pathway). Familial forms of Alzheimer's disease can result from mutations in the APP gene or the proteases that cleave the protein and further the amyloidogenic pathway. The APP protein gene is found on chromosome 21. People with Down syndrome have three chromosome 21s and produce a higher-than-normal level of APP. Early onset Alzheimer's is extremely common in these individuals, presumably because of the excess of APP. The mechanism for the age-dependent production of Aβ amyloid protein and neuritic plaque in sporadic Alzheimer's disease remains unclear. The APOE gene involved in cholesterol transport is associated with the risk of Alzheimer's disease. There are three alleles for the gene (e2, e3, e4). Inheriting the e4 allele increases one's risk (about 3-fold for one copy, about 10-fold for two copies) as compared to those having two copies of the e3 allele. About 3 percent of Americans have two copies of e4.

The diagnosis of Alzheimer's disease is made by excluding other conditions that can impair brain function, such as chronic infections of the nervous system or multiple strokes. Recently, specialized forms of MRI imaging and PET scans have become available that are highly predictive of the presence of the disease. Unfortunately, no specific treatment can arrest the relentless progression of the disease, although some drugs may be useful to improve cerebral function temporarily. One group of drugs (cholinesterase inhibitors) prolongs the activity of the acetylcholine in the brain by inhibiting the enzyme (cholinesterase) that breaks down acetylcholine, and other drugs may be helpful to improve the affected person's quality of life. A second drug (memantine), which inhibits a particular class of nerve cells in the brain that use glutamate to transmit impulses, has become available for treatment of moderate to severe Alzheimer's. Monoclonal antibodies (Leqembi and Kisunla) directed against amyloid plaques are available for treating early disease and may slow down disease progression. More drugs are being investigated, but no prevention or cure is yet available despite intensive research efforts.

Multiple Sclerosis

Multiple sclerosis (MS) is a chronic progressive autoimmune disease characterized by the development of focal areas of degeneration of the myelin sheaths of the nerve fibers in the brain and spinal cord. The lesions develop in multiple locations throughout the brain spinal cord and optic nerve. The areas of demyelination eventually heal by forming masses of glial scar tissue (**Figure 23-20**). The name of the disease is derived from the characteristic multiple areas of involvement that heal by sclerosis (a form of scarring characterized by thickening of the tissue and increased fiber production) The glial scarring in this disease is produced by astrocytes, and differs somewhat from the usual

Multiple sclerosis (MS) Chronic progressive autoimmune disease characterized by focal areas of demyelination in the central nervous system, followed by glial scarring.

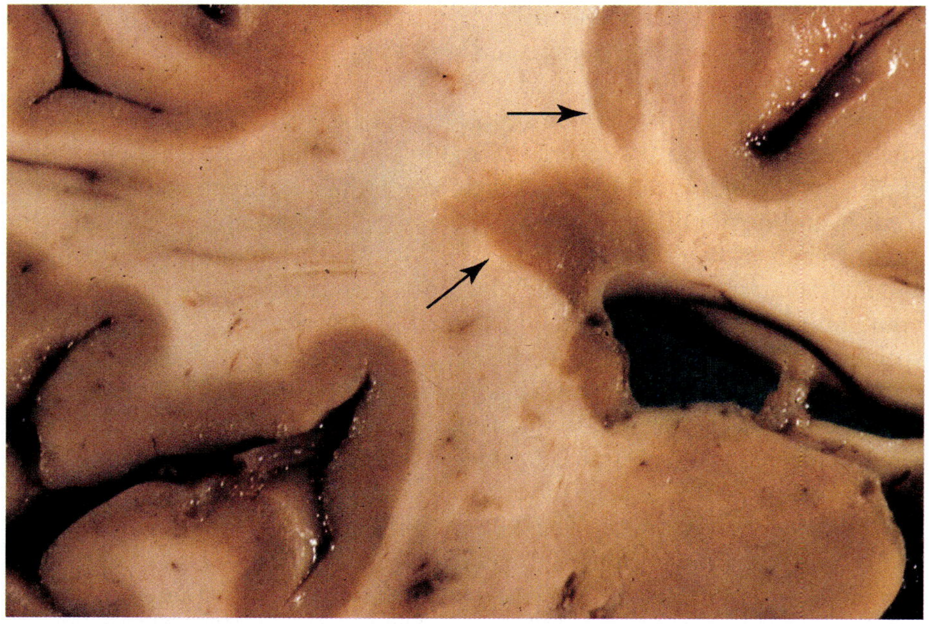

Figure 23-20 Coronal section of brain illustrating areas of glial scarring (*arrows*) adjacent to ventricle in multiple sclerosis. The demyelinated areas appear much darker than the adjacent normal white matter because of loss of myelin.

Courtesy of Leonard V. Crowley, MD, Century College.

fibrous scar produced by connective tissue cells. The discrete areas of myelin loss with glial scarring are termed "multiple sclerosis plaques" and are readily demonstrated within the nervous systems of affected individuals by means of magnetic resonance imaging (MRI, see Chapter 1). This diagnostic procedure is extremely useful for evaluating patients with neurologic disease in whom multiple sclerosis is suspected (**Figure 23-21**).

Multiple sclerosis is commonly diagnosed in young adults. The onset of symptoms before the age of 15 or after the age of 40 is rare. Clinically, the disease is characterized by periodic episodes of acute neurologic disturbances, the nature depending on the location of the demyelination. Each episode is followed by a period of recovery and remission. The progression of the disease is prolonged and quite unpredictable, with repeated acute episodes followed by remissions extending over many years. Eventually, the neurologic disabilities become permanent as a consequence of multiple areas of glial scarring, which impair conduction of nerve impulses in the brain and spinal cord. No specific treatment can arrest the progression of the disease. A number of measures, however, are available to relieve symptoms and minimize the neurologic disabilities. Corticosteroids and a variety of more potent anti-inflammatory and immunosuppressive agents are used to suppress the autoimmune response and to shorten the recovery from an acute episode.

Much evidence indicates that multiple sclerosis is an autoimmune disease, possibly initiated by a viral infection in a genetically predisposed individual that stimulates an abnormal immune response. Activated T lymphocytes and monocytes target myelin proteins and destroy the myelin insulation, and autoantibodies to myelin-related proteins are found in the cerebrospinal fluid.

The disease appears more frequent at high latitudes, suggesting a possible association with low vitamin D (as might occur with low solar exposure at high latitudes). High vitamin D levels are believed to be immunoprotective, but this remains speculative. There is also a genetic susceptibility to multiple sclerosis

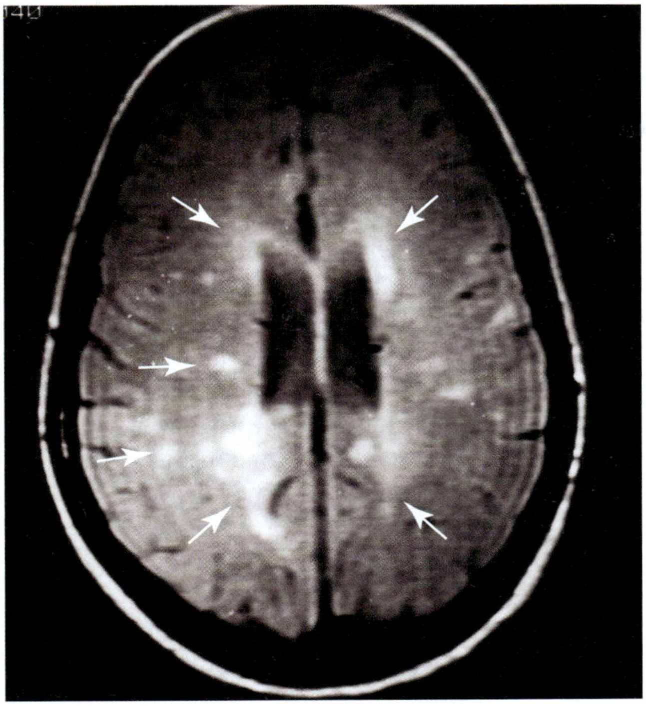

Figure 23-21 Multiple sclerosis demonstrated by MRI. The ventricular system is well demonstrated (*center*). Dense white areas adjacent to posterior horns of the ventricles and scattered throughout the brain lateral to the ventricles (*arrows*) are multiple sclerosis plaques.

that appears to be related to multiple genes, including genes that code for the individual's HLA antigens. (The relationship of HLA antigens to disease susceptibility is presented in Chapter 5.) As an example, a specific HLA antigen designated HLA-DRB1 is present in 60 percent of patients with multiple sclerosis but in only about 25 percent of those in a control group. The incidence of multiple sclerosis is higher than usual in people with a family history of the disease, probably because family members may share some of the same HLA and other susceptibility genes with the affected individual. Monozygotic twins show a 25 percent rate of concordance in having the disease, further supporting a role for genetics in susceptibility.

Parkinson's Disease

Parkinson's disease, a chronic disabling disease that occurs in about 1 percent of individuals over 60 years of age, reaching 5 percent by age 85, is characterized by rigidity of voluntary muscles and tremor of fingers and extremities, resulting from a progressive loss of neurons in the substantia nigra of the midbrain. The axons of these neurons synapse with neurons in the basal ganglia, where they release the neurotransmitter dopamine, one of the important connections of the extrapyramidal motor system. As a result of the progressive neuron loss in the substantia nigra, fewer fibers are available to release dopamine in the basal ganglia, allowing the concentration of dopamine in the basal ganglia to fall. The muscular rigidity, increased muscle tone, and abnormal repetitive involuntary movements, which are common manifestations of the disease, result from the deranged function of the extrapyramidal system.

Parkinson's disease
A chronic disease of the central nervous system characterized by rigidity and tremor, caused by decreased concentration of dopamine in the central nervous system.

As is the case with Alzheimer's disease, an accumulation of abnormal proteins within neurons is a characteristic of Parkinson's disease. For this reason,

Neurodegenerative proteinopathies General classification of diseases caused by misfolded abnormal proteins resulting in neural disease.

Lewy bodies Damaged neurites characteristic of Parkinson's disease.

both Alzheimer's and Parkinson's diseases, as well as Huntington's disease and amyotrophic lateral sclerosis, are sometimes termed **neurodegenerative proteinopathies**. In most cases, the cause of the particular disease is unknown (although there are uncommon inherited forms). There is some evidence that proteinopathies may show cell-to-cell transmission of the misfolded abnormal proteins, which act as "infectious agents" spreading within the neural tissue of the disease host and leading to additional neuronal injury and death. Parkinson's disease is characterized by the presence of **Lewy bodies**, damaged neurites containing intracellular inclusions that are rich in aggregates of α-synuclein, a neuronal protein of uncertain function. Although Parkinson's disease starts in the dopaminergic neurons of the midbrain, the disease (as characterized by the presence of Lewy bodies) spreads with time to higher cortical areas, and dementia begins to accompany the early motor symptoms.

In most cases, the cause of Parkinson's disease is unknown, although there is some evidence that exposure to pesticides, herbicides, and manganese in welding fumes increases the risk of disease. The use of the illicit drug MPTP also leads to a specific loss of dopaminergic neurons because of damage to mitochondrial proteins in those cells, resulting in a disease essentially identical to Parkinson's. About 10 percent of cases are genetic in origin and tend to occur in younger people with increased severity. Mutations in the SNCA gene, which codes for α-synuclein, and in the LRRK2 gene, which results in increased autophagy of mitochondria in neurites and leads to changes in neurite structure, are both associated with autosomal dominant disease, as are a number of additional gene mutations.

The manifestations of Parkinson's disease can be relieved by a drug termed L-dopa, which is converted within the brain into dopamine and raises the concentration of dopamine in the basal ganglia, thereby supplying the neurotransmitter that is deficient. Various other drugs also have been used successfully to control the manifestations of Parkinson's disease, including a class of drugs termed monoamine-oxidase-B (MAO-B) inhibitors. Drugs that potentiate the activity of dopamine (dopamine agonists) are also used. Drug therapy is usually successful for about 5 years. Some surgical procedures also are available to reduce the tremors associated with the disease when they are not controlled adequately by drugs. In such cases, electrodes may be implanted into specific areas of the brain. Electrical stimulation of the electrodes (using an implanted electronic device often located at the collarbone) improves motor function and reduces tremors in the patient. This technique has supplanted previously used surgical destruction of selected brain areas.

Treatment, however, does not arrest the progressive neuron loss in the substantia nigra, nor does it stop the progression of the disease. Attempts to transplant dopamine-producing cells into the brain of affected patients have largely been abandoned because these treatments had little effect.

Huntington's Disease

This is an uncommon but relatively well-known hereditary autosomal dominant disease characterized by progressive mental deterioration associated with abnormal jerky and writhing movements. The first manifestations in affected individuals occur between 30 and 50 years of age. The disease progresses slowly and is usually fatal within 15 to 20 years. Huntington's disease causes progressive atrophy of groups of neurons termed "basal ganglia," which are located deep within the cerebral hemispheres. These structures are part of the extrapyramidal motor system, which regulates smooth and coordinated muscle movements, and damage to the system gives rise to the abnormal movements characteristic of the disease. The cerebral cortex is also affected, which eventually leads to dementia as the disease progresses. CT scans of affected patients demonstrate the cortical and basal ganglia atrophy characteristic of the disease.

The normal form of the gene HTT located on chromosome 4 contains from 6 to 40 or more repeating groups of 3 nucleotides: cytosine, adenine, and guanine. These are termed CAG triplet repeating sequences (coding for glutamine), or simply "repeats." People with Huntington's disease have a larger number of repeats (generally 36 or more), and the greater the number, the earlier the onset of the disease. An expansion of triplets that disrupts gene function and leads to disease is also seen in fragile X syndrome (see Chapter 3). The number of repeats increases during gametogenesis, so the number of repeating sequences in the gene transmitted to the child may be greater than the number in the parent's gene, depending on which parent transmits the gene. In Huntington's disease, the expansion of triplet repeats increases during spermatogenesis, so the gene with expanded repeats comes from the affected father instead of the mother.

Although there is no way to arrest the progression of the disease, drugs are available to help control some of its manifestations. Children of people with Huntington's disease are offered genetic counseling and should be advised that they can be tested to determine whether they carry the abnormal gene. However, not all of the children of affected individuals want this information. Some prefer living with an uncertain future rather than being tested and possibly learning that they carry the abnormal gene and are destined to acquire the disease.

Spinocerebellar Degenerative Disease

A group of more than 25 diseases of genetic origin results in symptoms of cerebellar disturbance (ataxia, loss of control of body movements) as well as deficits in sensory and motor function as a result of neuronal death in corticospinal tracts and peripheral nerves. The **spinocerebellar ataxias (SCA)**, which are given numeric designations (SCA1, SCA2, etc.), have different modes of inheritance as well as different patterns of neuronal damage. Most SCAs are first noted in early middle age and result in a gradual loss of control of body movement over a period of years. The most common SCA, affecting 1 to 2 per 100,000 people, is Friedreich's ataxia (FA), which is distinctive in that it has an autosomal recessive pattern of inheritance of an excess of trinucleotide (GAA) repeats in the frataxin gene, resulting in a decrease in levels of this mitochondrial protein. Alleles that result in disease generally have between 600 and 900 repeats (normal alleles have 30 or fewer). Characteristically, FA becomes evident at about 13 years of age and is followed by loss of the ability to move over the next 15 years. Most individuals die by age 45.

Spinocerebellar ataxia (SCA) Cerebellar disturbances resulting in loss of control of body movements. Most common is Friedreich ataxia.

Motor Neuron Degenerative Disease (ALS)

One of the best known neuronal degenerative diseases is amyotrophic lateral sclerosis (ALS), also known as Lou Gehrig's disease. The disease affects both upper motor neurons projecting into the corticospinal tracts and the lower motor neurons in the brain stem and spinal cord. The loss of lower motor neuron function leads to weakness and eventual flaccid paralysis of muscles. The degeneration of the cortical neurons is followed by the secondary degeneration of the corticospinal tracts that descend to synapse with the lower motor neurons in the spinal cord. The disease is relentlessly progressive, with muscle atrophy and contractions leading to total disability (often without loss of intellectual capacity). Death results from respiratory failure, often 2 to 3 years after diagnosis. About 10 percent of ALS cases are clearly familial, and at least 10 percent of sporadic cases carry a mutation. Mutations in at least nine genes have been associated with inherited ALS. The most common mutated gene (C9orf72) results in the formation of RNA foci in neurons that are translated into abnormal polypeptides. Many of the mutations result in the formation of abnormal protein aggregates in neurons and may also result in abnormal RNA processing. The disease may be characterized as a proteinopathy, but the reason for neuronal death is uncertain.

Tumors of the Nervous System

Tumors of the nervous system may arise from three sites: peripheral nerves, meninges, or the cells of the brain and spinal cord. In addition, the brain is a common location for metastases that arise from malignancies in other organs. Metastatic tumors of the CNS are considerably more frequent than primary tumors.

Peripheral Nerve Tumors

Schwannomas A tumor of peripheral nerves deriving from the Schwann cells.

Neurofibromas Tumors that contain neoplastic Schwann cells and other cells; von Recklinghausen disease is an example.

Tumors of peripheral nerves, cranial nerves, and spinal roots derive from the Schwann cells that invest the nerve fibers and are termed **schwannomas**. These tumors may be either solitary or multiple, benign or (rarely) malignant. Most form discrete, well-circumscribed nodules attached to larger nerve trunks and usually can be dissected easily from the adjacent nerve (see Chapter 6).

Sometimes a schwannoma arises from one of the cranial nerves at the base of the brain or from one of the spinal nerves within the spinal canal. A tumor in either of these locations is much more difficult to remove. One of the more common locations for an intracerebral neuroma is the vestibulocochlear nerve (cranial nerve VIII), which is often called by its older name, the acoustic nerve. The tumor arising from this nerve is usually termed an acoustic schwannoma. Frequently, the tumor compresses the adjacent brain and the nearby cranial nerves as it grows and may also erode the adjacent temporal bone. Clinically, the tumor causes ringing in the ear (tinnitus) on the affected side. Compression of the nerve causes partial hearing loss on the affected side, and symptoms related to pressure on the adjacent cranial nerves and the brain stem also may be present. Although the tumor is benign, its inaccessibility makes surgical removal difficult.

Neurofibromas are distinct from schwannomas in that they contain neoplastic Schwann cells, fibroblasts, and other neural-associated cells. Multiple neurofibromas are associated with the autosomal dominant disease neurofibromatosis type 1 (NF-1), or von Recklinghausen disease. These tumors can be disfiguring and become a malignant neurofibrosarcoma about 5 percent of the time. Multiple café au lait spots, light brown pigment patches on the skin, occur in almost all affected individuals. There is no specific treatment for this disease. Large tumors that encroach on vital organs or are cosmetically disfiguring must be removed surgically. A Schwann cell sarcoma is treated by wide surgical excision, in the same way as any malignant tumor. Single neurofibromas that occur sporadically are not related to NF-1 and do not become sarcomatous.

Tumors of the Brain

Primary brain tumors may arise from the meninges, from the glial supporting tissues of the brain, from the cells lining the ventricular system, or (rarely) from other tissues such as the blood vessels within the brain. Tumors do not develop from neurons because adult nerve cells are no longer capable of cell division.

A tumor of the meninges is termed a **meningioma**. This is a well-circumscribed benign tumor arising from cells in the middle layer of the arachnoid and is firmly adherent to the dura. The tumor causes symptoms as a result of compression of the underlying brain and can be removed successfully if it is located in an accessible location because these tumors are not invasive. The tumors have a distinctive whorled or lamellar pattern when microscopically examined (**Figure 23-22**).

Any tumor of neuroglial origin is termed a **glioma**. These tumors are further classified according to the type of glial supporting cell from which the neoplasm arises. The most common type arises from astrocytes (**astrocytoma**). A special name, glioblastoma multiforme, is applied to a highly undifferentiated, rapidly growing astrocytoma (**Figure 23-23**). The name describes the primitive appearance of the neoplastic astrocytes (blast = primitive cell) and their great variability in shape and appearance (multiform = having many shapes). Gliomas arise less frequently from other supporting cells. Most astrocytomas are diffuse; they are highly malignant and readily infiltrate the brain tissue. Because they cannot be totally removed surgically, treatment combines radio- and chemotherapy, and prolonged survival is rare. Circumscribed astrocytomas

Meningioma A benign tumor arising from the meninges.

Glioma Any brain tumor arising from glial (supporting) cells of the brain.

Astrocytoma A neuroglial tumor arising from astrocytes; the most common type.

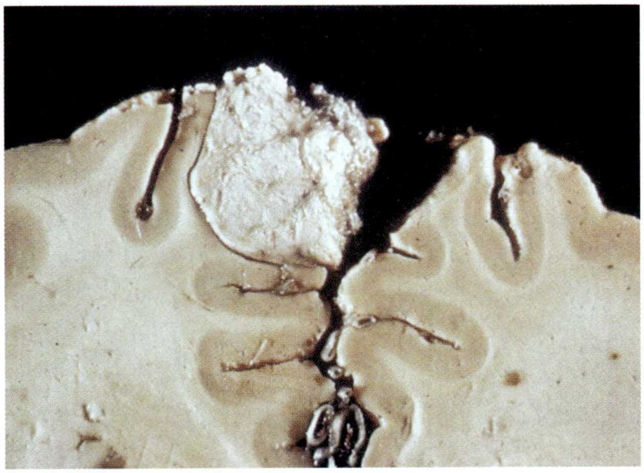

Figure 23-22 Meningioma arising from the dura, resulting in displacement but no infiltration of the brain.

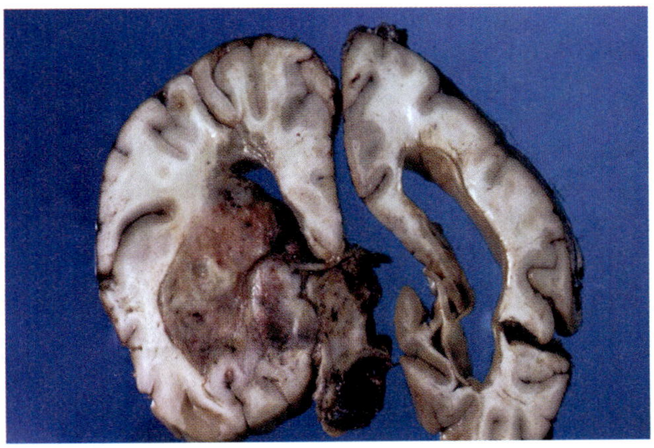

Figure 23-23 Glioblastoma. A large pink, tan, and hemorrhagic mass is infiltrating the left side of the brain. It is displacing the midline to the right and impeding the outflow of the ventricle. The right ventricle is greatly dilated, and the remainder of the tissue on the right is markedly atrophic due to the resultant hydrocephalus.

are generally found in young patients and are expansile but do not invade the body of the brain. They often can be totally resected and, if so, have a good prognosis. Oligodendromas arise from oligodendrocytes. Like most astrocytomas, they are highly invasive, but the prognosis is much better for patients with this type of tumor.

Two other types of tumors are often considered along with the gliomas. One is an uncommon malignant tumor arising from primitive cells in the cerebellum of young children (medulloblastoma). The tumor is malignant but also extremely radiation sensitive. The second is a tumor arising from the cells lining the ventricular system. These cells are termed ependymal cells, and the tumor is termed an ependymoma. Although some tumors can be totally resected, the tumors may spread broadly through the CSF.

Primary lymphomas also may arise within the central nervous system and are relatively common in patients who are immunosuppressed (such as patients with AIDS) or those who have undergone organ transplantation. These tumors do not often spread outside the nervous system. Interestingly, lymphomas arising outside the CNS generally do not invade the body of the brain but may be found in the CSF.

Primary central nervous system tumors do not normally spread outside the nervous system, but many carry a poor prognosis because they often lie deep within the brain and are infiltrative. Treatment consists of surgical resection of as much of the tumor as possible. In selected cases, surgery is followed by radiation and sometimes by anticancer chemotherapy as well.

The symptoms of a brain tumor depend on the size and location of the neoplasm. Headache is a common initial manifestation because the increased volume within the cranial cavity caused by the tumor raises the intracranial pressure. Growth of the tumor also disrupts nerve cells and fiber tracts within the brain, leading to various neurological disturbances, including seizures.

Peripheral Nerve Disorders

Demyelinating neuropathy Neural disease with the loss of the myelin sheath surrounding axons resulting in abnormal neural signal transmission.

Polyneuropathies An inflammation of multiple nerves.

Peripheral nerves and nerve roots may develop **demyelinating neuropathies** in which the axon is spared (much as is the case in demyelinating disease of the CNS). In such cases remyelination will occur to some degree as Schwann cells (and their precursors) proliferate. Neuronopathies affect the nerve body itself and result in varying degrees of secondary axon degeneration. Clinical manifestations depend on the degree of nerve degeneration and on which nerves are affected. Involvement of a single nerve is usually secondary to injury or external compression. Involvement of multiple nerves, termed "**polyneuropathies**" or sometimes "peripheral neuritis," is usually a manifestation of any of a large number of systemic diseases of inflammatory, infectious, or other etiologies.

Polyneuropathies (Peripheral Neuritis)

Polyneuropathy, also termed "peripheral neuritis," is characterized by progressive muscular weakness; numbness and tingling; tenderness; and pain in the parts of the body supplied by the peripheral nerves (termed "the distribution of the nerves"). Often, the muscles supplied by the involved nerves also exhibit some degree of atrophy. Usually, the neural damage is axonal, and the weakness and sensory disturbances affect the distal parts of the limbs, whereas strength and sensation remain relatively normal in the proximal parts of the extremities.

This "glove and stocking" pattern of sensory and motor dysfunction is quite characteristic of polyneuritis. Most cases result from systemic diseases such as long-standing diabetes or autoimmune diseases or from occupational exposure to toxic drugs, heavy metals, or industrial compounds. Alcoholism is another common cause of peripheral neuritis, which is probably related to a coexisting deficiency of B vitamins. Treatment of the underlying disease may produce some symptomatic improvement.

Guillain-Barré Syndrome

A special type of autoimmune inflammatory demyelinating polyneuropathy with characteristic clinical manifestations is the **Guillain-Barré syndrome**. The disease is characterized by widespread patchy demyelination of nerves and nerve roots with mild inflammatory changes and sometimes by axon degeneration as well. Onset is usually a few weeks after a mild influenza-like respiratory or other infection (notably the Zika virus) or (much less frequently) following immunizations. *Campylobacter jejuni* infection is one of the most common risk factors. The illness appears to be a type of autoimmune reaction to myelin or other neuronal components that is triggered by the preceding infection or immunization.

Clinically, the disease is characterized by muscular weakness that usually begins in the legs and often spreads rapidly to affect the muscles of the trunk and upper extremities. Sensory disturbances are infrequent. Severe respiratory distress may occur if the nerves supplying the intercostal muscles are involved. The muscular weakness generally progresses for 1 to 2 weeks, remains stationary for a time, and then gradually improves. The patient usually recovers rapidly if the nerve injury is limited to demyelination. Although the prognosis for this disease is good in general, some percentage of patients may die as a result of respiratory and cardiac failure; many who survive will suffer some degree of long-term disability. Replacement of patient plasma (plasmapheresis) may be beneficial because it removes damaging autoantibodies. Intravenous immunoglobulin, thought to have an anti-inflammatory effect, is also used in therapy.

Guillain-Barré syndrome A type of polyneuritis resulting from an autoimmune reaction.

Carpal tunnel syndrome A condition resulting from nerves in the hand being compressed on the anterior surface of the wrist.

Paresthesia An abnormal sensation, such as burning, prickling, or numbness.

Peripheral Nerve Injury

A peripheral nerve may be damaged in association with a deep laceration, a fracture, or a crushing injury. A common cause of a more chronic type of nerve injury is external compression by a fibrous band or ligament. This condition is often termed a nerve-entrapment neuropathy. The median nerve, which supplies sensory and motor fibers to the hand, is often involved in a condition termed "**carpal tunnel syndrome**." The nerve is usually compressed on the anterior surface of the wrist, within the confined space between the wrist bones and the overlying ligaments that cross the wrist joint and stabilize the positions of the flexor tendons. The nerve compression causes pain and **paresthesias** (abnormal sensations such as burning, numbness, and tingling) in the index and middle fingers, together with decreased sensation in the part of the hand supplied by the nerve. The small muscles of the hand at the base of the thumb, which are supplied by the nerve, may also undergo atrophy. Sometimes symptoms can be relieved by conservative measures such as injecting a corticosteroid mixed with a local anesthetic into the confined space (termed the carpal tunnel) in which the nerve is compressed. In many cases, however, it is necessary to relieve the compression surgically by resecting the part of the ligament that compresses the nerve.

Case 23-1

Estrella, an 18-month-old female child who lives in a small North Carolina town, is the only child in the family. Estrella's mother states she was born at home in the United States, but no documentation is available. Her parents are agricultural workers who also do home cleaning and repairs during the winter. Although Estrella has apparently not received pediatric medical care, her mother states that in the past she has always eaten well and been healthy. Estrella has been brought to a community-free medical clinic by her parents. Her mother states that on the previous day Estrella was irritable and turned away from bright light (had photophobia). She was unwilling to eat, vomited, and felt very warm. This morning Estrella had a convulsion and became lethargic (did not move much). Her parents became very concerned, prompting the visit to the clinic. The clinic was staffed by a physician assistant (PA), Jill.

Jill notes that Estrella's height and weight are age-appropriate, but her developmental stage is difficult to assess as she is in distress and poorly responsive. On examination, Jill noted that the child was lethargic but could be aroused. She had a fever of 103°F. She cried when her head was turned and appeared to have a stiff neck (nuchal rigidity). Although the "soft spot" on her skull (anterior fontanelle) was almost closed, there appeared to be some bulging of the brain tissue. Jill thought a petechial rash consisting of pinpoint-like purple spots was beginning to appear. Jill is concerned about possible signs of a neurological disease (and specifically bacterial meningitis, an infection of the meningeal layer of the brain), and these concerns are exacerbated by Estrella's socioeconomic background. To confirm Jill's suspicion, a lumbar puncture was required. Jill was inexperienced (and there are some risks to the patient), so the test was deferred until Estrella could be transferred to the pediatric infectious disease division of a regional hospital.

At the hospital, CSF obtained by lumbar puncture had elevated protein and reduced glucose, and neutrophils were detected (15 cells per microliter of CSF). Estrella also had an elevated neutrophil count in her blood. The gram-negative diplococci detected in her CSF was determined to be *Neisseria meningitides*, confirming a diagnosis of Neisseria meningitis. Estrella was admitted to the pediatric ICU, where she demonstrated signs of shock and was given IV fluids. She was immediately started on IV antibiotics (initially vancomycin and cefotaxime), which were continued for 10 days, after which she was discharged. Estrella's household contacts (parents) and children in her nursery were treated with prophylactic antibiotics.

Discussion

The classic symptoms of bacterial meningitis are demonstrated in the case: fever, meningeal signs (neck rigidity), bulging fontanelle, photophobia, convulsions, and (had Estrella been able to express herself) undoubtedly headache. Examination of the CSF demonstrated the signs of bacterial meningitis, reduced glucose (said to be related to bacterial consumption), and increased protein (as a result of acute inflammatory changes in the meningeal vasculature). In addition, an elevated blood neutrophil count was indicative of bacterial infection. Detection of Gram-negative diplococci in the CSF (and subsequent confirmation by culture) confirmed the organism to be *Neisseria*, which tends to cause a very rapidly progressive (and potentially lethal) disease. The bacteria colonize the respiratory system but can spread via the blood in non-immuned individuals. A bacterial endotoxin can result in disseminated intravascular coagulation (DIC) (see Chapter 12), a disastrous complication with a very high likelihood of death (or disability if the patient survives). The petechial rash is an indicator of DIC that results from platelet consumption, activation of the coagulation system, and capillary bleeding. Luckily for Estrella, the rash noted by Jill was not related to the disease. Rapid antibiotic therapy is life-saving, and the disease can be spread to contacts (hence, the use of prophylactic antibiotics in contacts). A vaccine is available but not generally used, as it has limited effectiveness in young children and is effective only against certain Neisseria strains. The vaccine is used in certain epidemic areas and in individuals who are housed in crowded circumstances (such as students in college dormitories) where it may be required. Another bacterial meningitis caused by *Haemophilus influenzae* type B (Hib) was formerly quite common in children under the age of 5. The incidence of this infection has sharply declined because of highly effective nearly universal childhood vaccination. Jill was concerned because she felt it unlikely that Estrella had been vaccinated for this bacterium (and she suspected it might be the causative agent).

Etiology and Pathogenesis

Bacterial infection with *Neisseria meningitides* and subsequent meningitis.

Questions

1. Jill had several specific concerns about Estrella's disease based on socioeconomic background. How would those concerns affect a potential diagnosis?
2. Jill's parents were agricultural (field) workers who lived in substandard housing. What additional etiologies might be suggested in an acutely sick child who came from such a background?
3. Assume that Estrella did, in fact, demonstrate DIC. What additional symptoms would she demonstrate? What laboratory tests might have been used to detect and monitor for DIC?
4. Under what circumstances might it be reasonable to require Hib immunization? Have you personally been immunized, and if so, why?
5. Several simple clinical tests can be used to demonstrate signs of meningeal disease. What are they, and how are they performed? (Hint: Investigate Brudzinski's sign.)

Questions for Review

1. Briefly describe the organization of the central nervous system. Describe the function and circulation of cerebrospinal fluid. What is meant by the following terms: upper motor neuron lesion, lower motor neuron lesion, flaccid paralysis, and spastic paralysis?
2. What are some of the possible effects of a severe blow to the head?
3. What is a stroke? What are the common causes of a stroke? What is a congenital aneurysm of the circle of Willis?
4. What are the common causes of hydrocephalus? How does a brain tumor cause hydrocephalus?
5. What is a neural tube defect? How can it be recognized before birth?
6. What is meant by the following terms: arachnoid, subdural hemorrhage, anencephaly, and meningioma?
7. What is a transient ischemic attack? How is it treated?
8. Describe the common tumors of the nervous system. What are their clinical manifestations?
9. What is the difference between a polyneuritis (peripheral neuritis) and Guillain-Barré syndrome?
10. Compare Creutzfeldt-Jakob disease and Alzheimer's disease.

References

Moini J. Chapters 11, 12, 13, 14. In *Anatomy and Physiology for Health Professionals*. 3rd ed. Jones & Bartlett Learning; 2020.

Loeffler AG, Hart MN. Central nervous system. In: *Introduction to Human Disease: Pathophysiology for Health Professionals*. 7th ed. Jones & Bartlett Learning; 2020.

Fuller GN, Goodman JC, Klintworth GK. The central nervous system. In: Rubin E, Reisner HM, eds. *Principles of Rubin's Pathology*. 7th ed. Wolters Kluwer; 2019.

- The area of neurobiology is complex, and no one text can do it justice. The first entry presents additional structural details of the nervous system in general and the CNS specifically. The illustrations are excellent. The second selection contains further information on the pathology of CNS disease. The third entry is a standard reference for the pathology of human organ systems written at a level appropriate for undergraduate medical school students. The chapter on the nervous system presents a more detailed view of the pathology of neurological disease and, in particular, CNS cancer.

Centers for Disease Control and Prevention. Neural Tube Defects. https://www.cdc.gov/ncbddd/birthdefects/facts-about-neural-tube-defects.html

The National Spina Bifida Patient Registry (NSBPR). Spina Bifida Association. https://www.spinabifidaassociation.org/about-our-research/national-spina-bifida-patient-registry/

Reghunath A, Ghasi RG, Aggarwal A. Unveiling the tale of the tail: An illustration of spinal dysraphisms. *Neurosurg Rev*. 2019. doi:10.1007/s10143-019-01215-z

- The first two references are good general introductions to the subject, with information on nutritional supplementation. The second is more detailed with additional resources. The third is a review of spinal development and defects.

Center for Disease Control and Prevention. Eastern Equine Encephalitis Virus, Historic Data (2003–2024). Last updated June 3, 2025. https://www.cdc.gov/eastern-equine-encephalitis/data-maps/historic-data.html#cdc_data_surveillance_section_2-explore-human-data-for-2003%e2%80%932024

The Global Statistics. West Nile Virus Death Rate in the US 2025. https://www.theglobalstatistics.com/west-nile-virus-death-rate/

- These two sources provide data on the two arboviruses.

Center for Disease Control and Prevention. About Prion Diseases. https://www.cdc.gov/prions/index.html

Wells C, et al. Prionoid proteins in the pathogenesis of neurodegenerative diseases. *Front Mol Neurosci*. 2019;12:271. https://www.ncbi.nlm.nih.gov/pmc/articles/PMC6861308/

Rivera NA, Brandt AL, Novakofski JE, Mateus-Pinilla N. Chronic wasting disease in cervids: Prevalence, impact and management strategies. *Vet Med (Auckl)*. 2019;10:123-129. https://www.ncbi.nlm.nih.gov/pmc/articles/PMC6778748/

- The first reference is a gateway to information on all human prion-based diseases. The second overlaps with references on neurodegenerative diseases, suggesting the role of prion-like agents in a variety of neurodegenerative diseases. The last should be read by all of those who hunt deer and love venison. Although emphasizing cervid disease, it is an excellent overview of the pathophysiology of prion agents.

Centers for Disease Control and Prevention. Stroke. http://www.cdc.gov/stroke

American Stroke Association. American Heart Association. https://www.stroke.org/en

- The CDC entry is a useful portal to a large source of material on stroke risk and prevention. An excellent starting point for additional detailed information. The American Heart Association provides a useful current guide to stroke therapy and care. Learn the F.A.S.T. warning signs of stroke.

Alzheimer's Association. 2019 Alzheimer's Disease Facts and Figures. https://www.alz.org/media/documents/alzheimers-facts-and-figures-2019-r.pdf

- An extensive review covering many aspects of Alzheimer's disease, such as many details of diagnosis not covered in the text.

Parkinson's Disease

NIH National Institute on Aging. Parkinson's Disease. https://www.nia.nih.gov/health/parkinsons-disease

Yang D, et al. The role of the gut microbiota in the pathogenesis of Parkinsons's disease. *Front Neurol*. 2019. doi:10.3389/fneur.2019.01155. https://www.ncbi.nlm.nih.gov/pmc/articles/PMC6851172/

- The first reference provides a useful overview. The second reviews one of the more mysterious aspects of Parkinson's disease: an apparent relation to early digestive problems. Some believe that gut microorganisms play an important role.

Huntington's Disease

NIH National Library of Medicine. Medline Plus. Huntington's Disease. https://ghr.nlm.nih.gov/condition/huntington-disease

Nordick K, Khalili YA. Genetics, Trinucleotide. StatPearls. Last updated August 14, 2023. https://www.ncbi.nlm.nih.gov/books/NBK545250/

- Much of the interest in Huntington's disease lies in it as a model of triplet-repeat diseases. The first reference presents a good general overview; the second covers a variety of triplet repeat diseases, including Huntington's.

Multiple Sclerosis

National Multiple Sclerosis Society. What is Multiple Sclerosis? https://www.nationalmssociety.org/What-is-MS

Stys PK, Tsutsui S. Recent advances in understanding multiple sclerosis. *F1000Res*. 2019. doi:10.12688/f1000research.20906.1. https://www.ncbi.nlm.nih.gov/pmc/articles/PMC6915812/

- The Multiple Sclerosis Society site is a good starting point for both current therapy and research. It describes the various clinical patterns of MS, which are not covered in the text. The second reference is an in-depth review of the clinical presentation, genetics, and pathology of the disease.

Amyotrophic Lateral Sclerosis

ALS Association. http://www.als.org/

Armon C. Amyotrophic Lateral Sclerosis. Medscape. Updated April 11, 2024. https://emedicine.medscape.com/article/1170097-overview#a1

- The ALS Association has an excellent review of the genetics of ALS as well as basic facts helpful in coping with the disease. The second is strong on the pathophysiology, etiology, and epidemiology.

Frosch MP, Anthony DC, De Girolami U. The central nervous system; tumors. In: Kumar V, Abbas AK, Aster JC. *Pathologic Basis of Disease*. 9th ed. Elsevier Saunders; 2014;1306-1317.

Kristensen BW, et al. Molecular pathology of tumors of the central nervous system. *Ann Oncol*. 2019;30(8):1265-1278. https://www.ncbi.nlm.nih.gov/pmc/articles/PMC6683853/

- Tumors of the CNS are an extremely complex (and rapidly changing) area best approached initially from pathology textbooks aimed at medical students and residents. The first reference here and Principles of Rubin's Pathology, 7th, listed previously, are both excellent starting points. The second reference covers important areas in the molecular characterization not addressed in the textbook chapters.

Noor A. Pediatric Bacterial Meningitis. Updated October 15, 2025. http://emedicine.medscape.com/article/961497_overview

- A useful review that was used in the case construction.

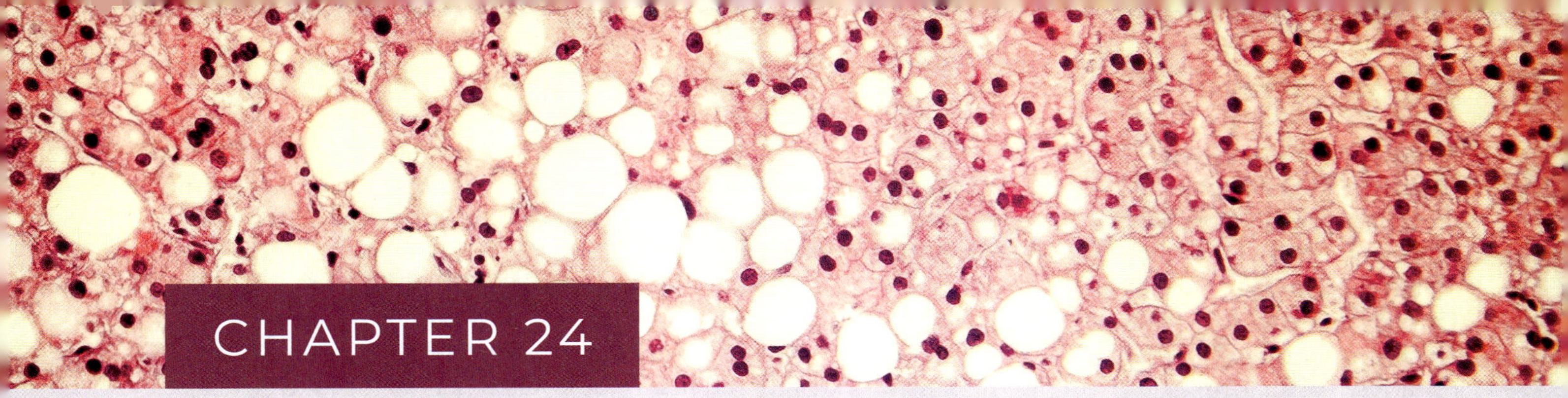

CHAPTER 24

The Musculoskeletal System

LEARNING OBJECTIVES

1. Describe the maturation process of bone.
2. Describe the process of bone remodeling.
3. List the major types of arthritis. Describe their pathogenesis and clinical manifestations, and explain the methods of treatment.
4. Describe the metabolic problems leading to gout.
5. Describe the process that occurs to repair a bone fracture.
6. Describe the causes and effects of osteoporosis, and name the methods of treatment.
7. Describe the manifestations, complications, and treatment of scoliosis.
8. Describe the structure of the intervertebral disks, and explain their function. Describe the clinical manifestations of a herniated disk.
9. Compare the pathogenesis and clinical manifestations of muscular atrophy and muscular dystrophy. Name and describe the common types of each.
10. Describe the pathogenesis, manifestations, and treatment of myasthenia gravis.
11. Understand the pathogenicity of scurvy and rickets, and describe treatment and prevention.

Structure and Function of the Skeletal System

The skeleton is the rigid supporting structure of the body, with all bones having the same basic structure. Bones are composed of an outer layer of compact bone (**cortical bone**) and an inner, spongy layer of bone (**cancellous bone**) arranged in a loose, meshed latticework of thin strands termed bone **trabeculae**. The spaces between the trabeculae contain the bone marrow, which consists of fat and blood-forming tissue. Cortical bone provides mechanical strength and makes up the majority of the skeleton. Cancellous bone contains a high number of bone cells and is responsible for changes in bone growth and structure.

Cortical bone Outer layer of compact bone.
Cancellous bone The inner, spongy layer of bone.
Trabeculae Thin strands of bone lattice work.

Individual bones vary in size and appearance. They may be long, short, flat, or irregular in shape. The typical long bone, such as those found in the upper and lower limbs, has a tubular shape with expanded ends. The shaft is the long cylindrical part, and the expanded ends of the shaft are termed the **epiphyses** (singular epiphysis). The center of the shaft is hollowed out to form the marrow cavity, which is filled with fat and bone marrow. This type of construction provides considerable strength without excessive weight. The parts of a typical long bone are referred to by specific terms. The ends of the bone, which are in contact with (articulate with) other bones, are the epiphyses, which extend from the cartilage component of the joint (articular cartilage) to the **epiphyseal plate** (composed of cartilage in children and critical to the ossification of and growth in length of the long bones). The **diaphysis** is the elongated central region of the shaft of the bone that blends into the more fluted region below the epiphyseal plate, the **metaphysis**. The metaphysis contains the cancellous bone and the active bone marrow (**Figure 24-1** and **Figure 24-2**).

Epiphyses The end parts of long bones, initially growing separately from the shaft.

Epiphyseal plate Cartilaginous end of epiphyses critical to ossification of long bones.

Diaphysis Elongated central region of the bone shaft.

Metaphysis Region below the epiphyseal plate containing cancellous bone and active bone marrow.

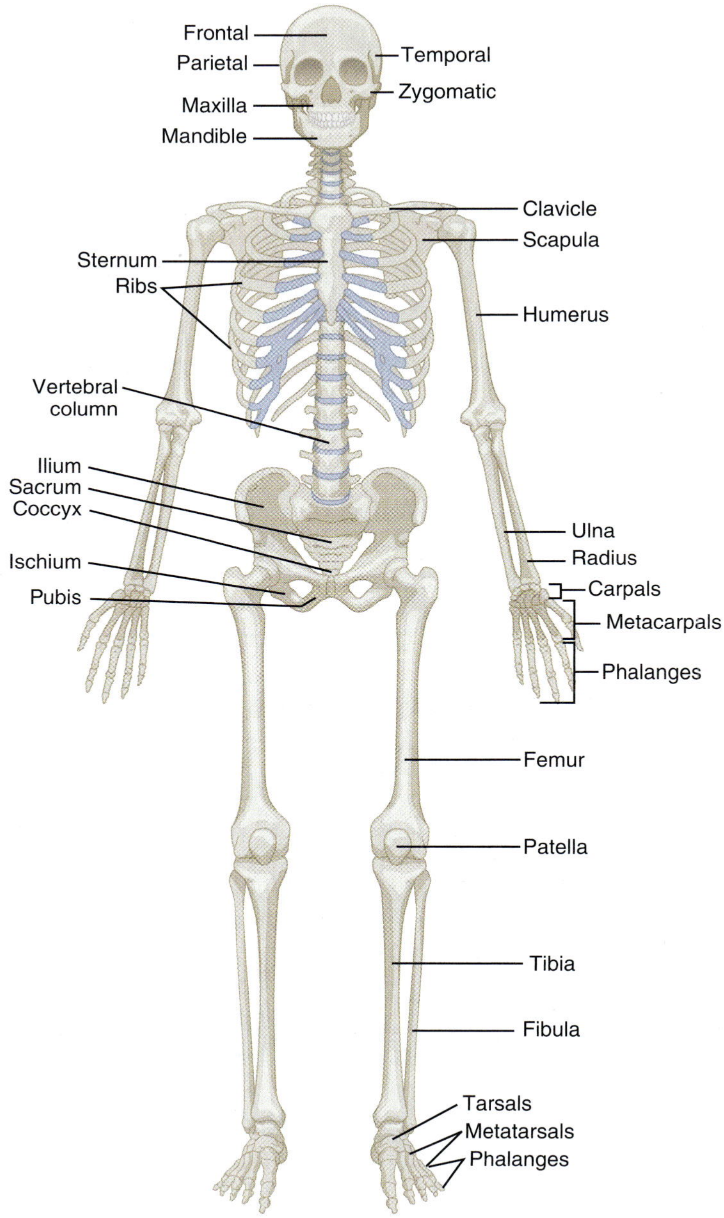

Figure 24-1 Major bones and joints of the body.

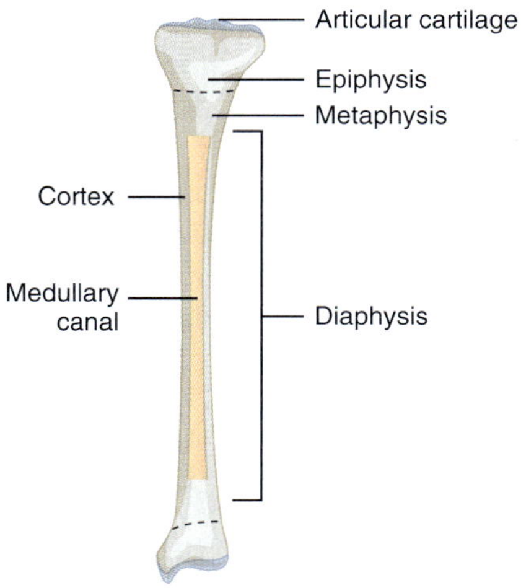

Figure 24-2 Structure of a long bone. The tibia is illustrated here.

Bone is a specialized type of connective tissue composed of a dense connective tissue framework composed mostly of type I collagen, which becomes impregnated with calcium phosphate salts (hydroxyapatite) along with smaller amounts of calcium carbonate and other minerals. Calcium salts in bone and calcium ions in the blood and body fluid are continuously interchanged. Three different types of cells are found in bone: **osteoblasts**, **osteocytes**, and **osteoclasts**. Osteoblasts are the active bone-forming cells that produce the collagenous bone matrix. They secrete an enzyme, alkaline phosphatase, that promotes deposition of calcium phosphate salts in the bone matrix to calcify the bone. As the bone matrix is formed and calcified, the osteoblasts become incorporated within the bone and differentiate into relatively inactive mature bone cells termed osteocytes. Osteoclasts, multinucleated cells related to macrophages, are concerned with bone resorption. They remove the bone matrix by phagocytosis, dissolve the bone salts, and release the calcium and phosphate ions into the circulation (**Figure 24-3**).

Osteoblasts/osteocytes/osteoclasts Types of cells in bone; active bone-forming cells, mature bone cells, and bone resorption cells, respectively.

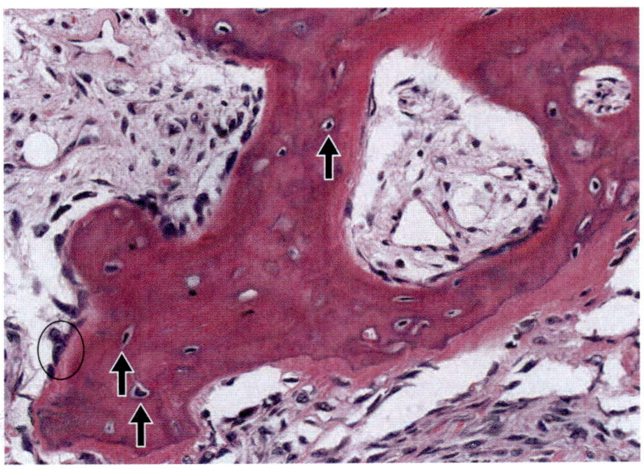

Figure 24-3 Bone repair at the site of a fracture. Examples of osteoblasts (*arrows*). The cells are surrounded by halos of matrix not yet calcified. Example of osteoclasts (*circle*), multinucleated cells remodeling the surface of a bone spicule. Osteocytes (not shown) appear similar to osteoblasts but are embedded in the bone matrix and are not surrounded by a clear halo.

Courtesy of Department of Pathology and Laboratory Medicine, University of North Carolina at Chapel Hill.

Disuse atrophy The reduction in structure or function of a body part when the use of that body part has diminished, and is often used in reference to bone or muscle.

Synovial joint Movable joint.

Syndesmosis A fixed joint joined by fibrous connective tissue.

Synchondrosis Cartilaginous joint.

Intramembranous bone formation Direct formation of bone by osteoblasts without prior formation of a cartilage model.

Endochondral bone formation The formation of bone, first as a cartilage model that is then reabsorbed and converted into bone.

In general, the strength and thickness of the bones depend on the activities of the individual. A person accustomed to strenuous physical labor has thicker, heavier bones than one who is normally engaged in light, sedentary activities. If an extremity is immobilized and is not allowed to bear weight, as after a fracture, the immobilized bone undergoes significant thinning and decalcification, termed **disuse atrophy**.

The bones of the skeleton are connected by joints. **Synovial joints** are movable, whereas synarthroses are relatively fixed. In fibrous fixed joints (a **syndesmosis**), such as occurs between the bones of the skull, the bones are firmly joined by fibrous tissue to form a firm union termed a suture line. In a cartilaginous joint (a **synchondrosis**), such as occurs between adjacent vertebral bodies in the spine and between the pubic bones of the pelvis (symphysis pubis), the ends of the bones are joined by cartilage, but there is no joint cavity or synovium. Joints of this type have very little mobility.

A synovial joint is a movable joint in which the ends of the bones that move against one another are covered by smooth hyaline cartilage, the articular cartilage (articulare = to connect). The ends of the bones are held together by dense fibrous bands (ligaments). The joint capsule is lined by a thin synovial membrane (the synovium), which secretes a small amount of mucinous fluid to lubricate the joint. **Figure 24-4** illustrates the structure of a typical movable joint. **Figure 24-5** illustrates the histologic appearance of the articular cartilage and underlying bone and the appearance of a normal synovium. In joint disease, the structures may be altered by inflammation (inflammatory arthritis) or degeneration (noninflammatory arthritis), leading to derangement in joint function.

Bone Formation

The two types of bone formation are fundamentally similar. In **intramembranous bone formation**, the embryonic connective tissue cells (mesodermal cells) differentiate into bone-forming cells (osteoblasts). The osteoblasts secrete a collagenous material termed osteoid, which eventually becomes calcified to form bone. The bones of the vertex of the skull, the facial bones, and a few other bones are formed in this manner. Most of the skeletal system, however, is formed by a process termed **endochondral bone formation** (endo = within + chondral = cartilage). In endochondral bone formation, the mesodermal cells differentiate first into immature cartilage cells (chondroblasts) and then mature into chondrocytes. The bones are formed initially as cartilaginous precursors. The cartilage is then absorbed and replaced by bone. Conversion of cartilage into bone is accomplished by vascular bone-forming mesoderm, which invades the cartilage.

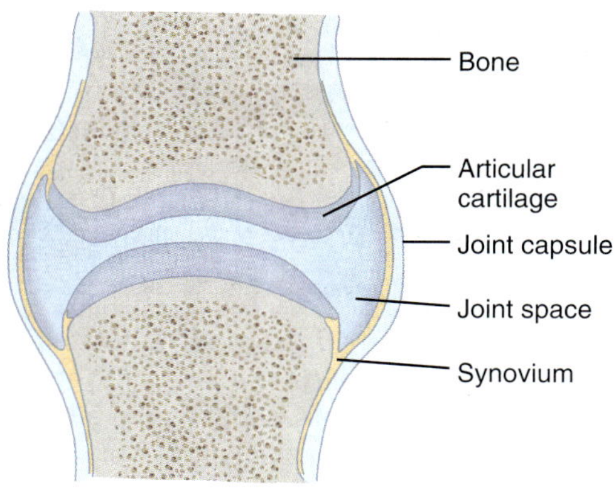

Figure 24-4 Structure of a movable joint.

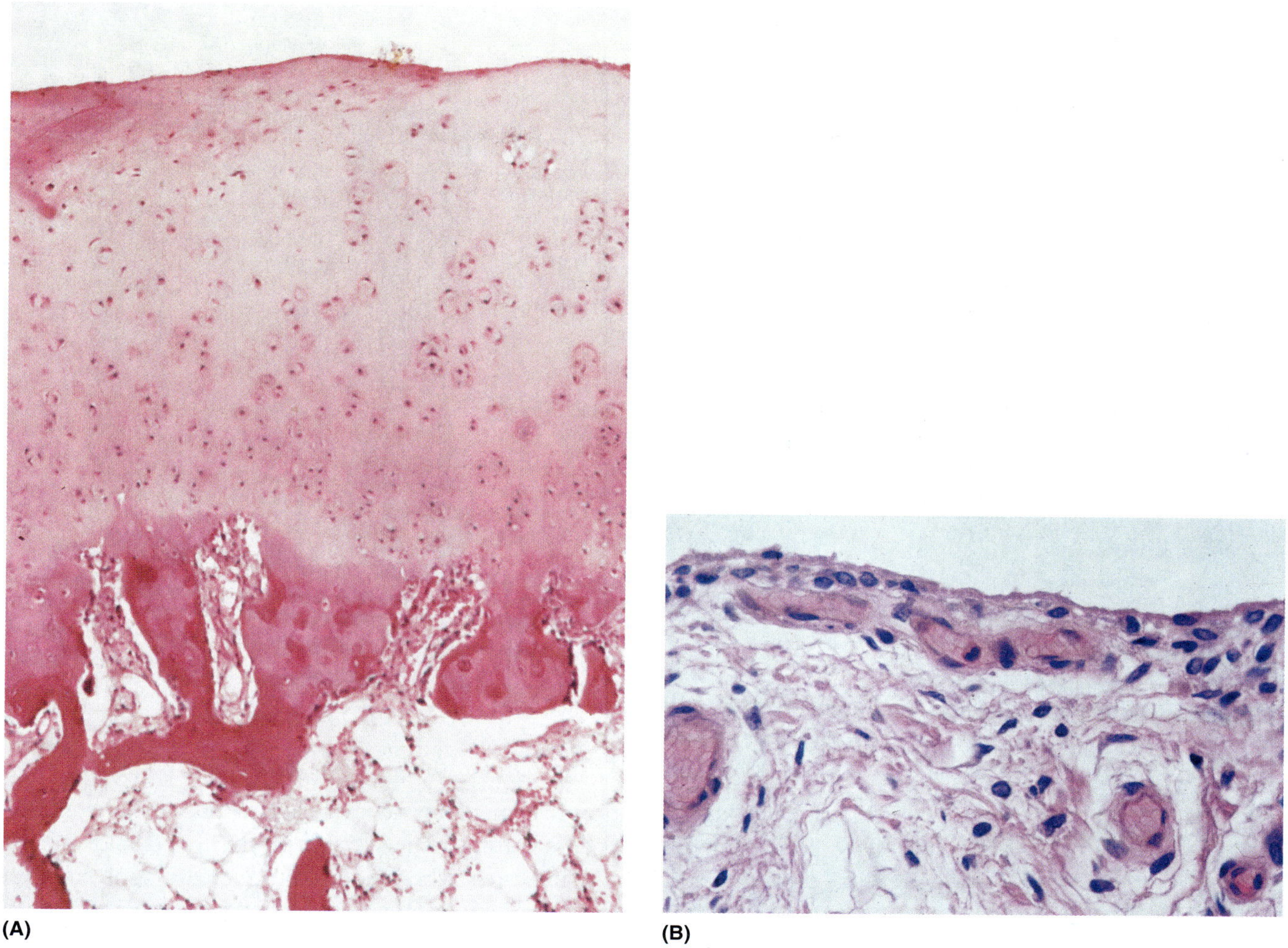

Figure 24-5 **(A)** A low-magnification photomicrograph of the cellular structure of a normal articular surface, illustrating articular cartilage (*top*), the junction of bone and cartilage (*middle*), and normal bone with fatty bone marrow (*bottom*) (original magnification x40). **(B)** Normal synovium composed of synovial cells (*top*) covering loose connective tissue.

Bones that have been preformed in cartilage undergo ossification at specific times throughout fetal and postnatal life. In the long bones, ossification begins first in the shaft diaphysis (primary ossification) and continues toward the ends of the bone; later, centers of ossification form at the ends (epiphyses) of the bone (secondary ossification). The actively growing zone of cartilage between the shaft and the epiphysis of a long bone is termed the epiphyseal plate (**Figure 24-6**).

Bone Growth and Remodeling

Bone grows in both length and thickness and is continually remodeled as it grows by absorption of bone in some areas and formation of new bone in others. Bone grows thicker by adding newly formed bone produced by the **periosteum** (a layer of specialized connective tissue cells surrounding the bone) to its external surface. The periosteal cells differentiate into osteoblasts, which in turn produce bone. Growth in the length of a bone is the result of the proliferation of cartilage at the epiphyseal plate, which is converted into bone. Growth in bone length continues into adolescence. Eventually, epiphyseal growth ceases, and the cartilaginous epiphyseal plate becomes converted into bone (closure of the epiphyses). Thereafter, no further growth in length of bone is possible.

Periosteum The tough, fibrous membrane that covers a bone, except for its articular surfaces.

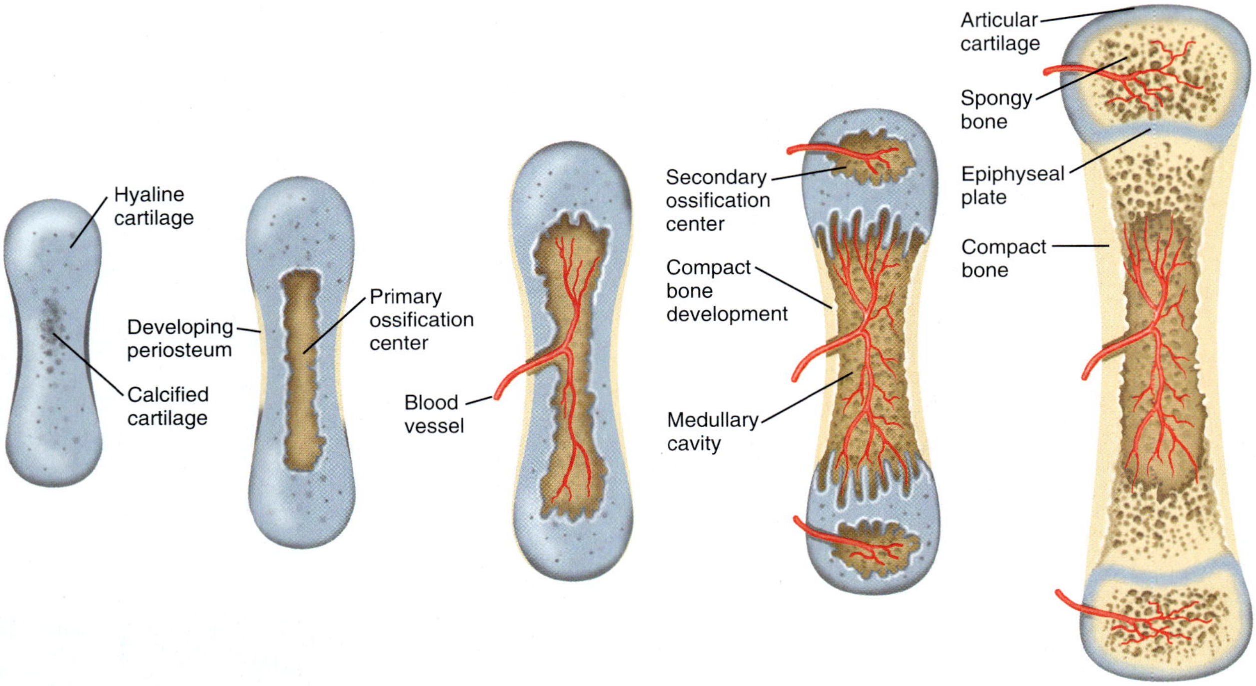

Figure 24-6 The major stages in the development of endochondral bone.

Data from Shier DN, Butler JL, Lewis R. Hole's Essentials of Human *Anatomy & Physiology*. 10th ed. New York, NY: McGraw-Hill Higher Education; 2009.

Bone breakdown and replacement by newly formed bone occur continuously. Bone remodeling occurs during bone growth in childhood and adolescence, during repair of bone fractures, when required to increase bone strength in response to greater weight-bearing requirements, and even in association with normal weight-bearing. Often, microscopic breaks occur in bone structure resulting from the stresses of daily weight-bearing, which are repaired or replaced by newly formed bone. Many other factors influence bone remodeling, including calcium, vitamin D, parathyroid hormone, and steroid hormones. Normally, bone breakdown and replacement occur concurrently so the strength and density of the skeletal system are not compromised. However, if bone loss exceeds replacement, the bone density falls, and the bones become more susceptible to fractures.

Normal bone growth and maturation require vitamin D, obtained by exposure of the skin to sunlight or from the diet in vitamin D–fortified milk and other foods. Calcium and phosphate are also needed to calcify the bone as it is formed; the parathyroid glands regulate the level of blood calcium and must function normally (see Chapter 22).

Rickets Impaired calcification of bone in a growing child caused by vitamin D deficiency, which leads to bowing of leg bones when weight-bearing is attempted.

Osteomalacia Impaired calcification of bone in an adult caused by vitamin D deficiency, which also contributes to bone loss caused by osteoporosis.

Bone Growth Disturbances Caused by Vitamin D Deficiency: Rickets and Osteomalacia

Rickets and **osteomalacia** refer to defects in bone mineralization in children and adults, respectively. Children lacking adequate vitamin D develop rickets, now an uncommon disease in industrialized countries as most children receive vitamin D supplements. If vitamin D is insufficient, calcium is not absorbed normally from the intestinal tract, and the blood calcium tends to fall. The parathyroid glands respond to the low calcium by increasing the secretion of parathyroid hormone, which raises blood calcium but also causes the level of phosphate in the blood to fall. As a result, the deposition of calcium phosphate

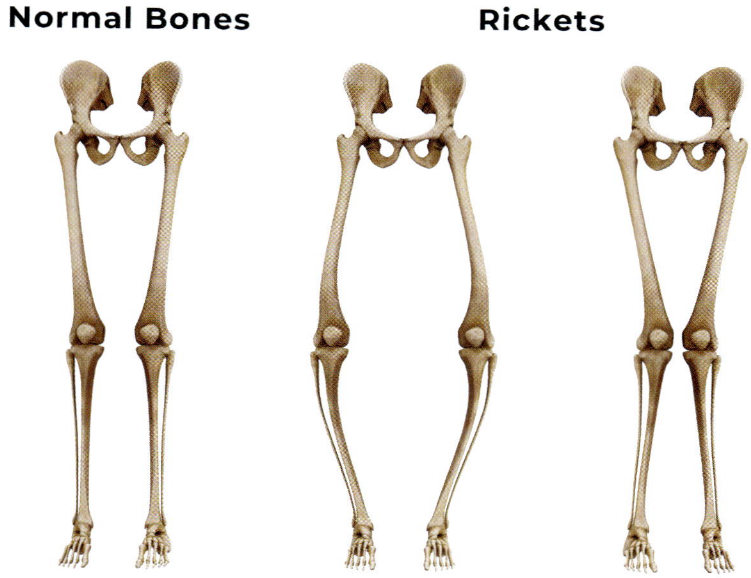

Figure 24-7 Comparison of normal bones and rickets.

in the bone matrix is impaired because there is not enough phosphate available to combine with calcium, so the bone matrix is not adequately calcified. Osteoid is formed in excess at the epiphyseal ends of the growing bones but lacks strength because it is so poorly calcified. Consequently, the weakened bones tend to become bowed when weight-bearing is attempted. Children who suffer from rickets often experience poor bone development and bony deformities such as bowlegs and knock-knees (**Figure 24-7**). Rickets can be divided into two categories: calcipenic rickets and phosphopenic rickets. Calcipenic rickets is mainly caused by inadequate calcium uptake, due to vitamin D deficiency (now uncommon) or defects in the metabolic pathway of vitamin D.

Phosphopenic rickets results from deficient/impaired intestinal phosphate absorption or abnormal renal excretion. Rickets also can be caused by autosomal recessive diseases that cause deranged vitamin D metabolism or a lack of a functional vitamin D cellular receptor (vitamin D–dependent rickets types I and II, respectively). However, the most common type of inherited rickets is X-linked hypophosphatemia (vitamin D-resistant rickets), which results from impaired phosphate uptake.

Rickets is curable, especially when diagnosed at early stages. Supplementing phosphate, calcium, and vitamin D and adequate sunlight exposure are effective in treating and preventing nutritional rickets.

Osteomalacia in adults is caused by defective intestinal absorption of vitamin D and calcium as a result of small intestine disease or liver disease. The reduced absorption is caused by diminished bile production (and hence reduced intestinal uptake of fat-soluble vitamin D).

Vitamin C Deficiency and Scurvy

Scurvy results from the lack of vitamin C, a condition that was first described in 1550 BCE Egyptian writings. The typical clinical presentations include swelling of the gums, petechiae, and bruising. In severe cases, patients may experience mucosal gastrointestinal bleeding. In terms of skeletal defects, scurvy inhibits osteoblast function, resulting in a lack of new bone growth and repair because of the inability of the osteoblasts to produce normal cross-linked collagen. The lack of vitamin C prevents the hydroxylation of proline and lysine residues in collagen, which is necessary for the collagen molecule to form its normal molecular structure.

The condition resulted from dietary insufficiency of vitamin C, chronic alcohol abuse, obesity, and chronic gastrointestinal disorders (such as IBS), which can result in a vitamin insufficiency.

Scurvy is typically treated with vitamin C supplements; this condition can be prevented by taking an adequate amount of vitamin C from dietary sources.

Genetic-Related Bone Growth Disturbances

Abnormal Bone Formation

Achondroplasia A genetic disorder that results from a mutation in the FGFR3 gene, which alters the cartilage to bone conversion during bone development.

Osteogenesis imperfecta A genetic disease with mutations involving collagen production causing bones to be excessivley brittle.

The two most important genetically determined diseases of the skeletal system that result from abnormal bone formation are **achondroplasia** and **osteogenesis imperfecta**. In achondroplasia, endochondral bone formation is faulty. When inherited, the abnormality is transmitted as Mendelian dominant; however, 80 percent of patients with the condition have a new mutation, and their parents are of normal height. The disease is the most common form of short-limbed dwarfism and is characterized by disturbed endochondral bone formation at the epiphyseal lines of the long bones, resulting in short, thick bones. The disturbance impairs growth of the extremities, causing a type of dwarfism in which the limbs are disproportionately short in relation to the trunk (achondroplastic dwarfism). The head is also abnormally formed because of disturbed endochondral ossification of the bones forming the base of the skull, and there is usually also an exaggerated curvature (lordosis) of the lumbar spine (**Figure 24-8**). Affected individuals have normal life spans and cognitive function.

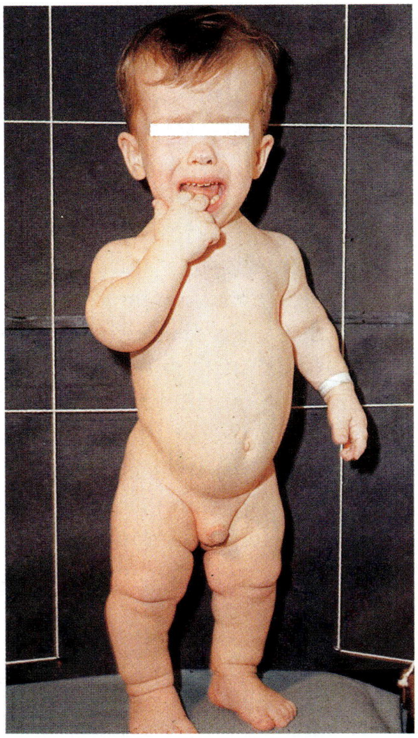

Figure 24-8 Characteristic appearance of a child with achondroplasia, illustrating the relatively large head and disproportionate shortening of the extremities.

Courtesy of Leonard V. Crowley, MD, Century College.

Osteogenesis imperfecta (meaning literally "imperfect bone formation") is characterized by the formation of very thin and delicate bones that are easily broken under very minimal stress. In the most severe cases, the infant is born with multiple fractures. Some fractures occur before birth, having been sustained as a result of the very minor stresses resulting from the movements of the fetus within the uterus; other fractures occur during delivery. The intrauterine fractures of the extremities usually heal in poor alignment, causing the limbs to appear bent and disproportionately short (**Figure 24-9**). In milder forms of the disease, the abnormal fragility of the bone may not become apparent until childhood or adolescence.

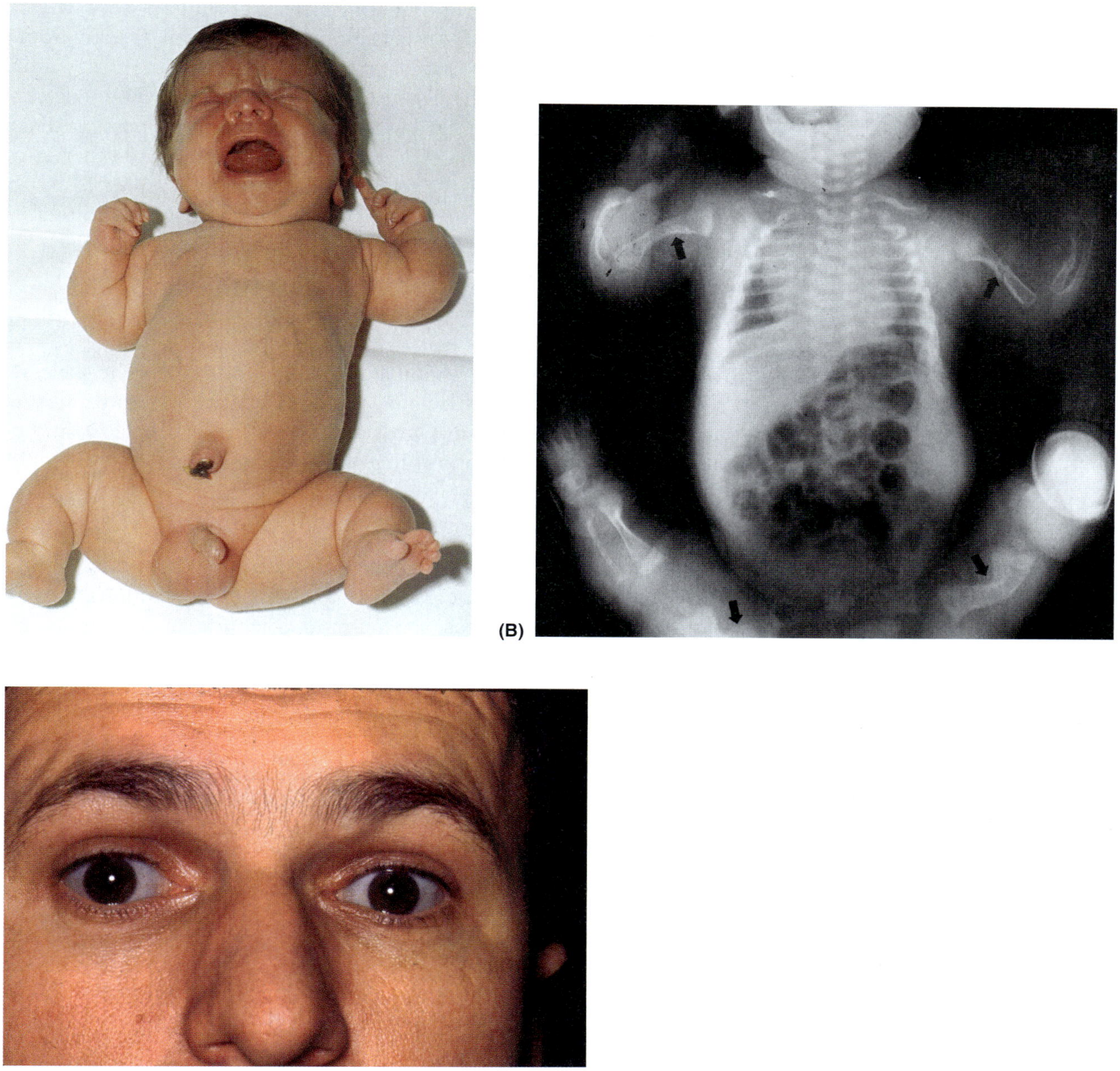

(A) (B) (C)

Figure 24-9 Severe form of osteogenesis imperfecta. **(A)** Shortening and bowing of the limbs resulting from multiple intrauterine fractures that have healed with poor alignment. **(B)** X-ray showing multiple fractures of ribs and limb bones, some showing poor alignment and evidence of healing. *Arrows* indicate the location of four fractures. **(C)** Blue sclerae of a person with osteogenesis imperfecta. The thin sclerae allows the black choroid layers to show through the sclera, which changes the scleral color from white to blue or blue-gray.

Courtesy of Leonard V. Crowley, MD, Century College.

The types of osteogenesis imperfecta differ in severity, ranging from mild to lethal, and differ in the age of onset and method of transmission but almost always involve mutations in genes involved in the synthesis of type I collagen. The newly formed bone is easily broken under very minimal stress in people who do not make enough type I collagen or who make such poor quality collagen that the bones cannot withstand normal stress. Other connective tissues containing type I collagen, such as ligaments and tendons, are not as strong as they should be, leading to excessive joint mobility. Even the connective tissue in the sclerae (the white outer layers of the eyes posterior to the corneas) is often affected. Because the sclerae are thinner than normal, the black pigmented choroid layers in the eyes under the sclerae show through the thin sclerae. As a result, the sclerae appear blue or blue-gray instead of white (**Figure 24-9C**).

The characteristic features of osteogenesis imperfecta vary greatly from person to person, even within the same family. The diagnosis of the disease is based on the clinical features and family history of the disease and genetic testing. Affected individuals are encouraged to lead as normal a life as possible. Exercise to maintain muscle strength is best achieved by swimming and other in-water activities to minimize the risk of exercise-induced fractures. Affected individuals may obtain limited benefit from some of the same drugs used to treat older adults with thinning bones caused by **osteoporosis**.

Osteoporosis Generalized thinning and demineralization of bone that tends to occur frequently in postmenopausal women but may occur in males as well.

Rheumatoid arthritis (RA) A systemic disease primarily affecting the synovium with major manifestations in the small joints.

Osteoarthritis A "wear and tear" degeneration of the major weight-bearing joints.

Arthritis

Arthritis is one of the most common and disabling diseases of the skeletal system. Although there are many different kinds of arthritis, the three most common in adults are **rheumatoid arthritis (RA)**, **osteoarthritis**, and gout. **Table 24-1** compares the major features of these conditions.

Rheumatoid Arthritis

Rheumatoid arthritis (RA) is a systemic disease affecting the connective tissues throughout the body, but the most pronounced clinical manifestations are in the joints. Clinically, the disease is a chronic, disabling, and often deforming

Table 24-1 Comparison of Major Features of Common Types of Arthritis

	Rheumatoid Arthritis	Osteoarthritis	Gout
Age and sex of the usual patient	Young and middle-aged, female	Adult, older persons, both sexes	Middle-aged to elderly, male
Major characteristic	Systemic inflammatory disease with major effects in joints; causes chronic synovitis	"Wear and tear" degeneration of articular cartilage	Disturbance of purine metabolism; acute episodes caused by crystals of uric acid in joints
Secondary effects of disease	Ingrowth of inflammatory tissue over cartilage destroys cartilage, leads to destruction of joint space; deformities common	Overgrowth of bone; thickening of periarticular soft tissues	Deposits of uric acid in joints with damage to joints (gouty arthritis); soft tissue tophi
Joints usually affected	Small joints of hands and feet	Major weight-bearing joints	Small joints; joint at base of great toe often affected
Special features	Autoantibodies against gamma globulin (rheumatoid factor) and modified self-proteins	No systemic symptoms or biochemical abnormalities	High blood level of uric acid

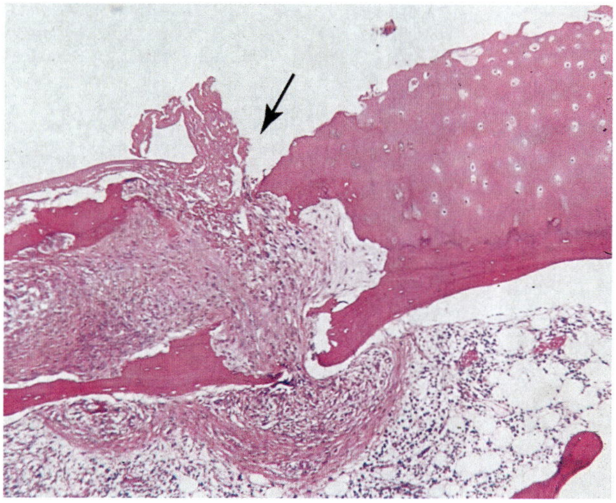

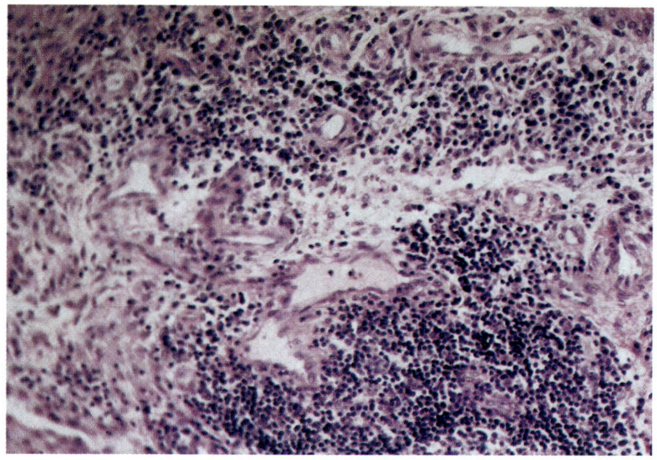

Figure 24-10 Rheumatoid arthritis. **(A)** Low-magnification photomicrograph illustrating destruction of articular cartilage by inflammatory reaction (*arrow*) extending from synovial surface (original magnification ×25). **(B)** Photomicrograph of chronic inflammatory reaction in synovium (original magnification ×100).

Courtesy of Leonard V. Crowley, MD, Century College.

arthritis affecting several joints. RA is encountered most frequently in young and middle-aged women, usually affecting the small joints of the hands and feet. In the joints, the arthritis is seen as a chronic inflammation and thickening of the synovial membrane. The inflammatory tissue (termed a pannus) extends over the surface of the articular cartilage, destroying the cartilage (**Figure 24-10**). The severe damage to the articular surfaces makes the joint unstable; this in turn leads to deviation or displacement of the bones owing to the pull of the surrounding ligaments and tendons (**Figure 24-11**). Fibrous adhesions often develop within the joint, and the ends of the adjacent bones may become completely fused. The end result of these various structural derangements is severe disability and conspicuous deformity of the affected joints (**Figure 24-12**).

The production of self-reactive antibodies (autoantibodies) to modified proteins is critical to the pathogenesis of rheumatoid arthritis. Arginine residues in proteins found in the lung and synovial tissue can be converted to citrulline (i.e., are deaminated) as a result of a number of environmental factors, including smoking and certain infectious agents. Up to two-thirds

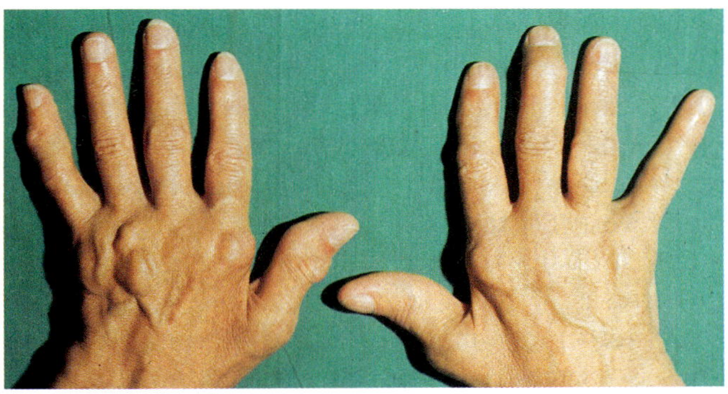

Figure 24-11 Rheumatoid arthritis. Early manifestations, illustrating swelling of knuckle joints (metacarpophalangeal joints) as a result of inflammation and ulnar deviation of fingers.

Courtesy of Leonard V. Crowley, MD, Century College.

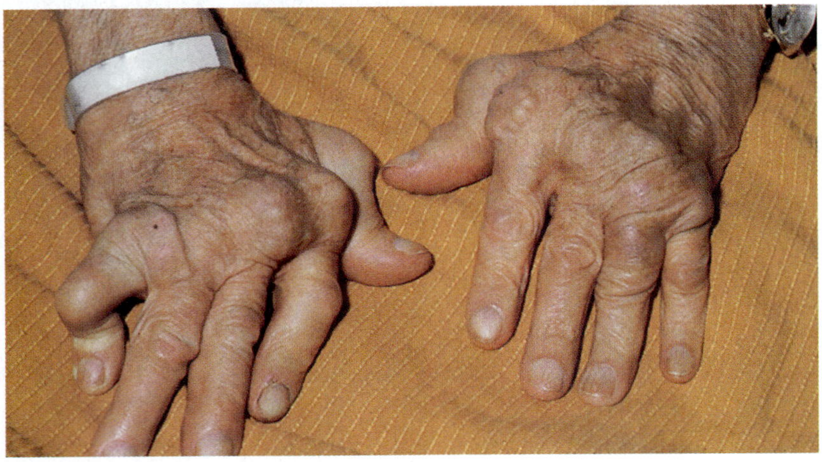

(A)

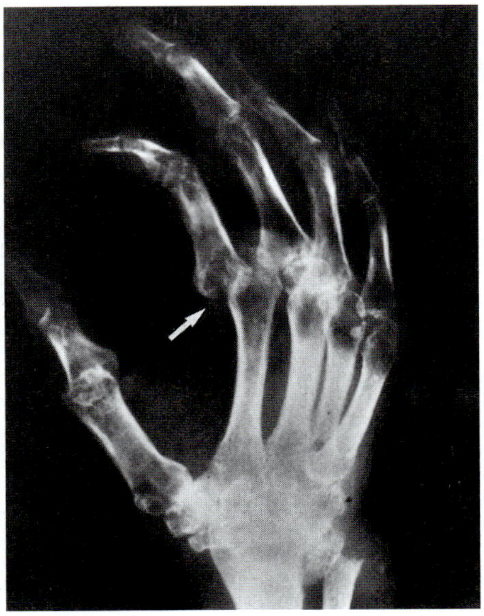

(B)

Figure 24-12 **(A)** Advanced joint deformities caused by rheumatoid arthritis. **(B)** Radiograph illustrating destruction of articular surfaces and anterior dislocation of base of index finger (*arrow*) as a result of joint instability.

of patients with RA have antibodies that react with citrullinated peptides (CP), and virtually all individuals with anti-CP antibodies develop RA. In fact, these antibodies may be found as a precursor to clinically evident disease. For this reason, anti-CP antibodies are an excellent serological test for RA. Additionally, the blood and synovial tissues of patients with rheumatoid arthritis often contain a substance termed rheumatoid factor (RF), an autoantibody of the IgM class produced by B lymphocytes, that is directed against the individual's own IgG. Although RF is present in many cases of RA (particularly when the disease is severe), it is not specific for the condition and is found in other autoimmune diseases and chronic infections where the formation of antibody-antigen complexes is likely to occur. Perhaps the previously mentioned anti-CP antibodies reacting with self-peptides provoke the formation of RF antibodies. Immune complexes, including those composed of RF and IgG (and possibly anti-CP and self-peptides), form within the joints, which activates complement and attracts inflammatory cells that damage the joints. The lymphocytes and macrophages (activated monocytes) in the synovial tissues also contribute to joint damage by secreting various injurious cytokines, including tumor necrosis factor and interleukin-1 (see Chapter 5). Much of the joint damage characteristic of rheumatoid arthritis is caused by tumor necrosis factor, which is a very destructive cytokine. Some RA patients also may demonstrate disease outside of joints, including dry mucosa (sicca syndrome), pericarditis, fatigue, and low-grade fevers. Because of the systemic nature of the disease and the presence of autoantibodies, rheumatoid arthritis is classified as one of the autoimmune diseases.

As with some other autoimmune diseases, a genetic susceptibility to rheumatoid arthritis is related to the individual's HLA antigens. About half of the people with rheumatoid arthritis have the HLA antigen HLA-DR4, which is present in only about 20 percent of a control group; this is considered a highly significant association. Patients with anti-CP antibodies show a very strong association with a particular set of HLA antigens (termed the HLA-DRB1 shared epitope alleles), presumably because those particular alleles are required for the immune recognition of CP-peptides (see Chapter 5).

Rheumatoid arthritis tends to fluctuate in severity. Periods in which the disease is active may alternate with periods in which it is inactive. Although there is no cure for rheumatoid arthritis, a number of measures can be used to control the disease and minimize its attending disability and deformity.

Treatment of Rheumatoid Arthritis

The primary objectives of treatment are reduction of joint inflammation and pain, maximal preservation of joint function, and prevention of joint deformity. Treatment consists of rest periods for several hours every day while the disease is active; stress-reduction physical therapy; and use of orthoses (braces and brace-like devices), crutches, and braces to aid weight-bearing. The affected joints are exercised gently and massaged mostly to preserve joint mobility and muscle strength.

Anti-inflammatory drugs such as aspirin and corticosteroids are prescribed to reduce inflammation within the joints early in the course of the disease to offer immediate relief. Disease-modifying antirheumatic drugs (DMARDs) slow the progression of the disease but often take several weeks or months to exert an effect, and all have some toxicity. Methotrexate (a cytotoxic immunosuppressive drug) is often used in combination with other drugs. Newer biological agents most commonly directed against tumor necrosis factor are critical in therapy. Many of these agents are monoclonal antibodies directed either against TNF or components of the immune system important in the inflammatory response. However, tumor necrosis factor also plays a role in protecting us from infections, so blocking its effect increases the risk of infection, which can lead to potentially serious complications. For example, patients who have been previously infected with the tubercle bacillus and have latent inactive infections can develop active pulmonary tuberculosis.

If severe joint deformities develop, surgical procedures can be performed to improve joint function. These measures include excision of thickened, inflamed synovium, surgical correction of joint dislocations, or even complete reconstruction of damaged joints.

Osteoarthritis

In contrast to rheumatoid arthritis, which is a systemic disease, osteoarthritis (primary osteoarthritis) is a result of "wear-and-tear" degeneration of one or more of the major weight-bearing joints (osteo = bone + arthro = joint + itis = inflammation). The disease is seen in older adults and may be considered a manifestation of the normal aging process. The primary change in osteoarthritis is degeneration of the articular cartilage, leading to roughening of the articular surfaces of the bones (**Figure 24-13**). As a consequence, the bones grate against one another when the joint moves instead of gliding smoothly. Degeneration of the cartilage sometimes leaves large areas of underlying bone exposed. Secondary overgrowth of bone frequently occurs in response to the trauma of weight-bearing (**Figure 24-14**), and some thickening of the synovium and adjacent soft tissues is also common. Secondary osteoarthritis may also result from a defect in bones and joints not related to aging and "wear and tear" but rather to an intrinsic defect that may be genetic in origin or relate to trauma or metabolic defects.

Clinically, people with osteoarthritis experience stiffness, creaking, and some pain with motions of the joints, but disability is usually not severe, and

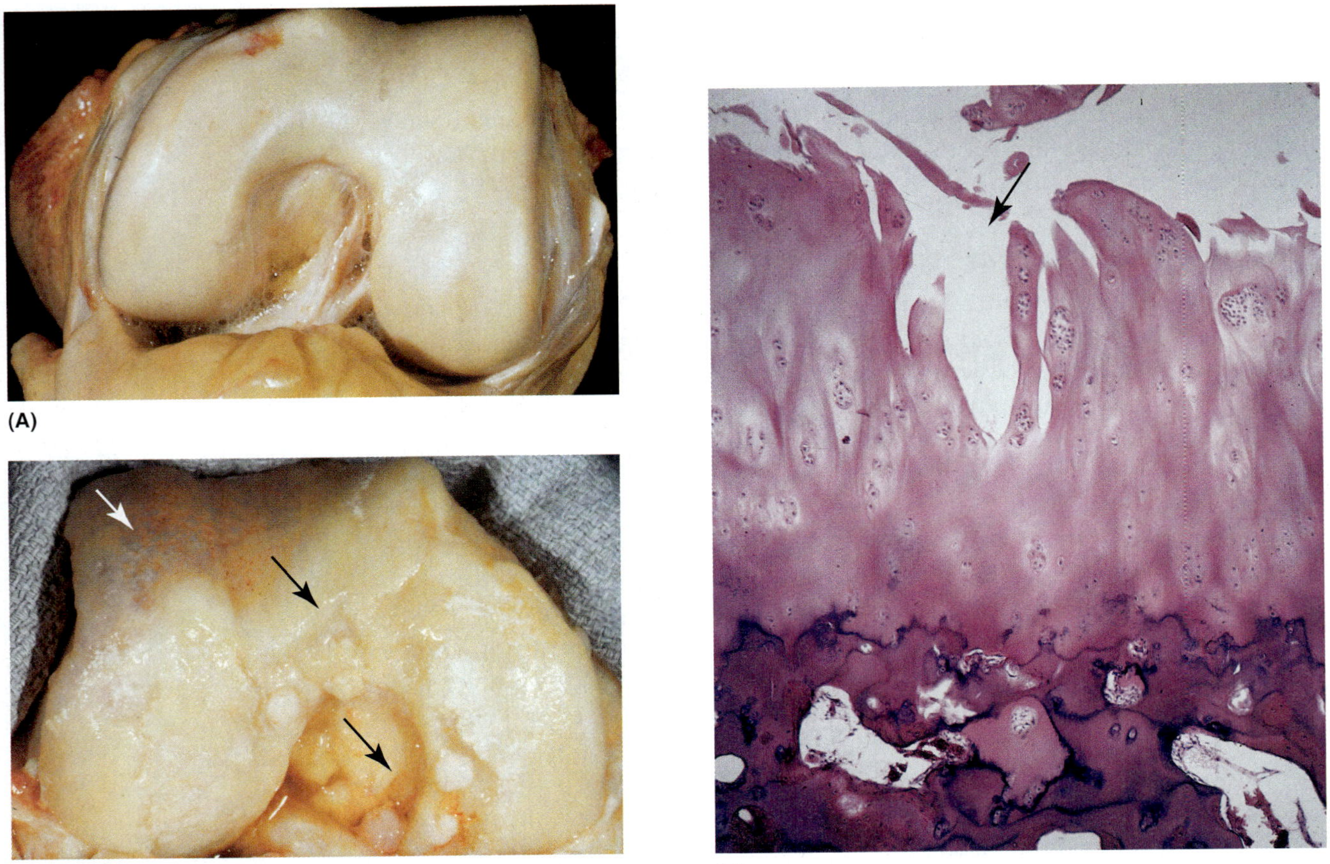

(A) (B) (C)

Figure 24-13 **(A)** Knee joint, illustrating the smooth articular surface of the femoral condyles. **(B)** Early histologic changes of osteoarthritis, illustrating splitting and fragmentation of articular cartilage (*arrow*) (original magnification ×160). Compare with normal articular cartilage in Figure 24-5A. **(C)** Advanced osteoarthritis, illustrating loss of art cular cartilage (*white arrow*) and nodular overgrowth of bone (*black arrows*).

Courtesy of Leonard V. Crowley, MD, Century College.

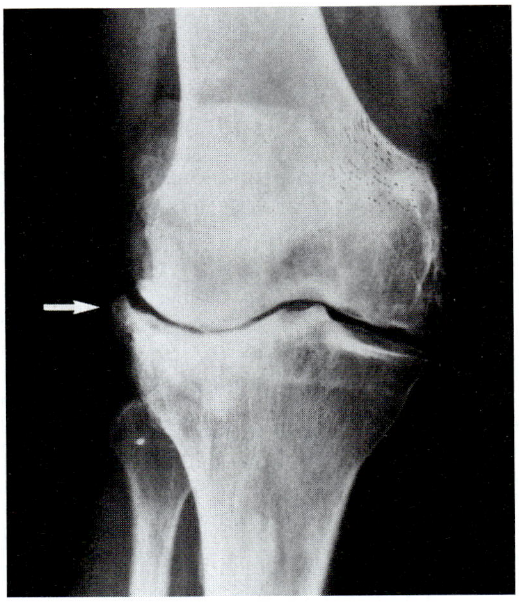

Figure 24-14 Osteoarthritis. The radiograph illustrates increased bone density of the femoral condyle (left side) and adjacent tibia, with overgrowth of bone at the margin of the tibia (*arrow*).

Courtesy of Leonard V. Crowley, MD, Century College.

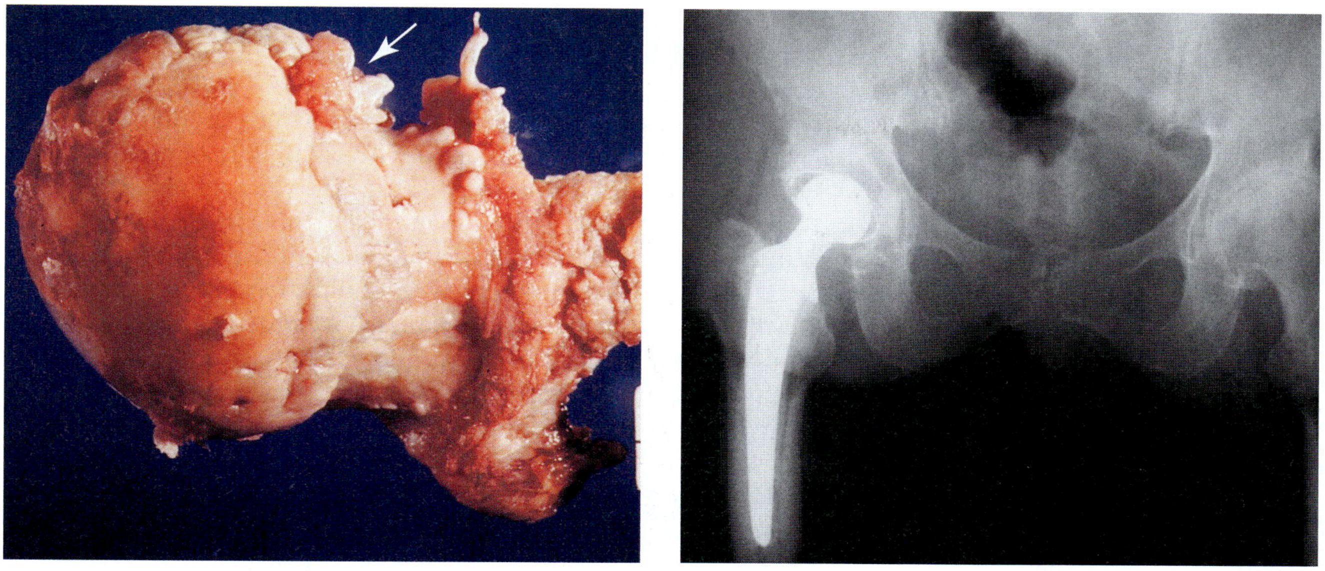

Figure 24-15 **(A)** Femoral head that was removed surgically and replaced by an artificial hip joint. Note the irregularity of the head and the overgrowth of bone at the margin of the femoral head (*arrow*). **(B)** X-ray illustrating total hip replacement.

Courtesy of Leonard V. Crowley, MD, Century College.

the joints are not destroyed. However, occasionally patients may experience considerable pain and disability from advanced arthritis affecting one or both hip joints. In these cases, it is possible to remove the affected femoral head and articular surface of the hip bone surgically and to replace them with an artificial hip joint. The procedure is termed a total hip joint replacement (**Figure 24-15**). Similar types of joint replacement procedures have been performed on the knee joint and some other joints as well. Joint replacement operations can provide excellent pain relief and greatly improved joint function in many patients.

Gout

Gout is a clinical syndrome associated with an elevated level of uric acid in the blood and body fluids (hyperuricemia), leading to precipitation of uric acid as sodium urate crystals in joints and other tissues. However, relatively few people with hyperuricemia develop gout. In most patients, hyperuricemia is caused by a metabolic disorder of purine metabolism, which leads to an overproduction of uric acid, an inadequate excretion of uric acid (most commonly), or a combination of both. This condition is sometimes termed **primary gout** to distinguish it from the much less common **secondary gout** in which the elevated uric acid is secondary to some other disease or condition, such as kidney failure or excessive breakdown of white blood cells in patients with leukemia.

Primary gout A metabolic disease caused by overproduction of uric acid, reduced excretion of uric acid, or a combination of both factors. Clinical manifestations are related to precipitation of uric acid in joints, kidneys, and other sites.

Secondary gout Elevated uric acid and clinical manifestations of gout not caused by the metabolic disease primary gout, but instead caused by some other disease that raises the blood uric acid excessively, such as kidney failure or excessive breakdown of white blood cells in patients with leukemia.

Primary Gout

Purines are double-ring nitrogen compounds used to form the nucleotides adenine and guanine. Along with the pyrimidine nucleotides, they make up the large DNA molecules within the nuclei of our cells. Although our body can produce purines from nonpurine precursor substances, most of the purines that we use to make nucleoproteins for new cells are salvaged (recycled) from our own worn-out cells when the cells are broken down. The purines that are not salvaged and recycled are converted into the end-product uric acid, which is excreted in the urine. Because uric acid is not very soluble in body fluids, any significant elevation may lead to precipitation of the uric acid in joints and other tissues.

Clinically, the person afflicted with gout experiences periodic episodes of extremely painful acute arthritis, usually involving initially only a single joint, often the joint at the base of the great toe (a condition termed podagra) (**Figure 24-16A**). The disease is by far most common in men (8:1, male: female), but in the elderly the condition becomes more common in women (3:1). The acute episodes are caused by crystallization of uric acid within the joint, which incites an intense inflammatory reaction. Gradually the symptoms of an acute attack subside, and joint function returns to normal until the next attack. If the disease is not treated, however, the attacks last longer, occur more frequently, and may involve several joints. Eventually, lumpy masses termed "gouty tophi" are deposited in the soft tissues around the joints (**Figure 24-16B**) and in other locations. The tophi consist of large masses of urate surrounded by macrophages, multinucleated giant cells, and fibrous tissue. When viewed under polarized light, the needlelike urate crystals have a characteristic appearance diagnostic of gout (**Figure 24-17**). In untreated patients, masses of urate crystals deposited in and around the articular surfaces of the joints damage the joint surfaces and adjacent bone; this is termed gouty arthritis (**Figure 24-18**).

In some people with gout, the disease also targets the kidneys and urinary tract. These people may develop uric acid kidney stones. The uric acid also may precipitate from the tubular filtrate within the kidney tubules, which blocks

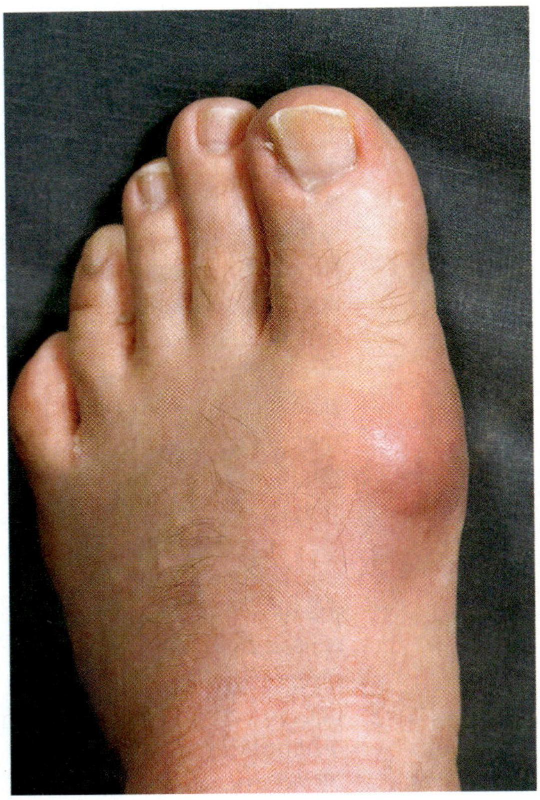

(A)

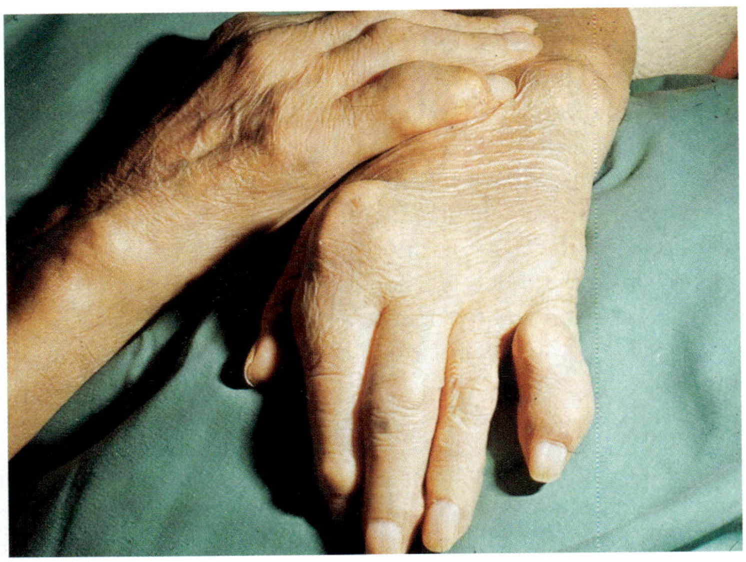

(B)

Figure 24-16 **(A)** Acute gout affecting the left great toe. **(B)** Deformities of hands caused by accumulation of uric acid crystals (tophi) in and around finger joints.

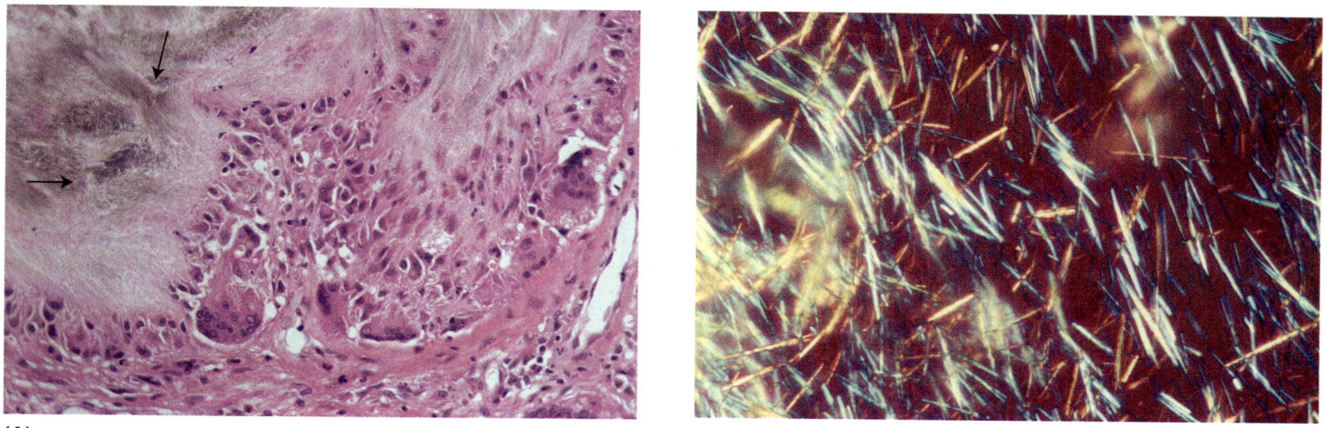

(A) (B)

Figure 24-17 **(A)** Margin of tophus illustrating mass of urate crystals (arrows) and adjacent zone of macrophages, multinucleated giant cells, and fibrous tissue formed in response to crystal deposits (original magnification ×250). **(B)** Characteristic histologic appearance of needlelike sodium urate crystals from tophus viewed under polarized light (original magnification ×400).

the tubules, damages the kidneys, and impairs renal function. This condition is termed urate nephropathy.

Gout is treated by administering drugs that reduce the concentration of uric acid in the blood by interfering with the formation of uric acid within the body or by promoting the excretion of uric acid by the kidneys. Patients are usually advised to avoid foods rich in nucleoproteins, such as liver, kidney, and pancreas, because they tend to raise uric acid levels. Heavy intake of alcohol also should be avoided because alcohol indirectly impairs excretion of uric acid by the renal tubules, causing the blood uric acid level to rise.

Patients also are advised to drink lots of fluids to maintain a high urine volume, so the urine is less concentrated, reducing the likelihood of kidney stones forming or of developing urate nephropathy. Acute attacks are treated with NSAIDs and corticosteroids. Colchicine, once a much-used agent, is not recommended. Several drugs, including allopurinol and febuxostat (which inhibit a key enzyme in the synthesis of urea from degraded nucleic acids), are used to help prevent and alleviate attacks.

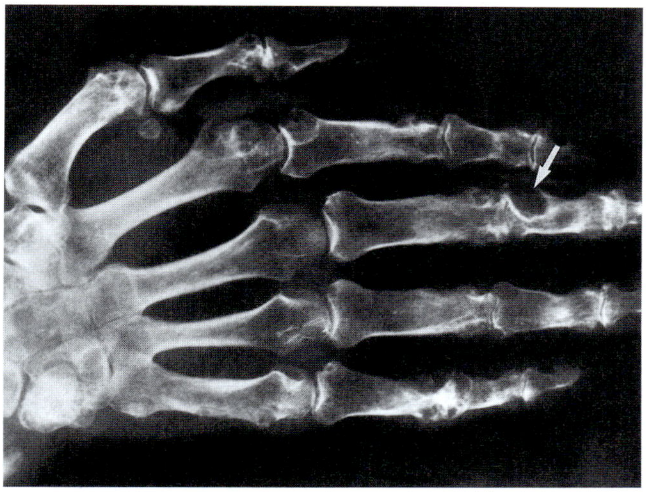

Figure 24-18 Radiograph of the right hand of a patient with gouty arthritis illustrating the area of bone destruction (*arrow*) caused by masses of uric acid crystals.

Secondary Gout

Other conditions also may raise blood uric acid, and at times, the level may be so high that the uric acid precipitates from the blood and produces the same manifestations as gout caused by the metabolic disorder of purine metabolism. The hyperuricemia results either from inadequate renal excretion of uric acid or from excessive nucleoprotein breakdown. This condition is often termed secondary gout because the elevated uric acid is secondary to some other disease. Patients with kidney failure may have high blood uric acid because the diseased kidneys are unable to excrete the uric acid efficiently, and some diuretics also may impair renal uric acid excretion. Hyperuricemia may be a problem in leukemia when patients have a greatly increased number of white blood cells, especially after treatment with drugs that destroy the leukemic cells and release large amounts of nucleoprotein from the disrupted cells. The breakdown of the nucleoprotein yields a large amount of uric acid. In these conditions, there is no underlying metabolic defect in purine metabolism. The use of a number of drugs (including some diuretics) may result in gout.

Fracture of Bone

A fracture is a break in a bone. In a simple fracture, the bone is broken into only two pieces. The term "comminuted fracture" is used when the bone is shattered into several pieces. A compound fracture is one in which the overlying skin has been broken. A compound fracture is more serious than the other types because of the possibility that bacteria may invade the fracture site and cause a secondary infection of bone (**osteomyelitis**).

Osteomyelitis An inflammation of bone.

After a fracture, the ends of the broken bone may remain aligned or may be displaced out of position (**Figure 24-19**). Reduction of a fracture refers to

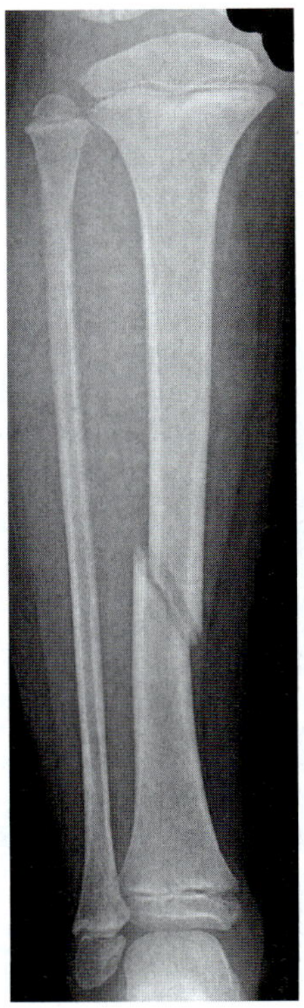

Figure 24-19 Displaced fracture of the tibia. Treatment by reduction of fracture and plaster cast.

Courtesy of Dr. Kirkland W. Davis, MD, Department of Radiology, University of Wisconsim School of Medicine and Public Health.

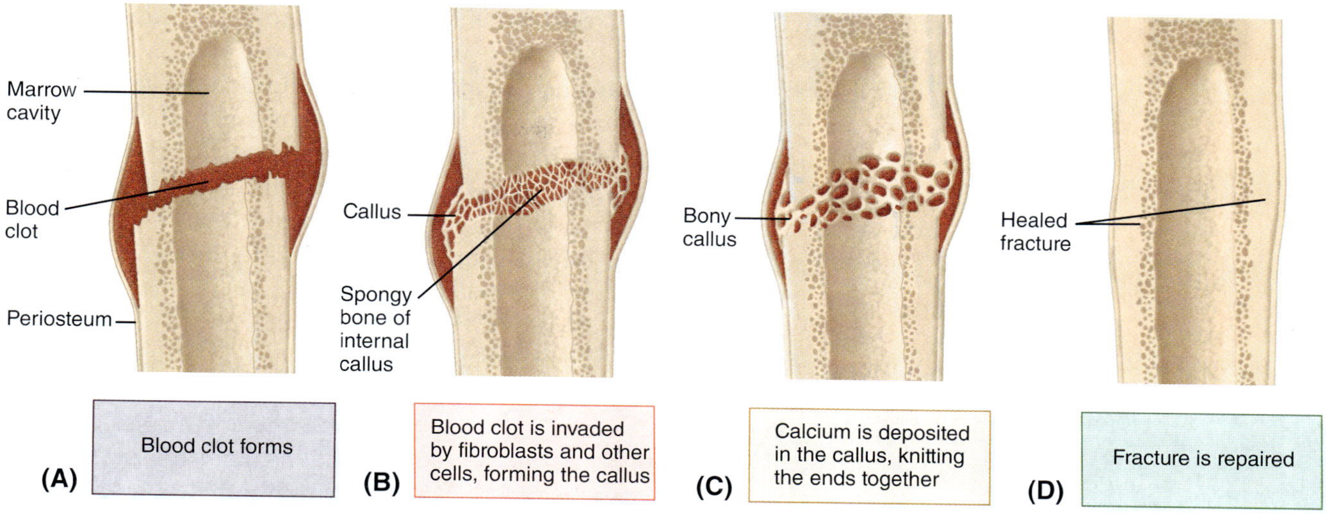

Figure 24-20 Stages in fracture repair.

realigning the ends of the broken bone so that the bone will heal in its normal anatomic position. Sometimes this can be accomplished by manipulating the injured extremity to realign the ends of the bone and then immobilizing it in a plaster cast. However, a surgical operation must sometimes be performed to reduce the fracture and hold it in position by means of a metal plate and screws or a similar device (an open reduction). Sometimes a bone may become so weakened by disease, such as a metastatic tumor, that it breaks after minimal stress (e.g., coughing or sneezing). A fracture of this type through a diseased area in a bone is termed a pathologic fracture.

The healing of fractures is a complex process involving several steps (**Figure 24-20**). Initially, within a few days of the fracture, bone necrosis occurs at the site of injury due to the disruption of blood supply to the bone. After about a week, reparative bone (woven bone) begins to appear at the margins of the injury. This is equivalent to the granulation tissue that forms during healing in other tissues. Ultimately, a **callus** containing newly synthesized bone (derived from stem cells in connective tissue and bone marrow) and newly formed blood vessels will join the two injured bones. This is the reparative phase. Once the fracture has been bridged, a slow process of remodeling of the newly formed bone occurs based on the stress and mechanical force to which the site of injury is subject. This remodeling phase may continue for years (even after the bone is strong enough to function properly).

Callus Newly synthesized bone repairing a break.

Infection of Bone

Osteomyelitis is an infection of bone and adjacent marrow cavity (osteo = bone + myelos = marrow + itis = inflammation) that is usually the result of staphylococci or various Gram-negative bacteria. The infecting organisms gain access to bone from a distant site by way of the bloodstream (hematogenous osteomyelitis) or are implanted directly in the bone from various causes.

Hematogenous Osteomyelitis

Hematogenous osteomyelitis is more common in children than in adults but also occurs in adult IV drug abusers. The bacteria are usually carried to the bone from a skin infection, such as a boil, from a kidney infection, or from an infection of some other distant site. In children, the organisms tend to lodge in the growing end of the bone on the diaphyseal side of the epiphyseal plate, where they proliferate and incite an acute inflammation. Local injury to bone near its very vascular growing end seems to favor localization of bacteria in the bone, probably because a small hemorrhage forms secondary to the injury, and the collection of blood provides conditions favorable for the growth of bacteria.

Once the infection is established, it tends to spread through the bone. In children, the epiphyseal plate cartilage generally prevents the infection from spreading into the adjacent joint. The infection may spread through the cortex, however, and pus may accumulate under the periosteum, stripping the periosteum away from the underlying cortex. Because much of the blood supply to the cortex comes from the periosteum, the part of the cortex deprived of its blood supply may undergo necrosis. Spread of the infection within the bone may also compress blood vessels that nourish bone, thereby further compromising the blood supply to the infected bone. In adults, hematogenous osteomyelitis is less frequent, and the periosteum is more firmly applied to the cortex than it is in children, tending to prevent pus from accumulating under the periosteum. However, the infection may instead spread to the end of the bone and break into the joint, causing a secondary infection in the adjacent joint. This condition is termed septic arthritis.

New bone formation proceeds concurrently with the inflammatory process, as the body attempts to repair the damage and localize the infection. Initial X-rays taken soon after the onset of the infection may show only swelling of the soft tissues surrounding the bone but no radiologic abnormalities in the affected bone at the site of infection. After the infection has been present for a time, however, evidence of bone destruction and new bone formation can be seen in the X-ray films.

Hematogenous osteomyelitis sometimes occurs in adults. Intravenous drug abusers are at risk because they often inject drugs with uncleaned needles and syringes that are contaminated with bacteria. Although hematogenous osteomyelitis may affect any bone, the infection frequently localizes in the vertebral bodies rather than in the long bones, probably because the stresses and trauma associated with weight-bearing predispose to localization in the spine.

Osteomyelitis as a Result of Direct Implantation of Bacteria

Various conditions may expose bone to direct infection, including compound fractures, gunshot wounds, or other severe injuries affecting bone. Various surgical procedures performed on bone, such as open reduction and internal fixation of fractures or total joint replacement, may also be complicated by osteomyelitis (**Figure 24-21**). Chronic ulcers of the feet, which sometimes develop in diabetic patients, may expose the small bones of the feet to chronic infection.

Clinical Manifestations and Treatment

Osteomyelitis is usually manifested as an acute febrile illness associated with localized pain, tenderness, and swelling over the affected bone. Sometimes, however, the inflammation is manifested only as chronic pain and localized tenderness over the affected bone. X-rays taken after the inflammation are well established to show characteristic changes.

Osteomyelitis is treated by a prolonged course of antibiotic therapy. In some patients, the infection may become chronic and may recur periodically. Chronic osteomyelitis is much more difficult to treat. In addition to intensive antibiotic treatment, surgical procedures may be required to remove infected degenerated bone and drain collections of pus in the bone.

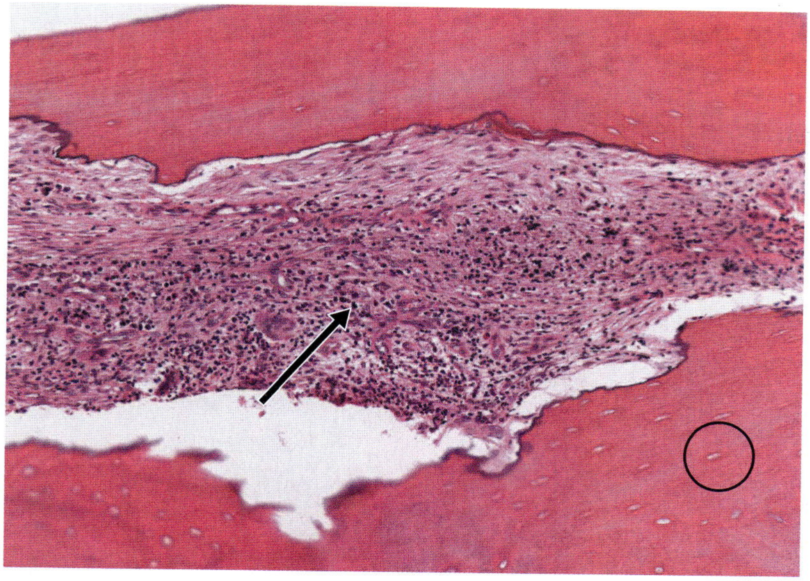

Figure 24-21 Chronic osteomyelitis in an amputated limb stump. The bone is necrotic. Note the empty lacunae, which formerly contained osteocytes (*circled*). A large area of chronic inflammation showing both mononuclear and multinucleated cells is present (*arrow*).

Courtesy of Department of Pathology and Laboratory Medicine, University of North Carolina at Chapel Hill.

Pathogenic fungi, tubercle bacilli, and various unusual opportunistic organisms may at times cause osteomyelitis, especially in immunocompromised adults. The infections are treated by appropriate antibiotics supplemented by various surgical procedures, if needed.

Tumors of Bone

Benign neoplasms and cystic lesions of bone are relatively common. **Non-ossifying fibroma**, a defect in the cortical bone of children, may be found in up to a quarter of the long bones of children during the first decade of life. These defects may not be true neoplasms, and they tend to regress with time. Although malignant tumors of the bone are uncommon and are most frequently metastases from other sites, primary bone tumors are significant because they tend to occur in youths and are often fatal if not appropriately treated. Malignant bone tumors most frequently are found in the long tubular bones, the distal femur and proximal tibia. The most common primary bone tumor, **osteosarcoma**, also termed **osteogenic sarcoma**, is most prevalent in males in their second decade. The tumor most commonly occurs near the knee and is characterized by the destruction of normal bone and the production of new (woven) bone by malignant osteoblast-like cells. The disease is first noted because of pain and swelling (sometimes mistaken as the result of an injury). There is a very characteristic radiographic pattern termed the "Codman triangle" that consists of newly formed bone extending toward and raising the periosteum (the connective tissue outer surface of the bone) (**Figure 24-22**). There is about a 75 percent 5-year survival rate for osteosarcoma when surgery (designed to spare the limb) and chemotherapy are combined. Formerly, rapid limb amputation was considered necessary to prevent metastatic disease.

Non-ossifying fibroma
A defect in the cortical bone of children.

Osteosarcoma/osteogenic sarcoma
Primary bone tumor.

Chondrosarcoma
A primary bone tumor occurring later in life.

The second most common primary tumor of bone is **chondrosarcoma** (**Figure 24-23**). Unlike osteosarcoma, the tumor is most likely to occur in the

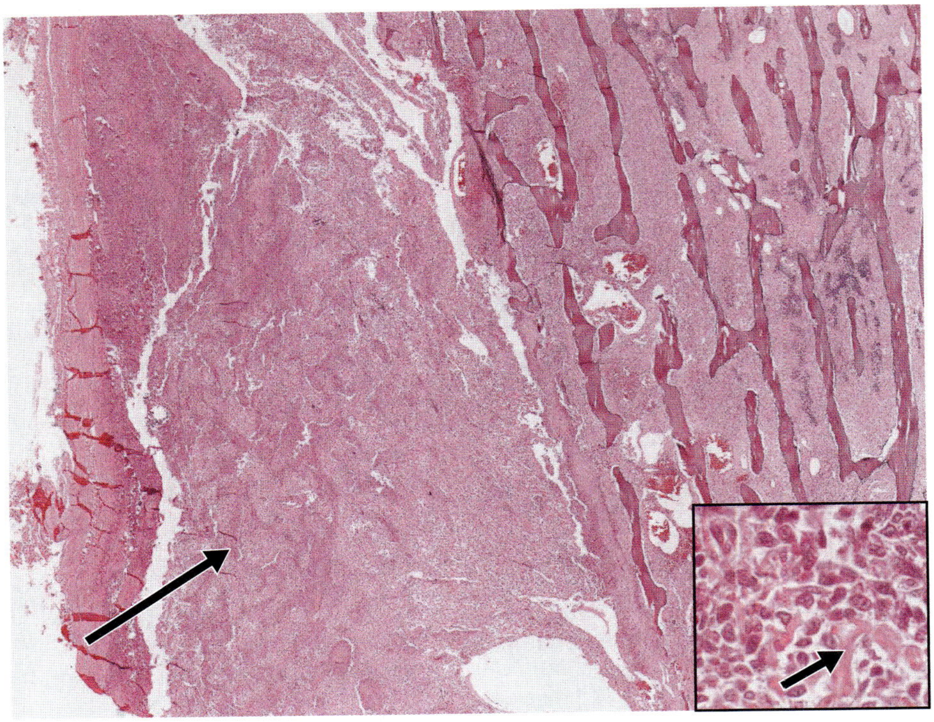

Figure 24-22 Osteosarcoma (microscopic view). There is a mass of tumor under the bone surface (*arrow*) and invading the body of the bone. A high-power view (*inset*) shows osteosarcoma cells and the small bone spicules they synthesize (*arrow*).

Courtesy of Department of Pathology and Laboratory Medicine, University of North Carolina at Chapel Hill.

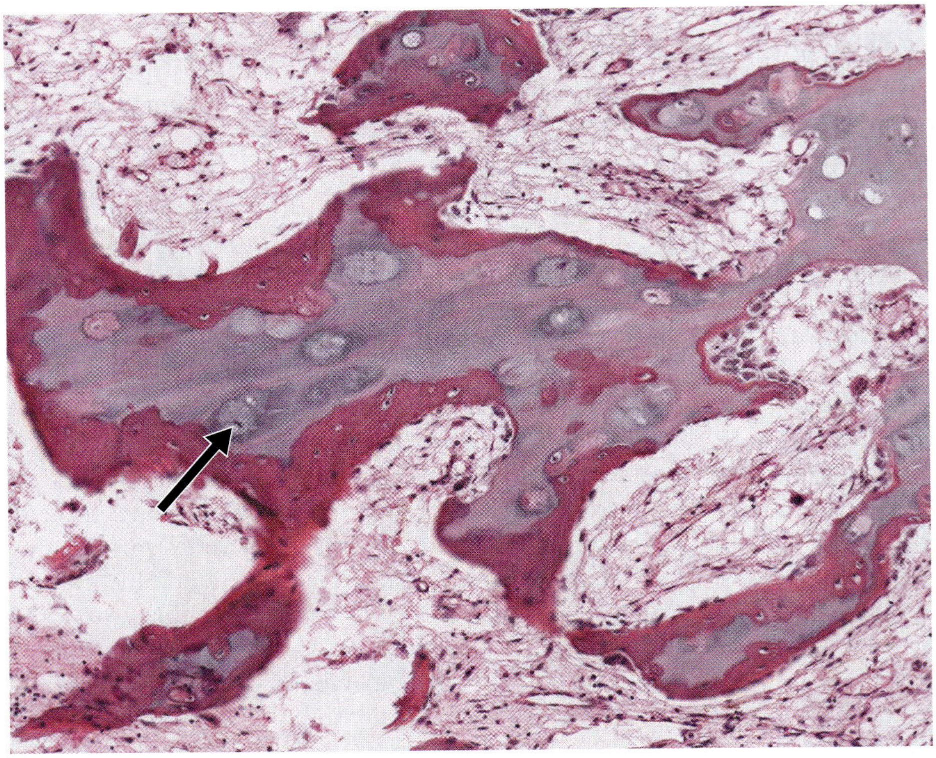

Figure 24-23 Chondrosarcoma (microscopic view). Neoplastic choncrocytes with bizarre nuclei are present in the cartilaginous matrix (*arrow*).

Courtesy of Department of Pathology and Laboratory Medicine, University of North Carolina at Chapel Hill.

fourth to sixth decade. This cartilaginous tumor most frequently derives from the medulla of bone, but there are many variants with very different prognoses depending on the tumor grade.

Bone is often affected by metastatic tumors. Carcinoma of breast or prostate, as well as many other tumors, frequently metastasize to bone.

Metabolic Bone Disease: Osteoporosis

Osteoporosis, literally meaning "porous bones," is a generalized thinning and demineralization of the entire skeletal system. It is the most common metabolic bone disease in the United States. Most cases are found in postmenopausal women, beginning in their 50s, and a significant degree of osteoporosis is said to be present in approximately one-fourth of all women in their 60s. Osteoporosis develops whenever bone resorption exceeds bone production. The incidence is high in postmenopausal women because the loss of ovarian function results in estrogen deficiency. Estrogen inhibits bone resorption, and the loss of estrogen accelerates the rate, which results in slowly progressive thinning of the bones. Osteoporosis also develops in older men, but it occurs at a much later age and is usually less severe than in women.

The osteoporotic bones can be quite fragile and susceptible to fracture (**Figure 24-24**). Fractures of vertebral bodies are frequent, either from the stress of weight-bearing or after minor exertion. These fractures produce back pain and tenderness and are often characterized by collapse of the anterior portions of the vertebral bodies (compression fractures). Collapse of vertebral bodies may compress the spinal nerve roots passing through the intervertebral foramina, causing pain to radiate along the course of the compressed nerve.

Maximum bone density is attained in young adults, and then slowly but steadily declines as the person ages. The greater the bone density as a young adult, the longer it will take before there is enough bone loss to increase the risk of fractures.

Bone loss can be retarded by regular weight-bearing exercises that help maintain bone density, by a high-calcium diet and calcium supplements if necessary to ensure an adequate calcium intake, and by an adequate intake of vitamin D, which is required to promote calcium absorption from the intestine and incorporation into bone. Hormone replacement therapy as a prophylactic treatment for peri-menopausal or post-menopausal women continues to be an area of discussion with differences in opinion evaluating the risk/benefit analyses. Further research is needed to continue to clarify these issues.

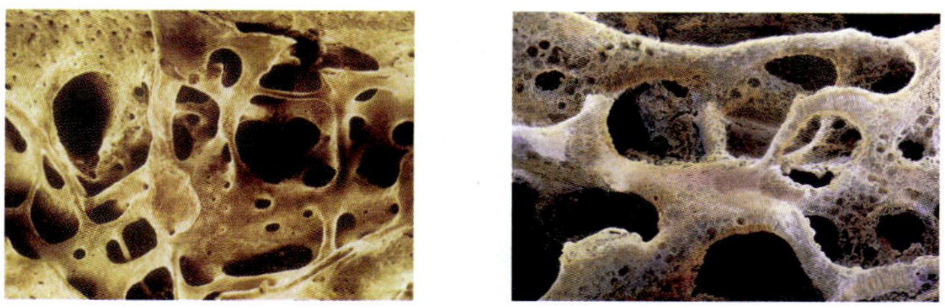

(A) (B)

Figure 24-24 Osteoporosis. This loss of estrogen or prolonged immobilization weakens bone. In these situations, the bone is dissolved and becomes brittle and easily breakable. **(A)** Normal bone. **(B)** Bone weakened by osteoporosis.

Once marked osteoporosis has developed and fractures occur, it is difficult to repair the changes in bone. A number of drugs are available to restore bone density. Each has advantages and disadvantages. Bisphosphonate drugs, which are usually taken orally, are the first-line agents recommended to treat osteoporosis. They act primarily by inhibiting bone resorption by osteoclasts. Over time, bisphosphonate drugs also may decrease bone turnover to such a degree that the skeleton has insufficient bone density to maintain skeletal strength, resulting in fractures. This is a particular concern with the most potent agents. Necrosis of the bones of the jaw may occur spontaneously or after dental procedures when using these drugs.

Selective estrogen receptor modulators (SERMs), such as raloxifene, function as estrogen-like drugs taken orally and inhibit bone resorption, like estrogens, but do not have the adverse effects of estrogen on the breast and uterus. Denosumab is a monoclonal antibody that prevents osteoclast formation and activity, thus decreasing bone breakdown. Calcitonin, a hormone produced by thyroid cells that inhibits the osteoclasts from breaking down bone, has been administered as a nasal spray but may be associated with an increased risk of cancer. Parathyroid hormone–like drugs used in daily injections increase bone density by stimulating osteoblasts, and the amount used is not enough to stimulate osteoclasts.

Significant loss of bone density also may occur in women athletes who engage in prolonged, intense physical activity, such as runners and gymnasts. The high level of physical activity triggers the hypothalamus and pituitary gland to increase adrenal corticosteroid output as an adaptation to the exercise-induced stress. This event, however, also is associated with a fall in the pituitary gonadotropic hormones that stimulate ovarian function. The ovaries, no longer adequately stimulated by pituitary gonadotropins, fail to produce adequate estrogen, which leads to cessation of menses, termed exercise-induced amenorrhea. In addition, the estrogen-deficient athlete is at risk of the same type of estrogen-deficiency osteoporosis that develops in postmenopausal women and is subject to the same osteoporosis-related complications.

Osteoporosis related to exercise-induced amenorrhea can be prevented by reducing the level of physical activity enough to reestablish normal menstrual cycles. Alternatively, the athlete who elects to continue the same level of exercise can reduce her risk of osteoporosis by taking supplementary estrogen and progesterone hormones (possibly in the form of low-dose birth control pills) to replace the missing ovarian hormones and by taking calcium supplements.

New X-ray and radioisotope methods are now available that make a quantitative assessment of a patient's bone density and compare the results with normal ranges established for people of the same age and sex. Bone mineral density measurement of the wrist using dual-energy X-ray absorptiometry (DXA) is recommended for all women over the age of 65 and for men over the age of 70. Those patients whose bones are losing mineral content to a greater extent or more rapidly than normal are at high risk of fractures and other complications related to osteoporosis. They should be treated vigorously to retard further bone demineralization.

Osteonecrosis (Avascular Necrosis)

Avascular necrosis Bone necrosis caused by interruption of its blood supply.

Occasionally, the growing cartilaginous ends of bone (epiphyses) undergo necrosis and degeneration, owing to interference with the blood supply to the epiphysis. Although the disease can occur at any age, **avascular necrosis** is most common between the ages of 30 and 50 years. Sometimes it follows an injury or is associated with excessive alcohol use or high-dose

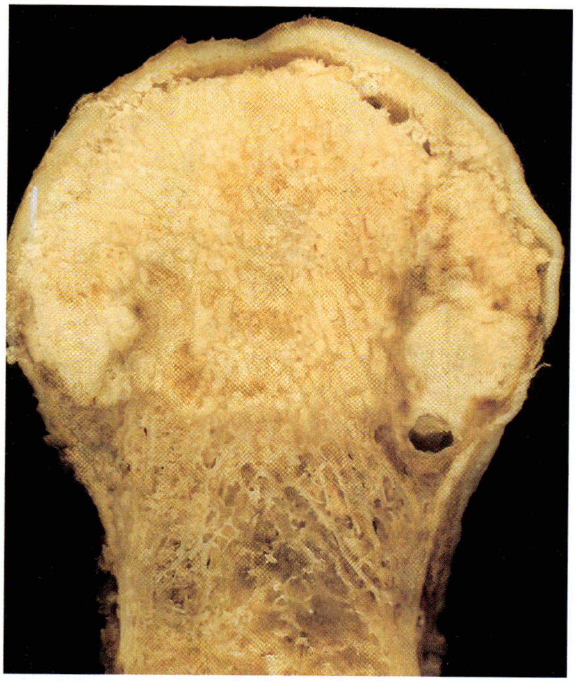

Figure 24-25 Avascular necrosis of femoral head. Articular cartilage has separated from the underlying bone, which appears dense and lacks a normal structural pattern. In contrast, bone of the femoral neck (lower area) appears normal. Treated by removal of femoral head and replacement with artificial hip joint.

Courtesy of Leonard V. Crowley, MD, Century College.

corticosteroid therapy, but in most cases the reason for the vascular disturbance is unknown. Common sites of avascular necrosis are the femoral head (**Figure 24-25**), the tibial tubercle, the articular surface of the femoral condyle, and occasionally, the small bones of the ankle and foot. Symptoms consist of pain and disability related to motion of the affected joint. Avascular necrosis may also occur in adults if the blood supply to a bone is interrupted for any reason, such as, for example, if the circulation to the femoral head is disrupted because of a hip fracture or dislocation.

Structure and Function of the Spine

The vertebral column forms the central axis of the body. It consists of a series of vertebrae joined by **intervertebral disks** and fibrous ligaments. The vertebral column has four curves. The cervical and lumbar curves arch forward. Those in the thoracic and sacral regions bend in the opposite direction (**Figure 24-26A**).

Intervertebral disk A fibrocartilaginous structure between adjacent vertebral bodies.

A typical vertebra has a large cylindrical body and a bony arch that encloses the spinal canal and protects the spinal cord. The parts of the arch that extend posteriorly from the body are termed the pedicles, and the parts that roof the spinal canal are termed the laminae (singular, lamina). A single midline spinous process projects posteriorly from the bony arch, and paired transverse processes extend laterally. Each vertebra also has two superior articular processes and two inferior articular processes. The superior processes articulate with the inferior processes of the vertebra above, and the inferior processes articulate with the superior processes of the vertebra below. The articulations form synovial joints that contribute to the mobility of the spine (**Figure 24-26B**).

When the vertebrae are viewed from the side, the superior and inferior margins of the vertebral pedicles appear concave. The spaces between the concave

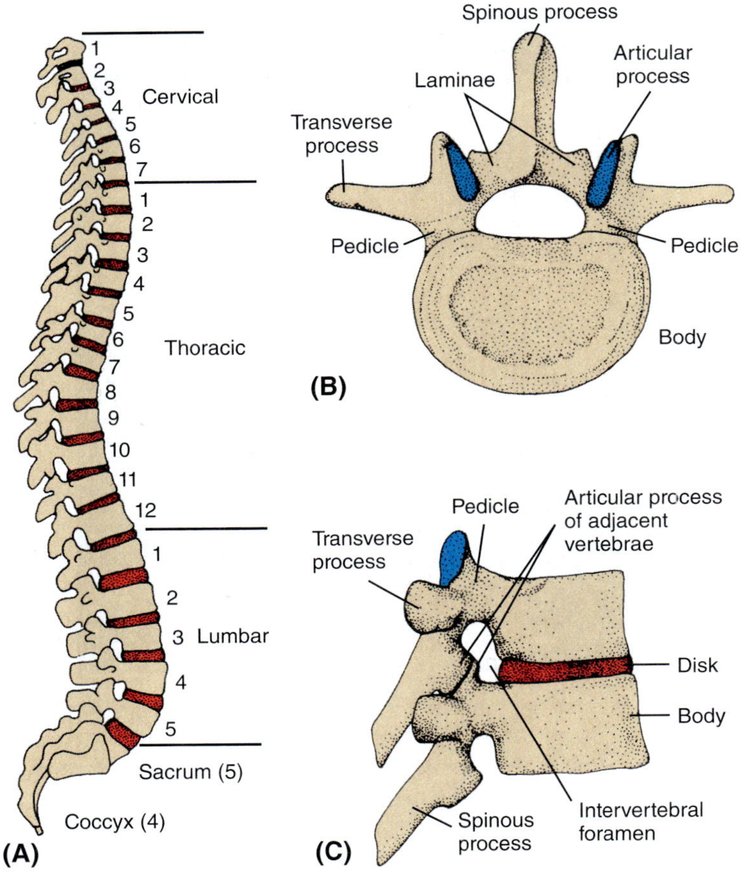

Figure 24-26 **(A)** Side view of the vertebral column illustrating normal curves. Vertebrae are numbered. **(B)** Structure of a typical vertebra viewed from above. The vertebral arch extends posteriorly from the vertebral body. The spinous process projects posteriorly from the arch, and the transverse processes project laterally. The articular processes of adjacent vertebrae articulate with each other by means of small synovial joints. **(C)** Side view of two vertebrae, illustrating the intervertebral disk, articular processes, and intervertebral foramen.

surfaces of the pedicles of adjacent vertebrae form oval openings termed intervertebral foramina (singular, foramen), through which the spinal nerves leave the spinal canal (**Figure 24-26C**).

Annulus fibrosus The dense peripheral ring of fibrocartilage making up the intervertebral disk.

Nucleus pulposus The soft elastic center of the intervertebral disk.

The intervertebral disks, interposed between adjacent vertebral bodies, consist of a peripheral fibrous ring, the **annulus fibrosus**, and a soft central **nucleus pulposus**. The annulus fibrosus ("fibrous ring") is structured as a ring of interlacing connective tissue bundles firmly adherent to adjacent vertebral bodies. Longitudinal bands of connective tissue, termed the anterior and posterior longitudinal ligaments, run the entire length of the vertebral column to reinforce the annulus. The nucleus pulposus ("pulpy nucleus") consists of a gelatinous material containing a carbohydrate substance termed a mucopolysaccharide and is about 80 percent water. Because of its very high water content, it is relatively incompressible.

The position of the nucleus pulposus within the disk changes slightly during flexion and extension of the spine. During flexion, as when one bends forward to pick up an object on the ground, compression forces are concentrated on the anterior parts of the vertebral bodies and cause the nucleus to shift slightly posteriorly, moving away from the compressing force. Conversely, when compression forces are concentrated on the posterior part of the vertebral bodies during extension, the nucleus pulposus tends to shift anteriorly.

Slight lateral movements of the nucleus also occur during lateral flexion of the spine. The intervertebral disks function somewhat like shock absorbers. Pressure applied to the disks is distributed evenly around the annulus by the soft nucleus pulposus, absorbing the forces of compression to some extent and preventing direct impact between adjacent vertebral bodies.

Scoliosis

Scoliosis, an abnormal lateral curvature of the spine, is a common abnormality estimated to occur in about 3 percent of people. A small percentage of cases result from a congenital abnormality of a spinal vertebra that disturbs the normal vertical alignment of the spinal vertebrae or result from a neurologic problem that disturbs the innervation of the muscles that maintain the spinal vertebrae in proper position. The majority of cases, however, occur during the growth spurt just prior to puberty for unknown reasons (idiopathic scoliosis).

The spinal curvatures lead to an asymmetry of the trunk, so one shoulder is higher than the other, and the pelvis is tilted so that one iliac crest is higher than its counterpart on the opposite side. Some degree of rotation of the vertebrae accompanies the curvatures, which may lead to some asymmetry of the ribs that attach to the thoracic vertebrae (**Figure 24-27**). Posterior protrusion of the ribs on one side of the thorax may cause a noticeable humplike deformity.

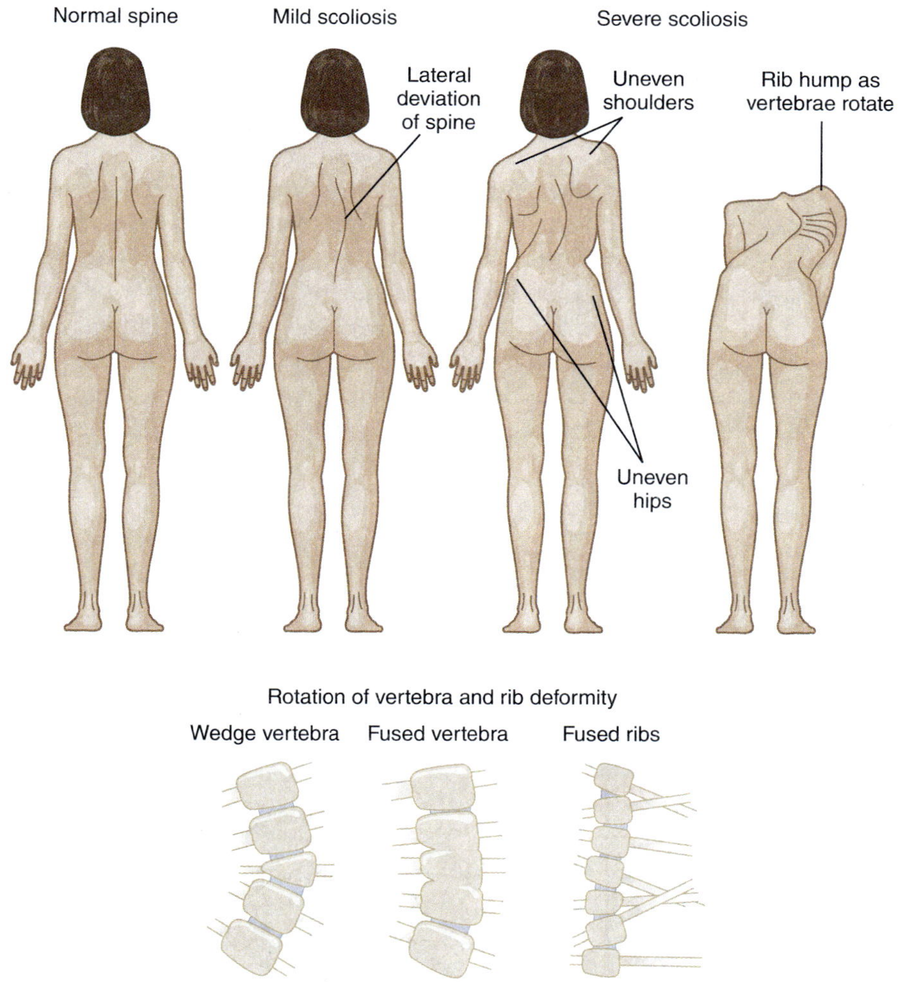

Figure 24-27 Scoliosis. The figure shows a normal spine, mild scoliosis, and two degrees of severe scoliosis.

Scoliosis can be identified by careful examination of the spine while the teenager is standing upright and while bending forward, as when touching the toes. If scoliosis is identified, X-rays are taken to measure the extent of the curvature. A small curvature may not require treatment, but the adolescent needs to be checked periodically because some curves may get worse as the adolescent grows. Usually, a curvature does not progress after the teenager stops growing, but a marked curvature may continue to get worse even after growth stops. Severe degrees of scoliosis may cause significant disability. A marked thoracic curvature greatly reduces the size of the thorax, which interferes with lung function (Figure 24-27).

Treatment depends on the degree of curvature. Slight curves may not require treatment. A growing teenager with a curvature that is getting worse is treated by means of a spinal brace to help maintain the normal position of the spine and stop the progression of the curvature. A marked scoliosis may require surgical treatment, and various surgical procedures are used to stabilize the spine and correct the curvature.

Intervertebral Disk Disease

With age, the intervertebral disks undergo a progressive wear-and-tear degeneration of both the nucleus and the annulus. The nucleus becomes more dense because its water content is reduced, and the annulus becomes weakened and thinned. When marked compression force is applied to the anterior part of the disk during flexion of the spine, the nucleus is forced posteriorly against the weakened annulus, and part of the nucleus may be forced into the spinal canal through a weak area or tear in the annulus (**Figure 24-28**). Most often, a disk protrusion occurs in the lumbosacral region because this is the part of the vertebral column where the disks are subject to the greatest mechanical compression during lifting. The disk usually protrudes in a posterolateral direction because the dense posterior longitudinal ligament reinforces the annulus in the midline, preventing a direct posterior protrusion.

Symptoms of disk protrusion (disk herniation or "slipped disk") in the lumbosacral region consist of sudden onset of acute back pain after an episode of lifting. Frequently, the pain is also felt in the leg and thigh on the side of the protrusion because the extruded disk material often impinges on lumbosacral nerve roots, causing pain to radiate along the course of the nerve compressed by

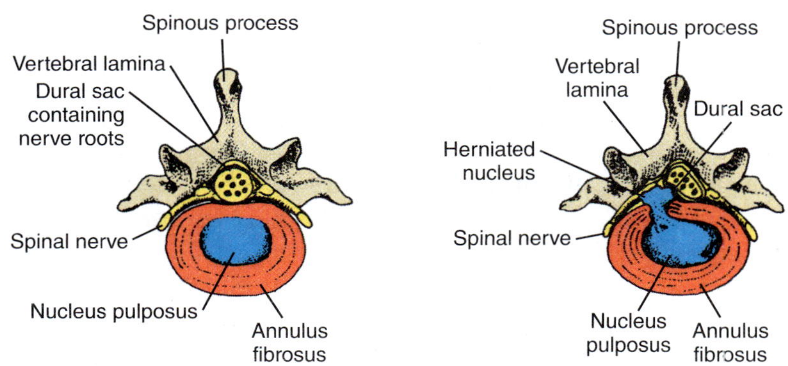

Figure 24-28 Cross section through the lumbar spine at the level of the intervertebral disk. **(A)** Normal relationships of intervertebral disk to spinal canal, dura, and spinal nerves. **(B)** Posterior protrusion of nucleus pulposus, impinging on dural sac and spinal nerve, exiting through the intervertebral foramen.

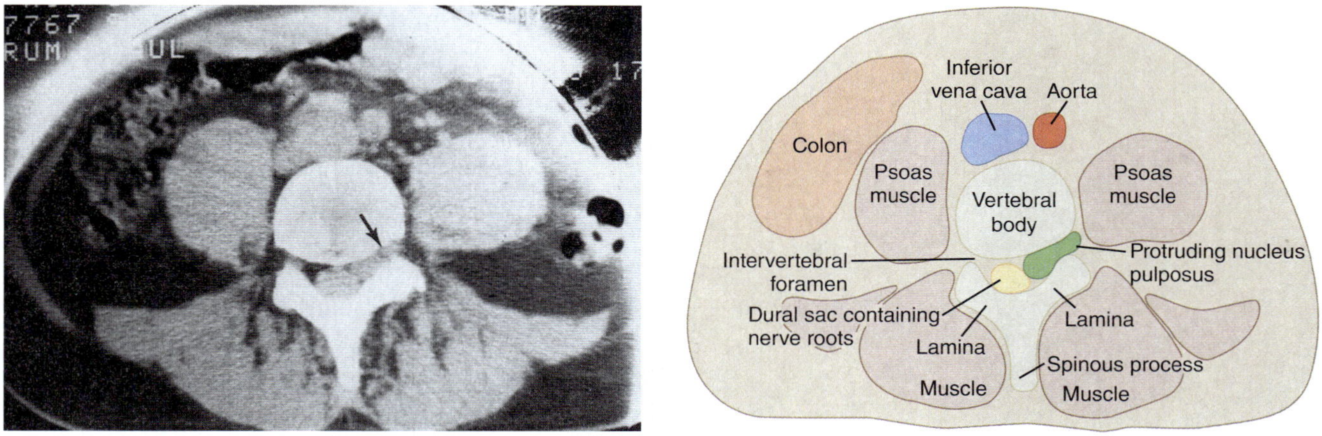

Figure 24-29 Demonstration of herniated nucleus pulposus ("slipped disk"). **(A)** CT scan of lumbar region. Protruding nucleus pulposus (*arrow*) is located adjacent to the dural sac and fills the intervertebral foramen (*arrow*). Compare with the appearance of the normal intervertebral foramen on the opposite side. **(B)** Schematic of anatomical structures and lesion as demonstrated on a CT scan.

(A) Courtesy of Leonard V. Crowley, MD, Century College.

the protruded nucleus pulposus. When nerve compression is severe, numbness of the inner thighs, back of legs, and around the anus may occur (saddle anesthesia). If the lowest region of the spinal cord nerve roots (the cauda equina) is compressed, loss of bladder and bowel function may occur, necessitating immediate surgical intervention. Treatment consists of bed rest and measures to minimize pain and disability, such as administration of anti-inflammatories or other pain-relieving medications, local application of heat, and use of muscle-relaxing drugs to relieve spasm of the back muscles that occurs after a disk protrusion and contributes to the disability. In some cases, local injection of corticosteroids may provide relief. Protruded disk material may be resorbed, and the tear in the annulus may be repaired by fibrous tissue. As noted, however, surgical removal of the protruded disk material may be required.

The protrusion of the disk material into the spinal canal can be demonstrated by computed tomography (CT) and magnetic resonance imaging (MRI) scans, noninvasive radiologic examinations described in Chapter 1 (**Figure 24-29**).

Structure and Function of the Thorax

The skeleton of the chest wall (thorax) consists of the thoracic spine posteriorly, the sternum anteriorly, and the ribs with their costal cartilages that connect them. The upper part of the sternum is termed the "manubrium," to which the first ribs attach by their costal cartilages. The body of the sternum is attached to the manubrium by a movable joint that acts as a hinge, allowing the sternal body to angle forward and the attached ribs to become more horizontal as the diaphragm descends during inspiration. The ribs articulate posteriorly with the thoracic vertebrae, and all except ribs 11 and 12 also attach to the sternum anteriorly by their costal cartilages. Below the sternal body is the small attached xiphoid process, which moves with the sternal body. The costal cartilages of ribs 3 through 5 attach to the body of the sternum so that the anterior surfaces of the costal cartilages and the body of the sternum form a uniform, relatively flat surface that is characteristic of the anterior surface of the chest wall. Ribs 6 and 7 attach to the lower part of the sternal body and xiphoid process (**Figure 24-30**).

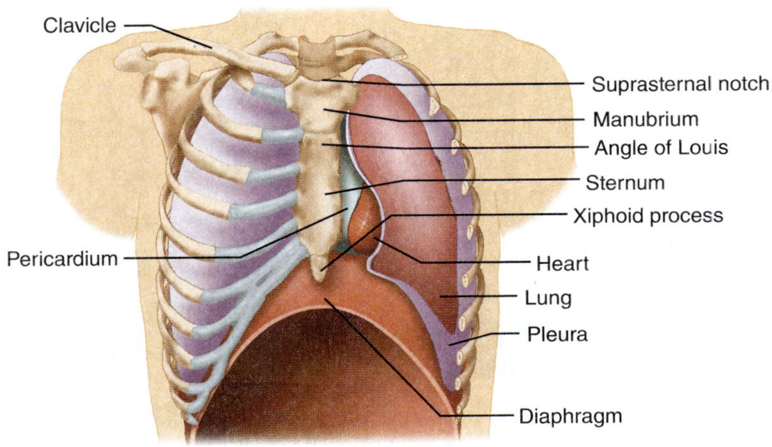

Figure 24-30 Thorax, illustrating borders and structures.

The ribs protect the lungs, and the sternum protects the heart, which is located in the mediastinum (the region between the lungs). However, the space available to the heart in the mediastinum is limited anteriorly by the sternum, and posteriorly by the vertebral bodies of the thoracic spine. Consequently, part of the left ventricle must project into the left pleural cavity to obtain additional space, which reduces slightly the space for expansion of the left lung during inspiration when compared to the size of the right pleural cavity.

Chest Wall Abnormalities

Chest wall abnormalities result from abnormal growth and attachment of the rib cartilages to the body of the sternum, which changes the position of the sternum. In the most common and clinically significant condition, the lower part of the sternum is displaced posteriorly, which is termed **pectus excavatum** (pectus = chest + excavatum = hollowed out), sometimes termed a "funnel chest." An anterior sternal protrusion, pectus carinatum (carina = prow of a ship), is much less frequent, and it is sometimes termed a "pigeon breast" because it resembles the anterior protrusion of the sternum in a bird.

Pectus excavatum Posterior displacement of the sternum caused by excessive growth of costal cartilages, which reduce the size of the retrosternal space available for the heart within the mediastinum.

Pectus Excavatum

In this condition, the lower two-thirds of the sternum is displaced posteriorly along with the lower costal cartilages, which curve inward to form a broad midline chest depression with the deepest depression in the lowest part of the sternum just above the xiphoid process. The posterior displacement of the sternum appears to be caused by excessive unbalanced growth of the lower costal cartilages 3 through 5, which pushes the sternum posteriorly. The sternal displacement also affects the position of the ribs, which may lead to some asymmetry of the thorax manifested as slight scoliosis. The manubrium and the attached first and second costal cartilages are unaffected. The abnormality usually becomes apparent soon after birth, progresses during childhood, and becomes even more pronounced during the rapid skeletal growth phase associated with adolescence but does not progress after skeletal growth ceases.

Pectus excavatum (PE) is a relatively common abnormality that occurs in about 1 in 250 White males, and possibly less often in White females (although this is disputed) and other ethnic groups. About 40 percent of affected individuals also have family members with PE, but the genetic basis has not yet been established.

Clinical Effects of Pectus Excavatum. A relatively minor posterior sternal depression may not encroach to a significant extent on the heart or the adjacent pleural cavities, but it can be a psychological problem to a teenager concerned about their body image. This is of particular concern in adolescent females because the condition results in breast asymmetry. Most cases of pectus excavatum show no functional defects. However, a marked posterior sternal depression can compromise both cardiac and pulmonary function, and exercise tolerance may be compromised, particularly with aging.

Treatment of Pectus Excavatum. Only a major degree of sternal depression is treated surgically, so it is important to document the severity of the deformity. X-ray or CT examinations can be used to determine the extent of the posterior sternal displacement, and other studies can assess its effects on cardiac and pulmonary function. Marked posterior sternal displacement is considered for surgical repair, especially if cardiac and pulmonary function studies are abnormal.

Pectus Carinatum

A less common chest wall abnormality is termed pectus carinatum because of the anterior, ridgelike projection of the sternum that has been compared to the prow of a ship (carina = ship's prow). Although the abnormality may be a concern to the individual, usually there are no associated disturbances of cardiac or pulmonary function. Braces worn by the patient have been used to push the sternum back into a more normal position, but they are not very effective. Surgical reconstruction of the chest wall can be performed if desired.

Connective Tissue Disease

The two important types of connective tissue are the widely distributed collagen fibers that provide strength but lack flexibility, and elastic tissue fibers that can stretch and return to their former shape when the stretching force ceases. Elastic fibers are abundant in blood vessels, where their elasticity permits the aorta and its branches to stretch and recoil in response to the blood pumped into the vessels during ventricular systole, and are present in many other tissues along with collagen fibers, where they perform various "stretchability" functions, including in the skin and subcutaneous tissues and in the eyes, where they attach the lens to the ciliary body in the correct position required for normal vision. Connective tissue fibers are constructed in part from a precursor protein termed "fibrillin-1" that forms structural microfibrils. The microfibrils serve a structural and force-bearing role in elastic and non-elastic connective tissue. A mutation of the gene coding for fibrillin (FBN1) gives rise to a group of abnormalities grouped together as a relatively common disease termed **Marfan syndrome** (**Figure 24-31**).

Its incidence is about 1 in 5000 people, and the condition usually is transmitted as a dominant trait. About 25 percent of the time, the disease results from a new spontaneous FBN1 gene mutation in the affected person. When the mutation is transmitted from a parent, its severity may differ among affected

Marfan syndrome A hereditary connective tissue disease characterized by excessive joint flexibility along with various skeletal and cardiovascular abnormalities.

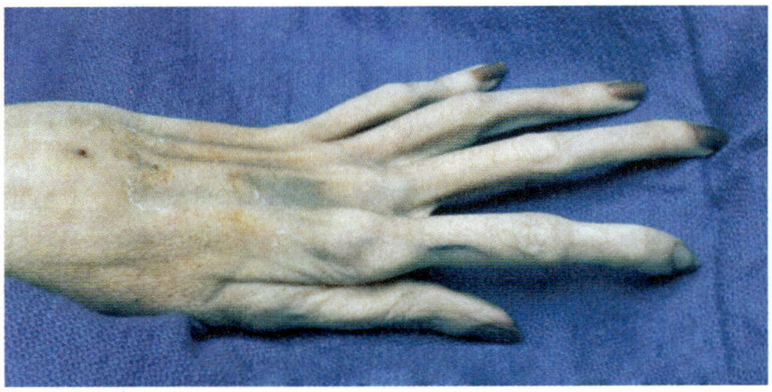

Figure 24-31 Marfan syndrome. This disorder used to be termed "arachnodactyly," literally "spider fingers."

individuals in the same family. The gene mutation leads to excessive growth in height; excessively long, thin fingers and toes with excessive joint flexibility; and various chest wall abnormalities, usually pectus excavatum. The fibers that hold the lens in the correct position behind the iris may not be able to maintain the lens in proper position, which leads to visual disturbances. However, the most serious complication of Marfan syndrome involves the cardiovascular system, which is caused by defective elastic fibers in the aorta. As a result, the aorta gradually dilates because the defective elastic fibers in the aortic wall are unable to maintain the normal shape of the aorta. Excessive dilation of the aorta may lead to a dissecting aneurysm of the aorta and its complications (described in Chapter 10). If the excessive dilation occurs in the ascending aorta, the cusps of the aortic valve, which are attached to the dilated aorta, are unable to fit closely together in diastole to close the aortic valve, which leads to aortic valve insufficiency. Mitral valve defects also occur. There is no specific treatment for the disease, although some antihypertensive agents may retard the rate of aortic dilation and reduce the risk of a dissecting aneurysm. Surgical procedures such as the use of prosthetic grafts are also available to treat the complications caused by dilation of the aorta, and prosthetic valves may be necessary to correct disturbed valve functions. Annual ultrasound examinations are recommended to monitor the progression of the aortic dilation, which may require eventual surgical repair to reduce the risk of a dissecting aneurysm or rupture of the aorta. Pectus excavatum often occurs in Marfan syndrome. In one series of cases, one-third of a group of patients treated for pectus excavatum were later confirmed to have Marfan syndrome.

Structure and Function of Skeletal Muscle

Muscle cells are highly specialized contractile cells. Three different types of muscle are recognized: smooth muscle, skeletal muscle, and cardiac muscle. Smooth muscle is found in the walls of the gastrointestinal tract, biliary tract, urogenital system, respiratory tract, and blood vessels. Skeletal muscle is attached to the skeleton by tendons and ligaments; it functions in voluntary muscular activity. Cardiac muscle closely resembles skeletal muscle but has certain special features related to its function of producing rhythmic contractions of the heart. Lesions in cardiac muscle can result in anatomical and physiological pathology associated with heart functioning (Chapter 9). Structural lesions of smooth muscles are rare. However, smooth muscle can be associated with benign and malignant neoplastic disease.

Contraction of Skeletal Muscle

Skeletal muscles are long, straplike fibers that measure as much as 30 cm in length. The cytoplasm (sarcoplasm) contains multiple nuclei located just beneath the cell membrane (sarcolemma). Filling the cytoplasm are long, threadlike myofibrils composed of the contractile myofilaments actin and myosin. The cytoplasm also contains many energy-rich organic compounds, ions, and enzymes required for the metabolic activity of the muscle cell (**Figure 24-32**).

Muscle cells contract in response to motor nerve impulses conveyed to the muscle. The area of communication between the nerve endings and the muscle cell is termed the neuromuscular junction, or **motor end plate**. The actual stimulation of the muscle cell is the result of a neurotransmitter termed "**acetylcholine**," which is released from the nerve endings at the neuromuscular junction and interacts with acetylcholine receptors on the surface of the muscle fibers. Acetylcholine initiates the biochemical chain of events that causes the actin microfilaments and myosin filaments to slide together, which leads to shortening of the muscle fiber. The duration of the chemical mediator is quite brief because this substance is rapidly broken down by the enzyme cholinesterase, which is present at the neuromuscular junction.

Motor end plate Neuromuscular junction between nerve and muscle.

Acetylcholine A neurotransmitter secreted by nerve endings that activates neurons or muscle cells.

Myasthenia gravis An autoimmune disease characterized by abnormal fatigability of muscle and caused by an autoantibody that damages the acetylcholine receptors at the neuromuscular junction.

Myasthenia Gravis

Myasthenia gravis is a chronic disease characterized by abnormal fatigability of the voluntary muscles as a result of an abnormality at the neuromuscular junction. Fatigue develops rapidly when the muscles are used and subsides

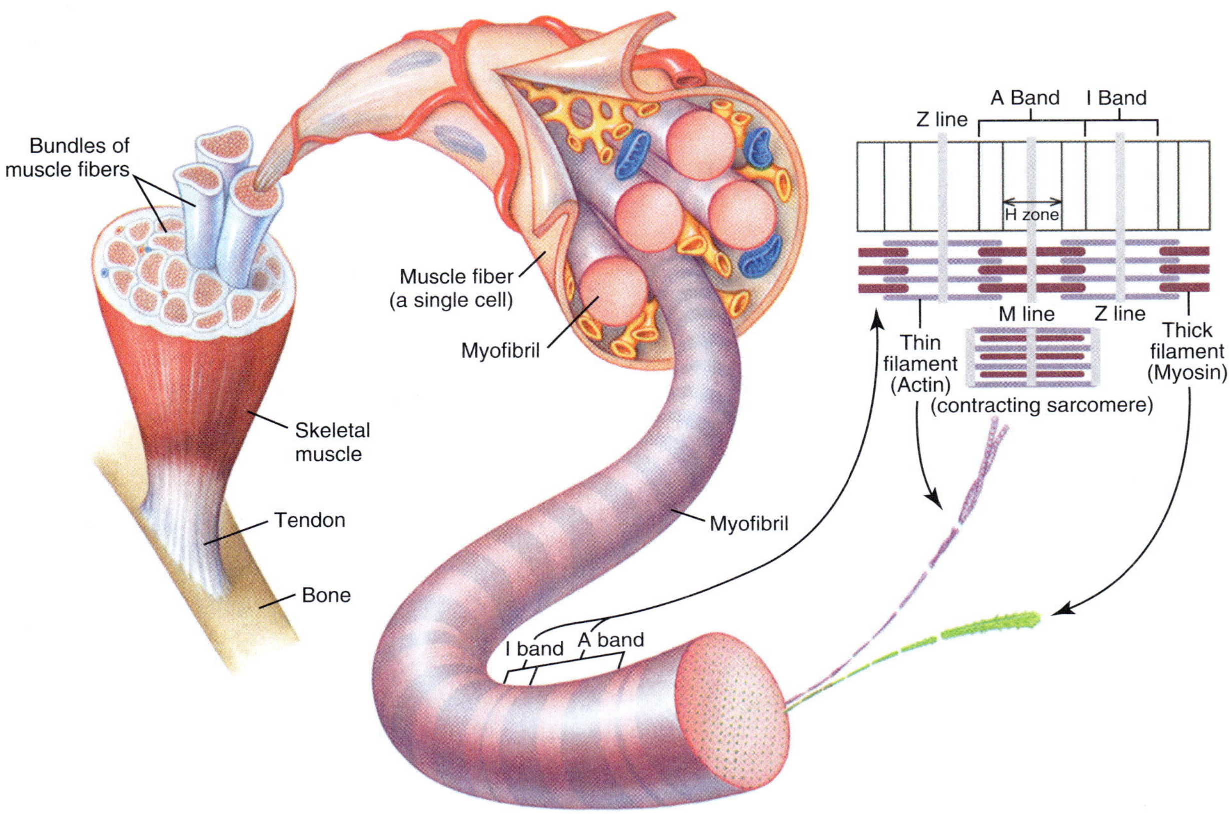

Figure 24-32 Structure of skeletal muscle fiber. Microanatomical details of the contractile apparatus are shown on the right of the figure.

when they are rested. Often, the dysfunction is most conspicuous in the small muscles of the face and in the muscles concerned with eye movement (extraocular muscles). Myasthenia gravis appears to be an autoimmune disease. The blood of affected patients contains an autoantibody directed against acetylcholine receptors on the surface of the muscle fibers at the neuromuscular junction. The manifestations of the disease occur because the antibody damages and greatly reduces the number of receptors available to interact with the acetylcholine liberated from motor nerve endings.

Symptoms can be relieved by drugs that inhibit the action of the enzyme cholinesterase. This prolongs the action of the chemical mediator acetylcholine so that it can continue to stimulate the reduced numbers of receptors for a longer time. Many patients with myasthenia gravis have either a tumor or a benign hyperplasia of the thymus gland that plays a role in the progression of the disease. Patients with hyperplasia or a tumor of the thymus gland are sometimes improved by removal of the thymus.

Factors Affecting Muscular Structure and Function

The normal structural and functional integrity of skeletal muscle depends on an intact nerve supply, normal transmission of impulses across the myoneural junction, and normal metabolic processes within the muscle cell. Skeletal muscles that are not used or muscles deprived of their nerve supply undergo marked **atrophy**, as discussed in Chapter 23 (**Figure 24-33**). Conversely, when additional work is required of the muscles, they undergo hypertrophy in response to the increased demands.

Atrophy Wasting of tissue due to underuse, typically due to the degeneration of cells.

Muscle cells contain a highly complex metabolic machinery capable of translating nerve impulses into muscle contractions. Any disturbance in the metabolism of the muscle cell leads to a disturbance in the function of the cell. The intracellular metabolic processes are also influenced by the

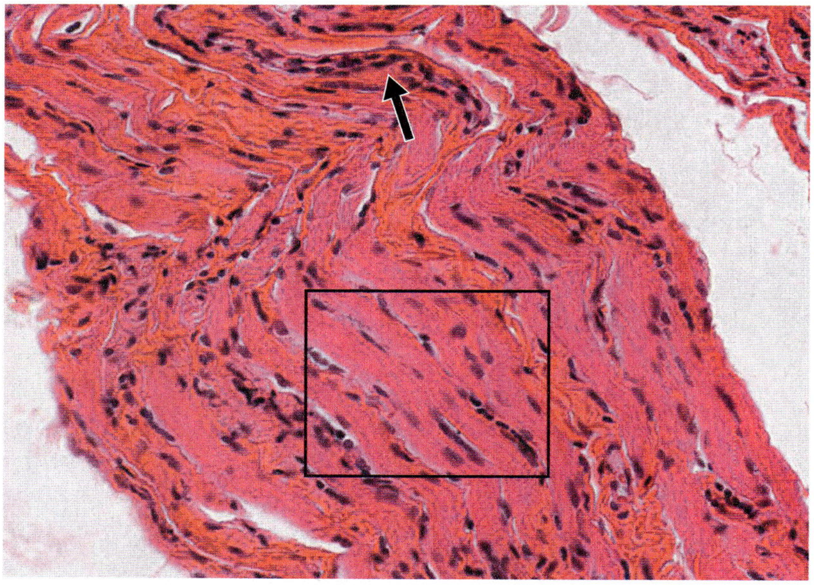

Figure 24-33 Muscle atrophy as a result of denervation (microscopic view). Necrotic muscle fibers being phagocytized by macrophages, termed lengthwise segmental necrosis (*arrow*). Area of necrotic muscle fibers that are anucleate and pale (*box*).

Courtesy of Department of Pathology and Laboratory Medicine, University of North Carolina at Chapel Hill.

endocrine glands that regulate the rate of metabolism within the muscle cell and affect the concentration of the various ions required for normal muscle contraction.

Diseases of skeletal muscle are uncommon. The principal disorders consist of inflammatory lesions, muscular atrophy, degeneration (dystrophy) of muscle, and disturbance of impulse conduction at the neuromuscular junction.

Inflammation of Muscle (Myositis)

Localized Myositis

Small areas of inflammation in skeletal muscle are encountered in many systemic diseases and have no major clinical significance. Inflammation of muscle (**myositis**) also may follow injury or muscular overexertion. The inflammation is secondary to necrosis and disruption of muscle cells and is associated with swelling and tenderness of the affected muscle. The inflammation gradually subsides as the muscle injury heals.

Myositis Inflammation of muscle.

Generalized Myositis

Generalized inflammations of skeletal muscle (inflammatory myopathy) are uncommon but serious systemic diseases believed to be of autoimmune etiology. They are characterized by widespread degeneration and inflammation of skeletal muscle and associated progressive weakness of muscles and, ultimately, muscle wasting. Dermatomyositis, a type of inflammatory myopathy associated with swelling and inflammation of the skin, affects both children and adults and is associated with autoimmune damage to capillaries and small vessels (microangiopathy) as a result of deposition of immune complexes in vessel walls (see Chapter 5). This results in ischemic damage to the muscle. Unlike dermatomyositis, polymyositis is limited to adults and is associated with T cell–mediated damage to muscles, although autoantibodies are also present and of unknown significance. Polymyositis is often associated with a systemic disease of connective tissue of multiple organs, particularly the lungs. Both forms of inflammatory myositis respond to corticosteroid therapy (**Figure 24-34**).

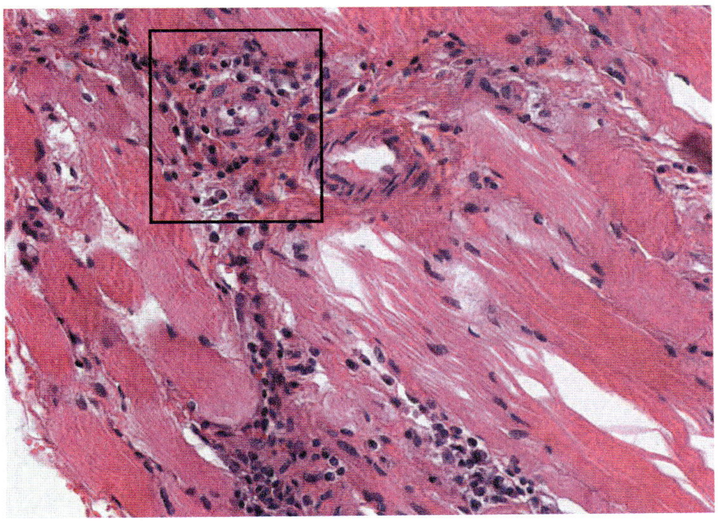

Figure 24-34 Dermatomyositis demonstrating perivascular inflammation (*box*). Microscopic view.

Courtesy of Department of Pathology and Laboratory Medicine, University of North Carolina at Chapel Hill.

Muscular Dystrophy

The muscular dystrophies are a group of relatively rare diseases characterized by progressive degeneration of skeletal muscle not primarily associated with inflammation. The muscle tissue shows necrosis and concomitant attempts at regeneration. Ultimately, muscle is replaced by fibrosis and fatty tissue. Many of the dystrophies are hereditary. Various clinical syndromes are recognized, depending on the muscle groups affected, the patterns of inheritance and gene(s) affected, and the rate of progression of the disease. In general, the diseases are characterized by progressive muscular weakness and gradually increasing disability, eventually terminating in death from paralysis of the respiratory muscles or superimposed respiratory infection.

In the muscular dystrophies, the nerve supply to the muscles is unaffected. The basic disturbance is an abnormality in the muscle fibers that causes them to degenerate. The most common and severe type is termed "Duchenne muscular dystrophy," and a milder form of muscular dystrophy is termed "Becker muscular dystrophy." Both forms result from the mutation of a large gene on the X chromosome, and the disease is transmitted as an X-linked trait to male children of women who carry the defective gene. The normal gene codes for a muscle protein termed "dystrophin," which is located on the inner surface of the sarcolemma; it plays a role in maintaining the structure and functions of the muscle fibers by aiding in connecting the muscle cell membrane to the external extracellular matrix.

As a result of the gene mutation, the absent or defective dystrophin is responsible for the manifestations of the disease, which appear first during early childhood and progress rapidly, leading to death in late adolescence or early adulthood. The muscles primarily affected are those of the lower extremities, trunk, hips, and shoulder girdle. Often, the extent of atrophy is visibly masked because the muscles are infiltrated by fat and fibrous tissue as they atrophy. The fat infiltration may at times be so extreme that the affected muscles appear hypertrophied, leading to the paradox of profound muscular weakness in an individual whose muscles appear (but are not) very well developed (**Figure 24-35**).

The less-severe Becker muscular dystrophy also is caused by a mutation of the same dystrophin-producing gene that causes Duchenne muscular dystrophy. Dystrophin is produced by the mutated gene but is either abnormal or produced in insufficient amounts. In both diseases, the muscle enzyme creatine kinase (CK) leaks from the abnormal muscle fibers, resulting in high levels of the enzyme in the blood of those who are affected. (This is similar to the enzyme that leaks from the heart muscle when the muscle is damaged, as described in Chapter 9.) The diagnosis of muscular dystrophy is made on the basis of the clinical features together with the very high CK blood concentration. Genetic testing reveals the gene mutation, and muscle biopsies reveal the absence of dystrophin in Duchenne dystrophy and an abnormal or reduced amount of dystrophin in Becker dystrophy.

Although the various types of muscular atrophy and muscular dystrophy are uncommon, they are of major concern, not only to the patient but also to the family, because of the hereditary nature of many of these illnesses. (See the case in this chapter.) Unfortunately, there is no way at present to arrest the relentless progression of the disease, although a recently introduced anti-inflammatory drug appears to slow muscle loss in early trials. Multiple trials using different forms of gene therapy to eventually allow insertion of replacement genes in muscle fibers to code for the synthesis of the missing or defective dystrophin are being actively investigated in clinical trials but to date have had limited success.

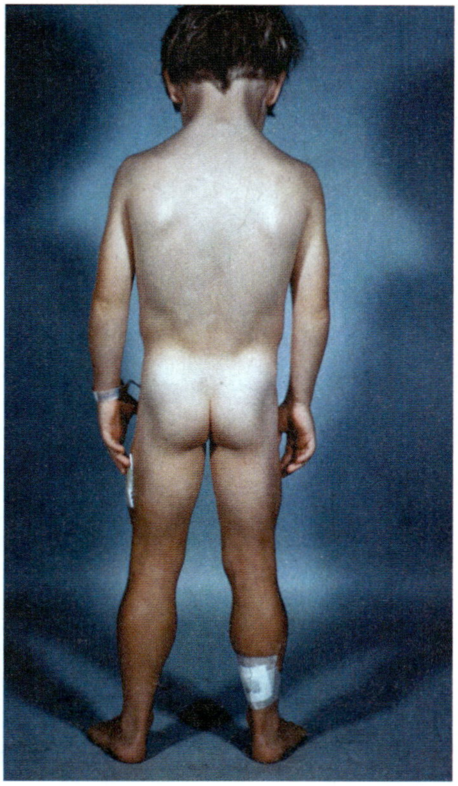

Figure 24-35 Duchenne muscular dystrophy. Note the "pseudohypertrophy" of the calves.

A controversial therapy (Exondys 51) promotes "skipping" of the mutation responsible for about 14 percent of Duchenne muscular dystrophy. Although it does increase the level of dystrophin in these patients (to levels still under 1 percent of normal), it has been associated with limited clinical benefit in early trials. Additional similar agents are awaiting approval, but the clinical utility remains in question, and the cost of the agents is very high.

Case 24-1

Charles was the first child in the family. When he was 4 years old, his parents became concerned about his unusual way of walking (gait). He appeared to "waddle." When Charles attempted to stand, he first got onto his knees and pushed himself up (Gower sign). He also seemed to occasionally walk on his toes. Concerned, his parents brought Charles to Dr. Jane, their pediatrician. Dr. Jane questioned Charles's mother, Annie, about her family history and, in particular, if any of her male relatives had muscle problems. Annie said that she was an adoptee and had no knowledge of her biological parents. Dr. Jane asked Annie if she had any unusual muscle weakness or had been diagnosed with any other medical problems. Annie said she had been in good health for the past several years. Dr. Jane noted that all of Charles's motor milestones were markedly delayed. She sent a sample of Charles's blood for a determination of creatine kinase level (found to be abnormally high). Suspecting that Charles had a dystrophic muscle disease, most likely muscular dystrophy, she referred Charles to a specialist in muscular diseases. The neuromuscular specialist obtained a muscle biopsy from Charles and ordered molecular analysis of his DMD gene.

(continues)

Case 24-1 *(Continued)*

Analysis of the muscle biopsy revealed a mixture of degenerating and regenerating fibers characteristic of a muscular dystrophy. Further analysis showed that Charles did have dystrophin, the protein product of the DMD gene present, but in reduced amount (about 50 percent of normal). However, the dystrophin did not have a normal structure; it was shorter than the normal protein. The specialist explained to Charles's parents that there are two types of muscular dystrophy that differ in severity and age of onset, but both are related to a mutation in the same DMD gene found on the X chromosome. Both are expressed in males, but females carry the disease and are sometimes affected. Duchenne muscular dystrophy (DMD) is the more common (about 1 in 3000 live male births). The disease usually shows up (presents) between 3 and 5 years of age and progresses with increased weakness for 6 to 7 years. The children become wheelchair bound and die of pulmonary and cardiac failure, usually in their early 20s. There is no current therapy, but corticosteroids delay the course of the disease by 1 to 2 years. Becker muscular dystrophy (BMD) is a less severe form of the disease. It is far less common (about 1 in 30,000 male births) and is very variable. Although sometimes symptoms may be found in a child of Charles's age, the disease usually is not diagnosed until a child is 11 or 12 years old. Most often BMD patients continue to walk until their late 20s and, on the average, live until the fifth decade of life, usually dying from cardiac failure. Charles's parents ask, "What about our son. Does he have DMD or BMD?" To answer, the specialist explains, he will have to do additional studies of the defect in Charles's DMD gene.

Discussion

Given the age of onset of the disease in Charles, DMD is most likely. However, the presence of a significant amount of dystrophin argues toward BMD. Mutations that result in very little or no dystrophin result in DMD. However, mutations in which a reduced amount of a "short" DMD molecule is made may function to some degree, but not always.

Why is this? Dystrophin is necessary to provide a stable structure in the muscle cell. The DMD gene is the largest gene found to date and takes up about 2 percent of the X chromosome. The protein dystrophin forms a "dumbbell" with two spherical areas (the amino and carboxy termini of the molecules) connected by a central rodlike domain. The protein bridges the contractile actin fibers in the muscle cell to the connective tissue on the outside of the muscle cell. The spherical areas on the ends of the molecule are the "connectors" to the actin and exterior connective tissue. The rodlike area links the two connectors. Many BMD patients have an "in-frame" mutation that deletes part of the central rodlike domain. The molecule is shorter (as was the case for Charles) but still has some ability to function as a bridge. Unfortunately, in Charles's case, the mutation was "in-frame" and deleted part of the central rod but also deleted an important part of the carboxy-terminal part of the molecule, which is necessary for it to connect to the extracellular matrix. (Note that this is a much simplified picture of the actual molecule.) Although Charles made a short dystrophin molecule, often characteristic of BMD, the molecule had no function in his muscle cells, meaning that Charles had DMD.

Etiology and Pathogenesis

Duchenne muscular dystrophy resulting from an in-frame mutation producing a nonfunctional dystrophin protein.

Questions

1. Why did the pediatrician start by asking Annie if she had male relatives with muscle problems? Would such problems be expected in the maternal

or paternal part of the family? Review sex-linked inheritance. Do you think Annie might show symptoms as she ages?

2. The case uses the term in-frame mutation. What is an in-frame mutation? Why are out-of-frame or truncating mutations more likely to result in DMD rather than BMD?
3. Predict the future; that is, make a prognosis. What are some potential approaches to therapy for DMD?
4. Often patients diagnosed with a particular disease show variability in severity and age of onset compared to others with the disease. What are some potential reasons?

Questions for Review

1. Describe the structure of the typical movable joint.
2. Describe the structure and function of the spine.
3. Describe the structure and function of the thorax.
4. What is the difference between a simple fracture and a compound fracture? What are the complications of a compound fracture? What is a comminuted fracture? A pathologic fracture?
5. What is a "slipped disk"? Why does it occur? Why does it sometimes produce pain radiating down the leg? How is it treated?
6. What is rheumatoid arthritis? What is its relationship to the immune system? How is it treated?
7. What are the types of muscle cells?
8. What is meant by the following terms: neuromuscular junction, acetylcholine, and myositis?
9. What is the difference between muscular atrophy and muscular dystrophy? What are the most common types of atrophic disease of the muscles? Of dystrophic disease?

References

Loeffler AG, Hart MN. Bones and joints and skeletal muscle and peripheral nerve. In: *Introduction to Human Disease*. 7th ed. Jones & Bartlett Learning; 2020.

Fritchie K, John I. Soft tissue and bone pathology; Thorne LB, Lee ET, Chahin N. eds. Neuromuscular pathology. In: Reisner HM. ed. *Pathology: A Modern Case Study*. 2nd ed. Lange McGraw Hill; 2019.

- Rheumatology, orthopedics, neurology, and neurosurgery all intersect in the study of diseases of the bone, muscle, and connective tissue. Loeffler presents a more detailed discussion of the areas covered in the chapter, and the last two chapters suggested are a good introduction. They serve as an advanced introduction to the etiology and pathogenesis of these diseases at the level of undergraduate medical education. The source is rich in illustrations and brief case studies.

Osteogenesis Imperfecta Foundation. OI Informational Fact Sheets. https://oif.org/informationcenter/factsheets/

NIH National Library of Medicine. Osteogenesis Imperfecta. https://ghr.nlm.nih.gov/condition/osteogenesis-imperfecta

- Osteogenesis imperfecta is an extremely complex disease with multiple types and degrees of severity. The two references outline the basic genetics and pathophysiology of the disease. The Osteogenesis Imperfecta Foundation has information on clinical care and coping with the disease.

Harrington J, Sochett E. The child with multiple fractures, what next? *Pediatr Clin North Am*. 2015;62(4):841-855.

- This is a problem that never goes away. A common defense for traumatic bone injury in cases of abuse is osteogenesis imperfecta, so what's next? A reference that is still very much worth reading.

National Institutes of Health, Office of Dietary Supplements. Vitamin D Fact Sheet for Health Professionals. https://ods.od.nih.gov/factsheets/VitaminD-HealthProfessional/

- An excellent resource for information on the function of vitamin D and appropriate vitamin D supplementation. This is an area rife with misinformation. This resource provides a wealth of current trustworthy information.

Stevenson J; Medical advisory council of the British Menopause Society. Prevention and treatment of osteoporosis in women. *Post Reprod Health*. 2023;29(1):11-14. doi:10.1177/20533691221139902. Epub 2022 Nov 10. PMID: 36357006; PMCID: PMC10009319.

- There are now recommendations for using HRT in selected groups of women. This reference gives a more balanced approach.

National Institutes of Health, National Institute of Arthritis and Musculoskeletal and Skin Diseases. Osteoporosis. http://www.niams.nih.gov/Health_Info/Bone/Osteoporosis/

U.S. Department of Health and Human Services Office on Women's Health. Osteoporosis. https://www.womenshealth.gov/a-z-topics/osteoporosis

- These two resources serve as a gateway to a wealth of material on the structure of bone (bone basics) and diseases of bone, including osteogenesis imperfecta, osteoporosis, and Paget disease (not discussed in the text). An excellent first place to look for additional trustworthy information in the area. The second entry is aimed at the area of women's health and is an excellent gateway to information on osteoporosis and also on nutrition and fitness.

van Delft MAM, Huizinga TWJ. An overview of autoantibodies in rheumatoid arthritis. *J Autoimmun*. 2020. doi:10.1016/j.jaut.2019.102392. https://www.sciencedirect.com/science/article/pii/S0896841119308194?via%3Dihub

- An overview of the source and role of autoantibodies that characterize rheumatoid arthritis. An area close to the heart of one of the text authors.

NIH National Library of Medicine. MedlinePlus. Arthritis. https://www.nlm.nih.gov/medlineplus/arthritis.html

- A portal for additional information on all aspects of arthritic disease, including osteoarthritis and gout.

Muscular Dystrophy Association (MDA). About Neuromuscular Diseases. https://www.mda.org/disease

Thangarajh M. The dystrophinopathies. *Continuum (Minneap Minn)*. 2019;25(6):1619-1639.

Wicklund MP. The muscular dystrophies. *Continuum (Minneap Minn)*. 2013;19:1535-1570.

- The MDA provides excellent summaries of a large number of neuromuscular diseases, many of which are not covered in the text. The second entry is an excellent overview of diseases associated with mutations of the dystrophin gene. Case studies are included. The third entry was used in part in the case construction. It reviews not only the more common muscular dystrophies but also several less common but distinctive conditions.

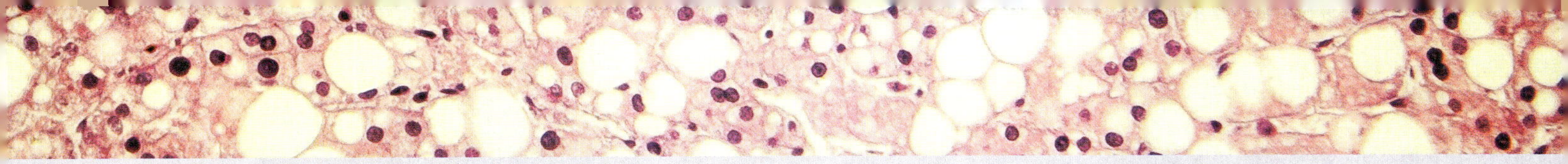

Glossary

A

ABO hemolytic disease A mild hemolytic disease in group A or B infants and group O mothers as a result of maternal anti-A and anti-B antibodies.

Abscess A localized accumulation of pus in tissues.

Acetylcholine A neurotransmitter secreted by nerve endings that activates neurons or muscle cells.

Achalasia Inability of a gastrointestinal sphincter to relax. Formerly known as cardiospasm.

Achondroplasia A genetic disorder that results from a mutation in the FGFR3 gene, which alters the cartilage to bone conversion during bone development.

Acinar cells The main functional units of the exocrine pancreas, responsible for producing, storing, and secreting crucial digestive enzymes.

Acini/acinar Acini are small grape-like clusters of glands composed of a cavity surrounded by secretory cells. "Acinar" means having the properties of acini.

Acquired immune deficiency syndrome (AIDS) An infection caused by the human immunodeficiency virus. The virus attacks and destroys helper T lymphocytes, which compromises cell-mediated immunity, leading to increased susceptibility to infection and some tumors.

Acromegaly A condition resulting from excessive secretion of growth hormone in the adult.

Actin Contractile protein, also referred to as a motor protein that enables muscle fibers to shorten and create contraction. Actin also contributes to non-muscle cell movement.

Actinic keratosis A precancerous scaly proliferation of squamous epithelial cells in sun-damaged skin.

Actin microfilament A cell framework filament made of globular proteins that polymerize, becoming filamentous actin. Actin is important in cell movement, cytoplasmic division, and muscle contraction.

Active transport Transfer of materials against a concentration gradient that is necessary to maintain proper concentration of intracellular and extracellular ions.

Acute calculous cholecystitis Mucosal injury from concentrated bile within the gallbladder.

Acute coronary syndrome (ACS) A broad classification of diseases arising from inadequate flow of blood to the heart, falling into one of three separate groups (unstable angina, myocardial infarction, and cardiac death). Subcategories of ACS are differentiated based upon ECG and other laboratory testing.

Acute hemorrhagic pancreatitis Severe pancreatic inflammation with necrosis of pancreatic ducts and release of pancreatic enzymes that damage the pancreas and blood vessels.

Acute inflammation Earliest phase of the inflammatory response.

Acute kidney injury (AKI) Injury to any part of the kidney. May also be defined as prerenal or postrenal.

Acute phase proteins Proteins produced by the liver in response to inflammation.

Adaptive immunity Immune response with the ability to mount an antigen specific reaction and establish immunologic memory.

Addison's disease A disease caused by chronic adrenal cortical hypofunction.

Adenosine triphosphate (ATP) A high-energy phosphate-containing compound that liberates energy to power numerous cellular metabolic processes when one phosphate group is removed.

Adhesion Band of fibrous tissue that form subsequent to the inflammatory response, which may include scar tissue formation binding adjacent tissues together.

Adipose tissue Loose, fibrous tissue containing fat cells.

Adjustable gastric banding A method for treating obesity by applying an adjustable gastric band to the stomach to reduce its capacity, thereby promoting weight loss.

Adjuvant chemotherapy Anticancer chemotherapy administered before or after surgical resection of a tumor in an attempt to destroy any small, undetected foci of metastatic tumor before they become clinically detectable.

Adrenal corticosteroid hormones/steroids Chemicals that suppress the inflammatory process.

Adrenocorticotropic hormone (ACTH) A hormone secreted by the anterior lobe of the pituitary that stimulates the adrenal cortex to manufacture and secrete adrenal cortical hormones.

Adult respiratory distress syndrome (ARDS)/ diffuse alveolar damage (DAD) A life threatening lung injury that causes fluid accumulating into the lungs.

Aerobic organisms Microbes that grow best in the presence of oxygen.

Affinity maturation Improvement in the ability of antibodies to bind specific antigen resulting from rapid mutation of antibody genes.

Akinetic/hypokinetic Lacking or showing reduced contraction.

Albumin-to-creatinine ratio (ACR) Measurement of urine albumin levels compared to amount of creatinine.

Alcoholic liver disease Long-term injury to the liver resulting from frequent and heavy alcohol consumption.

Aldosterone A steroid hormone produced by the adrenal cortex that regulates the rate of sodium absorption from the renal tubules.

Alkylating agent An anticancer drug that disrupts cell function by binding DNA chains together so they cannot separate.

Allele One of several related forms of a single gene.

Allogeneic/syngeneic/autologous Terms used to classify the relationship of donor cells to the patient: not from self/from an identical twin/from self.

Alpha-fetoprotein (AFP) Protein produced by fetal liver early in gestation. Sometimes produced by tumor cells. Level is elevated in amnionic fluid when fetus has a neural tube defect resulting in abnormally high levels in the maternal serum.

Alveoli/alveolus One of the terminal air sacs of the lung.

Amenorrhea Absence of menses.

Ampulla of Vater The area in the duodenum where the pancreatic duct and common bile duct come together, also known as the hepatopancreatic ampulla or hepatopancreatic duct.

Anaerobic organisms Microbes that grow best in the absence of oxygen.

Anaphylactoid reaction Immune response resembling an anaphylactic reaction but by direct action on mast cells or by activating complement.

Anaphylaxis A widespread systemic hypersensitivity reaction.

Anaplastic cell Type of tumor cell whose structure is so deranged as to make identification of origin difficult.

Anasarca Widespread edema.

Anastomosis A communication between two blood vessels or other tubular structures. Also refers to a surgical connection of two hollow tubular structures, such as the divided ends of the intestine or a blood vessel (surgical anastomosis).

Anemia A decrease in hemoglobin or red cells or both.

Anencephaly A congenital malformation considered to be a neural tube defect where parts of the brain, cranium and scalp may be missing.

Anergy Continued non-responsiveness of immune cells to a host or foreign antigen.

Aneuploidy Condition of having extra or missing chromosomes.

Aneurysm A dilatation of a structure, such as the aorta, a cerebral artery, or a part of the ventricular wall.

Angiogenesis The formation of new blood vessels.

Anicteric hepatitis Symptoms of hepatitis without the appearance of jaundice.

Anions Negatively charged ions.

Annulus fibrosus The dense peripheral ring of fibrocartilage making up the intervertebral disk.

Anthracosis Carbon pigment deposited in the connective tissue around the individual lobules of lung.

Antibody-dependent cellular cytotoxicity (ADCC) Recognition and destruction of cells coated with antibody.

Antibody Immunoglobulin molecules produced by B cells when activated by an antigen and secreted by B cells, which mature into plasma cells.

Antidiuretic hormone (ADH) Posterior lobe pituitary hormone that regulates urine concentration by altering the permeability of the renal collecting tubules.

Antigenic determinant/epitope Specific molecular region from an antigen that triggers immune response.

Antigen-presenting cell (APC) Cell that displays the foreign material.

Antigen Substance recognized by the immune system.

Antimetabolite A substance that competes with or replaces another substance (metabolite) required for cell metabolism.

Aortic valve Semilunar valve surrounding the orifices of the aorta.

Apoptosis Programmed cell death that does not provoke a host protective response.

Appendicolith A calcified stone in the appendix.

Arachnoid (mater) The middle of the three meninges that cover the brain.

Arnold-Chiari malformation Congenital condition with spinal cord defects and compression of the brain stem and cerebellum downward.

Aromatase inhibitor A drug that inhibits the conversion of adrenal androgenic steroids to estrogens, used to treat postmenopausal women with estrogen receptor-positive breast carcinoma.

Arrhythmia An irregularity of the heartbeat

Arthropod-borne virus/arbovirus Viruses that are transmitted to humans primarily through the bites of infected mosquitoes, ticks, sand flies, or midges.

Arthropod Invertebrate animal with jointed limbs and segmented body, such as insect and spider. Important arthropods that parasitize humans include the crab louse and the organism causing scabies.

Asbestosis A type of pneumoconiosis caused by inhalation of asbestos fibers.

Ascites The buildup of fluid in the abdomen, causing a swollen belly, most often occurring because of cirrhosis, a liver disease.

Astrocytes Participate in numerous physiological processes, such as regulation of axonal growth support, blood–brain barrier formation, and immune responses, as well as participating in higher cognitive functions, including memory.

Astrocytoma A neuroglial tumor arising from astrocytes; the most common type.

Asymptomatic Without symptoms.

Atelectasis Collapse of the lung, either caused by bronchial obstruction (obstructive atelectasis) or external compression (compression atelectasis).

Atheroma Formation of plaque with a necrotic core rich in lipids.

Atherosclerosis Formation of lipid-rich plaques in large and medium arteries, which result in stiffening of the vessel in the area of the plaque.

Atrioventricular (AV) valves The flaplike heart valves located between the atrium and the ventricle.

Atrium/atria Upper chambers of the heart.

Atrophy Wasting of tissue due to underuse, typically due to the degeneration of cells.

Attack complex Group of complement molecules that destroys the target micro-organism or abnormal cell.

Autoantibody An antibody formed against the host's own cells or tissue components.

Autocrine Cell signaling to itself by releasing products that act on signal receptors found associated with the cell.

Autoimmune disease A disease associated with formation of cell-mediated or humoral immunity against the subject's own cells or tissue components.

Autoimmunity Immunological activity against self-antigen markers.

Autophagy Process by which internal cellular components are degraded and recycled by the cells.

Autosomal chromosomes Chromosomes other than sex chromosomes. A human has 22 pairs of autosomes.

Autosomal dominant polycystic kidney disease Autosomal dominant disease characterized by the formation of multiple cysts throughout both kidneys.

Avascular necrosis Bone necrosis caused by interruption of its blood supply.

Axon Portion of the neuron that conducts impulses away from the neuronal cell body.

B

Bacillus Rod-shaped bacteria.

Barr body The inactivated X chromosome attached to the nuclear membrane in the female. Sex chromatin body.

Barrett esophagus Squamous lining changes to a more acid-resistant columnar mucosa.

Basal-like tumors Type of breast cancer cell demonstrating a specific gene expression profile with tumor cells look similar to the epithelial cells of the basal layer of the breast's milk ducts.

Basophil A cell that contains numerous variable-sized granules that stain intensely purple with basic dyes.

B cell A lymphocyte that differentiates into plasma cells and is associated with humoral immunity.

Bell-clapper defect Anatomic abnormality responsible for increased testicular mobility.

Benign Quality of neoplasms that do not invade surrounding tissue or spread to sites distant from their origin.

Bile A secretion of the liver containing bile salts, cholesterol, and other substances.

Bile canaliculi Small terminal bile channels located between liver cords.

Bile salts Derivatives of bile acids present in bile that act as emulsifiers to promote fat digestion and absorption.

Biliary cirrhosis Diffuse liver cell damage and scarring with the distortion of liver cell structure and function (cirrhosis) caused by obstruction of bile ducts.

Biliary colic Abdominal pain that results when a gallstone enters the biliary duct system.

Bilirubin One of the bile pigments derived from the breakdown of hemoglobin.

Bioinformatics A fast-evolving field that uses tools from multiple disciplines, such as computer science, mathematics, and statistics to collect, store, analyze, and interpret data in biological systems.

Biopsy Removal of a small sample of tissue for examination and diagnosis by a pathologist.

Blastocyst A stage of development of the fertilized ovum (zygote) in which a central cavity forms within the cluster of developing cells.

Blastomycosis A systemic fungus infection caused by the fungus *Blastomyces dermatiditis*.

Bleeding time Time needed for a small standardized skin incision to stop bleeding.

Blood agar plates Bacteria media incorporating red blood cells.

B lymphocyte A lymphocyte associated with humoral immunity that is capable of producing antibodies, which can differentiate into antibody-secreting plasma or memory cells.

Body stalk The structure connecting the embryo to the chorion. Eventually develops into the umbilical cord.

Borborygmi Loud bowel sounds.

Botulism Food poisoning caused by ingestion of a neurotoxin produced by an anaerobic spore-forming bacillus, *Clostridium botulinum*, growing in improperly canned or preserved food.

Bowman's capsule The cuplike expanded end of the nephron that surrounds the tuft of glomerular capillaries.

Bradykinin A chemical mediator of inflammation derived from components in the blood plasma.

Brain stem The brain stem is the elongated central portion of the brain connecting the cerebral hemispheres with the spinal cord. It controls the flow of messages to the rest of the body and is critical for autonomic functions such as breathing.

Brain ventricle A small hollow cavity in the brain.

Breast-conserving surgery Surgery designed to remove the minimal amount of breast tissue.

Bronchi/bronchus One of the large subdivisions of the trachea.

Bronchiectasis Dilatation of bronchi caused by a weakened airway wall as a result of infection.

Bronchiole One of the small terminal subdivisions of the branched bronchial tree.

Buccal plate Specialized attachment organ of hookworms. Also refers to a thin layer of bone in the mouth which supports teeth and facial structure.

Budd-Chiari syndrome Thrombosis of the hepatic vein.

C

Calcitonin A hormone that lowers blood calcium, produced by the interfollicular cells of the thyroid gland.

Calculi Stones formed within the body, as in the kidney or gallbladder.

Callus Newly synthesized bone repairing a break.

Cancellous bone The inner, spongy layer of bone.

Canker sore Small, painful ulcer developed in the oral cavity.

Capsid The protein covering the central nucleic acid core of a virus.

Capsomere One of the subunits that make up the protein shell (capsid) of a virus.

Capsular epithelium Outer layer of cells of Bowman's capsule. It is also termed the parietal layer of Bowman's capsule.

Carcinoembryonic antigen (CEA) A tumor-associated antigen that resembles the antigen secreted by the cells of the fetal gastrointestinal tract.

Carcinogenesis Development of cancer.

Carcinoma A malignant tumor derived from epithelial cells.

Carcinoma in situ Neoplasm occupying full thickness of the epithelium.

Cardiac arrest Complete cessation of cardiac activity.

Cardiac muscle Muscle found only in the heart; has features of both striated and smooth muscle.

Cardiac tamponade Fluid accumulation in the pericardial sac, which compresses the heart and impairs heart function.

Cardinal signs of inflammation Heat, swelling, redness, and pain observed at the site of injury.

Caries Tooth decay.

Carpal tunnel syndrome A condition resulting from nerves in the hand being compressed on the anterior surface of the wrist.

Cartilage A type of flexible connecting tissue in which cells are dispersed in a dense matrix.

Caseous Necrotic center of nodule characteristic of tuberculosis.

Catecholamines A class of molecules that act as neurotransmitters and hormones in various body regions. These chemical messengers include dopamine, norepinephrine (noradrenaline), and epinephrine (adrenaline), which are derived from the amino acid tyrosine.

Cations Positively charged ions.

Cell-mediated defense mechanism The defense against foreign antigens provided by a population of T lymphocytes that can attach and destroy the foreign antigens.

Cell-mediated immunity Immunity associated with population of sensitized lymphocytes.

Cell The basic living structural and functional unit of the body.

Cellular component Circulating blood cell part of acute inflammation.

Cellulitis An acute spreading inflammation affecting the skin or deeper tissues.

Central tolerance Part of the development of cellular and humoral immunity; cells reacting against self-antigen are removed during development; takes place in primary lymphoid organs.

Centrioles Short, cylindrical structures located adjacent to the nucleus that participate in the formation of spindle fibers during cell division.

Centromere The structure that joins each pair of chromatids formed by chromosome duplication.

Cerebellum Part of the brain regulating muscle tone, coordination, posture, and balance.

Cerebral cortex Receives sensory input and initiates voluntary motor activity.

Cerebral embolus A stroke caused by blockage of a cerebral artery by a blood clot that had formed elsewhere, a fat globule, or air bubble, which was transported in the bloodstream to the brain.

Cerebral hemorrhage A stroke caused by rupture of a cerebral artery, usually in a person with hypertension that allows blood to escape under high pressure into the brain.

Cerebral infarct Brain tissue that became necrotic after a stroke.

Cerebral thrombosis A stroke caused by thrombosis of an arteriosclerotic cerebral artery.

Cervical intraepithelial neoplasia (CIN) Precancerous condition characterized by cervical dysplasia in mucosa of cervix.

Chancre Small ulcer at site of syphilis inoculation.

Chemical mediators of inflammation Messenger molecule that acts on blood vessels, inflammatory cells, or other cells to contribute to an inflammatory response.

Chemotaxis Process of active movement of inflammatory cells to the site of the injury.

Cholecystitis Inflammation of the gallbladder.

Cholelithiasis Formation of gallstones.

Cholestasis Decreased bile flow and bile stasis.

Cholesterol A complex lipid (sterol) containing several hydrocarbon ring structures.

Chondrosarcoma A primary bone tumor occurring later in life.

Chordae tendineae Bands of fibrous tissue connecting the margins of the valves to papillary muscles.

Choriocarcinoma A malignant proliferation of trophoblastic tissue.

Chorionic villi Fingerlike columns of cells extending from the chorion that anchor the chorionic vesicle in the endometrium.

Chorion The layer of trophoblast and associated mesoderm that surrounds the developing embryo.

Chromatid One of two newly duplicate chromosomes held together by the centromere.

Chromatin Tightly wound DNA in the nucleus; formed in part from nucleosomes.

Chromophobe cells Anterior lobe pituitary epithelial cells containing sparse, poorly stained granules.

Chromosome Cell structure organizing the molecules of DNA; individual structural units of DNA which are best seen in dividing cells.

Chronic cholecystitis Ongoing irritation of the gallbladder by repeated bouts of acute disease.

Chronic inflammation Cellular reaction leading to repair.

Chronic obstructive pulmonary disease (COPD) Combination of emphysema and chronic bronchitis.

Cilia Specialized cytoplasmic processes on cells.

Cirrhosis of the liver A disease characterized by diffused intrahepatic scarring and circulatory disturbance within the liver.

Class switch A change in the immunoglobulin constant region using the same variable region.

Clear cell carcinoma Glycogen-rich tumors similar to endometrioid carcinoma.

Clinician Health care provider having direct contact with patients.

Clonal Derived from a single cell.

Coccidioidomycosis A disease caused by the pathogenic fungus *Coccidioides immitis*.

Coccus Spherical bacteria.

Codominant Products of both genes are expressed in the heterozygous state.

Colitis Inflammation restricted to colon.

Collagen fibers Fibers that are strong but do not stretch.

Collagen Main constituent of fibrous proteins in the human body.

Collateral circulation An accessory circulation capable of delivering blood to a tissue when the primary circulation is blocked, as by a thrombus or embolus.

Colloid Homogenous substances with particles dispersed throughout the substance and include gels, sols an emulsions. Colloidal osmotic pressure contributes to water balance throughout the body.

Colonoscopy Procedure for examination of the colon with an endoscope.

Columnar cells Tall, narrow cells.

Communicable disease A disease transmitted from person to person.

Complementary The relationship between the base sequence of the two strands in a DNA molecule. During DNA replication, either strand can make an exact copy of the other. Complementary DNA strands bind to each other by base pairing.

Complement Group of proteins interact to produce by-products, some of which act as mediators of inflammation or cytolysis.

Computed tomographic (CT) scan An X-ray technique producing detailed cross-sectional images of the body by means of an X-ray tube and detectors connected to a computer. Sometimes called a CAT scan.

Computerized tomography pulmonary angiography (CTPA) This is a specialized type of CT test in which a dye is injected into the vascular system to allow visualization of the blood vessels in the lung.

Concussion A temporary loss of consciousness caused by a head injury, often without any memory of the events that occurred shortly before or after the head injury.

Condyloma A warty, tumor-like overgrowth in the squamous epithelium of the anorectal or genital tract, caused by a virus that is spread by sexual contact.

Congenital Present at birth.

Conjoined twins Identical twins, historically known as Siamese twins, that are joined to one another and often share organs in common.

Conjugated bilirubin A more soluble form of bilirubin produced by the addition of two molecules of glucuronic acid to the bilirubin molecule.

Consumption coagulopathy A disturbance of blood coagulation within the blood vessel as a result of the uncontrolled activation of the coagulation mechanism.

Contusion Injury resulting from severe blunt force.

Coronary thrombosis Thrombus formation on the surface of a plaque blocking the coronary artery.

Cortex Outer layer of an organ.

Cortical bone Outer layer of compact bone.

Cortisol The major glucocorticoid.

Councilman/apoptotic bodies Cell shrinkage/apoptotic cell death in inflammation of the liver.

Crab louse A parasite of the pubic area; causes intense itching.

C-reactive protein Acute phase reactant associated with inflammation.

Creatinine clearance test A test of renal function that measures the ability of kidneys to remove (clear) creatinine from the blood and excrete it in the urine.

Crenate Descriptive term for cell shrinkage effected by a hypertonic solution. More generally, to form a scalloped or toothed edge.

Crescentic glomerulonephritis Form of glomerulonephritis in which Bowman's space (surrounding the glomerular capillary tuft) becomes filled with proliferating cells derived from the parietal epithelium of Bowman's capsule.

Cretinism Hypothyroidism in the infant.

Crigler-Najjar syndrome Lack of UGT, which causes a severe disease of early childhood.

Crohn's disease A type of chronic enteritis with the potential to impact any areas of the digestive tract. Most frequently involving the end of the small intestine and the beginning of the large intestine, inflammation often spreads to the deeper layer of the bowel.

Cuboidal cells Cube-shaped cells.

Cushing's disease Caused by an ACTH-producing tumor of the pituitary gland that stimulates the adrenal glands to enlarge.

Cyclooxygenase Enzyme needed for synthesis of prostaglandins.

Cystitis/pyelonephritis Urinary tract infections affecting only the bladder or upper urinary tract.

Cytokine A general term for any protein secreted by cells that functions as an intercellular messenger and influences cells of the immune system. Cytokines are secreted by macrophages and monocytes (monokines), lymphocytes (lymphokines), and other cells.

Cytomegalovirus One of the herpes viruses that causes an infectious mononucleosis-like syndrome in adults; may cause congenital malformation in fetuses (Chapter 16).

Cytoskeleton Protein tubules and filaments that form the structural framework of cells.

Cytotoxic Causing cell death.

D

Damage-Associated Molecular Patterns (DAMPs) Molecules that can initiate and perpetuate immune response in the noninfectious inflammatory response.

Daughter cell A cell resulting from the division of a single cell (called the parent cell).

Debride Remove dead, infected, and excess granulation tissue from the wound bed.

Decidua The endometrium of pregnancy.

Definitive host Organism in which a parasite reaches final maturity.

Delayed hypersensitivity A state of reactivity to a foreign material that takes time to develop.

Demyelinating neuropathy Neural disease with the loss of the myelin sheath surrounding axons resulting in abnormal neural signal transmission.

Dendrite Nerve process conducting impulses toward the nerve cell body.

Dental cavity A loss of tooth structure caused by the combined action of mouth bacteria and organic acids derived from bacterial fermentation of retained food particles.

Dental plaque Masses of bacteria, bacterial products, and salivary proteins adherent to teeth, which predispose to tooth decay.

Dentine Bony structure of the tooth.

Deoxyribonucleic acid (DNA) The nucleic acid present in the chromosomes of the nuclei of cells that carries genetic information.

Dermatophyte A fungus that causes a superficial infection of the skin.

Desensitization Treatment for allergy that induces the formation of IgG antibodies.

Diabetes insipidus A condition resulting from a deficiency of antidiuretic hormone, characterized by the excretion of a large volume of very diluted urine.

Diabetes mellitus A metabolic disease characterized by hyperglycemia and caused by insufficient insulin secretion or inefficient utilization of insulin.

Diabetic glomerulosclerosis Diffuse and nodular thickening of glomerular basement membranes, a common occurrence in patients with long-standing diabetes mellitus.

Diabetic ketoacidosis A disturbance of the body's acid–base balance (acidosis) caused by an inability to utilize glucose, which requires the body to use fat as an energy source. Fat metabolism generates excessive amounts of ketone bodies, which disrupts the normal alkalinity of body fluids.

Diagnosis The determination of the nature and cause of a patient's illness.

Diaphysis Elongated central region of the bone shaft.

Diastole Ventricular relaxation.

Diastolic heart failure Heart failure caused by inadequate filling of the ventricles during diastole, in contrast to systolic heart failure in which ejection of blood from the ventricles during systole is inadequate.

Differential diagnosis Consideration of the different diseases possible given the patient's symptoms.

Diffusion The passive movement of solutes in solution from an area of higher concentration to an area of lower concentration.

Dilatation and curettage (D&C) Procedure involving scraping the lining of the uterus; used to treat irregular bleeding.

Diploid Cell containing 2N (pairs) of each chromosome.

Disease Any disturbance of the structure or function of the body.

Disseminated intravascular coagulation syndrome (DIC) A rare but serious condition that causes blood clotting within the blood vessel and can be life threatening.

Disuse atrophy The reduction in structure or function of a body part when the use of that body part has diminished, and is often used in reference to bone or muscle.

Diverticula/diverticulum An outpouching from an organ, as from the mucosa of the colon, that projects through the muscular wall.

Diverticulitis An inflammation of a diverticulum.

Diverticulosis A condition characterized by outpouchings of the colonic mucosa through weak areas in the muscular wall.

DNA Deoxyribonucleic acid (DNA) is the molecule carrying the coding information for genes.

DNA repair gene Gene that normally functions to repair DNA.

Dominant gene A gene that expresses a trait in the heterozygous state.

Dopamine agonist A drug such as bromocriptine that binds to the dopamine receptors on the anterior pituitary cell and mimics the function of dopamine, producing effects such as inhibition of prolactin secretion.

Dopamine Chemical mediator released by some neurons of the central nervous system. Dopamine also serves as a neurotransmitter in the nervous system.

Dorsal Front surface.

Dosage effects Differing amounts of gene product in the heterozygous and homozygous states.

Down syndrome Condition resulting from trisomy for chromosome 21.

Ductal carcinoma in situ (DCIS) The precursor lesion to most breast cancer.

Ductal carcinoma Tumor arising from the epithelium of the ducts.

Dura (mater) The outer covering of the brain and spinal cord.

Dysmenorrhea Painful menstruation.

Dysphagia Difficulty swallowing.

Dysplasia Abnormal maturation of cells. Localized areas of dysregulated growth.

E

Ecchymosis Bruise.

Echocardiogram A record obtained from an ultrasound examination of the heart and related blood vessels; used to assist in the diagnosis of cardiovascular disease.

Eclampsia One or more convulsions in a pregnant woman with preeclampsia.

Ectoderm The outer germ layer in the embryo that gives rise to specific organs and tissues.

Ectopic pregnancy A pregnancy outside the endometrial cavity.

Edema Accumulation of excess fluid in the interstitial tissues.

Edematous Filled with fluid.

Effector T cell Activated T cell upon exposure to foreign substance.

Ejection fraction Percentage of the ventricular volume ejected during systole.

Elastic cartilage Contains elastic fibers.

Elastic fibers Fibers found in the extracellular matrix.

Elastin Protein made by several cell types that is capable of stretching.

Electrocardiogram (ECG) A technique for measuring the serial changes in the electrical activity of the heart during the various phases of the cardiac cycle. (Often termed ECG or EKG.)

Electrocardiogram (ECG)/electroencephalogram (EEG)/electromyogram (EMG) Tests analyzing the patterns of electrical impulses of different body parts used to evaluate function—ECG for heart, EEG for brain, and EMG for muscle. EMG only indirectly measures the nervous system.

Electrolyte Substance that can conduct electricity through the movement of ions, but not through the movement of electrons. They include many soluble salts, acids, and bases dissolved in a polar solvent like water.

Embolism A condition in which a blockage composed of a detached clot, mass of bacteria, or other foreign material (embolus) occludes a blood vessel.

Embryonal carcinoma A malignant testicular tumor in which the malignant cells have features resembling rapidly growing trophoblastic tissue.

Embryo Developing organism from fertilization until organogenesis. A human embryo is from conception until the beginning of the ninth week of gestation.

Emigration/diapedesis Movement of cells through walls of blood vessels.

Emphysema Disease in which the air spaces in the lung are enlarged and their walls destroyed.

Encephalitis An inflammation of the brain.

Encephalomalacia Cystic lesion of degenerated brain tissue as a result of obstruction of cerebral blood supply. Same as cerebral infarct.

Endochondral bone formation The formation of bone, first as a cartilage model that is then reabsorbed and converted into bone.

Endocrine Cell-to-cell communication by soluble mediators acting on cells that may be distant from the cell originating the signal.

Endocrine gland A gland that discharges its secretions directly into the bloodstream.

Endoderm The inner germ layer of the embryo that gives rise to specific organs and tissues.

Endometrial cyst An ovarian cyst lined by endometrium and filled with old blood and debris. A manifestation of endometriosis.

Endometrial intraepithelial neoplasia (EIN) Result of long-term nonatypical endometrial hyperplasia; a precursor lesion to cancer.

Endometrioid tumor Tumor epithelium resembles endometrium.

Endometriosis Presence of endometrial tissue in abnormal locations, such as in the ovary or pelvis.

Endoplasmic reticulum (ER) A mass of hollow tubular channels within the cytoplasm of the cell, frequently bordered by ribosomes. Depending on the type, ER may be associated with protein or lipid synthesis.

Endoscopy An examination of the interior of the body by means of various lighted tubular instruments. Method may also be used to obtain tissue samples.

Endothelium The internal lining of blood vessels and interior of the heart.

Enteritis Inflammation of the intestinal tract.

Enzymatic fat necrosis See fat necrosis.

Eosinophil A cell whose cytoplasm is filled with large, uniform granules that stain intensely red with acid dyes.

Epicardium/myocardium/endocardium Three layers of the heart moving from the external surface to the internal.

Epigenetics Mechanisms that control gene expression independent of the base code of DNA.

Epinephrine Is both a neurotransmitter in the autonomic nervous system and a hormone secreted by the adrenal medulla.

Epiphyseal plate Cartilaginous end of epiphyses critical to ossification of long bones.

Epiphyses The end parts of long bones, initially growing separately from the shaft.

Epithelioid macrophages Activated macrophages that resemble the appearance of epithelial cells.

Epstein-Barr (EB) virus A virus that causes infectious mononucleosis.

Erythrocyte Commonly known as red blood cells (RBCs), these are the most abundant blood cells, specifically designed to transport oxygen from the lungs to body tissues and carbon dioxide back, using the iron-rich protein hemoglobin.

Erythrocyte sedimentation rate (ESR) A laboratory test to measure the speed red cells settle out of the blood; used to detect inflammation.

Erythroplakia Depressed red lesions on the oral mucosa.

Eschar A layer of dead tissue that commonly forms over a wound or burn.

Esophageal varices Thin-walled vessels that can rupture.

Essential hypertension High blood pressure with no identifiable cause.

Estrogen receptors (ER)/progesterone receptors (PR) A protein on the surface of certain cells, which binds estrogen or progesterone. The presence or absence of the receptors is an important aspect of cancer diagnosis and treatment.

Etiology The cause of a disease.

Evidence-based medicine The scientific method to organize and apply current data to improve healthcare decisions.

Exchange transfusion Partial replacement of the patients blood with blood from another source in hemolytic disease of the newborn.

Exocrine gland A gland that discharges its secretions through a duct onto a mucosal surface.

Exome The totality of sequences in the genome that code for proteins.

Exophthalmic goiter A manifestation of Graves' disease, named for the protrusion of the eyes seen in many patients with this disease. It is also referred to as thyroid eye disease.

Exophytic Outward growing mass of tissue protruding from the wound.

Expression vector A set of DNA sequences necessary for the expression of a foreign gene in an organism, such as a plasmid. Often engineered to promote high levels of production of the gene product.

Extracellular matrix (ECM) Area where connective tissue cells and fibers are embedded.

Extravasation Leakage of plasma from dilated vessels.

Extrinsic pathway Clotting process needing substances outside the vascular system for activation.

Exudate The fluid, leukocytes, and debris that accumulate as a result of an inflammation.

F

False negative Negative test result, which should be positive.

False positive Positive test result, which should be negative.

Familial adenomatous polyposis (FAP) A genetic disease characterized by many polyps in the colorectal region.

Fat necrosis A specific form of inflammation that occurs after trauma (or other damage) to areas of the body rich in lipid.

Fatty casts Aggregated lipids that maintain the cylindrical shape of the tubule.

Fatty streak lesions Early sign of atherosclerosis as elongated flat accumulations of foam cells.

Fc receptor Cell surface receptor for the constant region of the immunoglobulin molecule.

Feedback mechanisms Biological control using levels of output, such as hormones, to control further production of substances.

Female Transition zone The junction of the ectocervix (the part of the cervix that protrudes into the vagina) and the endocervical canal (the inner part of the cervix)

Fertilization Penetration of the ovum by the sperm.

Fetal alcohol syndrome Developmental abnormalities related to heavy alcohol consumption during pregnancy.

Fetal deformation Structural changes noted at birth.

Fetal disruption Congenital abnormality caused by physical disruption of the fetus.

Fetal lung dysplasia Abnormal development of the lungs in a fetus.

Fetus The unborn offspring after eight weeks' gestation.

Fibrinogen A precursor in plasma converted into fibrin by thrombin during blood coagulation.

Fibrinolytic system Process of breaking down clots.

Fibrinous Fibrin-rich exudate.

Fibrin The meshwork of protein threads that form during the clotting of blood.

Fibrocartilage Contains many dense collagen bundles.

Fibrocystic change (FCC) Common benign cystic change in breast tissue.

Fibroma Benign tumor arising from the fibrous connective tissue of the ovary.

Fibrosis Scar formation.

Fibrous framework Layer of dense fibrous tissue located between the atria and the ventricles.

Fine-needle aspiration Sampling fluid and cells from a surface-accessible lesion.

Flagellum/flagella A whiplike process that propels an organism or sperm.

Fluorescent probes Artificial pieces of DNA labeled with a fluorescent dye.

Foamy macrophages Macrophages carrying lipids.

Focal segmental glomerulosclerosis (FSGS) Scar tissue in the filtering unit of the kidney.

Follicle-stimulating hormone (FSH) One of the gonadotropic hormones secreted by the anterior lobe of the pituitary; it stimulates the growth of ovarian follicles in females and sperm production in males.

Frozen section A method of rapid diagnosis of tumors used by the pathologist; tissue is frozen solid, cut into thin sections, stained, and examined microscopically.

G

Galactorrhea Secretion of milk by breast not associated with pregnancy or normal lactation.

Gametes Reproductive cells—egg and sperm cells—each containing 23 chromosomes, which unite during fertilization to form a zygote containing 46 chromosomes.

Gametogenesis The development of mature eggs and sperm from precursor cells.

Gangrene Tissue death caused by bacterial infection or lack of blood circulation.

Gastritis Inflammation of the stomach.

Gastroesophageal/cardiac sphincter Lower esophageal sphincter.

Gene amplification Generation of multiple copies of a gene, increasing gene activity.

Gene expression profile List of proteins synthesized by the cells, often used for diagnosis of cancer.

Gene expression The production of a product by a gene.

Gene mutation Change in the DNA sequence of the gene.

Gene therapy A process of editing a mutated gene in the cell with the objective of curing its associated diseases.

Genetic code The information carried by DNA molecules in chromosomes. The DNA basis of the phenotype/genotype.

Genetic mosaic Condition of having one or more cell populations with distinct genotype and phenotype. It can affect somatic cell, germ line cell, or both.

Genome All the genes contained in a cell's chromosomes.

Genome-wide association studies (GWAS) Process using tests of many SNPs (single nucleotide polymorphisms) to identify genes associated with particular diseases or traits.

Genomics Bioinformatic techniques applied to studies of human genome.

Genotype DNA/chromosome basis of inherited traits in an individual.

Germinal center Site in lymph node where selection for strong binding B cells occurs.

Germ layers The three layers of cells derived from the inner cell mass; each layer is destined to form specific organs and tissues in the embryo.

Gestational diabetes Elevated blood glucose caused by insulin resistance resulting from elevated hormones related to pregnancy. Blood glucose returns to normal postpartum, but the woman has an increased risk of diabetes later in life.

Gestational trophoblast disease A general term for all diseases characterized by abnormal trophoblast proliferation. Includes both hydatidiform mole and choriocarcinoma.

Gestation Duration of pregnancy from fertilization to delivery.

Ghon complexes Inactive tubercular lesions.

Gilbert syndrome Common inherited condition related to a mild lack of uridine diphosphate-glucuronyltransferase (UGT).

Gingivitis Gum inflammation.

Gliadin A protein component of gluten causing an adverse immune response that damages the small intestine.

Glial cells/neuroglia Supporting cells of tissue of the nervous system.

Glioma Any brain tumor arising from glial (supporting) cells of the brain.

Glomerular epithelium Layer of Bowman's cells closely applied to the capillaries. It is also termed the visceral layer of Bowman's capsule.

Glomerular filtration rate (GFR) Measure of the volume of body fluid cleared by the kidneys per unit of time.

Glomerulonephritis An inflammation of the glomeruli caused by either antigen–antibody complexes trapped in the glomeruli or by antiglomerular basement membrane antibodies.

Glucocorticoid An adrenal cortical hormone that regulates carbohydrate metabolism.

Gluten-sensitive enteropathy (GSE) Damage to intestinal villi in gluten-sensitive people caused by ingestion of gluten-containing food; characterized by passage of large, bulky stools containing a large amount of poorly absorbed fat.

Glycated hemoglobin test/hemoglobin A1c test A test that measures the amount of glucose permanently attached to hemoglobin, which is higher than normal in many people with diabetes.

Glycosaminoglycans (GAGs) Long, unbranched polysaccharides contributing to the ground substance.

Goiter Any enlargement of the thyroid gland.

Golgi apparatus A group of membrane-lined sacs found in the cytoplasm of the cell near the nucleus; functions with the endoplasmic reticulum to synthesize and package secretory granules.

Gonad A general term referring to either the ovary or the testis.

Gout A disorder of nucleoprotein metabolism characterized by elevated uric acid and deposition of uric acid in and around the joints.

Grade Term in cancer diagnosis describing how closely the neoplasm resembles host tissue.

Graft versus host disease Condition where a graft of immunologically active cells mounts a response to the host.

Gram stain Staining process used to differentiate the cell wall structure of bacterial cells.

Granulation tissue Normal part of the healing process.

Granulocytes Collective name for neutrophils, eosinophils, and basophils.

Granulosa cell tumor/thecoma An ovarian tumor arising from the estrogen-producing granulose cell of an ovarian follicle.

Graves' disease An autoimmune thyroid disease in which autoantibodies resembling thyroid-stimulating hormone stimulate an excessive output of thyroid hormone, causing hyperthyroidism.

Gray matter Part of the brain containing the neuronal cell bodies and many of the supportive glial cells.

Gross examination Study of diseased organ with the naked eye.

Ground substance Gel-like substance in the ECM in which fibers and cells are embedded.

Growth factor A soluble growth-promoting substance produced by cells that attaches to receptors on the cell membrane of other cells, which activates the receptors and initiates events leading to growth or division of the target cells.

Growth hormone (GH), or somatotropin An anterior lobe pituitary hormone that stimulates the growth of bone and other body tissues.

Guillain-Barré syndrome A type of polyneuritis resulting from an autoimmune reaction.

Gynecomastia Excessive development of the male breast.

H

Haploid Cell containing 1N of each chromosome, a gamete.

Hashimoto thyroiditis An autoimmune disease in which an autoantibody is directed against thyroid epithelial cells, causing progressive destruction of the thyroid gland, leading to chronic hypothyroidism.

Hayflick limit Fixed number of cell divisions possible for a normal cell.

Heavy chains (H chains) Longer of two types of chains making up an immunoglobulin molecule.

Hemarthrosis Arthritic condition caused by bleeding into the joint.

Hematemesis Bloody vomit, an indication of bleeding in upper GI, a medical emergency.

Hematoma Accumulation of blood within tissue.

Hematopoietic tissue Tissue that forms the blood cells.

Hemiplegia Paralysis of one side of the body.

Hemizygous A term applied to genes located on the X chromosome in the male.

Hemoglobin An oxygen transport protein within red cells composed of an iron-porphyrin complex (heme) combined with a protein chain (globin).

Hemolysis Destruction of blood cells.

Hemopericardium Hematoma between the heart and its pericardial lining.

Hemophilia A Bleeding disease caused by lack of active F.VIII.

Hemophilia B Bleeding disease caused by lack of active F.IX.

Hemorrhage Release of blood into surrounding tissue.

Hemorrhagic diathesis Variety of clinical disorders in which small injuries lead to unusual bleeding.

Hemorrhagic Red cell–rich inflammatory fluid.

Hemorrhoids Dilated veins around the anus and the rectum.

Hemostasis The body's biological processes to stop bleeding and prevent hemorrhage, including vasoconstriction, platelet plugging, and coagulation.

Hemothorax Hematoma within the chest.

Heparin An anticoagulant produced by the liver.

Hepatitis B core antigen (HBcAg) The antigen contained in the core of the hepatitis B virus.

Hepatitis B e-antigen (HBeAg) Antigen associated with active hepatitis B virus proliferation.

Hepatitis B surface antigen (HBsAg) The coating of the hepatitis B virus that is also found in great excess in the blood of infected patients.

Hepatitis Inflammation of the liver.

Hepatocellular carcinoma (HCC) Most common liver cancer.

Hernia A protrusion of a loop of bowel through a narrow opening, usually in the abdominal wall.

Herpes zoster A virus that causes chicken pox.

Heterochromatin Small dense mass of condensed chromatin appearing in inactivated X chromosomes.

Heterophile antibodies Antibodies that react with substances unrelated to the immunizing antigen.

Heterozygous Having two different alleles at a given gene locus on the homologous pair of chromosomes.

High-density lipoprotein (HDL) Plasma protein molecule carrying cholesterol away from the tissue.

High-grade disseminated cancer Cancer cells that are poorly differentiated (aggressive) and extensively spread throughout the body.

Hilus A depression in an organ from where the blood vessels enter or leave.

Histamine Chemical released by mast cells.

Histocompatibility The degree of being compatible between tissues of different individuals, such as donor and recipient, controlled by the HLA gene.

Histologic examination Study of disease using a microscope to examine tissue.

Histone A protein found in the nucleus, which is important in the packaging of DNA.

Histoplasmosis An infection caused by the fungus *Histoplasma capsulatum*.

HLA system The genes of the histocompatibility complex and the antigens that they determine on the surface of cells.

Hodgkin cell Abnormal mononucleated lymphocyte.

Hodgkin's lymphoma (HL) A form of lymphoma that occurs in young adults with Hodgkin and Reed-Sternberg cells mixed with other cell types.

Homeostasis A dynamic process where the body maintains stable internal conditions while reacting to changes in both the internal and external environments.

Homocysteine/homocysteinemia Sulfur-containing amino acid/excessive levels of homocysteine.

Homologous chromosomes A matched pair of chromosomes, one derived from each parent.

Homozygous Having the same alleles at a given gene locus on the homologous chromosome pair.

Host Individual infected with a disease-producing organism.

Human chorionic gonadotropin (hCG) A hormone made by the placenta in pregnancy with actions similar to pituitary gonadotropins. Same hormone is made by neoplastic cells in some types of malignant testicular tumors.

Human chorionic somatomammotropin (hCS) One of the hormones produced by the placenta that has properties similar to the pituitary growth hormone. Also termed human placental lactogen.

Human epidermal growth factor receptor 2 (HER-2) A protein on the surface of breast cells that can bind to the human epidermal growth factor.

Human papillomavirus (HPV) A virus that stimulates epithelial cell proliferation. Causes warts and genital tract condylomas.

Humoral immunity Immunity associated with the formation of antibodies produced by plasma cells.

Hyaline cartilage Most common type of cartilage; contains only a few fine collagen fibers.

Hydatidiform mole A neoplastic proliferation of trophoblast associated with the formation of large cystic villi.

Hydrocele An accumulation of excess fluid within the tunica vaginalis of the testis.

Hydrocephalus Dilatation of the cerebral ventricular system caused by pressure arising from accumulation of cerebrospinal fluid within the ventricles.

Hydronephrosis A dilatation of the urinary drainage tract proximal to the site of an obstruction.

Hydropic swelling Cell swelling as a result of excessive water uptake by a cell. Associated with failure of active transport of ions.

Hydrothorax Accumulation of fluid in the pleural cavity.

Hydroureter A dilatation of the ureter secondary to obstruction of the urinary drainage system, often associated with coexisting dilatation of the renal pelvis and calyces (hydronephrosis).

Hygiene hypothesis Hypothesis that lack of early childhood exposure to infectious agents, symbiotic microorganisms (such as the gut flora or probiotics), and parasites increases susceptibility to allergic reaction or response by suppressing the natural development of the immune system.

Hyperbilirubinemia High levels of unconjugated bilirubin in the newborn.

Hypercholesterolemia Elevated blood cholesterol.

Hyperemesis gravidarum Excess vomiting associated with pregnancy.

Hyperemia Increased blood flow through vessels.

Hyperglycemia Blood glucose levels higher than the normal range.

Hyperlipidemia Elevated blood lipids.

Hyperosmolar coma Coma resulting from neurologic dysfunction caused by hyperosmolarity of body fluids as a consequence of severe hyperglycemia.

Hyperplasia An increase in the number of cells.

Hypersensitivity reaction A state of increased abnormal reactivity to a foreign material.

Hypertension Excessively high systemic blood pressure.

Hypertonic solution A solution having a greater osmolarity than body fluids, which causes cells to shrink (crenate) in such a solution because water moves by osmosis from the cells into the hypertonic solution.

Hypertrophy An enlargement or overgrowth of an organ caused by an increase in the size of its constituent cells.

Hyphae Filamentous branching structures formed by fungi.

Hypoglycemia Lower than normal concentration of glucose in the blood.

Hyponatremia Lower than normal concentration of sodium ions in the plasma and extracellular fluid.

Hypospadias A congenital abnormality of penile development.

Hypotension Abnormally low blood pressure.

Hypotonic solution A solution having a lower osmolarity than body fluids, causing cells in the solution to swell because water moves by osmosis from the hypotonic solution into the cells.

I

Iatrogenic Disease resulting from a medical examination or treatment.

Idiopathic Disease of unknown origin.

Iliac crest Area of hip bone in abdomen.

Immune complex Combination of antibody and antigen forming a lattice.

Immune memory Enhanced and more rapid immune response upon secondary encounter with antigen in adaptive immunity.

Immunogen Antigen that can provoke an adaptive immune response by binding to antigen receptors.

Immunoglobulin The class of proteins that includes antibodies.

Immunological techniques Procedures using antibody or antigen preparations, usually with chemical labels.

Immunotherapy Treatment given to retard growth of a disseminated malignant tumor by stimulating the body's own immune defenses.

Inclusion bodies Spherical structures in the nucleus or cytoplasm of virus-infected cells or intracytoplasmic clusters of organisms such as Chlamydiae within a cell.

Infarction Cell and tissue death from impaired blood supply.

Infarct Necrosis of tissue caused by interruption of its blood supply.

Infection Invasion by pathogens, which stimulates the hosts immune and inflammatory processes.

Infectious mononucleosis A common viral disease, the most common cause of benign lymphocytosis.

Inferior vena cava syndrome This syndrome occurs with blockage or compression of the inferior vena cava and results in edema of the lower extremities.

Inflammation An early defensive reaction by the body to tissue damage and/or infection.

Innate immunity Immunity present at birth and lasting a person's entire life and the first response of the body's immune system to a harmful foreign substance, non specific, no immune memory involved.

Inner cell mass A group of cells derived from the fertilized ovum that are destined to form the embryo.

Insulin reaction/insulin shock Condition in which there is too much insulin in the blood.

Insulin resistance Condition when target tissues are relatively insensitive to the action of insulin.

Interferon A broad-spectrum antiviral agent produced by various cells in the body.

Interferon alpha A broad-spectrum antiviral agent produced by various cells in the body.

Interleukin A type of cytokine produced by leukocytes and other body cells, involved in activation and maturation of immune cells.

Interleukin-1 (IL-1) Pro-inflammatory cytokine, regulates immune response such as fever, leukocytes adhesion, and release of acute phase protein by the liver.

Interleukin-2 (IL-2) A lymphokine that stimulates growth of lymphocytes.

Intermediate filaments Small, tough filaments of high tensile strength within the cell cytoplasm and nucleus.

Intermediate host Organism that harbors an immature stage of a parasite.

Interstitial pneumonia Characterized by the thickening of supporting tissues between the air sacs of the lungs.

Intervertebral disk A fibrocartilaginous structure between adjacent vertebral bodies.

Intramembranous bone formation Direct formation of bone by osteoblasts without prior formation of a cartilage model.

Intraoperative During surgery.

Intrinsic pathway Clotting process needing only substances within the blood vessels.

Intussusception Telescoping of a bowel segment into an adjacent segment.

Invasive hydatidiform mole An aggressive hydatidiform mole that invades the uterine wall.

Invasive testing Test requiring a physical invasion of the body.

Invasive Tumor Type that infiltrates host tissue.

Irritable bowel syndrome (IBS) A condition characterized by frequent loose stools and excessive amounts of mucus. This umbrella term includes Crohn's disease and ulcerative colitis.

Ischemia Poor blood supply to cells of tissues that may lead to injury or death.

Islets of Langerhans Cluster of endocrine cells in the pancreas.

Isotonic solution A solution having essentially the same osmolarity as body fluids so that cells neither shrink nor swell when exposed to the solution.

J

Jaundice Yellow discoloration of skin and the white part of the eyes (sclera) resulting from an accumulation of bilirubin in the body.

Juxtacrine Cell-to-cell communication by direct contact or contact with the extracellular matrix.

Juxtaglomerular apparatus A specialized group of cells at the vascular pole of the glomerulus that regulates blood flow through the glomerulus of the kidneys.

K

Karyotype Chromosomes from a single cell arranged in pairs in descending order according to the size of the chromosomes and the positions of the centromeres used to visualize the chromosome composition of an individual.

Keratin An insoluble sulfur-containing protein that is the principal constituent of the hair and nails.

Keratin filament Type of filament in epithelial cells.

Keratinization Accumulation of a fibrous protein called keratin inside cells.

Kernicterus/bilirubin encephalopathy Severe brain damage caused by high levels of unconjugated bilirubin in the infant.

ketoacidosis A buildup of ketone bodies due to increased fat metabolism and decreased carbohydrate metabolism, often resulting in a decrease (acidification) of the plasma or other body fluids.

Ketone bodies Three related compounds (acetone, acetoacetic acid, and beta-hydroxybutyric acid) are produced during the metabolism of fats. These molecules are small and water-soluble.

L

Labile cell populations Cells that divide continually.

Laboratory medicine Analysis of clinical and biology specimens to aid in diagnosing disease.

Laceration An irregular jagged wound.

Lamin filament A protein involved in nuclear structure in all cells.

Laparoscope A long tubular telescope-like instrument passed through the abdominal wall to examine structures within the peritoneal cavity.

Latent autoimmune diabetes of adults (LADA) Subtype of type 1 diabetes first appearing in adults.

Latent tuberculosis Arrested tuberculosis infection containing viable organisms.

Lecithin A phosphorus-containing lipid (phospholipid) having detergent properties similar to bile salts.

Legionnaires' disease A type of pneumonia caused by an airborne bacterium called *Legionella pneumophila*.

Leiomyomas Benign, smooth muscle tumors in the uterus.

Lesion Any structural abnormality or pathologic change.

Leukemia A neoplastic proliferation of leukocytes.

Leukocyte Collective term for white cells.

Leukopenia An abnormally small number of leukocytes in the peripheral blood.

Leukoplakia A white patch of hyperplastic and usually atypical squamous epithelium on the oral mucosa or genital tract mucosa.

Leukotriene A prostaglandin-like mediator of inflammation.

Lewy bodies Damaged neurites characteristic of Parkinson's disease.

Light chains (L chains) Shorter of two types of chains making up an immunoglobulin molecule.

Liver lobule A histologic subdivision of the liver in which columns of liver cells converge toward a central vein and portal tracts are located at the periphery.

Lobular carcinoma Tumor of the breast arising from the lobules.

Locus The location of a gene on a chromosome.

Low-density lipoprotein (LDL) Plasma protein molecule carrying cholesterol to the tissue.

Luminal A/Luminal B Specific types of gene expression profiles found in breast cancer cells.

Lung lobule A small group of terminal bronchioles and their subdivisions.

Luteinizing hormone (LH) One of the gonadotropic hormones secreted by the anterior lobe of the pituitary; it triggers ovulation in females, and production of testosterone in males.

Lyme disease A tick-borne systemic infection caused by a spirochete, *Borrelia burgdorferi*, characterized by neurologic, joint, and cardiac manifestations.

Lymphadenitis An inflammation of lymph nodes draining a site of infection.

Lymphadenopathy Enlargement of one or more lymph nodes.

Lymphangitis An inflammation of lymph vessels draining a site of infection.

Lymphatic tissue Tissue that forms the lymphatic system.

Lymphocyte A mononuclear blood cell produced in lymphoid tissue that takes part in cell-mediated and humoral immunity.

Lymphoid leukemia Neoplasm of B-cell or T-cell lineage involving primarily the bone marrow and peripheral blood.

Lymphokine A soluble hormone-like substance liberated by lymphocytes.

Lymphoma A neoplasm of lymphoid cells limited to lymph nodes and sometimes spleen.

Lysosome A cytoplasmic organelle containing digestive enzymes with an acidic pH internal environment.

M

Macrophage-like cells (monocytes) Type of white blood cell important in the immune response.

Magnetic resonance imaging (MRI) A diagnostic procedure that yields computer-generated images based on the movement of hydrogen atoms in tissues subjected to a strong magnetic field.

Major histocompatibility complex (MHC) A group of proteins that bind to peptide fragments derived from pathogens and display and present them to corresponding T cells. In humans, the genes coded for MHC are located on chromosome 6.

Malformation Defect in development.

Malignant Quality of neoplasms that spread to sites distant from their origin.

Mallory body An irregular, red-staining structure in the cytoplasm of injured liver cells, usually resulting from alcohol-induced liver injury.

Mammary ridges Location of embryonic cells that develop into breasts.

Mammogram An X-ray image of the breast that helps to detect tumors and other abnormalities within the breast.

Mammography Technique used to create an X-ray image of the breast that helps to detect tumors and other abnormalities within the breast.

Marasmus Global deficiency of caloric intake in infants and children.

Marfan syndrome A hereditary connective tissue disease characterized by excessive joint flexibility along with various skeletal and cardiovascular abnormalities.

Mast cell A specialized connective tissue cell containing granules filled with histamine and other chemical mediators.

Mature teratomas/dermoid cyst A common type of benign cystic teratoma that commonly arises in the ovary.

McBurney's point Localization of pain to region of abdomen specific for appendicitis.

Media Solid, liquid, or gel-sol substances created to support the growth of organisms *in vitro*.

Mediastinum Middle compartment of the thorax.

Medulla Inner part of an organ.

Meiosis A special type of cell division resulting in gamete production (ova and sperm) in which the number of chromosomes is reduced by one-half.

Melanin-stimulating hormone (MSH) One of the hormones produced by the pituitary. Causes darkening of the skin.

Membranous glomerulopathy A slowly progressive disease of the glomeruli most often found in White and Asian patients between the ages of thirty and fifty.

Menarche Onset of menses.

Meninges The membranes covering the brain and spinal cord.

Meningioma A benign tumor arising from the meninges.

Meningitis Inflammation of the meninges.

Meningocele A protrusion of meninges through a defect in the spinal vertebral arches.

Meningoencephalitis A serious disease of the brain and its linings, which can be caused by amoebic infections from freshwater sources.

Meningomyelocele A type of spina bifida characterized by protrusion of meninges and cord through the defect in the vertebral arches.

Mesoderm The middle germ layer of the embryo, which gives rise to specific organs and tissues.

Mesothelium A layer of flat, squamous epithelial cells that covers the surfaces of the pleural, pericardial, and peritoneal cavities.

Metabolic acidosis Condition with decreased plasma pH resulting from a decrease in serum bicarbonate, often associated with loss of acidic gastric contents, overuse of certain diuretics, or endocrine disease.

Metabolic alkalosis Condition with elevated plasma pH resulting from increased bicarbonate level due to diseases in the endocrine system or loss of hydrogen ions.

Metabolic syndrome A syndrome characterized by obesity and insulin resistance often associated with nonalcoholic fatty liver disease.

Metaphysis Region below the epiphyseal plate containing cancellous bone and active bone marrow.

Metaplasia Conversion of one differentiated tissue type to another.

Metastasize The spread of cancer cells from the primary site of origin to a distant site within the body.

Metazoan parasite Complex multicelled animal parasite, such as worms and flukes.

Micelle Spherical structure formed by the aggregation of surfactant molecules. In aqueous solution the hydrophobic regions face inward and the hydrophilic areas interact with the aqueous solution.

Microcephaly Condition in which an infant's head circumference is smaller than normal, often due to failure of the brain to develop normally.

Microglia Macrophage-like cells that regulate brain development, maintenance of neuronal networks, and injury repair.

Micro-RNA (miRNA) Small RNA molecules that regulate the activity of sets of individual genes.

Microtubule Largest type of cell framework filament.

Miliary tuberculosis Multiple foci of tuberculosis throughout the body as a result of bloodstream dissemination of tubercle bacilli from a primary focus in the lung or peribronchial lymph nodes.

Milliequivalents (mEq) Measurement of the amount of an ion in body fluids.

Millimolar Concentration of one thousandth of a mole per liter of solvent.

Mineralocorticoid Adrenal cortical hormone that regulates salt and water metabolism.

Minimal change nephropathy Common kidney disease of young children that is generally idiopathic.

Mitochondria Bean-shaped structures in the cell capable of converting molecules into energy to power the cell.

Mitosis The type of cell division for somatic/body cells in which chromosomes from parent cells are duplicated and transferred to daughter cells. This type of cell division produces two daughter cells that are identical with each other and to the parent cell. The characteristic cell division found in all cells in the body except for the gametes.

Mitotic spindle Microtubule structure organized around the centriole during cell division.

Mitral valve AV valve, also called the bicuspid valve, separating the left atrium and ventricle.

Mnemonics Aids to memory.

Monoclonal antibodies Antibodies with a unique specificity for use in treating human disease, produced in tissue culture from a single clone of immune cells.

Monocyte The largest leukocyte, a phagocytic cell that forms part of the reticuloendothelial system.

Motor end plate Neuromuscular junction between nerve and muscle.

Mucinous tumor Ovarian tumor made of cells resembling the mucus-secreting epithelium of the endocervix.

Multifactorial pattern of inheritance Transmission of a trait, condition, or congenital anomaly that involves the likely interaction of multiple gene loci as well as probable environmental interactions. The inheritance pattern does not follow Mendelian genetic patterns.

Multiple myeloma A neoplasm of plasma cells characterized by production of M-protein.

Multiple sclerosis (MS) Chronic progressive autoimmune disease characterized by focal areas of demyelination in the central nervous system, followed by glial scarring.

Muscle tone The slight contractility (tension) present in resting muscles.

Mutation Alteration in the DNA sequence of the genome.

Myasthenia gravis An autoimmune disease characterized by abnormal fatigability of muscle and caused by an autoantibody that damages the acetylcholine receptors at the neuromuscular junction.

Mycelium Matted mass of hyphae forming a fluffy colony characteristic of fungi.

Myelin Lipid based molecule secreted by some glial cells the wraps around the axon of a neuron. It provides protection and increases the rate of signal transmission.

Myelitis An inflammation of the spinal cord.

Myelodysplastic syndrome Marrow disease with features of a "pre-leukemia."

Myeloid leukemia Characterized by rapid growth of abnormal white blood cells that accumulate in the bone marrow and interfere with the production of normal blood cells.

Myocardial infarct/heart attack Necrosis of heart muscle as a result of interruption of its blood supply. May affect full thickness of muscle wall (transmural infarct) or only part of the wall (subendocardial infarct).

Myocardial ischemia Inadequate blood flow through the coronary arteries to the heart muscle.

Myosin Contractile and motor protein that uses ATP to drive muscle cell contraction and relaxation cycles.

Myositis Inflammation of muscle.

Myxedema Hypothyroidism in the adult.

N

Natural killer (NK) cells Lymphocytes capable of destroying foreign or abnormal cells, although they have not had any prior antigenic contact with the cells.

Necrosis Unprogrammed cell death as a result of injury and subsequent structural changes. Often results in a host response.

Necrotizing fasciitis Destruction of subcutaneous tissues in beta streptococcal infection.

Neisseria gonorrhoeae Bacterium causing gonorrhea.

Neoadjuvant therapy Therapy used before primary cancer treatment.

Neoplasia A form of uncontrolled cell growth that may follow dysplasia and lead to formation of a tumor.

Nephrosclerosis Thickening and narrowing of the afferent glomerular arterioles.

Nephrosis Renal disease resulting from excessive protein loss in the urine, caused by various types of renal injury. Also referred to as nephrotic syndrome.

Nephrotic syndrome Characterized by severe loss of plasma protein into urine.

Neurodegenerative proteinopathies General classification of diseases caused by misfolded abnormal proteins resulting in neural disease.

Neurofibromas Tumors that contain neoplastic Schwann cells and other cells; von Recklinghausen disease is an example.

Neurofilament Type of filament in nerve cells.

Neuroglia Supporting cells of the nervous system that do not conduct electrical impulses.

Neuron A nerve cell, including the nerve cell body and its processes.

Neuropil The densely packed interworven areas of the central nervous system containing nerve and glial cells that form the gray matter.

Neutrophils A type of polymorphonuclear (PMN) leukocyte that is actively phagocytic; most abundant of all leukocytes.

Nonalcoholic fatty liver disease (NAFLD) Fatty liver without significant inflammation or scarring within the liver, which usually occurs in insulin-resistant obese people with lipid abnormalities.

Nonatypical endometrial hyperplasia Uterine condition characterized by unevenly distributed areas of increasing gland density in the uterus.

Noninvasive testing Diagnostic procedure requiring no physical invasion of the body.

Non-ossifying fibroma A defect in the cortical bone of children.

Non-steroidal anti-inflammatory drugs (NSAIDs) Drug such as ibuprofen and naproxen that inhibit the production of prostaglandins.

Norepinephrine Is both a neurotransmitter in the autonomic nervous system and a hormone secreted by the adrenal medulla.

Norovirus An extremely infectious RNA virus easily spread from person to person and by contaminated food or water.

Nuclear pleomorphism Irregular nuclear structures seen in groups of dysplastic cells.

Nucleoli Structure containing RNA in the nucleus.

Nucleosome A bead-like structure of DNA wrapped around histone and other nuclear proteins.

Nucleotide Basic structural unit of DNA or RNA consisting of a phosphate group linked to a five-carbon sugar, deoxyribose or ribose.

Nucleus pulposus The soft elastic center of the intervertebral disk.

O

Obstructive jaundice Symptom from a blocked common bile duct.

Occlusion Blockage or closing of an open blood vessel or hollow organ.

Oligodendroglia/Oligodendrocyte/Schwann cells Types of neurogila that wrap around nerve axons within the central and peripheral nervous sytems. They provide the myelin sheath that protect the axon and speeds up nerve transmission.

Oligohydramnios An insufficient quantity of amnionic fluid.

Oncofetal antigens Proteins normally synthesized only during fetal development and associated with neoplasia.

Oncogene An abnormally functioning gene that causes unrestrained cell growth leading to formation of a tumor. Results from mutation or translocation of a proto-oncogene.

Oncologist Physician specializing in treatment of cancer.

Oncosis Cell death due to swelling of epithelial cells caused by failure of pumping out Na+ ions. A type of necrosis.

Oncotic pressure Osmotic pressure exerted by a very large molecule such as blood proteins.

One-second forced expiratory volume (FEV_1) The maximum volume of air that can be expelled from the lungs in one second.

Oocyst Infectious form of a parasite that contains the zygote.

Oocyte Germ cells in a late stage of egg development.

Opportunistic host Accidental host of parasite, often humans.

Opportunistic infection Infection in an immunocompromised person caused by an organism that is normally nonpathogenic or of limited pathogenicity.

Opsonins Plasma proteins that attract neutrophils and macrophages to foreign material.

Organelle A small structure with specific functions present inside the cell.

Organs A group of different tissues, which perform a specific function.

Organ systems A group of organs that function together as a unit, such as the various organs of the gastrointestinal tract.

Osler-Weber-Rendu disease (OWRD)/hereditary hemorrhagic telangiectasia (HHT) Disease caused by hereditary defects in blood vessels leading to spontaneous bleeding.

Osmolarity A measure of the osmotic pressure exerted by a solution.

Osmosis The movement of water molecules from a dilute solution to a more concentrated one.

Osmotic activity/osmotic pressure "Water attracting" property of a solution.

Osteoarthritis A "wear and tear" degeneration of the major weight-bearing joints.

Osteoblasts/osteocytes/osteoclasts Types of cells in bone; active bone-forming cells, mature bone cells, and bone resorption cells, respectively.

Osteogenesis imperfecta A genetic disease with mutations involving collagen production causing bones to be excessivley brittle.

Osteomalacia Impaired calcification of bone in an adult caused by vitamin D deficiency, which also contributes to bone loss caused by osteoporosis.

Osteomyelitis An inflammation of bone.

Osteoporosis Generalized thinning and demineralization of bone that tends to occur frequently in postmenopausal women but may occur in males as well.

Osteosarcoma/osteogenic sarcoma Primary bone tumor.

Oxidizing agents Chemicals that will accept electrons from other chemicals. In the inflammatory response they can be synthesized by neutrophils that help destroy bacteria and fungi.

Oxytocin A hormone that is stored and released in the posterior lobe of the pituitary gland that causes uterine contractions during labor and ejection of milk from the breast lobules into the larger ducts.

P

Panhypopituitarism Failure of secretion of all anterior lobe pituitary hormones.

Papilloma Otherwise known as a wart, a neoplasm produced after human papilloma virus infection.

Pap smear A collection of cells from the cervix. Commonly used as a screening test for cervical cancer.

Paracrine Cell-to-cell communication by soluble mediators released from a cell and acting on nearby groups of cells.

Parasites Organism that lives in or on another organism, deriving nutrients at the host's expense.

Parenchymal cell The functional cell of an organ or tissue.

Parenchyma The functional cells of an organ, as contrasted with the connective and supporting tissue that forms its framework.

Paresthesia An abnormal sensation, such as burning, prickling, or numbness.

Parkinson's disease A chronic disease of the central nervous system characterized by rigidity and tremor, caused by decreased concentration of dopamine in the central nervous system.

Partial thromboplastin time (PTT) test A test that measures the overall efficiency of the blood coagulation process. Detects defects in intrinsic coagulation and is used to monitor heparin therapy.

Pathogen-Associated Molecular Patterns (PAMPs) Microbial products that stimulate innate immunity.

Pathogenesis Progression of the development of a disease.

Pathogens Disease-causing microorganisms.

Pathologist Person who studies the structural and functional changes in the body caused by disease.

Patient-centered medicine Practice of medicine providing care that is respectful of and responsive to individual preferences, needs, and values and ensuring that people's values guide all clinical decisions.

Pattern of inheritance Occurrence of detectable traits across generations in a family.

Pectus excavatum Posterior displacement of the sternum caused by excessive growth of costal cartilages, which reduce the size of the retrosternal space available for the heart within the mediastinum.

Pedigree Formal pattern displaying the inheritance of traits or gene products through generations of a family.

Pelvic inflammatory disease (PID) A general term for an infection affecting the fallopian tubes and adjacent pelvic organs.

Periapical abscess Infection of the tooth root.

Pericardium Fibrous sac enclosing the heart.

Periodontal disease Pockets of infection between teeth and gum.

Periosteum The tough, fibrous membrane that covers a bone, except for its articular surfaces.

Peripheral tolerance A process to further eliminate self-reactive T cells and B cells that escaped from central tolerance; takes place in secondary lymphoid organs.

Peripheral zone Part of the prostate that surrounds the other zones.

Peristalsis The wavelike contractions of the wall of a tubular anatomic structure such as the alimentary tract or ureter, which propel luminal contents forward.

Periumbilical Situated in the abdominal area near belly button.

Permanent Type of population of cells that have no ability to divide.

Peroxisome A cytoplasmic organelle containing various enzymes, including those that decompose potentially toxic compounds through the production of hydrogen peroxide.

Petechiae A small pinpoint hemorrhages caused by decreased platelets, abnormal platelet function, or capillary defect.

Phagocytic Capable of engulfing and destroying agents that are injurious to the cell.

Phagocytic vacuole Membrane-lined vacuole used to contain foreign material.

Phagocytosis Process by which the cell engulfs foreign material.

Phenotype Collection of inherited/phenotypic traits detectable in an individual.

Phenotypic traits Characteristics apparent in the individual.

Pheochromocytoma Catecholamine-secreting tumor of the adrenal medulla.

Philadelphia chromosome Chromosome translocation common in neoplastic cells of chronic myelogenous leukemia.

Phlebitis Inflammation of a vein.

Phocomelia A congenital reduction deformity where the limbs do not develop properly and the hands and/or feet are abnormally close to the trunk.

Phototherapy Fluorescent light treatment of jaundiced babies to reduce the concentration of unconjugated bilirubin in their blood.

Physiological adaptive change Cell or organ response to changing conditions.

Pia (mater) The innermost of the three membranes covering the brain and spinal cord.

Pinocytosis Process similar to phagocytosis but for the ingestion of extra-cellular fluid.

Pinworm A small parasitic worm infecting humans. Lives in the lower bowel and causes perianal pruritus.

Pituitary dwarfism Stunted growth caused by a deficiency of growth hormone in a child.

Pituitary gigantism A condition resulting from excessive secretion of growth hormone in the child.

Placenta Flat, disk-shaped structure that maintains the developing organism within the uterus.

Placenta previa Attachment of the placenta in the uterus such that it partially or completely covers the cervix.

Plasma oncotic pressure The likelihood of osmotic movement of water from the surrounding tissues into the plasma is mostly driven by the concentration of the plasma proteins in blood.

Plasmin Blood enzyme that degrades blood plasma proteins, including fibrin clots.

Plasminogen Precursor compound of plasmin in the blood.

Platelet A component of the blood; a roughly circular or oval disk formed from the plasma membrane of the megakaryocytes found in the bone marrow. Platelets are a key component in blood coagulation.

Platelet activation Release of active clotting components after adhesion of platelets.

Platelet agonists Substances promoting platelet function.

Pleura The mesothelial covering of the lung (visceral pleura) and chest wall (parietal pleura).

Pneumoconiosis An occupational lung disease caused by inhalation of injurious substances.

Pneumonia Inflammation of the lung.

Pneumothorax Accumulation of air in the pleural cavity.

Podocytes Cells with highly branched cytoplasmic processes covering the glomerular capillaries of the kidneys.

Point-of-care test Laboratory test that can be performed at the patient's bedside or in the physician's office.

Polyclonal antibodies Humoral response consisting of antibodies produced by a number of clones of B cells.

Polycystic ovary syndrome (PCOS) Common endocrine disorder and common cause of anovulatory infertility; associated with obesity, diabetes, and hirsutism.

Polycythemia An increase of red cells and hemoglobin above normal levels.

Polyhydramnios An excess of amnionic fluid.

Polymerase chain reaction (PCR) Technology used to amplify stretches of DNA.

Polymorphism Collection of common alleles for a single gene found in populations.

Polymorphonuclear leukocytes (PMN) A leukocyte having a multilobed nucleus whose cytoplasm is filled with fine granules.

Polyneuropathies An inflammation of multiple nerves.

Polyp/papilloma Wart-like benign tumor often associated with viral infection.

Porins Unique proteins on G-bacteria's outer membrane that contribute to resistance to antimicrobial agents.

Portal hypertension Characterized by increased resistance to blood outflow and impaired liver function.

Portal tract/triad Branches of the hepatic artery, portal vein, and bile duct are located at the periphery of liver lobule.

Positive/negative selection Selection of lymphocytes with receptors recognizing self MHC molecules (positive selection)/deletion of lymphocytes that strongly bind to self-antigen (negative selection).

Positron emission tomography (PET) scan Imaging using radioactive tracers that analyzes metabolic or biochemical functioning.

Posterior urethra The section of the male urethra encompassing the membranous urethra and the prostate urethra.

Postsinusoidal portal hypertension Hypertension resulting from thrombosis of the hepatic vein.

Precancerous Describing an area of dysplasia in early stages of cancer development.

Prediabetes Higher than normal blood glucose but not high enough to establish diagnosis of diabetes.

Preeclampsia A pregnancy-related complication characterized by hypertension and proteinuria that usually occurs after the twentieth week of gestation, thought to be caused by placental dysfunction.

Presinusoidal portal hypertension Portal hypertension resulting from occlusions in the portal vein.

Primary gout A metabolic disease caused by overproduction of uric acid, reduced excretion of uric acid, or a combination of both factors. Clinical manifestations are related to precipitation of uric acid in joints, kidneys, and other sites.

Primary hemostasis Part of hemostatic process that is mostly platelet-dependent.

Primary hemostatic plug Mass of aggregated platelets at site of injury.

Primary lymphoid organs Bone marrow and thymus.

Primary site Tissue of origin for neoplasm.

Primary tuberculosis Initial infection of tuberculosis.

Primary union Form of healing of a sutured wound.

Prion A protein infectious particle responsible for Creutzfeldt-Jakob disease and some other degenerative diseases of the nervous system, such as Kuru.

Progerias Diseases characterized by dramatic and premature aging.

Prognosis The probable outcome of a disease or disorder, the outlook for recovery.

Progressive primary tuberculosis Initial tubercular infection that does not go into remission.

Prolactin Hormone produced by the anterior lobe of the pituitary gland that stimulates milk secretion.

Proliferative phase Growth of endometrial cells lining the uterus.

Prone Lying on the back with feet toward the viewer.

Prostaglandin A series of derivatives of arachidonic acid that have widespread physiologic effects.

Prostatic-specific antigen (PSA) An antigen produced by prostatic epithelial cells that is often found in higher-than-normal concentrations in the blood of patients with prostatic cancer and other diseases of the prostate.

Proteoglycans/mucoproteins Extremely large molecules in connective tissue.

Prothrombin Clotting factor activated by factor X to release thrombin/FIIa.

Prothrombin time (PT) test A test that detects defects in extrinsic coagulation and is used to monitor warfarin-like anticoagulant therapy.

Proto-oncogenes A gene promoting cell growth, differentiation, or mitotic activity associated with neoplasia.

Protozoan parasite Simple one-celled animal parasite, such as the plasmodium causing malaria.

Proud flesh Growth of excessive granulation tissue that can gape above the wound.

Pseudoautosomal region (of the X chromosome) The region of the X chromosome containing genes which are not inactivated

Public health Area of medicine concerned with the health of populations.

Pulmonary congestion Pooling of blood in the lungs.

Pulmonary valve Semilunar valve surrounding the orifices of the pulmonary artery.

Pulpitis Inflammation of the dental pulp.

Purpura Bleeding under the skin or mucus membrane observed as large discolored areas on the skin.

Purulent Neutrophil-rich exudate, also called pus.

R

Radiograph An image taken with X-rays.

Radiologist Physician specializing in the use and analysis of imaging techniques and results.

Reactive oxygen species (ROS) Highly reactive molecules containing oxygen that can be either environmentally- or self-produced and can damage cells.

Receptor Cell signal receiver.

Receptor molecules/Pattern/Pathogen Recognition Receptors (PRRs) Receptors on cells recognizing molecular markers of disease-causing microorganism.

Recessive gene A gene that expresses a trait only when present in the homozygous state.

Recombinant DNA technology/genetic engineering/gene splicing Methods for combining a gene from one organism, such as a gene specifying insulin synthesis, with genes from another organism, such as a bacterium.

Reduction division Process occurring in meiosis reducing the 2N pairs of chromosomes to 1N.

Reed-Sternberg cell Abnormal multinucleated lymphocyte.

Reflux esophagitis Inflammation of the lining of the esophagus caused by reflux of acidic gastric secretions through an incompetent lower gastroesophageal sphincter.

Regulatory T cells Type of T cells that modulate the extent of immune response and prevent autoimmune activity.

Regurgitation Backward flow of blood in the heart because of a valve does not close properly.

Releasing hormones Hormone synthesized in the hypothalamus that act to stimulate release of specific hormones from the anterior pituitary.

Renal pelvis/major calyces Expanded upper end of the ureter and divisions of the renal pelvis.

Renin An enzyme secreted by the kidneys in response to a fall in blood pressure, blood volume, or sodium concentration.

Resolution Regression of an inflammatory process without significant tissue destruction and with return of the tissues to normal.

Respiratory acidosis Decreased plasma pH due to insufficient excretion of CO_2.

Respiratory alkalosis Elevated blood pH resulting from increased excretion of CO_2.

Respiratory unit A functional unit of the lung consisting of a cluster of respiratory bronchioles, alveolar ducts, and alveoli derived from a single terminal bronchiole. Another term for acinus.

Reticular fibers Very thin fibers made of collagen found in the bone marrow.

Reticular tissue A special type of connective tissue characterized by fine reticulin fibers.

Reye's syndrome Acute illness following mild viral infection in infants, children, and teens, characterized by brain swelling associated with aspirin consumption.

Rheumatic fever A disease caused by hypersensitivity to antigens of the Group A beta-hemolytic streptococcus, characterized by fever, joint pains, and inflammation of heart valves and muscle.

Rheumatoid arthritis (RA) A systemic disease primarily affecting the synovium with major manifestations in the small joints.

Ribonucleic acid (RNA) A type of nucleic acid contained in the nucleoli of cells. A component of messenger, transfer, and ribosomal RNA.

Ribosome A small cytoplasmic particle that serves as the site of protein synthesis. Ribosomes are usually attached to the endoplasmic reticulum but may be free in the cytoplasm.

Rickets Impaired calcification of bone in a growing child caused by vitamin D deficiency, which leads to bowing of leg bones when weight-bearing is attempted.

Rocky Mountain spotted fever Disease caused by rickettsial infection of endothelial cells.

Root canal treatment Replacement of tooth root canal with a filling material.

Rotavirus An RNA virus that is transmitted primarily through the oral-fecal route and causes severe gastroenteritis in children.

Rough endoplasmic reticulum (RER) Cell structure containing ribosomes and synthesizing protein.

S

Salpingitis Inflammation of the fallopian tubes.

Sarcoma A malignant tumor arising from connective and supporting tissues.

Schwann cells Cells making myelin for nerve fibers in the peripheral nervous system.

Schwannomas A tumor of peripheral nerves deriving from the Schwann cells.

Screening Examining a large asymptomatic population for signs of future disease.

Secondary gout Elevated uric acid and clinical manifestations of gout not caused by the metabolic disease primary gout, but instead caused by some other disease that raises the blood uric acid excessively, such as kidney failure or excessive breakdown of white blood cells in patients with leukemia.

Secondary hemostasis Process involving plasma coagulation factors.

Secondary hemostatic plug Formation of mature thrombus along with fibrin.

Secondary lymphoid organs Lymph nodes, spleen tonsils and adenoids, and mucosal-associated lymphoid tissue.

Secondary site Site of tumor following metastatic growth.

Secondary union Form of healing of a large unsutured wound.

Self-tolerance Selection process to remove ability to recognize self.

Semilunar valve The cup-shaped valve located between the ventricles and the aorta or pulmonary artery.

Seminoma One type of malignant tumor of the testis.

Sensitivity Classification of diagnostic tests in regard to percentage of patients with the disease who are classified as positive by the test.

Sentinel lymph node The lymph node that is located closest to a malignant tumor, which is examined to determine whether the tumor has spread to the node. If the sentinel node is not involved, additional lymph node dissection is not required.

Septicemia An infection in which large numbers of pathogenic bacteria are present in the bloodstream.

Seropositive Having antibodies to a pathogen.

Serotonin A vasoconstrictor mediator of inflammation released from platelets.

Serotype Immunologically detected pathogen strains.

Serous Fluid-rich exudate.

Serous tumor Ovarian tumor resembling cells in the fallopian tube.

Sex chromosomes The X and Y chromosomes that determine genetic sex. A human has one pair of sex chromosomes.

Sex-linked gene Gene present on the X or Y chromosome.

Sex-linked trait Product of gene present on X or Y chromosome.

Shingles Another name for herpes zoster flare in adults who were infected with chicken pox as children.

Shock A general term for any condition leading to receiving an inadequate amount of oxygen, most often caused by acute blood loss or severe infection (sepsis).

Shock wave lithotripsy A method for removing stones from the urinary tract by breaking them into small bits that can be excreted in the urine.

Signs Physical manifestations of disease.

Silicosis A type of occupational lung disease caused by inhalation of silica-rich rock dust.

Single nucleotide polymorphisms (SNPs) Minor variations in the nucleotides contained in the individual genes of different individuals.

Sinusoid Small, irregularly shaped blood vessel, which in the livers is found between the sheets of hepatocytes.

Smooth endoplasmic reticulum (SER) Cell structure containing enzymes and synthesizing lipids.

Smooth muscle Muscle that functions automatically.

Solid Tumor Type that is embedded in host tissue.

Somatostatin Hormone produced by the delta cells of the pancreas.

Spastic Describes muscle with excess tone that resists stretching.

Specificity Classification of diagnostic tests in regard to the percentage of patients without the disease who are classified as negative by the test.

Specific treatment Treatment of underlying cause of disease.

Spina bifida Incomplete closure of vertebral arches over the spinal cord, sometimes associated with protrusion of meninges and neural tissue through the defect (cystic spina bifida).

Spinocerebellar ataxia (SCA) Cerebellar disturbances resulting in loss of control of body movements. Most common is Friedreich ataxia.

Spontaneous depolarization The automatic change in cell membrane potential that occurs without stimulation from other cells.

Spores A unit of asexual reproduction found in life cycles of many plants, algae, fungi and protozoa that can remain viable even under extreme conditions.

Squamous cells Flat, platelike cells.

Squamous intraepithelial lesions (SILs) Precancerous results of infection with some HPV serotypes.

Stable angina Temporary chest pain during stress or exertion caused by partial chronic blockage of the coronary vasculature, usually relieved by rest or nitroglycerin.

Statins Drugs effective against the development of atherosclerosis.

Steatosis Abnormal storage of fat in the liver. Can result from alcoholic damage or some other cause.

Stem cells A self-renewing pool of cells that normally give rise to mature differentiated progeny.

Stenosis Abnormal narrowing of a passageway.

Stent Short tube often made of expandable metal mesh used to hold the blood vessel open.

Stillbirth Spontaneous abortion after twenty weeks' gestation.

Stomatitis Inflammation of the oral cavity.

Striated muscle Muscle that moves body parts under voluntary control.

Stroke/cerebrovascular accident (CVA) An injury to the brain resulting in a disturbance of cerebral blood flow caused by a cerebral thrombosis, cerebral embolism, or cerebral hemorrhage.

Stroma The tissue that forms the framework of an organ.

Subarachnoid space The space between the arachnoid and the pia, containing large blood vessels supplying the brain.

Subclinical hepatitis Liver inflammation resulting in few symptoms.

Sudden infant death syndrome (SIDS) Unexplained death of child under the age of one year.

Superantigens Antigens that cause widespread activation of T cells and release of cytokines.

Superior vena cava syndrome This syndrome occurs with blockage or compression of the superior vena cava, the vessel that carries blood from the head, neck, upper chest, and arms. This results in fluid accumulation in those areas.

Surfactant Substance which reduces the surface tension of a liquid, such as water. In the lungs, a lipid material secreted by type II pneumocytes that facilitates respiration by decreasing the surface tension of the fluid lining the pulmonary alveoli.

Sweat test Diagnostic test for cystic fibrosis.

Symptomatic treatment Treatment to alleviate symptoms rather than underlying cause of disease.

Symptoms Subjective manifestations of disease as reported by the person (patient) experiencing them.

Synapse Gap between connecting neurons.

Synchondrosis Cartilaginous joint.

Syndesmosis A fixed joint joined by fibrous connective tissue.

Syndrome Signs and symptoms often collectively associated with a disease or pathogenic process.

Synovial joint Movable joint.

Systolic heart failure Heart failure caused by inadequate ejection of blood from the ventricles during systole, in contrast to diastolic heart failure, in which filling of the ventricles in diastole is inadequate.

T

T cell A type of lymphocyte associated with cell-mediated immunity.

T cell help Requirement of a T cell to stimulate a B cell to deliver humoral response.

T cell–independent/T cell–dependent Whether T cells are needed or not needed for a response from B cells.

T cell receptor (TCR) Antigen recognition molecule on the surface of T cells.

Teratocarcinomas/malignant teratomas A malignant testicular tumor composed of many different types of malignant tissues.

Teratoma A tumor of mixed cell components.

Terminal duct lobular unit (TDLU) Lobe of the female breast, including the cluster of milk gland ducts and stromal tissue.

Tetany Spasm of skeletal muscles caused by a subnormal level of ionized calcium in the blood or certain bacterial toxins.

Thrombin A coagulation factor formed by activation of prothrombin in the process of blood coagulation.

Thrombin time test A laboratory test measurement that determines the concentration of fibrinogen in the blood by determining the clotting time of the blood plasma after addition of thrombin.

Thrombocytopenia A deficiency of platelets.

Thrombosis The formation of blood clots (thrombi plural, thrombus singular) within the vascular system.

Thrombotic stroke Reduction in blood flow in the brain due to thrombus.

Thrombus Clot within a blood vessel.

Thrush Superficial infection of mouth caused by *Candida albicans*.

Thyroglobulin A protein within the colloid of the thyroid follicles, which is a precursor of thyroid hormone.

Thyroid-stimulating hormone (TSH) Hormone secreted by the anterior lobe of the pituitary that regulates thyroid function.

Tissue A group of similar cells associated with each other to perform a specific function.

Tissue factor Protein that is a trigger for extrinsic coagulation.

Tissue transglutaminase Human enzyme target of antibodies detected in gluten sensitivity.

T lymphocyte/T cell A type of lymphocyte associated with cell-mediated immunity.

Toll-like receptors (TLRs) Cell surface and intracellular pathogen recognition receptors (PRRs) critical for sensing pathogens in innate immune responses.

Tonicity Measure of ionic concentration determined only by solutes that cannot cross the membrane.

TORCH complex Mnemonic for organisms causing maternal infections injurious to the developing fetus.

Toxic shock syndrome (TSS) Disease characterized by elevated temperature, vomiting and diarrhea, muscular aches, and a fall in blood pressure.

Toxoplasma gondii A small intracellular parasite of birds, animals, and humans. Causes the disease toxoplasmosis.

Trabeculae Thin strands of bone lattice work.

Tracheoesophageal fistula Abnormal connection between the esophagus and trachea.

Transient ischemic attack (TIA) Temporary cerebral dysfunction as a result of transient obstruction of a cerebral vessel by a bit of atheromatous debris or blood clot, usually embolized from an arteriosclerotic plaque in the carotid artery.

Transitional cell tumor/Brenner tumor Benign tumor containing nests of urothelial-like cells.

Transjugular intrahepatic portosystemic shunt A nonsurgical method used to lower portal vein pressure in a person with cirrhosis by connecting an intrahepatic branch of the portal vein to a hepatic vein branch.

Trauma Injury caused by a physical extrinsic agent.

Treponema pallidum The spiral organism causing syphilis.

Tricuspid valve AV valve separating the right atrium and ventricle.

Triglycerides Lipids used to store excess calories in fat cells.

Trigone Triangular area at the base of the bladder.

Triple-negative Breast cancer cell lacking ER, PR, and HER-2.

Triple therapy Treatment of ulcer with proton pump inhibitors combined with two antibiotics.

Trisomy The presence of an extra chromosome within a cell; having three of a given chromosome instead of the usual pair.

Trophoblast Cell derived from the fertilized ovum that gives rise to the fetal membranes and contributes to the formation of the placenta.

Trophozoite Active, motile vegetative phase of a parasite.

Tumor A benign or malignant overgrowth of tissues that serves no normal function, which is no longer under homeostatic control.

Tumor-associated antigen An antigen associated with growing tumor cells that serves as an indicator of tumor growth in the body.

Tumor necrosis factor alpha (TNF-a) Pro-inflammatory cytokine, regulates a large group of cellular responses to injury, infection, leading to necrosis or apoptosis.

Tumor suppressor gene Gene that normally functions to suppress abnormal cell growth.

Type 1 diabetes mellitus (T1DM) Diabetes resulting from a deficit in insulin production.

Type 2 diabetes mellitus (T2DM) Diabetes resulting from the resistance of target tissue to the effect of insulin with a compensatory oversecretion by the pancreas.

Type I membranoproliferative glomerulonephritis A more severe form of glomerulonephritis associated with infections of the heart, bone, and hepatitis C.

Type I pneumocytes/type II pneumocytes Cells lining the alveoli.

Tyrosine kinases A family of enzyme that produces multiple effects concerned with cell growth and cell division by phosphorylation of selected tyrosine residues in a protein.

U

Unstable angina Angina of prolonged duration resistant to therapy.

Urea A normal byproduct of protein metabolism excreted in the urine.

Uremia An excess of urea and other waste products in the blood, resulting from renal failure.

Urinalysis A commonly performed chemical and microscopic analysis of the urine.

V

Variable region Area on the immunoglobulin molecule specific for a particular pathogen. Amino-terminal end of the immunoglobulin chain; the part that recognizes the antigen.

Varicocele Varicose veins that develop within the spermatic cord veins.

Varicosities Outpouching and excessive tortuosity and dilation of blood vessels, often found in veins.

Vascular claudication Severe cramping leg pain due to atherosclerosis of arteries in the leg.

Vascular dementia/multi-infarct dementia Compromise of cerebral function caused by blockage of small cerebral blood vessels.

Vascular pole Site where the afferent arteriole enters the glomerulus and the efferent arteriole exits.

Vasodilator A substance that dilates blood vessels.

Vectors Transmission agents of a parasite; may be insects or other animals.

Velamentous insertion of umbilical cord Attachment of the umbilical cord to the fetal membranes rather than to the placenta.

Ventilation/perfusion scan (V/Q scan) Procedure used to detect a pulmonary embolus.

Ventricle One of two lower chambers of the heart.

Ventricular systole Period of ventricular contraction.

Vesicoureteral reflux Retrograde flow of urine from the bladder into the ureter during voiding.

Vimentin filament Type of filament in connective and muscle cells.

Viremia Presence of large numbers of viral particles in the bloodstream.

Virtual colonoscopy A high-resolution contrast CT image of the colon. May be substituted for colonoscopy in special cases.

Virulence Assessment of the ability of a pathogen to cause disease.

Virulence/virulent Ability to cause disease.

Vital capacity The maximum volume of air that can be forcefully expelled after a maximum inspiration.

Volvulus Rotary twisting of the bowel.

von Willebrand factor (vWF) A large protein that acts to adhere platelets to collagen.

Vulvar intraepithelial neoplasia (VIN) Cancer of the vulva.

W

Well-circumscribed Tumor with a clear border.

West Nile virus An arbovirus that infects birds, animals, and humans.

White matter Area of the CNS that contains a lot of nerve axons, many of which are myelinated, giving those areas a white appearance.

X

Xerostomia Dry mouth, which is lacking in saliva.

X-ray A form of electromagnetic radiation used to generate images of the internal structures of living organisms.

Y

Yolk sac A sac formed that will contribute to the gastrointestinal tract and other important embryonic structures.

Z

Zenker diverticulum Outpouching in the upper portion of the esophagus.

Zika virus An *Aedes* mosquito-borne flavivirus which can cause severe neurological damage in the developing fetus of an infected mother.

Zygote The fertilized ovum.

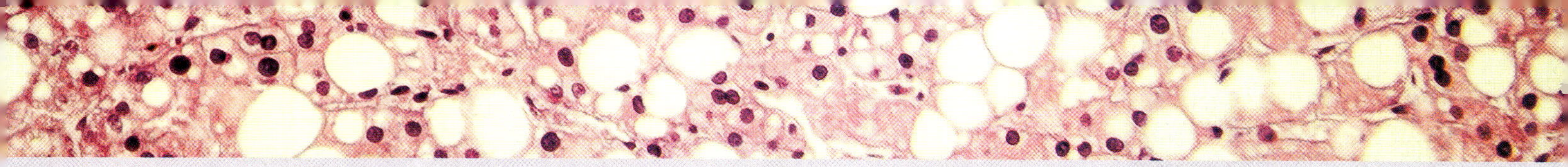

Index

NOTE: Page numbers followed by *f*, *t*, and *c* denote figures, tables, and cases, respectively.

A

B

C

F

G

H

I

J

K

L

M

N

O

P

Q

R

S

T

U

V

W

X

Y

Z